Cosmetic Dermatology

PRINCIPLES AND PRACTICE

SECOND EDITION

Cosmetic Dermatology

PRINCIPLES AND PRACTICE

SECOND EDITION

LESLIE BAUMANN, MD
Author and Editor
Director, University of Miami
Cosmetic Medicine and Research Institute
Professor of Dermatology
University of Miami
Miami Beach, FL

SOGOL SAGHARI, MD
Associate Editor
Department of Dermatology
University of Miami
Miami, FL
Private Practice
Los Angeles, CA

EDMUND WEISBERG, MS
Managing Editor
Center for Clinical Epidemiology and Biostatistics
University of Pennsylvania School of Medicine
Philadelphia, PA

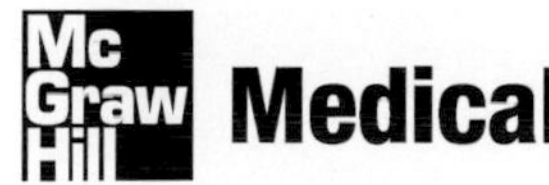

New York Chicago San Francisco Lisbon London
Madrid Mexico City Milan New Delhi San Juan
Seoul Singapore Sydney Toronto

The McGraw-Hill Companies

Cosmetic Dermatology: Principles and Practice Second Edition

1 2 3 4 5 6 7 8 9 0 CTP/CTP 0 9 9

ISBN 978-0-07-149062-7
MHID 0-07-149062-0

This book was set in StempelSchneidler by Aptara.
The editor was Anne M. Sydor.
The production supervisor was Sherri Souffrance.
Project management was provided by Aptara.
The interior designer was Alan Barnett.
The cover designer was Aimee Davis.
The index was prepared by Aptara.
China Translation & Printing, Inc. was printer and binder.

This book is printed on acid-free paper.

Library of Congress Cataloging-in-Publication Data

Baumann, Leslie.
Cosmetic dermatology / Leslie Baumann.—2nd ed.
p. ; cm.
Rev. ed. of: Cosmetic dermatology : principles and practice / Leslie Baumann. c2002.
Includes bibliographical references and index.
ISBN 978-0-07-149062-7 (hardcover)—ISBN 978-0-07-164128-9 (ebook)
1. Skin—Care and hygiene. 2. Cosmetics. 3. Dermatology. 4. Skin—Diseases—Treatment. I. Baumann, Leslie. Cosmetic dermatology. II. Title.
[DNLM: 1. Skin Diseases—therapy. 2. Cosmetic Techniques. 3. Skin Care—methods. WR 650 B347c 2009]
RL87.B365 2009
616.5—dc22

2008044457

Dedication

This book is dedicated to the three men in my life:

Roger Alexander Baumann
Thank you for encouraging me and being there to help me with all the technology and business aspects of my life. Your never- ending support has kept me sane over the years. Most of all, my thanks for dragging me out of the mud when times were tough like a good cutting horse does! You are an ideal husband, father, and friend. Here's to another 20 years together!

Robert Edward Baumann
I am so proud of what a good person you are growing up to be. You are kind, have a great sense of humor, and have a love for others that is truly refreshing. You have many talents, one of which is making me feel very special and proud to have you as a son.
Keep up the good work!

Maximilian Carl Baumann
When this book comes out, you will be 7 years old. It is hard to believe that you are growing up so fast; however, you will always be my baby. I am very proud of what a great student and person you are. I am so happy to have someone in the family who is so much like me and loves to read as much as I do.
Never stop snuggling!

Roger, Robert and Max,
You all brighten my life, remind me of what is important, and make it all worthwhile.
Thank you for loving me!

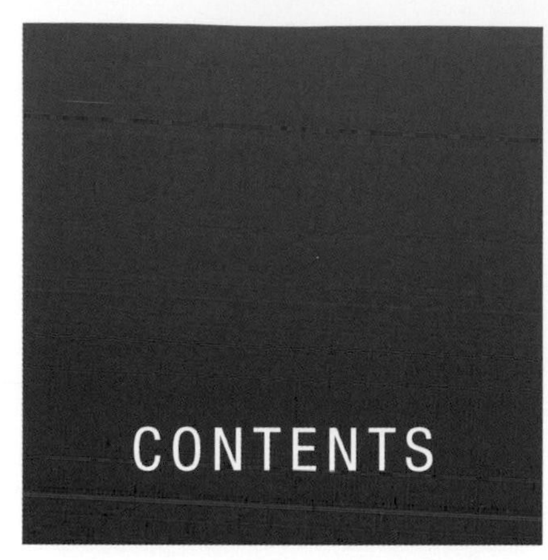

CONTENTS

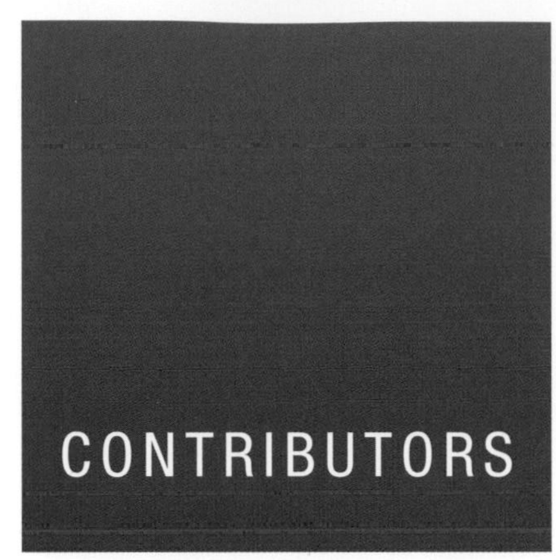

CONTRIBUTORS

Inja Bogdan Allemann, MD
Cosmetic Dermatology Fellow, Department of Dermatology and Cutaneous Surgery, Miller School of Medicine, University of Miami, Miami, Florida; Dermatologic Clinic, University Hospital of Zurich
Zurich, Switzerland
Chapters 33 and 34

K. P. Ananth
Chapter 31

Nidhi J. Avashia, BS
Miller School of Medicine, University of Miami, Miami, Florida
Chapter 29

Marianna L. Blyumin, MD
Dermatology Resident, Department of Dermatology and Cutaneous Surgery, Miller School of Medicine, University of Miami, Miami, Florida
Chapter 23

Angela S. Casey, MD
Assistant Professor, Dermatology and Mohs Surgery, University of Vermont College of Medicine, Fletcher Allen Health Care, Burlington, Vermont
Chapter 26

Maria Paz Castanedo-Tardan, MD
Department of Dermatology and Cutaneous Surgery, Miller School of Medicine, University of Miami
Miami, Florida
Chapters 29, 35, 38, and 39

Mohamed L. Elsaie, MD, MBA
Cosmetic Dermatology Fellow, Department of Dermatology and Cutaneous Surgery, Miller School of Medicine, University of Miami, Miami, Florida; Department of Dermatology and Venereology, National Research Center, Cairo, Egypt
Chapters 10 and 22

Lisa Danielle Grunebaum, MD
Assistant Professor, Division of Facial Plastic and Reconstructive Surgery, Department of Otolaryngology and Head and Neck Surgery, University of Miami, Miami, Florida
Chapter 22

Sharon E. Jacob, MD
Assistant Professor, Divisions of Medicine and Pediatrics (Dermatology), University of California, San Diego, San Diego, California
Chapter 18

H. Ray Jalian, MD
Resident Physician, Department of Medicine, Division of Dermatology, David Geffen School of Medicine at UCLA, Los Angeles, California
Chapter 4

Joely Kaufman, MD
Assistant Professor, Department of Dermatology and Cutaneous Surgery and Director of Laser and Light Therapy, University of Miamia Cosmetic Medicine and Research Institute, Miami, Florida
Chapter 24

Jonette Keri, MD, PhD
Assistant Professor, Miller School of Medicine, University of Miami, Miami, Florida;
Chief, Dermatology Service, Miami VA Hospital, Miami, Florida
Chapters 15 and 16

Jenny Kim, MD, PhD
Associate Professor, Department of Medicine and Division of Dermatology, David Geffen School of Medicine at UCLA, Los Angeles, California
Chapter 4

Suzan Obagi, MD
Assistant Professor of Dermatology, Director, The Cosmetic Surgery and Skin Health Center, University of Pittsburgh Medical Center, Pittsburgh, Pennsylvania
Chapters 3 and 26

Sogol Saghari, MD
Department of Dermatology, University of Miami, Miami, Florida; Private Practice, Los Angeles, California
Chapters 1, 2, 7, 13, 16, 19, 20, 21, 23, and 30

Susan Schaffer, RN
University of Miami, Cosmetic Medicine and Research Institute, Miami Beach, Florida
Chapter 21

Stuart Daniel Shanler, MD, FACMS
Private Practice, New York, New York
Chapter 16

Anita Singh, MS
Miller School of Medicine, University of Miami, Miami, Florida
Chapter 3

Kumar Subramanyan, PhD
Senior Manager, Consumer and Clinical Evaluation, Unilever Global Skin Research & Development
Shanghai, China
Chapter 31

Voraphol Vejjabhinanta, MD
Postdoctoral Fellow, Mohs, Laser and, Dermatologic Surgery, Department of Dermatology and Cutaneous Surgery, Miller School of Medicine,University of Miami, Miami, Florida; Clinical Instructor
Suphannahong Dermatology Institute, Bangkok, Thailand
Chapter 3

Edmund Weisberg, MS
Managing Editor, Center for Clinical Epidemiology and Biostatistics, University of Pennsylvania School of Medicine, Philadelphia, Pennsylvania
Chapters 9, 28, 36, 37, and 40

Heather Woolery-Lloyd, MD
Assistant Professor, Department of Dermatology and Cutaneous Surgery, Director of Ethnic Skin Care
University of Miami Cosmetic Medicine and Research Institute, Miami, Florida
Chapter 14

Larissa Zaulyanov-Scanlan, MD
Voluntary Faculty, University of Miami Cosmetic Medicine and Research Institute, Miami Beach, Florida; Private Practice, Delray Beach, Florida
Chapters 5 and 25

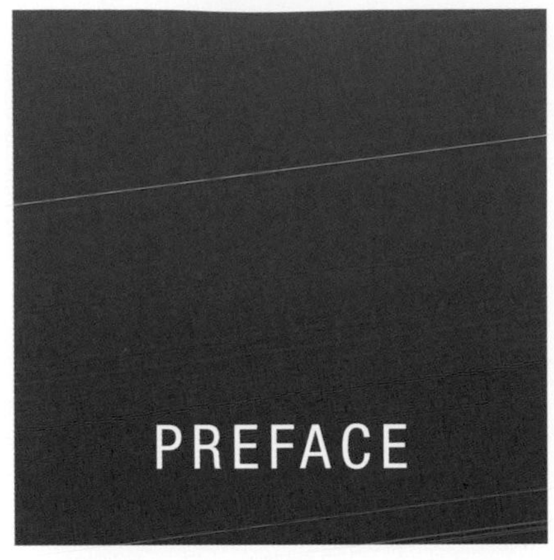

PREFACE

Cosmetic dermatology is a rapidly growing field that can attribute its popularity to aging baby boomers. Although many dermatologists perform cosmetic procedures and millions of dollars are spent each year on cosmetic products, there is a paucity of published research in this field. I was stimulated to write this text because I have found it challenging to conduct thorough research in preparation for my lectures and articles on cosmetic science as there exists no undisputed reference at the moment. Of the research performed by cosmetic scientists, much of it, unfortunately, is proprietary information owned by corporations and is not published or shared in any way for the immediate benefit of the medical community and other cosmetic professionals. This results in each company or cosmetic scientist having to "reinvent the wheel." My goal, with this book, is to create a link, featuring a better streaming flow of information, between the fields of dermatology and cosmetic science. This text is designed to help cosmetic dermatologists understand the available information on various cosmetic products and procedures. It should also help cosmetic chemists to understand the issues that cosmetic dermatologists deal with on a frequent basis. In addition, this text should fill the gap in knowledge among professionals such as aestheticians who need to know what to apply to patients' or clients' skin and about the products that people purchase over-the-counter and apply to their skin. This text should help these professionals answer the questions that their clients/patients ask about skin care products and their scientific validity. It is my hope that this text will encourage cosmetic dermatologists, cosmetic scientists and aestheticians to insist upon well researched cosmetic products and procedures. By working together in this way we can preserve the integrity of an exciting and rapidly developing field of study.

Research in the field of cosmetic dermatology should be encouraged for many reasons. Obviously, it is vital to maintain the hard earned integrity of the field of dermatology. In addition, the discoveries made though cosmetic dermatology research will likely benefit other fields of dermatology. For example, research into the anti-aging effects of antioxidants may lead to enhanced knowledge of chemopreventive techniques to be used to prevent skin cancer. Advances in acne therapy, vitiligo and other disorders of pigmentation are also possible. In fact, it is interesting to note that the development of Vaniqa™, a cream designed to slow hair growth in women with facial hair, has led to the availability of an intravenous treatment for African Sleeping Sickness, a major cause of death in Africa. Without the financial incentive to develop Vaniqa, which is used for purely aesthetic purposes, this life-saving drug would not be available. For many reasons, all pharmaceutical, medical device, and cosmetic companies should be encouraged to research their products.

Although there is much research performed by cosmetic companies on the effects of cosmetics on the skin, much of this data is proprietary and is not published nor shared with the rest of the scientific community. The reasons for this are numerous, but competition between companies and the desire to be the first to come out with a new "miracle product" are prominent among them. However, the issue is even more complex. The FDA has different definitions for drugs and cosmetics. Cosmetic products do not have to be researched in any standard way because FDA approval is not required. Instead, cosmetic products are voluntarily registered by the companies that develop them. However, drugs must undergo years of expensive trials establishing both safety and efficacy before receiving FDA approval (see Ch 28). This disparity means that a company is more reluctant to publish data that could cause their product to be labeled as a drug.

The dearth of published data on cosmetic products has forced physicians, aestheticians, and lay people to rely on sales people and marketing departments to obtain information about cosmetic formulations. This has led to much misinformation that has diminished the credibility of cosmetic products and the cosmetic field in general. Because an ever-increasing number of dermatologists and other physicians are practicing "cosmetic dermatology," it is imperative that the cosmetic dermatologist practice evidence-based medicine in order to distinguish efficacious treatments from mere marketing hype. This text sifts through the knowledge of the effects cosmetic products and procedures have on the skin and its appearance. The amount of research that should still be performed is daunting; however, the field is young and the rewards are great. I encourage everyone to join me in the exciting endeavor to find scientifically proven methods of improving the appearance of the skin.

Leslie Baumann, MD

"Don't worry if your job is small,
And your rewards are few.
Remember that the mighty oak,
Was once a nut like you."
Anonymous

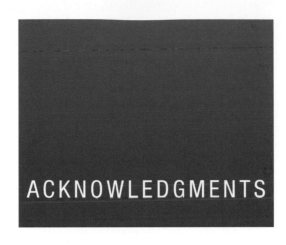

ACKNOWLEDGMENTS

The first edition of this book was printed in 4 languages and was the best-selling textbook on cosmetic dermatology worldwide (or so I have been told). There are many people to thank for this and the many wonderful things that have occurred in the last 6 years. First I would like to thank Dr. Stephen Mandy who took me in as a newly graduated resident in 1997, and let me and my husband live with him for two weeks while he taught me about the newly emerging field of cosmetic dermatology (I learned to inject collagen on his secretary!) That was the beginning of what has now been an 11-year friendship. Dr. Francisco Kerdel negotiated my first job and office space and he and Dr. William Eaglstein mentor me to this day. They were thanked in the first edition but I will never be able to thank them enough for what they have done for me.

This year, the University of Miami Miller School of Medicine decided to create the Cosmetic Medicine and Research Institute (CMRI), which consists of cosmetic dermatology, oculoplastic surgery, facial plastic surgery and nutrition. The role of this multi-specialty institute is to provide cutting edge dermatologic and surgical procedures to enhance appearance. By combining accomplished physicians from the various cosmetic specialties, the Institute can offer patients the expertise of many different types of physicians in order to achieve the best outcome. The mission of the Institute is to perform research in the area of cosmetic medicine, and many genetic initiatives to look for the genetic influences on appearance have begun. In addition, the CMRI will provide training to physicians on cosmetic dermatology and cosmetic procedures. (See www.derm.net for more information.)

I am very proud to announce that I have been selected to be the Director of the University of Miami Cosmetic Medicine and Research Institute. For this honor I would like to thank several people for believing in me and giving me this opportunity:

Pascal Goldschmidt MD, (the Dean of the University of Miami Medical School) – Dr. Goldschmidt is a true visionary and a leader in the field of the genetic influences in atherosclerosis. He opened the doors to basic science research for me and shared his genetic research team with me until I could find funding. In addition, he did the great honor of introducing me to Bart Chernow, MD and William O'Neil, MD (both of whom are Vice Deans at the University of Miami). The three of them appointed me Director of the University of Miami Cosmetic Medicine and Research Institute and gave me one of the most wonderful opportunities of my life. Dr. Chernow is a brilliant man and a true magician because he can pull all kinds of opportunities and ideas and innovations "out of his hat." I consider Bart and his wife Peggy good friends and I thank them both for their support.

I would like to thank David Seo, MD, my partner on the genetic trials, for his patience in getting me up to speed on genetic research. My fingers are crossed that we will discover great things together in the next 2 years. Thanks to the doctors who are a part of the CMRI and have chapters in this text. They have all taught me so much and are great to work with: Drs. Lisa Grunebaum, Joely Kaufman, Wendy Lee, Heather Woolery-Lloyd, and Larissa Zaulyanov-Scanlan. Thanks to Neal Shapiro for handling the financial aspect of the Institute so that I can concentrate on my true loves…seeing patients and performing research. Huge hugs and thanks to Susan Schaffer-RN who is my great friend, confidant, and Head of Nursing for the CMRI. She travels around the world with me, lecturing on cosmetic issues and helping to keep me sane. Edmund Weisberg-you are hilarious and fun to work with. I would never have written the first edition of this book without you! Stephanie and Fransheley- you have worked with me for many years and I have loved it and I look forward to MANY more.

I would like to thank Catherine Drayton and Richard Pine, my book agents for my NY Times bestselling book called "The Skin Type Solution" (Bantam 2005) (www.skintypesolutions.com). They negotiated an unprecedented book deal for me and are the best in the field. I first unveiled the Baumann Skin Typing System in this book. Catherine- Thanks for all the attention that you give to me in spite of the fact that we live on opposite sides of the world (and thanks for taking me sailing with you in Australia when I was there for the book launch-that was SO COOL!). I will never forget the support that Irwin Applebaum and his amazing team at Bantam Dell (a division of Random House) gave The Skin Type Solution when it launched. Phillip Rappaport is a great editor and friend.

I would like to thank my family, to whom this book is dedicated. My husband Roger and my sons Robert and Max are a constant source of joy and strength for me. I love cooking with them! I am fortunate to be very close with both my mother, Lynn McClendon, and my mother-in-law, Josie Kenin. They are great role models and friends and I am very lucky to have them. Thanks to my friends Jill Cooper, Melina Goldstein, Sofie Matz and Debbie Kramer for listening to me and keeping me calm.

Dr. Sogol Saghari, who was my fellow for one year and now has a dermatology practice in Los Angeles, made huge contributions to this book. She helped on the first draft of many of the chapters. She is a brilliant dermatologist and an incredibly nice person. I was so lucky to have her as a fellow. Thanks to all the doctors who contributed to the chapters in this book. Special thanks to Mohammed Lotfy, MD, who was available 24 hours a day helping me with literature searches and drawing the illustrations. He is one of the most dedicated dermatologists I have ever met. Inja Bogdan, MD and Maria Paz Castanedo-Tardan, MD were also fellows that contributed chapters and have great careers ahead of them.

And last but certainly not least-I would like to thank Anne Sydor for convincing me to write the second edition of this book. I never would have been able to get up at 5am and get this done if you had not encouraged me. Thanks for being my cheerleader and for lighting a fire in me to get this done . . . FINALLY! I am so proud of this book and poured my soul into it. I hope that all of you enjoy reading it as much as I enjoyed writing it.

Affectionately,

Leslie Baumann, MD

SECTION 1

Basic Concepts of Skin Science

CHAPTER 1

Basic Science of the Epidermis

Leslie Baumann, MD
Sogol Saghari, MD

The skin is composed of three primary layers: epidermis, dermis, and subcutaneous tissue. Each layer possesses specific characteristics and functions. Although research regarding skin layers continues, much is already known about the structure of each component. New discoveries about these components have already led to prenatal diagnoses of many inherited diseases and to improved therapies. In the future, study of these components will likely lead to an enhanced understanding of skin aging and the effects of topical products on the biologic function of the skin.

The epidermis is the most superficial layer of the skin. It is very important from a cosmetic standpoint, because it is this layer that gives the skin its texture and moisture, and contributes to skin color. If the surface of the epidermis is dry or rough, the skin appears aged. Knowledge of the basic structure of the epidermis best enables a practitioner to improve the appearance of patients' skin.

THE KERATINOCYTE

Keratinocytes, also known as corneocytes, are the cells that comprise the majority of the epidermis. Keratin filaments are major components of the keratinocytes, and provide structural support. There are two types of keratin filaments: acidic (type I, K10–20) and basic (type II, K 1–10). They both must be expressed for a keratin filament to develop.[1] In other words, an acidic type and a basic type are always expressed together and they form a keratin filament together. Keratinocytes are "born" at the base of the epidermis at the dermal–epidermal junction (DEJ). They are produced by stem cells, which are also called basal cells because they reside at the base, basal layer, of the epidermis. When the stem cells divide, they create "daughter cells," which slowly migrate to the top of the epidermis. This process of daughter cells maturing and moving to the top is called keratinization.

As these cells progress through the epidermis and mature, they develop different characteristics. The layers of the epidermis are named for these characteristic traits. For example, as mentioned, the first layer is the basal layer because it is located at the base of the epidermis. Basal cells are cuboidal in shape. The next layer is referred to as the spinous layer because the cells in this layer have prominent, spiny attachments called desmosomes. Desmosomes are complex structures composed of adhesion molecules and other proteins and are integral in cell adhesion and cell transport. The next layer is the granular layer, named so because these cells contain visible keratohyaline granules. The last, outermost layer is the stratum corneum (SC), a condensed mass of cells that have lost their nuclei and granules (Figs. 1-1 and Fig. 1-2). The SC is covered by a protein material called the cell envelope, which aids in providing a barrier to water loss and absorption of unwanted materials.

As keratinocytes migrate through the layers of the epidermis, their contents and functions change according to, or depending on, the specific epidermal layer in which they are moving. Although the functions of the keratinocyte have not been completely elucidated, many of them are understood. It is known that keratinocyte activity, such as the release of cytokines, can be affected by topical products administered to the skin. Keratinocytes and their components at each level of the epidermis starting at the basal layer and proceeding to the superficial layers of the epidermis are described below.

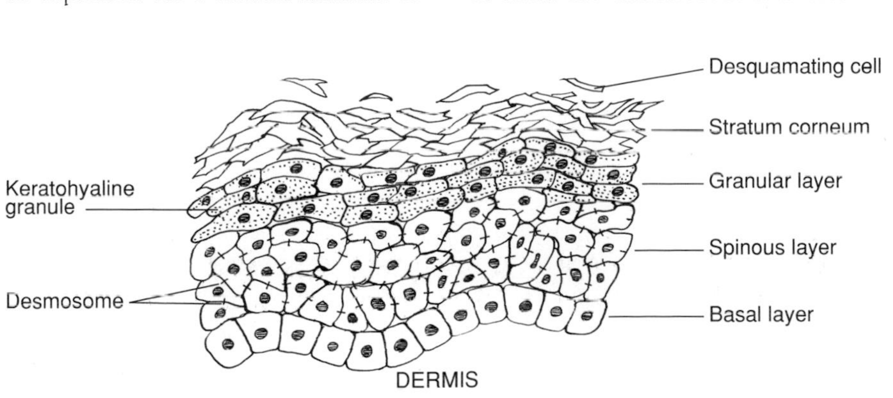

▲ **FIGURE 1-1** The layers of the epidermis.

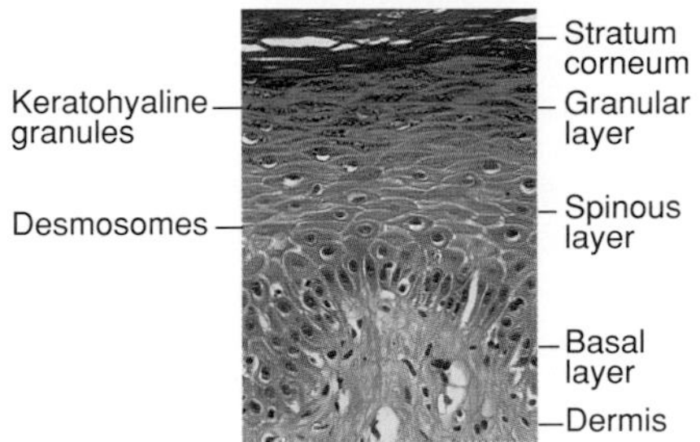

▲ **FIGURE 1-2** Histopathology of the epidermis demonstrating the four layers. (*Image courtesy of George Ioannides, MD.*)

Keratinocyte Function

THE BASAL LAYER (STRATUM BASALE)

Basal cells join with other basal and the overlying spinous cells via desmosomes, thus forming the basement membrane. These basal keratinocytes contain keratins 5 and 14, mutations in which result in an inherited disease called epidermolysis bullosa simplex. Keratins 5 and 14 are presumed to establish a cytoskeleton that permits flexibility of the cells. This flexibility allows cells to proceed out of the basal layer and migrate superficially, thus undergoing the keratinization process.

Basal cells are responsible for maintaining the epidermis by continually renewing the cell population. Of the basal layer, 10% of cells are stem cells, 50% are amplifying cells, and 40% are postmitotic cells. Normally, stem cells are slowly dividing cells, but under certain conditions such as wound healing or exposure to growth factors, they divide faster. They give rise to transient amplifying cells. Transient amplifying cells are responsible for most of the cell division in the basal layer and produce postmitotic cells, which undergo terminal differentiation and move superficially to become suprabasal cells that continue their upward migration to become granular cells and ultimately part of the SC (Fig. 1-3).

THE SPINOUS LAYER (STRATUM SPINOSUM)

Keratins 1 and 10 are first seen in this layer of suprabasal keratinocytes. These keratins form a more rigid cytoskeleton

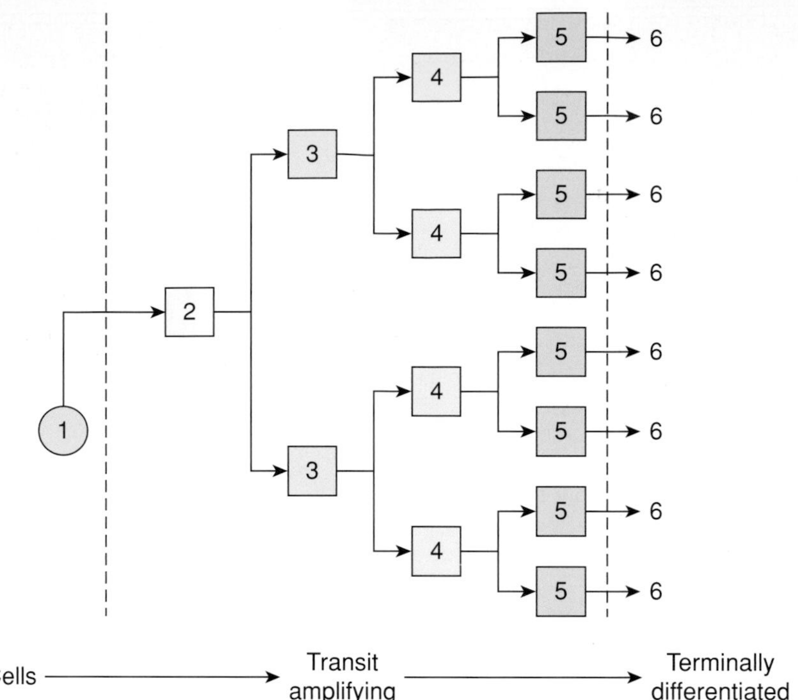

▲ **FIGURE 1-3** The stem cells divide and produce amplifying cells that greatly increase the number of keratinocytes. These in turn become the mature, terminal, and differentiated cells. The numbers indicate the cell generation.

that confers greater mechanical strength to the cell. It is worth mentioning that under hyperproliferative conditions such as actinic keratosis, wound healing, and psoriasis, keratins 6 and 16 are upregulated in the suprabasal keratinocytes.

Lamellar granules, which are considered the first sign of keratinization, first appear in this layer. They contain lipids such as ceramides, cholesterol, and fatty acids as well as enzymes such as proteases, acid phosphatase, lipases, and glycosidases. It has been recently shown that cathelicidin, an antimicrobial peptide, is also stored in the lamellar granules.[2] These granules migrate to the surface and expel their contents by exocytosis. The released lipids coat the surface, imparting barrier-like properties. Desmosomes are very prominent in this layer, thus accounting for the name "spinous layer."

The advanced stage of differentiation of suprabasal keratinocytes is conducive to staining for products not found on basal cells (i.e., sugar complexes and blood group antigens). The cytoplasm contains proteins not found in the lower layers such as involucrin, keratolinin, and loricrin. These proteins become cross-linked in the SC to confer strength to the layer.

THE GRANULAR LAYER (STRATUM GRANULOSUM) Granular layer keratinocytes reside in the uppermost viable layer of the epidermis. The "granules" represent keratohyaline granules, which contain profilaggrin, the precursor to filaggrin. The protein filaggrin cross-links keratin filaments providing strength and structure. The proteins of the cornified cell envelope (involucrin, keratolinin, pancornulins, and loricrin) are cross-linked in this layer by the calcium-requiring enzyme transglutaminase (TGase) to form the cell envelope. There are four types of transglutaminases present in the epidermis: TGase 1 or keratinocyte TGase, TGase 2 or tissue TGase, TGase 3 or epidermal TGase, and TGase 5. Only TGases 1, 3, and 5 participate in the development of the corneocyte envelope (CE) formation. TGase 2 has other functions including a role in apoptosis (programmed cell death). It is known that TGase activity increases with the elevation of Ca^{2+} levels in the medium of cultured keratinocytes.[3] This in turn results in the formation of the cornified cell envelope and differentiation of keratinocytes.[4,5] The active metabolite of vitamin D, known as 1,25-dihydroxyvitamin D_3 [1,25$(OH)_2D_3$], also plays a role in keratinocyte differentiation (Box 1-1). It enhances the Ca^{2+} effect on the keratinocytes, and increases transglutaminase activity as well as involucrin levels,[6] the combined effects of which induce CE formation.[7,8]

Calcium is known to be an inducer of differentiation and a suppressor of proliferation in epidermal keratinocytes.[9,10] It has been shown that in the state of low Ca^{2+} levels (0.05 mM), keratinocytes are in a proliferative stage, while increases in Ca^{2+} levels (0.10–0.16 mM) lead to expression of differentiation markers such as keratins 1 and 10, TGase, and filaggrin.[9]

Granular cells exhibit anabolic properties such as synthesis of filaggrin, cornified cell envelope proteins, and high molecular weight keratins. In addition, they show catabolic events such as dissolution of the nucleus and organelles.

THE HORNY LAYER (SC) The most superficial layer of the epidermis is the SC or horny layer, which is, on average, approximately 15-cell layers thick.[13,14] The keratinocytes that reside in this layer are the most mature and have completed the keratinization process. These keratinocytes contain no organelles and their arrangement resembles a brick wall. The SC is composed of protein-rich corneocytes embedded in a bilayer lipid matrix assembled in a "brick and mortar" fashion. The "bricks" are composed of keratinocytes and the "mortar" is made up of the contents extruded from the lamellar granules including lipids and proteins (Fig. 1-4). Cells of the midcornified layer have the most amino acid content and therefore have the highest capability for binding to water, while the

BOX 1-1

1,25-Dihydroxyvitamin D_3 [1,25$(OH)_2D_3$] stimulates differentiation and prohibits proliferation of the keratinocytes. It exerts its effects via the nuclear hormone receptor known as vitamin D receptor (VDR). VDR operates with the aid of coactivator complexes. There are two known coactivator complexes: vitamin D interacting protein complex (DRIP) and the p160 steroid receptor coactivator family (SRC/p160). It has been proposed that the DRIP mediator complex is involved in proliferation and early differentiation while the SRC/p160 complex is engaged in advanced differentiation.[11] The vitamin D receptors of undifferentiated keratinocytes bind to the DRIP complex, inducing early differentiation markers of K1 and K10.[12] The DRIP complex on the vitamin D receptor is then replaced by the SRC complex. The SRC complex induces gene transcription for advanced differentiation, which occurs with filaggrin and loricrin.[12] The replacement of the DRIP complex with the SRC complex on the vitamin D receptor is believed to be necessary for keratinocyte differentiation. It is important to realize that vitamin D levels are lower in older people and that this reduction may play a role in the slower wound healing characteristic in the elderly.

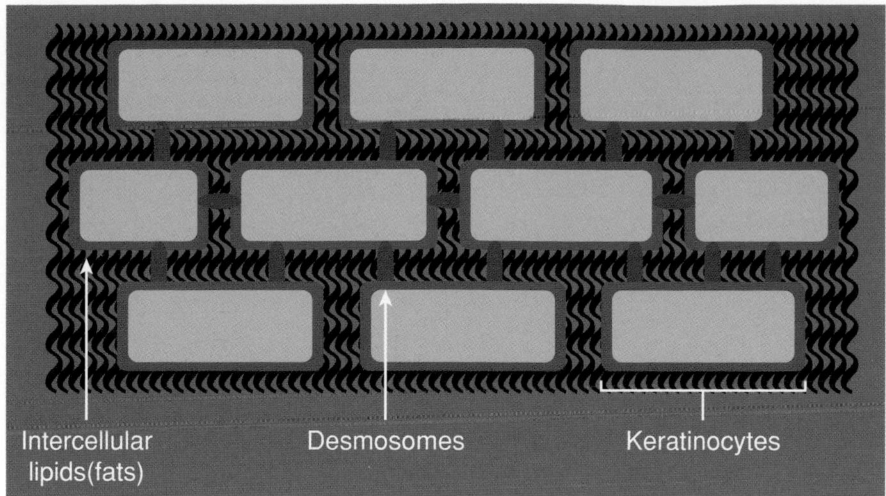

▲ **FIGURE 1-4** The desmosomes form attachments between the keratinocytes. The keratinocytes are surrounded by lipids. These structures form the skin barrier.

deeper layers have less water-binding capacity.[15] The SC is described as the "dead layer" of cells because these cells do not exhibit protein synthesis and are unresponsive to cellular signaling.[16]

The horny layer functions as a protective barrier. One of its protective functions is to prevent transepidermal water loss (TEWL). Amino acids and their metabolites, which are by-products formed from the breakdown of filaggrin, comprise a substance known as the natural moisturizing factor (NMF). Intracellularly-located NMF and lipids released by the lamellar granules, located extracellularly, play an important role in skin hydration, suppleness, and flexibility (see Chapter 11).

The Cell Cycle

The above keratinization process is also referred to as the "cell cycle." The normal cell cycle of the epidermis is from 26 to 42 days.[17] This series of events, known also as desquamation, normally occurs invisibly with shedding of individual cells or small clumps of cells. Disturbances of this process may result in the accumulation of partially detached keratinocytes, which cause the clinical findings of dry skin. Disease states may also alter the cell cycle. For example, psoriasis causes a dramatic shortening of the cell cycle, resulting in the formation of crusty cutaneous eruptions. The cell cycle lengthens in time as humans age.[18] This means that the cells at the superficial layer of the SC are older and their function may be impaired. Results from such compromised functioning include slower wound healing and a skin appearance that is dull and lifeless. Many cosmetic products such as retinol and alpha hydroxy acids are believed to quicken the pace of the cell cycle, yielding younger keratinocytes at the superficial layers of the SC, thus imparting a more youthful appearance to the skin.

GROWTH FACTORS

Growth factors can be classified into two groups: proliferative and differentiative factors. Proliferative factors engender more DNA synthesis and result in proliferation of the cells. Differentiative factors inhibit the production of DNA and suppress growth, thereby resulting in differentiation of the keratinocytes. Epidermal growth factor (EGF) is one of the integral chemokines in the regulation of growth in human cells. It binds to the epidermal growth factor receptor (EGFR) located on the basal and suprabasal cells in the epidermis and activates tyrosine kinase activity, which ultimately results in proliferation of the cells.[19] Keratinocyte growth factor (KGF), a member of the fibroblast growth factor family, also has a proliferative effect via the tyrosine kinase receptor on epidermal cells.[20] It has been shown that KGF contributes to and enhances wound healing.[21] In addition, KGF has been demonstrated to enhance hyaluronan synthesis in the keratinocytes.[22] Other important growth factors include the polypeptide transforming growth factors, which consist of two types: Transforming growth factor alpha (TGF-α) and transforming growth factor beta (TGF-β). They differ in both configuration and function. TGF-α is a proliferative factor, similar to EGF, and works by stimulating a tyrosine kinase response. TGF-β, which includes three subtypes (1–3), is a differentiative factor with a serine/threonine kinase receptor. TGF-β1 and TGF-β2 are present in small amounts in the keratinocytes. The presence of calcium, phorbol esters, as well as TGF-β itself increases the epidermal TGF-β level and promotes differentiation.[23] TGF-β has also been proven to have a role in scarring, and antibodies to this factor have been shown to decrease the inflammatory response in wounds and reduce scarring.[24, 25]

ANTIMICROBIAL PEPTIDES

Antimicrobial peptides (AMPs) have recently become an area of interest because of their involvement in the innate immune system of human skin. AMPs exhibit broad-spectrum activity against bacteria, viruses, and fungi.[26,27] The cationic peptide of the AMPs attracts the negatively charged bacteria, becoming pervasive in the bacterial membrane in the process, and ultimately eliminates the bacteria. Cathelicidin and defensin are the two major groups of AMPs believed to have an influence in the antimicrobial defense of the skin. Cathelicidin has been identified in the keratinocytes of human skin at the area of inflammation, as well as in eccrine and salivary glands.[28–30] In addition to antimicrobial activity, cathelicidin LL-37 demonstrates a stimulatory effect on keratinocyte proliferation in the process of wound healing.[31] Pig cathelicidin PR-39 has been shown to induce proteoglycans production (specifically, syndecan-1 and 4) in the extracellular matrix in wound repair.[32] Defensin is also expressed in the human keratinocytes[33] and mucous membranes.[34,35] β-Defensin 1 seems to promote differentiation in the keratinocytes by increasing expression of keratin 10.[36] Interestingly, UVB radiation has been shown to increase the levels of human β-defensin mRNA in the keratinocytes.[37]

AMPs have been demonstrated to be involved in several dermatologic conditions including atopic dermatitis, psoriasis, and leprosy,[27] as well as wound healing, all of which are beyond the scope of our discussion. The role of AMPs in the epidermal barrier will be discussed in Chapter 11.

MOISTURIZATION OF THE SC

The main function of the SC is to prevent TEWL and regulate the water balance in the skin. The two major components that allow the SC to perform this role are lipids and the NMF.

BOX 1-2

Filaggrin, named for *fil*ament *agg*regating prote*in*, derived its name from the fact that it binds keratin filaments to form a structural matrix in the SC. Genetic defects in the filaggrin gene are known to play a role in a subset of ichthyosis vulgaris cases.[38] Interestingly, filaggrin is not present in the superficial layers of the SC. Studies have shown that it is completely degraded into amino acids within 2 to 3 days of profilaggrin formation and its constituents are further metabolized to form the NMF.[40] This is nature's way of keeping its water-binding capabilities in the top layer of the SC where they are needed while preventing the lower layers of the SC from being disrupted by having too much water present. In addition, the level of NMF is regulated by the water activity present in the SC.

Natural Moisturizing Factor

Released by the lamellar granules, NMF is composed of amino acids and their metabolites, which are by-products formed from the breakdown of filaggrin (Box 1-2). NMF is found exclusively inside the cells of the SC and gives the SC its humectant (water-binding) qualities (Fig. 1-5). NMF is composed of very water-soluble chemicals; therefore, it can absorb large amounts of water, even when humidity levels are low. This allows the SC to retain a high water content even in a dry environment. The NMF also provides an important aqueous environment for enzymes that require such conditions to function. The importance of NMF is clear when one notes that ichthyosis vulgaris patients, who have been shown to lack NMF, manifest severe dryness, and scaling of the skin.[38] It has been demonstrated that normal skin exposed to normal soap washing has significantly lower levels of NMF when compared to normal skin not washed with surfactants.[39] NMF levels have also been reported to decline with age, which may contribute to the increased incidence of dry skin in the elderly population (see Chapter 11).

Lipids

In order of abundance, the composition of skin surface lipids includes triglycerides, fatty acids, squalene, wax esters, diglycerides, cholesterol esters, and cholesterol.[41] These lipids are an integral part of the epidermis and are involved in preventing TEWL and the entry of harmful bacteria. They also help prevent the skin from absorbing water-soluble agents. For decades it has been known that the absence of lipids in the diet leads to unhealthy skin (see Chapter 11). More recently, it has been shown that inherited defects in lipid metabolism, such as the deficiency of steroid sulfatase seen in X-linked ichthyosis, will lead to abnormal skin keratinization and hydration.[42] It is now known that SC lipids are affected by age, genetics, seasonal variation, and diet. Deficiency of these lipids predisposes the individual to dry skin. This has been demonstrated in mice with essential fatty acid deficiency (EFAD); when fed a diet deficient in linoleic acid these mice developed increased TEWL.[43] Interestingly, administration of hypocholesterolemic drugs has also been associated with dry skin changes.[44]

Skin lipids are produced in and extruded from lamellar granules as described above or are synthesized in the sebaceous glands and then excreted to the skin's surface through the hair follicle. The excretion of sebum by sebaceous glands is hormonally controlled (see Chapter 10). Lipids help keep the NMF inside the cells where it is needed to keep cells hydrated and aqueous enzymes functioning. Although this is less well characterized, lipids can themselves influence enzyme function.

ROLE OF LIPIDS IN TEWL

The major lipids found in the SC that contribute to the water permeability barrier are ceramides, cholesterol, and fatty acids.

Since the 1940s, when the SC was first identified as the primary barrier to water loss, many hypotheses have been entertained as to exactly which lipids are important in the SC. The research with the EFAD mice described above led to a focus on phospholipids because they contain linoleic acid. However, it was later found that phospholipids are almost completely absent from the SC.[40] In 1982, ceramide 1 was discovered. This lipid compound is rich in linoleic acid and is believed to play a major role in structuring SC lipids essential for barrier function.[45] Later, five more distinct types of ceramides were discovered and named according to the polarity of the molecule. Ceramide 1 is the most nonpolar and ceramide 6 is the most polar.

Although the ceramides were once thought to be the key to skin moisturization, studies now suggest that no particular lipid is more important than the others. It appears that the proportion of fatty acids, ceramides, and cholesterol is the most important parameter. This was demonstrated in a study in which after altering the water barrier with acetone, the application of a combination of ceramides, fatty acids, and cholesterol resulted in normal barrier recovery.[46] Application of each of the separate entities alone resulted in delayed barrier recovery. Manufacturers now include ceramides or a mixture of ceramides, cholesterol, and fatty acids in several available products as a result of these findings. However, the use of these mixtures to

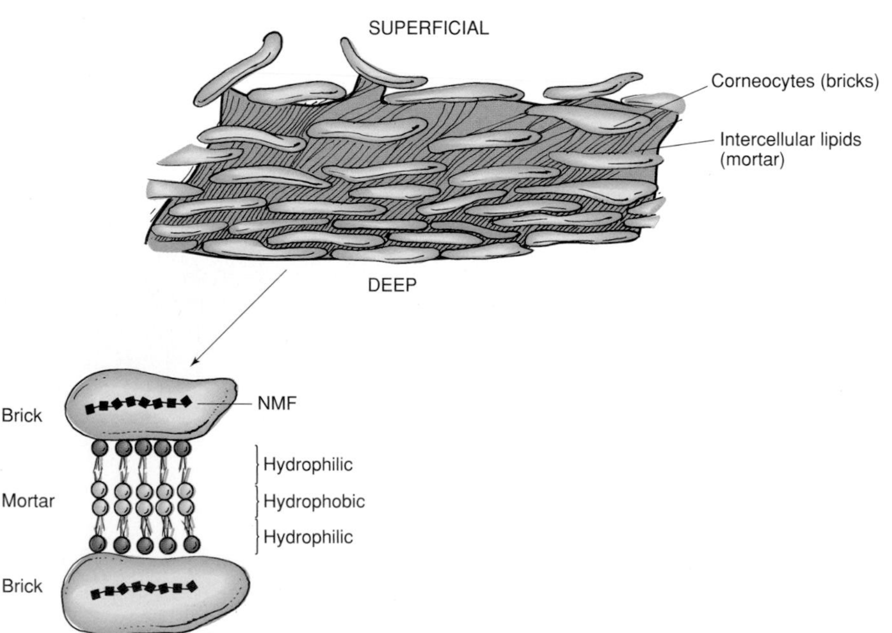

▲ **FIGURE 1-5** The keratinocytes are embedded in a lipid matrix that resembles bricks and mortar. Natural moisturizing factor (NMF) is present within the keratinocytes. NMF and the lipid bilayer prevent dehydration of the epidermis.

treat atopic dermatitis and other ichthyotic disorders has been disappointing.

SUMMARY

The epidermis is implicated in many of the skin complaints of cosmetic patients. It is the state of the epidermis that causes the skin to feel rough and appear dull. A flexible, well-hydrated epidermis is more supple and radiant than a dehydrated epidermis. The popularity of buff puffs, exfoliating scrubs, masks, moisturizers, chemical peels, and microdermabrasion attest to the obsession that cosmetic patients have with the condition of their epidermis. It is important to understand the properties of the epidermis in order to understand which cosmetic products and procedures can truly benefit patients as opposed to those that are based on myths or hype.

REFERENCES

1. Chu D. Overview of biology, development, and structure of skin. In: Wolff K, Goldsmith L, Katz S, Gilchest B, Paller A, Leffell D, eds. *Fitzpatrick's Dermatology in General Medicine*. 7th ed. New York, NY: Mcgraw-Hill; 2008:60.
2. Braff MH, Di Nardo A, Gallo RL. Keratinocytes store the antimicrobial peptide cathelicidin in lamellar bodies. *J Invest Dermatol*. 2005;124:394.
3. Li L, Tucker RW, Hennings H, et al. Inhibitors of the intracellular $Ca^{(2+)}$-ATPase in cultured mouse keratinocytes reveal components of terminal differentiation that are regulated by distinct intracellular Ca^{2+} compartments. *Cell Growth Differ*. 1995;6:1171.
4. Green H. The keratinocyte as differentiated cell type. *Harvey Lect*. 1980;74:101.
5. Eckert RL, Crish JF, Robinson NA. The epidermal keratinocyte as a model for the study of gene regulation and cell differentiation. *Physiol Rev*. 1997;77:397-424.
6. Su MJ, Bikle DD, Mancianti ML, et al. 1,25-Dihydroxyvitamin D_3 potentiates the keratinocyte response to calcium. *J Biol Chem*. 1994;269:14723.
7. Hosomi J, Hosoi J, Abe E, et al. Regulation of terminal differentiation of cultured mouse epidermal cells by 1 alpha, 25-dihydroxyvitamin D_3. *Endocrinology*. 1983;113:1950.
8. Smith EL, Walworth NC, Holick MF. Effect of 1 alpha,25-dihydroxyvitamin D_3 on the morphologic and biochemical differentiation of cultured human epidermal keratinocytes grown in serum-free conditions. *J Invest Dermatol*. 1986;86:709.
9. Yuspa SH, Kilkenny AE, Steinert PM, et al. Expression of murine epidermal differentiation markers is tightly regulated by restricted extracellular calcium concentrations in vitro. *J Cell Biol*. 1989;109:1207.
10. Sharpe GR, Gillespie JI, Greenwell JR. An increase in intracellular free calcium is an early event during differentiation of cultured human keratinocytes. *FEBS Lett*. 1989;254:25.
11. Oda Y, Sihlbom C, Chalkley RJ, et al. Two distinct coactivators, DRIP/mediator and SRC/p160, are differentially involved in VDR transactivation during keratinocyte differentiation. *J Steroid Biochem Mol Biol*. 2004;273:89-90.
12. Bikle D, Teichert A, Hawker N, et al. Sequential regulation of keratinocyte differentiation by $1,25(OH)_2D_3$, VDR, and its coregulators. *J Steroid Biochem Mol Biol*. 2007;103:396.
13. Christophers E, Kligman AM. Visualization of the cell layers of the stratum corneum. *J Invest Dermatol*. 1964;42:407.
14. Blair C. Morphology and thickness of the human stratum corneum. *Br J Dermatol*. 1968;80:430.
15. Proksch E, Jensen J. Skin as an organ of protection. In: Wolff K, Goldsmith L, Katz S, Gilchest B, Paller A, Leffell D, eds. *Fitzpatrick's Dermatology in General Medicine*. 7th ed. New York, NY: McGraw-Hill; 2008:383-395.
16. Egelrud T. Desquamation. In: Loden M, Maibach H, eds. *Dry Skin and Moisturizers*. 1st ed. Boca Raton, FL: CRC Press; 2000:110.
17. Proksch E, Jensen J. Skin as an organ of protection. In: Wolff K, Goldsmith L, Katz S, Gilchest B, Paller A, Leffell D, eds. *Fitzpatrick's Dermatology in General Medicine*. 7th ed. New York, NY: McGraw-Hill; 2008:87.
18. Yaar M, Gilchrest B. Aging of skin. In: Freedberg IM, Eisen A, Wolff K, Austen K, Goldmsith L, Katz S, Fitzpatrick T, eds. *Fitzpatrick's Dermatology in General Medicine*. 5th ed. New York, NY: McGraw-Hill; 1999.1697-1706.
19. Jost M, Kari C, Rodeck U. The EGF receptor—an essential regulator of multiple epidermal functions. *Eur J Dermatol*. 2000;10:505.
20. Miki T, Bottaro DP, Fleming TP, et al. Determination of ligand-binding specificity by alternative splicing: two distinct growth factor receptors encoded by a single gene. *Proc Natl Acad Sci U.S.A*. 1992,89.246.
21. Brauchle M, Fässler R, Werner S. Suppression of keratinocyte growth factor expression by glucocorticoids in vitro and during wound healing. *J Invest Dermatol*. 1995;105:579.
22. Karvinen S, Pasonen-Seppänen S, Hyttinen JM, et al. Keratinocyte growth factor stimulates migration and hyaluronan synthesis in the epidermis by activation of keratinocyte hyaluronan synthases 2 and 3. *J Biol Chem*. 2003;278:49495.
23. William I, Rich B, Kupper T. Cytokines. In: Wolff K, Goldsmith L, Katz S, Gilchest B, Paller A, Leffell D, eds. *Fitzpatrick's Dermatology in General Medicine*. 7th ed. New York, NY: McGraw-Hill; 2008:116.
24. Shah M, Foreman DM, Ferguson MW. Neutralisation of TGF-beta 1 and TGF-beta 2 or exogenous addition of TGF-beta 3 to cutaneous rat wounds reduces scarring. *J Cell Sci*. 1995;108:985.
25. Shah M, Foreman DM, Ferguson MW. Control of scarring in adult wounds by neutralising antibody to transforming growth factor beta. *Lancet*. 1992; 339:213.
26. Ganz T, Lehrer RI. Defensins. *Curr Opin Immunol*. 1994;6:584.
27. Izadpanah A, Gallo RL. Antimicrobial peptides. *J Am Acad Dermatol*. 2005; 52:381.
28. Frohm M, Agerberth B, Ahangari G, et al. The expression of the gene coding for the antibacterial peptide LL-37 is induced in human keratinocytes during inflammatory disorders. *J Biol Chem*. 1997;272: 15258.
29. Murakami M, Ohtake T, Dorschner RA, et al. Cathelicidin anti-microbial peptide expression in sweat, an innate defense system for the skin. *J Invest Dermatol*. 2002;119:1090.
30. Murakami M, Ohtake T, Dorschner RA, et al. Cathelicidin antimicrobial peptides are expressed in salivary glands and saliva. *J Dent Res*.2002;81:845.
31. Heilborn JD, Nilsson MF, Kratz G, et al. The cathelicidin anti-microbial peptide LL-37 is involved in re-epithelialization of human skin wounds and is lacking in chronic ulcer epithelium. *J Invest Dermatol*. 2003;120:379.
32. Gallo RL, Ono M, Povsic T, et al. Syndecans, cell surface heparan sulfate proteoglycans, are induced by a proline-rich antimicrobial peptide from wounds. *Proc Natl Acad Sci U S A*. 1994;91:11035.
33. Ali RS, Falconer A, Ikram M, et al. Expression of the peptide antibiotics human beta defensin-1 and human beta defensin-2 in normal human skin. *J Invest Dermatol*. 2001;117:106.
34. Mathews M, Jia HP, Guthmiller JM, et al. Production of beta defensin antimicrobial peptides by the oral mucosa and salivary glands. *Infect Immun*. 1999;67:2740.
35. Dunsche A, Acil Y, Dommisch H, et al. The novel human beta-defensin-3 is widely expressed in oral tissues. *Eur J Oral Sci*. 2002;110:121.
36. Frye M, Bargon J, Gropp R. Expression of human beta-defensin-1 promotes differentiation of keratinocytes. *J Mol Med*. 2001;79:275.
37. Seo SJ, Ahn SW, Hong CK, et al. Expressions of beta-defensins in human keratinocyte cell lines. *J Dermatol Sci*. 2001;27:183.
38. Sybert VP, Dale BA, Holbrook KA. Ichthyosis vulgaris: identification of a defect in synthesis of filaggrin correlated with an absence of keratohyaline granules. *J Invest Dermatol*. 1985;84:191.
39. Scott IR, Harding CR. Physiological effects of occlusion-filaggrin retention (abstr). *Dermatology*. 1993;2000:773.
40. Rawlings AV, Scott IR, Harding CR, et al. Stratum corneum moisturization at the molecular level. *J Invest Dermatol*. 1994; 103:731.
41. Downing DT, Strauss JS, Pochi PE. Variability in the chemical composition of human skin surface lipids. *J Invest Dermatol*. 1969;53:322.
42. Webster D, France JT, Shapiro LJ, et al. X-linked ichthyosis due to steroid-sulphatase deficiency. *Lancet*. 1978;1:70.
43. Prottey C. Essential fatty acids and the skin. *Br J Dermatol*. 1976;94:579.
44. Elias PM. Epidermal lipids, barrier function, and desquamation. *J Invest Dermatol*. 1983;80:44s.
45. Swartzendruber DC, Wertz PW, Kitko DJ, et al. Molecular models of the intercellular lipid lamellae in mammalian stratum corneum. *J Invest Dermatol*. 1989;92:251.
46. Man MQ, Feingold KR, Elias PM. Exogenous lipids influence permeability barrier recovery in acetone-treated murine skin. *Arch Dermatol*. 1993;129:728.

CHAPTER 2

Basic Science of the Dermis

Leslie Baumann, MD
Sogol Saghari, MD

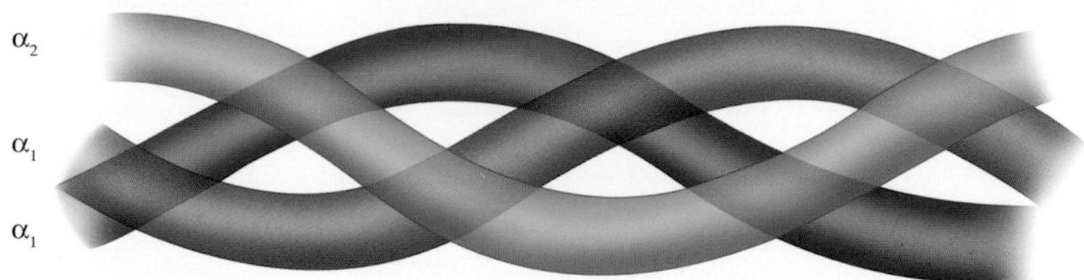

▲ **FIGURE 2-2** Collagen is formed when three chains come together to form a triple helix.

The dermis lies between the epidermis and the subcutaneous fat. It is responsible for the thickness of the skin, and as a result plays a key role in the cosmetic appearance of the skin. The thickness of the dermis varies over different parts of the body and the size doubles between the ages of 3 and 7 years and again at puberty. With aging, this basic layer decreases in thickness and moisture. The dermis, which is laden with nerves, blood vessels, and sweat glands, consists mostly of collagen. The uppermost portion of this layer, which lies beneath the epidermis, is known as the papillary dermis and the lower portion is known as the reticular dermis. Smaller collagen bundles, greater cellularity, and a higher density in its vascular elements characterize the papillary dermis as compared to the reticular dermis. Fibroblasts are the primary cell type in the dermis. They produce collagen, elastin, other matrix proteins, and enzymes such as collagenase and stromelysin. These structural components will be discussed individually because each exhibits significant characteristics that influence the function of the skin. Immune cells such as mast cells, polymorphonuclear leukocytes, lymphocytes, and macrophages are also present in the dermis.

The junction between the epidermis and dermis is known as the dermal–epidermal junction (DEJ) (Fig. 2-1). Much is known about the attachment proteins found in the basement membrane of the DEJ. At this point there are no known cosmetic implications for this area, as such a discussion is beyond the scope of this book. Instead, this chapter will focus on the components of the dermis that are known to be important in aging.

COLLAGEN

Collagen, one of the strongest natural proteins and the most abundant one in humans as well as in skin, imparts durability and resilience to the skin. It has been the focus of much antiaging research and the target of several skin products and procedures. The importance of collagen is emphasized in the literature regarding many of the topical agents that are touted to increase collagen synthesis such as glycolic and ascorbic acids. Resurfacing techniques such as the CO_2 laser and dermabrasion are intended to change collagen structure, thereby improving skin texture. Various forms of collagen are injected into the dermis to replace damaged collagen and to reverse the signs of aging. Finally, topical retinoids have been shown to reduce the collagen damage that occurs because of sun exposure. These sundry aspects of collagen health or replacement will be discussed separately in upcoming chapters; however, it is necessary first to gain an understanding of the structure and function of collagen.

"Collagen" is actually a complex family of 18 proteins, 11 of which are present in the dermis. Collagen fibers are always seen in the dermis in the final, mature state of assembly as opposed to elastin, the immature fibers of which are seen in the superficial dermis with the more mature fibers found in the deeper layer of the dermis. Each type of collagen is composed of three chains (Fig. 2-2). Collagen is synthesized in the fibroblasts in a precursor form called procollagen. Proline residues on the procollagen chain are converted to hydroxyproline by the enzyme prolyl hydroxylase. This reaction requires the presence of Fe^{++}, ascorbic acid (vitamin C), and α-ketoglutarate. Lysine residues on the procollagen chain are also converted to hydroxylysine; in this case, by the enzyme lysyl hydroxylase. This reaction also requires the presence of Fe^{++}, ascorbic acid, and α-ketoglutarate. It is interesting to note that a deficiency of vitamin C, which is an essential mediating component in these reactions, leads to scurvy, a disease characterized by decreased collagen production.

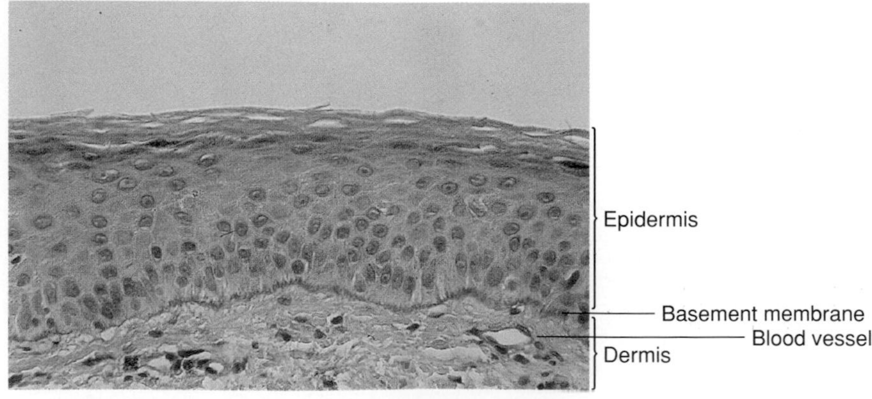

▲ **FIGURE 2-1** Histopathology of the dermal-epidermal junction. The basement membrane separates the epidermis and the dermis. (*Image courtesy of George Loannides, MD.*)

Collagen Glycation

Glycation of extracellular matrix (ECM) collagen and proteins plays an important role in the aging process. This is not to be confused with glycosylation of collagen, which is an enzyme-mediated process in the intracellular step of collagen biosynthesis. Glycation is a nonenzymatic series of biologic events that involves adding a reducing sugar molecule (such as glucose or fructose) to ECM collagen and proteins. This reaction is also known as the Maillard reaction. The sugar molecule mainly reacts with the amino group side chains

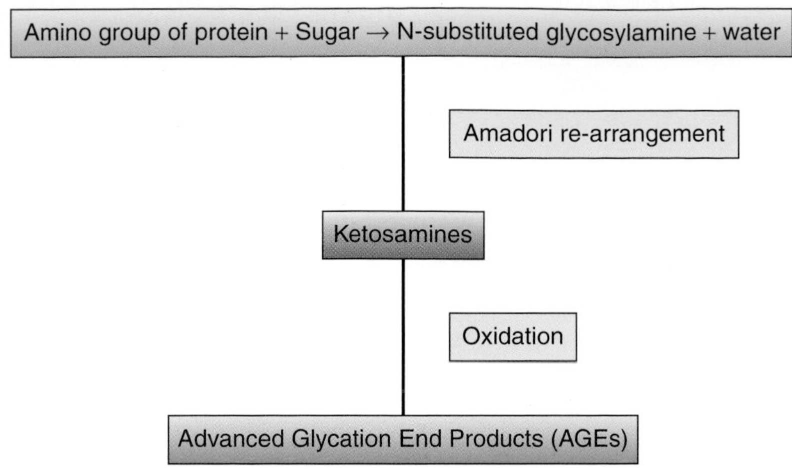

▲ **FIGURE 2-3** Glycation of proteins is thought to play a role in the aging process.

of lysine and arginine of collagen and ECM proteins. Subsequently, the product of this process undergoes oxidative reactions resulting in the formation of advanced glycation end products (AGEs) (Fig. 2-3). AGEs have been implicated in the aging process and age-related diseases such as diabetes mellitus,[1–3] chronic renal failure,[4,5] and Alzheimer's disease.[6–8] It is believed that with time, AGEs increase,[9] accumulate on human collagen[10] and elastin fibers,[11] and contribute to aging of the skin. As a result of glycation, collagen networks lose their ability to contract, and they become stiffer and resistant to remodeling. Fibroblasts are key elements for collagen contracture, as they apply contracture force on the collagen lattice via their actin cytoskeleton.[12] Glycated collagen modifies the actin cytoskeleton of the fibroblasts thereby diminishing their collagen contraction capacity.[13] Fibroblasts also secrete collagenase (MMP-1), which is essential for collagen turnover. Glycated collagen has been proven to decrease levels of collagenase I (MMP-1), leading to less tissue remodeling.[14] Studies have shown that UV exposure may also contribute to the production and function of AGEs. $N_e\epsilon$-(carboxymethyl) lysine (CML) is one of the AGEs in which the amino side chain of lysine is reduced. This product was shown to accumulate on elastin tissue of photoaged skin and proven to be higher in sun-exposed skin as compared to sun-protected skin.[11] In addition, it has been proposed that AGE-modified proteins act as endogenous photosensitizers in human skin via oxidative stress mechanisms induced by UVA light.[15]

The Key Types of Collagen Found in the Dermis (Table 2-1)

Type I collagen comprises 80% to 85% of the dermal matrix and is responsible for the tensile strength of the dermis. The amount of collagen I has been shown to be lower in photoaged skin, and to be increased after dermabrasion procedures.[16] Therefore, it is likely that collagen I is the most important collagen type in regard to skin aging. Type III is the second most important form of collagen in the dermis, making up anywhere from 10% to 15% of the matrix.[17] This collagen type has a smaller diameter than type I and forms smaller bundles allowing for skin pliability. Type III, also known as "fetal collagen" because it predominates in embryonic life, is seen in higher amounts around the blood vessels and beneath the epidermis.

The other types of collagen that are noteworthy for a cosmetic dermatologist are type IV collagen, which forms a structure lattice that is found in the basement membrane zone and type V collagen, which is diffusely distributed throughout the dermis and comprises roughly 4% to 5% of the matrix. Type VII collagen makes up the anchoring fibrils in the DEJ. Type XVII collagen is located in the hemidesmosome and plays an important structural role as well. The importance of these collagens and other structural proteins is evident in genetic diseases characterized by a lack of these structures and in acquired diseases characterized by antibody formation to these important structures. For example, patients with an inherited blistering disease known as dominant dystrophic epidermolysis have been shown to have a scarcity of type VII collagen with resulting abnormalities in their anchoring fibrils. An acquired bullous disease, epidermolysis bullosa acquisita (EBA), is caused by antibodies to this same collagen type VII. Although the discussion of these diseases is beyond the scope of this text, it is interesting that patients with chronic sun exposure have also been found to have alterations in collagen type VII. This may contribute to the skin fragility seen in elderly patients. Some investigators have postulated that a weakened bond between the dermis and epidermis caused by loss of the anchoring fibrils (collagen VII) may lead to wrinkle formation.[10] The importance of collagen and changes seen in aged skin will be discussed further in Chapter 6.

ELASTIN

Elastic fibers represent one of the essential components of the ECM of connective tissue (Fig. 2-4). They confer resilience

TABLE 2-1
Major Collagen Types Found in the Dermis

Collagen Type	Other Name	Location	Function	% of Dermis	Associated Diseases
I		Bone, tendon, skin	Gives tensile strength	80	
III	Fetal collagen	Dermis, GI, vessels	Gives compliance	15	
IV		Basement membranes	Forms a lattice		
V		Dermis, diffusely distributed	Unknown	4–5	epidermolysis bullosa
VII		Anchoring fibrils	Stabilizes DEJ		acquisita (EBA), dystrophic
XVII	BPAG2, BP 180	Hemidesmosome	?		epidermolysis bullosa (EB), bullous pemphigoid (BP), herpes gestationis

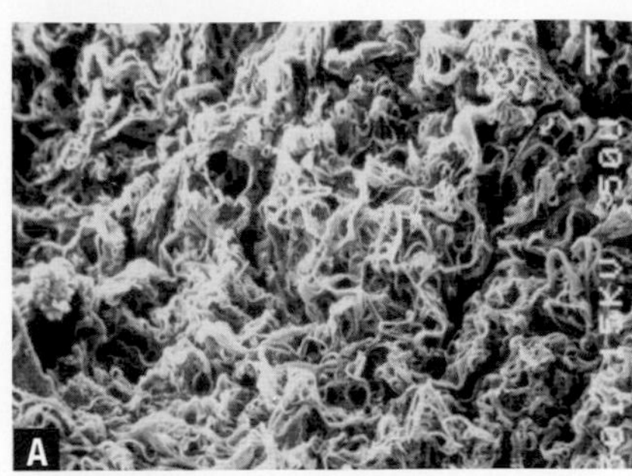

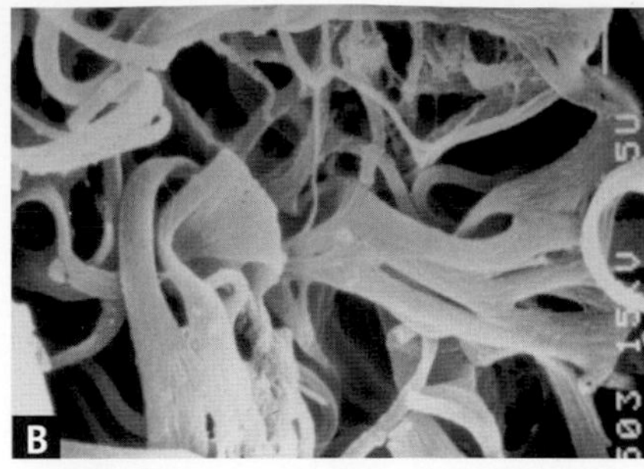

▲ **FIGURE 2-4** A and B. Scanning electron micrographs of the elastic fibers in human skin. Adapted from Fitzpatrick's Dermatology in General Medicine, seventh edition (McGraw Hill), page 532, with permission.

and elasticity to skin as well as other organs such as the lungs and blood vessels. Elastogenesis starts during fetal life and reaches its maximum near birth and the early neonatal period. It then decreases significantly and is virtually nonexistent by adult life. Elastic fibers have two components. Their main component is elastin, an amorphous, insoluble connective tissue protein. Elastin is surrounded by microfibrils, the second component. Elastin constitutes 2% to 3% of the dry weight of skin, 3% to 7% of lung, 28% to 32% of major blood vessels, and 50% of elastic ligaments.[19]

Elastin is produced from its precursor tropoelastin in the fibroblasts as well as endothelial cells and vascular smooth muscle cells. In contrast to collagen fibers, elastin fibers are present in the dermis in various levels of maturity. The least mature fibers are called oxytalan. They course perpendicularly from the DEJ to the top of the reticular dermis. More mature elastin fibers, called elaunin, then attach to a horizontal plexus of fibers found in the reticular dermis. Elaunin is more mature because it has more elastin deposited on the fibrillin mesh. The most mature elastin fibers are unnamed and are found deeper in the reticular dermis (Fig. 2-5).

Microfibrils play a very important role in elastogenesis and act as a scaffold for tropoelastin deposition and assembly.[20] Microfibrils are primarily composed of glycoproteins from the fibrillin family and microfibril-associated glycoprotein (MAGP)-1 and -2. Fibrillin-1 has been shown to be important in elastic fiber development[21] and wound repair.[22] Microfibrils are adjacent to tropoelastin-producing cells and parallel to the developing elastin fiber.[23] The microfibrils form a template on which tropoelastin is deposited. The tropoelastin polypeptides are then covalently cross-linked to form elastin. Tropoelastin polypeptides contain alternating hydrophilic and hydrophobic regions. The hydrophobic domains, which are rich in proline, valine, and glycine, are believed to be responsible for the elasticity of the elastin tissue.[24] The hydrophilic domains on the other hand are rich in alanine and lysine, and interact with the enzyme lysyl oxidase in the process of cross-linking.[25] The cross-linking of elastin is a complex process necessary for its proper function and stability. This process is mediated via the copper-requiring enzyme lysyl oxidase,[26] and the subsequent formation of desmosine and isodesmosine cross-links, which result in an insoluble elastin network.[27]

Elastin is fascinating and although much is known about it, its relevance in cosmetic dermatology is unclear. It seems certain that collagen, hyaluronic acid (HA), and elastin bind each other covalently and make up a three-dimensional structure that is impaired in aged skin. There is a commonly held belief that these three components must be increased in order to give skin a younger appearance. However, the trick is that de novo elastin production does not occur in adulthood. Trying to increase production of elastin in adults will surely be a focus of cosmetic dermatology research in the future.

The elastic fiber's structure provides clues about its ability to interact with HA and collagen. Mature elastic fibers contain an array of proteoglycans. Versican is one of the most widely studied proteoglycans[28] and is a member of the hyaluronan binding family that also includes aggrecan and neurocan. Versican contributes to cell adhesion, proliferation, and migration and can interact with multiple ECM proteins to mediate assembly. Mature elastic fibers are found at the periphery of collagen bundles, offering a clue that elastin has important interactions with collagen as well as with HA.

Elastic fibers are degraded by the elastolytic enzymes such as human leukocyte elastase (HLE). With significant levels of sun exposure, elastin degrades and is seen as an amorphous substance in the dermis when viewed by light microscopy. This resultant "elastosis" is a hallmark of photoaged skin. Interestingly, there are protective mechanisms in the skin preventing elastin degradation. Lysozymes are believed to play a protective role in this matter. They have been shown to increase and deposit on the elastin fibers of UV-exposed skin.[29] By binding to the elastin, the lysozymes prevent the proper interaction between elastase and elastin,[30] thereby inhibiting the proteolytic activity of the elastolytic enzymes.[30,31] It is also believed that damage to the elastin fibers leads to the decreased skin elasticity seen in aged skin.[32] Defects or damage to elastin may lead to wrinkles even in the absence of sun exposure and aging. Indeed, in one case, a child with "wrinkled skin syndrome" was shown to have a deficiency of elastin fibers,[33] which demonstrates the importance of elastin in skin integrity. Defective elastic fibers can give rise to multiple dermatologic diseases including cutis laxa, pseudoxanthoma elasticum

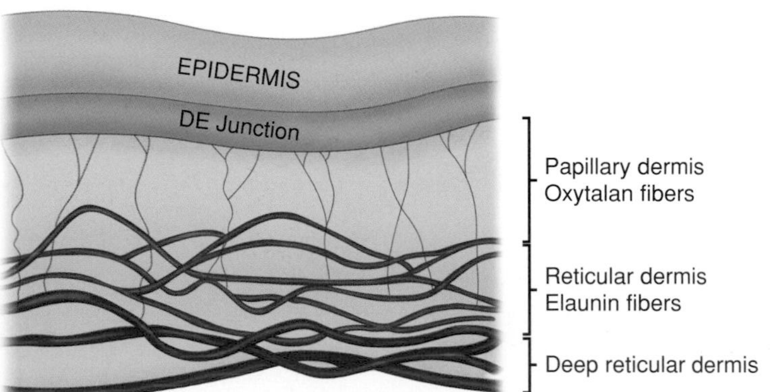

▲ **FIGURE 2-5** The elastic fiber network in the dermis consists of immature oxytalan fibers in the superficial dermis and the more mature elaunin fibers in the middle dermis. The most mature elastic fibers are unnamed and are found in the deep reticular dermis.

(PXE), elastosis perforans serpiginosa (also known as Lutz-Miescher's syndrome), and dermatofibrosis lenticularis (also known as Buschke-Ollendorf syndrome).

Studies have demonstrated a reduction in the elastin content in protected areas of the skin with aging. In a study performed on Egyptian subjects, the relative amount of elastin in the non-UV-exposed abdominal skin significantly decreased from 49.2% ± 0.6% in the first decade to 30.4% ± 0.8% in the ninth decade.[34] Another study on elastin content in the nonexposed buttock skin of 91 Caucasians between 20 and 80 years of age showed a reduction of 51% in elastin tissue.[31] Although UV exposure may result in elastosis and a higher content of elastin tissue, the elastic fibers are rendered structurally abnormal,[34] which is microscopically seen as thickened and twisted granular deposits of elastin in the dermis.

Replacing the elastin component of the ECM has always posed a challenge in skin rejuvenation approaches. Researchers have investigated the production of recombinant and cross-linked tropoelastin in great detail.[35] However, since it is very difficult to have elastin pass through human skin, stimulating the dermis to produce elastin may be an alternative option. Recently, zinc has become a subject of interest as an elastin tissue stimulator in the skin. Zinc has been shown to increase the epidermal growth factor (EGF) receptor signaling pathway.[36] It increases protein tyrosine phosphorylation by inhibiting protein tyrosine phosphatase (PTPase),[37] and activates mitogen-activated protein (MAP) kinases,[38] which are important for cosignaling in ECM production. Clinical studies have suggested improvement in the elasticity of periocular skin following use of a patented zinc complex topical preparation.[39] In a 4-week study of 27 female subjects with a zinc complex-containing eye product, overall improvement of the eye area was noted by 78%, reduction of fine lines by 74%, and firmer skin by 70% of the patients.[39] These studies, although promising, need to be conducted in a larger patient population.

GLYCOPROTEINS

Glycoproteins (GP) influence cell migration, adhesion, and orientation. Fibronectin and tenascin are the GPs most relevant in the dermis although vitronectin, thrombospondin, and epibolin are also present in the dermis. Fibronectin is a filamentous GP that mediates platelet binding to collagen, development of granulation tissue, and reepithelialization. Chemotactic for monocytes, fibronectin contains six binding sites including one for collagen, two for heparin, and a region that binds fibrin. Tenascin is abundant in developing skin but found only in the papillary dermis in adult skin. These matrix components play a significant role in tissue remodeling and are important in wound healing following cosmetic procedures.

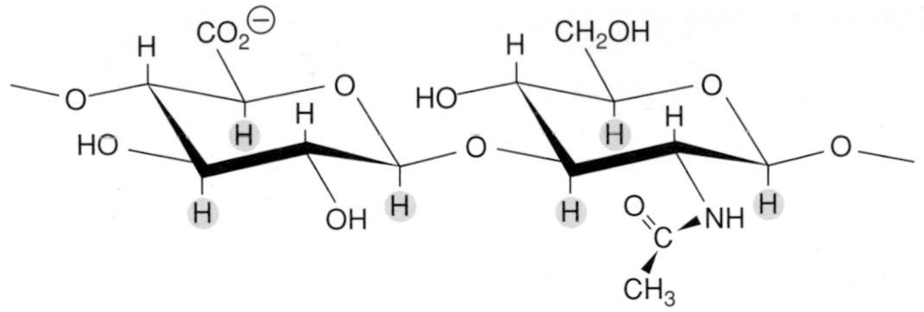

GLYCOSAMINOGLYCANS

Glycosaminoglycans (GAGs) are polysaccharide chains composed of repeating disaccharide units linked to a core protein. Together the GAGs and attached core protein form proteoglycans. All GAGs except for HA are synthesized in Golgi apparatus. HA is the only GAG that is not produced on a core protein; rather, it is synthesized by an enzyme complex of the plasma membrane.[40]

Although all the functions of GAGs are not understood, it is known that these compounds avidly bind water and may contribute to the maintenance of salt and water balance. GAGs are found in areas with a fibrous matrix where cells are closely associated but have little space for free movement. Most studies on human skin show an age-related decline in GAG content. The most abundant GAGs in the dermis are HA, which is the only nonsulfated GAG, and dermatan sulfate. The other GAGs include heparin sulfate, heparin, keratan sulfate, chondroitin-4, and chondroitin-6-sulfate.

HA is a very important component of the dermis that is responsible for attracting water and giving the dermis its volume. The name reflects its glassy appearance (the Greek word for glass is *hyalos*) and the presence of a sugar known as uronic acid. HA is known to be important in cell growth, membrane receptor function, and adhesion. Its structure is identical, whether it is derived from bacterial cultures, animals, or humans (Fig. 2-6). HA appears freely in the dermis and is more concentrated in areas where cells are less densely packed. In young skin, HA is found at the periphery of collagen and elastin fibers and at the interface of these types of fibers. These connections with HA are absent in aged skin.[41] HA is a popular ingredient in cosmetic products because it acts as a humectant. Several types are also available in an injectable version for the treatment of wrinkles (see Chapter 23). HA appears to also play a role in keratinocyte differentiation and formation of lamellar bodies via its interaction with CD44,[42] a cell surface glycoprotein receptor with HA binding sites.[43–45]

▲ FIGURE 2-6 HA is made of repeating dimers of glucuronic acid and N-acetyl glucosamine assembled into long chains.

Decorin is a member of the small leucine-rich proteoglycans (SLRPs) found in the extracelluar matrix protein. Its name is derived from its apparent "decorating" of collagen fibers. Decorin contains a core protein with a high content of leucine repeats and GAG chains of dermatan or chondroitin sulfate. It is shaped in a "horseshoe" pattern and binds to collagen fibrils, resulting in their proper organization.[46] Decorin-deficient mice have shown clinical skin fragility and irregular collagen fibrils with increased interfibrillar space on histology.[47] In addition to collagen fibrillogenesis, decorin interacts with fibronectin[48] and fibrinogen,[49] thereby playing a role in wound healing and hemostasis. Another interesting function of decorin is that it reduces the proliferation of cells in neoplasms by stopping their growth in the G_1 phase of the cell cycle.[50] Carrino et al.[51] studied the catabolic fragment of decorin in adult skin. They noted a higher content of the altered decorin in adult dermis as opposed to nonmeasurable amounts in fetal skin and named it "decorunt." Decorunt was shown to have a lower affinity for collagen fibrils. This finding may explain some of the changes related to collagen disorganization in aging skin.

MATRIX METALLOPROTEINASES

The ECM architecture of human skin is based on its continuous remodeling. This process requires ECM-degrading enzymes followed by synthesis and deposition of new molecules. The matrix metalloproteinases (MMPs), which include a large family of zinc-dependent endopeptidases, are crucial to the turnover of ECM components. Interstitial collagenase, or MMP-1, was the first enzyme discovered in this group. MMP-1 is secreted from the fibroblasts and is mainly involved in the degradation of collagen types I, II, and III, but has been shown to also cleave the anchoring fibrils of collagen VII.[52] Human neutrophil collagenase (MMP-8), another type of collagenase, is engaged in cleaving collagen types I and III. Collagenase 3 (MMP-13) is the third member of this group of enzymes, and it is known to fragment fibrillar collagens. It is also believed to have a role in scarless wound healing[53] by enhancing fibroblast proliferation and survival.[54] Gelatinases are another class of MMPs and consist of two types of enzymes, gelatinase A (MMP-2) and gelatinase B (MMP-9), that are responsible for attacking gelatin and collagen IV in the basement membrane. Other groups of MMPs include stromelysins, which are mainly involved in degradation of proteoglycans, laminins, collagen IV, and matrilysin, which is expressed on stromal tissue, fetal skin, and in the setting of carcinomas.[55]

The activity of MMPs is regulated by an endogenous tissue inhibitor of metalloproteinases (TIMPs). TIMPs are naturally produced proteins that specifically inhibit the MMPs. The balance between MMPs and their inhibition by TIMPs leads to proper tissue remodeling. TIMPs are regulated via expression of cytokines (such as IL-1), growth factors, and even retinoids.[56,57] Retinoids have been shown to provoke a two- to threefold increase in the biosynthesis of human fibroblast-derived TIMP in vitro.[58] Increased production of MMPs and decreased production of TIMPs have a role in the metastatic behavior of tumors. Synthetic inhibitors of MMPs are of interest to researchers especially in the area of cancer research. These inhibitors, such as hydroxamates, contain a zinc-chelating group that binds to the active site of MMPs leading to its inhibition. Currently, their use is mostly limited to research studies because of their side-effect profile. Certain medications such as doxycycline are also known for their inhibitory effect on MMPs and have been studied in myriad MMP-related conditions such as periodontal and atherosclerotic diseases.

HYPODERMIS

The hypodermis, or subcutis, located beneath the dermis, is composed mostly of fat, which is an important energy source for the body. This layer also contains collagen types I, III, and V. As humans age, some of the subcutaneous fat is lost or redistributed into undesired areas. This phenomenon contributes to the aged appearance. Fat injections have been employed to move fat from undesired areas into desired areas where fat has been lost, such as the lower face (see Chapter 23).

The adipocytes secrete a hormone called leptin, a product of the obesity (*ob*) gene. Leptin exhibits a regulatory effect on human metabolism and appetite and therefore affects adipose tissue mass. Leptin has been shown to be higher in the serum of obese patients, with commensurate levels found in body fat percentage.[59] It is believed that a higher percentage of body fat results in elevated leptin levels and the turning off of signals to the brain for appetite reduction. Recombinant leptin injections in mice have been associated with reduction of weight and body fat percentage.[60] However, more research is needed to ascertain the therapeutic potential of leptin in humans.

SUMMARY

Although the epidermis is the target of most topical cosmetic products because most do not penetrate to the dermis, the dermis is the target for many of the injectable treatments for aging. The dermis is an extremely important component in skin appearance because it is responsible for imparting thickness and suppleness to the skin. A thinner dermis and an altered DEJ are hallmarks of aged skin. Loss of collagen, elastin, and GAGs located primarily in the dermis contribute significantly to cutaneous aging. Various measures intended to prevent or retard aging target these key constituents of the dermis.

REFERENCES

1. Monnier VM, Kohn RR, Cerami A. Accelerated age-related browning of human collagen in diabetes mellitus. *Proc Natl Acad Sci U S A*. 1984;81:583.
2. Schnider SL, Kohn RR. Glucosylation of human collagen in aging and diabetes mellitus. *J Clin Invest*. 1980;66:1179.
3. Schnider SL, Kohn RR. Effects of age and diabetes mellitus on the solubility and nonenzymatic glucosylation of human skin collagen. *J Clin Invest*. 1981;67:1630.
4. Yamada K, Miyahara Y, Hamaguchi K, et al. Immunohistochemical study of human advanced glycosylation end-products (AGE) in chronic renal failure. *Clin Nephrol*. 1994;42:354.
5. Thornalley PJ. Advanced glycation end products in renal failure. *J Ren Nutr*. 2006;16:178.
6. Vitek MP, Bhattacharya K, Glendening JM, et al. Advanced glycation end products contribute to amyloidosis in Alzheimer disease. *Proc Natl Acad Sci U S A*. 1994;91:4766.
7. Yan SD, Chen X, Schmidt AM, et al. Glycated tau protein in Alzheimer disease: a mechanism for induction of oxidant stress. *Proc Natl Acad Sci U S A*. 1994;91:7787.
8. Takeuchi M, Kikuchi S, Sasaki N, et al. Involvement of advanced glycation end-products (AGEs) in Alzheimer's disease. *Curr Alzheimer Res*. 2004;1:39.
9. Dyer DG, Dunn JA, Thorpe SR, et al. Accumulation of Maillard reaction products in skin collagen in diabetes and aging. *J Clin Invest*. 1993;91:2463.
10. Verzijl N, DeGroot J, Odehinkel E, et al. Age-related accumulation of Maillard reaction products in human articular cartilage collagen. *Biochem J*. 2000;350: 381.
11. Mizutari K, Ono T, Ikeda K, et al. Photo-enhanced modification of human skin elastin in actinic elastosis by N(epsilon)-(carboxymethyl)lysine, one of the glycoxidation products of the Maillard reaction. *J Invest Dermatol*. 1997;108:797.
12. Tomasek JJ, Haaksma CJ, Eddy RJ, et al. Fibroblast contraction occurs on release of tension in attached collagen lattices: dependency on an organized actin cytoskeleton and serum. *Anat Rec*. 1992; 232:359.
13. Howard EW, Benton R, Ahern-Moore J, et al. Cellular contraction of collagen lattices is inhibited by nonenzymatic glycation. *Exp Cell Res*. 1996;228:132.
14. Rittie L, Berton A, Monboisse JC, et al. Decreased contraction of glycated collagen lattices coincides with impaired matrix metalloproteinase production. *Biochem Biophys Res Commun*. 1999;264:488.
15. Wondrak GT, Roberts MJ, Jacobson MK, et al. Photosensitized growth inhibition of cultured human skin cells: mechanism and suppression of oxidative stress from solar irradiation of glycated proteins. *J Invest Dermatol*. 2002;119:489.
16. Nelson B, Majmudar G, Griffiths C, et al. Clinical improvement following dermabrasion of photoaged skin correlates with synthesis of collagen I. *Arch Derm*. 1994;130:1136.
17. Oikarinen A. The aging of skin: chronoaging versus photoaging. *Photodermatol Photomed*. 1990;7:3.
18. Craven NM, Watson RE, Jones CJ, et al. Clinical features of photodamaged human skin are associated with a reduction in collagen VII. *Br J Derm*. 1997;137: 344.
19. Vrhovski B, Weiss AS. Biochemistry of tropoelastin. *Eur J Biochem*. 1998;258:1.

20. Robb BW, Wachi H, Schaub T, et al. Characterization of an in vitro model of elastic fiber assembly. *Mol Biol Cell.* 1999; 10:3595.
21. Kielty CM, Sherratt MJ, Shuttleworth CA. Elastic fibres. *J Cell Sci.* 2002;115: 2817.
22. Amadeu TP, Braune AS, Porto LC, et al. Fibrillin-1 and elastin are differentially expressed in hypertrophic scars and keloids. *Wound Repair Regen.* 2004;12: 169.
23. Mithieux SM, Weiss AS. Elastin. *Adv Protein Chem.* 2005;70:437.
24. Li B, Daggett V. Molecular basis for the extensibility of elastin. *J Muscle Res Cell Motil.* 2002;23:561.
25. Rosenbloom J, Abrams WR, Mecham R. Extracellular matrix 4: the elastic fiber. *FASEB J.* 1993;7:1208.
26. Smith-Mungo LI, Kagan HM. Lysyl oxidase: properties, regulation and multiple functions in biology. *Matrix Biol.* 1998;16:387.
27. Starcher BC. Determination of the elastin content of tissues by measuring desmosine and isodesmosine. *Anal Biochem.* 1977;79.11.
28. Wight TN. Versican: a versatile extracellular matrix proteoglycan in cell biology. *Curr Opin Cell Biol.* 2002;14:617.
29. Suwabe HA, Serizawa H, Kajiwara M, et al. Degenerative processes of elastic fibers in sun-protected and sun-exposed skin: immunoelectron microscopic observation of elastin, fibrillin-1, amyloid P component, lysozyme and alpha1-antitrypsin. *Pathol Int.* 1999;49: 391.
30. Park PW, Biedermann K, Mecham L, et al. Lysozyme binds to elastin and protects elastin from elastase-mediated degradation. *J Invest Dermatol.* 1996;106:1075.
31. Seite S, Zucchi H, Septier D, et al. Elastin changes during chronological and photo-ageing: the important role of lysozyme. *J Eur Acad Dermatol Venereol.* 2006;20:980.
32. Escoffier C, de Rigal J, Rochefort A, et al. Age-related mechanical properties of human skin: an in vivo study. *J Invest Dermatol.* 1989;93:353.
33. Boente MC, Winik BC, Asial RA. Wrinkly skin syndrome: ultrastructural alterations of the elastic fibers. *Pediatr Dermatol.* 1999;16:113.
34. El-Domyati M, Attia S, Saleh F, et al. Intrinsic aging vs. photoaging: a comparative histopathological, immunohistochemical, and ultrastructural study of skin. *Exp Dermatol.* 2002;11:398.
35. Mithieux SM, Wise SG, Raftery MJ, et al. A model two-component system for studying the architecture of elastin assembly in vitro. *J Struct Biol.* 2005;149:282.
36. Wu W, Graves LM, Jaspers I, et al. Activation of the EGF receptor signaling pathway in human airway epithelial cells exposed to metals. *Am J Physiol.* 1999; 277:L924.
37. Samet JM, Silbajoris R, Wu W, et al. Tyrosine phosphatases as targets in metal-induced signaling in human airway epithelial cells. *Am J Respir Cell Mol Biol.* 1999;21:357.
38. Samet JM, Graves LM, Quay J, et al. Activation of MAPKs in human bronchial epithelial cells exposed to metals. *Am J Physiol.* 1998;275:L551.
39. Baumann L, Weinkle S. Improving elasticity: the science of aging skin. *Cosm Dermatol.* 2007;20:168.
40. Uitto J, Chu M, Gallo R, Eisen A. Collagen, elastic fibers, and extracellular matrix of the dermis. In: Wolff K, Goldsmith L, Katz S, Gilchrest B, Paller A, Leffell D, eds. *Fitzpatrick's Dermatology in General Medicine.* 7th ed. New York, NY: McGraw Hill; 2008:539.
41. Ghersetich I, Lotti T, Campanile G, et al. Hyaluronic acid in cutaneous intrinsic aging. *Int J Dermatol.* 1994;33:119.
42. Bourguignon LY, Ramez M, Gilad E, et al. Hyaluronan-CD44 interaction stimulates keratinocyte differentiation, lamellar body formation/secretion, and permeability barrier homeostasis. *J Invest Dermatol.* 2006;126:1356.
43. Aruffo A, Stamenkovic I, Melnick M, et al. CD44 is the principal cell surface receptor for hyaluronate. *Cell.* 1990;61:1303.
44. Culty M, Miyake K, Kincade PW, et al. The hyaluronate receptor is a member of the CD44 (H-CAM) family of cell surface glycoproteins. *J Cell Biol.* 1990,111:2765.
45. Underhill C. CD44: the hyaluronan receptor. *J Cell Sci.* 1992;103:293.
46. Scott JE. Proteodermatan and proteokeratan sulfate (decorin, lumican/fibromodulin) proteins are horseshoe shaped. Implications for their interactions with collagen. *Biochemistry.* 1996;35: 8795.
47. Danielson KG, Baribault H, Holmes DF, et al. Targeted disruption of decorin leads to abnormal collagen fibril morphology and skin fragility. *J Cell Biol.* 1997; 136: 729.
48. Schmidt G, Robenek H, Harrach B, et al. Interaction of small dermatan sulfate proteoglycan from fibroblasts with fibronectin. *J Cell Biol.* 1987;104:1683.
49. Dugan TA, Yang VW, McQuillan DJ, et al. Decorin binds fibrinogen in a Zn2+-dependent interaction. *J Biol Chem.* 2003; 278:13655.
50. De Luca A, Santra M, Baldi A, et al. Decorin-induced growth suppression is associated with up-regulation of p21, an inhibitor of cyclin-dependent kinases. *J Biol Chem.* 1996;271:18961.
51. Carrino DA, Onnerfjord P, Sandy JD, et al. Age-related changes in the proteoglycans of human skin. Specific cleavage of decorin to yield a major catabolic fragment in adult skin. *J Biol Chem.* 2003; 278:17566.
52. Seltzer JL, Eisen AZ, Bauer EA, et al. Cleavage of type VII collagen by interstitial collagenase and type IV collagenase (gelatinase) derived from human skin. *J Biol Chem.* 1989;264:3822.
53. Ravanti L, Hakkinen L, Larjava H, et al. Transforming growth factor-beta induces collagenase-3 expression by human gingival fibroblasts via p38 mitogen-activated protein kinase. *J Biol Chem.* 1999; 274:37292.
54. Toriseva MJ, Ala-aho R, Karvinen J, et al. Collagenase-3 (MMP-13) enhances remodeling of three-dimensional collagen and promotes survival of human skin fibroblasts. *J Invest Dermatol.* 2006; 127:49.
55. Karelina TV, Goldberg GI, Eisen AZ. Matrilysin (PUMP) correlates with dermal invasion during appendageal development and cutaneous neoplasia. *J Invest Dermatol.* 1994;103:482.
56. Reynolds JJ, Hembry RM, Meikle MC. Connective tissue degradation in health and periodontal disease and the roles of matrix metalloproteinases and their natural inhibitors. *Adv Dent Res.* 1994; 8:312.
57. Wojtowicz-Praga SM, Dickson RB, Hawkins MJ. Matrix metalloproteinase inhibitors. *Invest New Drugs.* 1997;15:61.
58. Clark SD, Kobayashi DK, Welgus HG. Regulation of the expression of tissue inhibitor of metalloproteinases and collagenase by retinoids and glucocorticoids in human fibroblasts. *J Clin Invest.* 1987; 80:1280.
59. Considine RV, Sinha MK, Heiman ML, et al. Serum immunoreactive-leptin concentrations in normal-weight and obese humans. *N Engl J Med.* 1996; 334:292.
60. Pelleymounter MA, Cullen MJ, Baker MB, et al. Effects of the obese gene product on body weight regulation in ob/ob mice. *Science.* 1995;269:540.

CHAPTER 3

Fat and the Subcutaneous Layer

Voraphol Vejjabhinanta, MD
Suzan Obagi, MD
Anita Singh, MS
Leslie Baumann, MD

Subcutaneous tissue, or the hypodermis, is one of the largest tissues in the human body. The major components of this layer are adipocytes, fibrous tissue, and blood vessels. It is estimated that this layer represents 9% to 18% of body weight in normal-weight men and 14% to 20% in women of normal weight.[1] Fat mass can increase up to four fold in severe obesity, which may represent 60% to 70% of total body weight.[2] Although gaining fat in the body is undesirable for many, losing fat in the face has cosmetic implications as well. Adipose tissue gain and loss and volume changes contribute to the aged appearance of the face and body. This chapter will review the importance of the subcutaneous tissue and its various functions.

The subcutaneous tissue is usually not given as much attention as the dermis and epidermis because pathology at superficial layers is easier to detect or diagnose by a shave or small punch biopsy. Subcutaneous tissue usually must have an extensive defect before it is noticed, and in order to biopsy this area, an incision or large punch biopsy (e.g., 6 mm) is required. During histologic tissue processing of biopsy tissue, the triglyceride component, which is the major component of adipocytes, is removed by alcohol and xylol. For this reason, subcutaneous tissue has long been ignored. However, with advances in diagnostic methods and new treatments, much more has been learned about the subcutaneous layer (Box 3-1). It is important for dermatologists and cosmetically oriented physicians to pay close attention to this tissue because it has many roles in cosmetic dermatology and general appearance.

BOX 3-1 Functions of the Subcutaneous Tissue

- The largest repository of energy in the body.
- Stores fat-soluble vitamins (A, D, E, K), including their derivatives such as retinoic acids.
- Helps to shape the surface of the body, and form fat pads that act as shock absorbers.
- Helps distribute force or stress to mitigate damage to underlying organs.
- Protects against physical injury from excessive heat, cold, or mechanical factors.
- Fills up spaces between other tissues and helps to keep organs in place.
- Involved in thermoregulation by insulating the body from heat loss.
- Functions as a secretory organ that releases many cytokines.
- Plays a role in regulating androgen and estrogen levels.[3]

ADIPOCYTES

In the past, adipocytes in adults were considered stable, nondividing cells, like other mature cells. However, recent data reveal that adipocytes in adults have the potential to increase in number or revert back into stem cells. These stem calls can differentiate to other tissue, such as fibroblasts, collagen, elastic fibers, and hematopoietic stromal cells.[4] Fat cells are derived from undifferentiated fibroblast-like mesenchymal cells. Under certain conditions, these mesenchymal cells give rise to adipose cells. Adipose tissue is classified into two morphologic types: white and brown adipose tissue. White adipose tissue normally appears yellow because of the accumulation of β-carotene, while brown adipose tissue was named by its appearance derived from its rich vascular supply. Mature white adipocytes are called round unilocular fat cells. They have a copious supply of cytoplasm, which contains a single, large lipid droplet that pushes the nucleus to the border of the cell. Brown adipocytes, called polygonal multilocular fat cells, have multiple small lipid droplets.

When observed with an electron microscope, brown adipocytes demonstrably contain much more mitochondria and smooth endoplasmic reticulum than white adipocytes. In humans, brown adipocytes play a major role in nonshivering thermogenesis. Brown adipose tissue can be found during the fetal and early neonatal phases, while the majority of adipocytes in adults are white adipocytes. Some scientists have tried to elucidate the mechanism of how brown adipocytes convert fat to energy, in order to find a way to get rid of body fat by stimulating brown fat to return.[5]

In the past, it was believed that the number of adipocytes, which develop during the 30th week of gestation, does not increase after birth. However, newer evidence has shown that adipocytes can increase in number and size in certain situations or environments. In general, adipocytes are thought to have two periods of growth. The first period occurs from the embryonic stage to 18 months after birth, and the second period occurs during puberty. Changes in adipose tissue mass are determined by both size and number of adipocytes.[6] An increase in size (hypertrophy)[7] usually precedes an increase in the number of cells (hyperplasia).[8]

ANATOMY

Subcutaneous tissue, also known as the superficial fascia, is divided into three layers: apical, mantle, and the deeper layer. The apical layer is located beneath the reticular dermis surrounding sweat glands and hair follicles. It contains blood vessels, lymphatic vessels, and nerves. It is also rich in carotenoids and tends to be yellow in gross appearance. Damage to this layer can lead to hematoma, seroma, paresthesia, and full thickness skin necrosis. The mantle layer is composed of columnar-shaped adipocytes and is absent from eyelids, nail beds, bridge of the nose, and penis. It contributes to the ability to resist trauma by distributing pressure across a large field. The deeper layer is located under the mantle layer and its shape depends on gender, genetics, anatomic area, and diet. Adipocytes in this layer are arranged in lobules between septa as well as between fibrous planes. This layer is suitable for liposuction. Vertical extrusion and/or expansion of this layer can cause cellulite (Fig. 3-1).

Subcutaneous tissue is found throughout the body except for the eyelids, proximal nail fold, penis, scrotum, and the entire auricle of the external ear except the lobule. In particular, subcutaneous tissue is prominent at the temples, cheeks, chin, nose, abdomen, buttocks, and thighs, as well as infraorbital areas and very thick at the palms and soles. Age, gender, and lifestyle choices determine the distribution and density of adipose deposits. For example, in newborns

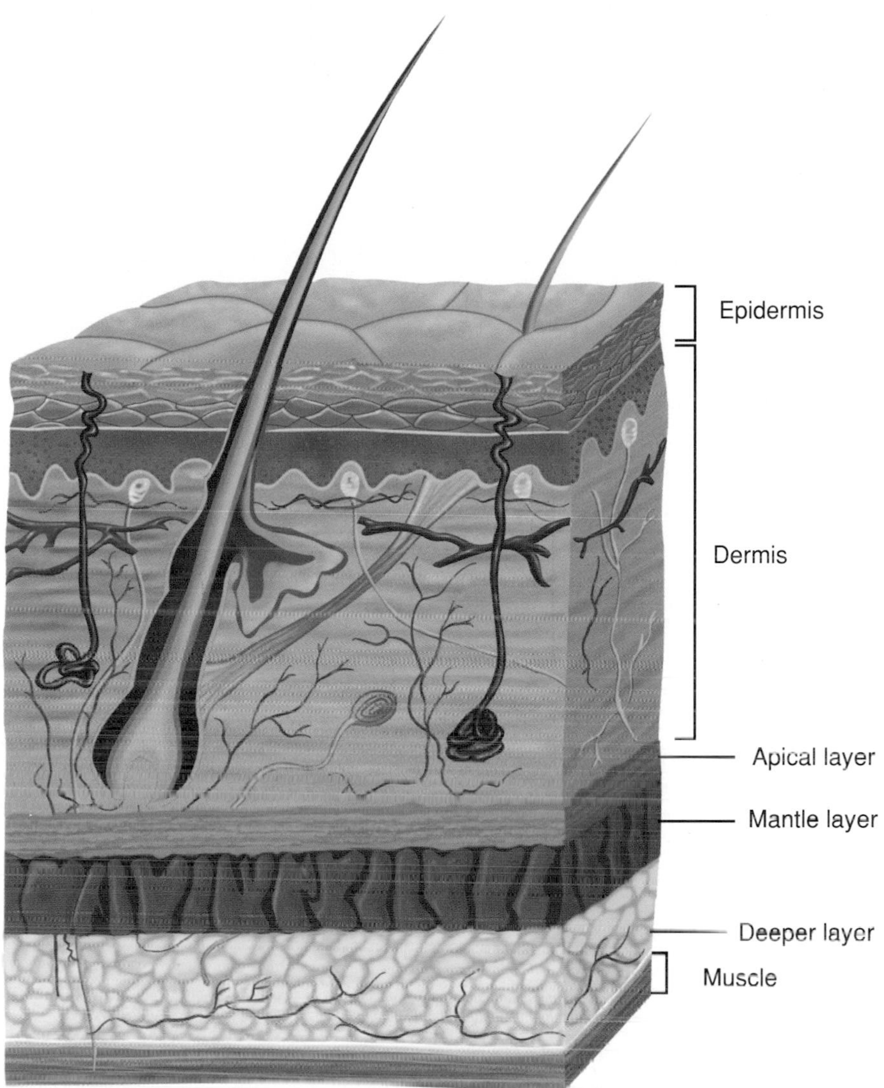

▲ **FIGURE 3-1** The three layers of the subcutaneous tissue.

adipose tissue has a uniform thickness throughout the body, while in adults the tissue tends to disappear from some areas of the body and increase in other areas under the influence of hormones.

Adipose tissue is distributed differently in men and women. Men tend to accumulate fat in an android or upper abdominal body distribution (apple shape). In contrast, women tend to accumulate fat in a gynoid or lower body distribution that predominantly involves the lower abdomen, hips, and thighs (pear shape) (Fig. 3-2).

In the elderly, hyper- or hypoaccumulation of fat occurs in various areas. For example, infraorbital eye bags, buccal fat pad accumulation (chipmunk feature), wattle of the anterior neck, loose skin and fat accumulation in the posterior arm, increase in breast size of males, and an increase in abdomen, buttock and thigh fat are common. Subcutaneous fat can also be lost in the malar fat pad during the aging process. This can lead to prominent flattening of the cheek/buccal area, sagging of the skin of the face, and prominent deep wrinkles, such as nasolabial folds and marionette lines or jowls.

Role of Lipids in the Human Body

Lipids can be found in different areas of the skin, not only in subcutaneous tissue. Lipids are constituents of phospholipids in the myelin sheaths of nerve tissue and cell membranes (lipid bilayers), play an important role in the skin barrier of the epidermis, and are essential for the production of steroids. They are water-insoluble organic molecules because they are nonpolar. However, after esterification (a condensation reaction between acid and alcohol), they are more water-soluble than their parent forms.

The most common lipids in the diet are triglycerides (triacylglycerol), which are composed of a glycerol subunit attached to three fatty acids (Fig. 3-3). Lipids can be saturated or unsaturated. Generally, an unsaturated fatty acid contains at least one double bond while saturated fatty acids do not. Unsaturated fatty acids provide slightly less energy during metabolism than saturated fatty acids with the same number of carbon atoms. In addition, saturated fatty acids are usually solids at room temperature

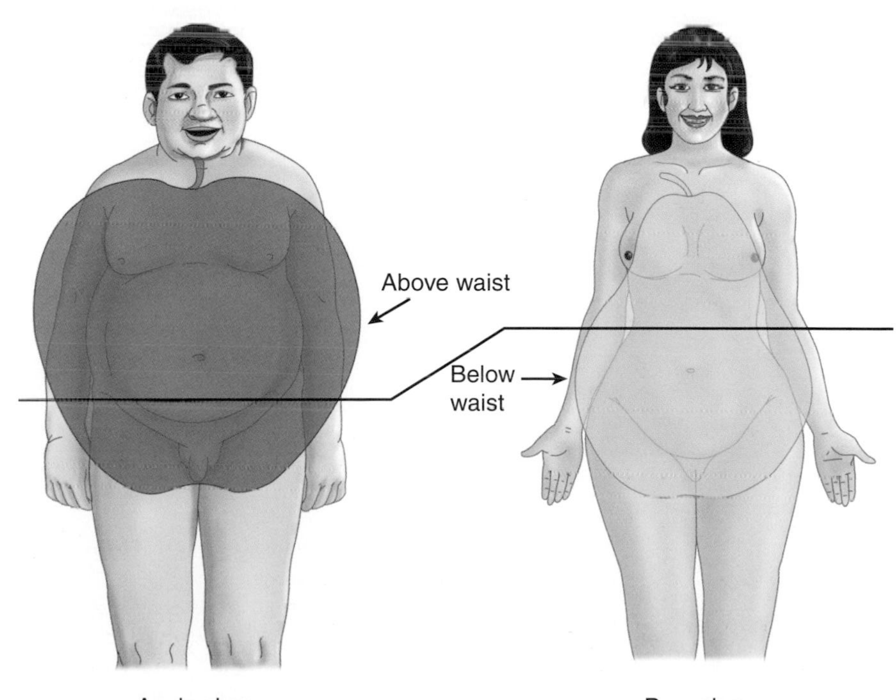

▲ **FIGURE 3-2** Android (apple) and gynoid (pear) fat distribution patterns in men and women.

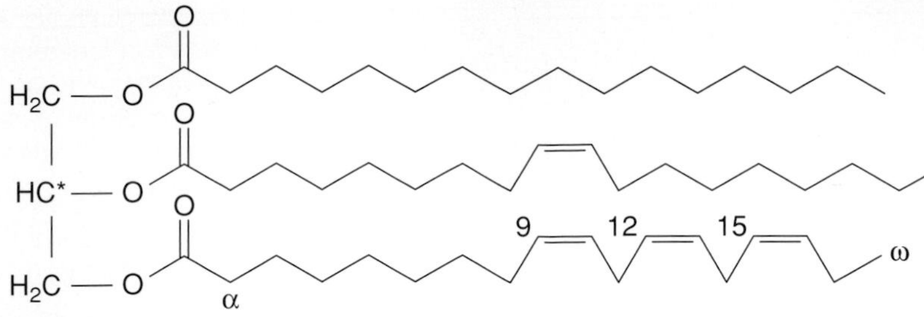

$$H_2C-O-C(=O)-\ldots$$

▲ **FIGURE 3-3** Triglyceride chemical structure.

TABLE 3-1
Body Mass Index (BMI) Categories

BMI	Weight Status
Less than 18.5	Underweight
18.5–24.9	Normal
25.0–29.9	Overweight
30.0 and greater	Obese

and unsaturated fats are usually liquids at room temperature.

Lipid Metabolism

During digestion, fats in the food are broken down in the duodenum by pancreatic lipase into free fatty acids and glycerol. The intestinal epithelium absorbs these substances and reesterifies them in the smooth endoplasmic reticulum into triglycerides. These triglycerides are then absorbed into the circulation and lymphatic system. When they arrive in the circulation they are combined with apoprotein to form a lipoprotein, which is called a chylomicron. Chylomicrons are exposed to lipoprotein lipase, which is synthesized by adipocytes and stored at the surface of endothelial cells. Lipoprotein lipase cleaves the chylomicron into free fatty acids and glycerol again. These free fatty acids pass into adipocytes and combine with intracellular glycerol phosphate to form triglycerides and are stored for energy.

Adipose tissue can also convert excessive glucose and amino acids into fatty acids when stimulated by insulin. This explains why people who consume a low-fat diet or fat-free diet still gain weight if they do not reduce the total amount of calories they consume or have a high-carbohydrate diet. High blood glucose can stimulate insulin synthesis and insulin can increase synthesis of lipoprotein lipase from adipocytes to help absorb triglycerides into the cells. People who want to control their weight should avoid any foods that have the ability to stimulate insulin production. Individuals with type II diabetes have high levels of insulin; therefore, they have a higher risk of becoming overweight or obese than nondiabetic individuals.

Lipoproteins

There are many different types of lipoproteins. Low-density lipoprotein (LDL) brings fat to the cells, while high-density lipoprotein (HDL) brings fat from the circulation to the liver for excretion in bile. High levels of LDL are associated with a high incidence of coronary artery disease and atherosclerosis. HDL, or the "good lipoprotein," can be elevated with exercise.

Lipid Synthesis

Triglycerides are derived from foods or synthesized from excessive glucose or amino acids. In humans, triglycerides are stored mainly in adipose tissue, which constitutes the body's reserve energy source. However, excessive consumption of calories can lead to the synthesis and accumulation of more fat in subcutaneous tissues. Unfortunately, fat storage is unlimited in the subcutaneous tissue, unlike glycogen storage in the liver and muscle. Therefore, excessive fat accumulation will not only change a person's cosmetic appearance but also increase their risk for osteoarthritis, diabetes, hypertension, as well as other diseases.

VOLUME EXCESS

Obesity

Obesity is defined as unhealthy, excessive fat mass. There are many regimens, products, and exercise programs available; however, there is still a rising pandemic in the United States[9] when compared to the past.[10] Obesity and hyperlipidemia are major risk factors and can lead to significant morbidity and mortality.

PATHOPHYSIOLOGY Obesity results from both environmental and genetic factors. Two genes that are known to have direct effects on obesity are the leptin (*ob gene*)[11,12] and proopiomelanocortin (POMC) genes.[13] These genes can control eating behavior and satiety. Defects in these genes can cause severe obesity. However, almost all people gain weight when they get older because of diminished physical activity and aging-induced changes in the chemical activity of hormones.

Body mass index [BMI: body weight divided by the square of height (kg/m^2)] is a popular index used for determining body weight status. The Centers for Disease Control and Prevention (CDC) and World Health Organization (WHO) use this index to classify adults into four groups (Table 3-1).

A normal BMI does not necessarily mean that a person has a "perfect" shape. Many people with a BMI less than 25 have fat accumulation in some area, such as the abdomen or buttocks.

IMPACT OF OBESITY ON THE SKIN Obesity is responsible for changes in skin barrier function by significantly increasing transepidermal water loss, which can lead to dry skin and impaired barrier function.[14] Hyperfunction of sebaceous glands due to high levels of androgen-like hormone or insulin-like growth factor hormone can aggravate severity of acne and hirsutism;[15,16] delay wound healing and collagen deposits in the wound healing process;[17] and disturb both blood and lymphatic circulation, which can cause angiopathy[18] and lymphedema, potentially precipitating chronic leg ulcers.[19] Rapid weight gain can cause striae distensae (stretch marks), which are challenging to treat.[20–23] In addition, in intertriginous areas such as the underarms, breasts, and groin, moisture accumulation can lead to candida infection (intertrigo).

It is widely known that obesity increases the risk of coronary heart disease, hypertension, hyperlipidemia, osteoarthritis, and diabetes. It is also known to be directly related to increased risk of sleep apnea; breast, endometrial, and colon cancer; gallbladder disease; musculoskeletal disorders; severe pancreatitis and diverticulitis; infertility;

TABLE 3-2
Classification of Overweight and Obesity by BMI

BMI	WEIGHT STATUS
25.0–29.9	Overweight
≥30.0	Obese
30.0–35.0	Moderate obesity (Class I)
35.0–40.0	Severe obesity (Class II)
≥40.0	Morbid obesity (Class III)

urinary incontinence; and idiopathic intracranial hypertension. Additionally, obesity has indirectly been related to anxiety, impaired social interaction, and depression.

Obesity is implicated in a wide spectrum of dermatologic diseases, including acanthosis nigricans, acrochordons, keratosis pilaris, hyperandrogenism and hirsutism, striae distensae, adiposis dolorosa, fat redistribution, lymphedema, chronic venous insufficiency, plantar hyperkeratosis, cellulitis, skin infections, hidradenitis suppurativa, psoriasis, insulin resistance syndrome, and tophaceous gout.[24]

To determine the severity of a person's obesity, BMI can be used. In fact, the more overweight a person is the higher the mortality rate (Table 3-2).

TREATMENT Dietary control is very important in the treatment of obesity. Patients must understand the principle of energy intake and expenditure. Weight reduction is usually not accomplished without exercise. However, exercise alone will usually produce little long-term benefit. The combination of exercise with dietary therapy can prevent weight being regained. In addition, regular exercise (30 min daily) will improve general health. The best results are obtained with education in well-motivated patients. Constant supervision by healthcare professionals and by family or friends can help to encourage compliance.

PREVENTION Prevention of obesity is key because once fat is gained and maintained over time, it is more difficult to lose. A high-fat diet can induce an increase in the number of adipocytes.[25,26] A low-fat and complex carbohydrate diet is recommended to reduce body weight. There is an important difference between preventing weight gain and producing weight loss. To prevent weight gain, portion size and composition of food are controlled. For weight loss, restriction of calorie intake is the most effective treatment.

Liposuction

Overweight patients frequently consult plastic surgeons and dermatologists for liposuction.[27–29] Liposuction is one of the most commonly performed cosmetic surgery procedures in the United States.[30] Physicians must inform their patients that liposuction is a modality for improving body contour and not for treatment of generalized obesity. In addition, excess fatty tissue will return if regular exercise and diet control are not maintained.

Large-volume liposuction may decrease weight and fat mass; however, there is controversy regarding whether or not it significantly improves insulin resistance and other obesity-associated metabolic abnormalities.[31–33] The most common areas treated are the neck, jowls, arms, abdomen, thighs, knees, and ankles. Other conditions that can be improved by liposuction include lipoma, gynecomastia, buffalo hump, and axillary hyperhidrosis.

There are strict guidelines from both the American Society of Dermatologic Surgery (ASDS) and the American Academy of Cosmetic Surgery (AACS) on the volume restrictions during liposuction. Tumescent liposuction is considered the safest method for performing the procedure. This technique relies on the infiltration of dilute anesthesia based on body weight, and the removal of limited amounts of adipose tissue during each operation. Tumescent anesthesia consists of very dilute lidocaine and epinephrine solutions ranging from 0.05% to 0.1% of lidocaine with 1:1,000,000 epinephrine and sodium bicarbonate. The total safe concentration of lidocaine that can be used in this formula is 35 to 55 mg/kg based on patient weight and any coexisting medical conditions. Table 3-3 is a synopsis of the 2006 ASDS guidelines of care for tumescent liposuction.[28]

LIPOSUCTION COMPLICATIONS While there have been reports of mortality with general anesthesia, there have been no reports of death with tumescent anesthesia alone. When practitioners adhere to the AACS and ASDS guidelines, tumescent liposuction is a safe outpatient procedure. Common complications are bruising, swelling, localized paresthesia, and irritated incision sites after liposuction. Other complications include hematomas, seromas, and infection. There are serious complications that the surgeon must be aware of, however, such as the development of a fat embolus,

TABLE 3-3
Synopsis of 2006 ASDS Guidelines of Care for Tumescent Liposuction

Indications
Aesthetic body contouring: most common regions include thighs, abdomen, hips, arms, back, buttocks, neck, breasts, and calfs
Other indications: treatment of lipomas, gynecomastia, lipodystrophy, axillary hyperhidrosis, axillary bromidrosis, and subcutaneous fat debulking during reconstructive procedures

Preoperative evaluation
History: diet patterns, exercise, unwanted regions, underlying disorders such as poor wound healing, bleeding abnormalities, diabetes mellitus, keloid formation, problems with past surgical procedures, personal or family history of thrombophlebitis, pulmonary emboli, and drugs that may interfere with blood coagulation or the metabolism of lidocaine
Explanation: procedure, risk and benefits, expected outcomes, needing a touch-up procedure
Physical examination: assessment of both general physical health and specific sites amenable to liposuction
Laboratory studies: may or may not be necessary for a given patient depending on the type and extent of anticipated liposuction procedure
Some surgeons may wish to obtain CBC, PT, PTT, LFT, UA, pregnancy test, screening for HIV, hepatitis B, and hepatitis C

Technique
Tumescent Anesthesia: consists of very dilute lidocaine and epinephrine solutions ranging from 0.05%–0.1% of lidocaine with epinephrine (around 1:1,000,000), sodium bicarbonate and +/− triamcinolone

Volume removal
Removal of more than 4 L of supranatant fat should be divided into more than one operative session
Monitoring: pulse oximetry, cardiac monitoring, and intermittent monitoring of BP, HR, and RR

Postoperative care
Use compression garments for 1 to 4 wk

visceral perforation, pneumothorax, deep vein thrombosis, congestive heart failure, and lidocaine toxicity. Fortunately, these complications are very rare during tumescent liposuction. The relative skills and experience level of the operating physician represent important contributing factors to the incidence of adverse events from liposuction.

Careful patient selection is the key to a successful outcome. Younger patients, those with good skin tone, and those close to their ideal weight tend to be the best candidates. Poor patient selection may lead to the development of rippling or poor skin contraction.

VOLUME LOSS

Normal Aging

The aging face shows characteristic changes, many of which were once solely attributed to the effects of gravity on skin, muscle, and fat. It is for this reason that the main approach to the aging face was to lift and reposition "ptotic" tissue. However, we now recognize that there are complex changes occurring in which volume loss is a significant contributor. These changes include muscle atrophy, bone resorption, and fat atrophy. There are some well-designed studies that look at the bony changes of the face and the change in the malar fat pad with time. The results of these studies show that the lower midfacial skeleton becomes retrusive with age relative to the upper face.[34] Study authors speculate that the skeletal remodeling of the anterior maxillary wall allows soft tissues to be repositioned downward thereby accentuating the nasojugal fold and malar mound. In a different study, some of the same authors describe the increasing incidence of a "negative vector face" as one ages.[35] A "negative-vector" patient is one in whom the bulk of the malar fat pads lies posterior to a line drawn straight down from the cornea to the orbital rim. With this change, the lower eyelid fat pads appear more prominent but are not truly hypertrophied.

In a magnetic resonance imaging (MRI) study by Gosain et al. the deepening appearance of the nasolabial fold with age seems to be a combination of ptosis and fat/skin hypertrophy.[36] They found a difference in the redistribution of fat within the malar fat pad by age, with older women exhibiting a relatively increased thickness of the midportion of the malar fat pad and overlying skin compared to younger females. More interestingly, they did not find an increase in the length or projection of the levator labii superioris muscle between young and old subjects.

A more recent cadaveric study considered the fat distribution of the face.[37] The authors found distinct facial fat compartments and subdivisions within these areas. The malar fat pad is composed of three separate compartments: medial, middle, and lateral temporal–cheek fat. The nasolabial fold was uniformly a discrete unit with distinct anatomic boundaries and little variation in size from one cadaver to the next. The forehead also consisted of three anatomic units: central, middle, and lateral temporal–cheek fat. Orbital fat is noted in three compartments determined by septal borders. However, the superior orbital fat did not connect to the inferior orbital fat. The jowl fat is the most inferior of the subcutaneous fat compartments and was found to be closely associated with the depressor anguli oris muscle.

One of the easiest ways for a cosmetic surgeon to begin to understand these changes in patients is by evaluating photographs of the patient both in youth and at the time of presentation for a consultation. This can be seen in the works of surgeons that have performed a great deal of volume restoration surgeries over the years.[38,39]

Autologous Fat Transplantation

Fat transplantation is the reinjection of aspirated adipocytes into an area that has lost volume as a result of aging, trauma, or after an inflammatory process. Autologous fat transplantation offers certain advantages over other fillers, most notably that it is an autograft with the same human leukocyte antigen therefore there is no allergic reaction or rejection via immune processes. Indications for fat transfer are volume loss anywhere in the face such as the nasolabial folds, lips, under eye hollow and tear trough deformity, submalar depressions, zygoma enhancement, chin augmentation, malar augmentation, congenital and traumatic defects, surgical defects, wide-based acne scarring, idiopathic lipodystrophy, facial hemiatrophy, rejuvenation of hands, body contour defects, depressions caused by liposuction or trauma, etc.[35,40,41] This technique can be divided into two processes: harvesting fat from the donor site, and reinjecting it into the recipient sites. The medical literature is replete with different techniques by which fat is harvested, prepared, and infiltrated into the tissue. The variation in these techniques probably accounts for why some surgeons find success with this modality and others do not achieve long-lasting results.[42]

Factors that influence survival of fat after injection include the anatomic sites of harvesting and placement, the degree of mobility in the recipient area, the vascularity of the recipient tissue, and the overall health and age of the patient.[43]

We found that fat aspirated from the lateral thigh lasts longer than fat taken from the abdomen. Even during harvesting, one will find a noticeable difference in the quality of the fat between the two areas. The fat of the upper arms, inner thighs, and abdomen tends to be softer and contain less connective tissue. Fat from the lateral thigh tends to be more dense and fibrous. Furthermore, placement of the fat into the tissues is critical to ensure viability. Adipocytes require a healthy and vascular bed in which to engraft. For this reason, fat must be placed in small parcels and in multiple layers, including in and under muscles. The less movement in the recipient site, the more that fat survives. Therefore, the malar and infraorbital areas do well while the nasolabial folds and lips require touch-ups to achieve the desired effect.

Complications

Complications are rare but include swelling, ecchymosis, hematoma, and infection. Known cases of blindness and cerebral strokes resulting after fat transplantation at the glabella[44–46] and paranasal areas[47] have been noted. In these cases, a sharp needle or large syringe were used to inject the fat. By using only blunt cannulas and 1 mL syringes, this complication has not been reported in the literature.

Fat Cells as a Source for Stem Cells and Collagen Stimulation

There is evidence that supports the utility of adipocytes for a potential stem cell role as well as collagen stimulation. First, it is known that even after puberty the human body can increase the number and size of fat cells. Second, subcutaneous tissue contains not only adipocytes but also fibrous tissue and blood vessels. These tissues are active cells and can proliferate when there is an increase in the size of subcutaneous tissue.[48] In addition, there is evidence demonstrating that aspirated fluid from liposuction contains cells that can differentiate into bone, cartilage, muscle, neurons, and adipocytes.[49–52]

In contrast to harvesting stem cells from the bone marrow, harvesting adipocytes from subcutaneous tissue is much easier and complications at the donor site can easily be visualized. In addition, adipocytes can be harvested from many areas and multiple times. Harvesting stem cells from fat will be an interesting topic in the future for tissue reengineering.

One intriguing observation noted both by the senior author (Suzan Obagi) and in her communications with other surgeons that frequently perform fat transfers is that the skin of patients continues to improve and show a reduction in rhytides and aging symptoms over time after autologous fat augmentation. This improvement is not seen in patients receiving synthetic fillers. This leads one to question whether the stems cells play a beneficial role in the skin.

MISCELLANEOUS ADIPOSE CONDITIONS

Cellulite

Cellulite occurs mainly in postadolescent women at the buttocks, abdomen, and thighs. Risk factors include lack of exercise; being female, overweight/obese, elderly, and having excess hormones and poor lymphatic drainage. It is characterized by dimpling and nodularity of the skin, where the skin looks and feels irregular, almost like an orange peel (Box 3-2). Cellulite largely results from changes in the dermis rather than changes in subcutaneous tissue. Although cellulite is frequently found in healthy, nonobese patients, it is aggravated by obesity.[53–55]

PATHOGENESIS The pathophysiology of cellulite is not completely understood, but many theories for the pathogenesis of cellulite have been postulated. One of the most important factors is the anatomy of this condition. There are morphologic differences of the fat lobes between males and females, which may explain the large frequency of cellulite in females and rare occurrence in males. Cellulite is thought to be formed from the breakdown of collagen in the reticular dermis, which leads to weakness in the dermis and herniation of subcutaneous fat into the dermis, as well as compression of the microcirculation of the dermis. Congestion of fluid and protein in the dermis is believed to lead to formation of fibrotic bands between the subcutaneous tissue and dermis resulting in retraction, dimpling, or nodularity.

TREATMENT This condition is considered normal in postadolescent women and is innocuous. Many people feel that it is cosmetically unappealing both visually and tactilely. This condition may not improve by weight reduction; however, weight control may improve the appearance of cellulite in some patients.

There are many modalities that propose to treat this condition by stimulation of collagen production in the dermis, such as infrared, diode laser, and radiofrequency.[56] These methods are new and the efficacy is unknown at this point. The most effective method to treat cellulite is to improve blood and lymphatic circulation and drainage of waste products with massage; however, the effects are temporary. Efforts to increase exercise can stimulate lymph flow and decrease fluid accumulation. A decrease in fat mass can also occur by lipolysis, such as with exercise and diet, liposuction, ultrasound-assisted lipolysis and mesotherapy. In severe dimpling lesions, minimally invasive procedures such as subcision can lead to improvement.[57] Many topical products claim to treat cellulite. The most effective of these contain caffeine and theophylline, which dehydrate the fat cells, temporarily shrinking them. Despite the many cellulite treatments on the market, none have been shown to be convincingly effective for more than 24 hours.

BOX 3-2 Hexsel Classification of Cellulite[a]

- At Stage 0, the skin's surface is not altered.
- At Stage I, skin is smooth when the individual is standing or lying down, but some cellulite appears if the skin is pinched.
- At Stage II, skin appears dimpled without any pinching or manipulation.
- At Stage III, skin appears both dimpled and raised in some areas.

[a]Personal communication with Doris Hexsel, Porto Allegre, Brazil.

Lipodystrophy

Lipodystrophy is a term describing abnormality with increasing subcutaneous fat (lipohypertrophy) or decreasing subcutaneous fat (lipoatrophy). It can be congenital or acquired, and generalized, partial, or localized. The two most common forms of lipodystrophy include lipodystrophy due to the aging process and HIV-associated lipodystrophy. Aging skin is characterized by a loss of subcutaneous tissue and laxity of the anterior supporting dermis. A decrease in supporting bone mass and loss of muscle tone can cause patients to look older. In HIV-associated lipodystrophy, most patients are treated with highly active antiretroviral therapy (HAART). This combination therapy contains nonnucleoside reverse transcriptase inhibitors that can hinder DNA polymerase leading to adipocyte apoptosis.

Common areas affected by lipodystrophy are the cheeks, forehead, temporal, infraorbital, and jowl fat compartments. Losing fat in some areas can affect the general appearance in other areas. For example, decreasing subcutaneous fat in the malar cheeks can cause a prominent nasolabial fold, or decreasing jowl fat can cause prominent marionette lines and jowls. Treatment can be performed by using synthetic filler agents or autologous fat transplantation. However, many HIV patients lack adequate fat for aspiration and transplantation or their fat is very fibrous, which makes harvesting difficult. Polylactic acid (Sculptra™, Dermik Laboratories, Berwyn, Pennsylvania), FDA-approved for the treatment of facial lipoatrophy in HIV patients, is a very useful product that works by stimulating collagen synthesis. The more recent use of higher dilutions and longer reconstitution times has led to a decrease in the formation of granulomas after injection of this agent (see Chapter 25).

FUTURE DIRECTIONS

Understanding the biology of adipocytes is important to the progress of lipolysis techniques and the possible usage of adipocytes as stem cells. In addition, various methods for fat removal are being investigated, including drugs or chemicals that can stimulate lipolysis (e.g., phosphatedylcholine, isoproterenal, theophylline, aminophylline, caffeine, carnitine, carbon dioxide, and herbal extracts) and device-assisted liposuction such as ultrasound (to burst fat cells) or 1064 nm Nd:YAG laser (to melt the fat cell). These new methods need to be evaluated for safety and efficacy.

SUMMARY

Adipocytes and subcutaneous tissue are important subjects to which the cosmetic dermatologist should pay attention. There are cosmetic concerns related to both excess and loss of fat for which the patient will seek cosmetic intervention. Advances in this field will be centered on more directed therapies of fat removal or disruption in heavy patients and on stem cell purification and injection in thinner patients. It is the role of the cosmetic dermatologist to remain abreast of these changes. Furthermore, cosmetic dermatologists and surgeons should take an active role in counseling patients on proper nutrition and weight management from both extremes (too thin or too heavy).

REFERENCES

1. Hausman DB, DiGirolamo M, Bartness TJ, et al. The biology of white adipocyte proliferation. *Obes Rev*. 2001;2:239.
2. Avram MM, Avram AS, James WD. Subcutaneous fat in normal and diseased states: 1. Introduction. *J Am Acad Dermatol*. 2005;53:663.
3. Bélanger C, Hould FS, Lebel S, et al. Omental and subcutaneous adipose tissue steroid levels in obese men. *Steroids*. 2006;71:674.
4. Wang B, Han J, Gao Y, et al. The differentiation of rat adipose-derived stem cells into OEC-like cells on collagen scaffolds by co-culturing with OECs. *Neurosci Lett*. 2007;421:191.
5. Avram MM, Avram AS, James WD. Subcutaneous fat in normal and diseased states 3. Adipogenesis: from stem cell to fat cell. *J Am Acad Dermatol*. 2007;56: 472.
6. Prins JB, O'Rahilly S. Regulation of adipose cell number in man. *Clin Sci*. 1997;92:3.
7. Faust IM, Miller HM Jr. Hyperplastic growth of adipose tissue in obesity. In: Angel A, Hollenberg CH, Roncari DAK, eds. *The Adipocyte and Obesity: Cellular and Molecular Mechanisms*. New York, NY: Raven Press; 1983:41-51.
8. Spiegelman BM, Flier JS. Adipogenesis and obesity: rounding out the big picture. Cell. 1996;87:377.
9. Manson JE, Bassuk SS. Obesity in the United States: a fresh look at its high toll. *JAMA*. 2003;289:229.
10. Kuczmarski RJ, Flegal KM, Campbell SM, et al. Increasing prevalence of overweight among US adults. The National Health and Nutrition Examination Surveys, 1960–1991. *JAMA*. 1994;272: 205.
11. Friedman JM, Halaas JL. Leptin and the regulation of body weight in mammals. *Nature*. 1998;395:763.
12. Montague CT, Farooqi IS, Whitehead JP, et al. Congenital leptin deficiency is associated with severe early-onset obesity in humans. *Nature*. 1997;387:903.
13. Krude H, Biebermann H, Schnabel D, et al. Obesity due to proopiomelanocortin deficiency: three new cases and treatment trials with thyroid hormone and ACTH4–10. *J Clin Endocrinol Metab*. 2003;88:4633.
14. Löffler H, Aramaki JU, Effendy I. The influence of body mass index on skin susceptibility to sodium lauryl sulphate. *Skin Res Technol*. 2002;8:19.
15. Deplewski D, Rosenfield RL. Growth hormone and insulin-like growth factors have different effects on sebaceous cell growth and differentiation. *Endocrinology*. 1999;140:4089.
16. Cappel M, Mauger D, Thiboutot D. Correlation between serum levels of insulin-like growth factor 1, dehydroepiandrosterone sulfate, and dihydrotestosterone and acne lesion counts in adult women. *Arch Dermatol*. 2005;141: 333.
17. Goodson WH III, Hunt TK. Wound collagen accumulation in obese hyperglycemic mice. *Diabetes*. 1986;35:491.
18. de Jongh RT, Serné EH, IJzerman RG, et al. Impaired microvascular function in obesity: implications for obesity-associated microangiopathy, hypertension, and insulin resistance. *Circulation*. 2004;109:2529.
19. Garcia-Hidalgo L. Dermatological complications of obesity. *Am J Clin Dermatol*. 2002;3:497.
20. Pribanich S, Simpson FG, Held B, et al. Low-dose tretinoin does not improve striae distensae: a double-blind, placebo-controlled study. *Cutis*. 1994;54:121.
21. Hernández-Pérez E, Colombo-Charrier E, Valencia-Ibiett E. Intense pulsed light in the treatment of striae distensae. *Dermatol Surg*. 2002;28:1124.
22. Jiménez GP, Flores F, Berman B, et al. Treatment of striae rubra and striae alba with the 585-nm pulsed-dye laser. *Dermatol Surg*. 2003;29:362.
23. Goldberg DJ, Sarradet D, Hussain M. 308-nm Excimer laser treatment of mature hypopigmented striae. *Dermatol Surg*. 2003;29:596.
24. Yosipovitch G, DeVore A, Dawn A. Obesity and the skin: skin physiology and skin manifestations of obesity. *J Am Acad Dermatol*. 2007;56:901.
25. Lemonnier D. Effect of age, sex, and sites on the cellularity of the adipose tissue in mice and rats rendered obese by a high-fat diet. *J Clin Invest*. 1972;51:2907.
26. Faust IM, Johnson PR, Stern JS, et al. Diet-induced adipocyte number increase in adult rats: a new model of obesity. *Am J Physiol*. 235:E279, 1978.
27. Coleman WP IV, Hendry SL II. Principles of liposuction. *Semin Cutan Med Surg*. 2006;25:138.
28. Svedman KJ, Coldiron B, Coleman WP III, et al. ASDS guidelines of care for tumescent liposuction. *Dermatol Surg*. 2006;32:709.
29. Coleman WP III, Glogau RG, Klein JA, et al. Guidelines of care for liposuction. *J Am Acad Dermatol*. 2001;45:438.
30. Dolsky RL. State of the art in liposuction. *Dermatol Surg*. 1997;23:1192.
31. Giese SY, Bulan EJ, Commons GW, et al. Improvements in cardiovascular risk profile with large volume liposuction: a pilot study. *Plast Reconstr Surg*. 2001;108: 510.
32. Klein S, Fontana L, Young VL, et al. Absence of an effect of liposuction on insulin action and risk factors for coronary heart disease. *N Engl J Med*. 2004;350:2549.
33. Giugliano G, Nicoletti G, Grella E, et al. Effect of liposuction on insulin resistance and vascular inflammatory markers in obese women. *Br J Plast Surg*. 2004;57: 190.
34. Pessa JE, Zadoo VP, Mutimer KL, et al. Relative maxillary retrusion as a natural consequence of aging: combining skeletal and soft-tissue changes into an integrated model of midfacial aging. *Plast Reconstr Surg*. 1998;102:205.
35. Obagi S. Autologous fat augmentation: a perfect fit in new and emerging technologies. *Facial Plast Surg Clin North Am*. 2007;15:221.
36. Gosain AK, Amarante MT, Hyde JS, et al. A dynamic analysis of changes in the nasolabial fold using magnetic resonance imaging: implications for facial rejuvenation and facial animation surgery. *Plast Reconstr Surg*. 1996;98: 622.
37. Rohrich RJ, Pessa JE. The fat compartments of the face: anatomy and clinical implications for cosmetic surgery. *Plast Reconstr Surg*. 2007;119:2219.
38. Donofrio LM. Fat distribution: a morphologic study of the aging face. *Dermatol Surg*. 2000;26:1107.
39. Coleman SR. Concepts of aging: rethinking the obvious. In: Structural Fat Grafting. St. Louis, MO: Quality Medical Publishing; 2004:xvii-xxiv.
40. Kranendonk S, Obagi S. Autologous fat transfer for periorbital rejuvenation: indications, technique, and complications. *Dermatol Surg*. 2007;33:572.
41. Narins RS. Fat transfer with fresh and frozen fat, microlipoinjection, and lipocytic dermal augmentation. In: Klein AW, ed. Tissue Augmentation in Clinical Practice. 2nd ed. New York, NY: Taylor and Francis; 2006:1-19.
42. Eremia S, Newman N. Long-term follow-up after autologous fat grafting: analysis of results from 116 patients followed at least 12 months after receiving the last of a minimum of two treatments. *Dermatol Surg*. 2000;26:1150.
43. Sommer B, Sattler G. Current concepts of fat graft survival: histology of aspirated adipose tissue and review of the literature. *Dermatol Surg*. 2000;26:1159.
44. Egido JA, Arroyo R, Marcos A, et al. Middle cerebral artery embolism and unilateral visual loss after autologous fat injection into the glabellar area. *Stroke*. 1993;24:615.
45. Teimourian B. Blindness following fat injections. *Plast Reconstr Surg*. 1988;82:361.
46. Dreizen NG, Framm L. Sudden visual loss after autologous fat injection into the glabellar area. *Am J Ophthalmol*. 1989;107: 85.
47. Danesh-Meyer HV, Savino PJ, Sergott RC. Case reports and small case series: ocular and cerebral ischemia following facial injection of autologous fat. *Arch Ophthalmol*. 2001;119:777.
48. Pinski KS, Coleman WP III. Microlipoinjection and autologous collagen. *Dermatol Clin*. 1995;13:339.
49. Strem BM, Hicok KC, Zhu M, et al. Multipotential differentiation of adipose tissue-derived stem cells. *Keio J Med*. 2005;54:132.

50. Mizuno H, Zuk PA, Zhu M, et al. Myogenic differentiation by human processed lipoaspirate cells. *Plast Reconstr Surg*. 2002;109:199.
51. De Ugarte DA, Morizono K, Elbarbary A, et al. Comparison of multi-lineage cells from human adipose tissue and bone marrow. *Cells Tissues Organs*. 2003;174:101.
52. Kokai LE, Rubin JP, Marra KG. The potential of adipose-derived adult stem cells as a source of neuronal progenitor cells. *Plast Reconstr Surg*. 2005;116:1453.
53. Draelos ZD, Marenus KD. Cellulite. Etiology and purported treatment. *Dermatol Surg*. 1997;23:1177.
54. Draelos ZD. The disease of cellulite. *J Cosmet Dermatol*. 2005;4:221.
55. Piérard GE. Cellulite: from standing fat herniation to hypodermal stretch marks. *Am J Dermatopathol*. 2000;22:34.
56. Alexiades-Armenakas M. Laser and light-based treatment of cellulite. *J Drugs Dermatol*. 2007;6:83.
57. Hexsel DM, Mazzuco R. Subcision: a treatment for cellulite. *Int J Dermatol*. 2000;39:539.

CHAPTER 4

Immunology of the Skin

H. Ray Jalian, MD
Jenny Kim, MD, PhD

Little is known about the relationship between immunology and skin appearance; however, it is certain that the immune system plays an important role in the health of the skin. Work is ongoing to help elucidate how this vital system interacts with the largest organ of the body. It is very likely that this segment of research, as it pertains to the cosmetic dermatology arena, will offer significant potential for discovery of new therapeutics and procedures in the next several years. This chapter will serve as a brief introduction to the skin as an immune organ and how the immune response plays a role in cosmetic dermatology.

In the past, the skin was viewed primarily as a barrier mechanism to prevent invading pathogens and other environmental toxins, including UV radiation, from penetrating into internal organs. However, we now know that the skin essentially acts as an immense and integral immune organ and first point of contact with the environment, capable of initiating an intricate series of events leading to host defense. A basic review of skin immunology, including the role of cytokines and growth factors, will be provided as an important part of this discussion. Mechanisms of various immune responses found in skin disease, the interplay between innate immunity and extracellular matrix synthesis, as well as emerging immune-based treatments will also be highlighted. Finally, the relevance of the local immune system and its relationship to skin aging, particularly photoaging, will be briefly reviewed.

SKIN—AN INNATE IMMUNE ORGAN

The immune response can be divided into innate and adaptive immunity. Innate immune response occurs rapidly and the cells of the innate immune system use pattern recognition receptors (PRRs) to secrete soluble factors that can lead to both inflammation and host defense. The adaptive immune response, on the other hand, occurs slowly and activation of adaptive immune cells, such as B and T cells, requires that receptors undergo gene rearrangements. The adaptive immune system can mount either humoral immunity (B cells, which make antibodies) or cell-mediated immunity (T cells). Furthermore, the adaptive immune system is also responsible for immune memory, which confers long-term protection to the host. Although the two systems appear distinct, they are not separate, and in fact can act synergistically, insofar as the innate immune system instructs the adaptive immune response and the adaptive immune system influences the innate system.

In the epidermis, the two main innate cells are the keratinocytes and Langerhans cells. In addition, neutrophils, macrophages, and dendritic cells present within the dermis also play a role in innate immunity. When a foreign substance is encountered, activation of innate cells occurs through PRRs, including the Toll-like receptors (TLRs), which are reviewed below. Upon activation, the innate cells become capable of inducing a direct antimicrobial response by producing factors that can help protect the host from external insults. These factors include reactive oxygen and nitrogen intermediates (also known as "free radicals") and antimicrobial peptides. In addition, activated innate cells produce cytokines and other inflammatory mediators that can instruct adaptive immunity. Paradoxically, the same innate immune response can induce proinflammatory cytokine production that can lead to inflammation and tissue injury, thereby facilitating disease pathology.

Cytokines and Growth Factors

Cytokines are soluble mediators of the immune system secreted by particular cell types in response to a variety of stimuli. They differ in molecular weight, structure, and mechanism of action. In general, secreted cytokines act locally in either an autocrine (effect on the producing cell itself) or paracrine (effect on adjacent cells) fashion. While there have been numerous cytokines identified to date, this section will focus on the common cytokines present in the skin and the changes that occur in expression profiles with aging.

In the epidermis, cytokines are primarily produced by keratinocytes, melanocytes, and Langerhans cells, while fibroblasts, endothelial cells, mast cells, macrophages, dendritic cells, lymphocytes, and other inflammatory cells are responsible for cytokine production within the dermis (Table 4-1 for a summary of cytokines present in the skin and the cells that produce them).

TABLE 4-1
Summary of Cytokines and Growth Factors Within the Skin and the Cells That Produce Them

	CELL TYPE
Cytokines	
Proinflammatory	
IL-1 (α, β)	Keratinocytes (IL-1α), Langerhans cells, melanocytes, fibroblasts, T cells, B cells, macrophages, neutrophils
TNF-α	Keratinocytes, Langerhans cells, melanocytes, fibroblasts, T cells, B cells, macrophages, neutrophils, eosinophils, basophils
IL-2	T cells
IL-4	T cells, mast cells, basophils, eosinophils
IL-5	Mast cells, T cells, eosinophils
IL-6	Keratinocytes, Langerhans cells, melanocytes, fibroblasts, T cells, B cells
IL-8	Keratinocytes, Langerhans cells, melanocytes, fibroblasts, T cells, B cells, macrophages, neutrophils, eosinophils, basophils
IL-12	Keratinocytes, Langerhans cells, macrophages, mast cells, B cells
Anti-inflammatory	
IL-10	T cells, mast cells, macrophages, B cells
Growth factors	
TGF-α	Keratinocytes, macrophages, eosinophils
TGF-β	Keratinocytes, melanocytes, fibroblasts, T cells, B cells, macrophages
EGF	Keratinocytes, eccrine ducts

PROINFLAMMATORY CYTOKINES Activation of the immune system is an important step in protecting the skin from pathogens and other environmental toxins; however, paradoxically, activation of the immune mechanism can also lead to inflammation, thus promoting disease and aging. Interleukin (IL)-1, a cytokine capable of being expressed by virtually any nucleated cells, including keratinocytes, exhibits a broad spectrum of biologic activity. Whereas IL-1β is predominantly expressed in most cells, IL-1α is expressed by keratinocytes.[1] IL-1 induces keratinocyte proliferation, promotes differentiation of B cells, activates neutrophils and macrophages, and initiates the expression of other proinflammatory cytokines. In addition, IL-1 is capable of enhancing the activation of T cells, and is involved in aspects of both humoral (B cells) and cellular immunity (T cells). IL-1 is continuously expressed at low levels in normal epidermis but is markedly enhanced when the skin barrier is disrupted. Furthermore, upon UV radiation, keratinocytes can secrete IL-1, which then initiates a cytokine cascade and the biologic sequelae may accelerate changes seen in photoaging.

Tumor necrosis factor (TNF)-α, although structurally unrelated to IL-1, shares similar biologic spectra. TNF-α is a potent inducer of inflammation and also induces prostaglandin synthesis in macrophages, further contributing to its proinflammatory nature. Within the skin, both IL-1 and TNF-α are expressed by keratinocytes and Langerhans cells. IL-6, produced by keratinocytes, Langerhans cells, and resident immune cells within the skin, synergizes with other cytokines, mainly potentiating the effects of TNF-α and IL-1.

Other members of the interleukin family are expressed by various cells within the skin and contribute to local innate and adaptive immunity. IL-2 is secreted by activated T cells within the skin and promotes clonal T cell proliferation as well as cytokine production, and is critical for activation of the adaptive immune response. IL-4, expressed by activated T cells, mast cells, and eosinophils, is important in allergic disease processes and has been shown to promote IgE production and the maturation of mast cells and eosinophils. IL-5, expressed by monocytes and eosinophils, serves mainly as an eosinophil growth and differentiation factor. IL-8, produced by keratinocytes and resident immune cells within the skin, is a potent chemotractant for neutrophils. IL-12, produced by antigen presenting cells, is a critical regulator of innate and adaptive immunity, and serves to potentiate cell-mediated immunity. It is also expressed by keratinocytes and Langerhans cells.

ANTI-INFLAMMATORY CYTOKINES Not all members of the interleukin family are proinflammatory. IL-10 inhibits the inflammatory immune response through various mechanisms. Specifically, it hinders antigen presenting cell function by downregulating major histocompatibility complex (MHC) class II expression. Along with T cells, macrophages, and B cells, keratinocytes express IL-10. Moreover, IL-10 disrupts cytokine production by immune effector cells and inhibits the generation of reactive oxygen species (via oxidative burst) and nitric oxide production. UV radiation enhances IL-10 production in keratinocytes, which can lead to immune dysregulation.[2] In addition, the production of IL-10 by nonmelanoma skin cancer can inhibit the function of tumor infiltrating lymphocytes and promote tumor growth.[3] Interestingly, the immune cells of older individuals have been shown to produce high levels of IL-10 in comparison to younger adults, suggesting that IL-10 is in part responsible for the immunosuppression observed in the elderly.[4]

GROWTH FACTORS Growth factors are proteins that have an effect on cellular proliferation and differentiation. While some cytokines can also be classified as growth factors, not all cytokines are considered growth factors (see Table 4-2 for a summary of the functions of cytokines and growth factors). There are numerous families of growth factors. The epidermal growth factor (EGF) family and the transforming growth factor (TGF)-β superfamilies will be discussed further.

TGF-α is a member of the EGF family of growth factors, which also consists of EGF, amphiregulin (AR), epiregulin, and neuregulin 1, 2, and 3. These growth factors are secreted by keratinocytes and bind to the EGF receptor in an autocrine manner to induce keratinocyte proliferation.[5] In addition to increasing epidermal thickness and contributing in a complex chain of events to the regulation of keratinocyte differentiation, EGF is important in wound healing.[6] Notably, EGF and TGF-α enhance migration of normal keratinocytes.[7] EGF accelerates wound healing in mice and enhances lateral migration of keratinocytes, wound closure, and subsequent reepithelialization.[8] Moreover, EGF stimulates fibroblast migration and proliferation and is critical for wound repair and dermal regeneration.[9,10]

Decreased responsiveness of EGF receptors is seen with increasing age, possibly because of a lower number and density of receptors, as well as to reduced ligand binding, receptor autophosphorylation, and internalization.[11] In addition,

TABLE 4-2
Summary of Function of Cytokines and Growth Factors

	FUNCTION
Cytokines	
Proinflammatory	
IL-1 (α, β)	Keratinocyte differentiation, B cell differentiation, activates neutrophils and macrophages
TNF-α	Similar to IL-1, prostaglandin synthesis in macrophages
IL-2	T-cell proliferation, cytokine production
IL-4	IgE production, mast cell and eosinophil maturation
IL-5	Eosinophil growth and differentiation
IL-6	Potentiates effects of TNF-α and IL-1
IL-8	Neutrophil chemoattractant
IL-12	Potentiates cell-mediated immunity
Anti-inflammatory	
IL-10	Downregulates MHC class II, disrupts cytokine production, inhibits production of reactive oxygen species and NO
Growth Factors	
TGF-α	Enhances keratinocyte migration and keratinocyte differentiation
TGF-β	Recruits monocytes, neutrophils, and fibroblasts, decreases matrix degradation
EGF	Enhances keratinocyte migration and keratinocyte differentiation, accelerates wound healing, stimulates fibroblast migration and proliferation

amphiregulin expression is downregulated in aged epidermis.[12] Diminished EGF activity and amphiregulin expression lead to a subsequent decrease in fibroblast migration and proliferation at the site of wound healing. These events result in the impaired wound healing that is observed in aged skin. Moreover, aged fibroblasts produce fewer matrix components,[13] yielding less dermal tissue and a thinner, weaker scar.

Many cosmeceuticals now contain various growth factors including EGF, insulin-like growth factor, platelet growth factor, and keratinocyte growth factor. Although these growth factors can theoretically induce keratinocyte differentiation and dermal remodeling, whether any of the products available to consumers demonstrate significant clinical effectiveness in preventing or reversing photoaging has not yet been established. Since cosmeceuticals are not subject to the same FDA regulatory requirements as drugs, well-controlled clinical studies that support the efficacy of cosmeceuticals are generally not available.

The TGF-β superfamily has a broad spectrum of functions dependent on the dosage and the target cell type. In the wound healing process, TGF-β is responsible for recruiting monocytes, neutrophils, and fibroblasts to the wound site. Higher concentrations of TGF-β activate monocytes to release numerous growth factors and stimulate fibroblasts to increase matrix synthesis and decrease matrix degradation.[14] The effects of TGF-β on keratinocytes are inconclusive with some studies showing an inhibitory role in growth, while others favoring keratinocyte chemoattraction and activation. This apparent discrepancy is perhaps linked to the temporal kinetics, dose of TGF-β administered, and also the dual activity TGF-β exerts on keratinocytes.

TGF-β is best known in cosmetic dermatology for its ability to promote the production of the extracellular matrix, notably the synthesis of procollagen.[15] TGF-β also serves as a growth factor for fibroblasts, the cells that produce collagen and play an important role in wound healing.[14] The subcutaneous injection of TGF-β into unwounded skin results in increased collagen deposition at the injection site.[16] Moreover, collagen synthesis is enhanced in animal models when TGF-β is administered locally or systemically.[17,18] Despite the encouraging results of TGF-β on collagen synthesis, its effects on reepithelialization are less predictable. In vivo studies have shown both accelerated and impaired reepithelialization in animal wound models,[19,20] echoing the contradictory effects of TGF-β on keratinocytes.

Loss of TGF-β function may be significant in photoaging. UV radiation impairs the TGF-β pathway via downregulation of TGF-β type II receptor (TGF-β RII). Loss of TGF-β RII occurs within 8 hours after irradiation and precedes the downregulation of type I procollagen expression,[21] which leads to reduced collagen production. Moreover, UV exposure decreases the expression of TGF-β, and upregulates Smad7, a negative regulator of TGF.[22] For this reason, TGF-β is included in skin care products. Whether the TGF-β and other growth factors contained in cosmeceuticals are stable, can be absorbed adequately, or exert a functionally significant outcome to induce dermal remodeling and reverse photoaging is unclear since well-controlled clinical studies are lacking.

Cytokines and Aging

Although the molecular mechanisms of photoaging and actinic damage have not been fully elucidated, skin-derived cytokines are likely involved in this process. UV radiation exposure, which is thought to be responsible for photoaging, results in inflammation, known as sunburn, and increased proinflammatory cytokines by resident skin cells, including IL-1, IL-6, and IL-8. These cytokines cause inflammation, but also initiate activation of keratinocytes, macrophages, and other immune cells that generate reactive oxygen species, resulting in cellular damage. In addition, these reactive oxygen species initiate the production of activator protein (AP)-1 and the formation of destructive enzymes such as collagenases that contribute to skin aging (see Chapter 6).[23]

UV exposure also increases the production of TGF-α from keratinocytes.[24] In addition, UVB irradiation of hairless mice has been shown to elevate levels of IL-1α, and TNF-α mRNA in skin.[25] Interestingly, UV-produced cytokines display opposing functions with regard to keratinocyte proliferation. UV exposure increases levels of IL-1, IL-6, and TGF-α, which are known to augment keratinocyte proliferation, while TNF-α is known to suppress keratinocyte growth.

Keratinocyte- and dermal-derived cytokines that result from UV exposure may also partially account for the dyspigmentation seen with photoaging. An experimental model has demonstrated that UVA-induced granulocyte monocyte colony stimulating factor from keratinocytes may play a role in melanocyte proliferation and thus result in UVA-induced pigmentation in the epidermis.[26] Further studies are needed to clarify the role of UV-induced cytokines on melanocyte growth and function.

Toll-like Receptors

The discovery of TLRs has created a new paradigm for how we view the innate immune system. Moreover, TLRs appear to play important roles in acne and other inflammatory skin diseases. Considering the partial proinflammatory nature of UV-induced photoaging, it is possible that TLRs factor into the aging process. Because TLRs are often activated early in the innate immune response resulting in cytokine production, part of the age-related cytokine aberration may be linked to changes in TLR expression and function. The background of TLRs and their known roles in skin disease and photoaging will be discussed in this section. In addition, the effect of retinoids on TLR expression and function will be explored.

The importance of innate immunity became clear with the discovery of TLRs a decade ago. The toll receptor, initially described in relation to drosophila, was shown to be crucial in preventing fungal infection in flies. Subsequently, it was demonstrated that TLRs play a role in human host defense.[27] To date, 10 human TLRs have been described and their role in innate immunity has greatly influenced our view on the immune system. TLRs are PRRs capable of recognizing a variety of conserved microbial motifs collectively referred to as pathogen-associated molecular patterns. Each TLR recognizes a unique microbial motif, such as bacterial cell wall components, fungal elements, viral RNA, and bacterial DNA. Moreover, individual TLRs can form dimers in order to increase specificity. A summary of TLRs and their respective ligands can be found in Fig. 4-1. Although their extracellular domains vary in specificity for their respective microbial ligands, the intracellular domains of TLRs are conserved and converge onto a common pathway. TLR signaling is thought to occur primarily in a MyD88-dependent pathway that ultimately leads to nuclear translocation of the transcription factor NF-κB. This in turn results in the transcription of immunomodulatory genes, including those that encode for various cytokines and chemokines.[28] In addition to a MyD88-dependent pathway, certain TLR activation can lead to MyD88-independent signaling resulting in an immune response.[29]

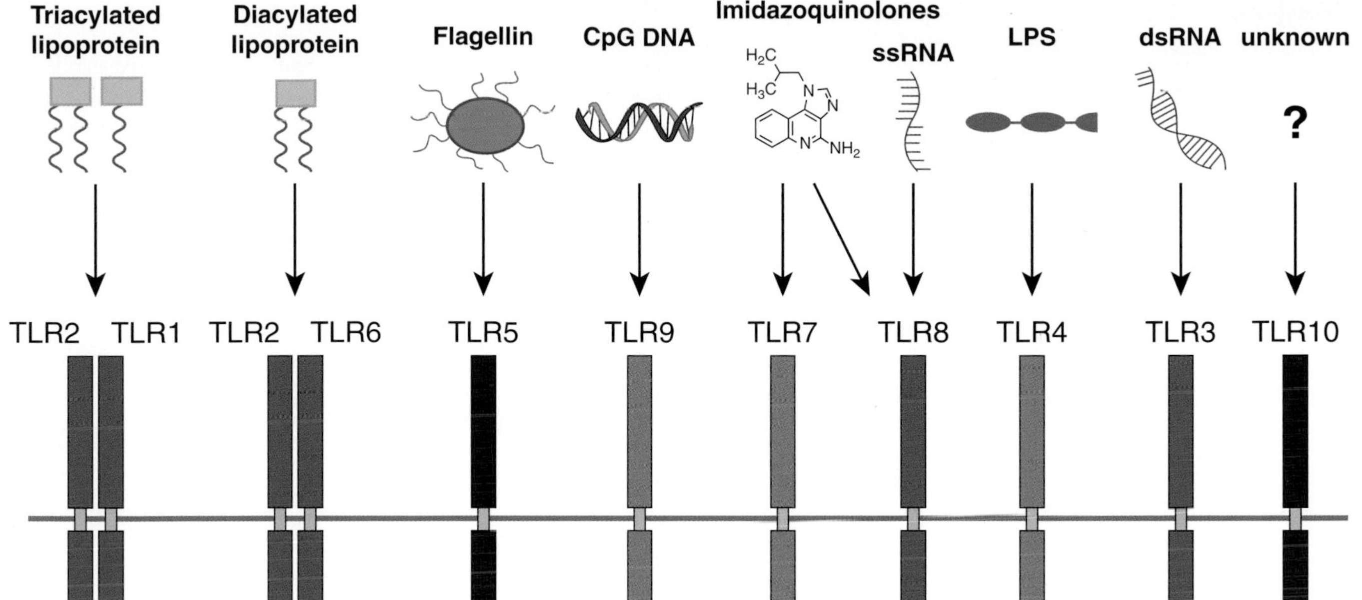

▲ **FIGURE 4-1** Toll-like receptors and their respective ligands.

TLRs are expressed by various cells of the innate immune system such as keratinocytes, neutrophils, monocytes, macrophages, dendritic cells, and mast cells. Moreover, as TLRs are key players in the innate response to pathogens, the expression and function of TLRs at sites of host-pathogen interaction are critical for host defense. It is therefore of little surprise that the skin, which is the first point of contact with cutaneous pathogens, exhibits functionally significant TLR expression. It is now known that keratinocytes express TLRs 1, 2, and 5, with TLR2 and 5 showing preferential staining in the basal keratinocytes.[30] In addition, other studies have identified expression of TLR4 in cultured human keratinocytes.[31] TLR9 has been shown to be preferentially expressed in keratinocytes found in the granular layer.[32] A more recent study has found that cultured keratinocytes constitutively express TLR1, 2, 3, 4, 5, 6, 9, and 10 mRNA, but not TLR7 or 8.[33,34] It has also been suggested that keratinocyte expression of TLR can be influenced by cytokines and growth factors, such as TGF-α.[32] Furthermore, TLR expression within the epidermis may correlate with keratinocyte maturation; as cells progress from the basal layer to the surface of the skin, patterns of TLR expression may change. TLRs are also expressed on fibroblasts. TLR1–9 are expressed and functionally active on cultured gingival fibroblasts.[35] TLR2 and 4 are also expressed in synovial fibroblasts.[36] Expression of TLRs on dermal fibroblasts has not been fully investigated, however.

Significantly, TLR expression and function have been demonstrated to change with aging. Studies evaluating the levels of TLR expression in murine macrophages in aged mice have shown significantly lower levels of expression of TLR. Moreover, when stimulated with known ligands to TLR2/1, 2/6, 3, 4, 5, and 9, significantly lower levels of IL-6 and TNF-α were produced, indicating a decline in function.[37] This supports the observation that increased susceptibility to pathogens and poor adaptive immunity in elderly individuals may be caused by a decline in TLR expression and function. A more recent study characterized TLR2/1 function in humans. TNF-α and IL-6 production from peripheral blood-derived monocytes were significantly reduced in those older than 65 years when compared to the cohort aged 21 to 30 years. Moreover, surface expression of TLR1 was decreased but TLR2 was unchanged as a function of aging.[38] While these studies have shown decreased TLR expression in monocytes, the effects of aging on keratinocyte TLR expression have not yet been described.

What role, if any, TLR expression and function have in photoaging and accumulation of actinic damage is uncertain. However, the importance of TLRs in skin has been gleaned through the study of various inflammatory skin diseases. For example, TLR2 has been implicated in the pathogenesis of acne vulgaris. *Propionibacterium acnes*, a gram-positive anaerobe that plays a *sine qua non* role in the pathogenesis of acne, induces the production of proinflammatory cytokines, such as IL-6 and IL-12, by binding TLR2.[39] Furthermore, TLR2 plays an important role in the production of key host defense components, such as antimicrobial peptides, which have been demonstrated to increase in culture systems when keratinocytes are stimulated with *P. acnes*.[40] Subtle variability in the expression of TLR1, 2, 5, and 9 has been described in psoriatic lesions when compared to normal skin, although these variances in TLR expression have not been linked to the etiology or pathogenesis of the disease.[30,41] Nevertheless, TLR2 is thought to be a key factor in host response to *Mycobacteria leprae*, the organism implicated in leprosy. The expression of TLR2 and TLR1 is markedly increased in tuberculoid leprosy (resistant form of leprosy) when compared to lepromatous leprosy (susceptible form of leprosy), suggesting that TLR2/1 is important for activating cell-mediated immunity.[42] Since TLR expression and function appear to play a role in the pathogenesis of various inflammatory and infectious skin conditions, modulation of the expression and function of these PRRs with pharmacologic agents appears to be a potential novel way in which certain dermatologic conditions can be treated.

Matrix Metalloproteinases

Recently, TLRs have been directly linked to collagen synthesis or breakdown by

TABLE 4-3
Types and Function of Select MMPs

Group	Enzyme	ECM Substrate	Other Select Substrates
Collagenases	MMP-1 (Collagenase-1)	Collagen I, II, III, VII, X	Pro-TNF, IL-1β, MMP-2, MMP-9
	MMP-8 (Collagenase-2)	Collagen I, II, III	
	MMP-13 (Collagenase-3)	Collagen I, II, III, IV, X	MMP-9
Gelatinases	MMP-2 (Gelatinase-A)	Gelatin I	IL-1β, MMP-1, MMP-9, MMP-13
		Collagen IV, V, VII, X	
		Fibronectin	
		Elastin	
	MMP-9 (Gelatinase-B)	Gelatin I, V	IL-1β
		Collagen IV, V	
		Fibronectin	
		Elastin	
Stromelysins	MMP-3 (Stromelysin-1)	Proteoglycans	IL-1β
		Fibronectin	
		Laminin	
		Gelatin I, III, IV, V	
	MMP-10 (Stromelysin-2)	Fibronectin	MMP-1, MMP-8
		Gelatin I, III, IV, V	
	MMP-11 (Stromelysin-3)	Fibronectin	IGF binding protein
		Gelatin	
		Laminin	
		Collagen IV	

mediating the expression of various metalloproteinases. Matrix metalloproteinases (MMPs) are a group of enzymes responsible for the breakdown of collagen and can be classified into four subfamilies: (1) Collagenases, (2) gelatinases, (3) stromelysins, and (4) membrane-type MMPs (Table 4-3 for a summary of the functions of the first three types). Initial breakdown of collagen depends on members of the collagenase family that are capable of cleaving native triple helical collagen. After the initial cleavage of collagen, the resultant fragments are further degraded by gelatinases and stromelysins.[43] The expression of MMPs is tightly regulated and regulation of the extracellular matrix involves a balance between synthesis of structural components and MMPs. MMPs are expressed primarily by fibroblasts, but also by macrophages and keratinocytes and the expression of MMPs is modulated by cytokines. For example, MMP-1 production from fibroblasts is stimulated by IL-1, IL-6, TNF-α, and TGF-β.[44–46] Moreover, other cytokines such as IL-4 inhibit MMP expression and are chemoattractant for fibroblasts, favoring collagen and fibronectin synthesis and matrix preservation.[47]

In addition to regulation at the transcriptional level, MMP activity is regulated by tissue inhibitors of metalloproteinase (TIMP). TIMPs, low molecular weight glycoproteins, are synthesized mainly in fibroblasts and macrophages,[48] and inhibit MMP activity by forming heat-stable 1:1 stoichiometric complexes. The expression of TIMPs is also regulated by cytokines and growth factors. For example, TIMP-1 is induced by IL-1, IL-6, and EGF.[45,49] Although both MMPs and TIMPs can be induced by similar stimuli, the expression can be regulated in both a coordinated and reciprocal manner. The critical balance between MMP and TIMP expression determines the balance between matrix degradation and matrix preservation. During periods of extracellular matrix homeostasis, the expression of MMP and TIMP is tightly coordinated providing for appropriate remodeling without excessive tissue breakdown. However, if the amount of MMP expression is increased relative to TIMP expression, excessive matrix degradation is thought to occur.

The role of MMPs in photoaging has been well documented. Both UVA and UVB radiation induce AP-1, a transcription factor important for the expression of MMP-1, 3, and 9.[50] It is then hypothesized that these MMPs are involved in collagen breakdown, and subsequent imperfect repair yields molecular scarring.[23] Cumulative UV exposure and the additive effect of molecular remodeling results in visible photoaging, characterized by wrinkles and decreased skin tone. Histologically, photoaged skin reveals disorganized dermal collagen fibrils and increased elastin.

In addition to their ability to induce cytokines and chemokines, TLRs have been implicated in the induction of MMPs. Several preliminary studies have shown that microbial agents are capable of inducing MMP expression through a TLR-dependent pathway. For example, in Lyme disease the causative agent *Borrelia burgdorferi* is capable of inducing MMP-9 through a TLR2-dependent mechanism.[51] Moreover, mycobacterial cell wall components are also thought to increase MMP-9 through TLR2.[52] More recently, CpG oligodeoxynucleotide, the ligand for TLR9, exhibited the capacity to induce MMP-9 expression in macrophages via a TLR9/NF-κB-dependent signaling pathway.[53]

Not all TLR pathways behave equally with regard to MMP regulation. Imiquimod, a TLR7 and 8 ligand, downregulates production of MMP-9 while simultaneously upregulating TIMP expression.[54] Clinical evidence to support the role of 5% imiquimod cream in the reversal of photoaging and actinic damage was recently described by Kligman and colleagues. The daily application of imiquimod cream for 5 days each week for 4 weeks resulted in a decrease in wrinkles, dyspigmentation, and hyperkeratotic pores. Histologically, reversal of epidermal atypia and atrophy were observed in posttreatment biopsies.[55] In this regard, imiquimod appears to have potential as a novel therapy for reversal of photoaging as well as the prevention of cutaneous neoplasms. The exact role imiquimod exerts in regulating the expression of MMP in vivo has not been determined and further studies are warranted in this area.

Retinoids

Retinoids, a class of vitamin A-derived compounds that bind various members of the retinoic acid receptor family, have long been used for the treatment of numerous inflammatory and hyperproliferative skin diseases. Given the anti-inflammatory nature of this class of compounds, retinoids are increasingly being used to counteract the effects of and prevent photoaging. Among the numerous mechanisms of action characterizing these vitamin A derivatives, it was recently shown that the retinoids exert their anti-inflammatory effect through downregulation of TLR2.[56] Because TLR2 has been implicated in the expression of MMPs, it is tempting to speculate that part of the mechanism of action of retinoids in photoaging is through the reduction of MMP expression via the downregulation of TLR2. Moreover, it has been well documented that retinoids directly affect MMP expression through negatively regulating AP-1 promoter activity,[57] thereby displaying utility in reversing photoaging. Retinoids have also been shown to increase TIMP expression, thus further promoting a matrix-preserving phenotype.

Retinoids are a common therapeutic agent for both the topical and systemic treatment of acne. In addition to their antiproliferative effects, recent evidence has emerged to partially account for the anti-inflammatory effect. The retinoid all-*trans* retinoic acid downregulates TLR2 and its coreceptor CD14 in monocytes. Also, the addition of retinoids to culture media reduces proinflammatory cytokine production stimulated by *P. acnes*.[56] MMPs have recently gained attention for their role in the pathogenesis of acne. MMP-1, 3, and 9 have been shown to be markedly increased in lesional skin when compared to donor-matched normal skin.[58,59] The overexpression of these MMPs may in part account for the scarring seen in acne. It is possible that retinoids partially target MMP expression as part of their therapeutic mechanism. Clinical evidence supports the role of retinoids in preventing scar formation and also for the treatment of both atrophic and hypertrophic scarring, perhaps indicating that retinoid regulation of MMPs may have important implications in the prevention and treatment of scarring.[60–62]

SUMMARY

We are beginning to see evidence that the immune system plays a role in skin appearance, factoring into the phenomena of aging and photoaging. While various hypotheses for aging exist, persistent inflammation has received much attention as one of the critical factors influencing aging in other organs, for example, in neurologic and cardiovascular conditions. Immune cells within the skin appear to respond to pathogens, UV radiation, and other environmental toxins to engender an immune response to protect the host. Yet the same mechanism through the activation of various receptors including the TLRs can lead to cytokine alterations and have important implications in cellular apoptosis, inflammation, and tissue injury. For example, the loss of TGF-β or decreased responsiveness to EGF leads to a decrease in collagen production, as well as the increased breakdown of collagen and hyaluronic acid, accounting for the dermal alterations characteristic of photoaging.

A better understanding of the mechanisms of skin aging, and photoaging in particular, from an immunologic perspective should lead to the development of improved novel therapies. Although currently there are no FDA-approved cytokine and growth factor therapies for photoaging, numerous cosmeceutical treatments containing these factors have been developed. It is important to note that for those who practice evidence-based medicine, not enough data are available to know if these products reverse or prevent photoaging and further studies are warranted. With the discovery of TLRs and their relationship to cytokine production as well as their indirect and direct links to collagen synthesis, it may be possible that TLRs could prove to be realistic targets for the prevention of photoaging. Furthermore, therapeutics that directly target downstream events of TLR activation such as modulators of MMPs and TIMPs may be of use. More research into the role of local immune response in skin aging should help provide physicians with tools to better treat and educate our patients.

REFERENCES

1. Bell TV, Harley CB, Stetsko D, et al. Expression of mRNA homologous to interleukin 1 in human epidermal cells. *J Invest Dermatol*. 1987;88:375.
2. O'Connor A, Nishigori C, Yarosh D, et al. DNA double strand breaks in epidermal cells cause immune suppression in vivo and cytokine production in vitro. *J Immunol*. 1996;157:271.
3. Kim J, Modlin RL, Moy RL, et al. IL-10 production in cutaneous basal and squamous cell carcinomas. A mechanism for evading the local T cell immune response. *J Immunol*. 1995;155:2240.
4. Uyemura K, Castle SC, Makinodan T. The frail elderly: role of dendritic cells in the susceptibility of infection. *Mech Ageing Dev*. 2002;123:955.
5. Cohen S. The stimulation of epidermal proliferation by a specific protein (EGF). *Dev Biol*. 1965;12:394.
6. Schultz GS, White M, Mitchell R, et al. Epithelial wound healing enhanced by transforming growth factor-alpha and vaccinia growth factor. *Science*. 1987;235:350.
7. Barrandon Y, Green H. Cell migration is essential for sustained growth of keratinocyte colonies: the roles of transforming growth factor-alpha and epidermal growth factor. *Cell*. 1987;50:1131.
8. Ando Y, Jensen PJ. Epidermal growth factor and insulin-like growth factor I enhance keratinocyte migration. *J Invest Dermatol*. 1993;100:633.
9. Blay J, Brown KD. Epidermal growth factor promotes the chemotactic migration of cultured rat intestinal epithelial cells. *J Cell Physiol*. 1985;124:107.
10. Carpenter G, Cohen S. Human epidermal growth factor and the proliferation of human fibroblasts. *J Cell Physiol*. 1976;88:227.
11. Reenstra WR, Yaar M, Gilchrest BA. Effect of donor age on epidermal growth factor processing in man. *Exp Cell Res*. 1993;209:118.
12. Ye J, Garg A, Calhoun C, et al. Alterations in cytokine regulation in aged epidermis: implications for permeability barrier homeostasis and inflammation. I. IL-1 gene family. *Exp Dermatol*. 2002;11:209.
13. Colige A, Nusgens B, Lapiere CM. Response to epidermal growth factor of skin fibroblasts from donors of varying age is modulated by the extracellular matrix. *J Cell Physiol*. 1990;145:450.
14. Sporn MB. The transforming growth factors-b. In: *Peptide Growth Factors and Their Receptors* (Handbook of Experimental Pharmacology), edited by AB Roberts. New York, NY: Springer-Verlag; 1990:419.
15. Edwards DR, Murphy G, Reynolds JJ, et al. Transforming growth factor beta modulates the expression of collagenase and metalloproteinase inhibitor. *EMBO J*. 1987;6:1899.
16. Roberts AB, Sporn MB, Assoian RK, et al. Transforming growth factor type beta: rapid induction of fibrosis and angiogenesis in vivo and stimulation of collagen formation in vitro. *Proc Natl Acad Sci U S A*. 1986;83:4167.
17. Beck LS, DeGuzman L, Lee WP, et al. One systemic administration of transforming growth factor-beta 1 reverses age- or glucocorticoid-impaired wound healing. *J Clin Invest*. 1993;92:2841.
18. Mustoe TA, Pierce GF, Thomason A, et al. Accelerated healing of incisional wounds in rats induced by transforming growth factor-beta. *Science*. 1987;237:1333.
19. Quaglino D Jr, Nanney LB, Kennedy R, et al. Transforming growth factor-beta stimulates wound healing and modulates extracellular matrix gene expression in pig skin. I. Excisional wound model. *Lab Invest*. 1990;63:307.
20. Hebda PA. Stimulatory effects of transforming growth factor-beta and epidermal growth factor on epidermal cell outgrowth from porcine skin explant cultures. *J Invest Dermatol*. 1988;91:440.
21. Quan T, He T, Kang S, et al. Solar ultraviolet irradiation reduces collagen in photoaged human skin by blocking transforming growth factor-beta type II receptor/Smad signaling. *Am J Pathol*. 2004;165:741.
22. Quan T, He T, Voorhees JJ, et al. Ultraviolet irradiation induces Smad7 via induction of transcription factor AP-1 in

human skin fibroblasts. *J Biol Chem.* 2005;280:8079.

23. Fisher GJ, Wang ZQ, Datta SC, et al. Pathophysiology of premature skin aging induced by ultraviolet light. *N Engl J Med.* 1997;337:1419.
24. James LC, Moore AM, Wheeler LA, et al. Transforming growth factor alpha: in vivo release by normal human skin following UV irradiation and abrasion. *Skin Pharmacol.* 1991;4:61.
25. Schwartz E, Sapadin AN, Kligman LH. Ultraviolet B radiation increases steady-state mRNA levels for cytokines and integrins in hairless mouse skin: modulation by topical tretinoin. *Arch Dermatol Res.* 1998;290:137.
26. Imokawa G, Yada Y, Kimura M, et al. Granulocyte/macrophage colony-stimulating factor is an intrinsic keratinocyte-derived growth factor for human melanocytes in UVA-induced melanosis. *Biochem J.* 1996;313:625.
27. Medzhitov R, Preston-Hurlburt P, Janeway CA Jr. A human homologue of the Drosophila Toll protein signals activation of adaptive immunity. *Nature.* 1997;388:394.
28. Takeda K, Kaisho T, Akira S. Toll-like receptors. *Annu Rev Immunol.* 2003;21:335.
29. Doyle SE, O'Connell RM, Miranda GA, et al. Toll-like receptors induce a phagocytic gene program through p38. *J Exp Med.* 2004;199:81.
30. Baker BS, Ovigne JM, Powles AV, et al. Normal keratinocytes express Toll-like receptors (TLRs) 1, 2 and 5: modulation of TLR expression in chronic plaque psoriasis. *Br J Dermatol.* 2003;148:670.
31. Pivarcsi A, Bodai L, Rethi B, et al. Expression and function of Toll-like receptors 2 and 4 in human keratinocytes. *Int Immunol.* 2003;15:721.
32. Miller LS, Sorensen OE, Liu PT, et al. TGF-alpha regulates TLR expression and function on epidermal keratinocytes. *J Immunol.* 2005;174:6137.
33. Mempel M, Voelcker V, Kollisch G, et al. Toll-like receptor expression in human keratinocytes: nuclear factor kappaB controlled gene activation by Staphylococcus aureus is toll-like receptor 2 but not toll-like receptor 4 or platelet activating factor receptor dependent. *J Invest Dermatol.* 2003;121:1389.
34. Lebre MC, van der Aar AM, van BL, et al. Human keratinocytes express functional Toll-like receptor 3, 4, 5, and 9. *J Invest Dermatol.* 2007;127:331.
35. Uehara A, Takada H. Functional TLRs and NODs in human gingival fibroblasts. *J Dent Res.* 2007;86:249.
36. Kim KW, Cho ML, Lee SH, et al. Human rheumatoid synovial fibroblasts promote osteoclastogenic activity by activating RANKL via TLR-2 and TLR-4 activation. *Immunol Lett.* 2007;110:54.
37. Renshaw M, Rockwell J, Engleman C, et al. Cutting edge: impaired Toll-like receptor expression and function in aging. *J Immunol.* 2002;169:4697.
38. van DD, Mohanty S, Thomas V, et al. Age-associated defect in human TLR-1/2 function. *J Immunol.* 2007;178:970.
39. Kim J, Ochoa MT, Krutzik SR, et al. Activation of toll-like receptor 2 in acne triggers inflammatory cytokine responses. *J Immunol.* 2002;169:1535.
40. Nagy I, Pivarcsi A, Koreck A, et al. Distinct strains of *Propionibacterium acnes* induce selective human beta-defensin-2 and interleukin-8 expression in human keratinocytes through toll-like receptors. *J Invest Dermatol.* 2005;124:931.
41. Curry JL, Qin JZ, Bonish B, et al. Innate immune-related receptors in normal and psoriatic skin. *Arch Pathol Lab Med.* 2003;127:178.
42. Krutzik SR, Ochoa MT, Sieling PA, et al. Activation and regulation of Toll-like receptors 2 and 1 in human leprosy. *Nat Med.* 2003;9:525.
43. Birkedal-Hansen H: Matrix metalloproteinases. *Adv Dent Res.* 1995;9:16.
44. Dayer JM, Beutler B, Cerami A. Cachectin/tumor necrosis factor stimulates collagenase and prostaglandin E2 production by human synovial cells and dermal fibroblasts. *J Exp Med.* 1985;162:2163.
45. Postlethwaite AE, Raghow R, Stricklin GP, et al. Modulation of fibroblast functions by interleukin 1: increased steady-state accumulation of type I procollagen messenger RNAs and stimulation of other functions but not chemotaxis by human recombinant interleukin 1 alpha and beta. *J Cell Biol.* 1988;106:311.
46. Wlaschek M, Heinen G, Poswig A, et al. UVA-induced autocrine stimulation of fibroblast-derived collagenase/MMP-1 by interrelated loops of interleukin-1 and interleukin-6. *Photochem Photobiol.* 1994;59:550.
47. Zhang Y, McCluskey K, Fujii K, et al. Differential regulation of monocyte matrix metalloproteinase and TIMP-1 production by TNF-alpha, granulocyte-macrophage CSF, and IL-1 beta through prostaglandin-dependent and -independent mechanisms. *J Immunol.* 1998;161:3071.
48. Stricklin GP, Welgus HG. Human skin fibroblast collagenase inhibitor. Purification and biochemical characterization. *J Biol Chem.* 1983;258:12252.
49. Edwards DR, Murphy G, Reynolds JJ, et al. Transforming growth factor beta modulates the expression of collagenase and metalloproteinase inhibitor. *EMBO J.* 1987;6:1899.
50. Herrlich P, Sachsenmaier C, Radler-Pohl A, et al. The mammalian UV response: mechanism of DNA damage induced gene expression. *Adv Enzyme Regul.* 1994;34:381.
51. Gebbia JA, Coleman JL, Benach JL. Selective induction of matrix metalloproteinases by *Borrelia burgdorferi* via toll-like receptor 2 in monocytes. *J Infect Dis.* 2004;189:113.
52. Elass E, Aubry L, Masson M, et al. Mycobacterial lipomannan induces matrix metalloproteinase-9 expression in human macrophagic cells through a Toll-like receptor 1 (TLR1)/TLR2- and CD14-dependent mechanism. *Infect Immun.* 2005;73:7064.
53. Lee S, Hong J, Choi SY, et al. CpG oligodeoxynucleotides induce expression of proinflammatory cytokines and chemokines in astrocytes: the role of c-Jun N-terminal kinase in CpG ODN-mediated NF-kappaB activation. *J Neuroimmunol.* 2004;153:50.
54. Li VW, Li WW, Talcott KE, et al. Imiquimod as an antiangiogenic agent. *J Drugs Dermatol.* 2005;4:708.
55. Kligman A, Zhen Y, Sadiq I, et al. Imiquimod 5% Cream reverses histologic changes and improves appearance of photoaged facial skin. *Cos Derm.* 2006;19:704.
56. Liu PT, Krutzik SR, Kim J, et al. Cutting edge: all-trans retinoic acid down-regulates TLR2 expression and function. *J Immunol.* 2005;174:2467.
57. Dedieu S, Lefebvre P. Retinoids interfere with the AP1 signalling pathway in human breast cancer cells. *Cell Signal.* 2006;18:889.
58. Kang S, Cho S, Chung JH, et al. Inflammation and extracellular matrix degradation mediated by activated transcription factors nuclear factor-kappaB and activator protein-1 in inflammatory acne lesions in vivo. *Am J Pathol.* 2005;166:1691.
59. Trivedi NR, Gilliland KL, Zhao W, et al. Gene array expression profiling in acne lesions reveals marked upregulation of genes involved in inflammation and matrix remodeling. *J Invest Dermatol.* 2006;126:1071.
60. Layton AM. Optimal management of acne to prevent scarring and psychological sequelae. *Am J Clin Dermatol.* 2001;2:135.
61. Janssen de Limpens AM. The local treatment of hypertrophic scars and keloids with topical retinoic acid. *Br J Dermatol.* 1980;103:319.
62. Mizutani H, Yoshida T, Nouchi N, et al. Topical tocoretinate improved hypertrophic scar, skin sclerosis in systemic sclerosis and morphea. *J Dermatol.* 1999;26:11.

CHAPTER 5

Hormones and Aging Skin

Larissa Zaulyanov-Scanlan, MD

It is well known that estrogen and testosterone play vital roles in the development of secondary sexual characteristics and are important for reproduction. There are also several ongoing investigations on the effects of these sex hormones in cardiovascular disease, neurodegenerative disease, mood, and cancer formation, as well as into their roles in adipogenesis and osteogenesis in women and men. With so many tissues expressing estrogen and androgen receptors, it is not surprising to find that several organ systems experience dramatic changes as sex hormone levels decline with advancing age. The first studies of sex hormone receptors in human skin and skin appendages began in the mid-1970s and examined estrogen receptors in breast cancer tissue,[1] and testosterone receptors in human hair follicles.[2] Since that time several studies have examined the roles of sex hormones in a variety of dermatologic and other disease states. While it has long been known that the skin has sex hormone receptors, the recent discovery of a second estrogen receptor (ER-β) has led to much interest in and new insights into the effects of sex hormones on various tissues including the skin. The aim of this chapter is to review the actions of sex hormones on the skin, specifically estrogen and testosterone, and to examine the roles of these hormones in skin aging.

SYNTHESIS OF SEX HORMONES AND THEIR DECLINE DURING AGING

Sex hormones are mainly synthesized in the gonads and the adrenal glands of humans. During puberty, both the male and female gonads begin to secrete testosterone. The prostate, a male secondary sex organ, can convert testosterone into the more potent dihydrotestosterone (DHT), which has an affinity 5 times as strong for the androgen receptor. During the female reproductive years, most of the testosterone produced by the ovaries is converted into estradiol (17β-estradiol), the physiologically active and most abundant estrogen during this time period.

TABLE 5-1
Types of Estrogen, Their Origin, and When Each Type Prevails

Estrogen Type	Stage of Production/Prevalence	Synthesized by	Relative Potency
Estradiol (E2)	Reproductive years	Ovaries	Most potent
Estriol (E3)	Pregnancy	Placenta	Least potent
Estrone (E1)	Postreproductive years	Fat cells, adrenal glands	

The other two types of physiologic estrogens are estrone and estriol. Estrone is the predominant estrogen after menopause, and estriol is synthesized by the placenta during pregnancy (Table 5-1). In the adrenal gland, the precursor to both estrogens and androgens is dehydroepiandrosterone (DHEA), a derivative of cholesterol. DHEA is converted into androstenedione in the adrenal gland. Both androstenedione and DHEA, which by themselves have weak androgenic activity, can enter the systemic circulation and be converted into testosterone or estrogen by peripheral target cells. The enzyme responsible for this conversion is aromatase. Both men and women have the ability to convert testosterone into estradiol via this enzyme. Besides the gonads, other tissues containing aromatase, and hence the ability to make estradiol or testosterone from DHEA, are bone, brain, vascular tissue, fetal liver, placenta, adipose tissue, and the skin[3,4] (Table 5-2).

As both men and women age, the levels of DHEA and DHEAS (its sulfate ester that can be measured in serum) produced by the adrenal glands begin to decline, so that by 70 to 80 years of age peak concentrations are only 10% to 20% of those found in young adults.[5] This steady decline in DHEA and DHEAS has been termed "*adreno*pause," for the associated decline in the adrenal secretion of DHEA/DHEAS,[5] although the levels of glucocorticoids and mineralocorticoids (other adrenal hormones) stay relatively constant throughout life. Since many age-related disturbances have been reported to begin with the decline of this hormone, there has been much interest in the use of DHEA (available as an over-the-counter supplement) as a replacement therapy in aging. In one randomized, double-blind, controlled trial examining men and women aged 60 to 88 years with low serum DHEAS levels, DHEA replacement therapy for 1 year improved hip bone mineral density;[6] however, most other studies examining the effects of DHEA administration in the elderly have displayed mixed results. Furthermore, the risks of DHEA supplementation and its specific mechanisms of action are unclear. *Adreno*pause, or a drop in DHEA and DHEAS, is independent from menopause. Menopause is the cessation of menses that occurs as ovarian follicles diminish over time, with a subsequent decline in serum estradiol levels. Men also have an age-associated decline in gonadal secretion of testosterone, termed "*andro*pause" for decline in androgen levels, and it is associated with various symptoms, such as sexual dysfunction, hypogonadism, and psychologic changes.[7] While menopause is a rapid decline in circulating estradiol and a subsequent abrupt onset of symptoms, in men testosterone begins to decrease gradually at an average rate of 1% per year, starting from age 19.[7] The reason(s) for this steady androgen decline in men are not as well understood as menopause in women, but the decline is attributed to decreased secretion of GnRH (gonadotropin-releasing hormone, secreted by the hypothalamus)[8] (Table 5-3).

TABLE 5-2
Tissues That Contain Aromatase

Gonads
Bone
Brain
Vascular tissue
Fetal liver
Placenta
Adipose tissue
Skin

TABLE 5-3
Menopause, Andropause, and Adrenopause. These Age-Related Conditions are Characterized by a Decline in the Hormones Listed

Condition	Hormone That Decreases
Menopause	Estrogen (Estradiol)
Adrenopause	DHEA/DHEAS
Andropause	Androgens

ESTROGEN AND ANDROGEN RECEPTORS IN THE SKIN

All steroid hormones, such as estradiol and testosterone, exert their biologic action by binding to nuclear receptors, thereby initiating transcription and translation of proteins. While the classic estrogen receptor (ER-α) was discovered in the 1970s, ER-β was discovered and isolated from human tissue in 1996.[9] Since then, studies have shown that ER-β is the predominant estrogen receptor in human skin and highly expressed in the epidermis, blood vessels, dermal fibroblasts, and outer root sheath of the hair follicle (the location of the bulge and stem cells). ER-α and the androgen receptor (which can bind testosterone or DHT) are expressed only in dermal papilla cells of the hair follicle.[10,11] All three receptors are also found in sebaceous glands.[10,11] In eccrine sweat glands, ER-β is highly expressed as are, to a lesser extent, androgen and progesterone receptors.[11] Recent studies of human adipose tissue found that sex hormone receptors differ by site, with ER-β being highly expressed in subcutaneous tissue.[12] With all these recent findings, it is clear that sex hormones are involved in the proliferation, differentiation, and function of the skin, adnexal structures, as well as fat, and that this regulation is far more intricate than previously thought. In addition, the recent description of the ER-β receptor (ER-β1–5) isoforms has made this subject more complex.[12]

SEX HORMONES AND ACNE

Both estrogen and androgen receptors are expressed in sebaceous glands,[10,11] and both hormones are known to have an effect on these structures. During puberty, the increase of androgenetic hormones triggers sebaceous gland growth with increased release of sebum. This sebum is a source of nutrition for skin bacteria such as *Propionibacterium acnes*. Proliferation of these bacteria leads to greater production of inflammatory factors, causing inflammation and pustule formation clinically seen as acne. Estrogens, however, demonstrate anti-inflammatory properties by decreasing neutrophil chemotaxis,[13] thereby counteracting the inflammatory effects of *P. acnes*. In contrast, androgens prolong inflammation,[14] and therefore compound their negative effects, resulting in worsened acne. This may help to explain why so many young women with acne benefit from the particular hormonal combinations found in oral contraceptives. These agents are especially useful for patients with the triad of acne, hirsutism, and abnormal menstrual periods. In fact, some oral contraceptives such as Ortho TriCyclen® and Yaz® have received FDA approval for use in the treatment of acne. These oral contraceptives can relieve the symptoms of acne by reducing the amount of circulating androgens. They also stimulate the production of sex hormone-binding globulin, thus reducing free and biologically active testosterone derived from both the ovaries and adrenal glands. At the same time, they suppress the ovarian production of testosterone by direct gonadotropin suppression.

Hormones also play a role in adult female acne. As women approach menopause and their estrogen levels decrease, the actions of androgens are unmasked. Testosterone stimulates the sebaceous glands to produce sebum, as is seen in puberty, leading to an increase in acne. Many female patients are surprised to find themselves with acne well into adulthood. Current studies demonstrate that androgen levels in patients with acne are higher than those in controls, and the fact that people with androgen insensitivity syndrome do not develop acne also points to androgens as the main culprit in this condition.[15] Local factors, other than androgen plasma levels, contribute to androgen levels in the skin and thus the development of acne. Since the skin contains enzymes such as aromatase, it can convert precursor hormones into more potent androgens such as testosterone and DHT at the cellular level. For a more extensive discussion on acne, (see Chapter 15).

SEX HORMONES AND HAIR GROWTH

The hair follicle cycle is characterized by a period of growth (anagen), followed by a period of regression and remodeling (catagen), and a period of rest (telogen). During pregnancy, there is an increase in the amount of anagen hairs secondary to the increase in estradiol. After giving birth, telogen effluvium is triggered by the rapid drop in estrogen, and is further suppressed in women who breastfeed because of the inhibitory effects of prolactin, a peptide hormone associated with lactation, on estrogen production. Postmenopausal women often experience a similar decrease in hair density owing to the decline in estradiol and the subsequent unmasking of androgen effects.

For many decades androgens have dominated hair growth research. A commonly prescribed drug for hair loss, finasteride (Propecia®), blocks the conversion of testosterone to DHT by inhibiting the enzyme 5-α-reductase type II. Regarding treatment of hair loss, finasteride is a pregnancy category X, thus contraindicated for women in their childbearing years who intend to have children. It is indicated for men with male pattern hair loss, and may be effective for the treatment of androgenetic alopecia, or male pattern hair loss, in postmenopausal women.[16] As both androgen and estrogen receptors are found in the hair follicles, theoretically either of them can be targeted for the treatment of patterned hair loss. Furthermore, as the aromatase enzyme is located in the hair follicle and the sebaceous gland, these tissues can be both target and source for estrogen or testosterone. While ER-β is found in the bulge region, ER-α and androgen receptors are found in the dermal papilla. The hair cycle is self-renewing because of the presence of stem cells in the bulge. It is thought that cells in the dermal papilla send a signal to the stem cells in the bulge to differentiate and ultimately restart the anagen phase. While it is known that the dermal papillae regulate hair growth and have receptors for androgens and ER-β, the sequence of signals that regulate hair growth has not been elucidated. What is clear is that estrogens and androgens are intimately involved in this process.

Gender differences in hair exist as evidenced in the commonality of androgenetic alopecia, which occurs but is much less common in women. This gender difference may be attributable more to the inherent enzyme content within hair follicles than to serum hormone levels. For instance, Sawaya and Price[17] examined the levels of 5-α-reductase types I and II, aromatase, and androgen receptors in hair follicles of women and men with androgenetic alopecia and found that the women had a six-fold greater aromatase level in frontal hair follicles than the men, giving them the ability to convert weaker sex hormone precursors into stronger ones. These authors also determined that the women had three- and three-and-a-half-fold less 5-α-reductase types I and II, respectively, in their hair follicles than the men did in their frontal hair follicles, thus reducing the women's ability to synthesize the more potent form of male hormone, DHT, which is responsible for hair miniaturization and eventual loss.[17] Sawaya and

Price[17] concluded that these differences in androgen receptor and steroid-converting enzymes may account for the different clinical presentations of androgenetic alopecia in women and men. A similar study examining androgen receptor and steroid-converting enzymes should be undertaken in women and men with normal hair growth as well as those with other hair growth disorders.

SEX HORMONES AND AGING SKIN

While skin quality deteriorates because of the synergistic effects of chronologic time, photoaging, and environmental factors such as smoking and poor nutrition, the results of hormonal decline with age on the quality of skin are also significant and worthy of examination. Young skin is often associated with acne, oiliness, and thick scar or keloid formation, while the clinically apparent changes associated with aging skin include skin thinning (notably, not in all layers) and atrophy, loss of elasticity, dryness, increased wrinkling, and poor wound healing but cosmetically better surgical scars. While androgen and estrogen receptors are found in the epidermis, sebaceous glands, and hair follicles, it is primarily ER-β that is localized in the fibroblasts of the dermis, and it is the fibroblasts that synthesize collagen, hyaluronic acid, elastin, and other components of the extracellular matrix.[10,11] Therefore, of the sex hormones, it is mainly estrogen that controls the fibroblast. Collagen is responsible for imparting strength and structure to the skin; elastin confers its elasticity; and hyaluronic acid content directly leads to an increase in water-holding capacity. Together, these constituents provide the resilience and fullness to the skin that is associated with youth, while the lack of these constituents leads to wrinkles, the feature most emblematic of aged skin.

In the fourth and fifth decades of life, many women begin to notice changes in their skin that are associated with changes seen in menopause. Most postmenopausal women complain of skin thinning and dryness, an increase in wrinkles, and decreased elasticity of the skin. In fact, studies have shown that as much as 30% of skin collagen (both type I, which confers strength to the skin, and type III, which contributes to the elasticity of skin) is lost in the first 5 years after menopause,[18] and total collagen levels are estimated to decline on an average of 2% per postmenopausal year over a period of 15 years.[19] In a study by Affinito et al. that evaluated the effects of aging and postmenopausal hypoestrogenism on type I and type III collagen content in the skin of premenopausal and postmenopausal women, a decrease in skin collagen was more closely related to years of postmenopause than to chronologic age.[18] While collagen content seems to quickly diminish with increased postmenopausal years, several studies demonstrate that postmenopausal women who start receiving hormone replacement therapy (HRT) with estrogen have an increase in skin collagen content,[19–22] with as much as a 6.5% increase in skin collagen content after 6 months of estrogen replacement.[21] In a study by Brincat et al. examining different regimens of estrogen replacement therapy in postmenopausal women, the authors found that all regimens of estrogen therapy under consideration increased skin collagen content and that estrogen replacement therapy is prophylactic in women who have higher skin collagen levels and both prophylactic and therapeutic in women with lower skin collagen levels.[19] Similarly, a study by Castelo-Branco et al. examining skin collagen changes and HRT in postmenopausal women at 0 and 12 months of treatment showed that various forms of HRT with estrogen-induced increases in skin collagen content in postmenopausal women, whereas the postmenopausal control group had significant decreases when assessed at the same time points[22] (Box 5-1). In another study by Brincat et al.[23] examining skin collagen changes in postmenopausal women receiving topical estradiol applied to the abdomen and thigh, the authors noted a strong correlation between the change in skin collagen content and the original skin collagen content, indicating that the change in response to estrogen therapy is dependent on the original collagen level, and that there is no further increase in collagen production once an "optimum" skin collagen level is reached. This study is particularly noteworthy insofar as it suggests that there is a therapeutic window in which estrogen exerts its maximal effect in stimulating collagen production.

Estrogen can also combat skin dryness by decreasing transepidermal water loss. In a study by Piérard-Franchimont et al. that examined transepidermal water loss in menopausal women, the authors found that women receiving transdermal hormone replacement with estrogen exhibited a significantly increased water-holding capacity of the stratum corneum as compared with menopausal women not receiving hormone replacement.[24] In addition, in a study examining changes in transepidermal water loss and cutaneous blood flow during the menstrual cycle, Harvell et al. found that transepidermal water loss was higher on the day of minimal estrogen/progesterone secretion as compared with the day of maximal estrogen secretion on both back ($p = 0.037$) and forearm ($p = 0.021$) skin in normal

BOX 5-1

Hormone replacement therapy (HRT), already in widespread use primarily to reduce the risk of osteoporosis, gained much attention, and some notoriety, when one of the studies in the Women's Health Initiative (WHI) was halted in 2002. The National Institutes of Health (NIH) National Heart, Lung, and Blood Institute (NHLBI) halted the Prempro phase (HRT phase) of the WHI during the summer of 2002 because of a higher than expected rise in breast cancer, heart attacks, strokes, and blood clots in the legs among this cohort as well as the failure of the expected benefits to materialize. The two studies consisted of an HRT phase, estrogen plus progestin in women with a uterus, and the estrogen replacement therapy (ERT) phase in women without a uterus. HRT is sometimes recommended for women who have undergone natural menopause; ERT is more appropriate for women whose menopause is surgically-induced. The ERT phase of the WHI ended in 2006. Follow-up of the women in both studies is scheduled to conclude in 2010. Over 16,000 women were randomized in the HRT phase to estrogen + progestin or placebo and approximately 10,000 women in the ERT phase were likewise randomized to estrogen or placebo. Few of the participants were taking HRT (13% in the HRT cohort and 6% in the ERT cohort), though the numbers that had ever used HRT were three-fold higher. It has been suggested that the results of these studies are not generalizable to premenopausal/perimenopausal women, who are more likely to be experiencing menopausal symptoms, because many of the women in the study may not have been experiencing menopausal symptoms any longer.

Women should decide on the appropriateness of HRT or ERT therapy in medical consultation based on the individual's specific risk factors and medical profile. See the NIH Web site (http://www.nhlbi.nih.gov/health/women/pht_facts.pdf) for more information.

women.[25] The use of topical estrogen has been shown to increase epidermal thickness in postmenopausal women.[26,27] However, whether the beneficial effects of estrogen on skin dryness are attributable to its influence on the fibroblast and an increase in hyaluronic acid content, with the concomitant increase in water-retaining capacity of the dermis, or a direct effect of estrogen on the epidermis remains unclear.

While the number of sebaceous glands remains the same during life, as androgen levels decline with advanced age, sebum levels tend to decrease.[28] Although the level of surface lipids falls with age owing to decreased sebaceous gland function, paradoxically the sebaceous glands become larger, rather than smaller, as a result of decreased cellular turnover.[28]

Subcutaneous fat is also important when it comes to maintaining the appearance of youth, and fat distribution is another area where sex hormones play a vital role. In postmenopausal women, the decrease in estrogen and the unmasking effects of systemic androgens lead to central fat accumulation. In a study by Dieudonne et al. examining androgen receptors in mature human adipocytes, androgen binding sites were found to differ by location, with twice as many androgen binding sites in intra-abdominal fat than in subcutaneous fat.[29] This finding was the same for fat deposits in men and women.[29] Another study by Dieudonne et al. investigating the location of estrogen receptors in mature human adipocytes of both men and women found that the predominant estrogen receptor was ER-α and that its level of expression was the same regardless of origin (intra-abdominal or subcutaneous fat).[30] These results suggest that the deposition of subcutaneous fat is mainly influenced by estrogen, while the deposition of abdominal fat is more androgen-dependent.

SEX HORMONES AND WOUND HEALING

Sex hormones also influence wound healing. It has recently been demonstrated that the mechanism by which estrogen can regulate the production of connective tissue molecules, namely collagen and hyaluronic acid, is by increasing the production of TGF-β,[31] a key modulator of wound healing. In a randomized, double-blind study by Ashcroft et al. that examined the effects of topical estrogen on cutaneous wound healing in healthy elderly men and women after receiving punch biopsies and related these effects to the inflammatory response and local elastase levels (a matrix metalloproteinase known to be upregulated in chronic wounds); it was found that compared to placebo treatment, estrogen treatment increased the extent of wound healing in both elderly males and females.[13] These authors further determined that estrogen treatment was associated with a decrease in wound elastase levels secondary to reduced neutrophil numbers and decreased fibronectin degradation. Similarly, an observational study showed that HRT recipients are approximately 30% to 40% less likely to develop a venous leg ulcer or a pressure ulcer than nonrecipients.[32] In contrast, androgens appear to prolong inflammation and inhibit wound healing.[14,33,34] Estrogen also promotes wound healing by increasing tissue expression of vascular endothelial growth factor (VEGF), an effect that is antagonized by androgens; therefore, estrogen can promote neovascularization that is necessary for wound healing while androgens inhibit it.[14]

As estrogen has a direct stimulatory role on dermal fibroblasts, it also affects scarring. Aged skin is associated with a reduced rate of cutaneous wound healing and improved quality of scarring, while young skin heals quickly but often with thick, visible scars. Keloids and hypertrophic scars are generally conditions of youth, owing to an increase in TGF-β production by dermal fibroblasts, while scarless wound healing is a characteristic of fetal skin that, like aged skin, has lower levels of TGF-β.[35] As estrogen is known to increase TGF-β, and is therefore profibrotic, antiestrogens such as tamoxifen have been shown to decrease TGF-β levels,[36,37] and are antifibrotic. Therefore, tamoxifen or other estrogen receptor modulators may be useful in improving scar cosmesis.

HORMONE REPLACEMENT THERAPY

The therapeutic benefits of HRT on easing postmenopausal symptoms or improving bone density have been known for many years. However, the benefits of HRT on skin aging and wound healing are just beginning to be explored. While many postmenopausal women would derive great cutaneous benefits from estrogen therapy, as estrogens are known to affect several organ systems, this subject is best addressed on a case-by-case basis and as part of a team approach with other physicians so that all risks and benefits are weighed. The primary risks associated with HRT are related to breast cancer and cardiovascular health; the primary benefits include relief of menopausal symptoms (such as vasomotor instability, sexual dysfunction, mood fluctuation, and skin atrophy) and a decrease in fracture risk. Current recommendations specify that HRT should only be used short term, for moderate to severe vasomotor symptoms, and primarily in younger women who are close to menopause (early menopause or first 5 years after menopause). It is important to note that estrogen-containing creams are contraindicated for women who have been diagnosed with estrogen-responsive cancers. Regarding the use of topical versus oral estrogens, topical estrogens are easily absorbed (hence the popularity of estrogen replacement in patch or gel form), but the cutaneous route avoids hepatic first-pass metabolism and high plasma levels of estrogen metabolites are associated with oral administration.

SUMMARY

For centuries, women have noted skin changes following menopause. Multiple studies show that women experience decreased skin thickness with a related reduction in the amount of skin collagen that occurs most rapidly in the first five postmenopausal years. Skin dryness may be related to decreased levels of hyaluronic acid as well as epidermal thinning. For these reasons, oral or topical HRT may be useful to prevent such changes in postmenopausal women. While men do not experience the same abrupt decline in sex hormones as women do with menopause, their characteristic hormonal composition also undergoes a decline with age, as witnessed by changes in their skin and other organ systems. Whether the skin of elderly men would benefit from hormone replacement, and in what combination, is another vast subject worthy of exploration. While estrogen promotes wound healing and testosterone seems to inhibit it, treating men with estrogens long term would certainly have a feminizing effect. Perhaps future research into sex hormones and aging skin should focus on hormone receptor or tissue enzyme modulators. Currently, most of these agents are being developed and utilized in the field of oncology.

Hormonal influences on the health and function of skin are an important topic in dermatology that warrant due consideration by the cosmetic practitioner in assessing health or prescreening patients' skin prior to performing corrective procedures. The beneficial effect of estrogen on collagen production and in the promotion of wound healing is clear. Future investigations into the effects of sex hormones on the skin and adnexa are likely to indicate that sex hormones constitute a promising target for therapeutic intervention in both cosmetic and medical dermatology.

REFERENCES

1. Liskowski L, Rose DP. Experience with a simple method for estrogen receptor assay in breast cancer. *Clin Chim Acta.* 1976;67:175-182.
2. Bassas E. Experimental studies on seborheic alopecia. III. Localization of testosterone receptors in human hairy follicles. *Med Cutan Ibero Lat Am.* 1975; 3:77-79
3. Bulun SE, Takayama K, Suzuki T, et al. Organization of the human aromatase p450 (CYP19) gene. *Semin Reprod Med.* 2004;22:5-9.
4. Simpson ER. Aromatase: biologic relevance of tissue-specific expression. *Semin Reprod Med.* 2004;22:11-23.
5. Genazzani AD, Lanzoni C, Genazzani AR. Might DHEA be considered a beneficial replacement therapy in the elderly? *Drugs Aging.* 2007;24:173-185.
6. Jankowski CM, Gozansky WS, Schwartz RS, et al. Effects of dehydroepiandrosterone replacement therapy on bone mineral density in older adults: a randomized, controlled trial. *J Clin Endocrinol Metab.* 2006;91:2989-2993.
7. Mooradian AD, Korenman SG. Management of the cardinal features of andropause. *Am J Ther.* 2006;13:145-160.
8. Keenan DM, Takahashi PY, Liu PY, et al. An ensemble model of the male gonadal axis: illustrative application in aging men. *Endocrinology.* 2006;147:2817-2828.
9. Mosselman S, Polman J, Dijkema R. ER–b: identification and characterization of a novel human estrogen receptor. *FEBS Lett.* 1996;392:49-53.
10. Thornton MJ, Taylor AH, Mulligan K, et al. Oestrogen receptor beta is the predominant oestrogen receptor in human scalp skin. *Exp Dermatol.* 2003;12: 181-190.
11. Pelletier G, Ren L. Localization of sex steroid receptors in human skin. *Histol Histopathol.* 2004;19:629-636.
12. Pedersen SB, Brunn JM, Hube F, et al. Demonstration of estrogen receptor subtypes alpha and beta in human adipose tissue: influences of adipose cell differentiation on fat depot localization. *Mol Cell Endocrinol.* 2001;182:27-37.
13. Ashcroft GS, Greenwell-Wild T, Horan MA, et al. Topical estrogen accelerates cutaneous wound healing in aged humans associated with an altered inflammatory response. *Am J Pathol.* 1999;155:1137-1146.
14. Kanda N, Watanabe S. Regulatory roles of sex hormones in cutaneou biology and immunology. *J Dermatol Sci.* 2005; 38: 1-7.
15. Dekkers OM, Thio BH, Romijn JA, et al. Acne vulgaris: endocrine aspects. *Ned Tijdschr Geneeskd.* 2006;150:1281-1285.
16. Trueb RM. Finasteride treatment of patterned hair loss in normoandrogenic postmenopausal women. *Dermatology.* 2004;209:202-207.
17. Sawaya ME, Price VH. Different levels of 5-alpha-reductase type I and II, aromatase, and androgen receptor in hair follicles of women and men with androgenetic alopecia. *J Invest Dermatol.* 1997; 109:296-300.
18. Affinito P, Palomba S, Sorrentino C, et al. Effects of postmenopausal hypoestrogenism on skin collagen. *Maturitas.* 1999;33:239-247.
19. Brincat M, Versi E, Moniz CF, et al. Skin collagen changes in postmenopausal women receiving different regimens of estrogen therapy. *Obstet Gynecol.* 1987; 70:123-127.
20. Patriarca MT, Goldman KZ, Dos Santos JM, et al. Effects of topical estradiol on the facial skin collagen of postmenopausal women under oral hormone therapy: a pilot study. *Eur J Obstet Gynecol Reprod Biol.* 2007;130:202-205.
21. Sauerbronn AV, Fonseca AM, Bagnoli VR, et al. The effects of systemic hormonal replacement therapy on the skin of postmenopausal women. *Int J Gynaecol Obstet.* 2000;68:35-41.
22. Castelo-Branco C, Buran M, Gonzalez-Merlo J. Skin collagen changes related to age and hormone replacement therapy. *Maturitas.* 1992;15:113-119.
23. Brincat M, Versi E, O'Dowd T, et al. Skin collagen changes in postmenopausal women receiving oestradiol gel. *Maturitas.* 1987;9:1-5.
24. Piérard-Franchimont C, Letawe C, Gofin V, et al. Skin water-holding capacity and transdermal estrogen therapy for menopause: a pilot study. *Maturitas.* 1995; 22:151-154.
25. Harvell J, Hussona-Saeed I, Maibach HI. Changes in transepidermal water loss and cutaneous blood flow during the menstrual cycle. *Contact Dermatitis.* 1992;27: 294-301.
26. Creidi P, Faivre B, Agache P, et al. Effect of a conjugated oestrogen (Premarin) cream on aging facial skin. A comparative study with a placebo cream. *Maturitas.* 1994; 19:211-223.
27. Fuchs KO, Solis O, Tapawan R, et al. The effects of an estrogen and glycolic acid cream on the facial skin of postmenopausal women: a randomized histologic study. *Cutis.* 2003;71:481-488.
28. Zouboulis CC, Boschnakow A. Chronological aging and photoaging of the human sebaceous gland. *Clin Exp Dermatol.* 2001;26:600-607.
29. Dieudonne MN, Pecquery R, Boumediene A, et al. Androgen receptors in human preadipocytes and adipocytes: regional specificities and regulation by sex steroids. *Am J Physiol.* 1998;274: C1645-C1652.
30. Dieudonne MN, Leneveu MC, Giudicelli Y, et al. Evidence for functional estrogen receptors alpha and beta in human adipose cells: regional specificities and regulation by estrogens. *Am J Physiol Cell Physiol.* 2004;286:C655-C661.
31. Ashcroft GS, Dodsworth J, van Boxtel E, et al. Estrogen accelerates cutaneous wound healing associated with an increase in TGF-beta1 levels. *Nat Med.* 1997;3:1209-1215.
32. Margolis DJ, Knauss J, Bilker W. Hormone replacement therapy and prevention of pressure ulcers and venous leg ulcers. *Lancet.* 2002;359:675-677.
33. Gilliver SC, Wu F, Ashcroft GS. Regulatory roles of androgens in cutaneous wound healing. *Thromb Haemost.* 2003; 90:978-985.
34. Fimmel S, Zouboulis CC. Influence of physiological androgen levels on wound healing and immune status in men. *Aging Male.* 2005;8:166-171.
35. Adzick NS, Lorenz HP. Cells, matrix, growth factors, and the surgeon. The biology of scarless fetal wound repair. *Ann Surg.* 1994;220:10-18.
36. Chau D, Mancoll JS, Lee S, et al. Tamoxifen downregulates TFG-beta production in keloid fibroblasts. *Ann Plast Surg.* 1998;40:490-493.
37. Mikulec AA, Hanasono MM, Lum J, et al. Effect of tamoxifen on transforming growth factor beta1 production by keloid and fetal fibroblasts. *Arch Facial Plast Surg.* 2001;3:111-114.

CHAPTER 6

Photoaging

Leslie Baumann, MD
Sogol Saghari, MD

As life expectancy has increased and "baby boomers" have begun to enter middle age, interest has increased in slowing the aging process. Implied in this escalating interest is the confidence that greater scientific knowledge and advancements in technology may allow us to control the physical manifestations of aging. In the meantime, more and more people are becoming aware of the external factors implicated in premature aging. Although dermatologists have discussed, since the end of the 19th century,[1] the notion that sunlight contributes to premature aging, there remains a great need for education to convince people of the hazards posed by sun exposure.

The consequences to the skin of chronic sun exposure are readily apparent when one compares the exposed skin of the face, hands, or neck to the unexposed skin of the buttocks, inner thigh, or inner arm (Fig. 6-1). This sun damage can be highlighted by using a Wood's lamp, blue light, or an ultraviolet camera system, rendering the epidermal pigment component more noticeable (Figs. 6-2, 6-3, and 6-4). Showing such results to sun-seeking patients can prove useful in convincing them of the havoc that the sun has wreaked on their skin.

The sun is not the sole source or cause of skin aging. It is the major external cause among several components, both endogenous and exogenous. This chapter will concentrate, though, on the role of the sun on the extrinsic aging process of the skin, also known as photoaging.

SKIN AGING

There are two main processes of skin aging, intrinsic and extrinsic. Intrinsic aging reflects the genetic background of an individual and results from the passage of time. It is inevitable and, thus, beyond voluntary control. Extrinsic aging is engendered by external factors such as smoking, excessive use of alcohol, poor nutrition, and sun exposure, which in many cases can be reduced with effort. This process, then, is not inevitable and, by definition, refers to premature skin aging. It is believed that as much as 80% of facial aging can be ascribed to sun exposure.[2]

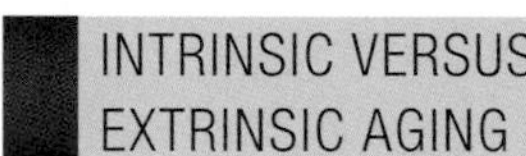

INTRINSIC VERSUS EXTRINSIC AGING

Intrinsically aged skin is smooth and unblemished, with exaggerated expression lines but preservation of the normal geometric patterns of the skin. Under the microscope, such skin demonstrates epidermal atrophy, flattening of the epidermal rete ridges, and dermal atrophy.[3] Collagen fibrils are not thickened but are elevated in number with an increase in the collagen III to collagen I ratio.[4]

Extrinsically aged skin appears predominantly in exposed areas such as the face, chest, and extensor surfaces of the arms. It is a result of the total effects of a lifetime of exposure to ultraviolet radiation (UVR). Clinical findings of photoaged skin include wrinkles and pigmented lesions such as freckles, lentigines, and patchy hyperpigmentation, and depigmented lesions such as guttate hypomelanosis (Fig. 6-5). Interestingly, a study in the *Journal of the American Medical Association* reported that children with the tendency to freckle developed 30% to 40% fewer freckles when treated with an SPF 30 sunscreen daily as compared to children not treated with a sunscreen.[5] This study illustrates the importance of sun protection in the prevention of these pigmented lesions that not only make the skin appear older, but also are known to be associated with an increased risk of melanoma. Other signs of skin aging include a loss of tone and elasticity, increased skin fragility, areas of purpura owing to blood vessel weakness, and benign lesions such as keratoses, telangiectasias, and skin tags (Fig. 6-6). Glogau developed a photoaging scale that is used to classify the extent of clinical photodamage (Table 6-1). Patients with a significant history

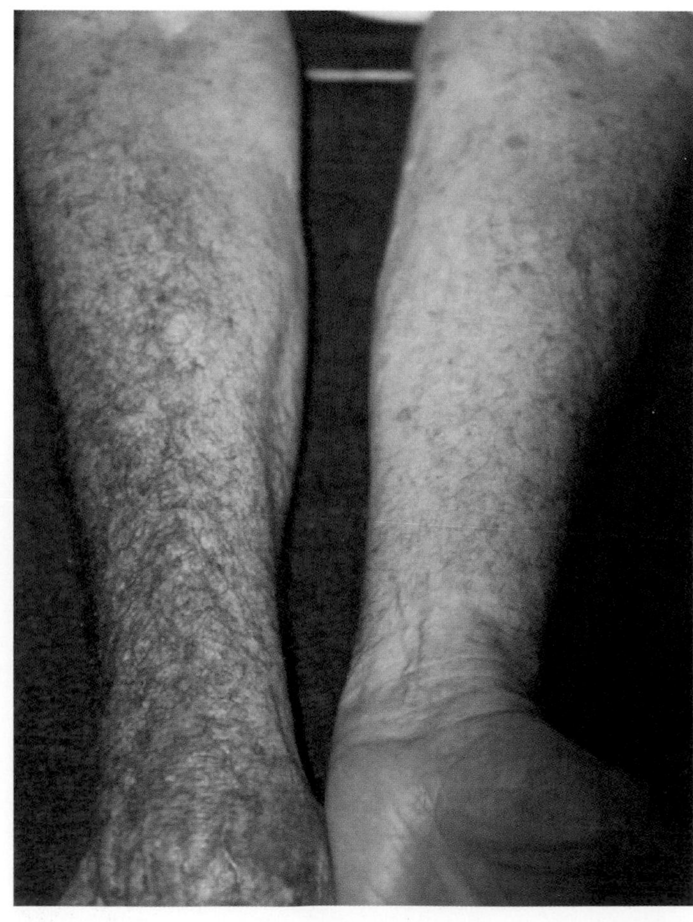

▲ **FIGURE 6-1** Comparing the sun-exposed surface of the forearm to the non-sun-exposed surface demonstrates the sun's ability to cause skin changes.

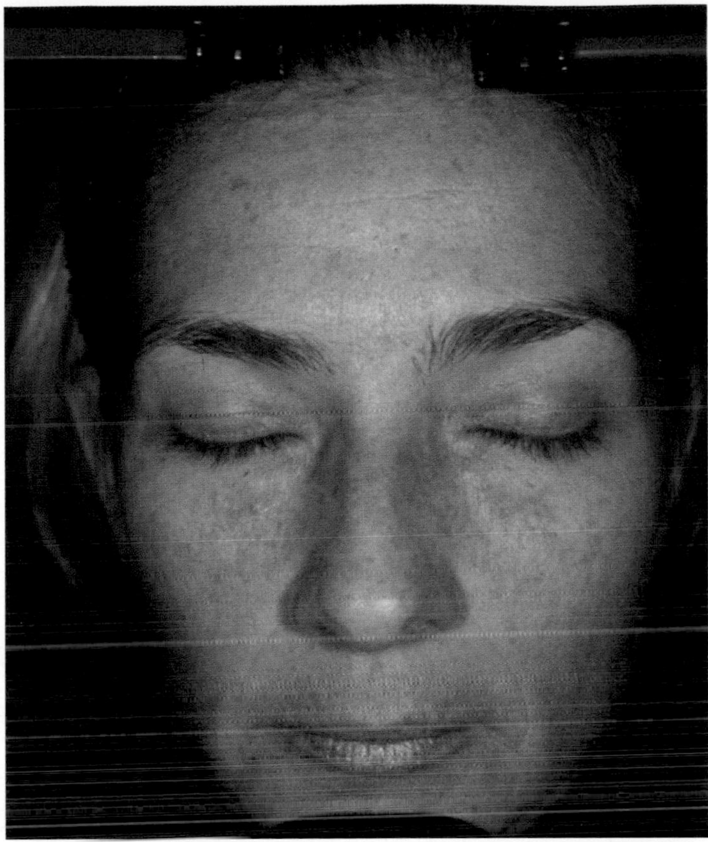

▲ **FIGURE 6-2** Facial skin of 25-year-old with normal lens. Sun damage is barely visible.

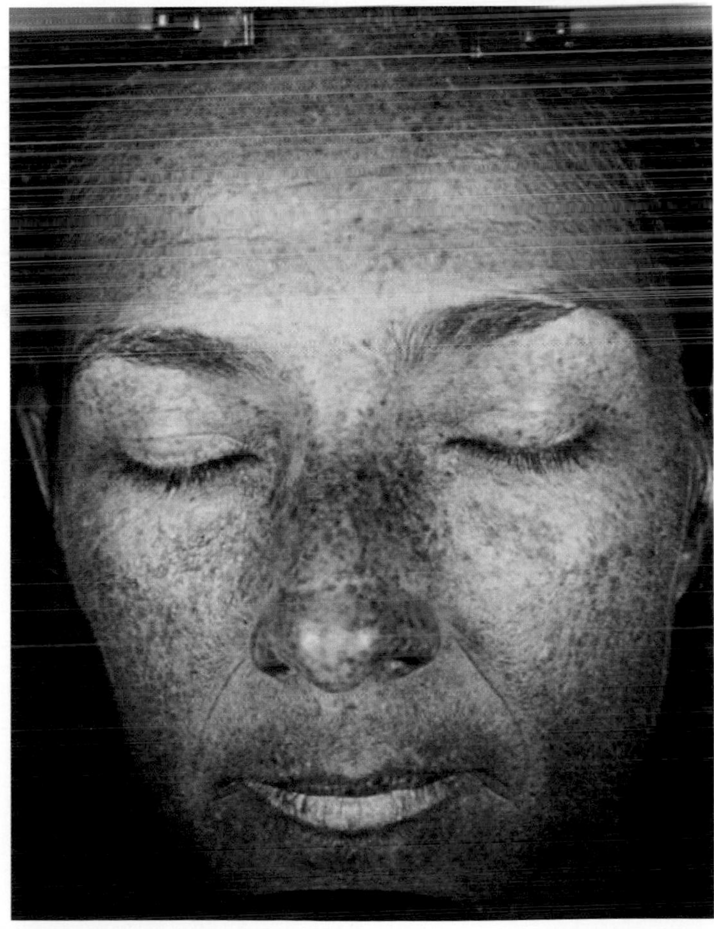

▲ **FIGURE 6-3** Photoaging is accentuated by using UV light.

of sun exposure may score higher on this scale than expected for their age, just as patients with a history of minimal sun exposure may achieve a score lower than expected for their age.

The histopathologic alterations in photoaged skin are easily distinguished and characterized by elastosis (Fig. 6-7). Photoaged skin is also marked by epidermal atrophy and discrete changes in collagen and elastic fibers. In severely photoaged skin, the collagen fibers are fragmented, thickened, and more soluble.[6] Elastic fibers also appear fragmented and may exhibit progressive cross-linkage and calcification.[7] These alterations in collagen and elastic fibers have been demonstrated to worsen with continued UV exposure.

CHARACTERISTICS OF AGED SKIN

Regardless of the etiology of skin aging, there are important characteristics of aged skin that must be considered. These changes occur throughout the epidermis, dermis, and subcutaneous tissue and can result in wide-ranging alterations in the topography of the skin.

Epidermis

Although age-related changes in the dermis are more pronounced than those in the epidermis, the epidermis does exhibit such alterations. Some studies suggest that aged skin displays a thinner epidermis,[6,8] but other studies do not bear such findings out.[9,10] Most studies are in agreement, though, that the thickness of the stratum corneum is unchanged with aging. One study demonstrated that the spinous layer of a wrinkle is thinner in the bottom or valley of the wrinkle than the spinous layer at the wrinkle's flanks.[11] This study also showed that fewer keratohyaline granules are present in the base of a wrinkle as compared to its flanks (Fig. 6-8).

Unlike the stratum corneum, the junction of the epidermis and dermis is altered in aged skin. Aged epidermis exhibits a flattening of the dermal–epidermal junction (DEJ) with a correspondingly smaller connecting surface area. One study of abdominal skin showed that the surface area of the DEJ decreased from 2.64 mm^2 in subjects aged 21 to 40 years to 1.90 mm^2 in subjects aged 61 to 80 years.[12] This loss of DEJ surface area may lead to the increased fragility of the skin and may

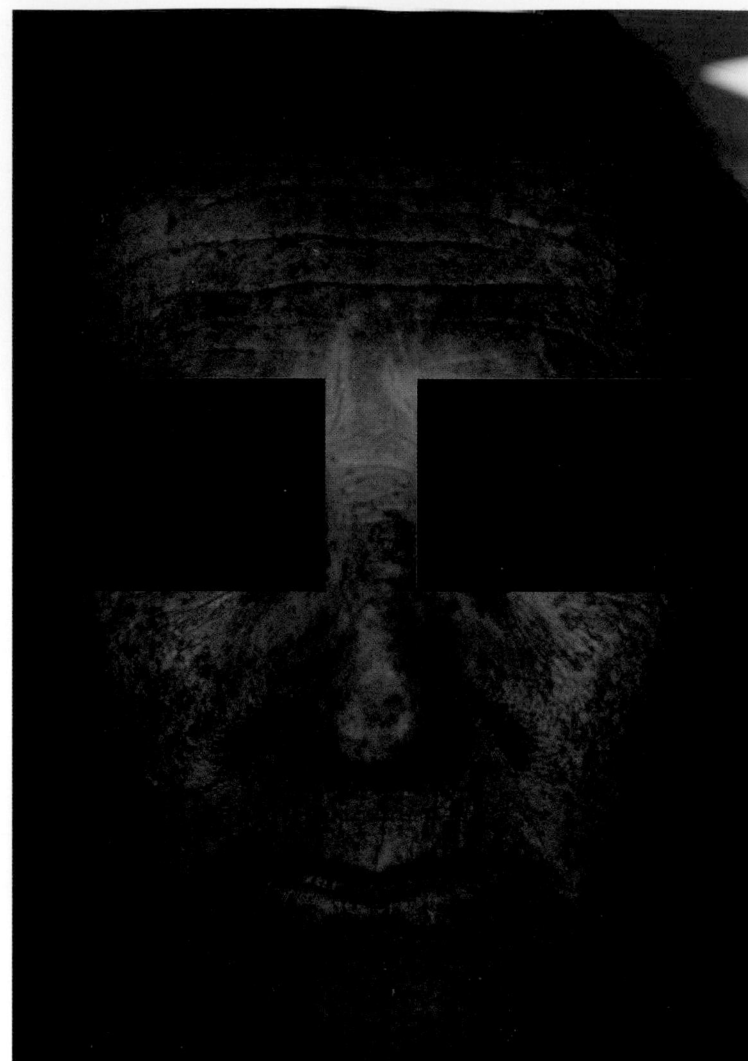

▲ **FIGURE 6-4** Photoaging as seen under blue light.

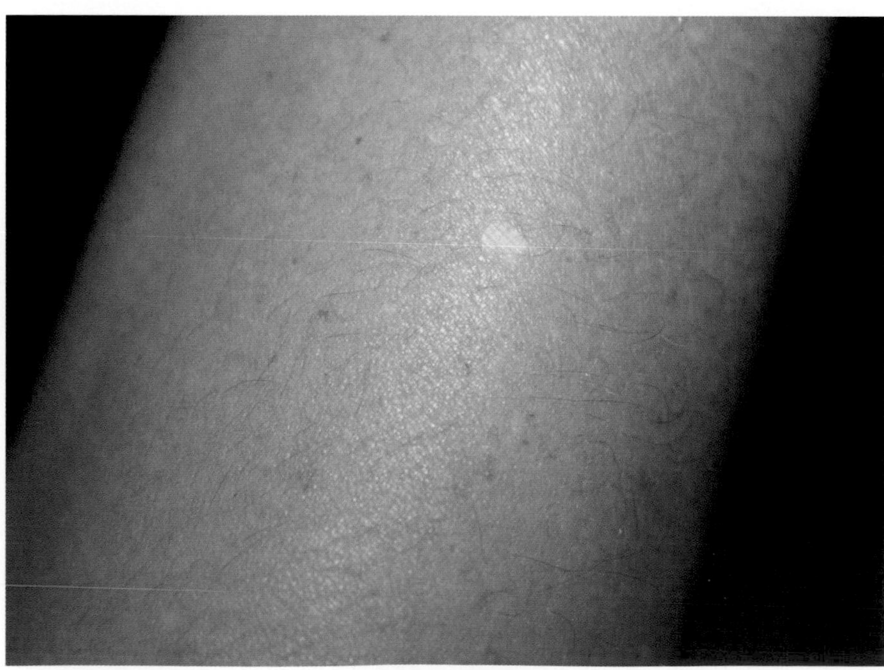

▲ **FIGURE 6-5** Photograph of idiopathic guttate hypomelanosis.

also result in less nutrient transfer between the dermis and epidermis.

DECREASED CELL TURNOVER The epidermal turnover rate slows from 30% to 50% between the third and eighth decades of life.[7] Kligman demonstrated that stratum corneum transit time was 20 days in young adults and 30 or more days in older adults.[13] This lengthening of the cell cycle corresponds to a prolonged stratum corneum replacement rate and decelerated wound healing. In fact, it has been shown that older patients take twice as long to re-epithelialize after dermabrasion resurfacing procedures when compared with younger patients.[14] The slow cell cycle is combined with less effective desquamation in many elderly individuals. The result is the development of heaps of corneocytes that render the skin surface dull and rough in appearance. Consequently, many cosmetic dermatologists employ products such as hydroxy acids or retinoids to "speed up" the cell cycle with the belief that a faster turnover rate will ameliorate skin appearance and accelerate wound healing after cosmetic procedures.

Dermis

Elderly individuals exhibit a loss of approximately 20% of dermal thickness.[14] Examination of the structure of the aged dermis reveals that it is relatively acellular and avascular.[3] Aged dermis is further characterized by changes in collagen production and the development of fragmented elastic fibers. The dermis that has been exposed to ultraviolet light also manifests disorganized collagen fibrils and the accumulation of abnormal elastin-containing material [15] (Fig 6-7). The three components of the dermis that have received the most attention in antiaging research are collagen, elastin, and glycosaminoglycans.

COLLAGEN Awareness of the importance of collagen in the aging process has led to the manufacture of many collagen-containing topical products as well as injectable materials such as Zyderm, Zyplast, CosmoDerm, CosmoPlast, and Evolence. Other components in targeted topical products, such as vitamin C and glycolic acid, owe some of their popularity to the claims that these agents can increase collagen synthesis. These products are usually labeled as "antiwrinkle creams." Although wrinkles are common, it is interesting that little is really known about their pathogenesis.[16] This may be due to

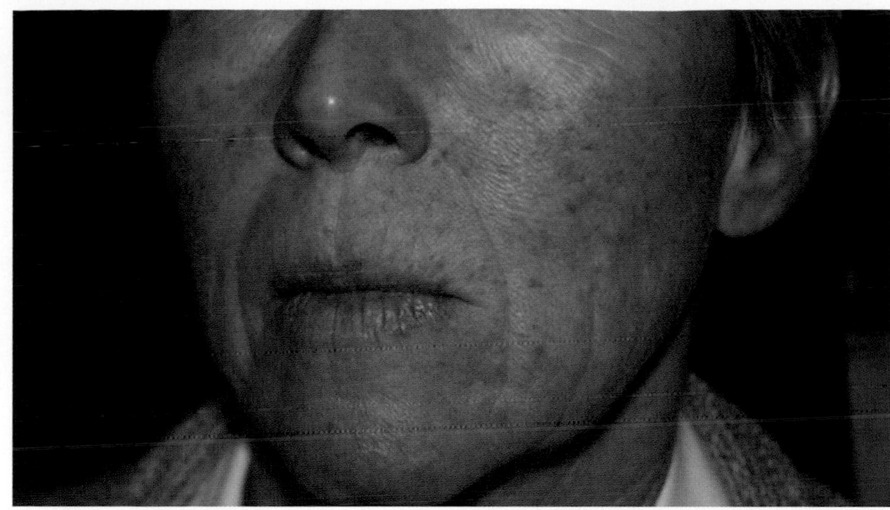

▲ **FIGURE 6-6** Photoaged skin shows telangectasias, solar lentigos, and wrinkles.

the fact that neither an animal model nor an in vitro model of wrinkling has been established. It is well established, however, that alterations in collagen seem to be important in the aging process, which accounts for the popularity of "antiaging," collagen-containing products.

Collagen constitutes 70% of dry skin mass.[17] The collagen in aged skin is characterized by thickened fibrils organized in rope-like bundles, which are in disarray as compared to the organized pattern seen in younger skin.[3] Type I collagen comprises 80% and type III collagen comprises approximately 15% of the total skin collagen of young skin. However, as the skin ages, the ratio of type III to type I collagen has been shown to increase (meaning that there is less type I collagen with aging).[18] Collagen type I levels were shown to decrease by 59% in irradiated skin;[15] this reduction was found to correlate with the extent of photodamage.[19] It is known that the overall collagen content per unit area of skin surface decreases approximately 1% per year.[20] Although type I collagen is the most abundant in the skin, the other types of collagen in the dermis may also be affected by aging.

Collagen IV, a key component in the DEJ, provides a framework for other molecules and is important in the maintenance of mechanical stability. Although studies have shown no difference in collagen IV levels in sun-exposed skin in comparison to nonexposed skin, a significant diminution of collagen IV was found in the bottom of wrinkles when compared to the flanks of wrinkles (Fig. 6-8). This loss of collagen IV may affect the mechanical stability of the DEJ and contribute to wrinkle formation.[11]

Anchoring fibrils, made of collagen VII, are important because they attach the basement membrane zone to the underlying papillary dermis. Patients with chronically sun-exposed skin have been characterized as having a significantly lower number of anchoring fibrils when compared to normal controls. The investigators who made this observation postulated that a weakened bond between the dermis and epidermis owing to loss of anchoring fibrils leads to wrinkle formation.[21] Interestingly, a more recent study demonstrated that this loss of collagen VII was more pronounced at the base of the wrinkle (similar to that seen with collagen IV in the same study)[11] (Fig. 6-8).

The mechanism of action of how UVR induces collagen damage has been well characterized in the last decade. It is now known that UVR exposure dramatically upregulates the production of several types of collagen-degrading enzymes known as matrix metalloproteinases (MMP). This occurs by the following mechanism: UV exposure causes an increase in the amount of the transcription factor c-jun (c-fos is abundant without UV exposure). These two transcription factors, c-jun and c-fos, combine to produce activator protein-1 (AP-1), which activates the MMP genes resulting in production of collagenase, gelatinase, and stromelysin. It has been demonstrated in humans that MMPs, specifically collagenase and gelatinase, are induced within hours of UVB exposure.[22] Fisher et al showed that multiple exposures to UVB yield a sustained induction of MMPs.[15] Because collagenase degrades collagen, long term elevations in collagenase and other MMPs likely result in the disorganized and clumped collagen seen in photoaged skin. These MMPs may represent the mechanism through which collagen I levels are reduced following UV exposure.

Mitogen-Activated Protein Kinases and Aging Mitogen-activated protein kinases (MAPKs) are serine–threonine protein kinases, meaning they phosphorylate the OH side chain of serine and threonine. Significantly, they are involved in signal transduction pathways for cell proliferation, differentiation, and apoptosis. Thus far, four groups of MAPKs have been identified: extracellular signal-regulated kinases (ERKs), c-Jun amino-terminal kinases (JNKs), also known as stress-activated protein kinases (SAPKs), p38 kinase, and ERK5. ERKs are activated via growth factors and play a role in cell proliferation and differentiation. JNKs, on

TABLE 6-1
Glogau Photoaging Classification

TYPE I NO WRINKLES	TYPE II WRINKLES IN MOTION	TYPE III WRINKLES AT REST	TYPE IV ONLY WRINKLES
Usually in age group 20s–30s	Usually in age group late 30s–40s	Usually in age group 50 or older	Usually in age group 60 or older
Early photoaging	Early-to-moderate photoaging	Advanced photoaging	Severe photoaging
Mild pigmentary changes	Early senile lentigines	Obvious dyschromias, telangiectasias	Yellow gray skin
No keratoses	Palpable but not visible keratoses	Visible keratoses	Prior skin malignancies
Minimal wrinkles	Parallel smile lines beginning to appear lateral to mouth	Persistent wrinkling	No normal skin

Adapted from Glogau RG. Chemical peeling and aging skin. *J Geriatric Dermatol.* 1994;2(1):31.

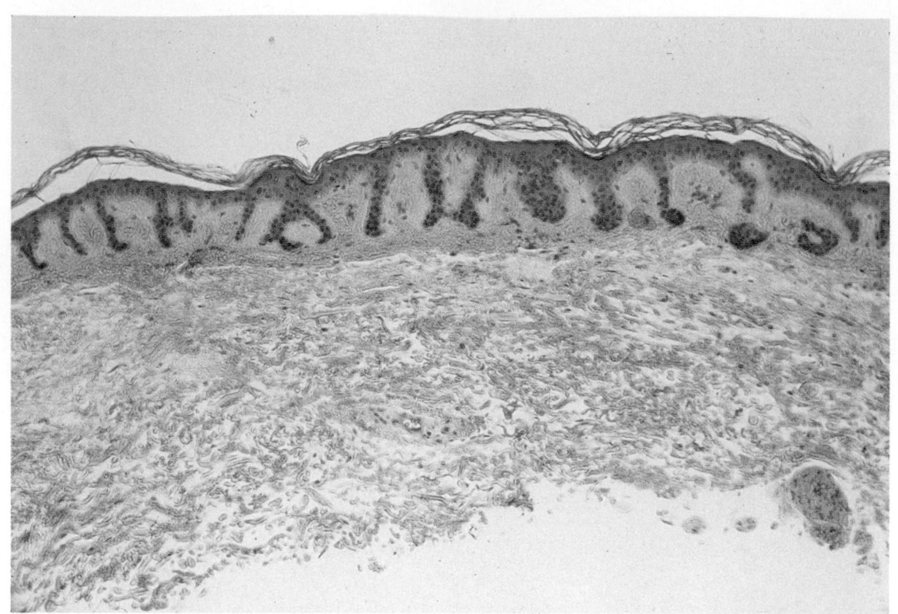

▲ **FIGURE 6-7** Hematoxylin and eosin (H and E) stain of sun-damaged skin demonstrates signficant elastosis in the dermis and multiple solar lentigos. (*Image courtsey of George Ioannides, MD.*)

the other hand, respond to stressful stimuli such as UV light, osmotic shock, or cytokines,[23] and are involved in cellular apoptosis.[24] In addition, p38 kinase is activated via stress-induced stimuli. It has been demonstrated that a synchronized inhibition of ERKs and activation of JNK/p38 must be present for cellular apoptosis, suggesting that a "balance" among these groups influences cell survival versus death.[25] The MAPKs have been implicated in both intrinsic and extrinsic aging of skin. Chung et al. demonstrated that JNK activity is higher and ERK activity lower in intrinsically aged skin.[26] As previously mentioned, the combination of UV-induced c-jun (through the JNK pathway), and naturally expressed c-fos produces AP-1, which promotes the degrading of collagen and the extracellular matrix by increasing MMPs.[27] AP-1 has an additional impact in collagen loss by decreasing collagen I gene expression.[28] Therefore, some collagen reduction in photoaged skin may be explained by the role of AP-1 in both increasing MMPs and decreasing collagen synthesis.

ELASTIN Changes in elastic fibers are so characteristic in photoaged skin that "elastosis," an accumulation of amorphous elastin material, is considered a hallmark of photoaged skin. Thickening and coiling of elastic fibers in the papillary dermis distinguish the alterations induced by UV exposure. Continued UV exposure leads to these same changes in the reticular dermis.[29] Electron microscopy examination of the elastic fibers reveals an increase in the complexity of the shape and arrangement of the fibers, a decrease in the number of microfibrils, a higher number of electron-dense inclusions, and more interfibrillar areas.[30] Elastin extracted from the skin of elderly patients has been shown to contain small amounts of sugar and lipids and an abnormally high level of polar amino acids.[3] The mechanism of these changes is not as well understood as it is in collagen; however, MMPs likely play a role because MMP-2 has been shown to degrade elastin.[31]

It is known that the initial response of elastic fibers to photodamage is hyperplastic, resulting in increased elastic tissue. The magnitude of this response depends on the degree of sun exposure. The second phase of response, seen in aged elastic fibers, is degenerative, resulting in reduced elasticity and resiliency of the skin.[32,33] Aged skin that has suffered this degenerative response manifests an alteration in the normal pattern of immature elastic fibers, called oxytalan, which are found in the papillary dermis. In young skin, these fibers form a network that ascends perpendicularly from the uppermost portion of the papillary dermis to just below the basement membrane (Fig. 2-5 in Chapter 2). As skin ages, this network gradually disappears.[34] In fact, a loss of skin elasticity has been shown to incrementally increase with age.[35] This loss of elasticity may account for much of the sagging often seen in the skin of elderly individuals.

GLYCOSAMINOGLYCANS Glycosaminoglycans (GAGs) are important molecules because they can bind water up to 1000 times their volume. The GAG family includes hyaluronic acid (HA), chondroitin sulfate, and dermatan sulfate, among many other constituents. Numerous studies report that GAGs, especially HA, are decreased in amount in photoaged skin.[36] However, some conflicting studies report no change in the amount of GAGs in aged skin.[37]

A study by Uitto demonstrated that photoaged skin exhibits a reduction in HA and an increase in chondroitin sulfate proteoglycans,[38] which, interestingly, is a pattern also seen in scars. In young skin, the HA is found at the

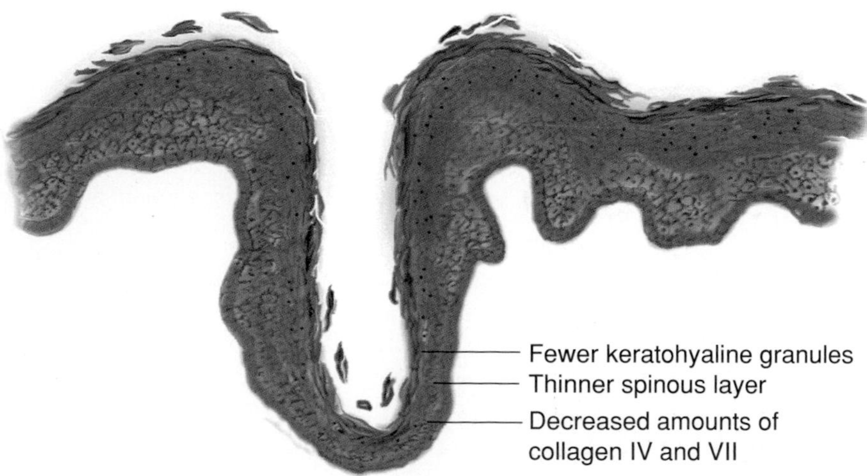

▲ **FIGURE 6-8** The spinous layer is thinner and there are fewer keratohyaline granules in the valley of the wrinkle. Levels of collagen IV and VII are also decreased in the valley of a wrinkle when compared to the flanks.

periphery of collagen and elastin fibers and at the interface of these types of fibers. Such connections with HA are absent in aged skin.[36] Decreases in the amount of HA, leading to its lack of association with collagen and elastin and decreased water binding, may play a role in the changes seen in aged skin including decreased turgidity, diminished capacity to support the microvasculature, wrinkling, and altered elasticity.

MELANOCYTES The number of melanocytes decreases from 8% to 20% per decade. This is displayed clinically by a reduction in the number of melanocytic nevi in older individuals.[3] Because melanin absorbs carcinogenic UV light, the skin of older patients is less able to protect itself from the sun and, consequently, is at greater risk for developing sun-induced cancers. It is for this reason that sun protection is important even for patients who feel it is "too late" to begin adding a sunscreen to their skin care regimens.

Vasculature

Many studies have shown that aged skin is relatively avascular. One particular study demonstrated a 35% reduction in the venous cross sectional area in aged skin as compared to young skin.[39] This reduction in the vascular network is particularly obvious in the papillary dermis with loss of the vertical capillary loops. Such a reduction of vascularity results in decreased blood flow, diminished nutrient exchange, impaired thermoregulation, lower skin surface temperature, and skin pallor.

Subcutaneous Tissue

Elderly skin displays both a loss and a gain of subcutaneous tissue that is site specific. Subcutaneous fat is decreased in the face, as well as the dorsal aspects of the hands and the shins. Other areas, however, such as the waist in women and the abdomen in men, accumulate fat with aging[3] (see Chapter 3).

UV IRRADIATION AND UROCANIC ACID ISOMERS

The cutaneous barrier is the initial line of defense, protecting other organs from external antigens, bacteria, and viruses, as well as UV light. Ultraviolet irradiation is a well-known contributor to decreased immunity of the skin, leading to less recognition of abnormal cells and eventually development of skin cancers. *Trans*-urocanic acid (*trans*-UCA), a metabolite of histidine, is commonly present in the epidermal skin layers. As discussed in Chapter 11, histidine is mostly derived from filaggrin in the epidermis and gets converted to *trans*-UCA, which plays an integral role in epidermal hydration. Following UV exposure, *trans*-UCA is photoisomerized into *cis*-urocanic acid (*cis*-UCA), a known photoreceptor for UV light (Fig. 6-9). *cis*-UCA is a well-recognized immunosuppressant in the skin. Impaired delayed hypersensitivity reaction and decreased function of epidermal antigen-presenting cells (Langerhans cells) occur following exposure to *cis*-UCA through TNF-α release.[40,41] Interestingly, the effect of *cis*-UCA is dose dependent.[42] In addition to UV irradiation dose, skin pigmentation is an important factor. Fair-skinned subjects have been shown to produce more *cis*-UCA with lower doses of UV light when compared to darker-skinned individuals.[43] It has been suggested that *cis*-UCA decreases the ability of APCs to present the abnormal cells and antigens to the immune system, thereby contributing to UV carcinogenesis.[44] However, the exact role of *cis*-UCA in skin cancers is not well understood and the few studies performed on this subject have not revealed a direct association between the total UCA levels and skin cancer. In a study by De Fine Olivarius et al. of the total UCA and percentage of *cis*-UCA in sun-exposed and sun-protected areas of skin in patients with a history of basal cell carcinoma (BCC), patients with malignant melanoma, and healthy subjects, the total UCA and *cis*-UCA levels did not differ among the three groups, while the percentage of *cis*-UCA was found to be higher in patients with a history of basal cell carcinoma (BCC) and melanoma as compared to healthy individuals.[45] Another study conducted by Snellman et al. also failed to demonstrate a statistically significant increase of UCA with UV exposure in subjects with a history of BCC and melanoma.[46]

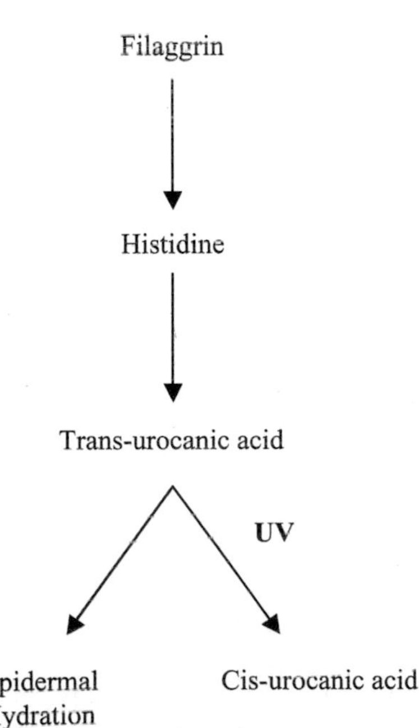

▲ **FIGURE 6-9** Filaggrin breaks down into *cis*-urocanic acid through the pathway shown.

THE ROLE OF FREE RADICALS IN PHOTOAGING

Free radicals, also known as reactive oxygen species, are composed of oxygen with an unpaired electron and are created by UV exposure, pollution, stress, smoking, and normal metabolic processes. They are suspected to be the cause, or at least a major contributor, to the aging process. There is evidence to suggest that free radicals induce changes in gene expression pathways that lead to the degradation of collagen and accumulation of elastin characteristic of photoaged skin.[31] Antioxidants neutralize these reactive oxygen species by providing another electron, which gives the oxygen ion an electron pair thereby stabilizing it (see Chapter 35).

It has been demonstrated that following a single dose of UV irradiation there is an initial decrease in expression and activity of antioxidant enzymes in the cultured fibroblasts of skin.[47] In this study, the antioxidant enzymes increased even to higher than pre-exposure levels in a few days, probably as a defense mechanism in preparation for more potential UV exposure.

TANNING AND ITS EFFECTS ON THE SKIN

UV light stimulates the production of melanin by causing α-melanocyte-stimulating hormone (α-MSH) to be secreted by keratinocytes. Redheads have a defect in the proopiomelanocortin (POMC) gene that prevents this tanning response from occurring. Data recently published in *Cell* showed that the tumor suppressor protein p53, when "stressed" by UV, activates the POMC gene, which leads to both tanning and an increase in β-endorphin.[48] This may explain why some people state that they feel good after tanning. Of course, many companies are looking at ways to safely stimulate p53 to create a "protective" tan but much more research is necessary.

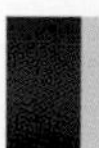

CHANGES IN SKIN APPEARANCE

Dry Skin

Elderly people often display dry scaled skin. This is due in part to the loss of barrier function that occurs with increasing age (see Chapter 11). Aged skin exhibits increased transepidermal water loss; therefore, it is susceptible to becoming dry in low-humidity environments. The recovery of damaged barrier function has been shown to be slower in aged skin leading to an increased susceptibility to dryness. This is caused by a combination of factors including lower lipid levels in lamellar bodies[49] and a reduction in epidermal filaggrin (see Chapter 11).[50] Roughness, wrinkling, skin pallor, and the appearance of dark and light spots also affect the appearance and texture of aged skin. In addition, aged skin is typically characterized by laxity, fragility, easy bruising, and benign neoplasms.

Benign Neoplasms in Aging Skin

The surface texture and appearance of skin can change dramatically through age with the emergence of acrochordons (skin tags), cherry angiomas, seborrheic keratoses, lentigos (sun spots), and sebaceous hyperplasias. It is not uncommon for cosmetic patients to request removal of these benign neoplasms. There are several different destructive treatment modalities available, such as hyfrecation, curettage, and laser.

TREATMENT

Many different topical agents and in-office procedures are used to treat photoaged skin. Most of these remedies function by "resurfacing" the epidermis. The goal is to remove the damaged epidermis and, in some instances, dermis, and allow them to be replaced with remodeled skin layers. There is some evidence that resurfacing procedures can induce the formation of new collagen with a normal staining pattern in contrast to the basophilic elastotic masses of collagen present in photoaged skin.[51] Although there are several treatments available for aged skin, prevention is still paramount and should be emphasized to all patients.

PREVENTION

It is well established that sun avoidance and sunscreen use are important adjuvants to antiaging regimens. Obviously, sun avoidance is not always possible and hardly a popular behavioral adjustment for many patients. However, patients should be discouraged from engaging in unnecessary sun exposure, particularly between 10 AM and 4 PM, and any exposure to tanning beds. Sunscreen should be recommended for use on a daily basis, even when the patient remains indoors. Patients should be reminded that UVA rays have the capacity to pass through glass, thus individuals are at risk of solar exposure even in their cars and homes as well as at work. UVA shields can be placed on windows, providing some protection. Sun protective clothing, such as a broad-brimmed hat and SPF 45 clothing, should be encouraged for patients planning any protracted exposure to the sun. Many patients believe that their sun exposure is minimal and does not warrant daily use of sunscreen. Use of a Wood's or a UV light to reveal solar damage is a helpful way to convince patients of the necessity of sun avoidance. Such a demonstration will also make them more likely to employ preventive measures, such as sunscreens, antioxidants, and retinoids, when sun avoidance is impractical. Sunscreens, antioxidants, and retinoids are discussed in upcoming chapters.

SUMMARY

Rough, dry skin, mottled pigmentation, and wrinkling epitomize the clinical appearance of photoaging. Extensive or severe photodamage can also be a precursor to skin cancer. Despite increasing awareness of the risks of prolonged sun exposure, too many people remain unaware that the proverbial "healthy tan" is, in fact, evidence of photodamage and indicative of premature aging. It is incumbent upon the dermatologist to educate patients on the ravages of the sun, the importance of sun avoidance and sun-protective behavior, and, as always, tailor treatments to individual patient needs.

REFERENCES

1. Unna PG. *Histopathologie der Hautkrankheiten.* Berlin, Germany: A. Herschwald; 1894.
2. Uitto J. Understanding premature skin aging. *N Engl J Med.* 1997;337:1463.
3. Fenske NA, Lober CW. Structural and functional changes of normal aging skin. *J Am Acad Dermatol.* 1986;15:571.
4. Lovell CR, Smolenski KA, Duance VC, et al. Type I and III collagen content and fibre distribution in normal human skin during ageing. *Br J Dermatol.* 1987;117: 419.
5. Gallagher RP, Rivers JK, Lee TK, et al. Broad-spectrum sunscreen use and the development of new nevi in white children: a randomized controlled trial. *JAMA.* 2000;283:2955.
6. Lavker RM. Structural alterations in exposed and unexposed aged skin. *J Invest Dermatol.* 1979;73:59.
7. Yaar M, Gilchrest B. Aging of skin. In: Freeberg I, Eisen A. Wolff K, et al., eds. *Fitzpatrick's Dermatology in General Medicine.* 5th ed. New York, NY: McGraw-Hill; 1999:1697.
8. Lock-Andersen J, Therkildsen P, de Fine Olivarius, et al. Epidermal thickness, skin pigmentation and constitutive photosensitivity. *Photodermatol Photoimmunol Photomed.* 1997;13:153.
9. Whitton JT, Everall JD. The thickness of the epidermis. *Br J Dermatol.* 1973;89: 467.
10. Sandby-Moller J, Poulsen T, Wulf HC. Epidermal thickness at different body sites: relationship to age, gender, pigmentation, blood content, skin type and smoking habits. *Acta Derm Venereol.* 2003;83:410.
11. Contet-Audonneau JL, Jeanmaire C, Pauly G. A histological study of human wrinkle structures: comparison between sun-exposed areas of the face, with or without wrinkles, and sun-protected areas. *Br J Dermatol.* 1999;140:1038.
12. Katzberg AA. The area of the dermo-epidermal junction in human skin. *Anat Rec.* 1985;131:717.
13. Kligman AM. Perspectives and problems in cutaneous gerontology. *J Invest Dermatol.* 1979;73:39.
14. Orentreich N, Selmanowitz VJ. Levels of biological functions with aging. *Trans NY Acad Sci.* 1969;31:992.
15. Fisher GJ, Wang ZQ, Datta SC, et al. Pathophysiology of premature skin aging induced by ultraviolet light. *N Engl J Med.* 1997;337:1419.
16. Kligman AM, Zheng P, Lavker RM. The anatomy and pathogenesis of wrinkles. *Br J Dermatol.* 1985;113:37.
17. Gniadecka M, Nielsen OF, Wessel S, et al. Water and protein structure in photoaged and chronically aged skin. *J Invest Dermatol.* 1998;111:1129.
18. Oikarinen A. The aging of skin: chronoaging versus photoaging. *Photo-dermatol Photoimmunol Photomed.* 1990; 7:3.
19. Griffiths CE, Russman AN, Majmudar G, et al. Restoration of collagen formation in photodamaged human skin by tretinoin (retinoic acid). *New Engl J Med.* 1993; 329:530.
20. Shuster S, Black MM, McVitie E. The influence of age and sex on skin thickness, skin collagen and density. *Br J Dermatol.* 1975;93:639.
21. Craven NM, Watson RE, Jones CJ, et al. Clinical features of photodamaged human skin are associated with a reduction in collagen VII. *Br J Dermatol.* 1997; 137:344.
22. Fisher GJ, Datta SC, Talwar HS, et al. Molecular basis of sun-induced premature skin ageing and retinoid antagonism. *Nature.* 1996;379:335.
23. Rosette C, Karin M. Ultraviolet light and osmotic stress: activation of the JNK cas-

cade through multiple growth factor and cytokine receptors. *Science*. 1996;274:1194.

24. Ham J, Babij C, Whitfield J, et al. A c-Jun dominant negative mutant protects sympathetic neurons against programmed cell death. *Neuron*. 1995;14:927.
25. Xia Z, Dickens M, Raingeaud J, et al. Opposing effects of ERK and JNK-p38 MAP kinases on apoptosis. *Science*. 1995;270:1326.
26. Chung JH, Kang S, Varani J, et al. Decreased extracellular-signal-regulated kinase and increased stress-activated MAP kinase activities in aged human skin in vivo. *J Invest Dermatol*. 2000;115: 177.
27. Fisher GJ, Voorhees JJ. Molecular mechanisms of retinoid actions in skin. *FASEB J*. 1996;10:1002.
28. Chung KY, Agarwal A, Uitto J, et al. An AP-1 binding sequence is essential for regulation of the human alpha2(I) collagen (COL1A2) promoter activity by transforming growth factor-beta. *J Biol Chem*. 1996;271:3272.
29. Mitchell RE. Chronic solar dermatosis: a light and electron microscopic study of the dermis. *J Invest Dermatol*. 1967;48: 203.
30. Tsuji T, Hamada T. Age-related changes in human dermal elastic fibers. *Br J Dermatol*. 1981;105:57.
31. Scharffetter-Kochanek K, Brenneisen P, Wenk J, et al. Photoaging of the skin from phenotype to mechanisms. *Exp Gerontol*. 2000;35:307.
32. Matsuoka L, Uitto J. Alterations in the elastic fibers in cutaneous aging and solar elastosis. In: Balin A, Kligman AM, eds. *Aging and the Skin*. New York, NY: Raven Press; 1989:141.
33. Lavker RM. Cutaneous aging: chronologic versus photoaging. In: Gilchrest BA. *Photodamage*. 1st ed. Cambridge, MA: Blackwell Science; 1995:128.
34. Montagna W, Carlisle K. Structural changes in aging human skin. *J Invest Dermatol*. 1979;73:47.
35. Escoffier C, de Rigal J, Rochefort A, et al. Age-related mechanical properties of human skin: an in vivo study. *J Invest Dermatol*. 1989;93:353.
36. Ghersetich I, Lotti T, Campanile G, et al. Hyaluronic acid in cutaneous intrinsic aging. *Int J Dermatol*. 1994;33:119.
37. Pearce RH, Grimmer BJ. Age and the chemical constitution of normal human dermis. *J Invest Dermatol*. 1972;58:347.
38. Bernstein EF, Underhill CB, Hahn PJ, et al. Chronic sun exposure alters both the content and distribution of dermal glycosaminoglycans. *Br J Dermatol*. 1996; 135:255.
39. Gilchrest BA, Stoff JS, Soter NA. Chronologic aging alters the response to ultraviolet-induced inflammation in human skin. *J Invest Dermatol*. 1982; 79:11.
40. Kurimoto I, Streilein JW. *cis*-urocanic acid suppression of contact hypersensitivity induction is mediated via tumor necrosis factor-alpha. *J Immunol*. 1992; 148:3072.
41. Kurimoto I, Streilein JW. Deleterious effects of cis-urocanic acid and UVB radiation on Langerhans cells and on induction of contact hypersensitivity are mediated by tumor necrosis factor-alpha. *J Invest Dermatol*. 1992;99:69S.
42. Ross JA, Howie SEM, Norval M, et al. Ultraviolet-irradiated urocanic acid suppresses delayed-type hypersensitivity to herpes simplex virus in mice. *J Invest Dermatol*. 1986;87:630.
43. de Fine Olivarius F, Wulf HC, Crosby J, et al. Isomerization of urocanic acid after ultraviolet radiation is influenced by skin pigmentation. *J Photochem Photobiol B*. 1999;48:42.
44. Beissert S, Mohammad T, Torri H, et al. Regulation of tumor antigen presentation by urocanic acid. *J Immunol*. 1997;159:92.
45. De Fine Olivarius F, Lock-Andersen J, Larsen FG, et al. Urocanic acid isomers in patients with basal cell carcinoma and cutaneous malignant melanoma. *Br J Dermatol*. 1998;138:986.
46. Snellman E, Jansen CT, Rantanen T, et al. Epidermal urocanic acid concentration and photoisomerization reactivity in patients with cutaneous malignant melanoma or basal cell carcinoma. *Acta Derm Venereol*. 1999;79:200.
47. Leccia MT, Yaar M, Allen N, et al. Solar simulated irradiation modulates gene expression and activity of antioxidant enzymes in cultured human dermal fibroblasts. *Exp Dermatol*. 2001;10:272.
48. Cui R, Widlund HR, Feige E, et al. Central role of p53 in the suntan response and pathologic hyperpigmentation. *Cell*. 2007; 128:853.
49. Ghadially R, Brown BE, Sequeira-Martin SM, et al. The aged epidermal permeability barrier. Structural, functional, and lipid biochemical abnormalities in humans and a senescent murine model. *J Clin Invest*. 1995;95:2281.
50. Tezuka T, Qing J, Saheki M, et al. Terminal differentiation of facial epidermis of the aged: immunohistochemical studies. *Dermatology*. 1994;188:21.
51. Nelson BR, Majmudar G, Griffiths CE, et al. Clinical improvement following dermabrasion of photoaged skin correlates with synthesis of collagen I. *Arch Dermatol*. 1994;130:1136.

CHAPTER 7

Cigarettes and Aging Skin

Leslie Baumann, MD
Sogol Saghari, MD

While there remains a good deal to learn about the mechanisms and factors related to intrinsic skin aging, scientists have a stronger grasp of the numerous exogenous factors implicated in the aging of skin, among them sun exposure and lifestyle choices such as smoking, drinking, and poor nutrition. Of course, the internal ramifications of smoking are much better known than are the external results, but more than two decades of epidemiologic research findings indicate that smokers indeed manifest greater facial aging and skin wrinkling than nonsmokers.[1] This chapter reviews the literature and discusses what is known about the effects on skin of chronic cigarette smoking.

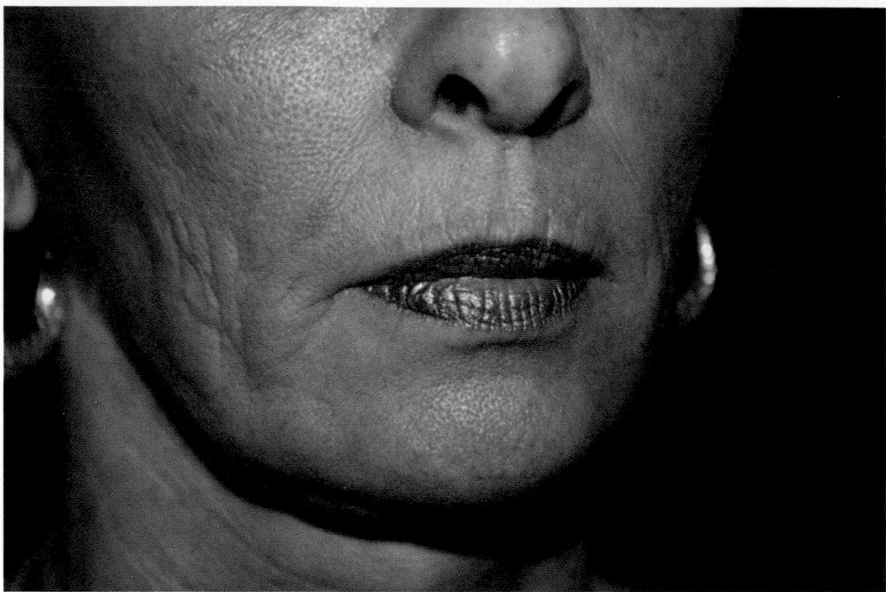

▲ **FIGURE 7-1** Smokers characteristically develop lines around the mouth.

HISTORICAL PERSPECTIVE

A relationship between smoking and skin wrinkling was observed as long ago as 1856.[1–3] Despite this relatively early recognition, scant research has focused on the effects of smoking on the skin and skin disease. Therefore, the effects of smoking on skin are not nearly as well understood as the strong correlation between smoking and lung cancer, emphysema, chronic bronchitis, heart disease, and other serious systemic conditions.[3,4] Recent studies have succeeded, though, in filling in significant gaps in knowledge regarding the typical cutaneous manifestations of the systemic alterations wrought by smoking, and the potential mechanisms behind such changes.

SYMPTOMS

The characteristics typically cited as evidence of "smoker's face" (Fig. 7-1) or "cigarette skin" include increased facial wrinkling; a slightly red/orange complexion; an ashen, pale, or gray overall skin appearance; puffiness; and gauntness.[2,3] A prematurely older appearance is also a typical symptom of chronic smoking. Boyd et al. reported that yellow, irregularly thickened skin forms from the breakdown of the skin's elastic fibers as a result of smoking.[2] In 1999, Demierre et al. noted that case–control studies and other reports suggest a higher prevalence of facial wrinkling among smokers and that smokers, more often than nonsmokers, appear older than their stated age.[1] A significant association between smoking and gray hair was also observed in a different study.[1]

A German literature review article from the mid-1990s concluded that smoking is at least culpable for promoting, if not actually causing, various skin changes.[5] This report noted the strong association between cigarette smoking and yellowed fingers as well as increased facial wrinkling, particularly in women. An elevated incidence of precancerous lesions and squamous cell carcinomas on lips and oral mucosa, as well as vasospasms and deterioration in large arteries and microvasculature were also linked to cigarette smoking in this report. In addition, smoking has recently been shown in an observational study to have a strong correlation with androgenetic alopecia by dint of a multifactorial array of mechanisms.[6]

HIGHLIGHTS OF SOME OF THE MAJOR STUDIES

Results of a 1998 study suggest that smokers do indeed incur a greater risk of facial wrinkling and that this risk is not mitigated by the introduction of hormone replacement therapy (HRT).[7] In this study, researchers set out to examine the combined effects on the skin of a protective factor (HRT) and a deleterious factor (smoking) by evaluating three different groups of postmenopausal women differentiated by smoking status: lifelong nonsmokers, current smokers, and former smokers. Results from direct questioning (on smoking and HRT status) and standardized visual assessment revealed a relative risk of moderate to severe wrinkling for current smokers to be over twice that for lifelong nonsmokers. Further, lifelong nonsmokers on HRT exhibited lower facial wrinkle scores than lifelong nonsmokers who had never received HRT, but HRT had little general effect on the facial wrinkle scores of current smokers.

Boyd et al. echoed these results in reporting that women seem to be more affected than men, and light skin more than dark skin. They also found that while sun exposure, age, weight change, and social status do not appear to play a role in cutaneous manifestations of smoking, the duration and amount of smoking are significant factors in wrinkle development. Further, in a study by Daniel, it was found that people who had smoked for less than 15 years and those who had smoked less than half a pack daily were just slightly more likely to exhibit salient wrinkling. These individuals were far less likely to be wrinkled than smokers of the same age and sex who had smoked a greater amount or over a longer period of time.[8] Daniel hypothesized that genetic predisposition may also play a role in increasing the likelihood that some smokers will develop facial wrinkling. He stated that the cutaneous vasculature of those who develop more wrinkles may be more susceptible to damage from the chemicals in tobacco products.[2] This, however has not yet been proven.

In a 1995 cross-sectional study of 299 subjects who never smoked, 551 former smokers, and 286 then-current smokers, aged 30 to 69 years, a positive association was observed between pack-years and facial wrinkling in women and men between the ages of 40 and 69 years. This finding buttressed previous evidence that facial wrinkling is more prominent among smokers than people who have never smoked.[9] In 1971, Daniel noted much greater facial wrinkling among smokers than nonsmokers across several demographic scales (age, sex, and sun-exposure groups), and concluded that smoking, more than sun exposure, was responsible for the subjects' facial wrinkling.[8] In a more recent study to evaluate the risk of premature facial wrinkling caused by cigarette smoking, investigators considered the cigarette smoking status, weight changes, average recreational and occupational sun exposure in 1 month, as well as past medical and facial cosmetic surgery as identified in self-questionnaires answered by 123 nonsmokers, 160 current smokers, and 67 past smokers, aged 20 to 69 years. In line with what has emerged as the prevailing sentiment regarding the cutaneous sequelae of smoking, current smokers exhibited a greater degree of facial wrinkling and average skin roughness as compared to nonsmokers and past smokers, even those past smokers who had smoked heavily at a younger age. Notably, microscopic superficial wrinkling was observed in the facial skin of young current smokers aged 20 to 39 years.[10]

In 1991, Kadunce et al. reported on a study of 132 adult smokers and nonsmokers. The researchers controlled for age, sex, skin pigmentation, and sun exposure and determined that sun exposure and pack-years of smoking were independently related to the observed prevalence of premature wrinkling, which increased with increased pack-years of smoking.[11] Those individuals considered heavy smokers (greater than 50 pack-years) were 4.7 times more likely to be wrinkled as compared with nonsmokers. The risk of excessive wrinkling was elevated over three-fold for those subjects with more than 50,000 lifetime hours of sun exposure. Kadunce et al., unlike Daniel, identified sun exposure as the greater risk factor for premature wrinkling, but also noted a multiplicative effect in subjects who smoked and absorbed significant sun exposure.[11]

In a 1999 study of 82 smokers who smoked more than 10 cigarettes per day and 118 nonsmokers who had smoked fewer than 100 lifetime cigarettes, O'Hare et al. found that smoking accounted for only 6% of the explained variance after controlling for solar risk behavior. The researchers concluded that if smoking is implicated in wrinkling, its role is minor and that other studies were unblinded or failed to consider potential confounding variables.[12] Conversely, Smith and Fenske had previously found that the weight of the evidence suggests that cigarette smoking causes premature aging and wrinkling.[3]

In a British study, investigators evaluated a random sample of 792 individuals aged 60 years or older (71 was the mean age of participants) registered with general practitioners in Wales, UK, to ascertain the key etiologic factors in skin wrinkling and assess the viability of using skin wrinkling as an objective measure of cumulative sun exposure. Researchers gathered data between 1988 and 1991 during home visit interviews, in which subjects were asked to estimate their average outdoor time during three periods of life, and via examination of the face, neck, and dorsal hand by an experienced dermatologist. Multiple logistic regression models revealed that chronologic age and daily cigarette smoking were the only factors significantly linked to visible cutaneous aging. In addition, the effects of smoking 20 cigarettes daily were deemed by the investigators to equate roughly to a decade of natural intrinsic aging.[13]

In a study of the effects of smoking on wrinkling and aging in males living in Northern Finland, where there is a low, cumulative sun exposure, eight panelists estimated the smoking status, age, and facial wrinkling of 41 smokers and 48 nonsmokers. Although clinical assessment and computerized image analysis revealed no significant differences in skin wrinkling, smokers appeared older than their age (an average of 2.1 years older) to the panelists, who were able to identify most of the smokers based solely on their facial features.[14]

In another study, investigators conducting a literature review on Medline covering articles published from 1966 to 2004 that pertained to the cutaneous effects of smoking found strong correlations between smoking and a wide array of dermatologic conditions, including wrinkling and premature skin aging, as well as poor wound healing, squamous cell carcinoma, psoriasis, hidradenitis suppurativa, hair loss, and oral cancers.[15] The same review also found that smoking affects the skin lesions associated with AIDS, diabetes, and lupus.

In a recent study, 82 subjects aged 22 to 91 years were assessed for the effects of smoking on photoprotected skin of the inner arm. Forty-one subjects (50%) had a history of previous or current smoking. Subjects were followed for 1 year and the evaluation was based on a 9-point scale in which 0 and 8 represented "no fine wrinkling" and "severe fine wrinkling," respectively. Results were studied by a multiple regression model in order to determine skin aging with controlling variables such as chronologic aging and hormone therapy. Packs of cigarettes smoked daily were found to be associated with wrinkling and to be a predictive variable of aging in photoprotected skin.[16]

SPECULATION ON ASPECTS OF MECHANISM OF ACTION

Several bodily tissues endure wide-ranging pharmacologic effects from the over 1500 ingredients of cigarette smoke. Although the clinical trials discussed above differed over the extent of the impact of smoking on skin, it is certain that smoking alters skin function and immune-mediated skin disease.[4] For example, lower stratum corneum water content has been reported in smokers,[17] likely because of the diuretic effect of nicotine.

Although little is known about the mechanism through which cigarette smoking manifests in facial wrinkling, the dynamic is probably multifactorial.[3] Matrix metalloproteinases (MMPs) likely play a significant role in the premature aging induced by cigarette smoking via the same mechanism that MMPs cause aging in patients with significant sun exposure (see Chapter 6). A recent study demonstrated that MMP-1 mRNA levels are significantly increased in the skin of smokers as compared to the skin of nonsmokers.[18] Because MMPs are known to degrade collagen, this finding may help explain the mechanism by which smoking causes premature aging. Other MMPs are known to affect elastic fibers; therefore, these MMPs likely play a role as well because the elastic fibers in the skin of non-sun-exposed smokers appear thicker and more fragmented than the elastic fibers in the skin of nonsmoking age-matched controls. These histopathologic findings are similar to those seen in sun-damaged skin, though the smoking-induced alterations occur deeper in the reticular dermis as opposed to the solar damage to the papillary dermis. In addition to the observed increased levels of MMPs noted in the skin of smokers, there are several other systemic and metabolic alterations induced by smoking.

Smoking appears to reduce facial stratum corneum moisture as well as vitamin A levels, the latter of which is important in fending off or neutralizing the free radicals thought to contribute to the etiologic pathway of aging. Of course, genetic factors also play a role in facial wrinkling because not all smokers exhibit the typical "smoker's face."

Many studies discussing the changes seen in the cutaneous microvasculature of smokers show that chronic smoking diminishes capillary and arterial blood flow, leading to local dermal ischemia.[18] This compromised blood flow leads to fewer nutrients and oxygen in the skin with a concomitant build-up of toxic waste products that can damage the skin. In fact, it is well known that smoking slows wound healing and that patients are strongly advised to stop smoking prior to any elective cosmetic surgery.[19] This is especially important in face-lifts, laser resurfacing, and dermabrasion procedures because a good blood supply to the skin is vital for a good surgical outcome.

Another confounding factor in the production of facial wrinkling is infrared radiation (IR). IR comprises 40% of the solar radiation that reaches the earth and has been associated with increasing the number and thickness of elastic fibers in exposed skin. The effects of IR are felt as heat, though the cutaneous results of such exposure are similar to the elastosis induced by UV exposure. This, along with the fact that several studies have suggested a link between exacerbated elastosis and chronic exposure to heat in the workplace, led investigators to conclude that the presence of a continuous source of heat such as a lit cigarette may have contributed to an increase in the elastosis observed in their patients who smoke.[19]

Facial Wrinkles and Chronic Obstructive Pulmonary Disease

Smoking is also the major risk factor for the development of chronic obstructive pulmonary disease (COPD). Not all cigarette smokers develop COPD; therefore, it is believed that individuals who develop COPD have a genetic susceptibility to the effects of cigarette smoke.[20,21] In 2006, researchers found that smokers with significant facial wrinkles were more likely to have COPD.[22] Collagen and elastin levels are affected in both facial wrinkling and COPD, so it is possible that these conditions share common mechanistic or genetic pathways. It has been suggested that smokers with significant facial wrinkles should be evaluated for COPD.

TREATMENT OF SKIN AGING INDUCED BY SMOKING

Of course, cessation of smoking should be the primary goal. There are many products available to help patients stop smoking, including nicotine patches and gum, as well as oral antidepressants such as Zyban™. All patients should stop smoking at least 1 month prior to any elective surgery to enhance wound healing. All cosmetic patients should be advised that sun exposure and smoking undermine efforts to look younger. However, if patients insist on smoking, the addition of an oral antioxidant vitamin formula (see Chapter 34) and a topical retinoid (see Chapter 30) may help prevent some of the deleterious effects of smoking, although this has not been studied or proven. The "smoker's wrinkles" around the mouth can be treated with dermal fillers such as CosmoPlast™, Juvéderm™, or Restylane™ (see Chapter 23), or with a very small amount of botulinum toxin (see Chapter 22). A more permanent improvement option for these patients is dermabrasion or laser resurfacing. However, perioral lines will rapidly reappear if the patient continues or resumes smoking.

SUMMARY

The preponderance of evidence suggests that cigarette smoking contributes to the exogenous aging of skin. Dermatologists are in a unique position to appeal to patients' vanity and to nudge them toward cessation of a habit that poses numerous risks and likely deleterious effects on their health. The cosmetic dermatologist may even have more leverage in suggesting to patients who smoke that continuation or resumption of smoking can seriously compromise the efficacy of any facial rejuvenation procedure. Although there are many treatments available for aging skin, there is no treatment as effective as prevention itself!

REFERENCES

1. Demierre MF, Brooks D, Koh H, et al. Public knowledge, awareness, and perceptions of the association between skin aging and smoking. *J Am Acad Dermatol.* 1999;41:27.
2. Boyd AS, Stasko T, King LE Jr., et al. Cigarette smoking-associated elastotic changes in the skin. *J Am Acad Dermatol.* 1999;41:23.
3. Smith JB, Fenske NA. Cutaneous manifestations and consequences of smoking. *J Am Acad Dermatol.* 1996;34:717.
4. Mills CM. Smoking and skin disease. *Int J Dermatol.* 1993;32:864.
5. Partsch B, Jochmann W, Partsch H. Tobacco and the skin. *Wien Med Wochenschr.* 1994;144:565.
6. Trüeb RM. Association between smoking and hair loss: another opportunity for health education against smoking? *Dermatology.* 2003;206:189.
7. Castelo-Branco C, Figueras F, Martinez de Osaba MJ, et al. Facial wrinkling in postmenopausal women. Effects of smoking status and hormone replacement therapy. *Maturitas.* 1998;29:75.
8. Daniel HW. Smoker's wrinkles. A study in the epidemiology of "crow's feet." *Ann Intern Med.* 1971;75:873.
9. Ernster VL, Grady D, Miike R, et al. Facial wrinkling in men and women, by smoking status. *Am J Public Health.* 1995;85:78.
10. Koh JS, Kang H, Choi SW, et al. Cigarette smoking associated with premature facial wrinkling: image analysis of facial skin replicas. *Int J Dermatol.* 2002;41:21.
11. Kadunce DP, Burr R, Gress R, et al. Cigarette smoking: risk factor for premature facial wrinkling. *Ann Intern Med.* 1991;114:840.
12. O'Hare PM, Fleischer AB Jr., D'Agostino RB Jr., et al. Tobacco smoking contributes little to facial wrinkling. *J Eur Acad Dermatol Venereol.* 1999;12:133.
13. Leung WC, Harvey I. Is skin ageing in the elderly caused by sun exposure or smoking? *Br J Dermatol.* 2002;147:1187.
14. Raitio A, Kontinen J, Rasi M, et al. Comparison of clinical and computerized image analyses in the assessment of skin ageing in smokers and non-smokers. *Acta Derm Venereol.* 2004;84:422.
15. Freiman A, Bird G, Metelitsa AI, et al. Cutaneous effects of smoking. *J Cutan Med Surg.* 2004;8:415.
16. Helfrich YR, Yu L, Ofori A, et al. Effect of smoking on aging of photoprotected skin: evidence gathered using a new photonumeric scale. *Arch Dermatol.* 2007;143:397.
17. Wolf R, Tur E, Wolf D, et al. The effect of smoking on skin moisture and surface lipids. *J Cosmet Sci.* 1992;14:83.
18. Lahmann C, Bergemann J, Harrison G, et al. Matrix metalloproteinase-1 and skin ageing in smokers. *Lancet.* 2001;357:935.
19. Silverstein P. Smoking and wound healing. *Am J Med.* 1992;93:22S.
20. Silverman EK, Chapman HA, Drazen JM, et al. Genetic epidemiology of severe, early-onset chronic obstructive pulmonary disease. *Am J Respir Crit Care Med.* 1998;157:1770.
21. McCloskey SC, Patel BD, Hinchliffe SJ, et al. Siblings of patients with severe chronic obstructive pulmonary disease have a significant risk of airflow obstruction. *Am J Respir Crit Care Med.* 2001;164:1419.
22. Patel BD, Loo WJ, Tasker AD, et al. Smoking related COPD and facial wrinkling: is there a common susceptibility? *Thorax.* 2006;61:568.

CHAPTER 8

Nutrition and the Skin

Leslie Baumann, MD

Food is the only medicine that the average healthy individual requires on a daily basis. Indeed, more than 2000 years ago, Hippocrates is said to have offered: "Let food be your medicine, and let medicine be your food."[1] It is from such a perspective—that good nutrition is a fundamental building block of good general health and healthy skin—that this discussion proceeds. Specifically, this chapter will focus on some of the key chemical components of a healthy diet that have been shown to confer benefits to the skin. In the process, cutaneous effects will be discussed in the context of vegetarianism, as well as the skin types of the Baumann Skin Typing System. Attention will first be focused on the effects of diet on acne, the most common dermatologic condition, and, finally, on oral supplementation.

There is copious research underway now on the direct effects on health from the consumption or supplementation of various nutrients. A significant proportion of such work focuses specifically on the potential benefits conferred to the skin through the intake of certain foods or supplements. For instance, in 2003, a cross-sectional study of 302 healthy men and women collected data on serum concentrations of nutrients, dietary consumption of nutrients, as well as various cutaneous measurements (including hydration, sebum content, and surface pH), revealing statistically significant relationships between serum vitamin A and cutaneous sebum content as well as surface pH as well as between skin hydration and dietary consumption of total fat, saturated fat, and monosaturated fat. The investigators concluded that such findings are evidence that the condition of the skin can be influenced by alterations in baseline nutritional status.[2]

DIET AND ACNE

Acne vulgaris is one of the most common conditions that prompt visits to a dermatologist. In 1998, it was believed that acne affected as many as 40 to 50 million people in the United States alone.[3] More recently, estimates of acne prevalence and incidence in Western populations, while remaining high, have come closer to 17 million in the United States[4,5] (see Chapter 15). Interestingly, recent epidemiologic studies in non-Westernized populations (i.e., Inuit, Okinawan Islanders, Ache hunter-gatherers, and Kitavan Islanders) in which acne is rare, indicate that dietary factors, including glycemic load, may play a role in the development of this condition, particularly since incidence of acne has risen in these communities in association with the adoption of Western lifestyles.[6–9]

Accordingly, Cordain, has argued persuasively for abandoning the traditional belief espoused in the dermatology community since the early 1970s that diet does not contribute to the pathophysiology of acne. In particular, he asserts that the dogma claiming that diet and acne are unrelated has been based on two fundamentally flawed studies from 1969 by Fulton et al. and 1971 by Anderson that lacked control groups, statistical data treatment, as well as blinding and/or placebos and were characterized by inadequate sample sizes and insufficient or absent baseline diet data, among other deficiencies.[6,10,11] Furthermore, Cordain contends that substantial evidence has been amassed since these two influential studies revealing that alterations in hormonal and cytokine homeostasis engendered by diet have emerged as the leading candidates for exogenous influences on acne development. Among such data is a study suggesting that the regular, long-term consumption of high glycemic meals, which raise insulin concentrations, may induce chronic hyperinsulinemia and insulin resistance, increasing levels of insulin-like growth factor 1 (IGF-1) and decreasing levels of insulin-like growth factor binding protein 3 (IGFBP-3), fostering keratinocyte proliferation and corneocyte apoptosis.[6,12,13] Other proximate causes of acne, such as androgen-mediated sebum production levels as well as inflammation, are also affected by diet. Cordain notes that insulin and IGF-1 incite the synthesis of androgens as well as sebum and inhibit the hepatic production of sex hormone-binding globulin, resulting in higher levels of circulating androgens.[6]

In 2007, Smith et al. investigated the effects of a low-glycemic-load diet on acne lesion counts in 43 males between the ages of 15 and 25 years. The experimental diet, over the 12-week, parallel design study with investigator-blinded skin evaluations, included 25% energy from protein and 45% from low-glycemic-index carbohydrates and the control group diet focused on carbohydrate-rich foods without regard to the glycemic index. The low-glycemic-load participants experienced larger reductions in the number of acne lesions, weight, and body mass index and a greater improvement in insulin sensitivity than the subjects consuming the control diet.[14] In the same cohort of patients, Smith et al. also compared the impacts from an experimental low-glycemic-load diet with those from a conventional high-glycemic-load diet on acne. Subjects following the intervention diet, which included recommendations to eat more fish, exhibited lower lesion counts than the high-glycemic control group after 12 weeks, and experienced greater reductions in weight and free androgen index in addition to elevated insulin-like growth factor binding protein-1 as compared to controls. While calling for additional research, the investigators concluded that these findings reflect an active role in acne etiology of nutritional choices.[15] While accepting this overarching argument by Smith and colleagues, Logan suggested in response that aspects other than a low glycemic index in the experimental diet, particularly its status as being lower in saturated fats as well as much higher in polyunsaturated fats and fiber, may account for hormonal alterations and inflammation that affect acne.[16] He added that greater consumption of fish, which contains anti-inflammatory omega-3 fatty acids, may have rendered the intervention diet higher in polyunsaturated fats and had a mitigating effect on acne. To further this work by Smith et al., Logan recommended research using high-fiber, high-omega-3 fatty acid, and low saturated-fat diets.

Such concerns were at least partially answered by a more recent report by Smith et al. An investigation using data on the same patients revealed a correlation between an elevated ratio of saturated to monounsaturated fatty acids of skin surface triglycerides and decreased acne lesion counts in the low-glycemic-load diet group as compared to controls after 12 weeks. An increase in monounsaturated fatty acids in sebum was also associated with greater sebum secretions. The authors concluded that desaturase enzymes may influence sebaceous lipogenesis and the emergence of acne, but suggest that more research is necessary on the interplay of sebum gland physiology and diet.[17] While additional research, particularly well controlled dietary intervention trials, is warranted and may prove revelatory in clarifying the contributory roles of specific foods in the etiologic pathway of acne, Cordain identifies increased consumption of foods high in omega-3 polyunsaturated fatty acids (PUFAs), thus reducing the ratio of omega-6 to omega-3 fatty acids, as important in attacking the inflammatory aspect of acne.[6]

Acne and Milk

The possibility of an association between dietary consumption of dairy products and acne has been long considered, though it has largely been overwhelmed by the dogma of the last few decades denying a connection between diet and acne eruptions.

In an assessment of Nurses Health Study II data of 47,355 women who completed questionnaires on high school diet in 1998 and teenage acne diagnosed by a physician as severe in 1989, Adebamowo et al. identified a positive relation between acne and consumption of total milk and skim milk, which they speculated might be attributed to the hormones and bioactive molecules present in milk.[18] In a critical response to this article, Bershad questioned the retrospective nature of the study, namely the accuracy of distantly recalled dietary habits. In addition, she suggested that the authors failed to control for the subjects' heredity, nationality, and socioeconomic status, and erred in ascribing a correlation to causation. Finally, she concluded that the most notable result of this study was not the purported link between milk consumption and acne, but the finding that acne is not caused by pizza, French fries, and sweets.[19] In a rebuttal, Adebamowo countered that the study population was similar socioeconomically by dint of job similarity. Furthermore, the study population comprised nurses of which 91.6% were non-Hispanic white women residing in the 14 most populous US states in 1989. While stipulating that socioeconomic status is a risk factor for acne development,[7] he noted that accounting for race and socioeconomic status in the study models did not significantly alter the study results. Adebamowo added that the methods of his team were well validated,[20] and that their findings of a positive relationship between milk consumption and acne and no observed association between certain foods and acne warrant further investigation.[19]

In 2006, Adebamowo et al. reported results of a prospective cohort study demonstrating a link between milk intake and acne in 6094 girls. The subjects were 9 to 15 years old in 1996, when they reported milk consumption on as many as three food frequency questionnaires from 1996 to 1998. In 1999, questionnaires were used to evaluate the presence and severity of acne. Again, they discerned a positive relationship between milk consumption and acne development, ascribing such cutaneous results to the metabolic effects of milk.[21]

More recently, Adebamowo et al., following a prospective cohort study of 4273 boys who also responded to dietary intake questionnaires from 1996 to 1998 and a teenaged acne questionnaire in 1999, reported a positive association between the consumption of skim milk and acne. The authors attributed these findings to hormonal components in skim milk, or factors that affect endogenous hormones.[22] Danby, a coauthor of Adebamowo on these studies, while acknowledging the unnatural aspect of humans, particularly in postweaned years, consuming copious amounts of another species' milk, has suggested that qualitative and quantitative research is necessary to ascertain the influence on acne pathogenesis of steroid hormones in all dairy products.[23] He also noted that Perricone's acne prescription diet is nearly devoid of dairy products,[23] and, in fact, focuses heavily on anti-inflammatory food ingredients and maintaining a low-glycemic load.[24] This may explain the success of Perricone's diet for the skin.

Acne and Iodine

In 1961, Hitch and Greenburg disproved the notion of a direct causal connection between acne and iodine intake as the largest quantities of fish and other seafood were consumed by adolescents who exhibited the lowest acne rates in their study.[25] However, in 1967, Hitch did establish that iodine consumption can aggravate acne.[26] In response to the Adebamowo et al. study on an association between dairy intake during high school and teenaged acne cited above, Arbesman indicated that the iodine content of milk may have also contributed to acne development in addition to the hormonal explanation proffered by the investigators.[27] He added that significant levels of iodine have been identified in milk in Denmark, Italy, Norway, the United Kingdom, and the United States, because of the use of iodine and iodophor at various stages of the production process, with variable levels of iodine in milk based on geography and season.[28–34]

In a reply to Arbesman, Danby counters that iodine deficiency poses a greater health risk than overdosage, and that iodine levels in milk appear to be comparable to those found in human mother's milk. Furthermore, he suggests that there are no data to uphold the notion that comedonal acne is caused by the ingestion of iodides.[35] The author has not observed an association between acne and iodine, either causally or as an exacerbating factor, but notes that Fulton, primary author of the 1969 study criticized by Cordain, argues that in individuals prone to acne, iodine excreted through the sebaceous glands may in the process irritate the pilosebaceous unit and contribute to a flare-up.

Acne and Chocolate

While Cordain and others[1] have exposed the flaws in the methodologies of the studies that denied a significant link between nutrition and acne, particularly the study by Fulton et al. that refuted a connection between chocolate and acne, such debunking has not undermined the basic truth happened upon more than 30 years ago regarding acne and chocolate. Cordain pointed out that the actual treatment variable in the Fulton study was an ingredient of the tested bittersweet chocolate candy bar, cacao solids, which were replaced with partially hydrogenated vegetable fat in the control bar. While suggesting that the only logical conclusion of this study was that cacao solids may not contribute to the causal pathway of acne, he also noted, among other criticisms, that because subjects also consumed their normal diets in addition to the 112-g test or control bar daily for 4 weeks with no baseline measurements, there was no way of determining the quantity of cacao solids consumed in either arm of the study.[6] Indeed, it is likely that it is the sugar that is added to various chocolate delicacies that engenders multiple deleterious health effects if consumed with regularity and over time, not the cacao or chocolate ingredient. Evidence suggests that sugar and sugar products may promote such cutaneous effects through the glycosylation of proteins in the skin,[36,37] ultimately leading to skin wrinkling and photoaging (see Chapters. 2 and 19).

Interestingly, rather than serving as a culprit in acne pathogenesis, chocolate has a history dating back at least since the 1500s as a component in the medical practices of the Olmec, Maya, and Aztec peoples.[38]

Not only does chocolate per se not directly cause acne (though a steady diet of highly-sugared chocolate products can certainly contribute to it), the Borba product line now includes a Clarifying Chocolate Bar made with Swiss dark chocolate that is touted for its patented formula that is said to have the opposite effect on skin—actually clearing skin or preventing breakouts. Of course, a healthy dose of skepticism regarding the potential contributory effects of a particular food toward acne is just as appropriate toward the notion of consuming a supposedly healthier item to exert the opposite effect. A consistent pattern of good nutrition is likely the optimal choice for overall health, total cutaneous health, and reducing the risk of developing acne. It has long been known that a diet rich in fruits and vegetables is ideal. Much has been learned in recent decades, though, regarding the chemical constituents in such foods that may play direct roles in health, including the health of the skin. The beneficial activities exhibited by certain chemical ingredients in foods have, in turn, been harnessed in various medications to exert more direct effects. For instance, retinoids are a form of vitamin A, which has long been known to play a role in acne. Notably, carotenoids are one of the best dietary sources of vitamin A.

CAROTENOIDS

Certain plant constituents have been established as exerting photoprotective effects as antioxidants, including carotenoids, flavonoids and other polyphenols, tocopherols, and vitamin C. In a recent study, Stahl et al. demonstrated that consumption of lycopene, which is the primary carotenoid in tomatoes and is also present in apricots, papaya, pink grapefruit, guava, and watermelon, was effective in preventing or curbing sensitivity to ultraviolet (UV)-induced erythema formation in volunteers consuming lycopene-rich products over 10 to 12 weeks.[39]

Stahl et al. previously investigated whether the use of dietary tomato paste, a rich source of lycopene, could deliver a protective effect against UV-induced erythema in humans. A solar simulator was used to induce erythema in the scapular area at the outset of the study and after weeks 4 and 10. For a period of 10 weeks, 9 volunteers ingested 40 g of tomato paste with 10 g of olive oil while 10 controls ingested olive oil only. Carotenoid levels were equivalent between the two groups at the beginning of the study and there were no significant differences between the groups at week 4. There was neither change in serum carotenoids in the control group by week 10 nor in other carotenoids but lycopene in the experimental group, but those consuming tomato paste exhibited higher serum levels of lycopene accompanied by scapular erythema development 40% less than controls.[40] In subsequent experiments that involved daily ingestion of tomato paste (16 mg/d) for 10 weeks, Stahl and Sies demonstrated similar results, with increases measured in serum levels of lycopene and total carotenoids in skin and significantly less erythema formation after 10 weeks. They also determined that there is an optimal level of protection associated with each carotenoid micronutrient.[41]

In a placebo-controlled, parallel study involving some of the same investigators, the protective effects against erythema of beta-carotene (24 mg/d) were compared to those of the same dose of a carotenoid combination of beta-carotene, lutein, and lycopene (8 mg/d each) or placebo for 12 weeks. Erythema intensity before and 24 hours after irradiation with a solar light simulator was recorded at baseline and following 6 and 12 weeks of supplementation. Researchers noted diminished intensity in erythema 24 hours after exposure (at weeks 6 and 12) in both experimental groups, with substantially less erythema formation after 12 weeks in comparison to baseline. While there were no observed changes in the control group, serum carotenoid levels increased significantly also, three- to four-fold in the beta-carotene group and one- to three-fold in the mixed carotenoid group.[42] In a more recent study by several of the same investigators, the photoprotective effects of synthetic lycopene were compared to the effects of a tomato extract (Lyc-o-Mato) and a beverage containing solubilized Lyc-o-Mato (Lyc-o-Guard-Drink) after 12 weeks of supplementation. Significant increases were observed in all groups in terms of serum levels of lycopene and total skin carotenoids and a protective effect against erythema formation was seen in all groups as well, but it was substantially larger in the Lyco-o-Mato and Lyc-o-Guard groups. The researchers speculated that the carotenoid phytofluene and carotenoid precursor phytoene may have assisted in providing this additional photoprotection.[43]

Finally, lutein and zeaxanthin, found in leafy green vegetables, were supplemented for 2 weeks in the diets of female hairless Skh-1 mice to determine the cutaneous response to UVB. Investigators observed significant reductions in the edematous cutaneous response as well as decreases in the UVB-induced elevation in hyperproliferative markers.[44]

POLYPHENOLS

Comprising a broad range of more than 8000 naturally-occurring compounds, polyphenols are secondary plant metabolites that exert varying degrees of antioxidant activity. All of these diverse substances share a definitive structural component, a phenol or an aromatic ring with at least one hydroxyl group. Polyphenols are an exceedingly important part of, and the most copious antioxidants in, the human diet, and found in a vast spectrum of vegetables, fruits, herbs, grains, tea, coffee beans, propolis, and red wine[45,46] (Table 8-1). Flavonoids are the most abundant polyphenols in the human diet as well as the most studied polyphenols, and can be further divided into several categories. These subclasses include flavones

TABLE 8-1
Foods with Significant Polyphenol Levels[45,46]

VEGETABLES	FRUITS	MISCELLANEOUS
Artichokes	Apples/pears	Cocoa
Broccoli	Apricots	Coffee beans
Cabbage	Berries (various)	Flaxseed/flaxseed oil
Eggplant	Cherries	Grains (e.g., wild rice)
Lettuce	Citrus fruits	Nuts
Olives	Currants (red and black)	Propolis
Onions	Grapes	Red wine
Soybeans	Peaches	Tea (green and black)
Spinach	Plums	

TABLE 8-2
Subclasses of the Most Abundant Polyphenols, Flavonoids, and Food Sources of Each Class[46–48]

Flavones	Flavonols	Flavanones	Isoflavones	Flavanols (catechins)	Anthocyanins	Proanthocyanidins
Celery	Apples	Oranges	Soy	Apples	Blackberries	Apples
Fresh parsley	Broccoli	Grapefruit		Cocoa	Cherries	Dark chocolate
Sweet red pepper	Olives			Dark chocolate	Currants (black and red)	Grapes
	Onions			Tea (black and green)	Grapes	Pears
	Tea (black and green)				Plums	Red wine
					Raspberries	Tea (black and green)
					Strawberries	

(e.g., apigenin, luteolin); flavonols (e.g., quercetin, kaempferol, myricetin, and fisetin); flavanones (e.g., naringenin, hesperidin, eriodictyol); isoflavones (e.g., genistein, daidzein); flavanols or catechins (e.g., epicatechin, epicatechin 3-gallate, epigallocatechin, epigallocatechin 3-gallate, catechin, gallocatechin); anthocyanins (e.g., cyanidin, pelargonidin); and proanthocyanidins (e.g., pycnogenol, leukocyanidin, leucoanthocyanin)[46–48] (Table 8-2). Among the many other polyphenols there are stilbenes (e.g., resveratrol, found in red wine), lignans (e.g., enterodiol, found in flaxseed and flaxseed oil), tannins (e.g., ellagic acid, found in pomegranates, raspberries, strawberries, cranberries, and walnuts), hydroxycinnamic acids, and phenolic acids, among which caffeic and ferulic acids are frequently found in foods. A survey of the research associated with many of these compounds and their sources is beyond the scope of this chapter, as such a discussion could fill volumes. Some of the most widely disseminated results involving polyphenols pertain to the identified efficacy of various topical applications of green tea catechins, ferulic acid, resveratrol, and other ingredients, which are discussed elsewhere in this textbook.

One recent experimental success with the oral ingestion of a polyphenolic compound resulting in benefits to the skin involved an as yet unmentioned food source. In an investigation of the antiaging effects of red clover isoflavones, which in high levels in diets have already been shown to contribute to low incidence of menopausal symptoms as well as osteoporosis, researchers orally administered red clover extract containing 11% isoflavones to ovariectomized rats for 14 weeks. Their findings revealed that collagen levels increased significantly in the treatment group as compared to the control group and epidermal thickness and keratinization was normal in the treated group, but diminished in the control group. The researchers concluded that skin aging engendered by estrogen depletion can be mitigated by regular dietary consumption of red clover isoflavones.[49] (See the Pigmented vs. Nonpigmented section below for additional studies on the cutaneous effects of orally administered polyphenols found in pomegranates and grapes.)

ESSENTIAL FATTY ACIDS AND VEGETARIAN/VEGAN DIETS

Nearly 25 years ago, investigators measured the omega-6 and omega-3 fatty acids (also known as n-6 and n-3 fatty acids, respectively) in the plasma phospholipids of 41 adults with atopic eczema and 50 normal controls and found the omega-6 linoleic acid (LA) to be significantly elevated, with all of its metabolites likewise reduced, and the omega-3 α-linolenic acid (ALA) elevated, but not significantly, with all of its metabolites substantially decreased. The researchers identified a link between atopic eczema and abnormal metabolism. Oral evening primrose oil (EPO) treatment partly rectified the abnormal metabolism of omega-6, but did not alter omega-3 levels.[50] Subsequently, Galland noted data indicating an association between poor desaturation of linoleic and linolenic acids by delta-6 dehydrogenase and atopic eczema and other allergic conditions, as well as the alleviation of atopic eczema symptoms through dietary supplementation with essential fatty acids.[51] Twenty years ago, investigators conducting a 12-week, double-blind study of the effects of dietary supplementation with n-3 fatty acids in patients with atopic dermatitis found that the experimental group taking eicosapentaenoic acid (EPA) experienced overall less subjective severity and pruritus than the control group taking a placebo.[52] It appears that supplementation with n-3 fatty acids may ameliorate symptoms of eczema in the short term. Notably, levels of n-3 fatty acids are depressed in vegetarians and vegans. Not all physicians embrace the utility of dietary modifications in the treatment of eczema. Of course, patient recommendations should include advice on bathing and skin moisturization (see Chapters 11 and 32) as well as dietary recommendations.

The dietary research in the 1980s helped form the theoretical framework that undergirds current studies of suitable sources for adjunct or alternative therapies for atopic eczema, such as hemp seed oil (which is rich in omega-6 and omega-3 fatty acids),[53] EPO,[54] and borage oil,[55] as well as the significance of varying levels of essential fatty acids for individuals with vegetarian or vegan diets as compared to omnivores.

An examination over a decade ago of lipid metabolism in 81 healthy lacto- and lacto-ovovegetarians and 62 nonvegetarians buttressed previous studies that revealed higher total serum polyunsaturated acid concentrations, particularly linoleic and linolenic acids, in vegetarians compared to nonvegetarians. Significantly higher plasma levels of vitamin C, beta-carotene, and selenium as well as vitamin E-to-cholesterol and vitamin E-to-triacylglycerol ratios (indicators of LDL and fatty acid protection, respectively) were observed.[56] (See Table 8-3 for a summary of potential nutritional deficits according to diet style.)

In an interesting matched-pair study two decades ago, Melchert et al. compared serum fatty acid content in 108 vegetarians (62 females, 40 males) and 108 nonvegetarians (70 females, 38 males). Palmitoleic (omega-7), vaccenic (omega-7), and docosahexaenoic (omega-3) acids were higher in nonvegetarians, and very low in vegetarians, and vegetarians exhibited higher levels of LA.[57] More supportive evidence was established in a study of essential fatty acids and lipoprotein lipids in female Australian vegetarians and omnivores, as investigators found that the vegetarians had significantly lower levels of n-6 and n-3 PUFAs and a lower ratio of n-3 to n-6 PUFAs.[58] It is also important to

TABLE 8-3
Potential Nutritional Deficiencies Based on Diet

	Vitamin D	Omega-3 Fatty Acids	Polyphenols	Cholesterol[a]
Vegetarian		X		X
Vegan	X	XX		X
Lactovegetarian		XX		X
Lacto-ovovegetarian	X	XX		X
Typical Western diet			X	
Atkins diet followers			XX	
South Beach diet followers			X (in first 2 wk)	

X, likely deficient; XX, must supplement.
[a]Low levels of cholesterol lead to dry skin. Topical, but not oral, supplementation is suggested (see Chapters. 11 and 32).

TABLE 8-4
Foods that may Mitigate or Improve Dry Skin[53–56,60]

Avocados
Borage seed oil
Canola oil
Evening primrose oil
Fish (particularly albacore tuna, lake trout, mackerel, menhaden, and salmon)
Flaxseed oil
Hempseed
Nuts
Olive oil
Olives
Peanuts
Safflower oil (high-oleic)
Soy
Sunflower oil (high-oleic)
Walnuts

note, PUFAs are known to inhibit the synthesis of eicosanoids derived from arachidonic acid, and are thus effective against allergic diseases.[59]

More recently, Davis and Kris-Etherton have indicated that vegetarian, particularly vegan, diets have been shown to deliver lower levels of ALA than LA, and especially low, if any, levels of EPA and docosahexaenoic acid (DHA), resulting in lower tissue levels of long-chain n-3 fatty acids. Given such low EPA and DHA levels as well as the inefficient conversion of ALA to the more active longer-chain metabolites EPA and DHA, they suggest that vegetarians may exhibit a greater dependence on ALA conversion to its metabolites and a corresponding greater need for n-3 acids than nonvegetarians.[60] In 2005, investigators conducted a cross-sectional study of 196 omnivore, 231 vegetarian, and 232 vegan men in the United Kingdom to compare plasma fatty acid concentrations in order to ascertain if the proportions of EPA, docosapentaenoic acid (DPA), and DHA relied on strict dietary adherence (data on which was obtained through a questionnaire) or to the proportions of LA and ALA in plasma. While only minor differences were observed in DPA levels, investigators noted reduced EPA and DHA levels in vegetarians and vegans, whose DHA levels were inversely correlated with plasma LA. Interestingly, they found that duration of adherence to dietary regimens was not significantly related to plasma n-3 levels. The researchers suggested that the endogenous synthesis of EPA and DHA is low but yields stable n-3 plasma levels in individuals whose diets exclude animal foods.[61] Such findings support the notion of vegetarian/vegan diets providing sufficient n-3 fatty acid concentration for survival. To optimize cutaneous health and appearance, though, vegetarians and vegans may benefit from adding supplemental EPA and DHA. It is worth noting that topically applied EPA has also been found to exert photoprotective and antiaging effects to the skin.[62]

Vegetarians Versus Nonvegetarians

As stated previously, vegetarians exhibit lower levels of serum cholesterol, ALA, EPA, and DHA and higher levels of antioxidants than nonvegetarians. (For example, a study of vegetarians estimated lipid parameters in four different groups of vegetarians, and noted higher levels of vitamin C in the blood of all four groups.[63]) Furthermore, individuals on a vegan diet for an extended period may have little to no serum cholesterol. Vegans also tend to have drier skin than vegetarians.

The main dietary fat should be derived from foods and oils rich in monounsaturated fat. When monounsaturated fats predominate, saturated fats, *trans*-fatty acids, and n-6 fatty acids are counterbalanced, and the ratio of n-6 to n-3 fatty acids improves as the proportion of omega-3 acids increases. Nuts (except for walnuts and butternuts), peanuts (a legume), olive oil, olives, avocados, canola oil, high-oleic sunflower oil, and high-oleic safflower oil all contain appreciable levels of monounsaturated fats. (See Table 8-4 for a summary of foods that may have an impact in ameliorating dry skin.) Monounsaturated fats are better to consume through whole foods as compared to oils, or supplements, because whole foods deliver several other nutrients to the diet. Certain seeds, nuts, and legumes (flaxseed, hempseed, canola, walnuts, and soy) as well as the green leaves of plants, including phytoplankton and algae, are the primary sources of dietary ALA. As stated above, fish, fish oil, and seafood are the best sources of dietary EPA and DHA. For lacto-ovovegetarians, eggs provide an adequate amount of DHA (≤50 mg/egg) but minimal EPA. Microalgae and seaweed are the only plant sources of long-chain n-3 fatty acids.

Although vegetarian diets are generally lower in total fat, saturated fat, and cholesterol compared to nonvegetarian diets, they deliver comparable levels of essential fatty acids. Clinical studies have shown that tissue levels of long-chain n-3 fatty acids are typically depressed in vegetarians, particularly so in vegans. However, vegetarians consume approximately one-third less saturated fat (vegans approximately one-half) and approximately one half as much cholesterol (vegans consume none) as omnivores.[60]

EPA/DHA, Immunoresponse and Psoriasis

DHA has been shown to inhibit inflammation and immunoresponses in the contact hypersensitivity reaction in mice. Investigators fed dietary DHA as well as EPA to mice sensitized with 2,4-dinitro-1-fluorobenzene. They found that 24 hours after the contact hypersensitivity challenge, ear swelling was reduced by DHA ethyl ester, but not EPA ethyl ester. DHA also diminished the infiltration of $CD4^+$ T lymphocytes into the ears, and minimized the expression of interferon-gamma, interleukin (IL)-6, IL-1beta, and IL-2 mRNA in the ears. The researchers concluded that the immunosuppressive activity associated with fish oil should be ascribed primarily to DHA and not its fellow n-3 PUFA.[64] However, in clinical trials, EPA and DHA in fish oils have, combined with medication, been shown to ameliorate the skin lesions, reduce the hyperlipidemia caused by etretinates (which were removed from the Canadian market in 1996 and the US market in 1998 because of elevated risks of birth defects), and lower cyclosporin toxicity in patients with psoriasis.[65] Furthermore, in a 14-day double-blind, randomized, parallel group multicenter study in which 83 patients hospitalized for chronic plaque-type psoriasis (with a Psoriasis Area and Severity Index [PASI] score of at least 15) were randomized to receive daily intravenous administration of either an omega-3 fatty acid-based lipid emulsion or an omega-6 emulsion, investigators observed greater improvements in the omega-3 group in terms of diminished psoriasis severity, which was echoed by patient self-assessment. The researchers concluded that chronic plaque-type psoriasis could be effectively treated with intravenous omega-3 fatty acids.[66]

MATCHING DIETARY NEEDS WITH SKIN TYPE

The Baumann Skin Typing System (BSTS), introduced in *The Skin Type Solution* (Bantam 2005), is a novel approach to classifying skin type (see Chapter 9). The BSTS score, derived from a self-administered questionnaire, is based on the understanding that skin can be assessed according to four major parameters: oily versus dry (O/D), sensitive versus resistant (S/R), pigmented versus nonpigmented (P/N), and wrinkled versus tight (W/T). Sixteen different skin type permutations are possible. The discussion of dietary needs based on skin type proceeds according to the four major parameters. The center of the spectrum is ideal for both the O/D and S/R parameters. Dietary interventions appear to be possible to render skin less oily or dry, as well as less sensitive, but not less resistant. Sensitive skin will be discussed briefly in "the OSNW Skin Type" section below, but primarily in the context of comparing vegetarian and nonvegetarian diets and nutritional approaches to curbing inflammation, which is a fundamental presentation of all sensitive skin subtypes. Regarding the P/N and W/T parameters, the N and T poles are the ideals. While various photoprotective behaviors are recommended to achieve these ends, particularly regarding the W/T spectrum, there appear to be dietary interventions that will promote or support these skin types.

Dry Skin

Fifteen years ago, investigators studied 79 vegetarians (51 females, 28 males) and 79 age- and sex-matched nonvegetarians to assess the relative antioxidant/atherogenic risks. Plasma alpha-tocopherol and corresponding cholesterol values were found to be significantly lower in the vegetarians as was their risk for atherosclerosis, but their tocopherol-to-cholesterol molar ratio was significantly increased.[67] Such results explain the higher incidence of dry skin in vegetarians. Cholesterol is an important substance in maintaining a balance in the oily–dry continuum. With more vitamin E and less cholesterol, vegetarians are more likely to experience dry skin (see Chapters 11 and 32).

In a 6-week study of the mechanisms and efficacy of n-3 PUFA for the treatment of atopic dermatitis (AD), investigators administered various formulas of ALA in NC/Nga mice with AD, and found that concentrations of n-3 fatty acids increased and n-6 fatty acids decreased in the red blood cell membranes, prostaglandin E(2) production was decreased, and skin blood flow was altered, increasing in the ear of mice treated with the highest dose of ALA. The researchers, noted, however, that AD development was not prevented.[59]

Oily Skin Types

In the adjusted models of the cross-sectional study of 302 healthy men and women cited above, serum vitamin A acted as a predictor of sebum content and surface pH, with a higher level of vitamin A associated with a lower sebum level.[2] Such findings suggest that individuals with oily skin would benefit from eating foods rich in vitamin A. Indeed, dietary consumption of plants and fish oil, high in PUFAs, is thought to be useful in treating inflammatory skin conditions because PUFAs are known to inhibit lipid inflammatory mediators[68] (see Chapter 10).

The OSNW Skin Type

Each of the Baumann Skin Types has specific dietary needs. Because of space constraints, each of the diets for the 16 Baumann Skin Types cannot be discussed here. However, as an example of the utility in knowing the patient's Baumann Skin Type, the oily, sensitive, nonpigmented, wrinkled (OSNW) skin type will be briefly discussed. Individuals with OSNW skin are at an increased risk of developing nonmelanoma skin cancer (basal cell or squamous cell carcinoma). The dietary guidelines that the author suggests for such patients to help them reduce cutaneous inflammation as well as the proclivity to wrinkle may also help decrease their risk for skin cancer, though.[69] Generally, the diet for individuals with OSNW skin should be focused on inhibiting oil secretion, decreasing inflammation, and preventing photodamage and skin cancer.

Dietary vitamin A has been demonstrated to exhibit an association with reduced oil gland secretion.[2] Therefore, a diet rich in foods that contain vitamin A, such as cantaloupe, carrots, dried apricots, egg yolks, liver, mangoes, spinach, and sweet potatoes, is recommended. Several foods have also long been fortified with vitamin A, including milk, some margarine, instant oats, breakfast cereals, and meal replacement bars. In addition, carotenoids, which can be converted into vitamin A, have been demonstrated to exhibit inhibitory activity against skin cancer.[70] Two of the most protective carotenoids are lycopene, found abundantly in tomatoes, and lutein, found especially in spinach, kale, and broccoli.[71,72] A diet rich in other antioxidants, in addition to carotenoids, is also recommended, including a wide variety of fruits, vegetables, and green tea. Antioxidants have been demonstrated to help reduce the production of free radicals and destructive enzymes that promote skin aging. In addition, olive oil has been shown to exhibit protective properties, especially imported extra virgin olive oil.[73]

A diet rich in fish and fish oils is also recommended for OSNWs, due to the high level of omega-3 fatty acids found in such food sources. As stated previously, omega-3 fatty acids appear to confer some anticancer and anti-inflammatory effects.[64,69] Because vegetarians, particularly vegans, have been shown to manifest low levels of serum omega-3 fatty acids,[60] vegetarian or vegan OSNWs should try to add seaweed, one of the best plant sources of omega-3 fatty acids, to their diet. (As stated previously, though, vegetarians and, particularly vegans, are more likely to tend toward dry skin.) Individuals with OSNW skin who suffer from rosacea, particularly facial flushing, are advised to abstain from alcohol, hot (in temperature) foods, and spicy food. In addition, such patients should be counseled to keep a record or diary of foods that exacerbate their condition, so that they have a clear idea of specific dietary triggers to avoid.

Pigmented Versus Nonpigmented Skin Types

One focus of altering one's susceptibility to develop pigmentary changes (melasma, solar lentigos) is the study of endogenous agents that have the potential to impart whitening or lightening activity. For example, vitamins C and E have been reported to suppress the spread of UV-induced hyperpigmentation in the skin of hairless mice.[74] (See Chapter 33 for more information on these agents.)

In a recent double-blind, placebo-controlled trial, investigators examined the various effects of dietary ellagic acid-rich pomegranate extract on skin pigmentation after UV irradiation in 13 women in their 20s to 40s. Volunteers were randomly assigned to one of three groups (high dose [200 mg/d ellagic acid], low dose [100 mg/d] or placebo [0 mg/d]) for the 4 week study. Subjects completed questionnaires regarding the condition of their skin prior to and after completing the dietary intervention. Based on the minimum erythema dose (MED) value recorded the previous day, a 1.5 MED dose of UV was administered to each participant on the inner right upper arm. Based on baseline recordings and assessments at weeks 1, 2, 3, and 4, investigators found that in the high ellagic acid dose group and the low-dose group in comparison to the control group declining luminance rates were inhibited by 1.73% and 1.35%, respectively. Questionnaire results indicated that the subjects observed improvements such as greater brightness and diminished pigmentation. The investigators concluded that the oral consumption of ellagic acid-rich pomegranate extract exerts inhibitory activity against moderate pigmentation engendered by UV exposure.[75] Previously, several of the same investigators reported that an ellagic acid-rich pomegranate extract displayed inhibitory properties against mushroom tyrosinase in vitro, comparable to the known skin-whitening agent arbutin. In addition, they demonstrated that oral administration of the pomegranate extract inhibited UV-induced skin pigmentation in brownish guinea pigs, comparable in skin-whitening effect to the use of L-ascorbic acid, although the number of DOPA-positive epidermal melanocytes was reduced by the ellagic-rich pomegranate extract but not by vitamin C. The investigators concluded that oral pomegranate extract may be a suitable skin-whitening agent, likely by dint of suppressing melanocyte proliferation and melanin production by tyrosinase in melanocytes.[76]

To determine the lightening activity of orally administered grape seed extract, which is laden with the potent polyphenolic antioxidant proanthocyanidin, Yamakoshi et al. fed diets containing 1% grape seed extract or 1% vitamin C for 8 weeks to guinea pigs with UV-induced pigmentation. No changes were seen in the vitamin C or control groups, but a lightening effect was manifested in the pigmented skin of the guinea pigs in the grape seed extract group, with a reduction in the number of DOPA-positive melanocytes, among other key parameters. In addition, grape seed extract was reported to have disrupted mushroom tyrosinase activity and melanogenesis without suppressing cultured B16 mouse melanoma cell growth. The researchers concluded that orally administered grape seed extract has the capacity to lighten pigmentation in guinea pig skin engendered by UV exposure, possibly through the inhibition of melanin production by tyrosinase in melanocytes as well as free radical fueled melanocyte proliferation.[74] More recently, in a 1-year open design study, Yamakoshi et al. evaluated the effectiveness of proanthocyanidin for the treatment of melasma. Between August 2001 and January 2002, proanthocyanidin-rich grape seed extract was orally administered to 12 Japanese female melasma patients and to 11 of these 12 subjects between March and July 2002. Improvements in the melasma of 10 of the 12 women were noted during the first period of the study and in 6 of the 11 patients during the second period, with lightening values increasing and the melanin index significantly decreasing. The investigators concluded that the polyphenolic grape seed extract is effective in diminishing the hyperpigmentation associated with melasma, with optimal results seen after 6 months of oral administration and additional supplementation perhaps helping to prevent exacerbation of the condition during the summer.[77] As is often the case, more research is necessary, but these preliminary animal study results support the notion of pomegranate and grape seed consumption or supplementation for combating the pigmentation tendency.

Pycnogenol is a standardized pine bark extract containing strong polyphenolic constituents with established antioxidant activity. Research has suggested that this patented botanical extract formulation is more potent than vitamins C and E and has the capacity to recycle vitamin C, regenerate vitamin E (as does vitamin C), and promote the activity of endogenous antioxidant enzymes.[78] The efficacy of Pycnogenol in protecting against UV radiation inspired a 30-day clinical trial of 30 women with melasma in which patients took one 25 mg tablet of Pycnogenol at each meal, 3 times daily. Researchers noted that the average surface area of melasma significantly decreased, suggesting that Pycnogenol is an effective and safe treatment for this condition.[78]

Wrinkled Skin Types

More than a decade ago, investigators estimated the levels of certain vitamins (i.e., A, C, E, and beta-carotene) and trace elements (i.e., copper, selenium, and zinc) in the blood of 67 vegetarian nonsmokers and 75 nonvegetarians (all between the ages of 34 and 60 years) living in the same geographical region. The average length of vegetarianism (lacto- or lacto-ovovegetarianism) was 6.2 years. The investigators found that vegetarians had higher plasma levels of all the tested vitamins and minerals, all of which play important roles as antioxidants or in activating antioxidant enzymes.[79] In turn, such compounds are associated with various salubrious effects, including a photoprotective effect against aging, exemplified most frequently by wrinkles.

In a recent double-blind, placebo-controlled trial assessing the effects of soy isoflavone aglycone on the skin, particularly the extent of linear and fine wrinkles at the lateral angle of the eyes, of 26 women in their late 30s and early 40s, the volunteers were randomly assigned to incorporate into their daily diets for 12 weeks either the experimental food containing soy (40 mg daily) or a placebo. Investigators observed statistically significant improvements of malar skin elasticity at week 8 and fine wrinkles at week 12 in the soy group, as compared to the control group, and concluded that the daily dietary consumption of 40 mg of soy isoflavone aglycones contributes to the amelioration of cutaneous signs of aging in middle-aged women.[80]

In a fascinating study of a possible association between dietary intake and skin wrinkling in sun-exposed areas, Purba et al. used questionnaires and cutaneous microtopographic measurements to evaluate diet and skin wrinkling in 177 Greek-born individuals living in Melbourne, Australia, 69 Greek subjects residing in rural Greece, 48

Anglo-Celtic Australian elderly individuals living in Melbourne, Australia, and 159 Swedish elderly participants living in Sweden. Investigators identified the Swedish elderly as exhibiting the least wrinkling in sun-exposed areas, followed by the Greek-born in Melbourne, rural Greek elderly, and then Anglo-Celtic Australians. Correlation and regression analyses revealed significant data that led the investigators to conclude that diet may very well influence skin wrinkling. Generally, they found that individuals that consumed more vegetables (especially green leafy vegetables, spinach specifically, as well as asparagus, celery, eggplant, garlic, and onions/leeks), olive oil, monounsaturated fat, and legumes and lower levels of milk and milk products, butter, margarine, and sugar products manifested fewer wrinkles in sun-exposed skin (Table 8-5). Significantly, the authors suggested that diets high in monounsaturated acids may raise the monounsaturated fatty acid levels in the epidermis, which resist oxidative damage, whereas the PUFAs are more susceptible to oxidation. They speculated that this might explain the correlation of monounsaturated olive oil and less wrinkling as well as the higher level of wrinkling associated with the consumption of polyunsaturated margarine. Specifically, the investigators identified positive associations between photodamage and dietary intake of full-fat milk (but not skim milk, cheese, or yogurt), red meat, potatoes, soft drinks/cordials, and cakes/pastries. Conversely, less actinic damage was associated with vegetables and legumes, as mentioned above, as well as apples/pears, cherries, dried fuits/prunes, jam, eggs, melon, multigrain bread, nuts, olives, tea, water, and yogurt. Finally, they noted that less photodamage was correlated with a higher intake of the following nutrients: total fat, especially monounsaturated fat, vitamins A and C, calcium, phosphorus, magnesium, iron, and zinc.[81]

TABLE 8-5
Foods to Consume and Avoid to Help Keep Wrinkles at Bay[81]

Eat	Avoid
Asparagus	Butter
Celery	Margarine
Eggplant	Milk and milk products
Garlic	Red meat
Legumes	Sugar products
Leeks/onions	
Monounsaturated fat	
Olive oil	
Spinach (and other green leafy vegetables)	

LIMITS TO ENDOGENOUS PHOTOPROTECTION

It is worth noting that in a review of the literature regarding the relationship of nutrient intake and the skin, particularly the photoprotective effects of nutrients, the influences of nutrients on cutaneous immune responses, and therapeutic actions of nutrients in skin disorders, investigators found that supplementation with the nutrients of focus (i.e., vitamins, carotenoids, and PUFAs) rendered protection against UV light, but not as much as topical sunscreens.[68] Oral supplements should be combined with sunscreen use (Chapter 29) and sun avoidance.

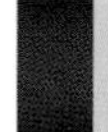

ORAL SUPPLEMENTS AND THE SKIN: FROM A TO Z

The following is a brief guide to some of the most common nutritional supplements currently used or under study in the beauty and skin care realm. The focus here is on the effects that such products confer on the skin. Several of these compounds provide broad systemic effects. Of course, it is incumbent upon practitioners to remind patients that they should always discuss the use of new supplements with their physician, particularly when pregnant, breastfeeding, or undergoing treatment for any medical conditions.

Alpha Lipoic Acid

Small amounts of alpha lipoic acid are produced naturally by the human body, but when present in excess (as a result of a supplement, for example), it may help prevent various diseases. Among these, alpha lipoic acid is said to help smooth skin and combat the cutaneous signs of aging. Significantly, perhaps, alpha lipoic acid was once considered an antioxidant, but a recent report has called such a designation into question.[82] While alpha lipoic acid seems to exert a positive impact on energy, and on several health conditions, the author does not recommend it for skin-related concerns. More research is required to better understand the protective role of alpha lipoic acid and its potential applications for the skin.

Antioxidants

Several of the supplements in this list qualify as antioxidants (see Chapter 34). This particular entry, though, refers to products that contain a blend or combination of antioxidants. For example, Imedeen Time Perfection tablets include antioxidants such as vitamin C and grape seed extract. Antioxidants are substances that protect cells from oxidative damage caused by exogenous factors such as UV light, air pollution, ozone, cigarette smoke, and even oxygen itself. In addition, antioxidants protect cells from endogenously generated oxidative stress, a natural by-product of cellular energy production. Oxidative stress, whether its origin is external or internal, contributes to inflammatory pathways mediated by the formation of free radicals, which are molecules with an uneven number of electrons and are thus highly reactive. Left unchecked, free radicals can cause damage to cell membranes, lipids, proteins, and DNA, thus contributing to skin aging, among a cascade of other deleterious effects on health. Indeed, the cumulative effects of free radicals over time form the basis of "The Damage Accumulation Theory of Aging."[83] Antioxidants scavenge and eliminate free radicals and are crucial to the success of a skin care regimen. The convenience of antioxidant products also renders them easy to use on a regular basis. Good dietary sources of antioxidants include berries; larger fruits; vegetables; beans; roots and tubers; cereals; as well as nuts, seeds, and dried fruits.[84] (See Table 8-6 for specific foods high in antioxidants.)

Recently, investigators conducted a prospective study among 1001 randomly chosen Australian adults to evaluate the relationship between consumption of antioxidants and risk of basal cell carcinomas (BCCs) and squamous cell carcinomas (SCCs). Histologically verified cases of skin cancer were recorded between 1996 and 2004 after antioxidant intake was estimated in 1996. In individuals with a baseline skin cancer history, dietary consumption of the carotenoids lutein and zeaxanthin was correlated with a lower incidence of SCC. However, a positive association was seen with various antioxidants and BCC development in those with and without a history of skin cancer, including individuals with a specific history of BCC. The researchers concluded that their findings supported prior evidence of divergent etiologic pathways for these types of skin cancer.[85] It is important to note that such results do not undermine the efficacy of antioxidants; rather, these findings reinforce the notion that evidence trumps hype.

TABLE 8-6
Dietary Sources of Antioxidants[84]

Berries	Larger Fruits	Vegetables	Beans	Roots and Tubers	Cereals (Wholemeal Flours of)	Nuts, Seeds, Dried Fruits
Black currant	Clementine	Artichoke	Broad beans	Ginger	Barley	Dried apricots
Blackberry	Date	Brussels sprouts	Groundnut	Red beets	Buckwheat	Dried prunes
Blueberry	Grape	Chili pepper	Pinto beans		Common millet	Sunflower seeds
Cloudberry	Grapefruit	Kale	Soybeans		Oats	Walnuts
Cowberry/cranberry	Kiwi	Parsley				
Crowberry	Lemon	Pepper				
Dog rose	Pineapple	Red cabbage				
Rowanberry	Plum	Spinach				
Sour cherry	Pomegranate					
Strawberry	Orange					

Antioxidants are not panaceas for all health problems. They offer significant benefits, but much additional research is required to grasp the full range of their capacities. While several antioxidants impart wide-ranging ameliorative effects, it appears likely that greater benefits are bestowed by the synergistic activity of several antioxidants. For example, the oral supplement DermaVite™ consists of a combination of, in descending order of concentration of a marine protein complex, alpha lipoic acid, vitamin C, red clover extract, tomato extract, pine bark extract, vitamins E and B_3, soya extract, zinc, vitamin B_5, and copper, that has demonstrated clinical efficacy in the treatment of cutaneous aging symptoms (e.g., fine and coarse wrinkles, roughness, and telangiectasia) in a randomized, double-blind, placebo-controlled study.[86]

Arnica

The use of the *Arnica montana* plant has been promoted by homeopathic practitioners for hundreds of years. Arnica is used as a supplement for its anti-inflammatory properties, which have been attributed to its constituent sequiterpene lactones.[87] Its primary skin care application is in the treatment and prevention of bruises (see Chapter 21). While taking arnica regularly offers little benefit to the skin, the author suggests it to patients before cosmetic procedures such as soft tissue augmentation. Four homeopathic arnica pills labeled with 30x dilution taken 4 to 6 hours before a cosmetic procedure is recommended. In a recent double-blind study of 29 patients given perioperative homeopathic *A. montana* or placebo after undergoing rhytidectomy, smaller areas of ecchymosis were measured on the 4 postprocedural observation days, with statistically significant reductions identified on 2 of the 4 days.[88] It is important to caution patients that high doses of oral arnica can be harmful, so this dose and potency should not be exceeded. If a mild rash develops, the patient is likely sensitive to the compound helenalin, a key constituent found in arnica. In this case, arnica use should be halted. While not falling into the category of nutritional supplements, topical creams with arnica, like Donell Super Skin K-Derm Gel and Boiron Arnica Cream, are used in the author's practice to accelerate the pace of bruise healing.

Beta-Carotene

Beta-carotene is a member of the carotenoid family, highly pigmented (red, orange, yellow), lipid-soluble substances naturally present in several fruits, grains, oils, and vegetables (such as apricots, carrots, green peppers, spinach, squash, and sweet potatoes). Notably, in a systematic study of antioxidants in dietary plants, carrots were found to have the lowest content of antioxidants of the array of roots and tubers screened.[84] Because it can be converted into active vitamin A (retinol), beta-carotene is a provitamin, as are alpha- and gamma-carotene. Beta-carotene has received substantially more attention than the other carotenoid compounds because it has been shown to contribute much more to human nutrition as compared to its related substances.[68]

In 2006, Stahl and Krutmann reported that the systemic use of beta-carotene in dosages of 15 to 30 mg/d for 10 to 12 weeks had been shown to impart protection against UV-induced erythema, but was insufficient in terms of offering full protection against UVR.[89] More recently, investigators reviewed the literature up to June 2007 in PubMed, ISI Web of Science, and the epidermolysis bullosa acquisita Cochrane Library in conducting a meta-analysis of supplementation studies of dietary beta-carotene as protection against sunburn. Meta-analysis of the seven studies identified revealed that beta-carotene supplementation did indeed confer protection against sunburn in a time-dependent fashion, with a minimum of 10 weeks of supplementation necessary.[90] Indeed, in September 2007, Stahl and Sies clarified that dietary carotenoids such as beta-carotene and lycopene, as well as flavonoids, contribute to the prevention of UV-induced erythema formation after ingestion and dispersal to light-exposed areas, including the skin and eyes. Specifically, these micronutrients reduced sensitivity to UV-induced erythema in volunteers after 10 to 12 weeks of dietary intervention.[91] Clearly, there are limits to the protection afforded by beta-carotene. In a large-scale randomized, double-blind, placebo-controlled 12-year primary-prevention trial of beta-carotene supplementation with follow-up, investigators found that supplementing with 50 mg of beta-carotene on alternate days in apparently healthy male physicians from 40 to 84 years of age in 1982 (n = 22,071) did not influence the development of a first basal cell or squamous cell carcinoma.[92] It is worth noting that beta-carotene supplementation has been demonstrated to contribute to elevating the risk of developing lung cancer in smokers and those exposed to asbestos.[93]

There are minor risks inherent in taking too much beta-carotene and other provitamin A compounds. Superficially, the tint of one's skin can be rendered more yellow by consuming excess carotenoids. Because of the inefficiency in the conversion of beta-carotene into retinol, there is less risk posed by beta-carotene supplementation in comparison to vitamin A supplementation. The author prefers to see patients derive the benefits of beta-carotene primarily from diet, but it can be a useful supplement for those living in warm climates where frequent sun exposure is more likely and whose diets do not include enough of this carotenoid.

Biotin

Also known as vitamin B_7, biotin has been shown to increase nail thickness by up to 25% in patients with brittle nails while minimizing nail breakage or flaking.[94] Nail strength can also be augmented through supplementation with biotin.[95] The author recommends a 2.5-mg daily dose of biotin to all patients whose nails are especially susceptible to breaking or splitting with little provocation. Indeed, brittle nail syndrome has been demonstrated to improve with this dosage.[96]

Borage Seed Oil

Borage seed oil is an omega-6 fatty acid rich in gamma-linolenic acid (GLA), which cannot be synthesized by human skin from the precursor LA. GLA is thought to assist in hydrating the skin. As an oral supplement, borage seed oil is thought to be effective for soothing skin inflammation and redness. It is also touted as an ingredient for moisturizing and strengthening the skin barrier. In a study of the effects of dietary supplementation with borage seed oil, 29 healthy elderly people, with an average age of nearly 69, were given daily doses of 360 or 720 mg for 2 months. A statistically significant improvement in the barrier function of the skin was observed, with reductions in transepidermal water loss and dry skin complaints. Investigators also noted decreases in saturated and monounsaturated fats, and concluded that fatty acid metabolism alterations and skin function amelioration resulted from borage seed oil consumption.[97]

Bromelain

The stem of the pineapple plant, *Ananas comosus*, is the source of bromelain, a term used to designate its constituent family of sulfhydryl-containing proteolytic enzymes.[98] It is indicated for cutaneous purposes because of its anti-inflammatory properties, although it is usually administered orally to aid digestion. In one study, patients with long bone fractures who received systemic bromelain manifested significantly less postoperative edema than the placebo group.[99] In addition to its use as a digestive aid, bromelain is commonly employed to treat inflammation and soft tissue injuries. The proteolytic enzymes of bromelain have imparted various wound-healing benefits, such as alleviating bruising, edema, and pain.[100] In fact, the presurgical administration of bromelain is associated with accelerated healing after surgical procedures and other trauma,[101] especially given its ability to potentiate antibiotics.[102] However, anecdotal reports suggest that using bromelain prior to a procedure will increase bruising. For this reason, the author recommends 500 mg of bromelain twice daily for 3 days to all patients *after* procedures such as dermal filling, to minimize bruising (see Chapter 21). In addition, it is worth suggesting the use of bromelain to patients that bruise easily. Bromelain is contraindicated in patients using anticoagulant agents such as warfarin. Other contraindications include children, individuals with allergies to pineapple or bee stings, and people with a history of heart palpitations.

Caffeine

The best-known ingredient of coffee, caffeine is found naturally in the leaves, seeds, or fruits in several plants, and is present in tea, chocolate, soda, and other products. Consumed in popular beverages such as coffee and tea, caffeine or its metabolites are thought to confer significant anticarcinogenic and antioxidant properties.[103–106] For example, a 23-week period of oral administration of green tea or black tea to SKH-1 mice at high risk of developing skin cancer because of twice weekly exposure to UVB (30 mJ/cm^2) yielded a lower incidence of tumors/mouse, decreased parametrial fat pad size, and decreased thickness of the dermal fat layer away from and directly under tumors. Decaffeinated teas exhibited little or no effect, but the restoration of caffeine restored the inhibitory effects.[107] Significant anticarcinogenic activity has also been displayed through the topical application of caffeine to SKH-1 hairless, tumor-free mice pretreated with UVB twice weekly for 20 weeks.[108] In topical products (e.g., La Roche-Posay Rosaliac and Replenix Cream CF), caffeine is an effective anti-inflammatory and constricts veins to reduce facial flushing. The anti-inflammatory and anticarcinogenic benefits of orally administered caffeine are compelling. Caffeine is also dehydrating and should be enjoyed with moderation, ideally along with water but without unhealthy condiments such as cream and sugar. The dehydrating effects of caffeine make it a popular additive in cellulite creams, where its effects can last around 24 hours.[109] Patients that are predisposed to facial flushing should be advised to consider iced beverages, as hot ones may exacerbate facial redness.

Coenzyme Q10

Ubiquinone, more familiarly referred to as coenzyme Q10 (CoQ10), is a potent antioxidant found in all human cells that assists with energy production. Good dietary sources of CoQ10 include fish, shellfish, spinach, and nuts. CoQ10, which is a fat-soluble compound, is thought to prevent oxidative stress-induced apoptosis by inhibiting lipid peroxidation in plasma membranes, thereby suppressing free radical development. In the mitochondria of each cell of the body, CoQ10 plays a significant role in the energy-producing adenosine triphosphate pathways. Energy production is an important aspect of cellular metabolism, the efficiency of which is thought to decrease with age. CoQ10 levels also coincidentally decline with age.[110] Supplementation with ubiquinone is believed to decelerate the reduction in energy production associated with senescence and illness. Recently, Ashida et al. found that CoQ10 intake augmented the epidermal CoQ10 level in 43-week-old hairless male mice, which, coupled with their previous finding that extended CoQ10 supplementation in humans lowered the wrinkle area rate and wrinkle volume per unit area around the corner of the eye, led them to conclude that CoQ10 supplementation may have the potential to reduce wrinkles and confer additional cutaneous benefits.[111] It is also worth noting that topical CoQ10 has been demonstrated to penetrate the viable layers of the epidermis and decrease the level of oxidation measured by weak photon emission, and reduce wrinkle depth. In the same study, CoQ10 inhibited collagenase expression in human fibroblasts after UVA irradiation. The investigators concluded that topical CoQ10 may be effective in preventing the deleterious effects of UV radiation exposure.[112] CoQ10 supplements impart a caffeine-like stimulatory effect. Therefore, the author recommends daily use in the morning, typically 200 mg. Individuals taking cholesterol-lowering statin drugs should be counseled to consider this supplement, as statins reduce natural CoQ10 levels. Low CoQ10 levels are associated with fatigue and muscle cramping. Those on cholesterol lowering drugs should consider taking 400 mg every morning.

Evening Primrose Oil

Derived from the seeds of evening primrose (*Oenothera biennis*), a hardy biennial member of the Onagraceae family noted for its fragrant flowers that open at dusk during the summer, EPO is an omega-6 fatty acid that contains both LA and GLA). In fact, it is one of the best sources of GLA, a polyunsaturated essential *cis*-fatty acid important in the production of prostaglandins, which play a role in the functioning of most bodily systems. LA is used by the body to synthesize GLA. In addition, LA imparts significant benefits to the skin, maintaining stratum corneum cohesion and reducing transepidermal water loss[113] (see Chapter 11). Overall, though, the health benefits of EPO are attributed to GLA. In a double-blind trial assessing the effects of oral EPO on atopic eczema, researchers found a statistically significant improvement among the EPO patients in overall severity of symptoms, including reductions in percentage of body surface involvement, inflammation, xerosis, and pruritus. While patients receiving placebo experienced less inflammation, EPO patients demonstrated a significantly greater reduction and a significant increase in plasma levels of dihomogammalinolenic acid.[114] Consequently, some authors have speculated that supplementing with products high in GLA, such as EPO, may be effective for patients with atopic eczema.[115] EPO taken as an oral supplement is judged a valuable source of essential fatty acids. It is approved in Germany for eczema and PMS and other uses. In 2004, it was found in a survey of more than 21,000 adults to be the most commonly used oral supplement.[116] In addition, EPO combined with zinc has been used to soothe dry eyes, ameliorate brittle nails, and to treat acne and sunburn. Overall, this supplement may be effective in helping to hydrate the skin, as well as easing inflammation and irritation. The author particularly recommends EPO to patients who experience frequent skin irritation.

Glucosamine

Typically derived from the shells of shellfish (although synthetic versions are also available), glucosamine and its derivative N-acetyl glucosamine are amino-monosaccharides that serve several significant biological roles, particularly in the production of cartilage. Both act as substrate precursors for hyaluronic acid (HA) as well as proteoglycans synthesis. Given its role in HA production, it is not surprising that glucosamine has been demonstrated to confer various cutaneous benefits, such as enhancing hydration, reducing wrinkles, and accelerating wound healing.[117] In addition to anti-inflammatory and chondroprotective properties, glucosamine has been shown to be effective in treating hyperpigmentation because it inhibits tyrosinase activation thereby suppressing melanin synthesis.[117] In a randomized, controlled, single-blind 5-week study with 53 female volunteers who were given an oral supplement containing glucosamine, amino acids, minerals, and various antioxidant compounds, investigators found a statistically significant reduction (34%) in the number of visible wrinkles and a reduction (34%) in the number of fine lines in the treatment group as compared to the 12-person control group.[118] Oral glucosamine supplementation has also been demonstrated to ameliorate symptoms and decelerate the development of osteoarthritis in animals as well as in clinical trials in humans, and its list of indications is expanding.[117] In a retrospective survey of the nonvitamin, nonmineral dietary supplements used among an elderly cohort between 1994 and 1999, glucosamine emerged as the most frequently used supplement.[119] The author recommends 1500 mg/d, particularly to patients older than 35 years. Glucosamine supplements have been demonstrated to assist in rebuilding cartilage, in which HA is an important component. Evidence suggests that the effects of glucosamine supplementation, namely, increased skin fullness and decreased wrinkles, can be seen in as little as 4 to 6 weeks.

Horse Chestnut Seed Extract

Of the various species of horse chestnuts, trees as well as bushes, the European horse chestnut (*Aesculus hippocastanum*) is the one used most often for medicinal purposes. In its oral form, horse chestnut seed extract (HCSE) has been shown to effectively enhance circulatory problems such as varicose veins and leg cramping. Indeed, researchers conducting a thorough literature review of double-blind, randomized controlled trials of oral HCSE for patients with chronic venous insufficiency in Medline, EMBASE, BIOSIS, CISCOM, and the Cochrane Library (until December 1996) found that HCSE was superior to placebo in all cases.[120] In addition, they noted reductions in lower-leg volume, leg circumference at the calf and ankle, and improvement in symptoms including leg pain, pruritus, fatigue, and tension, with only rare mild adverse reactions. The same investigators, along with a third, subsequently conducted a broad database search of Medline, EMBASE, the Cochrane Library, CISCOM, and AMED (until October 2000) on complementary and alternative medicine and found additional cogent evidence for the effectiveness of oral HCSE for the treatment of chronic venous insufficiency.[121] HCSE has been proven to improve inflammation and circulatory discomfort in its oral form. Patients taking anticoagulant drugs should be advised not to supplement with HCSE.

Hyaluronic Acid

One of the three primary constituents of the dermis, HA, also known as hyaluronan, is the most abundant glycosaminoglycan in the human dermis. HA, which has the capacity to bind water up to 1000 times its volume, plays an important role in cell growth, membrane receptor function and adhesion. Its main biologic function in the intercellular matrix is to stabilize intercellular structures and form the elastoviscous fluid matrix in which collagen and elastin fibers are firmly enveloped.[122,123] HA holds onto moisture, as well, and helps provide fullness and radiance to the skin. While HA is the main component of several effective and popular dermal filling agents, and has also demonstrated efficacy as an intra-articular injection agent for knee osteoarthritis,[124] oral HA supplements are also available. These products are touted for combating the decline of HA, which occurs with age. However, HA is metabolized in the stomach; therefore, the author does not believe there is any evidence demonstrating the effectiveness of these supplements.

Iron

Found in every cell of the body, iron is an important mineral for all-around good health and is essential in the production of hemoglobin, the blood component that distributes oxygen throughout the body. Low iron levels have been associated with hair loss.

Supplementation could help control or resolve this condition. Iron deficiency may also manifest in the fingernails, as white spots or vertical ridges. Physicians should check a patient's ferritin levels prior to recommending an iron supplement. Excess iron can generate free radicals, which attack vital skin constituents, such as collagen and elastin, and accelerate cutaneous aging. Iron supplements should be recommended to patients only if it is determined that they have low iron levels. Good dietary sources of iron include dried beans, dried fruits, egg yolks, salmon, tuna, whole grains, and other foods.

Lycopene

Naturally present in human blood and tissues, lycopene is a non-provitamin A carotenoid best known as the pigment mainly responsible for the characteristic red color of tomatoes. During the last decade, lycopene has garnered much attention for its potent antioxidant activity.[125,126] Lycopene may play a role in reducing oxidative damage to tissues, as suggested by a placebo-controlled study that examined the effects on plasma and skin concentrations of beta-carotene and lycopene from ingesting a single 120-mg dose of beta-carotene. The effects from UV light exposure were also examined. Lycopene levels in plasma and skin, which are comparable or greater than those of beta-carotene, were unaffected by beta-carotene ingestion, but beta-carotene levels increased. Furthermore, a single intense exposure (3 times the MED) of solar-simulated light on a small area of the volar arm resulted in a 31% to 46% decrease in skin lycopene concentration, but no significant changes in skin beta-carotene, which led the investigators to conclude that lycopene may contribute to absorbing or mitigating the effects of UV radiation and other forms of oxidative insult.[127] Recently, protection against erythema development after UV exposure has been demonstrated as a result of increasing lycopene intake by daily consumption of tomato paste for a 10-week period.[125] Consequently, Sies and Stahl, who conducted the study, have deemed lycopene an effective oral sun protectant that can play an important role in maintaining the health of the skin. In work published by these and additional investigators in the same year, supplementation for 12 weeks with 24 mg/d of a carotenoid formulation including beta-carotene, lutein, and lycopene was found in a placebo-controlled, parallel study design to exert a comparable improvement in mitigating UV-induced erythema in humans as 24 mg of beta-carotene alone.[42] More recent work by some of the same investigators has further buttressed the evidence showing the photoprotective effects of lycopene supplementation, with significant increases measured in lycopene serum levels and total skin carotenoids; erythema was also demonstrably prevented after UV irradiation.[43] More research is necessary, but lycopene, through oral supplementation or topical administration, is also considered a potential chemopreventive agent of nonmelanoma skin cancer.[126]

Niacin

Also known as vitamin B_3 or nicotinic acid, niacin has long been known to be essential for the healthy functioning of the skin and nervous system. Niacinamide (also called nicotinamide) is the amide form of niacin. The terms nicotinic acid and nicotinamide are used less frequently because they sound similar, though unrelated, to nicotine. Neither niacin nor niacinamide are synthesized in the human body; therefore, they must be supplied through the diet, topical application or oral supplementation. Peanuts, brewer's yeast, fish, and meat are the best dietary sources of niacin. The deficiency of niacin and niacinamide appears to play a role in the development of several types of cancer, including skin cancer, and niacin deficiency is also associated with pellagra, a disease characterized by diarrhea, dermatitis, and dementia. Mice given oral niacin or topical niacinamide exhibited a 70% decrease in UV-induced skin cancers and near-complete prevention of photoimmunosuppression.[128]

For several years, niacinamide has been used both topically and orally to treat inflammatory diseases. For example, Berk et al. described the use of oral niacinamide plus tetracycline for the treatment of bullous pemphigoid.[129] Rosacea is also among the indica-tions for niacinamide treatment.[130] The use of oral or intravenous niacin has been described for the treatment of migraines and tension-type headaches, though randomized controlled trials are lacking.[131] Indeed, niacin is well known for exhibiting vasodilatory activity.[131] Patients who take oral niacin for a long-term to control hypertension tend to develop bothersome flushing. Because of this, topical products may be more desirable, though the recently introduced extended-release 1000 mg niacin ER tablet has been shown to reduce the frequency, duration, and intensity of niacin-induced flushing.[132] Although niacin supplements may be prescribed for various conditions, there is no skin-related reason to take more than what would be derived from a typical multivitamin. Niacinamide, in contrast, imparts no cutaneous side effects and is a very effective ingredient in topical formulations for treating photodamage, inflammation, hyperpigmentation, and dry skin. Niacinamide is found in the Olay brand products such as Total Effects, Regenerist, and Definity. The brand Nia24 contains an ingredient very similar to niacinamide.

Omega-3 Fatty Acids

Although they are not synthesized naturally in the body, omega-3 fatty acids are a family of polyunsaturated fatty acids (also referred to as n-3 PUFAs or PUFAs) that are crucial components of cell membranes and key constituents in the skin barrier. ALA, EPA, and DHA are the primary essential omega-3 fatty acids. The anti-inflammatory activities of these compounds are well established, as several studies have demonstrated their efficacy in combating erythema and irritation associated with cutaneous conditions such as psoriasis and rosacea. Significant anti-inflammatory activity displayed by EPA and DHA, from oily extracts of three Mediterranean fish species, against UVB-induced erythema has been demonstrated recently in vivo in human volunteers.[133] The hydrating qualities of omega-3 fatty acids also serve to add volume to the skin, minimizing the appearance of fine lines. Good dietary sources of the omega-3 fatty acid ALA include canola oil, walnuts, and "omega-3 eggs" (which provide much more than the typical level of omega-3 as a result of the special diet fed to the hens); for the omega-3 fatty acids EPA and DHA, fish and other seafood, as well as "omega-3 eggs" are good dietary sources.[134] The fish that contain significant levels of omega-3 fatty acids are fatty predatory fish, including albacore tuna, lake trout, mackerel, menhaden, and salmon[68] (Table 8-7). It is important to note that such fish do not synthesize these acids but accumulate them through their diet, which may also include toxic substances. For this reason, particularly in the case of mercury toxicity in albacore tuna, the FDA recommends limiting consumption of selected predatory fish species. Supplementing

TABLE 8-7
Good Dietary Sources of Omega-3 Fatty Acids[60,68,134]

Canola oil
Fish (and other seafood)
Albacore tuna
Lake trout
Mackerel
Menhaden
Salmon
Flaxseed/flaxseed oil
Hempseed
"Omega-3 eggs"
Seaweed
Walnuts

with fish oil has become an increasingly popular alterative. Cod liver oil and other fish oils are also good sources of n-3 PUFAs.[68] While noting the natural dietary sources of such nutrients, particularly fish, it is important to make dietary choices with environmental sensitivity. In particular, fish should be selected with this in mind, as several species may be endangered (e.g., cod) or approaching such status.

Sies and Stahl contend that omega-3 fatty acids are among the various micronutrients that exhibit the capacity to deliver systemic photoprotection against UV-induced damage.[135] In addition, Black and Rhodes suggest that there is a wide array of experimental and clinical studies indicating an important role for omega-3 fatty acids in preventing nonmelanoma skin cancer, as manifested in evidence of increasing tumor latency periods, decreasing tumor number, increasing the UV radiation-mediated erythema threshold in humans, and significantly reducing proinflammatory and immunosuppressive prostaglandin E synthase type 2 [PGE(2)] levels in human skin exposed to UVB.[136]

In a recent report in the *Journal of the American Medical Association*, MacLean et al. conducted a literature review, and consulted experts in the neutraceutical field regarding unpublished studies, to sift through mixed results on the capacity of omega-3 fatty acids to lower the risk of developing cancer. Thirty-eight articles were ultimately considered in their evaluation, yielding the conclusion that dietary supplementation with omega-3 fatty acids does not likely prevent cancer.[137] However, Chen et al. countered that none of the 38 studies reviewed took into account the measurement of fatty acid composition in patients. In addition, they suggested that in reviewing dietary data, it is important to note that some fish (particularly farm-raised fish) are inadequate sources of omega-3 fatty acids. Chen et al. suggested that it remains uncertain, but is not unlikely, as to whether omega-3 fatty acids confer a preventive effect against cancer.[138] While more research is clearly needed regarding the diverse effects of dietary omega-3 fatty acids, several benefits have been patently established. The author recommends incorporating as many sources of omega-3 fatty acids into one's diet as desired and supplementing with 1000 mg/d.

Polypodium Leucotomos

Derived from the fern family, the extract of *Polypodium leucotomos* has been used to treat inflammatory conditions and shown, in vitro and in vivo, to display immunomodulating activity.[139] It is also thought to exhibit potent antioxidant activity and is considered a viable oral photoprotectant.[140,141]

In 2004, Middelkamp-Hup et al. assessed whether oral *Polypodium leucotomos* extract (PLE) could diminish the clinical and histologic phototoxic damage to human skin caused by psoralen with ultraviolet A (PUVA) treatment. Ten healthy patients with skin types II to III were exposed to PUVA alone and PUVA accompanied by 7.5 mg/kg of oral PLE. After 48 to 72 hours, clinical results revealed consistently lower phototoxicity in PLE-treated skin, with pigmentation reduced 4 months after treatment. Histologic examination indicated significantly fewer sunburn cells, and reductions in vasodilatation and the tryptase-positive mast cell infiltration, in addition to preservation of Langerhans cells in PLE-treated skin. The authors found that PLE effectively protected the skin against the known deleterious effects of PUVA.[142] Although this was a small study, the results spurred the team to additional study of PLE. In research reported later in 2004 by the same group, nine healthy individuals, with skin types II to III were exposed to various doses of artificial UVR radiation without or following oral administration of 7.5 mg/kg PLE. Investigators assessed erythematous reactions 24 hours after exposure and obtained paired biopsy specimens from PLE-treated skin and untreated skin. Significantly less erythema was noted in the PLE-treated skin. In the biopsy specimens, researchers recorded fewer sunburn cells, cyclobutane pyrimidine dimers, and proliferating epidermal cells as well as less mast cell infiltration. Preservation of Langerhans cells was also achieved. The team's previous findings were supported by this study, which prompted them to conclude that oral PLE effectively protects the skin against UV insult.[143]

In a study by Middelkamp-Hup et al. of the potential of oral PLE in the treatment of vitiligo vulgaris, 50 patients were randomly administered 250 mg of oral PLE or placebo 3 times daily, combined with the first-line therapy (narrow-band UVB) twice weekly for 25 or 26 weeks. Investigators identified a definite trend in repigmentation in the head and neck area, particularly in light skin types, with the combined narrow-band UVB and oral PLE therapy.[144] PLE is most widely available in a capsule supplement known as Heliocare. It is expensive, but it helps protect the skin against UV damage, and reduces erythema caused by sun exposure. The author recommends one capsule taken in the morning when sun exposure is anticipated, two capsules if the exposure is expected to be prolonged.

Selenium

An important antioxidant, selenium is a trace mineral found naturally in the body and various foods, particularly Brazil nuts. Some seafood, meat, cereals, and dairy products contain selenium as do several plant foods, depending on the selenium content of the soil in which they are grown. Selenium is essential to good health, but required in only small amounts.[145] A properly functioning thyroid is also dependent on selenium. In addition, the protective activity characteristic of the immune cells is supported by the synergistic cooperation of various vitamins and minerals, including selenium.[146] Although a capacity to protect against skin cancer has been recently disproved, selenium remains among the list of potential oral or topical chemopreventive agents against other forms of cancer,[126] and it is considered an important contributor to antioxidant defense.[135,147] However, in a recent prospective case-cohort study of the link between arsenic-related premalignant skin lesions and prediagnostic blood selenium levels in 303 cases newly diagnosed from November 2002 to April 2004 and 849 subcohort members randomly selected from the 8092 subjects in the Health Effects of Arsenic Longitudinal Study, investigators found that dietary selenium intake may lower the incidence of arsenic-related premalignant skin lesions among susceptible populations (those exposed to arsenic from drinking water).[148] In addition, it is thought to exhibit potent anti-inflammatory and antiaging properties and, in oral form, appears to mitigate UV-induced skin damage. Although more research is necessary, selenium in both oral and topical form appears to impart several benefits to the skin. It is used as a topical water to treat psoriasis, eczema, and other inflammatory skin conditions in the La Roche-Posay spa in France dedicated to the treatment of these skin conditions. Most multivitamins typically contain a sufficient amount of selenium. The recommended daily allowance of selenium for adults is 55 μg, and overdose can be harmful (generally, more than 400 μg/d). In fact, excessive amounts of selenium can lead to hair loss.

Vitamin A

Retinol, also known as vitamin A, has such status because it is not synthesized in the human body. The term "retinoids" refers to vitamin A and all its natural and synthetic derivatives including retinol. Carotenoids such as carrots, cantaloupes, sweet potatoes, and spinach are among the best dietary sources of vitamin A.[149] Milk, margarine, eggs, beef liver, and fortified breakfast cereals are also important dietary contributors of vitamin A.[150] The retinoids exhibit several important biologic effects, such as regulating growth and differentiation of epithelial cells, inhibiting tumor promotion during experimental carcinogenesis, diminishing malignant cell growth, decreasing inflammation, and enhancing the immune system[151] (see Chapter 30). Retinoids have also been shown to improve the appearance of striae and improve skin discoloration.[152] Vitamin A is also particularly beneficial for individuals with acne, as it helps diminish oil levels in the skin. In addition, retinoic acid, or tretinoin, is known to reverse the signs of photoaging by diminishing wrinkles, actinic keratoses, and lentigines as well as smoothing skin texture.[153] In cooperation with several other vitamins and minerals, including vitamins C and E, as well as zinc, vitamin A contributes to enhancing skin barrier function as well as immune cell protective activity.[146]

Vitamin A is an important part of any diet, but consuming or taking excessive amounts poses risks, including a greater susceptibility to bone fracture. There is rarely a reason to take more than what is found in a good multivitamin. It is healthier, however, to derive one's necessary vitamin A through diet, particularly by eating leafy greens, carrots, cantaloupes, sweet potatoes, spinach, broccoli, squash, and mangoes.

Vitamin C

Known historically for its role in the prevention of scurvy, vitamin C is abundantly available in citrus fruits. In fact, by the 18th century, sailors knew that eating citrus fruits prevented this condition associated with dental abnormalities, bleeding disorders, characteristic purpuric skin lesions, and mental deterioration. In the 1930s, researchers confirmed that vitamin C is the key ingredient in citrus fruit that fends off scurvy, and dubbed it ascorbic acid (*scobutus* is Latin for *scurvy*). Currently, vitamin C is considered a potent antioxidant and is used effectively as an antiaging and anti-inflammatory agent.

In the skin, vitamin C plays an integral role in the metabolism of collagen, where it is essential for the hydroxylation of lysine and proline in procollagen (see Chapter 2). Vitamin C has also been demonstrated to augment collagen synthesis in both neonatal and adult fibroblasts when added to culture medium.[154] Aging skin is characterized by decreased collagen production (see Chapter 6). Consequently, it is thought that increasing collagen production in the skin with vitamin C should theoretically contribute to preventing or even reversing some of the signs of cutaneous aging.[155] The stimulatory effects of vitamin C on collagen synthesis are believed to be effective in preventing and treating striae alba (stretch marks). This important role in collagen synthesis indicates the relevance of vitamin C in wrinkle prevention.

In a literature review of the photoprotective effects of vitamins C and E, investigators found that topical applications of each individual antioxidant performed significantly better than their orally administered counterparts. The photoprotective effects of vitamin C and E combinations, along with other antioxidants, proved to be markedly more effective than monotherapies in delivering cutaneous protection against UVB.[156]

In a 3-month study of the effects of oral administration of a combination of vitamins C and E, investigators found significant decreases in the sunburn response to UVB exposure, with substantially fewer thymine dimers induced by UV radiation, implying a protective effect against DNA damage conferred by the antioxidant combination.[157] In a more recent study of the effects of the oral administration of a mixture combining the antioxidants vitamins C and E, Pycnogenol, and EPO on UVB-induced wrinkle formation, female SKH-1 hairless mice received the test mixture or control vehicle for 10 weeks along with UVB irradiation 3 times weekly, with graduated increases in UVB intensity. Investigators found that UVB-induced wrinkle formation was significantly inhibited, with substantial reductions also seen in epidermal thickness as well as UVB-engendered acanthosis, hyperplasia, and hyperkeratosis.[158]

Many physicians, including the author, recommend that patients take oral vitamin C 500 mg twice daily. This way they enjoy the benefits of vitamin C without the irritation and expense of topical formulations, which are difficult to stabilize. Other than an upset stomach, there is no risk of taking too much vitamin C.

Vitamin D

Perhaps best known as the vitamin skin produces when exposed to ultraviolet light, vitamin D_3, often shortened to vitamin D, is actually a hormone, and a potent antioxidant. Besides sun exposure, vitamin D can be obtained through the diet, especially by consumption of fatty fish.[159] Through the metabolic process, vitamin D is converted into 25-hydroxyvitamin D (25(OH)D) by the liver and 1,25-dihydroxyvitamin D(1,25(OH)2D) by the kidneys.[159] It has been known for several years that UVB exposure induces epidermal keratinocytes to convert 7-dehydrocholesterol into vitamin D_3. In addition, the metabolites of vitamin D_3, particularly calcitriol, are known to confer significant benefits, such as antiproliferative and prodifferentiating activity as well as regulating cellular activity in keratinocytes and immunocompetent cells.[160]

In addition to imparting benefits to most bodily organ systems, vitamin D plays a significant role in psoriasis treatments, including the drug Dovonex. Like all antioxidants, vitamin D exhibits the capacity to decelerate aspects of cutaneous aging. Cutaneous vitamin D_3 synthesis declines with age. Consequently, vitamin D deficiency is not uncommon in the elderly, the demographic group most in need of taking oral vitamin D supplements. Low vitamin D status is a factor in the development of osteoporosis. Vitamin D insufficiency is also associated with rickets, certain types of cancer, and various other diseases.[161]

Vitamin D deficiency can lead to an elevation in serum parathyroid hormone, contributing to bone resorption, osteoporosis, and fractures. Supplementation with vitamin D has been shown to inhibit serum parathyroid hormone, increase bone mineral density, and may reduce the incidence of fractures, particularly in the elderly.[159] In a 12-week randomized clinical study in a psychogeriatric nursing home comparing the effects of UV radiation and oral vitamin D_3 on the vitamin D status and parathyroid hormone concentration in elderly nursing home patients, investigators found UVB to be as effective as oral vitamin D_3 in raising serum 25(OH)D and serum calcium as well as inhibiting secondary hyperparathyroidism.[162]

Research has also shown that vitamin D analogs may have a role to play in the medical therapy of melanoma, even though avoiding exposure to UV remains the best protection against melanoma and nonmelanoma skin cancers.[163] In addition, research has shown that obesity-related vitamin D insufficiency likely results from the diminished bioavailability of vitamin D_3 from cutaneous and dietary sources due to deposition in body fat.[164]

More than a decade ago, vitamin D became the subject of controversy when claims emerged that the use of sunscreen led to vitamin D deficiency.[165] Despite mounting evidence to the contrary, this remains a controversial topic. Interestingly, Gilchrest cites evolutionary changes in countering the argument for controlled exposure to UV to obtain sufficient vitamin D levels. Specifically, she suggests that when the human capacity to photosynthesize vitamin D emerged, the lifespan for human beings was considerably shorter than it is today, and the effects of long-term photodamage, or the modern option of purchasing oral vitamin D, could not be part of the equation.[166]

Currently, the tolerable upper intake level (UL) for vitamin D_3 stands at 50 μg/d (2000 IU/d) in North Americans and Europeans, but several studies suggest that metabolic utilization of vitamin D_3 would be optimized at a UL as high as twice this level, particularly to ameliorate vitamin D status in the elderly.[161,167,168] The challenge with vitamin D is balancing the mounting evidence that cutaneous vitamin D production helps prevent various diseases, including some cancers, with the understanding that prolonged sun exposure greatly increases the risk of skin cancer and other photodamage. Oral vitamin D supplementation in place of UV exposure appears to be the safest approach, and may be particularly appropriate for certain populations. For instance, individuals at high risk for skin cancer (e.g., those who have red hair and freckles, or a family history of skin cancer) should be advised to avoid unprotected sun exposure and to obtain vitamin D in oral supplement form and diet. Mushrooms have been found to be a good source of vitamin D. Blood levels of vitamin D should be checked in all patients. If levels are low, vitamin D supplementation and the addition of mushrooms to the diet should be recommended along with *limited* sun exposure. It takes only a few minutes of solar exposure each day to stimulate vitamin D synthesis. Patients should be reminded of this and advised that there is never a good reason to bake in the sun all day.

Vitamin E

Vitamin E includes the tocopherols and the tocotrienols. It is the most significant lipid-soluble antioxidant and it is found naturally in many vegetables, especially spinach, avocados, corn, vegetable oils, sunflower seeds, soy, whole grains, nuts, and margarine. Usually referred to as alpha-tocopherol, its most biologically active form, vitamin E is also found in some meat and dairy products. In humans, vitamin E naturally occurs in the membranes of cells and organelles. It protects cell membranes from peroxidation and scavenges free radicals. Consequently, vitamin E is thought to help prevent cardiovascular disease and the "aging" of the arteries. It is also effective in mitigating skin dryness, particularly in those taking oral retinoids.

Vitamin E has also been shown to exert anti-inflammatory effects on the skin through the inhibition of chemical mediator synthesis and release. In addition to stabilizing lysosomes, vitamin E influences prostaglandin E2 production (decreasing it) as well as interleukin-2 production (increasing it). Anti-inflammatory and immunostimulatory effects are the result.[151] An important component of sebum, vitamin E is found in greater supply in individuals with oily skin. This may correlate with less skin aging and less skin cancer. The lips, which have no oil glands and are thus devoid of vitamin E, are more susceptible to skin cancer than many other areas of the skin surface. Antitumorigenic, photoprotective, and skin barrier-stabilizing activities have been associated with topical and oral vitamin E.[169]

In a hairless mouse model of photocarcinogenesis induced by UVB expression, investigators showed that oral administration of alpha-tocopherol resulted in significant inhibitory effects on tumor incidence and number.[170] However, in a study assessing the capacity of orally administered vitamin E and beta-carotene to diminish markers of oxidative stress and erythema in response to UV exposure in 16 healthy participants who took either of the lipid-soluble antioxidants for 8 weeks, results revealed that such supplementation had no effect on skin sensitivity, though the vitamin E group experienced significant decreases in cutaneous malondialdehyde. No other measures of oxidative stress in basal or UV-exposed skin were influenced by the supplementation, suggesting that neither conferred photoprotection.[171]

While results remain conflicting over the relative photoprotective effects of oral vitamin E, the evidence strongly indicates significant photoprotective effects from the orally administered combination of vitamins C and E. In a single-blind controlled clinical trial examining the photoprotective effects of vitamins C and E, 45 healthy volunteers were divided into three groups, one receiving oral vitamin C, one receiving oral vitamin E, and one receiving an oral mixture of the two antioxidants. Daily treatments lasted 1 week. The MED was ascertained before and after treatment, with the median MED increasing the most in the combination group, suggesting that d-alpha-tocopherol combined with ascorbic acid yielded better photoprotective effects than either of the antioxidants alone.[172] For more information on just a few of the several reports on the success of this combination, see section "Vitamin C" above. This combination of antioxidants currently represents one of the skin's best defenses against photodamage, including photocarcinogenesis and photoaging.

Vitamin E is an important part of any diet, but there is a risk from taking too much. The author recommends 400 IU, in gel cap form, per day. Vitamin E can increase the likelihood of bruising if taken in large doses. Indeed, doses greater than 3000 mg daily when taken over a long period may cause such side effects. Patients undergoing surgical procedures should avoid doses of vitamin E greater than 4000 IU.[151] In addition, vitamin E should be discontinued 10 days prior to surgical procedures, soft tissue augmentation, or Botox injections in order to minimize the risk of bruising.

Vitamin-fortified Beverages

Various "enhanced water" products have been recently introduced onto the market. As an occasional treat, they represent a much better choice than soda, which offers no health benefits. At least these products provide a few vitamins. Ersatz water products are not a substitute for a good multivitamin, however, and do not include common supplements such as glucosamine or biotin. In addition, these products often contain high levels of sugar, which can contribute to various health outcomes and, in the cutaneous realm, foster wrinkling caused by glycation as well as acne eruptions.

The appeal of this market has resulted in the emergence of sugar-free and nutrient-added formulations. For example, Coca-Cola recently launched a product called Enviga, a sugar-free beverage that contains green tea, one of the most potent and best-researched antioxidants available. In addition, the Borba product line features nutrient-fortified waters specifically formulated for the skin. (These have no added sugar and zero calories.) Not surprisingly, only proprietary in-house studies are available on such products. While it remains to be seen whether these products confer any health benefits, there is no reason to think that they would be harmful or unhealthy. Another way to derive cutaneous benefits from liquid nutrients, other than red wine and green and other teas, is a "water booster." These formulations, packaged in dropper-style bottles, can be added to any beverage. The author recommends Dr. Brandt Anti-Oxidant Water Booster/Pure Green Tea. Liquid supplements to be placed on the tongue such as Dr. Andrew Weil for Origins™ Plantidote™ Mega-Mushroom Supplement are also popular, but unproven. These products should be combined, more importantly, with a well-rounded diet, exercise, and a good multivitamin. Finally, pomegranate juice does note require any vitamin fortification. As long as no sugar is added, pomegranate juice packs a potent antioxidant punch.

Zinc

Zinc is an essential trace element found in, but not produced by, the human body. It is present in various foods, particularly high-protein meats such as lean beef, chicken, and fish. A vegetarian diet often contains less zinc than a meat-based diet. Good vegetarian sources of zinc include beans, dairy products, lentils, nuts, seeds, particularly pumpkin seeds, whole grain cereals, and yeast.[173] Only known as an essential dietary factor for 40 years, zinc is now also thought to exhibit antioxidant and anti-inflammatory activity.[174] In addition, zinc assists other micronutrients in bolstering the function of the skin barrier as well as the protective actions of immune cells.[146] Zinc is also necessary for synthesizing retinol binding protein, which transmits vitamin A. Although there are no areas in the body where zinc is stored, the essential mineral is found in muscle (60%), bone (30%), skin (5%), and other organs.[173,175]

The beneficial effects on immunity are typically cited as the reason for the inclusion of zinc in various cold and flu over-the-counter remedies. Indeed, antiviral effects are now being considered. In a placebo-controlled trial reported on in 2002, investigators found oral zinc sulfate at a dose of 10 mg/kg daily to be successful for the treatment of recalcitrant viral warts after a follow-up of 2 to 3 months.[176] The overlapping, protective roles of the skin and the immunity system appear to be reflected in the activity of zinc. In a recent study of the effects on the allergic response of zinc deficiency in a DS-Nh mouse model of atopic dermatitis, investigators fed male mice a zinc-deficient diet for 4 weeks and found that zinc deficiency affects the skin barrier and immune systems, and aggravated atopic dermatitis.[177]

With age, zinc absorption declines and zinc deficiency is not uncommon in the elderly, particularly individuals older than 75 years.[175] Zinc supplementation has been shown to reverse the plasma zinc reductions, plasma oxidative stress marker increases, and elevated production of inflammatory cytokines seen in the elderly.[174] The adult recommended daily amount (RDA), now referred to as the reference nutrient intake (RNI), for zinc is 15 mg/d for men and 12 mg/d for women, though pregnant women require more zinc. It is important to note that only 20% of the zinc present in the diet is actually absorbed by the body. In addition, zinc absorption is often impaired in patients with chronic GI inflammation. For oral mineral supplements, the amounts of zinc and iron should be equivalent so that they do not interfere with absorption. Zinc is lost primarily through feces, urine, hair, skin, sweat, semen, and menstrual blood.

DIET AND THE SKIN

Diet plays a crucial role in the appearance of the skin and plays a role in everything from skin hydration, redness, and acne to cutaneous aging. Even broken blood vessels on the face can be caused by diet. Based on the studies reviewed above, certain dietary principles can be gleaned and formulated into suggestions for patients regarding general cutaneous health as well as specific concerns such as which foods to eat or avoid in an antiaging or acne treatment regimen. The following discussion provides some general dietary guidelines for healthy skin (Box 8-1) as well as some specific recommendations that depend on skin type (Box 8-2). The following dietary recommendations are long-term interventions intended for good overall health and the prevention of future wrinkles, not as treatment for already extant wrinkles.

Fish and Omega-3 Fatty Acids

As stated above, predatory fish such as albacore tuna, lake trout, mackerel, menhaden, and salmon are high in omega-3 fatty acids. Salmon, in particular, is highly regarded and readily available, as is tuna. Salmon contains omega-3 and omega-6 fatty acids that help human skin hold onto water, inhibiting transepidermal water loss. The numerous omega-3 fatty acids in salmon (particularly EPA and DHA) are also anti-inflammatory; therefore, eating salmon may help curb acne and facial redness. Patients should be advised to select wild salmon because it may have a greater abundance of omega-3 fatty acids and fewer contaminants, such as PCB, as compared to farmed salmon. The author recommends eating salmon at least 3 times a week.

Omega-3 fatty acids as well as omega-6 fatty acids are essential for healthy human growth and development. The typical Western diet had a typical ratio of omega-6 to omega-3 fatty acids of 10:1 during the mid-1990s,[178] which has now increased to a range of approximately 15:1 to 16.7:1.[179] A healthy ratio is thought to be closer to 4:1.[178] A high ratio of omega-6 to omega-3 fatty acids has been associated with a greater risk for depression and various inflammatory diseases.[180] Omega-3 fatty acids exhibit significant anti-inflammatory activity. Good sources of omega-3 fatty acids, in addition to the fish mentioned above, are cod liver oil, fish oil, flaxseeds, and flaxseed oil. Crushed or ground flaxseeds can make a healthy complement to yogurt or oatmeal. Flaxseed oil

BOX 8-1 General Dietary Recommendations in Brief

1. Eat salmon at least 3 times per week.
2. Add flaxseeds to your diet or use flaxseed oil as a salad dressing.
3. Eat foods high in antioxidants, such as a wide variety of berries and pomegranates.
4. Eat a wide variety of fruits, vegetables, and legumes—what nutritionists have been advising for decades. In particular, eating fruits and vegetables that are in season is more nutritious.
5. Use spices such as oregano, ginger, and basil, all of which exhibit antioxidant properties.
6. Drink 2 to 4 cups of green tea per day.
7. Drink plenty of water (1 to 2 L a day, depending on level of exertion, humidity conditions, and individual need).
8. Supplement with CoQ10, at least one 200 mg gel cap in the AM.
9. Drink a moderate amount of red wine, which contains the polyphenolic antioxidants resveratrol and grape seed extract, both of which confer significant antiaging benefits. Consumption of too much alcohol leads to free radical formation, which ages the skin.
10. Limit or avoid calorie-dense refined sugars, saturated fats, and processed foods. Sugar can contribute to acne and accelerate aging by causing the glycosylation of necessary proteins.
11. Following the premise that what is good for the digestion is good for the skin, eat smaller portions (the typical American diet, particularly as evidenced by restaurant portions, overdoes this considerably), and chew slowly (ideally not while reading, watching TV, or otherwise distracted).

It is important to note that these are general guidelines. Individual dietary needs may vary. In fact, the BSTS system is founded on the notion that skin care needs vary according to skin type. (See Table 8-8 for oral supplementation guidelines by BSTS.) Accordingly, some dietary needs or restrictions can be categorized by skin type. It is worth noting that ancient medical systems that continue in the present day—traditional Chinese medicine and Ayurveda, from the Indian subcontinent—base nutritional advice on evaluations of an individual's constitution and their relative deficits upon examination. Ultimately, as we are learning in the West, one healthy diet plan does not fit all—individual tailoring is necessary.

For Vegetarians: To achieve the optimal level of essential fatty acid intake, vegetarians should follow these practical guidelines: (1) Make a wide variety of whole plant foods the foundation of the diet. (2) Derive the majority of fat from whole foods—nuts, seeds, olives, avocados, and soy foods. (3) If using concentrated fats and oils, select those rich in monounsaturated fats, such as olive, canola, or nut oils. Oils rich in omega-3 fatty acids can also be used but should not be heated. Moderate use of oils rich in omega-6 fatty acids is advised. (4) Limit or avoid intake of processed foods and deep-fried foods rich in trans and omega-6 fatty acids. (5) Reduce intake of foods rich in saturated fat. (6) Include foods rich in omega-3 fatty acids in the daily diet (ideally consuming 2–4 g ALA/d). (7) Consider using a direct source of DHA, ideally 100 to 300 mg/d.

TABLE 8-8
Oral Supplement Recommendations by BSTS Parameter

Skin Type Parameter	Supplement
Dry	Borage seed oil Cholesterol Evening primrose oil Glucosamine Omega-3 fatty acids
Oily	Vitamin A
Sensitive	Fish oils, marine oils (omega-3 fatty acids, particularly eicosapentaenoic acid and docosahexaenoic acid)
Resistant	NA
Pigmented	Pycnogenol Vitamin C Soy
Nonpigmented	NA
Wrinkled	Coenzyme Q10 Green tea Pomegranate Pycnogenol Vitamin C Vitamin E
Tight	NA

used as a salad dressing is a very healthy approach to keeping a healthy dish healthy—many standard salad dressings are high in sugar. Omega-3 fatty acids may also assist in skin hydration, as these compounds have been shown to contribute to improving eczema.

Antioxidants

Antioxidants impart protection to cells from oxidative damage caused by exogenous factors such as UV light, air pollution, ozone, cigarette smoke, and even oxygen itself, as well as from endogenous insult. The expression "antioxidant" is more of a reflection of the activity exhibited by the substance rather than its chemical family or constituency. Antioxidants include carotenoids, polyphenols, vitamins, and other classes of compounds. A diet rich in various antioxidants is strongly advised.

Skin Hydration

Skin hydration is a very important factor in achieving and maintaining healthy skin. The enzymes in the skin that perform a variety of functions need water to work. Without water skin will age quicker and be more likely to itch and get red. EPO, black currant oil, and borage oil are all good sources of the omega-6 fatty acid GLA, which helps prevent water evaporation from the skin. Humans tend to lose approximately 2.5 liters of water per day. This is partly replenished through food intake. The level of water consumption varies by individual, one's level of activity, and climate, but 1 to 2 liters is probably a reasonable estimate. One must drink water to prevent becoming dehydrated. However, as far as skin is concerned it is not how much water you drink but how well the skin holds onto the water and keeps it from evaporating. Skin needs adequate levels of fatty acids, ceramides, and cholesterol to hold onto water (see Chapter 11). This is why vegans and people on low-cholesterol diets or cholesterol-lowering drugs often have dry skin. Any liquid can provide skin hydration; however, water consumption should be increased when drinking caffeine and alcohol, which can cause dehydration.

Caloric Restriction

During the last several years, one focus of antiaging research has included examinations oriented toward determining whether the lifespan and healthspan of human beings can be increased. In the process, caloric restriction (CR) has been shown to prolong the mean and maximum lifespan in various species.[181] It is not yet known whether CR can extend the average and maximum lifespan or the healthspan of human beings. However, available epidemiologic evidence appears to suggest that CR has already contributed to increased lifespan, average and maximum, in one human population—in Okinawa, Japan.[182] It is important to note that restricting caloric intakes to the extremes (as high as 60%) as performed

BOX 8-2—Dietary Quick Fixes

Alterations to one's lifestyle to ensure long-term improvements are not easy to implement. Patients are often in the market for short-term solutions for longer-term problems. Dietary guidelines for overall health as well as cutaneous health and enhancement are geared toward long-range benefits, and can withstand or blunt the effects of occasional lapses. For the patient who seeks to see a relatively quick change in the appearance of the skin through nutrition alone, however, a few immediate steps can be taken, with the understanding that the skin's individual needs must also be taken into account. The following suggestions, based on skin type or dietary restrictions, may be helpful:

For *dry skin,* increase omega-3 fatty acids, such as those in salmon, and other fatty acids and a small amount of cholesterol to remain hydrated, and increase water consumption.

For *oily skin,* increase consumption of green leafy vegetables (e.g., kale and spinach), butternut squash, cantaloupe, carrots, mangoes, pumpkins, and sweet potatoes, which are high in vitamin A and will help decrease oil production.

For *sensitive skin,* as manifested through redness and facial flushing, add omega-3 fatty acids, fish in particular, as discussed above and antioxidants, which have anti-inflammatory effects.

For *sensitive skin with the acne subtype,* attention should be paid to concentrating on eating a diet with a low glycemic load. In addition to consuming the foods just cited, foods high in vitamin A are particularly beneficial. Fruits and vegetables have lower glycemic loads than most foods. Interestingly, given the reports and studies linking milk consumption and acne, dairy foods have lower glycemic loads than fruits and vegetables.[6] (The potential role of milk in the etiologic pathways of acne appears to involve other factors, however.) Grain products, and processed foods in general, are to be avoided.

For *sensitive skin with the rosacea subtype,* add omega-3 fatty acids, particularly through fish, but also cut out hot (temperature) foods, spicy foods, alcohol, and caffeine.

For *vegans*: Add flaxseed oil to the diet. This will help hydrate the skin, reduce redness, and puff out fine lines, restoring skin radiance. Skin radiance results from reflection of light off of a smooth surface.

in animal studies is not recommended for human beings.[182] But CR at an 8% level has been demonstrated to confer benefits on some biochemical and inflammatory biomarkers.[183]

While much more research is necessary on the viability of expanding the life- and healthspan of humans, one of the cultural practices on Okinawa—to "...eat until you are 80% full" (or hara hachi-bu)[182]—is sound advice alone to help stem the obesity epidemic that is afflicting an increasing proportion of the global population, particularly in the West. Such a practice would also likely benefit the skin if the individual consumes a healthy diet.

SUMMARY

Nutrition has long been ignored or given short shrift in the Western medical community, particularly in medical school education. This has also filtered into the practice of dermatology, perhaps most saliently in the treatment of acne as manifested by dermatologists' decades-long attempts to debunk popular myths regarding certain foods and the eruption of acne. While the two seminal, and admittedly flawed studies, that Cordain cited played an influential role in dermatologists' approaches to disabusing patients and/or their parents of the myths linking certain foods to acne, the myth itself has often been misinterpreted by the public and physicians have still offered sound basic nutritional advice (i.e., recommending generous portions of fruits and vegetables) even while trying to refute misinformation. That is to say, in the public mind, the myth took on an all-or-none implication that either chocolate, greasy foods, or other culprits directly caused acne. We know now that the correlation between diet and the skin is more convoluted. One chocolate bar will not lead to acne eruptions, but unhealthy eating patterns can certainly contribute to the etiologic pathway of acne.

Cosmetic dermatologists, while on the front lines in terms of treating the most conspicuous disorders and, in many cases, diagnosing systemic conditions with cutaneous manifestations, are increasingly expected to help patients endogenously and exogenously maintain the appearance, and health, of the skin and forestall the cutaneous symptoms of aging. With ever-evolving technology, practitioners are better and better equipped to offer procedures as well as oral and topical products that meet patients' health needs and cosmetic desires. But to further carry the banner of Hippocrates, and to take a broader look at cutaneous health and antiaging approaches, we must consider food, the only "medicine" that all individuals require on a daily basis. While the official or curricular attitudes toward nutrition are slowly changing, more rapidly accruing evidence suggests that nutrition has a varied and complex role to play in overall health as well as the health of the skin. Of course, much more research is necessary, but enough data exist to suggest that the old saw "you are what you eat" has been venerated for a reason. The food that we consume does exert far-reaching systemic influences that have the potential to result in cutaneous manifestations.

REFERENCES

1. Wolf R, Matz H, Orion E. Acne and diet. *Clin Dermatol.* 2004;22:387.
2. Boelsma E, van de Vijver LP, Goldbohm RA, et al. Human skin condition and its associations with nutrient concentrations in serum and diet. *Am J Clin Nutr.* 2003;77:348.
3. White GM. Recent findings in the epidemiologic evidence, classification, and subtypes of acne vulgaris. *J Am Acad Dermatol.* 1991;24:495.
4. Berson DS, Chalker DK, Harper JC. Current concepts in the treatment of acne: report from a clinical roundtable. *Cutis.* 2003;72:5.
5. Health Topics Questions and Answers About Acne: NIDDK. http://www.wrongdiagnosis.com/artic/health_topics_questions_and_answers_about_acne_niddk.htm. Accessed February 7, 2008.
6. Cordain L. Implications for the role of diet in acne. *Semin Cutan Med Surg.* 2005;24:84.
7. Cordain L, Lindeberg S, Hurtado M, et al. Acne vulgaris—a disease of Western civilization. *Arch Dermatol.* 2002;138:1584.
8. Schaefer O. When the Eskimo comes to town. *Nutr Today.* 1971;6:8.
9. Steiner P. Necropsies on Okinawans: anatomic and pathologic observations. *Arch Pathol.* 1946;42:359.
10. Fulton JE, Plewig G, Kligman AM. Effect of chocolate on acne vulgaris. *JAMA.* 1969;210:2071.
11. Anderson PC. Foods as the cause of acne. *Am J Fam Pract.* 1971;3:102.
12. Edmondson SR, Thumiger SP, Werther GA, et al. Epidermal homeostasis: the role of the growth hormone and insulin-like growth factor systems. *Endocr Rev.* 2003;24:737.
13. Nam SY, Lee EJ, Kim KR, et al. Effect of obesity on total and free insulin-like growth factor (IGF)-1, and their relationship to IGF-binding protein (BP)-1, IGFBP-2, IGFBP-3, insulin, and growth hormone. *Int J Obes Relat Metab Disord.* 1997;21:355.
14. Smith RN, Mann NJ, Braue A, et al. A low-glycemic-load diet improves symptoms in acne vulgaris patients: a

randomized controlled trial. *Am J Clin Nutr.* 2007;86:107.
15. Smith RN, Mann NJ, Braue A, et al. The effect of a high-protein, low glycemic-load diet versus a conventional, high glycemic-load diet on biochemical parameters associated with acne vulgaris: a randomized, investigator-masked, controlled trial. *J Am Acad Dermatol.* 2007; 57:247.
16. Logan AC. Dietary fat, fiber, and acne vulgaris. *J Am Acad Dermatol.* 2007;57: 1092.
17. Smith RN, Braue A, Varigos GA, et al. The effect of a low glycemic load diet on acne vulgaris and the fatty acid composition of skin surface triglycerides. *J Dermatol Sci.* 2008;50:41.
18. Adebamowo CA, Spiegelman D, Danby FW, et al. High school dietary dairy intake and teenage acne. *J Am Acad Dermatol.* 2005;52:207.
19. Bershad SV. Diet and acne—slim evidence, again [author reply 1103]. *J Am Acad Dermatol.* 2005;53:1102.
20. Spiegelman D, McDermott A, Rosner B. Regression calibration method for correcting measurement-error bias in nutritional epidemiology. *Am J Clin Nutr.* 1997;65:1179S.
21. Adebamowo CA, Spiegelman D, Berkey CS, et al. Milk consumption and acne in adolescent girls. *Dermatol Online J.* 2006;12:1.
22. Adebamowo CA, Spiegelman D, Berkey CS, et al. Milk consumption and acne in teenaged boys. *J Am Acad Dermatol.* 2008 January 12 [Epub ahead of print].
23. Danby FW. Acne and milk, the diet myth, and beyond. *J Am Acad Dermatol.* 2005;52:360.
24. Perricone N. *The Acne Prescription: The Perricone Program for Clear and Healthy Skin At Every Age.* New York, NY: Harper Collins; 2003.
25. Hitch JM, Greenburg BG. Adolescent acne and dietary iodine. *Arch Dermatol.* 1961;84:898.
26. Hitch JM. Acneform eruptions induced by drugs and chemicals. *JAMA.* 1967; 200:879.
27. Arbesman H. Dairy and acne—the iodine connection. *J Am Acad Dermatol.* 2005;53:1102.
28. Rasmussen LB, Larsen EH, Ovesen L. Iodine content in drinking water and other beverages in Denmark. *Eur J Clin Nutr.* 2000;54:57.
29. Girelli ME, Coin P, Mian C, et al. Milk represents an important source of iodine in schoolchildren of the Veneto region, Italy. *J Endocrinol Invest.* 2004;27: 709.
30. Dahl L, Opsahl JA, Meltzer HM, et al. Iodine concentration in Norwegian milk and dairy products. *Br J Nutr.* 2003; 90:679.
31. Dahl L, Johansson L, Julshamn K, et al. The iodine content of Norwegian foods and diets. *Public Health Nutr.* 2004;7:569.
32. Brantsæter AL, Haugen M, Julshamn K, et al. Evaluation of urinary iodine excretion as a biomarker for intake of milk and dairy products in pregnant women in the Norwegian Mother and Child Cohort Study (MoBa). *Eur J Clin Nutr.* 2007 December 5 [Epub ahead of print].
33. Lee SM, Lewis J, Buss DH, et al. Iodine in British foods and diets. *Br J Nutr.* 1994;72:435.
34. Pearce EN, Pino S, He X, et al. Sources of dietary iodine: bread, cow's milk, and infant formula in the Boston area. *J Clin Endocrinol Metab.* 2004;89:3421.
35. Danby FW. Acne and iodine: reply. *J Am Acad Dermatol.* 2007;56:164.
36. Vliegenhart JF, Casset F. Novel forms of protein glycosylation [Review]. *Curr Opin Struct Biol.* 1998;8:565.
37. Freitas JP, Filipe P, Guerra Rodrigo F. Glycosylation and lipid peroxidation in skin and in plasma in diabetic patient. *C R Seances Soc Biol Fil.* 1997;19:837.
38. Dillinger TL, Barriga P, Escárcega S, et al. Food of the gods: cure for humanity? A cultural history of the medicinal and ritual use of chocolate. *J Nutr.* 2000;130: 2057S.
39. Stahl W, Heinrich U, Aust O, et al. Lycopene-rich products and dietary photoprotection. *Photochem Photobiol Sci.* 2006;5:238.
40. Stahl W, Heinrich U, Wiseman S, et al. Dietary tomato paste protects against ultraviolet light-induced erythema in humans. *J Nutr.* 2001;131:1449.
41. Stahl W, Sies H. Carotenoids and protection against solar UV radiation. *Skin Pharmacol Appl Skin Physiol.* 2002;15: 291.
42. Heinrich U, Gartner C, Wiebusch M, et al. Supplementation with beta carotene or a similar amount of mixed carotenoids protects humans from UV-induced erythema. *J Nutr.* 2003;133:98.
43. Aust O, Stahl W, Sies H, et al. Supplementation with tomato-based products increases lycopene, phytofluene, and phytoene levels in human serum and protects against UV light-induced erythema. *Int J Vitam Nutr Res.* 2005;75:54.
44. González S, Astner S, An W, et al. Dietary lutein/zeaxanthin decreases ultraviolet B-induced epidermal hyperproliferation and acute inflammation in hairless mice. *J Invest Dermatol.* 2003; 121:399.
45. Svobodvá A, Psotová J, Walterová D. Natural phenolics in the prevention of UV-induced skin damage. A review. *Biomed Papers.* 2003;147:137.
46. Scalbert A, Williamson G. Dietary intake and bioavailability of polyphenols. *J Nutr.* 2000;130:2073S.
47. Ross JA, Kasum CM. Dietary flavonoids: bioavailability, metabolic effects, and safety. *Annu Rev Nutr.* 2002;22:19.
48. Grove K. Catechins are the major source of flavonoids in a group of Australian women. *Asia Pac J Clin Nutr.* 2004;13(suppl):S72.
49. Circosta C, De Pasquale R, Palumbo DR, et al. Effects of isoflavones from red clover (Trifolium pretense) on skin changes induced by ovariectomy in rats. *Phytother Res.* 2006;20:1096.
50. Manku MS, Horrobin DF, Morse NL, et al. Essential fatty acids in the plasma phospholipids of patients with atopic eczema. *Br J Dermatol.* 1984;110:643.
51. Galland L. Increased requirements for essential fatty acids in atopic individuals: a review with clinical descriptions. *J Am Coll Nutr.* 1986;5:213.
52. Bjørneboe A, Soyland E, Bjørneboe GE, et al. Effect of dietary supplementation with eicosapentaenoic acid in the treatment of atopic dermatitis. *Br J Dermatol.* 1987;117:463.
53. Callaway J, Schwab U, Harvima I, et al. Efficacy of dietary hempseed oil in patients with atopic dermatitis. *J Dermatolog Treat.* 2005;16:87.
54. Morse NL, Clough PM. A meta-analysis of randomized, placebo-controlled clinical trials of Efamol evening primrose oil in atopic eczema. Where do we go from here in light of more recent discoveries? *Curr Pharm Biotechnol.* 2006;7:503.
55. Kanehara S, Ohtani T, Uede K, et al. Undershirts coated with borage oil alleviate the symptoms of atopic dermatitis in children. *Eur J Dermatol.* 2007;17:448.
56. Krajcovicova-Kudlackova M, Simoncic R, Bederova A, et al. Lipid and antioxidant blood levels in vegetarians. *Nahrung.* 1996;40:17.
57. Melchert HU, Limsathayourat N, Mihajlovic H, et al. Fatty acid patterns in triglycerides, diglycerides, free fatty acids, cholesteryl esters and phosphatidylcholine in serum from vegetarians and non-vegetarians. *Atherosclerosis.* 1987;65:159.
58. Li D, Ball M, Bartlett M, et al. Lipoprotein(a), essential fatty acid status and lipoprotein lipids in female Australian vegetarians. *Clin Sci (Lond).* 1999;97:175.
59. Suzuki R, Shimizu T, Kudo T, et al. Effects of n-3 polyunsaturated fatty acids on dermatitis in NC/Nga mice. *Prostaglandins Leukot Essent Fatty Acids* 2002;66:435.
60. Davis BC, Kris-Etherton PM. Achieving optimal essential fatty acid status in vegetarians: current knowledge and practical implications. *Am J Clin Nutr.* 2003;78:640S.
61. Rosell MS, Lloyd-Wright Z, Appleby PN, et al. Long-chain n-3 polyunsaturated fatty acids in plasma in British meat-eating, vegetarian, and vegan men. *Am J Clin Nutr.* 2005;82:327.
62. Kim HH, Cho S, Lee S, et al. Photoprotective and anti-skin-aging effects of eicosapentaenoic acid in human skin in vivo. *J Lipid Res.* 2006; 47:921.
63. Krajcovicova-Kudlackova M, Simoncic R, Babinska K, et al. Lipid parameters in blood of vegetarians. *Cor Vasa.* 1993;35: 224.
64. Tomobe YI, Morizawa K, Tsuchida M, et al. Dietary docosahexaenoic acid suppresses inflammation and immunoresponses in contact hypersensitivity reaction in mice. *Lipids.* 2000;35:61.
65. Simopoulos AP. Omega-3 fatty acids in health and disease and in growth and development. *Am J Clin Nutr.* 1991;54: 438.
66. Mayser P, Mrowietz U, Arengerger P, et al. Omega-3 fatty acid-based lipid infusion in patients with chronic plague psoriasis: results of a double-blind, randomized, placebo-controlled, multicenter trial. *J Am Acad Dermatol.* 1998;39: 539.
67. Pronczuk A, Kipervarg Y, Hayes KC. Vegetarians have higher plasma alpha-tocopherol relative to cholesterol than do nonvegetarians. *J Am Coll Nutr.* 1992;11:50.
68. Boelsma E, Hendriks HF, Roza L. Nutritional skin care: health effects of

micronutrients and fatty acids. *Am J Clin Nutr*. 2001;73:853.

69. Liu G, Bibus DM, Bode AM, et al. Omega 3 but not omega 6 fatty acids inhibit AP-1 activity and cell transformation in JB6 cells. *Proc Natl Acad Sci U S A*. 2001;98:7510.
70. Hata TR, Scholz TA, Ermakov IV, et al. Non-invasive Raman spectroscopic detection of carotenoids in human skin. *J Invest Dermatol.* 2000;115:441.
71. Conn PF, Schaleh W, Truscott TG. The singlet oxygen and carotenoid interaction. *J Photochem Photobiol*. 1991;11:41.
72. Lee EH, Faulhaber D, Hanson KM, et al. Dietary lutein reduces ultraviolet radiation-induced inflammation and immun osuppression. *J Invest Dermatol*. 2004; 122:510.
73. Fielding JM, Sinclair AJ, DiGregorio G, et al. Relationship between colour and aroma of olive oil and nutritional content. *Asia Pac J Clin Nutr*. 2003;12(suppl): S36.
74. Yamakoshi J, Otsuka F, Sano A, et al. Lightening effect on ultraviolet-induced pigmentation of guinea pig skin by oral administration of a proanthocyanidin-rich extract from grape seeds. *Pigment Cell Res*. 2003;16:629.
75. Kasai K, Yoshimura M, Koga T, et al. Effects of oral administration of ellagic acid-rich pomegranate extract on ultraviolet-induced pigmentation in the human skin. *J Nutr Sci Vitaminol (Tokyo)*. 2006;52:383.
76. Yoshimura M, Watanabe Y, Kasai K, et al. Inhibitory effect of an ellagic acid-rich pomegranate extract on tyrosinase activity and ultraviolet-induced pigmentation. *Biosci Biotechnol Biochem*. 2005;69:2368.
77. Yamakoshi J, Sano A, Tokutake S, et al. Oral intake of proanthocyanidin-rich extract from grape seeds improves chloasma. *Phytother Res*. 2004;18:895.
78. Ni Z, Mu Y, Gulati O. Treatment of melasma with Pycnogenol. *Phytother Res*. 2002;16:567.
79. Krajcovicova-Kudlackova M, Simoncic R, Babinska K, et al. Selected vitamins and trace elements in blood of vegetarians. *Ann Nutr Metab*. 1995;39:334.
80. Izumi T, Saito M, Obata A, et al. Oral intake of soy isoflavone aglycone improves the aged skin of adult women. *J Nutr Sci Vitaminol (Tokyo)*. 2007;53:57.
81. Purba M, Kouris-Blazos A, Wattanapen paiboon N, et al. Skin wrinkling: can food make a difference? *J Am Coll Nutr*. 2001;20:71.
82. Lin JY, Lin FH, Burch JA, et al. Alpha-lipoic acid is ineffective as a topical antioxidant for photoprotection of skin. *J Invest Dermatol*. 2004;123:996.
83. Rattan SI. Theories of biological aging: genes, proteins, and free radicals. *Free Radic Res*. 2006;40:1230.
84. Halvorsen BL, Holte K, Myhrstad MC, et al. A systematic screening of total antioxidants in dietary plants. *J Nutr*. 2002;132:461.
85. Heinen MM, Hughes MC, Ibiebele TI, et al. Intake of antioxidant nutrients and the risk of skin cancer. *Eur J Cancer*. 2007;43:2707.
86. Thom E. A randomized, double-blind, placebo-controlled study on the clinical efficacy of oral treatment with Derma Vite on ageing symptoms of the skin. *J Int Med Res*. 2005;33:267.
87. Wagner S, Suter A, Merfort I. Skin penetration studies of Arnica preparations and of their sesquiterpene lactones. *Planta Med*. 2004;70:897.
88. Seeley BM, Denton AB, Ahn MS, et al. Effect of homeopathic Arnica montana on bruising in face-lifts: results of a randomized, double-blind, placebo-controlled clinical trial. *Arch Facial Plast Surg*. 2006;8:54.
89. Stahl W, Krutmann J. Systemic photoprotection through carotenoids. *Hautarzt*. 2006;57:281.
90. Köpcke W, Krutmann J. Protection from sunburn with beta-carotene—a meta-analysis. *Photochem Photobiol*. 2007 December 15 [Epub ahead of print].
91. Stahl W, Sies H. Carotenoids and flavonoids contribute to nutritional protection against skin damage from sunlight. *Mol Biotechnol*. 2007;37:26.
92. Frieling UM, Schaumberg DA, Kupper TS, et al. A randomized, 12-year primary-prevention trial of beta carotene supplementation for nonmelanoma skin cancer in the physicians' health study. *Arch Dermatol*. 2000;136:179.
93. Huang HY, Caballero B, Chang S, et al. Multivitamin/mineral supplements and prevention of chronic disease. *Evid Rep Technol Assess (Full Rep)*. 2006;139:1.
94. Hochman LG, Scher RK, Meyerson MS. Brittle nails: response to daily biotin supplementation. *Cutis*. 1993;51:303.
95. Iorizzo M, Pazzaglia M, M Piraccini B, et al. Brittle nails. *J Cosmet Dermatol*. 2004;3:138.
96. Scheinfeld N, Dahdah MJ, Scher R. Vitamins and minerals: their role in nail health and disease. *J Drugs Dermatol*. 2007;6:782.
97. Brosche T, Platt D. Effect of borage oil consumption on fatty acid metabolism, transepidermal water loss and skin parameters in elderly people. *Arch Gerontol Geriatr*. 2000;30:139.
98. MacKay D, Miller AL. Nutritional support for wound healing. *Altern Med Rev*. 2003;8:359.
99. Kamenicek V, Holan P, Franek P. Systemic enzyme therapy in the treatment and prevention of post-traumatic and postoperative swelling. *Acta Chir Orthop Traumatol Cech*, 2001;68:45.
100. Maurer HR. Bromelain: biochemistry, pharmacology and medical use. *Cell Mol Life Sci*. 2001;58:1234.
101. Rico MJ. Rising drug costs: the impact on dermatology. *Skin Therapy Lett*. 2000; 5:1.
102. Orsini RA. Bromelain. *Plast Reconstr Surg*. 2006;118:1640.
103. Lu YP, Lou YR, Li XH, et al. Stimulatory effect of oral administration of green tea or caffeine on ultraviolet light-induced increases in epidermal wild-type p53, p21(WAF1/CIP1), and apoptotic sunburn cells in SKH-1 mice. *Cancer Res*. 2000;60:4785.
104. Huang MT, Xie JG, Wang ZY, et al. Effects of tea, decaffeinated tea, and caffeine on UVB light-induced complete carcinogenesis in SKH-1 mice: demonstration of caffeine as a biologically important constituent of tea. *Cancer Res*. 1997;57:2623.
105. Gómez-Ruiz JA, Leake DS, Ames JM. In vitro antioxidant activity of coffee compounds and their metabolites. *J Agric Food Chem*. 2007;55:6962.
106. Devasagayam TP, Kamat JP, Mohan H, et al. Caffeine as an antioxidant: inhibition of lipid peroxidation induced by reactive oxygen species. *Biochem Biophys Acta* 1996;1282:63.
107. Lu YP, Lou YR, Lin Y, et al. Inhibitory effects of orally administered green tea, black tea, and caffeine on skin carcinogenesis in mice previously treated with ultraviolet B light (high-risk mice): relationship to decreased tissue fat. *Cancer Res*. 2001;61:5002.
108. Lu XP, Lou YR, Xie JG, et al. Topical applications of caffeine or (−)-epigallocatechin gallate (EGCG) inhibit carcinogenesis and selectively increase apoptosis in UVB-induced skin tumors in mice. *Proc Natl Acad Sci USA*. 2002;99:12455.
109. Velasco MV, Tano CT, Machado-Santelli GM, et al. Effects of caffeine and siloxanetriol alginate caffeine, as anticellulite agents, on fatty tissue: histological evaluation. *J Cosmet Dermatol*. 2008;7:23.
110. Willis R, Anthony M, Sun L, et al. Clinical implications of the correlation between coenzyme Q10 and vitamin B6 status. *Biofactors*. 1999;9:359.
111. Ashida Y, Yamanish H, Terada T, et al. CoQ10 supplementation elevates the epidermal CoQ10 level in adult hairless mice. *Biofactors*. 2005;25:175.
112. Hoppe U, Bergemann J, Diembeck W, et al. Coenzyme Q10, a cutaneous antioxidant and energizer. *Biofactors*. 1999;9:371.
113. Berbis P, Hesse S, Privat Y. Essential fatty acids and the skin. *Allerg Immunol (Paris)*. 1990;22:225.
114. Schalin-Karrila M, Mattila L, Jansen CT, et al. Evening primrose oil in the treatment of atopic eczema: effect on clinical status, plasma phospholipid fatty acids and circulating blood prostaglandins. *Br J Dermatol*. 1987;117:11.
115. Levin C, Maibach H. Exploration of "alternative" and "natural" drugs in dermatology. *Arch Dermatol*. 2002;138:207.
116. Harrison RA, Holt D, Pattison DJ, et al. Who and how many people are taking herbal supplements? A survey of 21923 adults. *Int J Vitam Nutr Res*. 2004;74:183.
117. Bissett DL. Glucosamine: an ingredient with skin and other benefits. *J Cosmet Dermatol*. 2006;5:309.
118. Murad H, Tabibian MP. The effect of an oral supplement containing glucosamine, amino acids, minerals, and antioxidants on cutaneous aging: a preliminary study. *J Dermatolog Treat*. 2001; 12:47.
119. Wold RS, Lopez ST, Yau CL, et al. Increasing trends in elderly persons' use of nonvitamin, nonmineral dietary supplements and concurrent use of medications. *J Am Diet Assoc*. 2005;105:54.
120. Pittler MH, Ernst E. Horse-chestnut seed extract for chronic venous insufficiency. A criteria-based systematic review. *Arch Dermatol*. 1998;134:1356.
121. Ernst E, Pittler MH, Stevinson C. Complementary/alternative medicine in dermatology: evidence-assessed efficacy of two diseases and two treatments. *Am J Clin Dermatol*. 2002;3: 341.
122. Piacquadio D, Jarcho M, Goltz R. Evaluation of hylan b gel as a soft-tissue augmentation implant material. *J Am Acad Dermatol*. 1997;36:544.

123. Comper WD, Laurent TC. Physiological function of connective tissue polysaccharides. *Physiol Rev*. 1978;58:255.
124. Petrella RJ. Hyaluronic acid for the treatment of knee osteoarthritis: long-term outcomes from a naturalistic primary care experience. *Am J Phys Med Rehabil*. 2005;84:278.
125. Sies H, Stahl W. Non-nutritive bioactive constituents of plants: lycopene, lutein and zeaxanthin. *Int J Vitam Nutr Res*. 2003;73:95.
126. Wright TI, Spencer JM, Flowers FP. Chemoprevention of nonmelanoma skin cancer. *J Am Acad Dermatol*. 2006; 54:933.
127. Ribaya-Mercado JD, Garmyn M, Gilchrest BA, et al. Skin lycopene is destroyed preferentially over beta-carotene during ultraviolet irradiation in humans. *J Nutr*. 1995;125:1854.
128. Gensler HL, Williams T, Huang AC, et al. Oral niacin prevents photocarcinogenesis and photoimmunosuppression in mice. *Nutr Cancer*. 1999;34:36.
129. Berk MA, Lorincz AL. The treatment of bullous pemphigoid with tetracycline and niacinamide. A preliminary report. *Arch Dermatol*. 1986;122:670.
130. Kademian M, Bechtel M, Zirwas M. Case reports: new onset flushing due to unauthorized substitution of niacin for nicotinamide. *J Drugs Dermatol*. 2007;6: 1220.
131. Prousky J, Seely D. The treatment of migraines and tension-type headaches with intravenous and oral niacin (nicotinic acid): systematic review of the literature. *Nutr J*. 2005;26:4.
132. Cefali EA, Simmons PD, Stanek EJ, et al. Improved control of niacin-induced flushing using an optimized once-daily, extended-release niacin formulation. *Int J Clin Pharmacol Ther*. 2006;44:633.
133. Puglia C, Tropea S, Rizza L, et al. In vitro percutaneous absorption studies and in vivo evaluation of anti-inflammatory activity of essential fatty acids (EFA) from fish oil extracts. *Int J Pharm*. 2005;299:41.
134. Bourre JM. Dietary omega-3 fatty acids for women. *Biomed Pharmacother*. 2007;61:105.
135. Sies H, Stahl W. Nutritional protection against skin damage from sunlight. *Annu Rev Nutr*. 2004;24:173.
136. Black HS, Rhodes LE. The potential of omega-3 fatty acids in the prevention of non-melanoma skin cancer. *Cancer Detect Prev*. 2006;30:224.
137. MacLean CH, Newberry SJ, Mojica WA, et al. Effects of omega-3 fatty acids on cancer risk: a systematic review. *JAMA*. 2006;295:403.
138. Chen YQ, Berquin IM, Daniel LW, et al. Omega-3 fatty acids and cancer risk. *JAMA*. 2006;296:282.
139. González S, Pathak MA, Cuevas J, et al. Topical or oral administration with an extract of Polypodium leucotomos prevents acute sunburn and psoralen-induced phototoxic reactions as well as depletion of Langerhans cells in human skin. *Photodermatol Photoimmunol Photomed*. 1997;13:50.
140. Gombau L, García F, Lahoz A, et al. Polypodium leucotomos extract: antioxidant activity and disposition. *Toxicol In Vitro*. 2006;20:464.
141. Gonzalez S, Alonso-Lebrero JL, Del Rio R, et al. Polypodium leucotomos extract: a nutraceutical with photoprotective properties. *Drugs Today (Barc)*. 2007;43:475.
142. Middelkamp-Hup MA, Pathak MA, Parrado C, et al. Orally administered Polypodium leucotomos extract decreases psoralen-UVA-induced phototoxicity, pigmentation, and damage of human skin. *J Am Acad Dermatol*. 2004;50:41.
143. Middelkamp-Hup MA, Pathak MA, Parrado C, et al. Oral Polypodium leucotomos extract decreases ultraviolet-induced damage of human skin. *J Am Acad Dermatol*. 2004;51:910.
144. Middelkamp-Hup MA, Bos JD, Rius-Diaz F, et al. Treatment of vitiligo vulgaris with narrow-band UVB and oral Polypodium leucotomos extract: a randomized double-blind placebo-controlled study. *J Eur Acad Dermatol Venereol*. 2007;21:942.
145. Thomson CD. Assessment of requirements for selenium and adequacy of selenium status: a review. *Eur J Clin Nutr*. 2004;58:391.
146. Maggini S, Wintergerst ES, Beveridge S, et al. Selected vitamins and trace elements support immune function by strengthening epithelial barriers and cellular and humoral immune responses. *Br J Nutr*. 2007;98:S29.
147. Klotz LO, Kroncke KD, Buchczyk DP, et al. Role of copper, zinc, selenium and tellurium in the cellular defense against oxidative and nitrosative stress. *J Nutr*. 2003;133:1448.
148. Chen Y, Hall M, Graziano JH, et al. A prospective study of blood selenium levels and the risk of arsenic-related premalignant skin lesions. *Cancer Epidemiol Biomarkers Prev*. 2007;16:207.
149. Harrison EH. Mechanisms of digestion and absorption of dietary vitamin A. *Annu Rev Nutr*. 2005;25:87.
150. U.S. Department of Health and Human Services. Advance Data from Vital and Health Statistics Dietary Intake of Selected Vitamins for the United States Population: 1999–2000. Centers for Disease Control and Prevention. National Center for Health Statistics. Number 339, 2004.
151. Keller KL, Fenske NA. Uses of vitamins A, C, and E and related compounds in dermatology: a review. *J Am Acad Dermatol*. 1998;39:611.
152. The Evolving Role of Retinoids in the Management of Cutaneous Conditions. New York, New York; USA; May 2–4, 1997. Conference proceedings. *J Am Acad Dermatol*. 1998;39:S1.
153. Kligman AM. Cosmetics. A dermatologist looks to the future: promises and problems. *Dermatol Clin*. 2000;18:699.
154. Geesin JC, Darr D, Kaufman R, et al. Ascorbic acid specifically increases type I and type III procollagen messenger RNA levels in human skin fibroblast. *J Invest Dermatol*. 1988;90:420.
155. Phillips CL, Combs SB, Pinnell SR. Effects of ascorbic acid on proliferation and collagen synthesis in relation to the donor age of human dermal fibroblasts. *J Invest Dermatol*. 1994;103:228.
156. Eberlein-König B, Ring J. Relevance of vitamins C and E in cutaneous photoprotection. *J Cosmet Dermatol*. 2005;4:4.
157. Placzek M, Gaube S, Kerkmann U, et al. Ultraviolet B-induced DNA damage in human epidermis is modified by the antioxidants ascorbic acid and D-alpha-tocopherol. *J Invest Dermatol*. 2005;124: 304.
158. Cho HS, Lee MH, Lee JW, et al. Anti-wrinkling effects of the mixture of vitamin C, vitamin E, pycnogenol and evening primrose oil, and molecular mechanisms on hairless mouse skin caused by chronic ultraviolet B irradiation. *Photodermatol Photoimmunol Photomed*. 2007;23:155.
159. Lips P. Vitamin D physiology. *Prog Biophys Mol Biol*. 2006;92:4.
160. Lehmann B, Querings K, Reichrath J. Vitamin D and skin: new aspects for dermatology. *Exp Dermatol*. 2004;13:11.
161. Zitterman A. Vitamin D in preventive medicine: are we ignoring the evidence? *Br J Nutr*. 2003;89:552.
162. Chel VG, Ooms ME, Popp-Snijders C, et al. Ultraviolet irradiation corrects vitamin D deficiency and suppresses secondary hyperparathyroidism in the elderly. *J Bone Miner Res*. 1998;13:1238.
163. Bialy TL, Rothe MJ, Grant-Kels JM. Dietary factors in the prevention and treatment of nonmelanoma skin cancer and melanoma. *Dermatol Surg*. 2002;28: 1143.
164. Wortsman J, Matsuoka LY, Chen TC, et al. Decreased bioavailability of vitamin D in obesity. *Am J Clin Nutr*. 2000; 72:690.
165. Marks R, Foley A, Jolley D, et al. The effect of regular sunscreen use on vitamin D levels in an Australian population. Results of a randomized controlled trial. *Arch Dermatol*. 1995;131:415.
166. Gilchrest BA. Sun protection and Vitamin D. three dimensions of obfuscation. *J Steroid Biochem Mol Biol*. 2007; 103:655.
167. Vieth R. Critique of the considerations for establishing the tolerable upper intake level for vitamin D: critical need for revision upwards. *J Nutr*. 2006; 136: 1117.
168. Heaney RP. Barriers to optimizing vitamin D3 intake for the elderly. *J Nutr*. 2006;136:1123.
169. Thiele JJ, Ekanayake-Mudiyanselage S. Vitamin E in human skin: organ-specific physiology and considerations for its use in dermatology. *Mol Aspects Med*. 2007;28:646.
170. Kuchide M, Tokuda H, Takayasu J, et al. Cancer chemopreventive effects of oral feeding alpha-tocopherol on ultraviolet light B induced photocarcinogenesis of hairless mouse. *Cancer Lett*. 2003;196: 169.
171. McArdle F, Rhodes LE, Parslew RA, et al. Effects of oral vitamin E and beta-carotene supplementation on ultraviolet radiation-induced oxidative stress in human skin. *Am J Clin Nutr*. 2004;80: 1270.
172. Mireles-Rocha H, Galindo I, Huerta M, et al. UVB photoprotection with antioxidants: effects of oral therapy with d-alpha-tocopherol and ascorbic acid on the minimal erythema dose. *Acta Derm Venereol*. 2002;82:21.
173. Vegetarian Information Sheet. http://www.vegsoc.org/info/zinc.html. Accessed February 16, 2008.
174. Prasad AS. Clinical, immunological, anti-inflammatory and antioxidant roles of zinc. *Exp Gerontol*. 2007 November 1 [Epub ahead of print].

175. Miyata S. Zinc deficiency in the elderly. *Nippon Ronen Igakkai Zasshi*. 2007;44:677.
176. Al-Gurairi FT, Al-Waiz M, Sharquie KE. Oral zinc sulphate in the treatment of recalcitrant viral warts: randomized placebo-controlled clinical trial. *Br J Dermatol*. 2002;146:423.
177. Takahashi H, Nakazawa M, Takahashi K, et al. Effects of zinc deficient diet on development of atopic dermatitis-like eruptions in DS-Nh mice. *J Dermatol Sci*. 2008;50:31.
178. Sugano M. Characteristics of fats in Japanese diets and current recommendations. *Lipids*. 1996;31:S283.
179. Simopoulos AP. Evolutionary aspects of diet, the omega-6/omega-3 ratio and genetic variation: nutritional implications for chronic diseases. *Biomed Pharmacother*. 2006;60:502.
180. Kiecolt-Glaser JK, Belury MA, Porter K, et al. Depressive symptoms, omega-6:omega-3 fatty acids, and inflammation in older adults. *Psychosom Med*. 2007;69:217.
181. Carter CS, Hofer T, Seo AY, et al. Molecular mechanisms of life- and health-span extension: role of calorie restriction and exercise intervention. *Appl Physiol Nutr Metab*. 2007;32:954.
182. Willcox DC, Willcox BJ, Todoriki H, et al. Caloric restriction and human longevity: what can we learn from the Okinawans? *Biogerontology*. 2006;7:173.
183. Dirks AJ, Leeuwenburgh C. Calorie restriction in humans: potential pitfalls and health concerns. *Mech Ageing Dev*. 2006;127:1.

SECTION 2

Skin Types

CHAPTER 9

The Baumann Skin Typing System

Leslie Baumann, MD
Edmund Weisberg, MS

The modern cosmetic and skin care product market began to take shape in 1915 amidst the intense rivalry between the burgeoning cosmetics entrepreneurs Helena Rubinstein and Elizabeth Arden, both of whom opened salons that year that would grow into powerful business empires. Since that period, the categories "dry," "oily," "combination," and "sensitive" have been used to characterize what Helena Rubinstein identified as the four fundamental skin types. While these designations were the virtually undisputed standards for understanding skin type, the skin care product and cosmetics markets were growing exponentially, evolving into an innovative multibillion dollar industry, and spawning a new category of products known as "cosmeceuticals," unregulated cosmetic formulations that may impart some alteration to the biologic function of skin. In fact, these products have become so popular that relatively recent sales figures indicated that $6.4 billion in sales of skin care cosmeceuticals were projected in the US in 2004, an increase of 7.3% from the previous year.[1] Such sales expectations have since been exceeded, as by spring 2006, sales of cosmeceuticals in the US had mushroomed to the $12 billion level.[2]

While the skin care product market has changed significantly and undergone rapid expansion during the past century, relatively few advances have been made in the understanding or classification of skin type. Indeed, the traditional skin-type designations have, in practice, come to be seen as insufficient characterizations particularly in terms of their capacity to guide physicians and consumers toward identifying the most appropriate products. This is especially noteworthy given that more and more products are marketed and designed for specific skin types, often dry or sensitive skin. When a person has dry or sensitive skin, are those individual descriptors the only or defining features? The skin types identified by Rubinstein do not address several other features of skin that have been clinically observed, such as oiliness, resistance, or propensities toward pigmentation or wrinkling. The Baumann Skin Typing System (BSTS) is an innovative approach to classifying skin type that is based on four main skin parameters:

1. Oily versus Dry;
2. Sensitive versus Resistant;
3. Pigmented versus Nonpigmented;
4. Wrinkled versus Tight (Unwrinkled).

Because these four parameters are not mutually exclusive, evaluating the skin based on all four parameters yields 16 potential skin-type permutations (Table 9-1). The Baumann Skin Type (BST) classification is determined from a questionnaire designed to ascertain baseline skin type identifications as well as assessments after significant life changes, since skin type is not necessarily static.[3]

The BSTS is especially useful as it provides specific guidance for physicians and patients/consumers to identify the most suitable skin products for the patient's BST.[4] For example, significantly different skin care products would be indicated for an individual with dry, resistant, pigmented, wrinkled skin (DRPW), as seen in Figure 9-1, compared to a person with oily, sensitive, pigmented, tight skin (OSPT), as seen in Figure 9-2. The BST is determined by a questionnaire that is constantly updated and improved as new data are collected. The questionnaire and a complete description of each skin type including product recommendations for each BST can be found in the book *The Skin Type Solution*, which is available in various countries and several languages. Physicians and skin care specialists can join the effort to collect skin-type data worldwide and can access the most up-to-date version of the Baumann Skin Type Indicator (BSTI) questionnaire online by registering at www.SkinIQ.com. The BSTI is available in 10 languages at this Web site. Once registered on the site, the skin care specialist can e-mail the link to the questionnaire to patients, so that patients can self-administer the examination. The result, the patient's BST, is available in a report to the physician or aesthetician. They can determine not only an individual's skin type, but also which skin types are most prevalent in their practice. More importantly, skin care specialists and dermatologists can use this information to help determine which products and procedures are most appropriate for their patient populations. The questionnaire (BSTI) is frequently updated following the evaluations of the most recent incoming data by statisticians. In addition, new questions are developed as a result of this vetting process. The nonidentifying data collected from the site should serve to expand knowledge of skin-type prevalence around the world.

This chapter will discuss the four parameters on which the BSTS is based, briefly focusing on their defining characteristics and pertinent basic science. In the process, the 16 skin-type variations will be described. Each of the four skin parameters has a

TABLE 9-1
The 16 Baumann Skin Types

	Oily, Pigmented	Oily, Nonpigmented	Dry, Pigmented	Dry, Nonpigmented	
Sensitive	OSPW	OSNW	DSPW	DSNW	Wrinkled
Sensitive	OSPT	OSNT	DSPT	DSNT	Tight
Resistant	ORPW	ORNW	DRPW	DRNW	Wrinkled
Resistant	ORPT	ORNT	DRPT	DRNT	Tight

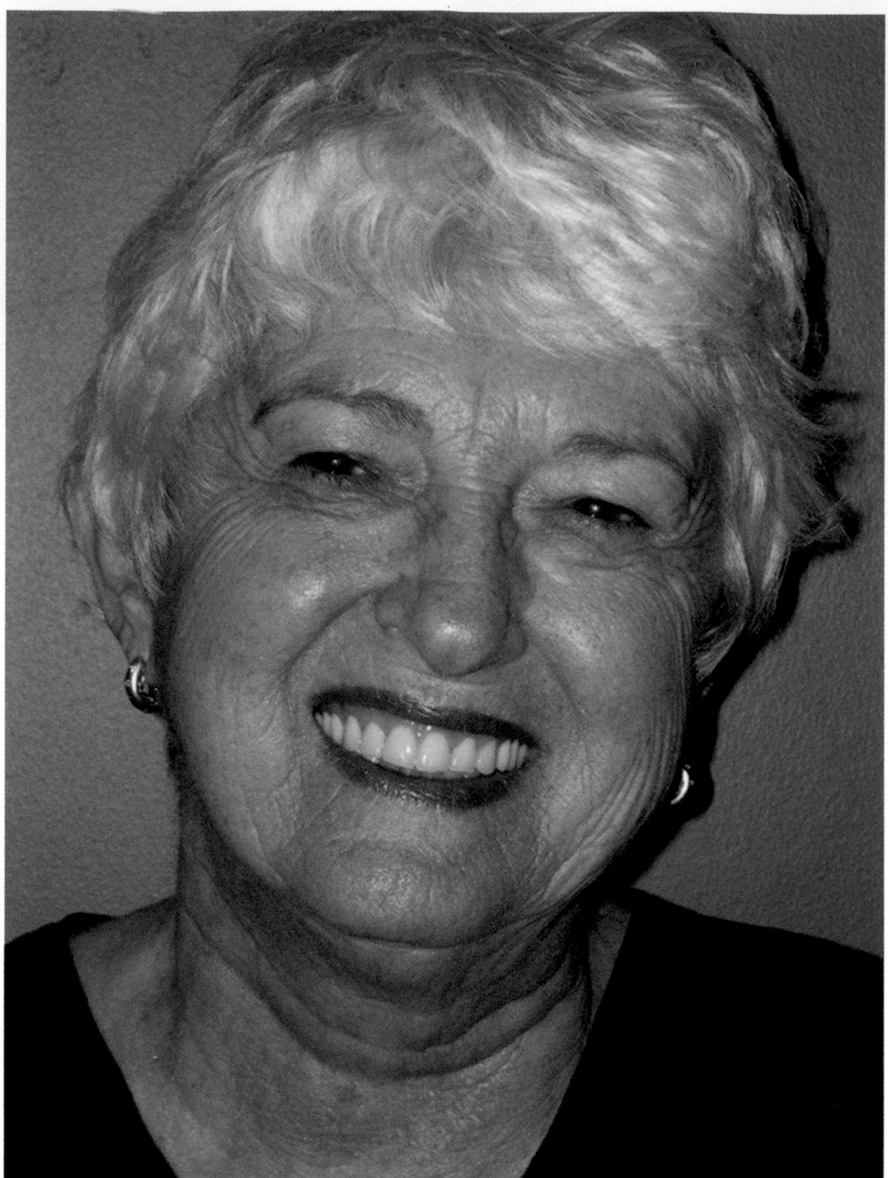

▲ **FIGURE 9-1** This patient played tennis for many years. She has no history of skin sensitivity. Her DRPW skin needs strong ingredients such as hydroxy acids, antioxidants, retinoids, and heavy moisturizers. If patients are on cholesterol-lowering drugs, add a coenzyme Q10 vitamin supplement. Of course, a daily sunscreen that does not burn eyes during tennis is a must.

separate set of questions and a score is assigned to that parameter. For example, the oily and dry questions determine if the user is an "O" or a "D" and assigns them an O/D score (Fig. 9-3). Once the score is known, skin care advice can easily be given. Treatment options or skin care approaches linked to the BST will also be covered with an emphasis on noninvasive, primarily topical therapies.

SKIN HYDRATION

The Spectrum of Oily (O) to Dry (D)

Dry skin is characterized by either an impaired barrier, lack of natural moisturizing factor, or decreased sebum production (see Chapter 11). Oily skin exhibits increased sebum production (see Chapter 10). Although patients can complain of combination skin, dry on the cheeks and oily in the T-zone, they often fall on one end of the spectrum. Knowing their O/D status helps simplify their skin care. In the BSTS, a higher score corresponds with increased sebum production, while a low score corresponds with decreased skin hydration. Skin that falls in the middle of this dichotomy would be considered "normal" skin (Fig. 9-4).

Skin Care for the O to D Parameter

Oily skin types are difficult to treat because there are no effective topical agents that significantly reduce sebum secretion. In addition, sunscreens, which are often soluble in oil, may increase skin greasiness (see Chapter 10). Oily skin is best treated with a cleanser directed to oily types. Foaming cleansers and cleansers with salicylic acid can be used on these patients. Toners may be used in this skin type, if desired, as well. Moisturizers are often unnecessary in oily skin types. If they are used, lighter forms such as lotions should be chosen. Sebum contains high levels of vitamin E, so oily skin types manifest a high degree of antioxidant protection. Most oily skin types are under the age of 40 years and may suffer from acne as well. Gel and serum formulations are preferred over creams in oily skin types. Layering a powder over sunscreen may help reduce the greasiness that occurs in these patients with sunscreen use.

Dry skin types need nonfoaming cleansers that will not strip protective lipids from the skin surface. While the skin is still damp, moisturizers should be applied to trap water on the skin's surface. Toners should not be used in dry skin types. Moisturizers should be chosen based on their ability to decrease transepidermal water loss and repair the skin's permeability barrier (see Chapter 32). Extremely dry types with a very low O/D score should avoid facial scrubs because friction is known to impair the skin's permeability barrier. There are many lotion and cream sunscreens on the market that are appropriate for dry skin types.

Normal skin types who fall in the middle of the O/D scoring system will fare well with a lotion formulation rather than a gel or a cream formulation. "Normal" skin types may change to dry skin types in low-humidity environments or in cold weather.

SKIN SENSITIVITY

The Spectrum of Sensitive (S) to Resistant (R)

A high score on the S/R spectrum correlates with sensitive skin, while a low score represents resistant skin. Sensitive skin is characterized by inflammation and manifests as acne, rosacea, burning and stinging, or skin rashes (see Chapter 12). The higher the "S" score is, the greater is the likelihood that the patient has several types of sensitive skin. For example, a patient with rosacea only will have a lower score than a patient with rosacea and symptoms of burning and stinging. These S scores can be used to

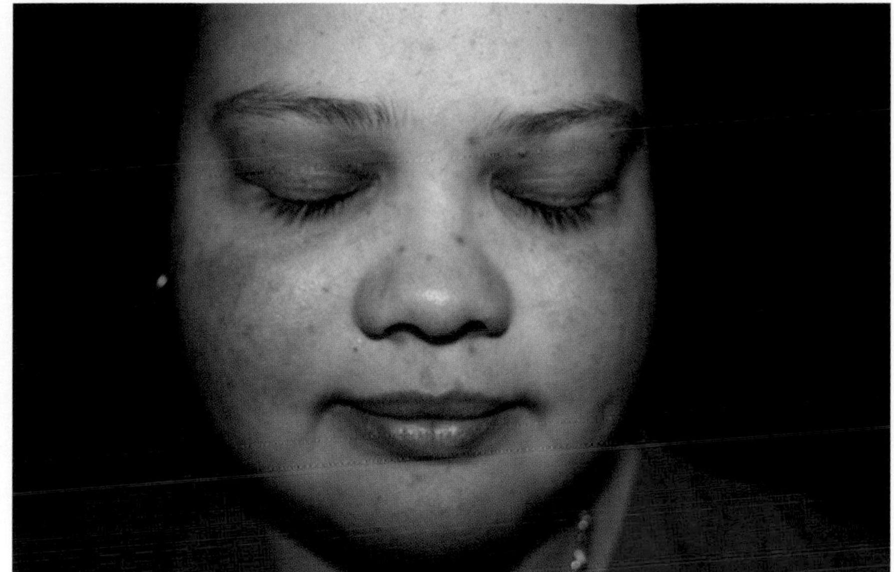

▲ **FIGURE 9-2** This OS[1,2] PT patient has a history of facial flushing, redness, and acne (S1 and S2 refers to the fact that she has acne and rosacea-sensitive skin types 1 and 2). She tries to avoid sun but lives in Miami and sunscreens usually make her sting or breakout. Her skin regimen should consist of a salicylic acid or selenium sulfide cleanser, a serum with anti-inflammatory ingredients, a topical antibiotic, and a sunscreen with micronized zinc oxide and titanium dioxide. Intense Pulsed Light treatments will improve her solar lentigos and facial redness. Antioxidant supplements such as vitamin C 500 mg twice a day and Pycnogenol 50 mg every day may help decrease the inflammation she experiences. Mild salicylic acid chemical peels are an option as well.

determine what skin treatments are necessary and which to avoid. Resistant skin is characterized by a robust stratum corneum (SC) that strongly protects the skin from allergens, other environmental irritants, and water loss. Individuals with resistant skin rarely experience erythema or acne (Fig. 9-5). In general, they can be treated with stronger skin care products and in office procedures, such as chemical peels, than can those with sensitive skin (Box 9-1).

BOX 9-1 Types of Sensitive Skin

S1—Acne
S2—Rosacea
S3—Burning and stinging
S4—Susceptibility to contact and irritant dermatitis

Skin Care for the S to R Parameter

Individuals with resistant "R" skin can use most skin care products without fear of incurring adverse reactions (e.g., acne, rashes, or a stinging response). On the other hand, the same qualities that protect resistant skin from most formulations also render many products ineffective because these patients exhibit an exceedingly high threshold for product ingredient penetration. In other words, resistant types have a strong skin barrier. Therefore, people with resistant skin may not benefit from weaker products, which are unable to penetrate the SC of such individuals to deliver the intended results. Resistant patients are the ones who should be treated with higher levels of glycolic acid and will require longer incubation periods with Levulan prior to photodynamic therapy. They are less likely to develop allergic reactions to skin care products that sensitive types cannot tolerate.

Individuals with sensitive skin share one quality in common: inflammation. Treatment is geared toward preventing

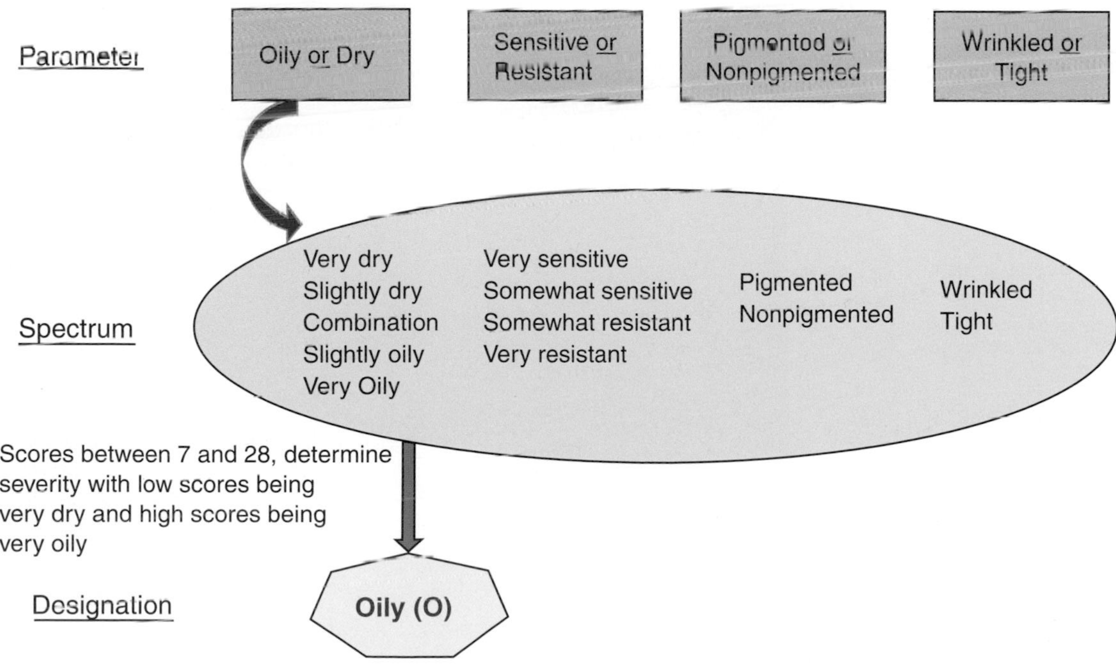

▲ **FIGURE 9-3** Algorithm for assessing oily skin according to the BSTI.

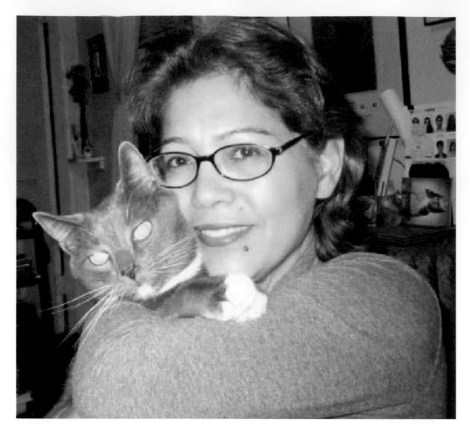

▲ **FIGURE 9-4** Oily skin types often show a light reflection or facial shine in photographs. People with these skin types should use serums and gels rather than creams. If skin is combination (oily in the T zone), then lotions are a good choice. Retinoids in the gel form are a good option for oily skin types.

and reducing irritation and inflammation through the use of anti-inflammatory products (see Chapter 35). Because there are four distinct types of sensitive skin that can overlap, skin care recommendations depend on which type of sensitive skin or which combination of types the patient exhibits. The issues to take into consideration when choosing a skin care regimen are discussed in the corresponding sensitive skin Chapters 15 to 18. In general, those with sensitive skin should avoid facial scrubs because friction impairs the skin barrier and can worsen acne.

SKIN PIGMENTATION

The Spectrum of Pigmented (P) to Nonpigmented (N)

Skin color is not the focus here. Although darker skin types are more likely to exhibit the "P" (pigmented) skin type, this parameter does not refer to ethnicity (Fig. 9-6). Rather, the P/N parameter measures the tendency to develop hyperpigmentation. This segment of the BSTS determines those with a history or current presentation of pigmentary alterations that can be prevented or improved with skin care products as well as dermatologic procedures, and includes conditions such as ephelides, melasma, postinflammatory hyperpigmentation, and solar lentigos (Fig. 9-7). Skin lesions that require excision or treatment beyond skin care (e.g., congenital nevi and seborrheic keratoses) fall beyond the scope of the BSTS.

An individual with a propensity to develop unwanted pigmentary changes is classified as having the "P" skin type in the BSTS system; a person not exhibiting this tendency has type "N" skin (Fig. 9-8). Knowing the "P" score of a patient will help alert the physician to the change of hyperpigmentation, and chemical peel strengths and laser settings can be adjusted accordingly to prevent postinflammatory hyperpigmentation in those with high "P" scores. Patients with the "N" skin type often have light skin and an inability to tan; however, individuals with red hair, who have a tendency to freckle, are designated as "P" skin types.

Skin Care for the P to N Parameter

Individuals with "N" type skin do not require any special skin care products. However, the "P" skin types benefit from

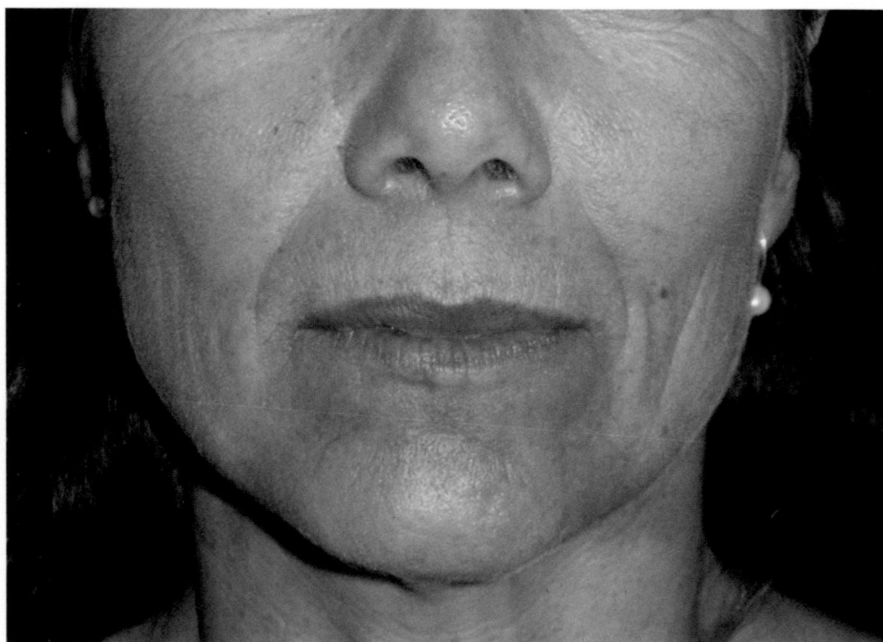

▲ **FIGURE 9-5** Resistant skin types have strong epidermal barriers. Skin may appear thickened or "weathered." This patient has the DRPW skin type. Daily sunscreen, alpha hydroxy acid moisturizers, retinoids, and topical antioxidants should be added to her regimen. Australians, Latin Americans, and others that live in a hot climate often have this skin type. This patient is an ideal candidate for a series of chemical peels, dermal fillers, and botulinum toxin.

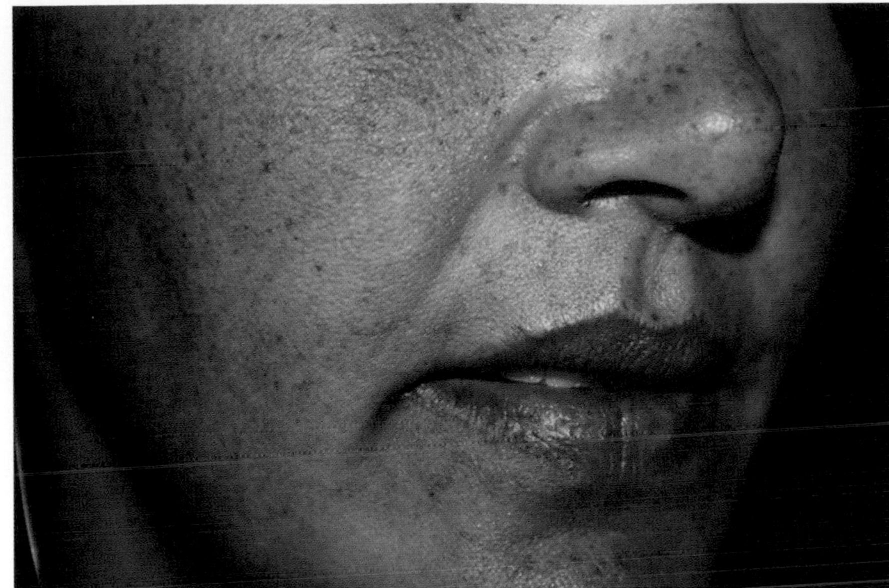

▲ **FIGURE 9-6** Pigmented skin types develop solar lentigos, melasma, and postinflammatory hyperpigmentation. Although darker skin types are more likely to be pigmented types, this is not always the case. This patient is a DRPT skin type. She avoids sun exposure and smoking and her skin tone may provide some protection from skin aging. The skin care recommendations include daily sunscreen, moisturizers, and skin-lightening agents. Light chemical peels can be used with caution to even out skin tone. IPL cannot be safely used because of her skin coloring; however, the Fraxel laser may be a good option when used by a physician experienced with skin of color. Asians and Latin Americans frequently have this skin type.

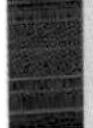

skin lightening ingredients such as arbutin, hydroquinone, and kojic acid. Products with niacinamide and active soy may help prevent unwanted pigmentation. These ingredients are discussed at length in Chapter 33. Causes of skin pigmentation are discussed in Chapter 13. Intense pulsed light and Fraxel treatments are useful additions for many patients with the pigmented BST to help remove unwanted solar lentigos or melasma.

SKIN AGING

The Spectrum of Wrinkled (W) to Tight (T)

This portion of the BSTS identifies the risk for wrinkles. The questionnaire asks about habits such as sun exposure, smoking, and tanning bed use. In addition, it asks questions about the skin of ancestors to ascertain the genetic influence on wrinkled skin. The "W" types may not necessarily have wrinkles at the time that they complete the BSTI, but in time they will need to begin prevention methods because they are at risk. Individuals with lighter skin are more likely to manifest "W" type skin than those with dark skin. Retinoids, sunscreen, and antioxidants should be used in those who test out as a "W" type.

SKIN TYPE COMBINATIONS AND CHANGES

As stated previously, evaluating the four skin parameters together results in a characterization of the simultaneous state or proclivities of the skin along four different spectra, yielding 16 different possible skin-type permutations. The BSTS can lend valuable assistance in the process of treating particular skin problems and selecting the most appropriate OTC products as well as dermatologic procedures for an individual's particular skin type. A person with dry, sensitive, nonpigmented, tight skin (DSNT), for example, would benefit from formulations with ingredients designed to repair the skin barrier (see Chapter 32). Products containing retinoids and antioxidants would be most suitable for an individual with oily, sensitive, nonpigmented, wrinkled skin (OSNW) because these individuals often have acne and a tendency to wrinkle (see Chapters 30 and 34). Product selection should also be made with the understanding that particular skin traits, tendencies, or conditions are associated with certain skin types. For example, a person with pigmented, wrinkled (PW) skin is more likely to have a history of chronic sun exposure, manifesting in wrinkles and solar lentigos. Dark skin is more common in people identified as having pigmented, tight (PT) skin, whereas light skin is more typical in individuals characterized as having nonpigmented, wrinkled (NW) skin. In addition, eczema is more often noted in people with dry, sensitive (DS) skin, while acne is associated with oily, sensitive (OS) skin. Rosacea is often observed in individuals with the OSNW skin type.

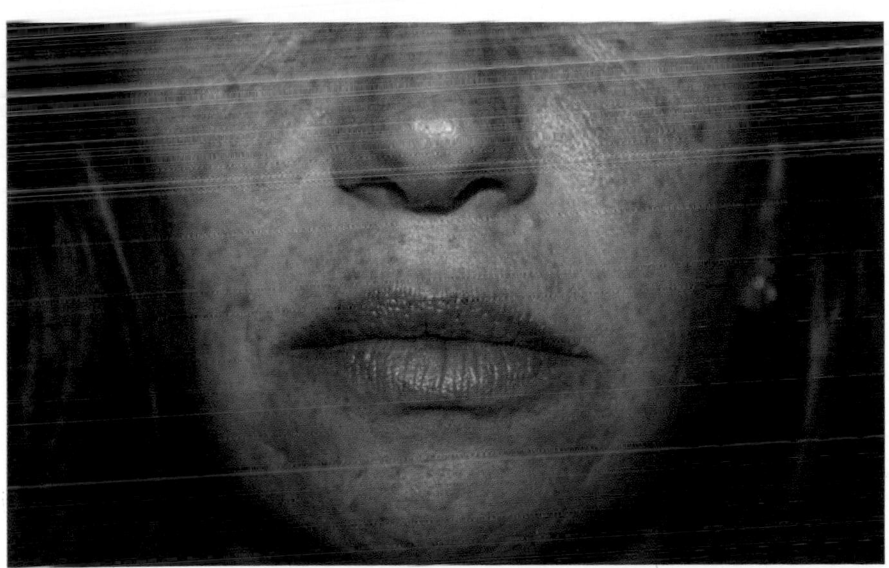

▲ **FIGURE 9-7** This patient is an ORPW skin type. A history of sun exposure and light skin color make her more susceptible to wrinkling; therefore, she is designated as a "tendency to wrinkle" type even though significant wrinkling is not present. The vitamin E in her sebum may have offered some protection from her frequent sun exposure. The best skin care regimen would include daily sunscreen, alpha hydroxy acid cleansers, skin lighteners, retinoids, and oral and topical antioxidants. The IPL or Fraxel laser would be great therapeutic options.

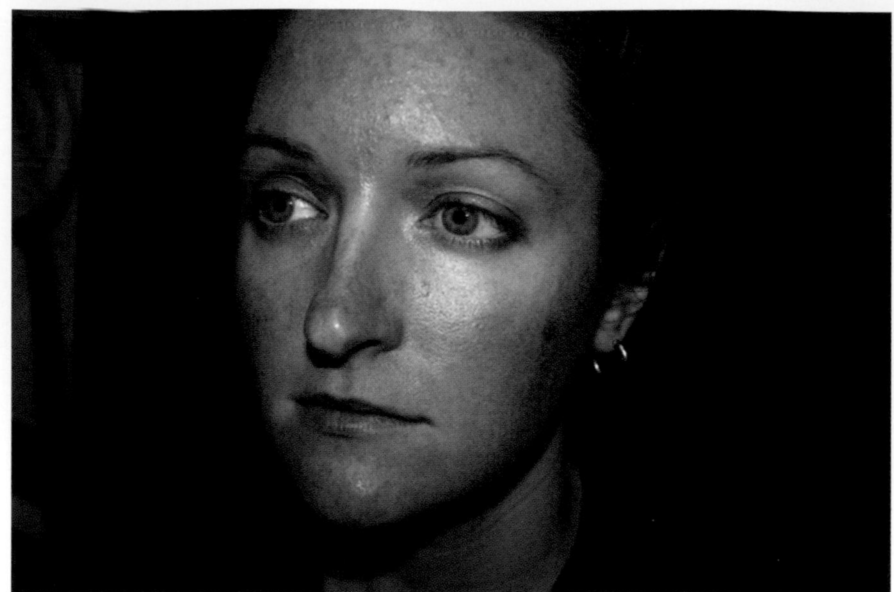

▲ **FIGURE 9-8** This patient is an OS^2NW skin type (the S^2 means "rosacea type"). She has light eyes and skin and does not tan easily. She has facial flushing and redness. Those of Irish and English ancestry often have this skin type. Skin care should be geared toward treating inflammation with anti-inflammatory cleansers and serums containing ingredients such as feverfew, green tea, caffeine, and licorice extract. Topical azelaic acid or metronidazole are good adjuncts. Oral antibiotics may be necessary. This Baumann Skin Type should avoid chemical peels, facial scrubs, and microdermabrasion, which can increase skin sensitivity. IPL and vascular laser are ideal for this skin type.

Finally, it is recommended that individuals take a baseline BSTI questionnaire and retake the test at times of stress, change, or when experiencing cutaneous symptoms because skin types are not necessarily static. Skin type alterations can be elicited by stress or marked fluctuations in stress, pregnancy, menopause, exposure to variable climates or moving to a different climate, or various other significant exogenous or endogenous changes.

SUMMARY

Significant innovation and exponential growth have characterized the skin care product market since the days of Helena Rubinstein and Elizabeth Arden. Now the plethora of skin care products on the market is overwhelming. The marketing claims by companies are often exaggerated and confusing. The BSTI, a self-administered questionnaire to determine the BST, can be used to simultaneously collect data and provide accurate skin care product and procedure recommendations. The BSTI assesses skin according to four dichotomous spectra, oily or dry, sensitive or resistant, pigmented or non-pigmented, and wrinkled or tight (unwrinkled), yielding a four-letter code for skin type. Each letter of the skin type designation indicates an individual's tendency to develop that skin concern. A patient's BSTI score provides physicians and aestheticians with substantial information that can facilitate recommending the most suitable OTC topical skin care formulations and dermatologic procedures for that patient. The BSTI score also enables the individual consumer to make more informed decisions in selecting the most appropriate topical treatments for their skin type. Most cutaneous needs of the 16 skin types can be met by the wide array of available topical skin products and dermatologic procedures available on the market. Support for aestheticians, physicians, and patients using the system can be found at www.skintypesolutions.com.

REFERENCES

1. Tsao A. The changing face of skin care. *Business Week* online, November 30, 2004. http://www.businessweek.com/bwdaily/dnflash/nov2004/nf20041130_0962_db035.htm. Accessed January 18, 2008.
2. Packaged Facts Web site. http://www.packagedfacts.com/ type care-market-c1554/. Accessed January 18, 2008.
3. Baumann L: *The Skin Type Solution*. New York, NY: Bantam Dell; 2005.
4. Baumann L. Cosmetics and skin care. In: K Wolff K, Goldsmith L, Katz S, Gilchrest B, Paller A, Leffell D, eds. *Fitzpatrick's Dermatology in General Medicine*. 7th ed. New York, NY: McGraw-Hill; 2008:2357-2364.

CHAPTER 10

Oily Skin

Mohamed L. Elsaie, MD
Leslie Baumann, MD

Sebum production plays an important role in skin hydration by producing glycerol, which is necessary for an intact skin barrier. In addition, sebum supplies lipids to the surface of the epidermis that may aid in preventing transepidermal water loss (TEWL) (see Chapter 11). Excess sebum production produces oily skin, and in many cases, contributes to acne. With continuing advances in understanding the physiology and molecular biochemistry of sebaceous glands (SGs) and lipid metabolism, dermatologists may soon be able to elucidate the underlying aspects of sebum secretion and oily skin. This chapter will focus on the various known causes of oily skin and their implications, a new classification approach for determining the oily skin type, and the available treatments for oily skin as well as the efficacy of these treatments.

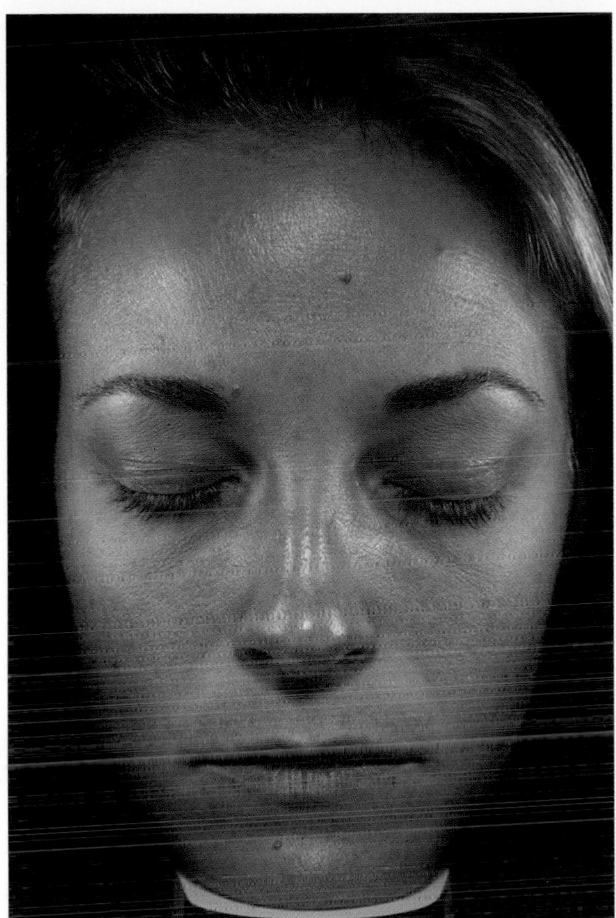

▲ **FIGURE 10-1** Oily skin often appears shiny in the T-zone area in photographs.

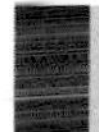

COSMETIC IMPLICATIONS OF OILY SKIN

Oily skin is a common complaint,[1-7] especially in the adolescent age group.[2] Those with moderate to severe oily skin complain of having to wash their face several times a day, looking shiny a few hours after washing, frequent streaking of facial foundation, and an inability to find a sunscreen that does not worsen perceived skin oiliness. These features of oily skin are disturbing to women and men alike and are perceived to be a serious cosmetic problem leading to a negative self-perception and possibly affecting social interactions. Clinically, oily skin presents as lipid-laden secretions resulting in a shiny appearance mostly over the T-zone area (forehead, nose, and chin)[4] (Fig. 10-1). SGs become large leading to a condition known as sebaceous hyperplasia, which is characterized by 0.5 to 1.5 mm umbilicated papules found in the T-zone area of the face (Fig. 10-2). In addition, many patients with oily skin complain of large pores.[8]

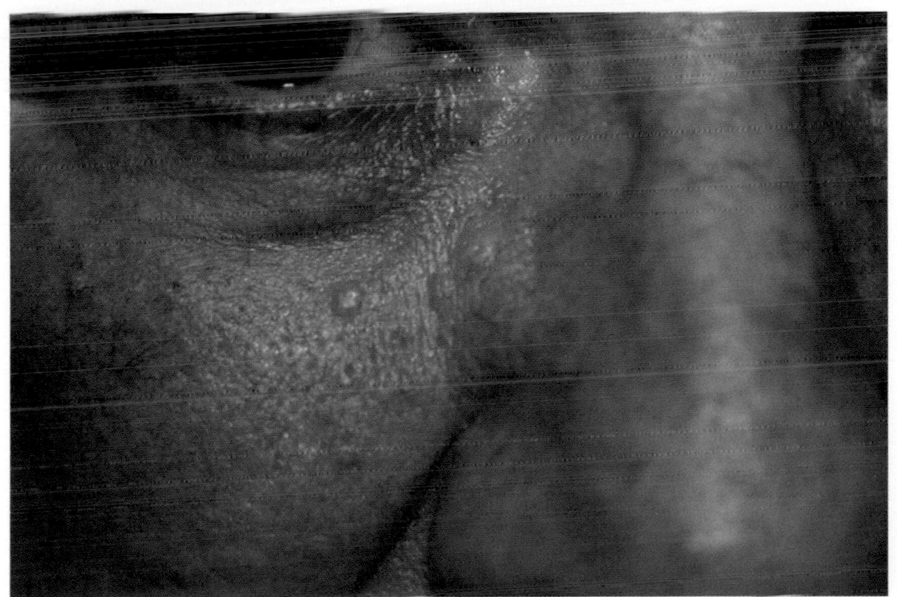

▲ **FIGURE 10-2** Sebaceous hyperplasias are enlarged oil glands that look like a small papule with a central umbilication. They can be confused with basal cell carcinoma.

SEBACEOUS GLANDS

SGs are uni- or multilobular entities usually associated with hair follicles that, with hair follicles, form a structure known as the pilosebaceous unit. The number of SGs remains approximately the same throughout life, whereas their size tends to increase with age. SGs vary in size and are located throughout the body except the palms and soles. The highest concentration of SGs is found on the face and scalp, but few are found on the lips. (This is important because the lips have lower vitamin E levels than the rest of the face because of the lack of sebum.) Although they are most frequently associated with hair follicles, SGs are found in some nonhair-bearing or glabrous areas such as the eyelids, where they are called "meibomian glands" (Table 10-1).

Functions of Sebum

The exact function of sebum is not fully understood. Current knowledge indicates that the functions of the SG are more complex than previously thought. Sebum is now known to play important roles in the three-dimensional organization of skin surface lipids (SSL), the glycerol production necessary for skin hydration, and as an occlusive moisturizing agent. Sebum protects the skin against oxidative stress because it contains vitamin E, a powerful antioxidant.[9] Moreover, sebum also exhibits innate antimicrobial activity because it contains IgG, which is thought to help prevent infection.[10] Similarly, the active cells of the sebaceous gland, sebocytes, express both pro- and anti-inflammatory properties, are able to utilize cholesterol as a substrate for complete steroidogenesis, present a regulatory program for neuropeptides, and selectively control the action of hormones and xenobiotics on the skin. The importance of both the SG and sebum production in skin homeostasis is further evidenced by the numerous skin disorders associated with their aberrant activity.[11–18] Of course, the most common of such disorders is acne (Table 10-2).

TABLE 10-2
Sebaceous Gland Functions

- Production of sebum[11]
- Integrity of skin barrier[12]
- Regulation of steroidogenesis[12–14]
- Expression of pro- and anti-inflammatory properties[12,17,18]
- Selective control on the action of cutaneous hormones[13]
- Regulation of neuropeptides[15]
- Transports antioxidants to skin surface in the form of vitamin E[16]
- Protects keratinocytes against UVB irradiation[16]
- Innate antimicrobial activity[10]

SG Count

SG count can reach as high as 400 to 900 glands per cm^2 on the face and less than 100 glands per cm^2 elsewhere in the body.[19] Several studies have used different techniques to evaluate SG count. Early studies that documented SG numbers used either of two techniques: the indirect or the direct. Benfenati and Brilliantini,[20] in their earliest study in 1939, and Powell and Beveridge,[21] in 1970, used the indirect technique. The number of lipid-producing orifices per cm^2 of skin surface was measured using osmium tetroxide at room temperature to visualize the small areas of lipids on a collecting paper left over the skin surface for 7 minutes. Adding the osmium tetroxide produced tiny black spots that were counted under a dissecting microscope. The direct technique was used by Cunliffe et al. in 1974 using a surface microscope.[22] They used a technique that involved staining the skin with Oil Red O (a lipophilic stain) and visualizing with a Leitz MZ surface microscope, which had a graticule attached to the eyepiece allowing the diameter of the pilosebaceous duct exit to be measured. A summary of the techniques and results is displayed in Table 10-3. As stated above, the number of SGs remains almost constant throughout life, whereas the size tends to increase with age.

TABLE 10-4
Composition of Human Sebum Compared to Epidermal Lipids

Lipid	Sebum Weight (%)	Epidermal Surface Lipid Weight (%)
Triglycerides, diglycerides, and free fatty acids	57	65
Wax esters	26	–
Squalene	12	–
Cholesterol	2	20

Sebaceous Structure and Secretion

Synthesis and discharge of the lipid content of the sebocytes takes more than a week. The turnover of SGs is slower in older individuals than in young adults. The SG is composed of two types of cells: the lipid-producing cells (sebocytes) and the stratified squamous cells lining the ductal epithelium. Sebocytes pass through three stages to attain a full mature size, namely, the undifferentiated, differentiating, and mature stages. As the sebocytes pass through the different maturation stages, the sebaceous cells increase in size because of accumulation of lipids and may undergo a 100- to 150-fold increase in volume.[24] The secretion mechanism of SGs is holocrine via rupture of individual sebocytes releasing the sebum,[25] which is discussed below. Sebum is the excretory product of the SGs. It is a mixture of nonpolar lipids synthesized by the SGs. Human sebum contains cholesterol, cholesterol esters, fatty acids, diglycerides, and triglycerides in addition to two constituents that are unique to sebum and not produced anywhere else in the body: wax esters and squalene[26–29] (Table 10-4 for the composition of human sebum as compared to other epidermal surface lipids).

TABLE 10-1[5,12]
Sebaceous Glands Found in Nonhairy Areas of the Skin

Location	Name
Eyelids	Meibomian glands
Nipples	Montgomery's glands
Genitals	Tyson's glands
Oral epithelium	Fordyce's spots

TABLE 10-3
Number of SGs per cm^2 of Skin in the Forehead of the Human Body

Study and Year	Number of Subjects	Number of SGs per cm^2	Technique Used for Sebaceous Count
Benfenati and Brilliantini[20]	4	560 ± 42	Indirect (osmium tetroxide)
Powell and Beveridge[21]	10	518 ± 91	Indirect (osmium tetroxide)
Cunliffe et al.[23]	120	334 ± 20	Direct (surface microscope)

Quantitative Evaluation of Sebum

As a determinant of the oiliness and greasiness of skin, evaluation of sebum has long been a target of interest. Sebum evaluation is performed on the skin surface; however, not all SSLs are sebum and, hence, understanding what SSLs are and taking them into consideration is crucial for an accurate estimation of sebum.

SSLs have a dual origin, resulting in a mixture of epidermal components (secreted by the mature corneocytes and composed mainly of cholesterol, cholestryl esters, triglycerols, ceramides, and hydrocarbons) and sebaceous components.[30] Because SSLs are not equally distributed over the surface of the body, the ratio of epidermal lipids to sebaceous lipids depends on the body region from which the sample is collected. In 1936, Emanuel reported regional variations of SSL concentrations in different regions of the body.[31] Body regions where the SSLs are comprised mainly of the sebaceous component (sebum) are the forehead, scalp, the upper part of the trunk, and thorax; the epidermal component only accounts for 3% to 6% in these areas, making such sites the most suitable for the evaluation of sebum parameters with minimal interference of epidermal lipids.[32–35]

Sebum quantities present on the skin surface may be as high as 100 to 500 μg/cm², compared with quantities as low as 25 to 40 μg/cm² of epidermal lipids.[31,33] Two parameters are used for measurement of sebum: *the casual level* and the *sebum excretion rate*. Both parameters express only quantitative information and do not give sebum qualitative (constituent) information, hence chromatographic techniques are required for subsequent constituent evaluation. A summary of both parameters is concisely highlighted in Table 10-5. Other significant evaluation parameters include the Sebum Replacement Time, Follicular Excretion Rate, and the sustainable Sebum Excretion Rate. (Box 10-1 for a summary of sebum collection techniques.)

TABLE 10-5
Parameters of Sebum Measurement

PARAMETER	CASUAL LEVEL	SEBUM EXCRETION RATE
Type of parameter	Static	Dynamic
Skin area involved	Done on untreated skin[36]	Sebum collected from degreased skin over a period of time[39]
Measurement	μg/cm²[2,37]	μg/cm²/min[36]
Requirement	Collection method to be fixed over skin for variable amounts of time sufficient to allow full greasing, e.g., forehead (5–6 h)[38]	Collection method fixed to skin; however, newer techniques of collection allow for rates to be obtained after 1 h[36]

BOX 10-1

Several sebum collection techniques have been used in studies based on the above parameters. Because of the large number of methods employed during more than 50 years of research, some of the methods that contributed to the basic knowledge of sebum are mentioned here; special attention should be focused on the newly developed techniques that meet the expectations of current and future research.

Extraction: The earliest sebum collection technique. Based on the dissolution of SSLs in an applied solvent to the skin, followed by the solvent evaporation and the lipid residue analysis.[40,41]

Cigarette paper techniques: Ether-soaked cigarette papers applied in four sheets on the forehead and kept in place by a rubber band. This was followed by gravimetric measurement of sebum.[40,42]

Sebutape method: A more accurate and faster technique using a polymer film for lipid absorption. The polymer tape absorbs SSLs and becomes transparent to light afterwards. Sebutape can be analyzed in many ways, the easiest of which is the visual scoring of the tapes on a 1 to 5 scale[43] (Fig. 10-3).

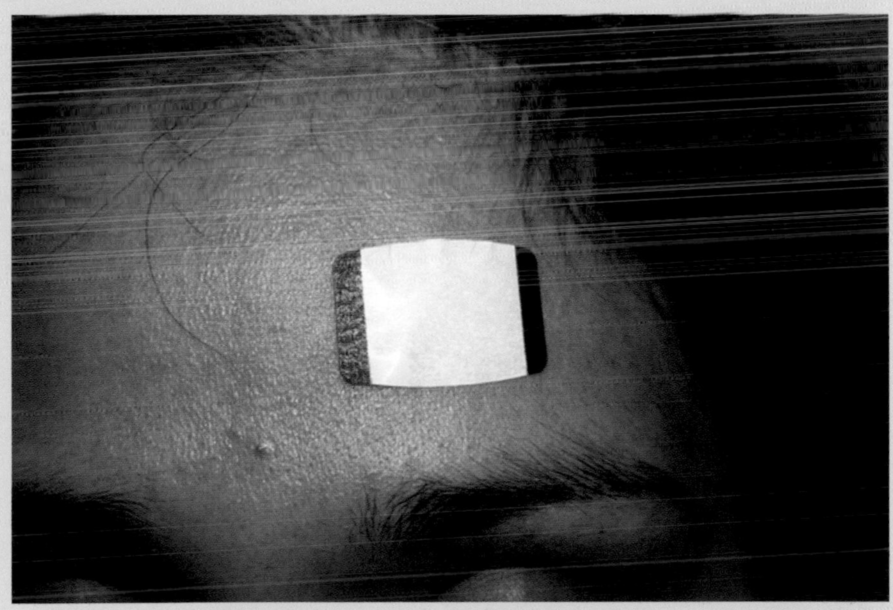

▲ **FIGURE 10-3** Sebutape being used to evaluate sebum excretion.

Lipometre: A photometric instrument designed by a group from L'Oréal that utilized a diode light energy for evaluation of sebum lipids that proved fast; however, proper calibration of the device is required for optimal results.[44]

Sebumeter: A more recent device to become commercially available. The measuring principle is based on increased transparency of a ground-glass slide after application of lipids. The sampling period is as short as 30

BOX 10-1 continued

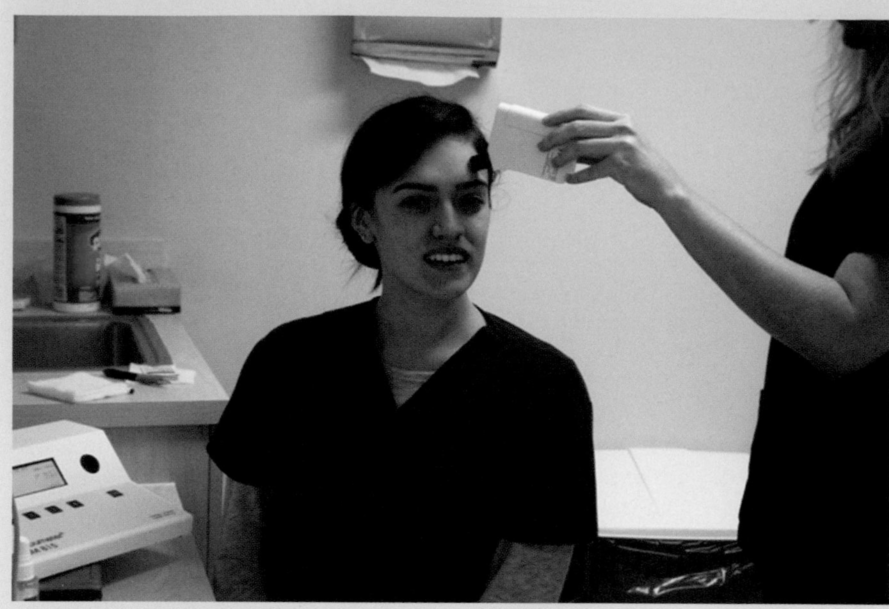

seconds. The device can be interfaced with a computer for data management[45] (Fig. 10-4).

In comparing the Lipometre with the Sebumeter, the latter is more practical. The Lipometre has to be washed between each application, whereas the Sebumeter procedure uses a new strip with each measurement. Moreover, the Sebumeter can be interfaced with a computer. The Sebumeter and Sebutape are both universally accepted as convenient instruments. Although these devices do not directly measure sebum, they are still useful as a research aid to extrapolate sebum levels.[46]

▲ **FIGURE 10-4** The Sebumeter provides a numeric value for sebum secretion.

FACTORS PREDISPOSING TO OILY SKIN

The exact mechanisms of sebum production have not been elucidated but the influential factors are thought to be multifactorial. Retinoids, hormones, and growth factors affect SG activity and differentiation. Androgens have long been thought to play a role in this process because sebum secretion increases when puberty begins and women with polycystic ovarian disease exhibit acne. Acne breakouts tend to occur right before a woman's menstrual cycle and a recent study showed that menstruation is accompanied by dilatation of the pilosebaceous ducts reaching its maximum during ovulation and exhibiting the maximum amount of sebum secretion.[8] However, the exact role of hormones in acne is confusing as studies are conflicting. Testosterone is not thought to be directly related to sebum secretion because although men have much higher levels of testosterone than women do, their sebum secretion rates are only slightly higher.[47] The weak androgen dihydroepiandrosterone sulfate (DHEAS) may play a role in acne. DHEAS is converted to testosterone by several enzymes that are found in the SGs, including type 1 5-α-reductase. However, a type 1 5-α-reductase inhibitor was not found to be effective in the treatment of acne.[48] Estrogens, insulin, glucocorticoids, and prolactin are also thought to influence SG function, but the mechanisms of action are poorly understood. Insulin growth factor-1 (IGF-1) expression is thought to play an important role in sebum production by stimulating SG lipogenesis.[49] IGF-1 increases expression of a transcription factor called sterol response element-binding protein-1 (SREBP-1). SREBP-1 regulates numerous genes involved in lipid biosynthesis and its expression stimulates lipogenesis in sebocytes.[50] Several recently discovered receptors such as the liver X receptors (LXRs) and the peroxisome proliferator-activated receptors (PPARs) have been shown to influence lipid metabolism and increase sebum production by such receptor agonists.[51,52] As research technologies improve, more insight into the processes that govern sebum secretion will likely be gleaned.

STRESS AND SEBUM PRODUCTION

In early 1972, stress was shown to be associated with an increase in the amount of free fatty acids on the skin.[53] Since then, much work has been accomplished to evaluate the role of stress in sebum production and acne. Corticotropin-releasing hormone (CRH), also known as a stress hormone, has been found in the SGs as has its receptor CRH-R.[54] CRH directly induces lipid synthesis and enhances the conversion of DHEAS to testosterone in sebocytes.[13,15] It is thought to play an important role in the link between stress and sebum production.[55] The SG also possesses receptors for substance P, which is a neuromediator released in response to stress.[56] In vitro, substance P stimulates sebaceous secretion.[57] It is postulated that substance P plays a role in acne as a response to stress.

SEBUM AND GENETICS

Interestingly, sebum production is also affected by genetic make up. In 1989, Walton et al. suggested in one study that acne development is *mediated* by genetic factors and only *modified* by environmental factors.[58] Their study of 20 pairs of homozygous twins versus 20 pairs of heterozygous twins demonstrated equal sebum excretion in the 20 identical pairs; however, the identical twins exhibited different acne severity showing an environmental influence in acne development. Conversely, the acne severity and sebum excretion parameters in the 20 nonidentical pairs of twins were significantly different. This study suggested that sebum excretion is under genetic control, but that environmental factors play a role in acne development. In 2002, a study that examined 458 pairs of monozygotic twins and 1099 pairs of dizygotic twins implied a strong genetic component in acne.[59] This study did not consider sebum secretion rates; however, many studies have demonstrated increased sebum rates in acne patients.[60]

Predominance of an allele of the gene cytochrome P450 has been recently reported in patients with hyperseborrhea. Cytochrome P450 is a large supergene family of enzymes involved in the metabolism of a wide range of endogenous and foreign compounds. A mutation of cytochrome P450 could lead to accelerated degradation of natural retinoids, which could cause disordered SG maturation and secretion leading to oily skin.[61]

More recently, B lymphocyte-induced maturation protein 1 (Blimp1), a transcription factor, was identified within the cells of the sebaceous glands. One study revealed that Blimp1 acted by repressing c-myc gene expression in mice. Mice without Blimp1 c-myc expression demonstrated an increased number of sebaceous gland-containing cells that divided more frequently. Moreover, these SGs were enlarged, which in turn enhanced the numbers of sebum producing sebocytes. The Blimp1-containing cells were shown to be the progenitors for the entire sebaceous gland, and Blimp1 somehow controls this progenitor population, regulating how many cells are allowed into the gland. Blimp1 is thought to act as an inhibitor for SG formation and secretion through repressing the c-myc gene. This study strongly supports the genetic basis of sebum secretion rates.[62,63]

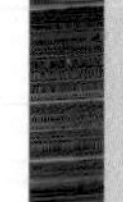

SUBJECTIVE VERSUS OBJECTIVE MEASUREMENTS OF SKIN OILINESS

When consumers shop for skin care products, they are often faced with choosing among products designed and marketed for oily, combination, or dry skin. They are obligated to determine their skin's barrier status and sebum secretion rates without any available objective measurements. In other words, they are forced to guess their skin type. Such subjective classification is often incorrect. One study enrolled 94 women for skin-type evaluation and compared the findings with the subjects' own preconceived skin types. The results showed that the subjective skin type does not match the amount of sebum secreted. The amounts of sebum secretion measured by the Sebumeter were relatively higher than what was expected by the study subjects. Moreover, for those who preconceived their skin type as dry, their skin type was determined to be oily by using the Sebumeter.[64] As mentioned above, patients' estimation of their skin type is subject to many biases. In addition, seasonal variations in sebum secretion can confuse the issue.[65]

Simple characterization, such as oily, dry, combination, and sensitive, based on subjective assessments is not a very useful tool for classifying skin types. The data available on the various skin types by the early skin classification systems have been inconsistent. No one system of classification was able to identify any prevalence or characterization of a specific skin type.[1] In 2005, a novel approach for assessment and categorization of skin types was published. This method utilizes a validated questionnaire, known as the Baumann Skin Type Indicator (BSTI), to determine skin type[66] (see Chapter 9).

THE BAUMANN SKIN TYPING SYSTEM AND DETERMINING OILY SKIN

The BSTI is a comprehensive, self-administered questionnaire divided into four parts. The first part of the questionnaire determines the occurrence and severity of oily skin based on historical data. Answers for each of the 11 questions are translated into a point system and accordingly the skin type is designated as either an oily (O) or a dry (D) type and assigned a score that determines severity of oiliness or dryness (Fig. 10-5).

BSTS and Ethnic Skin Variations

Many endogenous and exogenous factors, as indicated earlier, are known to affect sebum secretion and skin oiliness. Ethnic differences in sebum secretion have not been well studied. Most of the available reports on oily skin are based on the Caucasian human model; therefore, less is known about sebum secretion in darker skin types. In spite of this, many myths abound that darker skin types have increased sebum secretion. In the few studies performed, this has not been shown to be the case. One study by Grimes et al. compared instrumental measurements for sebum, pH, corneometry (skin moisture), or transepidermal water loss (barrier function) and found no difference between African Americans and Caucasians.[67]

A recent study at the University of Miami used the BSTS to look for ethnic differences in skin type. This unpublished study included 399 subjects of four different ethnic groups: Caucasians, African Americans, Hispanics, and Asians. Categorization of skin type according to the BSTS was used and each of the study subjects was designated a skin type. The percentage of oily skin subjects among each ethnic group was in ascending manner: Caucasians (47.13%), Hispanics (55.88%), Asians (57.70%), and African Americans (61.9%). This study was the first to use the BSTS to compare ethnic differences and demonstrates some variability in skin types by ethnicity. Although it reports an increased incidence of oily skin among African Americans, it is important to realize that all subjects were being treated in a general dermatology clinic in Miami and therefore may not be representative of the general population.

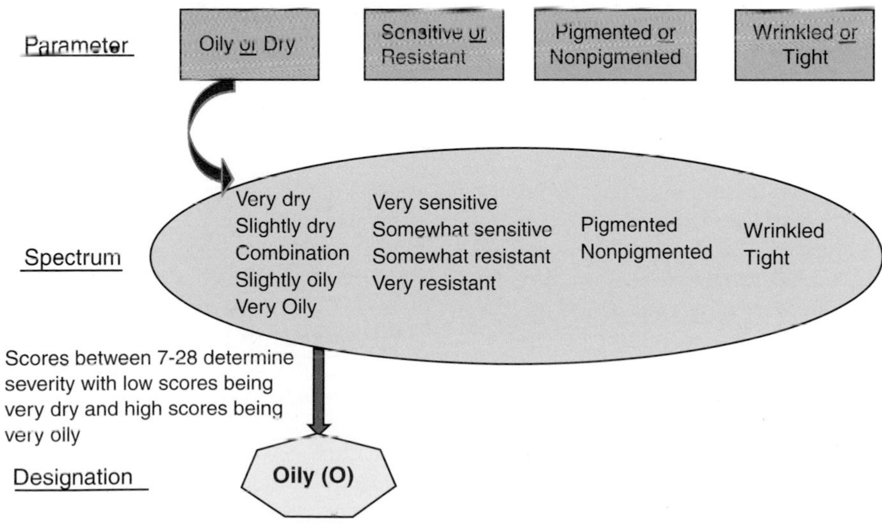

▲ **FIGURE 10-5** The BSTI is used to determine whether skin is very dry, slightly dry, combination, slightly oily, or very oily.

Other studies have shown black subjects to have 60% to 70% more lipids in their hair compared with white subjects. Another study suggested an increased pore number and sebaceous secretion among African Americans compared to other racial groups.[68] Ethnic skin differences in skin lipids remain inconclusive given the discrepancies in study results. Despite the paucity of available data on ethnic skin differences and surface lipid variations among different ethnic groups, the majority of available studies suggest an existing disparity in skin of color as compared to lighter skin tones. Further research is needed to be able to identify the exact areas of differences in order to develop optimum regimens for targeting ethnic skin conditions.

CHANGE IN SEBUM PARAMETERS IN PATIENTS WITH ACNE

It is generally and scientifically accepted that the severity of acne correlates, and is directly proportional, to the sebum secretion level.[69] However, the correlation of sebum excretion rates and acne has been a subject of debate since the early 1960s when Fry and Ramsay measured sebum excretion in 17 acne patients and reported that there was no direct relation of the sebum excretion rate to acne severity.[70] Cunliffe and Shuster, using a better collection technique in the late 1960s, demonstrated that sebum excretion is directly related to the severity of acne.[71] Many recent studies have indicated that sebum levels are indeed higher in the acne population. Piérard et al. demonstrated a higher overall sebum excretion rate in acne subjects when studying it on the forehead using the Lipometre.[5] Piérard-Franchimont et al. noted a change in the rate of sebum excretion directly proportional to the severity of acne.[72] Harris et al. used disks of fine Dacron mesh embedded in fresh clay to report that inflammatory acne patients had a higher sustainable rate of sebum excretion.[73] Recently, Kim et al. confirmed increased sebum secretion rates in subjects with acne using the Sebumeter in a study on 36 Asian patients.[74] However, it is important to realize that even though acne is associated with high sebum rates, all patients with high sebum rates do not develop acne. Patients with high sebum rates and no acne are classified as oily resistant types in the BSTS (see Chapter 9).

Acne vulgaris is a disease of the pilosebaceous unit. Acne is a multifactorial condition with distinct pathologic factors including increased sebum production, ductal hypercornification, colonization of ducts by *Propionibacterium acnes* (*P. acnes*), and inflammation.[2] For a full review on acne vulgaris, refer to Chapter 15. PPARs α, β, and γ may play a role in acne and increased sebum production. These receptors have been identified in sebocytes, with the γ form being the most important. Free fatty acids, linoleic acid, and androgens activate these receptors, which bind to RXR retinoid receptors (in the formation of heterodimers) inducing modifications of sebocyte proliferation and differentiation as well as the synthesis of free fatty acids. PPARs are therefore involved in the maturation of the SGs and initiation of the inflammatory reaction in acne. The PPARs present in the SGs of hyperseborrheic patients are at a higher level, suggesting a disordered effect on the natural retinoids and leading to the development of acne.[68]

SEASONAL SKIN TYPE: MYTH OR REALITY?

Many patients self-report seasonal variability in self-perceived "oily skin." Strauss et al. suggested that there is no evidence for seasonal changes in SG activity, although the skin may appear oilier in hot weather because of changes in the viscosity of SSLs, making the skin feel oilier.[19] In addition, sebum excretion rates have been shown to be increased with exposure to higher temperatures; however, this measure may reflect a change in sebum collection methods (increased uptake of sebum on collection paper) used to measure sebum production rather than an actual increase in sebum production.[75] In 2005, Youn et al. observed regional and seasonal variations in sebum secretion that led to changes of skin type from dry to oily, resulting in what they termed a "combination skin type."[65] This was the first study to show sebum changes throughout different seasons. Forty-six patients were included in the study and their sebum secretion was measured over an entire year. They reported that summer was the only season in which a significant increase in sebum secretion was seen. In addition, a reduction in the dry skin type and an increase in the oily type based on their categorization system was recorded in the summer.

SEBOSUPPRESSIVE AGENTS

Topical Agents

Although many products claim to inhibit sebum production, very few, if any, have been conclusively proven to work. Most oil control products on the market contain talc and other oil-absorbing components that mask or absorb oil rather than function as sebum production inhibitors. Antiandrogens such as ketoconazole and spironolactone have shown some effects.[76,77] Progesterone has demonstrated a short-term effect (2–3 months) when applied topically in women. However, it has not reduced sebum excretion rates in men.[78] Corticosteroids, erythromycin-zinc complex, elubiol (dichlorophenyl imidazoldioxolan), and recently an extract from saw palmetto, sesame seeds, and argan oil have all been used for this purpose.[79–82] Notably, topical retinoids have not been shown to decrease sebum secretion.[83]

Systemic Agents

The most potent pharmacologic inhibitor of sebum secretion is the retinoid isotretinoin (13-*cis* retinoic acid). Reductions in sebum excretion rates can be reduced by 90% as early as 2 weeks after initiating treatment with isotretinoin. Its exact mechanism of action has not been fully described or understood yet, but histologically it shrinks the SG size and the sebocytes lose their characteristic interior accumulation of lipids.[2,84] Hypothesized mechanisms of action of 13-*cis* retinoic acid in reducing sebum are listed in Table 10-6.

In-office Procedures

In a 2006 study, chemical peels using 30% glycolic acid solution and Jessner's solution were not shown to decrease

TABLE 10-6
Hypothesized Mechanisms by Which Isotretinoin Suppresses Sebum

Affect on the cell cycle progression, differentiation, cell survival, and apoptosis by inhibiting G1/S phase of cell cycle and inhibiting DNA synthesis.[84]
Inhibition of 3-alpha-hydroxysteroid activity of retinol dehydrogenase leading to decreased steroid in vivo synthesis.[2]
It may act in a receptor-independent manner, influencing cellular signaling pathways by either direct protein interactions, as demonstrated with other retinoids, or by enzyme inhibition.[85]

sebum secretion rates as measured by a Sebumeter.[86] Photodynamic therapy using blue light and 5-ALA (aminolevulinic acid) failed to demonstrate changes in sebum excretion rates, although improvement was observed in ace lesions, as reported in 2007.[87] Microdermabrasion has not been shown to decrease sebum excretion rates. Further, it is important for practitioners and patients alike to understand that at this time, there are no known in-office procedures that reduce sebum excretion rates.

SUMMARY

Oily skin is not an uncommon condition. It presents in varying degrees in both men and women. Excessive sebum secretion (hyperseborrhea) is influential in the ascertainment of skin type. The condition ranges from a mild cosmetic burden to a true skin disease manifesting as acne. Improvements in genetic research, objective skin typing, and more accurate measurement of sebum levels will lead to an enhanced understanding of sebum and the mechanisms that affect its excretion rates.

REFERENCES

1. Nouveau-Richard S, Zhu W, Li YH, et al. Oily skin: specific features in Chinese women. *Skin Res Technol.* 2007; 13:43.
2. Clarke SB, Nelson AM, George RE, et al. Pharmacologic modulation of sebaceous gland activity: mechanisms and clinical applications. *Dermatol Clin.* 2007;25:137.
3. Chicq FS, Zaouati DC, Wolkenstein P, et al. Development and validation of a questionnaire to evaluate how a cosmetic product for oily skin is able to improve well-being in women. *J Eur Acad Dermatol Venereol.* 2007;21:1181.
4. Thiboutot D. Regulation of human sebaceous glands. *J Invest Dermatol.* 2004;123:1.
5. Piérard G, Piérard-Franchimont C, Lê T, et al. Patterns of follicular sebum excretion rate during lifetime. *Arch Dermatol Res.* 1987;279:S104.
6. Daniel F. The seborrheic skin. *Rev Prat.* 1985;35:3215.
7. Lasek RJ, Chren MM. Acne vulgaris and the quality of life of adult dermatology patients. *Arch Dermatol.* 1998;134:454.
8. Roh M, Han M, Kim D, et al. Sebum output as a factor contributing to the size of facial pores. *Br J Dermatol.* 2006;155:890.
9. Thiele JJ, Weber SU, Packer L. Sebaceous gland secretion is a major physiologic route of vitamin E delivery to skin. *J Invest Dermatol.* 1999;113:1006.
10. Gebhart W, Metze D, Jurecka W. Identification of secretory immunoglobulin A in human sweat and sweat glands. *J Invest Dermatol.* 1989;92:648.
11. Zouboulis CC, Fimmel S, Ortmann J, et al. Sebaceous glands. In: Hoath SB, Maibach HI, eds. *Neonatal Skin:Structure and Function.* New York, NY: Marcel Dekker; 2003:59-88.
12. Zouboulis CC. Human skin: an independent peripheral endocrine organ. *Horm Res.* 2005;54:230.
13. Fritsch M, Orfanos CE, Zouboulis CC. Sebocytes are the key regulators of androgen hemostasis in human skin. *J Invest Dermatol.* 2001;116:793.
14. Thiboutot D, Jabara S, McAllister JM, et al. Human skin is a steroidogenic tissue. *J Invest Dermatol.* 2003;120:905.
15. Zouboulis CC, Seltmann H, Hiroi N, et al. Corticotropin-releasing hormone: an autocrine hormone that promotes lipogenesis in human sebocytes. *Proc Natl Acad Sci U S A.* 2002;99:7148.
16. Zouboulis CC. Acne and sebaceous gland function. *Clin Dermatol.* 2004;22: 360.
17. Zouboulis CC. Is acne vulgaris a genuine inflammatory disease? *Dermatology.* 2001;203:277.
18. Bohm M, Schiller M, Stander S, et al. Evidence of expression of melanocortin-1 receptor in human sebocytes in vitro and in situ. *J Invest Dermatol.* 2002; 118:533.
19. Strauss J, Downing FJ, Ebling ME, Stewart ME. Sebaceous glands. In: Goldsmith LA, ed. *Physiology Biochemistry and Molecular Biology of the Skin.* New York. NY: Oxford University Press; 1991:712-740.
20. Benfenati A, Brilliantini F. Solla distribuzione delle ghiandole sabacee nella cute del corpho humano. *Arch Ital Derm Siflogr Venereal.* 1939;15:33.
21. Powell E, Beveridge GW. Sebum excretion and sebum composition in adolescent men with and without acne vulgaris. *Br J Dermatol.* 1970,82:243.
22. Cunliffe WJ, Forster RA, Williams M. A surface microscope for clinical and laboratory use. *Br J Dermatol.* 1974;90:619.
23. Cunliffe WJ, Perera WD, Thackray P, et al. Pilosebaceous duct physiology. *Br J Dermatol.* 1976;97:153.
24. Tosti A. A comparison of the histodynamics of sebaceous glands and epidermis in man: a microanatomic and morphometric study. *J Invest Dermatol.* 1974; 62:147.
25. Jenkinson D, McEwan HY, Elder I, et al. Comparative studies of the ultrastructure of the sebaceous gland. *Tissue Cell.* 1985;17:683.
26. Rajaratnam RA, Gylling H, Miettinen TA. Serum squalene in postmenopausal women with and without coronary artery disease. *Atherosclerosis.* 1999;146: 61.
27. Pochi PE, Strauss JS, Downing DT. Age-related changes in sebaceous gland activity. *J Invest Dermatol.* 1979;73:108.
28. Stewart ME, Downing DT. Proportions of various straight and branched fatty acid chain types in the sebaceous wax esters of young children. *J Invest Dermatol.* 1985;84:501.
29. Stewart ME, Quinn MA, Downing DT. Variability in the fatty acid composition of wax esters from vernix caseosa and its possible relation to sebaceous gland activity. *J Invest Dermatol.* 1982;78:291.
30. Clarys P, Barel A. Quantitative evaluation of skin surface lipids. *Clin Dermatol.* 1995;13:307.
31. Saint-Léger D. Quantification of skin surface lipids and skin flora. In: Leveque JL, ed. *Cutaneous Investigation in Health and Disease: Non-invasive Methods and Instrumentations.* New York, NY: Basel, Marcel Dekker; 1989:153-182.
32. Blume U, Ferracin J, Verschoore M, et al. Physiology of the vellus hair follicle: hair growth and sebum excretion. *Br J Dermatol.* 1991;124:21.
33. Greene RS, Downing DT, Pochi PE, et al. Anatomical variation in the amount and composition of human skin surface lipid. *J Invest Dermatol.* 1970;54:240.
34. Vantrou M, Venencie PY, Chaumeil JC. Skin surface lipids in man: origins, synthesis and regulation. *Ann Dermatol Venereol.* 1987;114:1115.
35. Verschoore M. Hormonal aspects of acne. *Ann Dermatol Venereol.* 1987;114: 439.
36. Saint-Leger D, Cohen E. Practical study of qualitative and quantitative sebum excretion on the human forehead. *Br J Dermatol.* 1985;113:551.
37. Muti P, Celentano E, Panico S, et al. Measurement of cutaneous sebum: reproduceability at different cleansing conditions. *J Appl Cosmetol.* 1987;5:131.
38. Saint-Leger D, Leveque JL. A comparative study of refatting kinetics on the scalp and forehead. *Br J Dermatol.* 1982;106:669.
39. Cunliffe WJ, Shuster S. The rate of sebum excretion in man. *Br J Dermatol.* 1969;81:697.
40. Piérard GE, Piérard-Franchimont C, Marks R, et al. EEMCO guidance for the in vivo assessment of skin greasiness. *Skin Pharmacol Appl Skin Physiol.* 2000;13:372.
41. Lavrijsen AP, Higounenc IM, Weerheim A. Validation of an in vivo extraction method for human stratum corneum ceramides. *Arch Dermatol Res.* 1994;286: 495.
42. Chivot M, Zeziola F, Saurat JH. The rate of sebum excretion in man. A study on the reproducibility and the accuracy of the gravimetric method. *Br J Dermatol.* 1981;105:701.
43. Serup J. Formation of oiliness and sebum output–comparison of a lipid-absorbant and occlusive-tape method with photometry. *Clin Exp Dermatol.* 1991;16:258.
44. Saint-Leger D, Berrebi C, Duboz C, et al. The lipometre: an easy tool for rapid quantitation of skin surface lipids (SSL) in man. *Arch Derm Res.* 1979;265:79.
45. Cunliffe WJ, Kearney JN, Simpson NB. A modified photometric technique for measuring sebum excretion rate. *J Invest Dermatol.* 1980;75:394.
46. Dikstein S, Zlotogorski A, Avriel E, et al. Comparison of sebumeter and lipometre. *Bioeng Skin.* 1987;3:197.
47. Nelson AM, Thiboutot DM. Biology of sebaceous glands. In: Wolff K, Goldsmith LA, Katz SI, Gilchrest BA, Paller AS, Leffell DJ, eds. *Fitzpatrick's Dermatology in General Medicine.* 7th ed. New York, NY: McGraw-Hill; 2007:689.
48. Leyden J, Bergfeld W, Drake L, et al. A systemic type 1 5 alpha-reductase inhibitor is ineffective in the treatment

of acne vulgaris. *J Am Acad Dermatol.* 2004;50:443.

49. Smith TM, Cong Z, Gilliland KL, et al. Insulin-like growth factor-1 induces lipid production in human SEB-1 sebocytes via sterol response element-binding protein-1. *J Invest Dermatol.* 2006;126:1226.
50. Smith TM, Gilliland K, Clawson GA, et al. IGF-1 induces SREBP-1 expression and lipogenesis in SEB-1 sebocytes via activation of the phosphoinositide 3-kinase/Akt pathway. *J Invest Dermatol.* 2007 Nov 8 [Epub ahead of print].
51. Schmuth M, Elias PM, Hanley K, et al. The effect of LXR activators on AP-1 proteins in keratinocytes. *J Invest Dermatol.* 2004;123:41.
52. Rosenfield RL, Kentsis A, Deplewski D, et al. Rat preputial sebocyte differentiation involves peroxisome proliferator-activated receptors. *J Invest Dermatol.* 1999;112:226.
53. Kraus SJ. Stress, acne and skin surface free fatty acids. *Psychosom Med.* 1970;32:503.
54. Kono M, Nagata H, Umemura S, et al. In situ expression of corticotropin-releasing hormone (CRH) and proopiomelanocortin (POMC) genes in human skin. *FASEB J.* 2001;15:2297.
55. Krause K, Schnitger A, Fimmel S, et al. Corticotropin-releasing hormone signaling is receptor-mediated and is predominant in the sebaceous glands. *Horm Metab Res.* 2007;39:166.
56. Singh LK, Pang X, Alexacos N, et al. Acute immobilization stress triggers skin mast cell degranulation via corticotropin releasing hormone, neurotensin, and substance P: a link to neurogenic skin disorders. *Brain Behav Immun.* 1999;13:225.
57. Toyoda M, Morohashi M. Pathogenesis of acne. *Med Elextron Microsc.* 2001;34:29.
58. Walton S, Wyatt EH, Cunliffe WJ. Genetic control of sebum excretion and acne—a twin study. *Br J Dermatol.* 1988;118:393.
59. Bataille V, Snieder H, MacGregor AJ, et al. The influence of genetics and environmental factors in the pathogenesis of acne: a twin study of acne in women. *J Invest Dermatol.* 2002;119:1317.
60. Stewart ME, Grahek MO, Cambier LS, et al. Dilutional effect of increased sebaceous gland activity on the proportion of linoleic acid in sebaceous wax esters and in epidermal acylceramides. *J Invest Dermatol.* 1986;87:733.
61. Paraskevaidis A, Drakoulis N, Roots I, et al. Polymorphisms in the human cytochrome P-450 1A1 gene (CYP1A1) as a factor for developing acne. *Dermatology.* 1998;196:171.
62. Horsley V, O'Carroll D, Tooze R, et al. Blimp1 defines a progenitor population that governs cellular input to the sebaceous gland. *Cell.* 2006;126:597.
63. Arnold I, Watt FM. c-Myc activation in transgenic mouse epidermis results in mobilization of stem cells and differentiation of their progeny. *Curr Biol.* 2001;11:558.
64. Youn SW, Kim SJ, Hwang IA, et al. Evaluation of facial skin type by sebum secretion: discrepancies between subjective descriptions and sebum secretion. *Skin Res Technol.* 2002;8:168.
65. Youn SW, Na JI, Choi SY, et al. Regional and seasonal variations in facial sebum secretions: a proposal for the definition of combination skin type. *Skin Res Technol.* 2005;11:189.
66. Baumann L. *The Skin Type Solution.* New York, NY: Bantam Dell; 2006.
67. Grimes P, Edison BL, Green BA, et al. Evaluation of inherent differences between African American and white skin surface properties using subjective and objective measures. *Cutis.* 2004;73:392.
68. Rawling AV. Ethnic skin types: are there differences in skin structure and function? *Int J Cosm Sci.* 2006;28:79.
69. Youn SW, Park ES, Lee DH, et al. Does facial sebum excretion really affect the development of acne? *Br J Dermatol.* 2005;153:919.
70. Fry L, Ramsay CA. Tetracycline in acne vulgaris. Clinical evaluation and the effect of sebum production. *Br J Dermatol.* 1966;78:653.
71. Cunliffe WJ, Shuster S. Pathogenesis of acne. *Lancet.* 1969;1:685.
72. Piérard-FranchimontC, Piérard GE, Saint-Léger D, et al. Comparison of the kinetics of sebum secretion in young women with and without acne. *Dermatologica.* 1991;183:120.
73. Harris HH, Downing DT, Stewart ME, et al. Sustainable rates of sebum secretion in acne patients and matched normal control subjects. *J Am Acad Dermatol.* 1983;8:200.
74. Kim MK, Choi SY, Byun HJ, et al. Comparison of sebum secretion, skin type, pH in humans with and without acne. *Arch Dermatol Res.* 2006;298:113.
75. Cunliffe WJ, Burton JL, Shuster S. The effect of local temperature variations on the sebum excretion rate. *Br J Dermatol.* 1970;83:650.
76. Brown M, Evans TW, Pyner T, et al. The role of ketoconazole 2% shampoo in the treatment and prophylactic management of dandruff. *J Dermatol Treat.* 1990;1:177.
77. Yamamoto A, Ito M. Topical spironolactone reduces sebum secretion rates in young adults. *J Dermatol.* 1996;23:243.
78. Simpson NB, Bowden PE, Forster RA, et al. The effect of topically applied progesterone on sebum excretion rate. *Br J Dermatol.* 1979;100:687.
79. Lévêque JL, Piérard-Franchimont C, de Rigal J, et al. Effect of topical corticosteroids on human sebum production assessed by two different methods. *Arch Dermatol Res.* 1991;283:372.
80. Piérard-Franchimont C, Goffin V, Visser JN, et al. A double-blind controlled evaluation of the sebosuppressive activity of topical erythromycin-zinc complex. *Eur J Clin Pharmacol.* 1995;49:57.
81. Piérard GE, Ries G, Cauwenbergh G. New insight into the topical management of excessive sebum flow at the skin surface. *Dermatology.* 1998;196:126.
82. Dobrev H. Clinical and instrumental study of the efficacy of a new sebum control cream. *J Cosmet Dermatol.* 2007;6:113.
83. Cunliffe WJ, Macdonald-Hull S. Lack of effect of topical retinoic acid on sebum excretion rate in acne. *Lancet.* 1988;2:503.
84. Nelson AM, Gilliland KL, Cong Z, et al. 13-cis Retinoic acid induces apoptosis and cell cycle arrest in human SEB-1 sebocytes. *J Invest Dermatol.* 2006;126:2178.
85. Sequin-Devaux C, Hanriot D, Dailloux M, et al. Retinoic acid amplifies the host immune response to LPS through increased T lymphocytes number and LPS binding protein expression. *Mol Cell Endocrinol.* 2005;245:67.
86. Lee SH, Huh CH, Park KC, et al. Effects of repetitive superficial chemical peels on facial sebum secretion in acne patients. *J Eur Acad Dermatol Venereol.* 2006;20:964.
87. Akaraphanth R, Kanjanawanitchkul W, Gritiyarangsan P. Efficacy of ALA-PDT vs blue light in the treatment of acne. *Photodermatol Photoimmunol Photomed.* 2007;23:186.

CHAPTER 11

Dry Skin

Leslie Baumann, MD

Dry skin, also known as xerosis, can be a congenital or acquired condition. It can be so mild that it is hardly noticed or so severe that it leads to skin breakdown, severe itching, and infection. Mild dry skin is a condition that affects many patients and is often a complaint of cosmetic patients in particular. Billions of dollars a year are spent worldwide on moisturizing skin care products. It is important, therefore, for the cosmetic dermatologist and cosmetic scientist to understand the underlying causes of dry skin and how current therapies treat this condition.

There are so many products on the market to treat skin dryness that one can become easily overwhelmed. This chapter will discuss what is known about the causes of dry skin with an eye toward elucidating issues that must be understood in order to identify the most effective products or the ones best suited to particular skin types.

WHAT IS DRY SKIN?

Dry skin is characterized by the lack of moisture in the stratum corneum (SC). Water is the major plasticizer of the skin, and when levels are low, cracks and fissures occur.[1] For the skin to appear and feel normal, the water content of the SC must be greater than 10%.[2] The increase in transepidermal water loss (TEWL) that leads to dry skin results when a defect in the permeability barrier allows excessive water to be lost to the atmosphere. This barrier perturbation is caused by several different factors such as harsh detergents, acetone and other contactants, and frequent bathing. When skin becomes too dry, the outer skin layers stiffen and may develop cracks. The cracks become fissures into the skin that become irritated, inflamed, and itchy. The condition is worse in areas of the body with relatively few oil glands such as the arms, legs, and trunk (Box 11-1).

Alterations in the epidermal lipid component of the skin can also cause xerosis. Some dermatologists believe that the incidence of dry skin has increased in recent years because people bathe and shower frequently using hot water, foaming cleansers, fragranced bubble baths, and bath salts, which impair the skin's barrier by stripping away important lipids. Soap, detergents, and hard water can wash off the healthy and normal barrier of the skin.

The preponderance of people who complain of having dry skin do not have an underlying disease but, rather, lack the ability to cope with environmental elements that adversely affect the water-binding capacity of the SC. Table 11-1 lists agents in the environment that can cause dry skin. Generally, as people age their skin tends to become drier and less oily. Dry skin occurs more during the fall and winter months because of low humidity and excessive bathing in hot water. Xerosis is often called "winter itch" because it is at its worst during that season.

BOX 11-1 Transepidermal Water Loss

Kligman discussed his observations on the efficiency of the epidermal water barrier as a structure to prevent TEWL in a text in 1964.[3] He described covering the orifice of an inverted vial of water with a sheet of SC. This sheet of SC tissue prevented water evaporation. TEWL is now used as a measure of the integrity of the SC. TEWL is defined as insensible water loss through the skin. It is not the same as active perspiration. TEWL is measured in two ways. The first is using a device called an evaporimeter, which calculates the gradient of the humidity at the skin's surface. The second way to gauge TEWL is to use devices that measure capacitance or conductance. Specifically, these devices measure the electrical capacitance in the skin that is altered by skin hydration. This is actually a measure of hydration of the SC rather than a measure of TEWL; however, the rate of water loss can be extrapolated using capacitance measurements. In order to increase the validity of the results, it is very important to perform both of these types of measurements in climate-controlled conditions with minimal air currents. Skin hydration is most accurately assessed using several methods including clinical correlation.

TABLE 11-1
Environmental Agents That Can Lead to Dry Skin

Hot water
Detergents
Friction from clothing
Frequent air travel
Pollution
Other chemicals
Air conditioning

Clinical Signs

The first clinical sign of skin dryness is a dull, gray white color and increased topographic skin markings[4] (Fig. 11-1). As the drying worsens, the loss of water causes a loss of cohesiveness between the corneocytes and abnormal retention of desmosomes. The edges of the corneocytes curl up much like shingles on a roof curl up in extremely arid conditions. The loosening of entire sheets of corneocytes results in scaling and flaking. The entire skin surface feels rough. Its appearance is dull because a rough surface is less able to refract light than a smooth surface. The skin may feel less pliable with stretching and bending; cracks and fissures can occur as a result of this reduced elasticity. Xerosis and impaired epidermal barrier can also be components in genetic disorders or conditions with genetic predisposition, including ichthyosis and atopic dermatitis (Box 11-2).

Dry or Oily Skin?

Many patients describe themselves as having either dry or oily skin. In reality, however, these two processes are not mutually exclusive. Dry skin is caused by a lack of moisture in the SC. Oily skin is caused by increased secretion of the sebaceous glands. It is possible to have dry skin on parts of the face and oily skin in the T-zone area. This is commonly called combination skin. In addition, one may have oily skin on the face and dry skin on the body because of a lack of sebaceous glands on the arms and legs.

ETIOLOGY OF DRY SKIN

Dry skin is a result of decreased water content in the SC, which leads to abnormal desquamation of corneocytes.[5] SC hydration is largely a property of corneocytes within the outer SC (stratum disjunctum), because corneocytes within the lower SC (stratum compactum) are relatively dehydrated and unable to absorb water when exposed to hypotonic

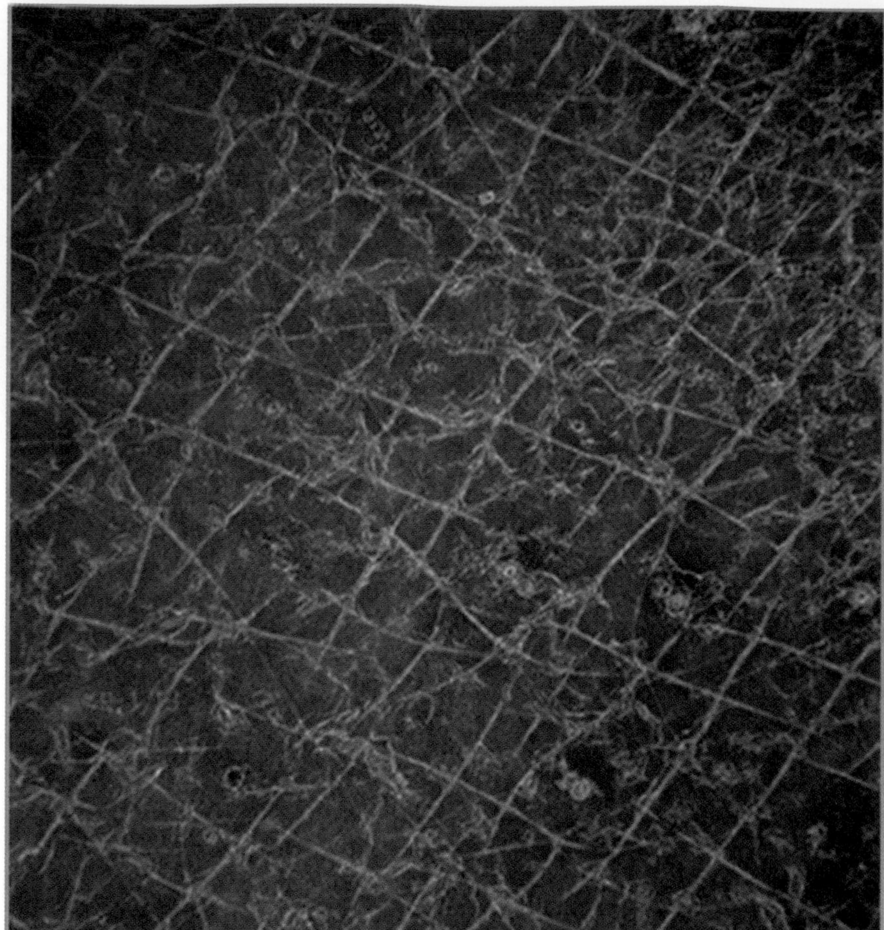

▲ **FIGURE 11-1** Dry skin exhibiting the characteristic overlying white scale.

BOX 11-2 Atopic Dermatitis

Atopic dermatitis is a multifactorial disorder characterized by dry skin. Multiple studies have suggested that an insufficiency of ceramides in the skin is an important pathophysiologic factor in this condition.[37] However, in a study that looked at patients with "xerosis," the deficiency in water-holding properties was not accompanied by an insufficiency of ceramides.[38] Researchers also found that sebum levels did not play a significant role in the etiology of xerosis when studied in atopic patients. They hypothesized that xerosis could be caused by an aberration of the lamellar structures of intracellular lipids in the SC.

Interestingly, mutations in the filaggrin gene have been described in patients with atopic dermatitis.[39,40] In fact, filaggrin mutation is the first strong genetic factor identified in atopic dermatitis. A defect in filaggrin would result in a structural cutaneous defect because it normally aggregates with keratin filaments in the stratum granulosum to form macrofilaments that impart strength to this layer.[41] In addition, a defect in filaggrin would lead to a decrease in NMF, a by-product of filaggrin that has hygroscopic properties. A decrease in secretions of lamellar bodies, which would lead to a decrease in fatty acids and ceramides, has been reported in atopic dermatitis patients.[42]

stress.[6,7] Rawlings et al. demonstrated that desmosomes remain intact at higher levels of the SC and desmoglein I levels remain elevated in the superficial SC of individuals with dry skin as compared to controls.[8] This occurs because the enzymes necessary for desmosome digestion are impaired when the water level is insufficient, which leads to abnormal desquamation resulting in visible "clumps" of corneocytes that cause the skin to appear rough and dry[9] (Fig. 11-2A and B). These clumps of corneocytes lead to the phenotype known as dry or scaled skin. In darker skin types, this perturbation of desquamation is associated with a grayish skin color and is labeled "ashy skin." Essentially, ashy skin is dry skin in a dark-skinned person.

The skin barrier resembles a brick and mortar type structure with the bricks representing the keratinocytes and the mortar mimicking the lipids that surround the keratinocytes in a protective coating. The lipids are arranged in lipid bilayers as illustrated in Figure 11-3. The skin barrier exhibits several important functions such as preventing evaporation of water, which is known as TEWL. The barrier also helps keep out unwanted compounds such as allergens and irritants. Injured barriers render one more susceptible to contact and irritant dermatitis. Lastly, the barrier displays a defensive role or mechanism against infections and this SC defense depends on corneocyte function and the surrounding extracellular matrix.[10]

THE SKIN BARRIER

Cornified Cell Envelope

The cornified cell (CE) envelope that encases the corneocyte is a 10-nm insoluble layer composed of several highly crossed proteins. Loricrin, the main component of this envelope, and other proteins such as involucrin, small proline-rich proteins, desmoplakin, and periplakin are cross-linked by the calcium (Ca^{2+})-dependent tranglutaminase 1 (TG-1) enzyme to form this structure.[11] Defects in CE envelope proteins or the TG-1 enzyme result in genetic disorders with impaired cornification, resulting in the phenotype of severely dry skin. Lamellar ichthyosis and Vohwinkel's syndrome are examples of TG-1 and loricrin defects, where impaired skin barrier is clearly present.

Extracellular Matrix and SC Lipids

The extracellular matrix surrounding the corneocyte is a lipid-rich component necessary for maintaining the epidermal barrier. Lamellar bodies that are secretory organelles located in the stratum granulosum play a key role in forming this lipid bilayer barrier by releasing their contents in the junction of the stratum granulosum and SC. They contain a mixture of lipids (ceramides, cholesterol, and fatty acids), lipid-processing enzymes, proteases (responsible for epidermal desquamation), and their inhibitors.

This extracellular lipid of the SC is well known to be responsible for that layer's water barrier function.[12] The lipid mixture that is delivered by lamellar bodies is composed of 50% ceramides, approximately 15% fatty acids, and approximately 25% cholesterol.[13] It has been stated that alterations in any of these three components can cause a

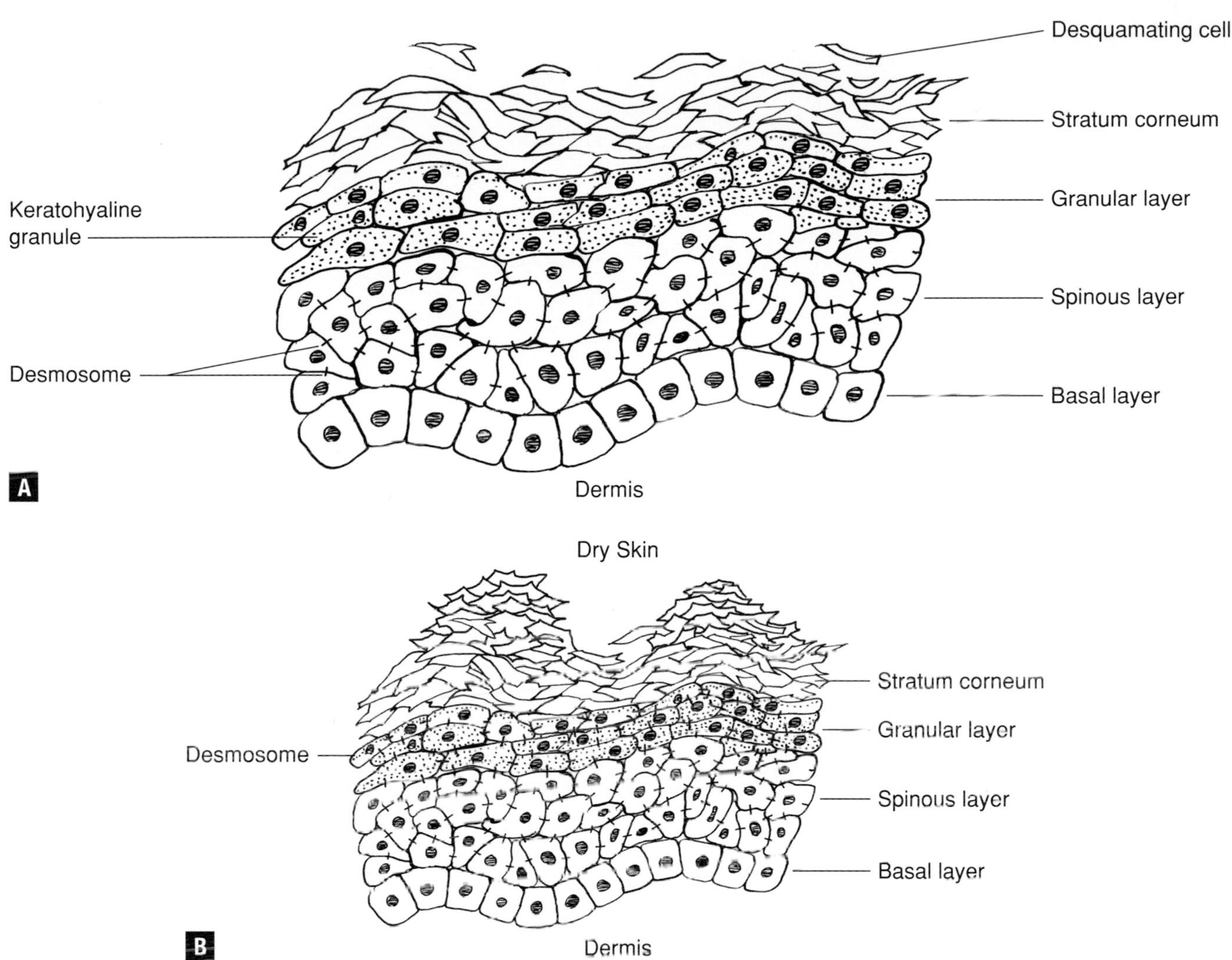

▲ **FIGURE 11-2 A.** Normal desquamation of corneocytes leads to a smooth skin surface and radiance because of good light reflectance. **B.** Corneocytes in dry skin cling together leading to heaps and valleys that give skin a dull appearance and rough texture.

disruption in barrier function. There are three rate-limiting enzymes involved in the synthesis of the main lipids of epidermal skin (Fig. 11-4) They include 3-hydroxy-3-methylglutaryl coenzyme A (HMG-Co A) reductase (the rate-limiting enzyme in cholesterol synthesis), acetyl Co-A carboxylase (ACC), and the fatty acid synthase involved in the synthesis of free fatty acids and palmitoyl transferase (SPT), which is the regulatory enzyme for the synthesis of ceramides.[14,15] As expected, when skin barrier disruption occurs, the activity of these enzymes is enhanced in order to compensate for barrier dysfunction.[15] In addition, a group of transcription factors known as sterol regulatory element binding proteins (SREBPs) regulate cholesterol and fatty acid synthesis. When decreased epidermal sterols are noted, the SREBPs are activated via proteolytic processes, enter the cell nucleus, and activate genes leading to increased synthesis of cholesterol and FA synthesis enzymes.[10,16] There are three known types of SREBPs: SREBP-1 a, -1 c, and SREBP-2. In human keratinocytes, SREBP-2 has been shown to be the predominant one and involved in regulating cholesterol and FA synthesis.[17] Interestingly, the ceramide pathway is not affected by the SREBPs.

CHOLESTEROL Basal cells are capable of absorbing cholesterol from the circulation; however, most cholesterol is synthesized from acetate in cells such as the keratinocytes. The synthesis of cholesterol is increased when the epidermal barrier is impaired.[18] Peroxisome proliferator-activated receptors (PPARs) and retinoid X receptors have been found to play a role in transporting cholesterol across keratinocyte cell membranes by increasing expression of ABCA1, a membrane transporter that regulates cholesterol efflux.[19]

CERAMIDES Ceramides constitute 40% of the SC lipids in humans[20]; however, they are not found in significant amounts in lower levels of the epidermis such as the stratum granulosum or basal layer. This suggests that terminal differentiation is a key factor in the production of ceramides. There are at least nine classes of ceramides in the SC classified as Ceramides 1 to 9. In addition, there are two protein-bound ceramides classified as Ceramides A and B, which are covalently bound to cornified envelope proteins such an involucrin[21] (Fig. 11-5). In 1982, Ceramide 1 was the first ceramide identified. Subsequently, additional types of ceramides were found and named according to the polarity and composition of the molecule. The basic ceramide structure is a fatty acid covalently bound to a sphingoid base. Different classes are based on arrangements of sphingosine (S) versus phytosphingosine (P) versus 6-hydroxysph-

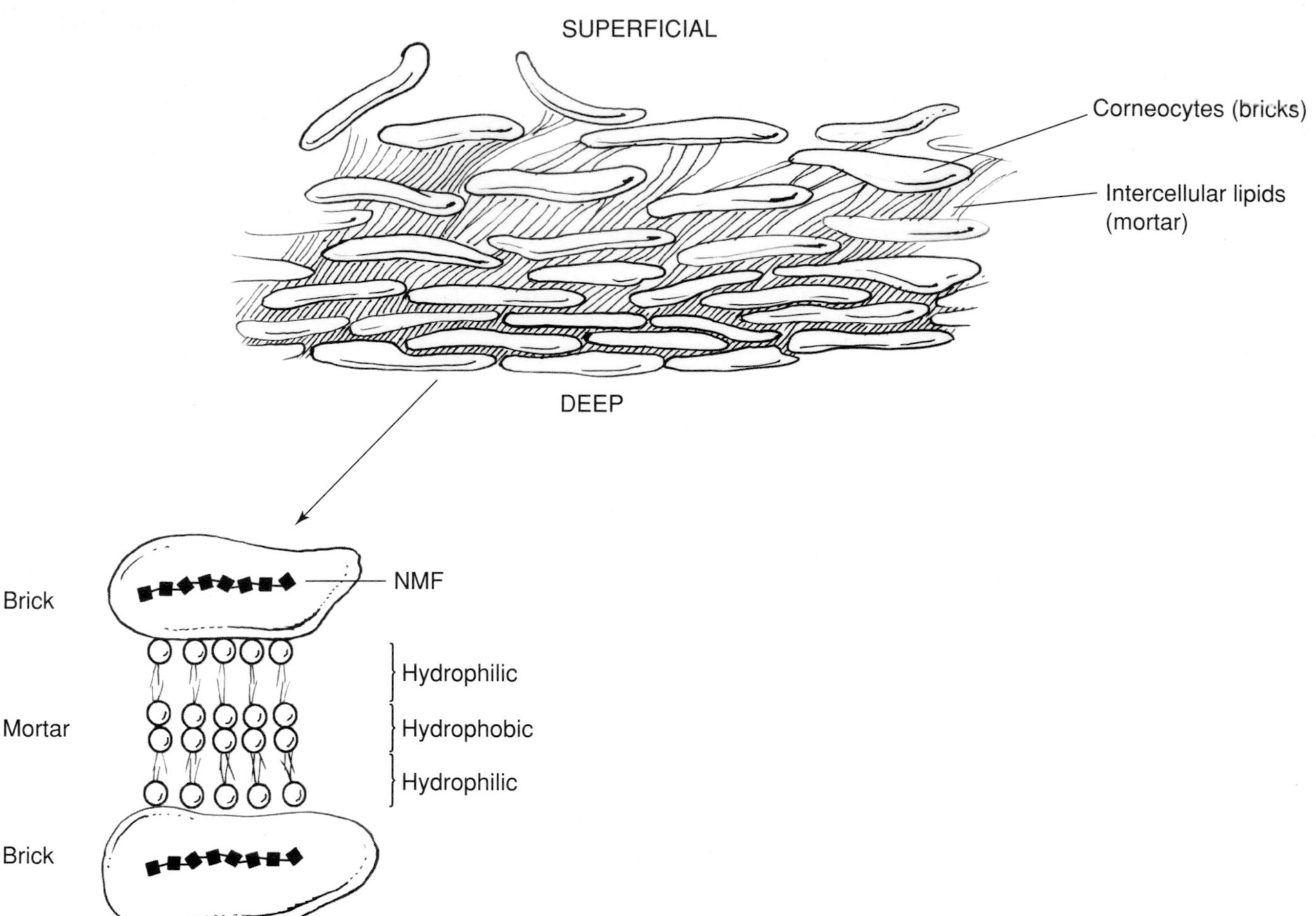

▲ **FIGURE 11-3** The keratinocytes are embedded in a lipid matrix that resembles bricks and mortar. Natural moisturizing factor (NMF) is present within the keratinocytes. NMF and the lipid bilayer prevent dehydration of the epidermis.

ingosine (H) bases, to which an α-hydroxy (A) or nonhydroxy (N) fatty acid is attached, as well as the presence or absence of a distinct ω-esterified linoleic acid residue.[22] Ceramide 1 is unique because it is nonpolar and contains linoleic acid (a fatty acid). It is believed that the unique structure of Ceramide 1 gives it a special function in the SC. Many have proposed that this unique structure allows it to function as a molecular rivet to bind the multiple bilayers of the SC.[20] This sort of interaction can account for the stacking of lipid bilayers that is observed. Ceramides 1, 4, and 7 play a vital role in epidermal integrity by serving as the main storage areas for linoleic acid, an essential fatty acid with key functions in the epidermal lipid barrier.[23] Although all epidermal ceramides are generated from a lamellar body-derived glucosylceramide precursor, sphingomyelin-derived ceramides (Ceramides 2, 5) are also necessary for the integrity of the epidermal barrier.[24] Alkaline pH inhibits the activity of β-glucocerebrosidase and acid sphingomyelinase.[25] Therefore, alkaline soaps may contribute to poor barrier formation.

The regulatory enzyme for ceramide synthesis (SPT) is increased via exposure to UVB radiation and cytokines.[26] A study by L'Oréal researchers showed that total ceramide levels (especially Ceramide 2) are decreased in skin xerosis.[27] They did not see a difference in total lipid amount between xerotic patients and controls.

A study by Unilever demonstrated that exogenously applied sphingoid precursors (specifically tetraacetyl phytosphingosine or TAPS) increased ceramide levels in keratinocytes.[28] Another study by Unilever showed that TAPS combined with the fatty acids 1% linoleic acid and 1% juniperic acid further increased these ceramide levels.[29] In the second study, barrier integrity was also assessed and shown to be improved in patients treated with TAPS, and even more improved in those treated with TAPS as well as linoleic and juniperic acids. These results suggest that topically applied lipid precursors are incorporated into ceramide biosynthetic pathways in the epidermis, increasing SC ceramide levels and thereby improving barrier integrity.

FATTY ACIDS The skin contains free fatty acids and fatty acids bound in triglycerides, glycosylceramides, ceramides, and phospholipids. The free fatty acids in the SC are predominantly straight chained, with 24 to 24 carbon chain lengths being the most abundant.[18] Acetyl Co-A carboxylase (ACC) and fatty acid synthase are the rate-limiting enzymes in fatty acid synthesis. Barrier disruption increases the mRNA and activity levels of both of these enzymes resulting in de novo fatty acid synthesis. (The increase in activity of these enzymes is likely caused by an increase in SREBPs.) Essential fatty acids such as linoleic acid can only be obtained through diet or by topical application.

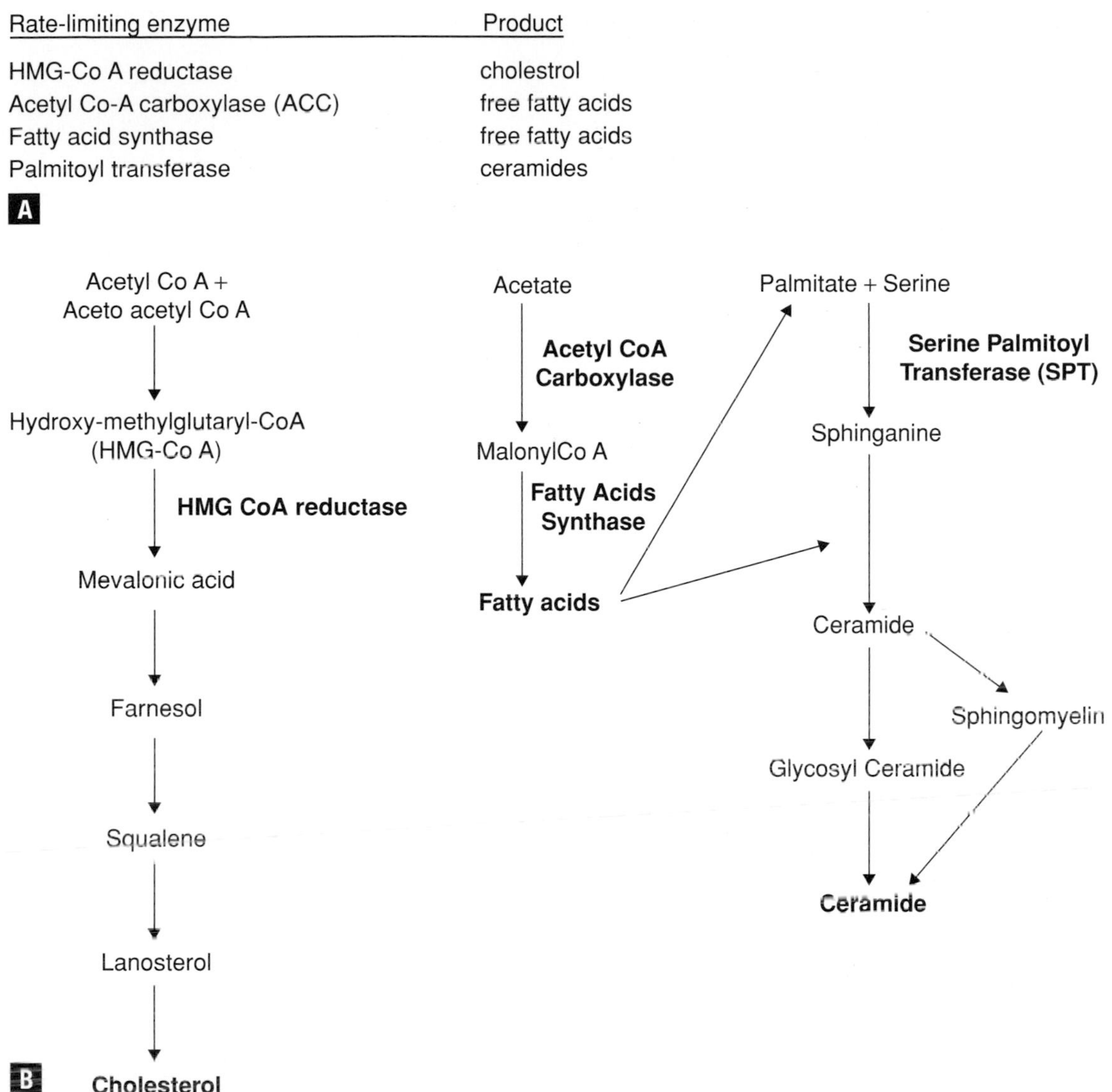

▲ **FIGURE 11-4** **A.** Rate-limiting enzymes involved in the synthesis of the main lipids of epidermal skin. **B.** Synthesis of fatty acids, ceramides, and cholesterol. (*Adapted from Elias PM. Stratum corneum defensive functions: an integrated view. J Invest Dermatol. 2005;125(2):183-200.*)

Changes in any of the three lipid components (ceramides, cholesterol, and fatty acids) or their regulatory enzymes result in impairment of the epidermal barrier. For example, lovastatin, an inhibitor of cholesterol synthesis (HMG-Co A reductase), slows barrier recovery,[30] and induces a defect in barrier function when applied topically.[31] Also, feeding mice with essential fatty acid deficiency (EFAD) a diet lacking in linoleic acid leads to barrier disruption, likely by lowering ceramide levels.[32] Therefore, it is clear that essential fatty acids and cholesterol play an integral role in dry skin conditions. It is currently believed that no single lipid alone mediates barrier function, and that normal levels of ceramides, cholesterol, and fatty acids, in the correct ratio, are necessary to achieve an intact barrier. Studies support this notion.[33] Man et al. showed that after altering the barrier with acetone, reapplication of ceramides, and fatty acids alone, or a combination of ceramides and fatty acids, further delayed barrier recovery. Only the application of a combination of all three components, ceramides, fatty acids, and cholesterol, resulted in normal barrier recovery.

OTHER COMPONENTS THAT PLAY A ROLE IN DRY SKIN

Natural Moisturizing Factor

SC hydration is highly regulated by the natural moisturizing factor (NMF), a mixture of low molecular weight- and water-soluble by-products of filaggrin. Corneocytes are anucleated with no lipid content. They are composed of keratin filaments and filaggrin and encased by a cornified cell envelope. Filaggrin, also known as filament aggregating protein, plays an interesting role in epidermal barrier function and hydration. In lower levels of the skin, filaggrin plays a structural role; however, higher up in the skin, it is broken down into amino acids that are hygroscopic and strongly bind water. Histidine, glutamine, and arginine are metabolites of filaggrin in the SC. Following deamination of the mentioned three amino acids to *trans*-urocanic acid, pyrrolidone carboxylic acid, and citrulline, respectively, an osmotically active compound that regulates skin hydration, known as NMF, is produced[10,34] (Fig. 11-6A and B).

As previously mentioned, *trans*-urocanic acid, pyrrolidone carboxylic acid, and citrulline, all derived from filaggrin, generate an inward gradient of water into the SC. Other components of NMF are lactic acid and urea, also functioning

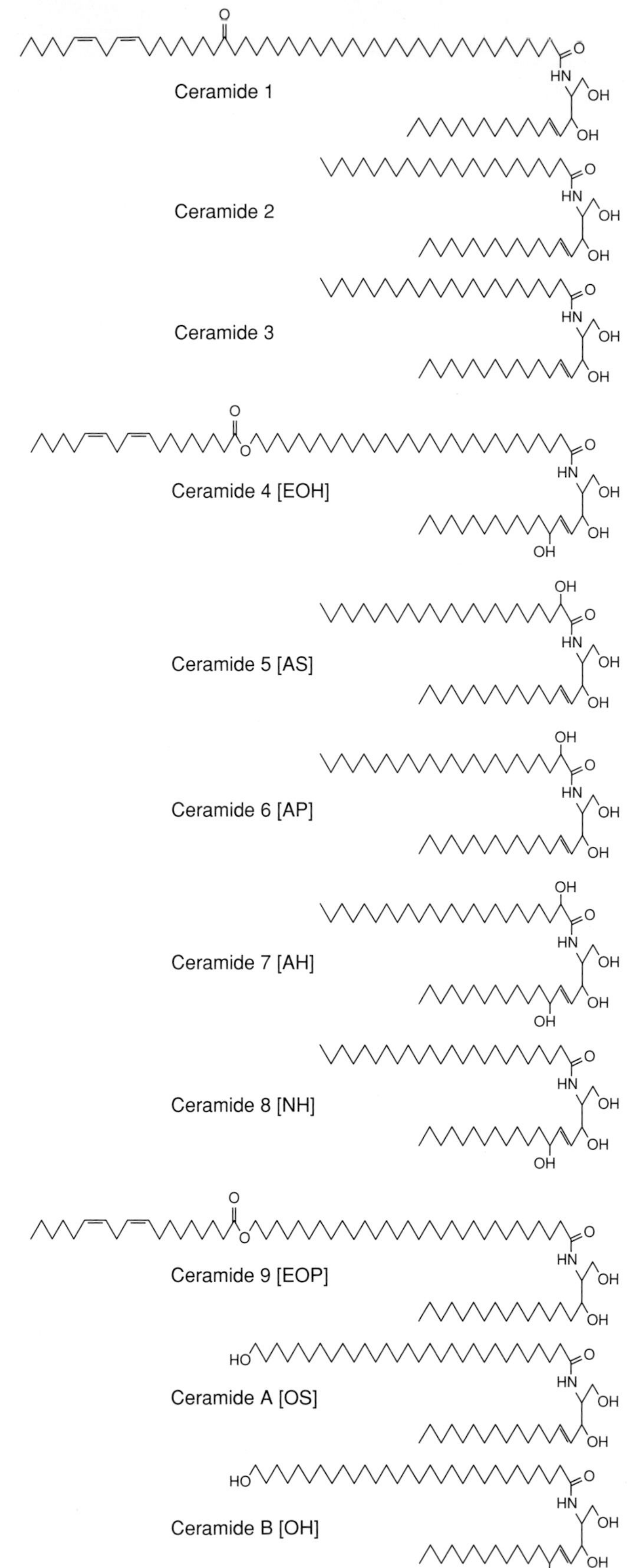

▲ **FIGURE 11-5** The chemical structures of free fatty acid, cholesterol, the nine unbound ceramides found in the SC as well as the two protein-bound ceramides, Ceramides A and B.

as humectants, and inorganic ions such as sodium, potassium, calcium, and chloride, which contribute to epidermal hydration. The osmotically active and humectant properties of NMF allow the epidermis to retain hydration even in dry environments. Extraction of NMF components results in a decrease in the moisture accumulation rate (MAT) of the epidermis,[35] emphasizing the importance of NMF in skin hydration. Interestingly, NMF components undergo seasonal changes. While amino acid components of NMF have been shown to increase during winter, lactic acid, potassium, sodium, and chloride were significantly lower compared to their levels in summer.[36] Although there are many products on the market simulating the NMF, formulating a product identical to it has been a challenge to researchers. This may be because of the natural adaptation of the NMF to different environments, in every person.

AQUAPORINS AND THE EPIDERMIS

Water is well known to permeate through the lipid bilayers of epidermal skin. Until recently, simple diffusion was the only presumed mechanism for water conduction through epidermis. Aquaporins (AQPs), which are a form of water channel, are integral membrane proteins that facilitate water transport in various organs such as skin, renal tubules, eyes, the digestive tract, and even the brain. In 2003, Peter Agre and Roderick MacKinnon received the Nobel Prize in chemistry for discovering aquaporins and for their structural studies of ion channels, respectively. There are 13 isoforms of aquaporins found in mammals, classified as AQP 0 to 12. In the cell membrane they are arranged as homotetramers. Each subunit of the tetramer consists of six α helical domains and contains a distinct aqueous pore (Fig. 11-7). Functionally, they can be classified into two subtypes: AQPs 1, 2, 4, 5, and 8, which only transport water, and AQPs 3, 7, 9, and 10, which are able to conduct other substances such as glycerol or urea in addition to water.[43] AQP-3 is the predominant water channel found in human epidermis, and is permeable to both water and glycerin. Glycerin has been implicated as an endogenous humectant contributing to SC hydration.[44] Studies have shown that defects in AQP-3 in mice models result in epidermal dryness, as well as decreased SC hydration and glycerol content of the epidermis, followed by decreased elasticity and impaired skin barrier recovery.[45,46] These studies have accentuated the importance of glycerol in skin hydration. Aquaporin is thought to facilitate transport of water, glycerol, and solutes between keratinocytes.

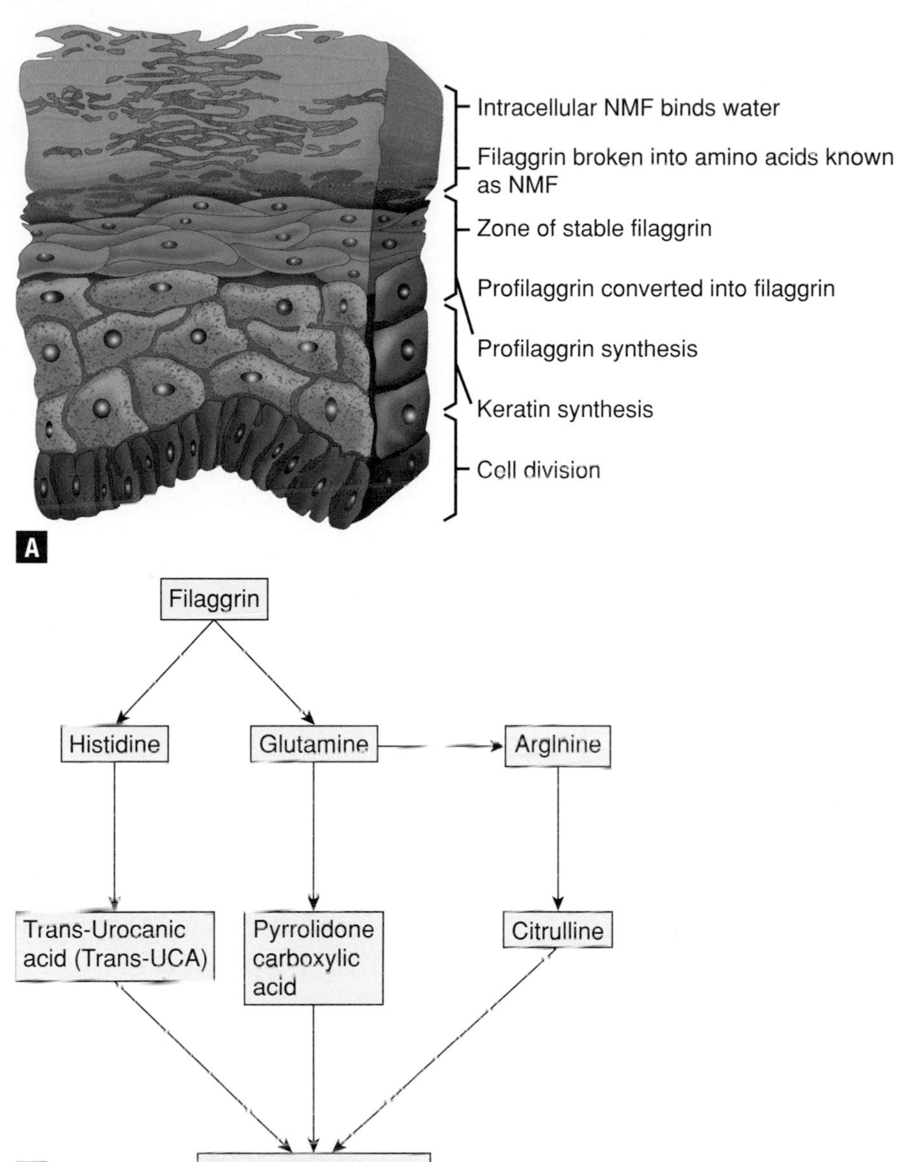

▲ **FIGURE 11-6** **A.** Filaggrin has multiple functions depending on where in the epidermis it is found. It has a structural role in lower layers and a hydration role in upper layers. **B.** Trans-UCA, pyrrolidone carboxylic acid and citrulline provide osmolarity regulating skin hydration. (*Adapted from Elias PM. Stratum corneum defensive functions: an integrated view. J Invest Dermatol. 2005;125(2):183-200.*)

SEBUM

Sebum-derived lipids may also play a part in dry skin pathophysiology by preventing water loss through forming lipid films on the skin's surface that function as an emollient. However, low levels of sebaceous gland activity have not been consistently correlated with the occurrence of dry skin and the impact of sebum on dry skin conditions is poorly understood.[20] Choi et al. compared sebum production and SC hydration and found that even though males had sebum secretion levels 30% to 40% higher than women, the males did not show greater SC hydration on the sebaceous gland enriched forehead sites than did females. They also showed that prepubertal children whose sebaceous glands have not reached maximal function demonstrated normal levels of SC hydration. They did, however, find a correlation with glycerol levels and SC hydration that can help explain the role of the sebaceous glands in dry skin. The sebaceous glands utilize large amounts of triglycerides, leading to the production of glycerol. Supplying glycerol for skin hydration may be an important role for sebaceous glands.[44] This theory is supported by the fact that mice with hypoplastic sebaceous glands have poor SC hydration and low SC glycerol levels.[47] However, glycerol can come from sources other than the sebaceous glands, which would explain the normal SC hydration in prepubertal children. Glycerol can be transported from the circulation into the basal cells via the AQP-3 channels.[45] The importance of glycerol is highlighted by the fact that topical glycerol restores hydration to asepia mice while topical sebaceous lipids do not.[47]

ANATOMICAL VARIATION IN WATER LOSS

Various body parts are known to regulate water loss differently. For example, the soles and palms regulate water loss poorly, while facial skin is relatively water impermeable. While the functions of the SC lipids are not fully understood, evidence supports the notion that lipids play a critical role in skin permeability. One study found no relationship between barrier function and the thickness or the number of cell layers in the SC.[48] However, an inverse relationship was discovered between lipid weight percent and permeability. Researchers found that the lipid weight percent was higher in the face (less permeable) and lower in the plantar SC (more permeable). Another study was conducted to identify the components of this "lipid weight percent" and how they vary site to site.[49] Investigators compared characteristics from the abdomen, leg, face, and sole, and found that the areas with superior barrier properties contained a higher percent of neutral lipids and lower amount of sphingolipids. In other words, the neutral lipid to sphingolipid ratio was proportional to the known permeability of each site. Interestingly, the plantar surface, known to be the most permeable, contained the highest amounts of sphingolipids.

ANTIMICROBIAL PEPTIDES AND THE EPIDERMAL BARRIER

Antimicrobial peptides (AMPs) are components of the innate immune system of the skin. They exhibit a broad spectrum of antimicrobial activity against bacteria, viruses, and fungi. Defensins and cathelecidins are two major groups of AMPs. Defensins are cysteine-rich cationic AMPs present in mammalians that are categorized into two subgroups: α-defensins and β-defensins. α-defensins are mostly found in neutrophils[50,51] and panteh cells of small intestines.[52] β-defensins, on the other hand, are present in the epidermis,[53,54] and possess antimicrobial activity against gram-positive and -negative bacteria, *Candida albicans,* and fungi.[54–50]

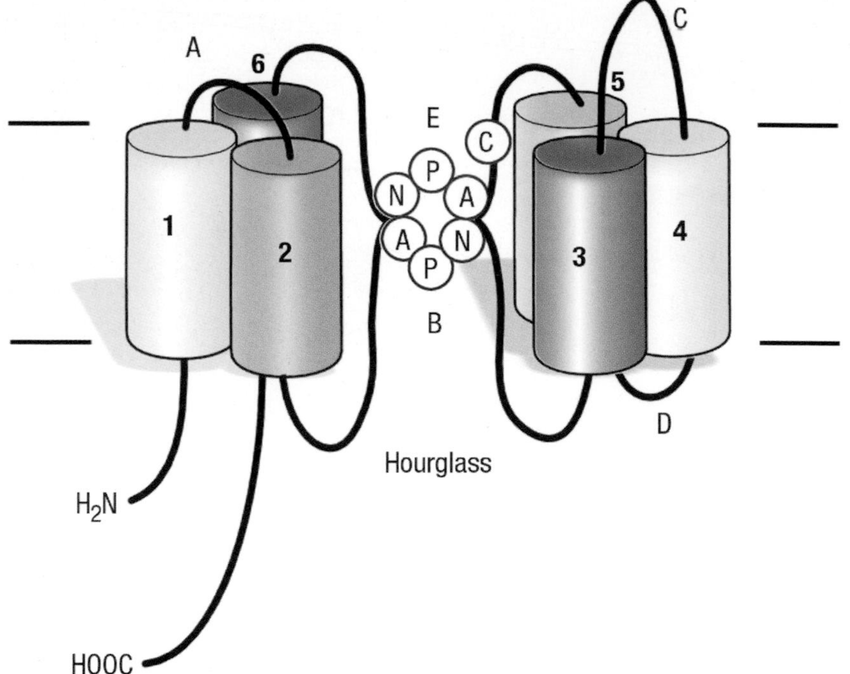

▲ **FIGURE 11-7** Hourglass model for aquaporin-1 membrane topology. Each aquaporin-1 subunit contains six bilayer-spanning domains composed of two obversely symmetric structures (TMI-3, hemipore 1; and TM4–6, hemipore 2). When NPA [formed by amino acids asparagine (N), proline (P), and alanine (A)] motifs in loops B and E are juxtaposed, they form a single aqueous channel spanning the bilayer (the "hour-glass") flanked by the mercury-sensitive residue (C189). (*Redrawn with permission from the Annual Review of Biochemistry. Volume 68 ©2999 by Annual Reviews. http://www.annualreviews.org.*)

Cathelecidins are another family of AMPs containing a C-terminal cationic segment with antimicrobial activity.[59] There is only one member of the cathelecidin family identified in humans, known as LL-37, which has been shown to be especially important against viral skin infections.[60] LL-37 has been demonstrated to increase in the keratinocytes of inflamed skin such as psoriasis and nickel allergy.[61,62] Patients with atopic dermatitis have been reported to have lower levels of LL-37 and human β-defensin 2 peptide in their epidermis,[63] which may explain their vulnerability toward viral, including herpetic,[60] and staphylococcal infections.

DRY SKIN AND INFLAMMATION

Disruption of skin barrier function stimulates the production of epidermal cytokines,[64] especially interleukin (IL)-1α.[65] This is amplified in low-humidity conditions, which may help explain why exacerbations of atopic dermatitis, skin itching, hyperproliferation, and inflammation are seen in winter and in low-humidity environments.[66] IL-1α has been shown to be preformed, stored, and released immediately when the barrier is disturbed.[67] Once IL-1α is expressed, it may also induce other cytokines or proinflammatory molecules such as IL-6, IL-8, granulocyte/macrophage colony-stimulating factor, and intercellular adhesion molecule-1. Ashida et al. showed that exposure to low humidity increased epidermal IL-1α synthesis and stimulated IL-1α release from the preformed pool in the epidermis after tape stripping. Interestingly, the increase of IL-1α seen in low humidity only lasted for 4 days after which the skin was able to adapt to the low-humidity environment by unknown mechanisms.

STRESS AND THE SKIN BARRIER

Psychologic stress has long been known to be associated with skin conditions, such as atopic dermatitis, psoriasis, and seborrheic dermatitis. Immune and neuroendocrine mechanisms likely play a role in these diseases, but studies have also shown that barrier disruption occurs during stress, leading to the exacerbation of dry skin and other skin conditions. Studies have also demonstrated that glucocorticoids lead to disruption of the skin barrier.[68] Glucocorticoids inhibit lipid synthesis resulting in decreased production and secretion of lamellar bodies. "Stress hormones" are glucocorticoids produced in response to stress. It follows then that stress would lead to barrier disruption by increasing glucocorticoid levels. Choi et al. showed that psychologic stress led to a decrease of lipid synthesis as well as disruption of lamellar body formation, and was corrected by applications of exogenous physiologic lipids[69] (Box 11-3).

BOX 11-3 How the Skin Responds to Changes in the Environment

The skin is able to adjust to changes in humidity. This process takes several days, so skin may be dry and inflamed during the first few days of exposure to decreased humidity, but several mechanisms seem to allow skin to adjust to these environmental changes. Epidermal permeability function is increased in a low-humidity environment.[70]

It has been found that changes in hydration status signal several downstream responses, including epidermal DNA synthesis and catabolism of filaggrin into deiminated carboxylic acid metabolites.[71,72] NMF production is increased in low-humidity environments as well.[73,74]

HOW THE EPIDERMIS RESPONDS TO EPIDERMAL BARRIER INSULT

Acute disruption of the epidermal barrier initiates a homeostatic repair response that results in the rapid recovery of permeability barrier function.[75] This repair mechanism is inhibited if the skin is covered with an occlusive dressing. Grubauer et al. showed that TEWL triggers lipid synthesis resulting in a repaired skin barrier. As TEWL decreases, lipid synthesis returns to normal levels.[76] Once triggered, this repair response begins within minutes with the rapid secretion of the contents of the lamellar bodies from the outer stratum granulosum cells. A marked decrease (50%–80%) of preexisting lamellar bodies is seen in the stratum granulosum cells initially but is soon followed by newly formed lamellar bodies. Accelerated lipid synthesis and lamellar body secretion continues until permeability barrier function returns toward normal.[77]

A calcium gradient seems to play a role in triggering the lamellar body secretion. High levels of extracellular calcium are found in the upper epidermis surrounding the stratum granulosum cells.[78]

Immediately after barrier disruption, the increased water movement through the compromised SC carries calcium outward toward the skin surface. This leads to a reduction in calcium concentration around the stratum granulosum cells, which triggers lamellar body secretion.[79] It is postulated that skin calmodulin-related factor (SCARF) acts as a Ca^{2+} sensor, by binding target proteins and leading to barrier repair.[80] The important role of calcium flux is demonstrated when exogenous calcium is supplied to a disturbed barrier, lamellar body secretion does not occur, and permeability barrier repair is not initiated.[81] If the calcium surrounding the stratum granulosum cells is decreased experimentally by iontophoresis or sonophoresis, secretion of lamellar bodies is stimulated even if the barrier is undisturbed.[82]

Other factors likely play a role in lamellar body secretion as well. Keratinocytes are able to produce large amounts of cytokines and a store of IL-1α and IL-1β is kept available in the keratinocyte. In response to acute barrier disruption, IL-1α is released[83] and an increase in the expression of TNF, IL-1, and IL-6 on messenger RNA and protein levels is seen.[67,64] Mice deficient in IL-1, IL-6, and tumor necrosis factor-α signaling exhibit a delay in permeability barrier repair after acute barrier disruption, a role for these cytokines in regulating permeability barrier homeostasis.[84]

Each of these factors is thought to play an important role in barrier repair, and topical therapies using cytokines, growth factors, and calcium modulators are being studied.

TREATMENT

The symptoms of dry skin can be treated by increasing the hydration state of the SC with occlusive or humectant ingredients and by smoothing the rough surface with an emollient. Moisturizers are products designed to increase hydration of the skin. They often contain lipids such as ceramides, fatty acids, and cholesterol. In addition, glycerin is a common component. The commonly used moisturizers are oil-in-water emulsions, such as creams and lotions, and water-in-oil emulsions such as hand creams. For more information on the range of topical dry skin treatment options, see Chapter 32.

Supplements, Diet, and Dry Skin

Lipids comprise only approximately 10% of the total weight of the SC, but their role in constructing a watertight barrier is crucial for survival. The epidermis is the main site of sterol and fatty acid synthesis and most lipids found in the epidermal barrier are produced in the epidermis itself and not derived by diet. In fact, lipid synthesis occurs independently of serum sterol levels and amount of dietary cholesterol.[76] Linoleic acid is a very important essential fatty acid that must be supplied through diet or topical application because it is not made in the epidermis. It is a component of phospholipids, glucosylceramides, and Ceramides 1, 4, and 9.[85] In essential fatty acid deficiency, when linoleate is not present, it is replaced with oleate, which results in marked abnormalities in cutaneous permeability barrier function.[86,87] These observations indicate that essential fatty acids are required for the normal structure and permeability barrier function of the SC. α-linoleic acid is an ω-3 fatty acid and is found in salmon and fish oils such as cod liver oil. Although no skin changes have been associated with a deficiency of ω-3 fatty acids, it is widely believed that they play an important role in regulating inflammation.

SUMMARY

Patients usually present with primary complaints other than dry skin, but often add, incidentally, that their skin feels dry. Mild dry skin is a condition that affects many patients plenty of whom try OTC products before seeking medical advice. Once the complaint of dry skin reaches the dermatologist, it is best that the practitioner be able to knowledgeably discuss the implications of "dry skin" and the spectrum of effective treatment options, and match such products to a patient's skin conditions.

REFERENCES

1. Takahashi M, Kawasaki K, Tanaka M, et al. The mechanism of stratum corneum plasticization with water. *Bioeng Skin.* 1981;67-72..
2. Draelos ZD. Therapeutic moisturizers. *Dermatol Clin.* 2000;18:597.
3. Kligman A. The biology of the stratum corneum. In: Montagna W, Jr. Lobitz W, eds. *The Epidermis.* New York, NY: Academic Press; 1964:387-433.
4. Chernosky ME. Clinical aspects of dry skin. *J Soc Cosmet Chem.* 1976;65:376.
5. Wildnauer RH, Bothwell JW, Douglass AB. Stratum corneum biomechanical properties. I. Influence of relative humidity on normal and extracted human stratum corneum. *J Invest Dermatol.* 1971;56:72.
6. Bouwstra JA, de Graaff A, Gooris GS, et al. Water distribution and related morphology in human stratum corneum at different hydration levels. *J Invest Dermatol.* 2003;120:750.
7. Richter T, Peuckert C, Sattler M, et al. Dead but highly dynamic—the stratum corneum is divided into three hydration zones. *Skin Pharmacol Physiol.* 2004;17: 246.
8. Rawlings A, Hope J, Rogers J, et al. Skin dryness What is it? *J Invest Dermatol.* 1993;100:510.
9. Orth D, Appa Y. Glycerine: a natural ingredient for moisturizing skin. In: Loden M, H Maibach H, eds. *Dry Skin and Moisturizers.* Boca Raton, FL, CRC Press; 2000:214.
10. Elias PM. Stratum corneum defensive functions: an integrated view. *J Invest Dermatol.* 2005;125:183.
11. Kalinin A, Marekov LN, Steinert PM. Assembly of the epidermal cornified cell envelope. *J Cell Sci.* 2001;114:3069.
12. Elias PM, Menon GK. Structural and lipid biochemical correlates of the epidermal permeability barrier. *Adv Lipid Res.* 1991;24:1.
13. Feingold KR. Thematic review series: skin lipids. The role of epidermal lipids in cutaneous permeability barrier homeostasis. *J Lipid Res.* 2007;48:2531.
14. Bigby M, Corona R, Szklo M. Evidence-based dermatology. In: Wolff K, Goldsmith LA, Katz SI, Gilchrest BA, Paller AS, Leffell DJ, eds. *Fitzpatrick's Dermatology in General Medicine.* 7th ed. New York, NY: McGraw-Hill; 2007:13
15. Holleran WM, Feingold KR, Man MQ, et al. Regulation of epidermal sphingolipid synthesis by permeability barrier function. *J Lipid Res.* 1991;32:1151.
16. Brown MS, Goldstein JL. Sterol regulatory element binding proteins (SREBPs): controllers of lipid synthesis and cellular uptake. *Nutr Rev.* 1998;56:S1.
17. Harris IR, Farrell AM, Holleran WM, et al. Parallel regulation of sterol regulatory element binding protein-2 and the enzymes of cholesterol and fatty acid synthesis but not ceramide synthesis in cultured human keratinocytes and murine epidermis. *J Lipid Res.* 1998;39: 412.
18. Wertz PW. Biochemistry of human stratum corneum lipids. In: Elias PM, Feingold KR, eds. *Skin Barrier.* New York, NY: Taylor and Francis; 2006:33-42.
19. Proksch E, Jensen J-M. Skin as an organ of protection. In: Wolff K, Goldsmith LA, Katz SI, Gilchrest BA, Paller AS, Leffell DJ, eds. *Fitzpatrick's Dermatology in General Medicine.* 7th ed. New York, NY: McGraw-Hill; 2007:386-387.
20. Downing D, Stewart M. Wertz P, et al. Skin lipids: an update. *J Invest Dermatol.* 1987;88:2 s.
21. Bouwstra JA, Pilgrim K, Ponec M. Structure of the skin barrier. In: Elias PM, Feingold KR, eds. *Skin Barrier.* New York, NY: Taylor and Francis; 2006:65.
22. de Jager MW, Gooris GS, Dolbnya IP, et al. Novel lipid mixtures based on synthetic ceramides reproduce the unique stratum corneum lipid organization. *J Lipid Res.* 2004;45:923.
23. Elias PM, Brown BE, Ziboh VA. The permeability barrier in essential fatty acid deficiency: evidence for a direct role for linoleic acid in barrier function. *J Invest Dermatol.* 1980;74:230.

24. Uchida Y, Hara M, Nishio H, et al. Epidermal sphingomyelins are precursors for selected stratum corneum ceramides. *J Lipid Res.* 2000;41:2071.
25. Hachem JP, Man MQ, Crumrine D, et al. Sustained serine proteases activity by prolonged increase in pH leads to degradation of lipid processing enzymes and profound alterations of barrier function and stratum corneum integrity. *J Invest Dermatol.* 2005;125:510.
26. Farrell AM, Uchida Y, Nagiec MM, et al. UVB irradiation up-regulates serine palmitoyltransferase in cultured human keratinocytes. *J Lipid Res.* 1998;39:2031.
27. Nappé C, Delesalle G, Jansen A, et al. Decrease in ceramide II in skin xerosis. *J Invest Dermatol.* 1993;100:530.
28. Carlomusto M, Pillai S, Rawlings AV. Human keratinocytes in vitro can utilize exogenously supplied sphingosine analogues for sphingolipid biosynthesis. *J Invest Dermatol.* 1996;106:871.
29. Davies A, Verdejo P, Feinberg C, et al. Increased stratum corneum ceramide levels and improved barrier function following topical treatment with tetraacetylphytosphingosine. *J Invest Dermatol.* 1996;106:918.
30. Feingold KR, Man MQ, Menon GK, et al. Cholesterol synthesis is required for cutaneous barrier function in mice. *J Clin Invest.* 1990;86:1738.
31. Feingold KR, Man MQ, Proksch E, et al. The lovastatin-treated rodent: a new model of barrier disruption and epidermal hyperplasia. *J Invest Dermatol.* 1991; 96:201.
32. Prottey C. Essential fatty acids and the skin. *Br J Dermatol.* 1976;94:579.
33. Man MQ, Feingold KR, Elias PM. Exogenous lipids influence permeability barrier recovery in acetone-treated murine skin. *Arch Dermatol.* 1993;129:728.
34. Scott IR, Harding CR, Barrett JG. Histidine-rich protein of the keratohyalin granules. Source of the free amino acids, urocanic acid and pyrrolidone carboxylic acid in the stratum corneum. *Biochim Biophys Acta.* 1982;719:110.
35. Visscher MO, Tolia GT, Wickett RR, et al. Effect of soaking and natural moisturizing factor on stratum corneum water-handling properties. *J Cosmet Sci.* 2003;54:289.
36. Nakagawa N, Sakai S, Matsumoto M, et al. Relationship between NMF (lactate and potassium) content and the physical properties of the stratum corneum in healthy subjects. *J Invest Dermatol.* 2004; 122:755.
37. Imokawa G, Abe A, Jin K, et al. Decreased level of ceramides in stratum corneum of atopic dermatitis: an etiologic factor in atopic dry skin? *J Invest Dermatol.* 1991;96:523.
38. Akimoto K, Yoshikawa N, Higaki Y, et al. Quantitative analysis of stratum corneum lipids in xerosis and asteatotic eczema. *J Dermatol.* 1993;20:1.
39. Weidinger S, Illig T, Baurecht H, et al. Loss-of-function variations within the filaggrin gene predispose for atopic dermatitis with allergic sensitizations. *J Allergy Clin Immunol.* 2006;118:214.
40. Irvine AD, McLean WH. Breaking the (un)sound barrier: filaggrin is a major gene for atopic dermatitis. *J Invest Dermatol.* 2006;126:1200.
41. Chu DH. Development and structure of skin. In: Wolff K, Goldsmith LA, Katz SI, Gilchrest BA, Paller AS, Leffell DJ, eds. *Fitzpatrick's Dermatology in General Medicine.* 7th ed. New York, NY: McGraw-Hill; 2007:61.
42. Fartasch M, Bassukas ID, Diepgen TL. Disturbed extruding mechanism of lamellar bodies in dry non-eczematous skin of atopics. *Br J Dermatol.* 1992;127: 221.
43. Takata K, Matsuzaki T, Tajika Y. Aquaporins: water channel proteins of the cell membrane. *Prog Histochem Cytochem.* 2004;39:1.
44. Choi EH, Man MQ, Wang F, et al. Is endogenous glycerol a determinant of stratum corneum hydration in humans? *J Invest Dermatol.* 2005;125:288.
45. Hara-Chikuma M, Verkman AS. Selectively reduced glycerol in skin of aquaporin-3-deficient mice may account for impaired skin hydration, elasticity, and barrier recovery. *J Biol Chem.* 2002; 277:46616.
46. Hara-Chikuma M, Verkman AS. Glycerol replacement corrects defective skin hydration, elasticity, and barrier function in aquaporin-3-deficient mice. *Proc Natl Acad Sci U S A.* 2003;100:7360.
47. Fluhr JW, Mao-Qiang M, Brown BE, et al. Glycerol regulates stratum corneum hydration in sebaceous gland deficient (asebia) mice. *J Invest Dermatol.* 2003; 120:728.
48. Elias PM, Cooper ER, Korc A, et al. Percutaneous transport in relation to stratum corneum structure and lipid composition. *J Invest Dermatol.* 1981;76: 297.
49. Lampe MA, Burlingame AL, Whitney J, et al. Human stratum corneum lipids: characterization and regional variations. *J Lipid Res.* 1983;24:120.
50. Rice WG, Ganz T, Kinkade JMJ. Defensin-rich dense granules of human neutrophils. *Blood.* 1987;70:757.
51. Harwig SSL, Park ASK, Lehrer RI. Characterization of defensin precursors in mature human neutrophils. *Blood.* 1992;79:1532.
52. Porter E, Liu L, Oren A, et al. Localization of human intestinal defensin 5 in Paneth cell granules. *Infect Immun.* 1997;65:2389.
53. Fulton C, Anderson GM, Zasloff M, et al. Expression of natural peptide antibiotics in human skin. *Lancet.* 1997;350:1750.
54. Harder J, Bartels J, Christophers E, et al. A peptide antibiotic from human skin. *Nature.* 1997;387:861.
55. Sahly H, Schubert S, Harder J, et al. Activity of human β-defensins 2 and 3 against ESBL-producing Klebsiella strains. *J Antimicrob Chemother.* 2006;57: 562.
56. Meyer JE, Harder J, Gorogh T, et al. Human β-defensin-2 in oral cancer with opportunistic Candida infection. *Anticancer Res.* 2004;24:1025.
57. Harder J, Bartels J, Christophers E, et al. Isolation and characterization of human β-defensin-3, a novel human inducible peptide antibiotic. *J Biol Chem.* 2001; 276:5707.
58. Zanetti M, Gennaro R, Romeo D. Cathelicidins: a novel protein family with a common proregion and a variable C-terminal antimicrobial domain. *FEBS Lett.* 1995;374:1.
59. Niyonsaba F, Ushio H, Nakano N, et al. Antimicrobial peptides human β-defensins stimulate epidermal keratinocyte migration, proliferation and production of proinflammatory cytokines and chemokines. *J Invest Dermatol.* 2007;127:594.
60. Howell MD, Jones JF, Kisich KO, et al. Selective killing of vaccinia virus by LL-37: implications for eczema vaccinatum. *J Immunol.* 2004;172:1763.
61. Frohm M, Agerberth B, Ahangari G, et al. The expression of the gene coding for the antibacterial peptide LL-37 is induced in human keratinocytes during inflammatory disorders. *J Biol Chem.* 1997;272:15258.
62. Frohm NM, Sandstedt B, Sørensen O, et al. The human cationic antimicrobial protein (hCAP-18), a peptide antibiotic, is widely expressed in human squamous epithelia and colocalizes with interleukin-6. *Infect Immun.* 1999;67:2561.
63. Ong PY, Ohtake T, Brandt C, et al. Endogenous antimicrobial peptides and skin infections in atopic dermatitis. *N Engl J Med.* 2002;347:1151.
64. Wood LC, Jackson SM, Elias PM, et al. Cutaneous barrier perturbation stimulates cytokine production in the epidermis of mice. *J Clin Invest.* 1992;90:482.
65. Barker JN, Mitra RS, Griffiths CE, et al. Keratinocytes as initiators of inflammation. *Lancet.* 1991;337:211.
66. Ashida Y, Ogo M, Denda M. Epidermal interleukin-1 α generation is amplified at low humidity: implications for the pathogenesis of inflammatory dermatoses. *Br J Dermatol.* 2001;144:238.
67. Wood LC, Elias PM, Calhoun C, et al. Barrier disruption stimulates interleukin-1 α expression and release from a preformed pool in murine epidermis. *J Invest Dermatol.* 1996;106:397.
68. Kao JS, Fluhr JW, Man MQ, et al. Short-term glucocorticoid treatment compromises both permeability barrier homeostasis and stratum corneum integrity: inhibition of epidermal lipid synthesis accounts for functional abnormalities. *J Invest Dermatol.* 2003;120:456.
69. Choi EH, Brown BE, Crumrine D, et al. Mechanisms by which psychologic stress alters cutaneous permeability barrier homeostasis and stratum corneum integrity. *J Invest Dermatol.* 2005;124:587.
70. Denda M, Sato J, Masuda Y, et al. Exposure to a dry environment enhances epidermal permeability barrier function. *J Invest Dermatol.* 1998; 111:858.
71. Denda M, Sato J, Tsuchiya T, et al. Low humidity stimulates epidermal DNA synthesis and amplifies the hyperproliferative response to barrier disruption: implication for seasonal exacerbations of inflammatory dermatoses. *J Invest Dermatol.* 1998;111:873.
72. Sato J, Denda M, Chang S, et al. Abrupt decreases in environmental humidity induce abnormalities in permeability barrier homeostasis. *J Invest Dermatol.* 2002;119:900.
73. Katagiri C, Sato J, Nomura J, et al. Changes in environmental humidity affect the water-holding property of the stratum corneum and its free amino acid content, and the expression of

filaggrin in the epidermis of hairless mice. *J Dermatol Sci.* 2003;31:29.
74. Scott IR, Harding CR. Filaggrin breakdown to water binding compounds during development of the rat stratum corneum is controlled by the water activity of the environment. *Dev Biol.* 1986;115:84.
75. Proksch E, Holleran WM, Menon GK, et al. Barrier function regulates epidermal lipid and DNA synthesis. *Br J Dermatol.* 1993;128:473.
76. Grubauer G, Elias PM, Feingold KR. Transepidermal water loss: the signal for recovery of barrier structure and function. *J Lipid Res.* 1989;30:323.
77. Menon GK, Feingold KR, Mao-Qiang M, et al. Structural basis for the barrier abnormality following inhibition of HMG CoA reductase in murine epidermis. *J Invest Dermatol.* 1992;98:209.
78. Menon GK, Elias PM. Ultrastructural localization of calcium in psoriatic and normal human epidermis. *Arch Dermatol.* 1991;127:57.
79. Lee SH, Elias PM, Proksch E, et al. Calcium and potassium are important regulators of barrier homeostasis in murine epidermis. *J Clin Invest.* 1992;89:530.
80. Hwang J, Kalinin A, Hwang M, et al. Role of Scarf and its binding target proteins in epidermal calcium homeostasis. *J Biol Chem.* 2007;282:18645.
81. Menon GK, Elias PM, Feingold KR. Integrity of the permeability barrier is crucial for maintenance of the epidermal calcium gradient. *Br J Dermatol.* 1994;130:139.
82. Lee SH, Choi EH, Feingold KR, et al. Iontophoresis itself on hairless mouse skin induces the loss of the epidermal calcium gradient without skin barrier impairment. *J Invest Dermatol.* 1998;111:39.
83. Wood LC, Feingold KR, Sequeira-Martin SM, et al. Barrier function coordinately regulates epidermal IL-1 and IL-1 receptor antagonist mRNA levels. *Exp Dermatol.* 1994;3:56.
84. Wang XP, Schunck M, Kallen KJ, et al. The interleukin-6 cytokine system regulates epidermal permeability barrier homeostasis. *J Invest Dermatol.* 2004;123:124.
85. Uchida Y, Hamanaka S. Stratum corneum ceramides: function, origins, and therapeutic implications. In: Elias PM, Feingold KR, eds. *Skin Barrier.* New York, NY: Taylor and Francis; 2006:43.
86. Elias PM, Brown BE. The mammalian cutaneous permeability barrier: defective barrier function is essential fatty acid deficiency correlates with abnormal intercellular lipid deposition. *Lab Invest.* 1978;39:574.
87. Hansen HS, Jensen B. Essential function of linoleic acid esterified in acylglucosylceramide and acylceramide in maintaining the epidermal water permeability barrier. Evidence from feeding studies with oleate, linoleate, arachidonate, columbinate and α-linolenate. *Biochim Biophys Acta.* 1985;834:357.

CHAPTER 12

Sensitive Skin

Leslie Baumann, MD

Sensitive skin is a condition characterized by hyperreactivity to environmental factors. Individuals experiencing this condition report exaggerated reactions to topical personal care products that may or may not be associated with visible symptoms. Approximately 50% of patients with sensitive skin manifest their uncomfortable symptoms without accompanying visible signs of inflammation.[1] Sensitive skin can be very distressing to those who have it. Affected individuals often have to travel with their own skin care products because they cannot use the skin care products provided in a hotel. These patients are the ones who should not experiment with skin care products, but should find what works for them and stick with it. Cosmetic companies realize the importance of avoiding marketing products with ingredients that aggravate sensitive skin. Most of the larger well-known companies conduct skin sensitivity testing of their products prior to launch; however, occasionally, a product will sneak through undetected that causes symptoms in sensitive skin types. This is a significant problem for companies when it occurs because 78% of consumers who have sensitive skin state that they have avoided a particular product or brand because of past skin reactions.[2] Those with frequent skin reactions learn to limit their use of skin products to the few that do not cause irritation in order to avoid the annoyance of redness and itching that can interfere with everyday activities. Those with frequent skin reactions report a decrease in quality of life and frustration is a common complaint. In a French study of more than 2000 individuals, it was found that those with sensitive skin reported a poorer quality of life compared to those without sensitive skin using the SF-12 questionnaire.[3] However, depressive symptoms were no more common in those with sensitive skin as compared to those with "normal" skin.

PREVALENCE

Epidemiologic surveys show a high prevalence of sensitive skin. In a phone survey of 800 ethnically diverse women in the US, 52% described having sensitive skin.[2] In a UK mail survey of 2058 people, 51.5% of the women and 38.2% of the men reported having sensitive skin.[4] Sensitive skin is most commonly reported on the face. However, one study showed that 85% of the 400 subjects evaluated described sensitive skin on the face, while 70% reported sensitive skin in other areas: hands (58%), scalp (36%), feet (34%), neck (27%), torso (23%), and back (21%).[5]

TYPES OF SENSITIVE SKIN

Sensitive skin has been difficult to characterize in the past because it is often self-perceived, is not accompanied by visible skin changes, and testing can show inconsistent results. In the attempt to characterize sensitive skin, several classification systems have been described. Yokota et al. classified sensitive skin into three different types based on their physiologic parameters.[6] Type 1 was defined as the low-barrier function group. Type 2 was defined as the inflammation group with normal barrier function and inflammatory changes. Type 3 was termed the "pseudohealthy group" in terms of normal barrier function and no inflammatory changes. In all of the Yokota sensitive skin types, a higher content of nerve growth factor was observed in the stratum corneum (SC). In both types 2 and 3, the sensitivity to electrical stimuli was high. These data suggest that the hypersensitive reaction seen in these types is closely related to nerve fibers innervating the epidermis.

Pons-Guiraud divided sensitive skin into three subgroups.[7] "Very sensitive skin" was described as reactive to a wide variety of both endogenous and exogenous factors. This type was associated with both acute and chronic symptoms and a strong psychologic component. The second type was called "environmentally sensitive" and was described as clear, dry, thin skin with a tendency to blush or flush in reaction to environmental factors. The final group was "cosmetically sensitive skin," which was transiently reactive to specific and definable cosmetic products.

Muizzuddin and others from the Estée Lauder companies defined three sensitive skin subgroups as well.[8] The first subgroup was called "delicate skin," distinguished by easily disrupted barrier function not accompanied by a rapid or intense inflammatory response. The second subgroup was "reactive skin," characterized by a strong inflammatory response without a significant increase in transepidermal water loss. The third group was known as "stingers" (a term coined by Kligman in 1977), which was described as a heightened neurosensory perception to minor cutaneous stimulation.

The Baumann Skin Typing System is determined by historical data gathered in a questionnaire form.[9] It divides sensitive skin into four types based on diagnosis (Table 12-1). Type 1 sensitive skin is prone to developing open and closed comedones and pimples and is known as the acne type or S1 type. Type 2 sensitive skin is characterized by facial flushing because of heat, spicy food, emotion, or vasodilation of any cause and is known as the flushing rosacea type or as the S2 type. Type 3 sensitive skin, or the S3 type, is characterized by burning, itching, or stinging of any cause. Type 4 sensitive skin is the phenotype that is susceptible to develop contact dermatitis and irritant dermatitis. The S4 type is often associated with an impaired skin barrier (see Chapters 15–18). An individual may suffer from combinations of the sensitive skin subtypes. For example, a person may burn and sting and develop acne from certain skin care products. In this case, they would be designated as an S1S3 sensitive skin type.

Acne

Baumann S1 sensitive skin is characterized by acne breakouts manifesting as open or closed comedones as well as papules and pustules (Figs. 12-1 and 12-2). This subtype was termed "acne cosmetica" by Kligman and Mills in 1972.[10] Ingredients in skin care and hair care products such as coconut oil and isopropyl myristate may contribute to acne. Blushes, lipstick, and other color cosmetics that contain D & C (Drug & Cosmetic) red dyes, which are coal

TABLE 12-1
Baumann Sensitive Skin Classification

Type 1	Pimples and comedones
Type 2	Flushing
Type 3	Burning and stinging or itching
Type 4	Impaired barrier, contact and irritant dermatitis

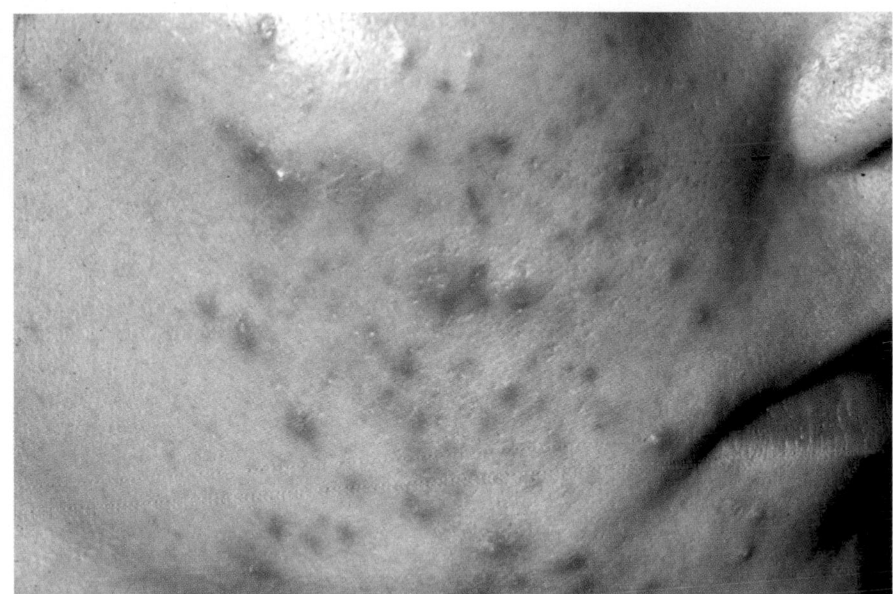

▲ **FIGURE 12-1** Inflammatory pustules seen in acne.

tar derivatives, are comedogenic (Table 12-2). Sunscreen ingredients have been known to cause acneiform eruptions as well.[11] For a detailed explanation of acne see Chapter 15.

Rosacea

Baumann S2 sensitive skin is manifested by flushing and facial redness (Fig. 12-3). Not all individuals who fall in this category have true rosacea; however, they all suffer from facial flushing that may be a predictor of future rosacea. Patients that fall into this category should be treated with anti-inflammatory skin care products to reduce inflammation (see Chapters 16 and 34).

Burning and Stinging

Baumann S3 sensitive skin is characterized by burning and stinging upon application of skin care products or exposure to environmental factors such as wind, cold, or heat. These subjective signs are usually not accompanied by facial flushing unless the subject also suffers from Baumann S2 sensitive skin with a tendency to flush (see Chapter 17).

Contact Dermatitis and Irritant Dermatitis

Baumann S4 sensitive skin is exhibited by individuals who have a history of frequent scaling, redness or irritation to allergens and irritants. Atopic dermatitis sufferers would fall into this category. These patients are more susceptible to react to substances that are not commonly considered irritants, likely caused by an impaired barrier. These substances include many cosmetics ingredients such as: dimethyl sulfoxide, benzoyl peroxide preparations, salicylic acid, propylene glycol, amyldimethylaminobenzoic acid, and 2-ethoxyethyl methoxycinnamate. The current theory is that an impaired skin barrier allows the entrance of chemicals into the skin, leading to vasodilatation, itching, scaling, and other symptoms. Many studies have supported the idea that an impaired barrier predisposes an individual to develop this type of sensitive skin. One elegant study used methyl nicotinate (MN), a water-soluble compound widely used to investigate transcutaneous penetration. Topical application of MN in humans induces vasodilatation because of the action of the drug on smooth muscle cells.[15] This study demonstrated that lactic acid stingers and those that showed susceptibility to SLS patch-testing irritation were more likely to develop vasodilatation when MN was

TABLE 12-2
Topical Ingredients in Skin Care and Hair Care Products That May Cause Acne[12–14]

Avocado oil
Butyl stearate
Ceteareth 20
Cocoa butter
Coconut oil
Decyl oleate
Evening primrose oil
Isocetyl stearate
Isopropyl isostearate
Isopropyl isothermal
Isopropyl myristate
Isopropyl palmitate
Isostearyl neopentanoate
Lanolin
Laureth 4
Lauric acid
Myristyl myristate
Octyl palmitate
Octyl stearate
Oleth-3
PPG myristyl propionate
Putty stearate
Red dyes
Soybean oil
Stearic acid

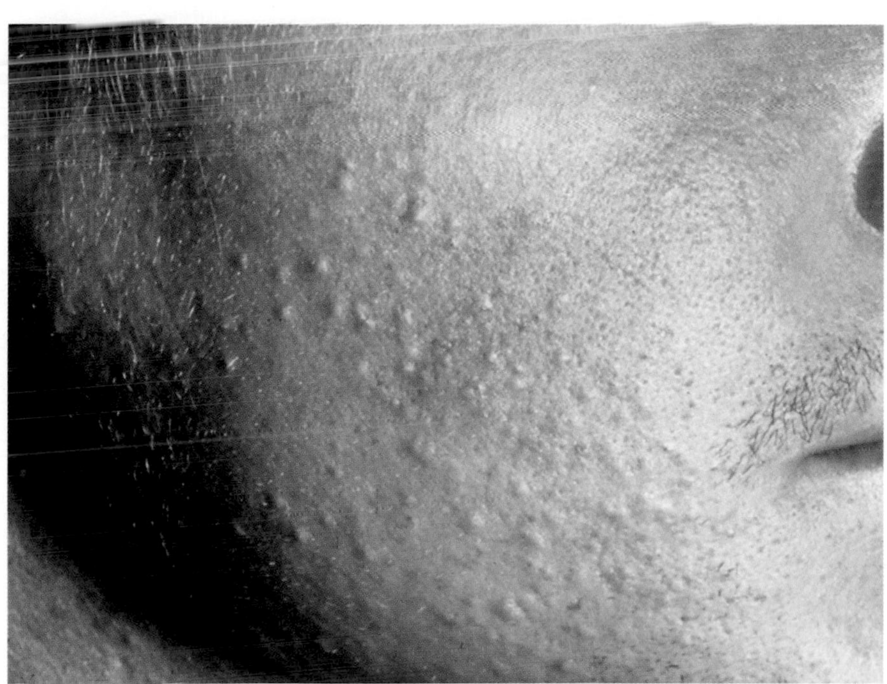

▲ **FIGURE 12-2** Comedones seen in acne subtype.

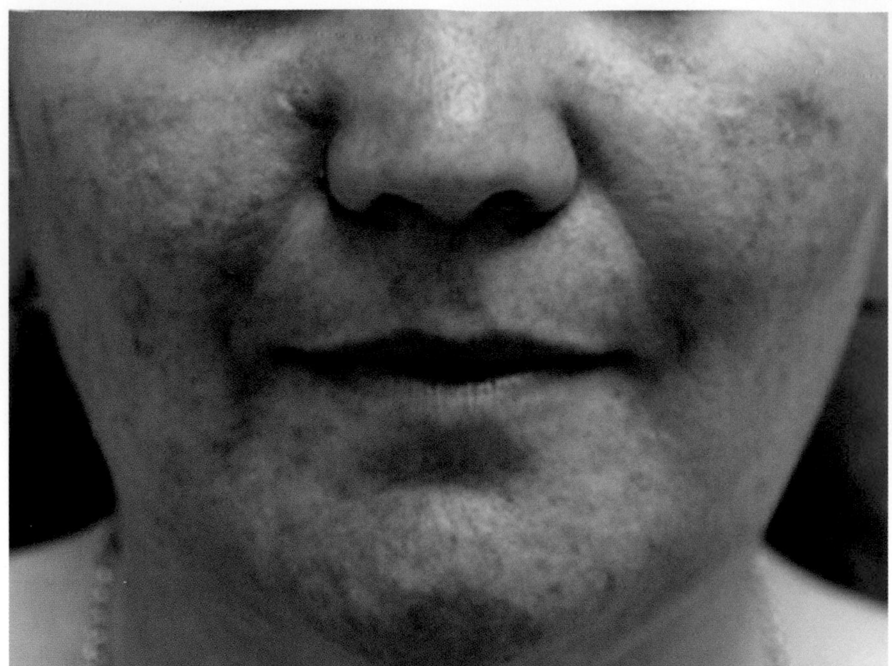

▲ **FIGURE 12-3** Facial redness in the rosacea type patient.

applied, revealing increased transcutaneous absorption in those labeled as sensitive skin types or "reactors."

SEASONALITY AND GENDER EFFECTS ON SENSITIVE SKIN

"Sensitive skin" of the burning, stinging, and itching type was found to be more frequent during the summer than the winter in one study.[3] In this same study, women were found to be more likely than men to have sensitive skin. This may reflect the fact that women have a much higher exposure, in terms of frequency and variety, to personal care products than do men. The thickness of the epidermis was observed to be greater in males than in females, which may mean that men have a stronger barrier to entry of irritants and allergens.[16] Hormonal differences may produce increased inflammatory sensitivity in females.[17]

ETHNICITY AND SENSITIVE SKIN

Studies suggest that blacks are less reactive and Asians are more reactive than whites, but no studies are conclusive.[18,19] A French study based on questionnaires showed that a fair skin type was more commonly associated with sensitive or very sensitive skin.[3] An American study, by Jourdain et al., used telephone surveys of approximately 200 each of African Americans, Asians, European Americans, and Hispanics and did not find any differences in the prevalence of sensitive skin among ethnic groups.[2] In a German–Japanese study, Japanese women reported subjective feelings of skin irritation more frequently than German women. This study demonstrated that Japanese women report skin stinging of greater severity than Caucasian women do.[20]

A normal SC, as measured in Caucasians, has been reported to consist of around 15 cell layers.[21,22] The SC appears to be equally thick in black and white skin.[23,24] However, African Americans have been shown to have a higher lipid content in the SC, more SC cell layers, and required more tape strips to remove the SC as compared to Caucasians.[25,26] This was purported to be the reason that several studies have reported decreased erythema in blacks after topical application of known irritants.[27–29] Large-scale global studies looking at the ethnic differences in incidence of the various types of sensitive skin have not been performed. At this time, the precise role of ethnicity in skin sensitivity remains to be elucidated.

TESTING FOR SENSITIVE SKIN

Baumann S1 Type Skin

For years, the rabbit ear model was used to test cosmetic ingredients for their potential to cause comedones.[30,31] Based on the rabbit ear model, it appeared that many ingredients used in cosmetics evoked a comedogenic response in animals. As animal testing fell into disfavor, new methods of comedogenicity testing were developed. Subsequently, Mills and Kligman published a study exploring the effects of these chemicals in human beings and found that the results were dissimilar from those observed in the rabbit ear model.[32] Human models of comedogenicity are currently used.[13]

Baumann S2 Type Skin

Vasoreactive tests examine vasodilatation of the skin to ascertain susceptibility to flush. The most popular test uses methyl nicotinate, a potent vasodilator. MN is applied to the upper third of the ventral forearm in concentrations varying between 1.4% and 13.7% for a period of 15 seconds. The vasodilatory effect is assessed by observing the induced erythema and measuring it with various devices such as a spectrometer or laser Doppler velocimeter (LDV). Another test used to measure the propensity for facial flushing is the red wine provocation test; however, this test is not very specific. Susceptible patients report a sense of warmth beginning around the head or neck area and moving upward on the face 10 to 15 minutes after ingestion of six ounces of red wine. Within 30 minutes, flushing becomes clinically evident.[33] The disadvantage of this test, though, is that it lacks specificity for S2 sensitive skin types; it may be positive when other conditions, such as alcohol dehydrogenase syndrome, are present.

Baumann S3 Type Skin

The sensory reactivity test focuses on the neurosensory component of the sensitive skin response. The most popular has been the sting test,[34] in which lactic acid or other agents including capsaicin, ethanol, menthol,[35] sorbic acid, and benzoic acid[36] are applied to the skin (see Chapters 17 and 38).

Baumann S4 Type Skin

To test for this type of skin, an irritant reactivity test is performed. This is also called a "patch test." In this test, an irritant or allergen is applied to the skin for a certain amount of time, usually 48 to 72 hours, and objective measures of irritation such as erythema and scaling are gauged. Primary irritants such as SLS or suspected allergens may be applied (see Chapter 18).

SUMMARY

Sensitive skin is a very common complaint globally. It has several presentations that have led to different classification systems. The Baumann Skin Typing System divides those with sensitive skin into four unique subtypes, which are discussed at length in other chapters. Using this system can help provide insights into the causes of these various subgroups of sensitive skin, including the potential roles of gender and ethnicity pertaining to subtype, and should help lead to advances in the treatment of these subtypes.

REFERENCES

1. Simion FA, Rau AH. Sensitive skin. *Cosmet Toilet*. 1994;109:43.
2. Jourdain R, de Lacharrière O, Bastien P, et al. Ethnic variations in self-perceived sensitive skin: epidemiological survey. *Contact Dermatitis*. 2002;46:162.
3. Misery L, Myon E, Martin N, et al. Sensitive skin: psychological effects and seasonal changes. *J Eur Acad Dermatol Venereol*. 2007;21:620.
4. Willis CM, Shaw S, De Lacharrière O, et al. Sensitive skin: an epidemiological study. *Br J Dermatol*. 2001;145:258.
5. Saint-Martory C, Roguedas-Contios AM, Sibaud V, et al. Sensitive skin is not limited to the face. *Br J Dermatol*. 2008;158:130.
6. Yokota T, Matsumoto M, Sakamaki T, et al. Classification of sensitive skin and development of a treatment system appropriate for each group. *IFSCC Mag*. 2003;6:303.
7. Pons-Guiraud A. Sensitive skin: a complex and multifactorial syndrome. *J Cosmet Dermatol*. 2004;3:145.
8. Muizzuddin N, Marenus KD, Maes DH. Factors defining sensitive skin and its treatment. *Am J Contact Dermat*. 1998; 9:170.
9. Baumann L. Cosmetics and skin care in dermatology. In: Wolff K, Goldsmith LA, Katz SI, Gilchrest BA, Paller AS, Leffell DJ, eds. *Fitzpatrick's Dermatology in General Medicine*. 7th ed. New York, NY: McGraw-Hill; 2007:2357-2364.
10. Kligman AM, Mills OH. Acne cosmetica. *Arch Dermatol*. 1972;106:893.
11. Foley P, Nixon R, Marks R, et al. The frequency of reactions to sunscreens: results of a longitudinal population-based study on the regular use of sunscreens in Australia. *Br J Dermatol*. 1993;128:512.
12. Betterhealthyskin.com, LLC. http://www.betterhealthyskin.com/lets-talk-cosmetics-james-e-fulton-jr-md-phd.aspx, Accessed January 2, 2008.
13. Draelos ZD, DiNardo JC. A re-evaluation of the comedogenicity concept. *J Am Acad Dermatol*. 2006;54:507.
14. Nguyen SH, Dang TP, Maibach HI. Comedogenicity in rabbit: some cosmetic ingredients/vehicles. *Cutan Ocul Toxicol*. 2007;26:287.
15. Berardesca E, Cespa M, Farinelli N, et al. In vivo transcutaneous penetration of nicotinates and sensitive skin. *Contact Dermatitis*. 1991;25:35.
16. Sandby MJ, Poulsen T, Wulf HC. Epidermal thickness at different body sites: relationship to age, gender, pigmentation, blood content, skin type and smoking habits. *Acta Derm Venereol*. 2003;83:410.
17. Farage MA. Vulvar susceptibility to contact irritants and allergens: a review. *Arch Gynecol Obstet*. 2005;272:167.
18. Modjtahedi SP, Maibach HI. Ethnicity as a possible endogenous factor in irritant contact dermatitis: comparing the irritant response among Caucasians, blacks and Asians. *Contact Dermatitis*. 2002;47:272.
19. Berardesca E, Maibach H. Ethnic skin: overview of structure and function. *J Am Acad Dermatol*. 2003;48:S139.
20. Aramaki J, Kawana S, Effendy I, et al. Differences of skin irritation between Japanese and European women. *Br J Dermatol*. 2002;146:1052.
21. Christophers E, Kligman AM. Visualization of the cell layers of the stratum corneum. *J Invest Dermatol*. 1964;42:407.
22. Blair C. Morphology and thickness of the human stratum corneum. *Br J Dermatol*. 1968;80:430.
23. Freeman RG, Cockerell EG, Armstrong J, et al. Sunlight as a factor influencing the thickness of epidermis. *J Invest Dermatol*. 1962;39:295.
24. Thomson ML. Relative efficiency of pigment and horny layer thickness in protecting the skin of Europeans and Africans against solar ultraviolet radiation. *J Physiol*. 1955;127:236.
25. Weigand DA, Haygood C, Gaylor JR. Cell layers and density of Negro and Caucasian stratum corneum. *J Invest Dermatol*. 1974;62:563.
26. Reinertson RP, Wheatley VR. Studies on the chemical composition of human epidermal lipids. *J Invest Dermatol*. 1959;32:49.
27. Weigand DA, Gaylor JR. Irritant reaction in Negro and Caucasian skin. *South Med J*. 1974;67:548.
28. Marshall EK, Lynch V, Smith HV. Variation in susceptibility of the skin to dichlorethylsulphide. *J Pharmacol Exp Ther*. 1919;12:291.
29. Weigand DA, Mershon GE. The cutaneous irritant reaction to agent O-chlorobenzylidene malonitrile (CS). Quantitation and racial influence in human subjects. *Edgewood Arsenal Technical Report 4332*. February, 1970.
30. Kligman AM, Kwong T. An improved rabbit ear model for assessing comedogenic substances. *Br J Dermatol*. 1979; 100:699.
31. Morris WE, Kwan SC. Use of the rabbit ear model in evaluating the comedogenic potential of cosmetic ingredients. *J Soc Cosmet Chem*. 1983;34:215.
32. Mills OH, Kligman AM. Human model for assessing comedogenic substances. *Arch Dermatol*. 1982;118:903.
33. Mills OH, Berger RS. Defining the susceptibility of acne prone and sensitive skin populations to extrinsic factors. *Dermatol Clin*. 1991;9:93.
34. Frosch P, Kligman AM. Method for appraising the sting capacity of topically applied substances. *J Soc Cosmet Chem*. 1977;28:197.
35. Marriott M, Holmes J, Peters L, et al. The complex problem of sensitive skin. *Contact Dermatitis*. 2005;53:93.
36. Seidenari S, Francomano M, Mantovani L. Baseline biophysical parameters in subjects with sensitive skin. *Contact Dermatitis*. 1998;38:311.

CHAPTER 13

Skin Pigmentation and Pigmentation Disorders

Leslie Baumann, MD
Sogol Saghari, MD

Pigmentation disorders and tanning play a significant role in skin appearance and the sense of well being. Many people feel that they look better with tanned skin, even though achieving such an appearance may be contributing in the long term to the formation of pigment disorders. In some cultures, such as in Asia, pigmentation concerns outweigh worries about developing wrinkles. Like acne, disorders of pigmentation cause significant stress and embarrassment, so the treatment options should be understood by every cosmetic physician. In this chapter, the mechanisms known to be involved in pigment formation will be explained and the pigmentary conditions most likely to be seen by a cosmetic dermatologist will be discussed. There is a wide array of rare dyschromias that are more pathologic in nature and that are beyond the scope of this chapter. Cosmetic dermatologists are often faced with patients presenting with melasma, solar lentigos, postinflammatory hyperpigmentation, and circles under the eyes. This group of conditions will be focused on here, in addition to some treatment options. Depigmenting agents will be discussed in greater detail in Chapter 33.

SKIN COLOR

Skin color results from the incorporation of the melanin-containing melanosomes, produced by the melanocytes, into the keratinocytes in the epidermis and their ensuing degradation. Although other factors contribute to skin color, such as carotenoids or hemoglobin,[1] the amount, quality, and distribution of melanin present in the epidermis is the main source responsible for human skin color. The number of melanocytes in human skin is equal in all races, thereby rendering melanocyte activity and interaction with the keratinocytes as the accountable factors for skin color.[2] In darker-pigmented individuals, melanocytes produce more melanin; the melanosomes are larger and more heavily melanized, and they undergo degradation at a slower rate than in lighter-skinned individuals.[3] Skin of color will be further discussed in Chapter 14.

Production of Melanin

Melanin pigment is produced in the melanosome, an organelle located in the cytoplasm of the melanocytes. Melanosomes in human skin undergo four stages of development while inside the melanocyte. In stage I, premelanosomes are characterized by their spherical structure and amorphous matrix. During stage II, they become more oval shaped with no apparent melanin. In stage III, following tyrosinase activity, melanin production starts and the melanization continues to stage IV, at which point the organelle contains high concentrations of melanin. The melanosomes are then transferred along microtubules to the dendritic structures of melanocytes and transferred to the keratinocytes.

The process of melanin production in the melanosomes is conducted via a pathway that begins with the hydroxylation of tyrosine to 3,4-dihydroxyphenylalanine (DOPA) using the enzyme tyrosinase, which subsequently oxidizes DOPA to dopaquinone, leading to the formation of melanin[4] (Fig. 13-1). Two types of melanin are produced: eumelanin and pheomelanin. The relative amounts of these two types determine hair color and skin tone. Individuals with darker skin tones have mostly eumelanin and a lesser amount of pheomelanin, while the opposite is true in people with a light skin color. Based on the levels of cysteine and sulfhydryl components such as glutathione, dopaquinone may be converted to cysteinyl-Dopa, giving rise to pheomelanin or DOPA chrome, which leads to eumelanin production.

Tyrosinase is the rate-limiting step for melanin production. Tyrosinase is stimulated by ultraviolet (UV) radiation, by DNA fragments such as thymidine dinucleotides that form as a result of UV radiation,[5] and other factors such as melanocyte-stimulating hormone (MSH), as well as growth factors such as bFGF and endothelin. Protein kinase C[6] and the cyclic adenosine monophosphate (cAMP) ± protein kinase A pathway[5] play a role in increasing melanin production as do prostaglandins D2, E2, and F2, tumor necrosis factor (TNF)-α, interleukins 1α, IL1β, and IL6.[7] Vitamin D may also play a role in stimulating melanogenesis.[8]

Once the melanin is synthesized within the melanosomes, it migrates into the dendrite tips of the melanocytes via microtubules and using myosin V filaments[9] and a dynein "motor."[10] Each melanocyte is in contact with an average of 36 keratinocytes, forming an "epidermal melanin unit"[1,11] (Fig. 13-2). The melanin in the melanocytes is then incorporated into other keratinocytes of the epidermal melanin unit or into the dermis by a process that is still poorly understood. Several mechanisms have been proposed for this transfer of melanin to the neighboring keratinocytes. The first involves phagocytosis. Melanin is released into the dermis following damage to melanocytes in the basal layer and is then phagocytized by melanophages. Another proposed mechanism of melanin transfer is endocytosis. This process would involve the melanosomes being discharged directly into the intercellular spaces followed by endocytosis by the keratinocytes. The final hypothesis is that the melanin transfer occurs by keratinocyte-melanocyte membrane fusion.[12] Although the exact process of melanin transfer is not completely understood, new discoveries are rapidly being made in this area. For example, Sieberg et al. found that the protease-activated receptor 2 (PAR-2), expressed on keratinocytes, is important in regulating the ingestion of melanosomes by keratinocytes in culture.[12] PAR-2 is a G-protein-coupled receptor that is activated by a serine protease cleavage,[13] and is able to enhance the capacity of keratinocytes to ingest melanosomes. The PAR-2 can be up- or downregulated, and is upregulated by UV radiation.[14] It is thought to be important in hyperpigmentation disorders because it has been found that serine protease inhibitors that interfere with PAR-2 activation induce depigmentation by reducing melanosome transfer and distribution.[15] Soybeans, which contain the serine protease inhibitors soybean trypsin inhibitor (STI) and Bowman-Birk protease inhibitor (BBI), have been shown to inhibit melanosome transfer, resulting in an improvement of mottled facial pigmentation.[16] In addition, activation of

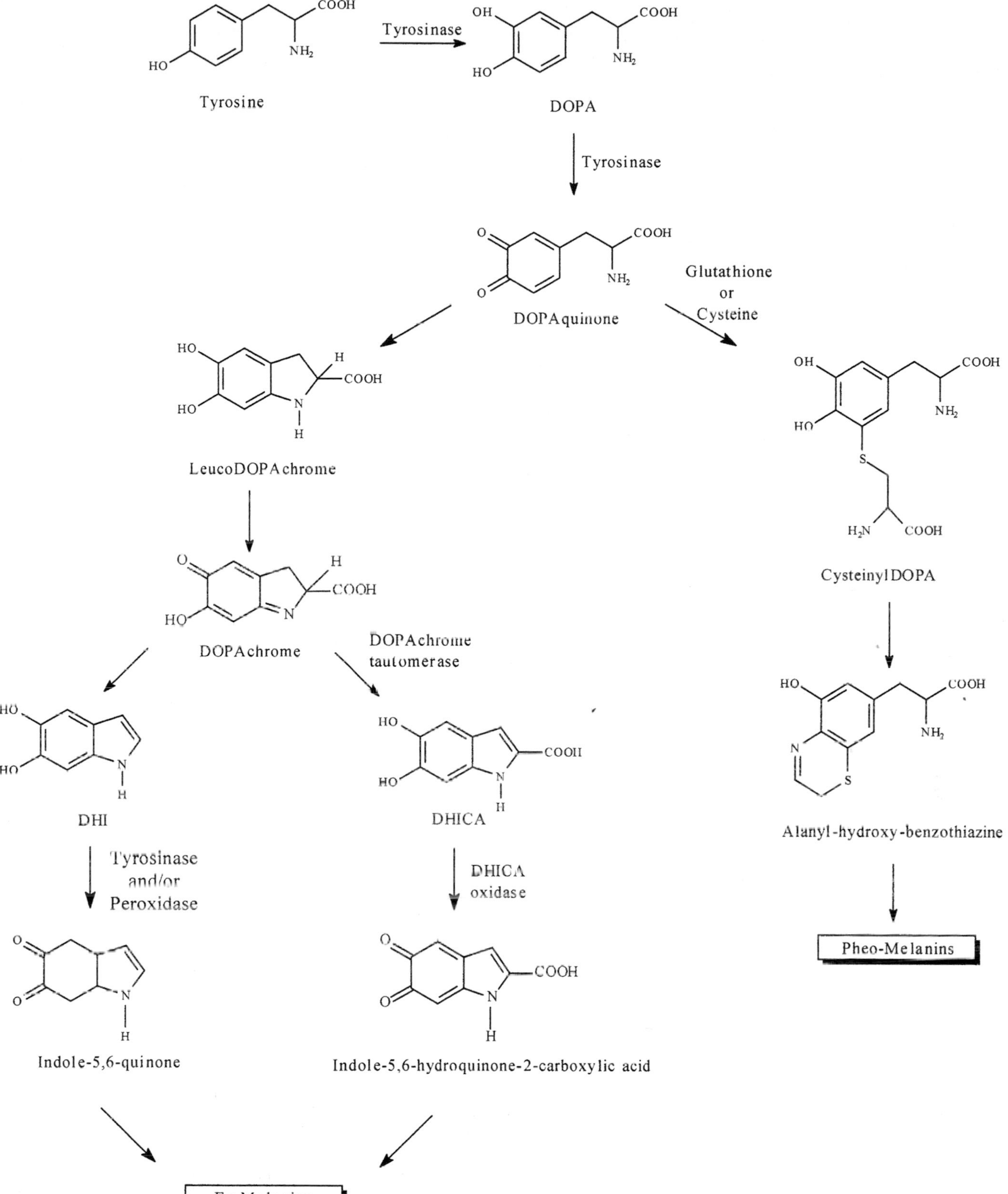

▲ **FIGURE 13-1** The melanin biosynthesis pathway. Most depigmenting agents work by inhibiting tyrosinase.

PAR-2 with trypsin and other synthetic peptides has been shown to result in visible skin darkening.[15]

Other systems play a role in melanosome transfer as well. For example, the soluble portion of the N-terminal of β-amyloid precursor protein (APP), called sAPP, is a newly detected epidermal growth factor that has been shown to increase the release of melanin as well as enhance the movements of the melanocyte dendritic tips.[17] Keratinocyte growth factor (KGF/FGF7) also promotes melanosome transfer by stimulating the phagocytic process.[18] Several different factors affect melanosome transfer and play a role in the complex pigmentation process.

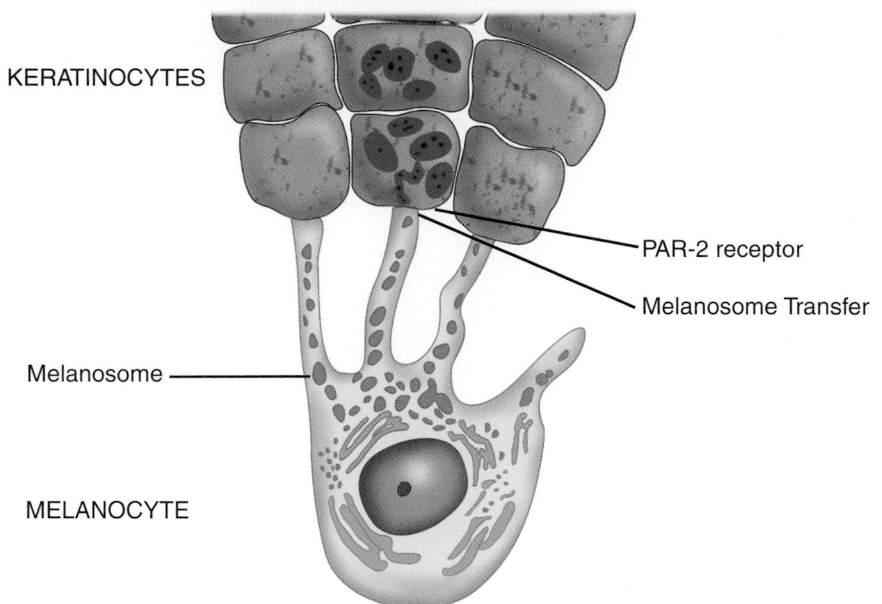

▲ **FIGURE 13-2** Epidermal—melanin unit. One melanocyte can intercalate with many keratinocytes.

MELANOCYTE-STIMULATING HORMONE AND PIGMENTATION

As discussed, many factors play a role in the formation and transfer of melanin; however, the role of MSH deserves a separate discussion. MSH is derived from the proopiomelanocortin (POMC) gene. Among the three forms of MSH (α, β, and γ), αMSH is the most active form in the human body. Melanocortin 1 receptor (MC1R) is the receptor for MSH commonly located on the melanocytes. The binding of MSH to MC1R leads to activation of adenylate cyclase, which increases cAMP levels. cAMP stimulates the activity of tyrosinase, leading to production of eumelanin. In cases in which MC1R is mutated or not functioning properly, the pathway switches to production of pheomelanin. MC1R mutation, and therefore a higher presence of pheomelanin, is seen in individuals with red hair[19] (Fig. 13-3). This pathway is interesting for several reasons. First, MSH has been found to be a factor in the tanning mechanism. Individuals with red hair have a defect in the MC1R and are poor tanners.[20] The role of MSH in tanning is discussed in the upcoming section on tanning. Second, MSH plays a role in the hyperpigmentation seen in endocrine disorders such as pituitary tumors and Cushing's syndrome. In addition, adrenocorticotropic hormone (ACTH) levels increase with stress; therefore, stress can lead to an increase in MSH. In fact, one study demonstrated increased tanning in stressed mice when exposed to UVB. This enhanced tanning response was inhibited when the mice were treated with corticostatin, an ACTH inhibitor.[21] MSH may contribute to the exacerbation of melasma and other pigmentary disorders in stressed patients, as well as in tanning.

ULTRAVIOLET LIGHT AND SKIN COLOR

UV irradiation is a major source of environmental influence and damage to the skin. Two expressions have been used to explain the particular skin tone for an individual that, out of necessity, address the issue of UV. *Constitutive skin color* (CSC) refers to the genetically influenced color and melanin production of someone without the impact of UV light

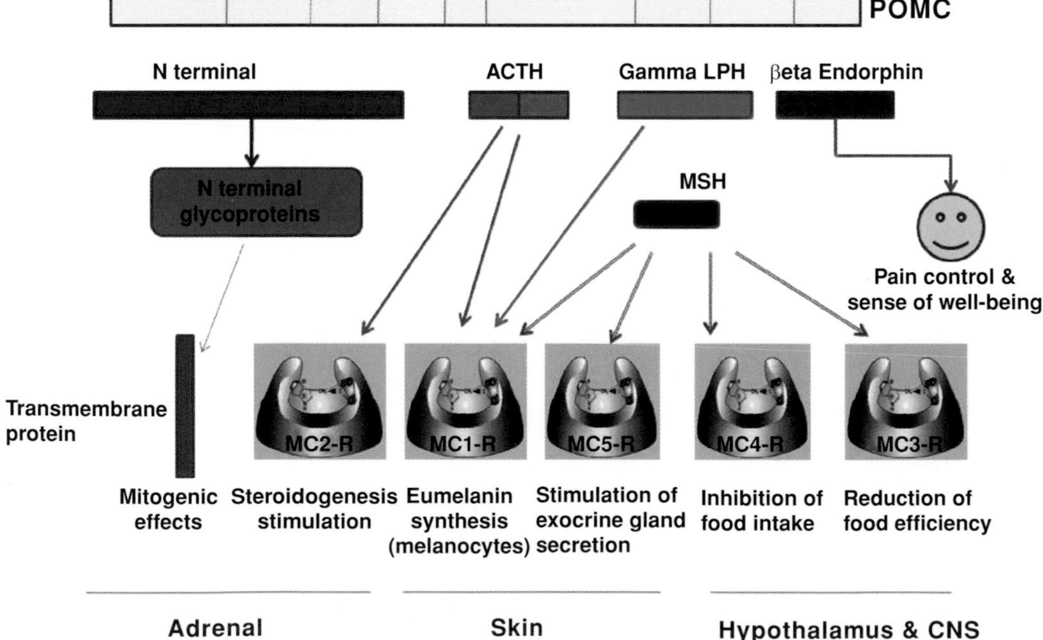

▲ **FIGURE 13-3** The POMC gene is found in keratinocytes, adrenal tissue, the hypothalamus, and CNS. When POMC is activated, it transcribes four main sequences: the N terminus, adrenocorticotrophin (ACTH), gamma lipotrophin (gamma LPH), and β-endorphins. These sequences subsequently lead to activation of the melanocortin receptors as shown. Activation of the MC1R receptor leads to melanogenesis.

or environmental factors, whereas *facultative skin color* (FSC) denotes the color influenced by UV light and hormones.[22] When exposed skin is subjected to UV light, melanogenesis or "tanning" occurs, representing the skin's major defense against further UV damage. This darkening results when the UV radiation provides a positive signal to the exposed epidermal melanin units. Subsequent to UVA exposure, the skin develops an *immediate pigmentary darkening* provoked by the oxidation of the existing melanin. This effect appears within a few minutes of exposure to UVA and lasts for approximately 6 to 8 hours. Both UVB and UVA are involved in the process of *delayed tanning*. It is seen 2 to 3 days after exposure and lasts for approximately 10 to 14 days. In this process, tyrosinase enzyme activity and the number of melanocytes that are actively producing melanin increase. In addition, melanosome transfer from the melanocytes to the keratinocytes is enhanced.[23] The resulting increase in melanin protects against further UV damage by surrounding the cell nucleus and absorbing UV photons and UV-generated free radicals before they can react with DNA and other critical cellular components. Research by Gilchrest et al. has demonstrated that DNA damage or DNA repair intermediates can stimulate melanogenesis in the absence of UV light.[24] In fact, small, single-stranded DNA fragments such as thymidine dinucleotides (pTT) are able to stimulate tanning through activation of p53.[5,25] A tumor suppressor and transcription factor, p53 is known to mediate the response to DNA damage. Once DNA damage occurs, p53 induces cell-cycle arrest and facilitates DNA repair or, when the DNA damage is irreparable, it triggers apoptosis. A link between tanning and p53 has been found that may explain the positive sensations, or endorphins, reported by tanners.[26] When p53 is stimulated by UV, transcription of the POMC gene is activated. This results in production of both MSH (leading to pigmentation) and β-endorphin, which is in the opiate family. These findings may lend credence to the theory that some individuals develop an addiction to tanning[27] (Fig. 13-4).

Once activated by adenylate cyclase, cAMP plays a role in the tanning process as well by mediating the effects of αMSH.[28] When MC1R is activated by MSH, adenylate cyclase is stimulated to form cAMP, which then stimulates melanogenesis, melanocyte differentiation, and the transfer of melanosomes to keratinocytes. Increasing activity of cAMP may lead to a tanning response. This theory is supported by a trial in mice. In this study, a topical formulation containing forskolin, a root extract of *Plectranthus barbatus* (also called *Coleus forskohlii*), was applied to MC1R-deficient mice. Forskohlii activates adenylate cyclase, which upregulates cAMP. In the mice, topical application induced melanogenesis and production of eumelanin. However, this effect was not seen in swine, likely because of greater skin thickness and therefore a stronger barrier to penetration. The tanning seen in the mice occurred without activation of MC1R and thus, it did not require sun exposure.[29] This study illustrates the importance of cAMP and may provide promise or insight into mechanisms for developing a "protective tan."

Although tanned skin is considered beautiful by many, stimulating the pigmentary system is not always desirable. In many Asian countries, for example, tanning is not commonplace and untanned skin is preferred. In addition, development of pigmentary disorders such as melasma and solar lentigos is undesirable. Understanding the mechanisms of the pigmentary system will help increase the understanding of the following pigmentary disorders.

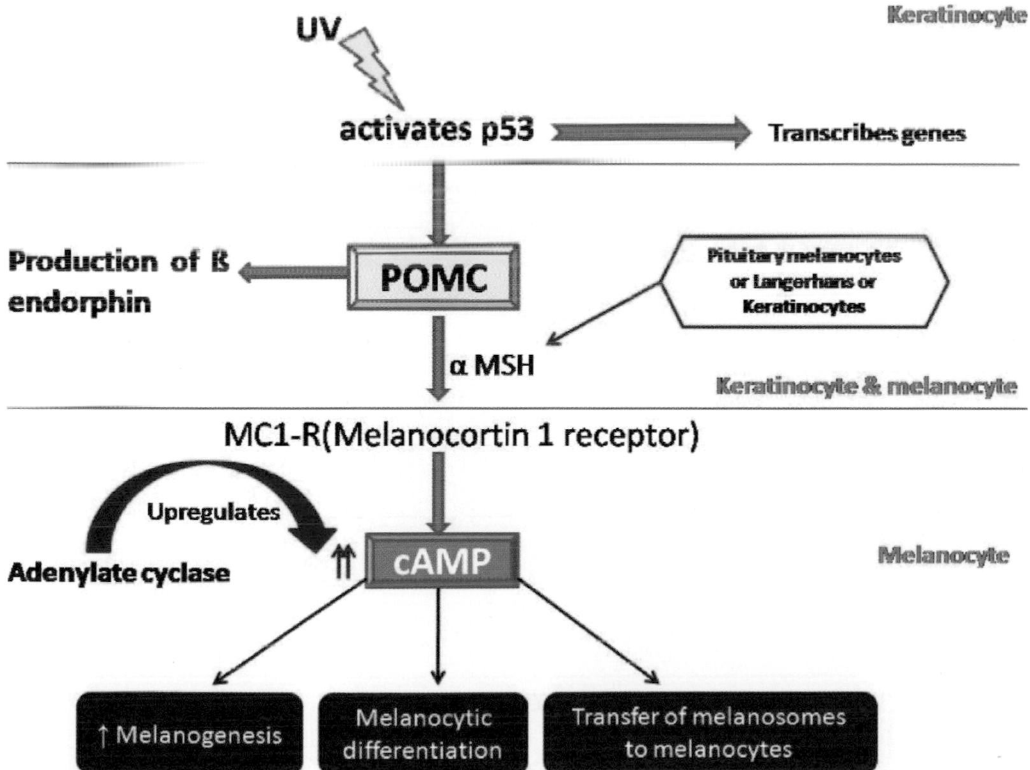

▲ **FIGURE 13-4** UV radiation activates p53, which stimulates the POMC gene to transcribe alpha melanocyte-stimulating hormone. αMSH binds the MC1-R receptor located on the melanocytes, which triggers adenylate cyclase to produce cAMP. cAMP then stimulates tyrosinase to produce melanin. Interestingly, when POMC transcription is stimulated, β-endorphin production also increases, leading to the "tanning high" reported by sun seekers.

MELASMA

Melasma, also known as chloasma or the "mask of pregnancy," is a very common condition usually seen in women of childbearing age (Fig. 13-5). It is a chronic disorder that can be frustrating to patients and physicians alike because it is very difficult to treat. Melasma presents as irregularly shaped, but often distinctly defined, blotches of light- to dark-brown pigmentation. These patches are usually seen on the upper lip, nose, cheeks, chin, forehead, and, sometimes, the neck. There are three typical patterns of distribution—most common is centrofacial, involving the cheeks, forehead, upper lip, nose, and chin.[30] The malar pattern, which affects the nose and cheeks, and mandibular pattern, are less common. It is most commonly seen in areas that receive sun exposure; however, melasma has been reported on the nipples and around the external genitalia.[31,32]

Etiology

Melasma is a fairly typical, physiologic occurrence seen most often during pregnancy or oral contraceptive use. It can occur at any time during a woman's reproductive years, and is more common in women of darker skin types. Although there have been many suggested causative factors, estrogen and UV light seem to be the most prominent culprits. Melasma is so common in pregnancy that it has been dubbed the "mask of pregnancy." It is currently unknown how increased estrogen levels lead to melasma; however, recent studies have suggested that estradiols may play an important role in the etiology. 17 β-Estradiol, which is known to affect other cells of neural crest origin, has been shown to significantly increase the activity of tyrosinase when added to melanocyte cultures.[33] However, melasma also occurs in men in approximately 10% of cases, most often in those of Middle Eastern, Caribbean, or Asian descent. Solar exposure is well known to exacerbate the condition and seems to be necessary for its development.[4,34] In fact, melasma has been reported to be less noticeable in the winter months when sun exposure is typically lower.[4]

The other proposed causes of melasma include genetic predisposition, nutritional deficiency, and influence from hormones such as progesterone, although the exact etiology remains vague.[31,32] In addition, the antiepilepsy drugs Hydantoin and Dilantin have been implicated in contributing to melasma in both women and men.[32,35] Approximately one-third of cases in women and most cases in men are idiopathic.[32] Some authors have hypothesized an endocrine, causal mechanism,[32] but no such mechanism has been established.[35] Although there have been a few familial cases reported, the evidence that melasma can be inherited is sparse.[35] Heat may play a role in melasma as well. Many women develop melasma on the upper lip after hot wax has been used as a hair removal method. Although this may represent a coincidence, it is so commonly reported by patients that the author believes that heat may play a role in melasma as it does in erythema *ab igne*. (Erythema *ab igne* is a reticulated erythematous hyperpigmented eruption that occurs after chronic exposure to heat.)

Several authors have noted that melasma most often appears in young women who are using oral contraceptives.[31,32] Melasma is also common among pregnant women and together these two conditions comprise the majority of melasma cases. Menopausal and premenstrual presentations occasionally occur as well. Although estrogen is thought to play a major role in the etiology of melasma, there is also a low incidence of melasma cases among postmenopausal women on estrogen replacement therapy.[4] Although melasma may diminish in the months following a patient's pregnancy or after the patient discontinues oral contraceptives, the condition often persists, taking up to 5 years to resolve.[32,35] The course of the condition varies significantly from patient to patient and within individual women, even from pregnancy to pregnancy.[4] Increased incidence of melasma also coincides with some ovarian disorders. Unfortunately, once patients develop melasma, they have a high chance of experiencing recurrence of this difficult disorder.

It is always important to consider the possibility of pigmented contact dermatitis (Riehl's melanosis) in response to cosmetic products when evaluating a patient for treatment of melasma, since avoidance of the specific allergen will improve the clinical picture (see Chapter 18 for more information about contact dermatitis). As mentioned earlier, stress hormones such as ACTH and MSH are involved in skin pigmentation. It has been previously shown that human keratinocytes are capable of synthesizing and secreting POMC-derived peptides such as ACTH and MSH.[36] Inoue et al. demonstrated that pretreatment of stressed mice, exposed to UV light, with an ACTH-inhibitor reduced the numbers of dopa-positive melanocytes.[21] More structural studies are needed to evaluate the effect of stress in induction or aggravation of melasma in humans.

Another influence in melasma is the stem cell factor, which is the ligand for c-kit located on the melanocytes. Stem cell factor is secreted by dermal fibroblasts and keratinocytes.[37] One study showed that there is increased expression of stem cell factor in the dermis and c-kit of lesional skin of patients with melasma.[38] The authors of this study proposed that UV light activates the

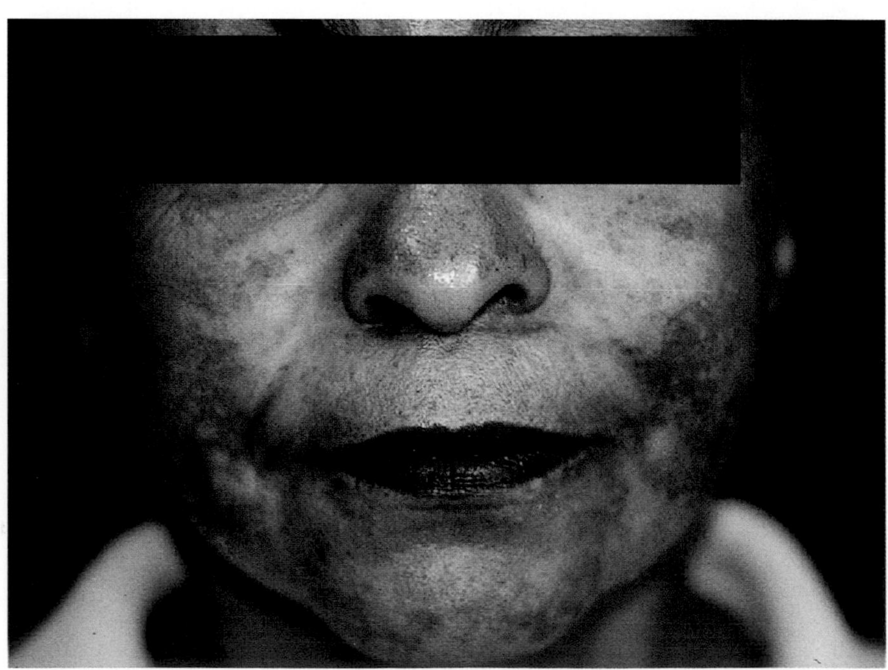

▲ **FIGURE 13-5** Patient with diffuse melasma. The patient has not improved despite multiple therapies including depigmenting agents, chemical peels, and good sun protection.

dermal fibroblasts, which leads to increased levels of soluble stem cell factor and activation of epidermal melanocytes. The role of stem cell factor in melasma is poorly understood at this time.

Histopathology

In the epidermal form of melasma, which appears light or dark brown or black clinically, the basal and suprabasal layers have a higher than normal level of melanin, which can also be present throughout the epidermis.[31,4] The melanocytes also appear larger with more noticeable dendritic processes; however, the number of melanocytes is equal to the number in unaffected skin.[39] In the dermal type of melasma, which appears blue-gray clinically, melanin-laden macrophages emerge in a perivascular arrangement in the superficial and middle level of the dermis. A mixed form, with both epidermal and dermal components, also commonly occurs.

Electron microscopy of skin from patients with melasma shows increased melanosomes and dendritic processes in the hyperpigmented area of the skin.[39] Dopa reaction has shown increased melanin production within the increased number of melanocytes.[34]

Epidermal Versus Dermal Disease

Epidermal melasma is easier to treat than dermal melasma because the melanin is at a higher level in the skin and therefore can be more easily reached by topically applied products. Because the epidermal component is amenable to treatment while the dermal component is usually not, it is helpful to determine the extent of the dermal component of the condition in order to accurately predict a patient's treatment response and to provide the patient with the proper expectations. A Wood's light or blue light can be used to examine the face at the initial visit to ascertain the extent of the dermal component[34] (Fig. 13-6). In the epidermal type, the epidermal component will appear darker under Wood's light examination. The dermal component will be less visible when observed under a Wood's light.[40] In other words, if the lesions are more pronounced with Wood's light examination, there is a better chance for clinical improvement. However, the Wood's light examination did not help to predict the clinical response to peels in a study by Lawrence.[41] The investigators felt that this occurred because there was such a high number of patients with a mixed epidermal/dermal form of melasma. However, the consensus remains that patients in whom epidermal melasma predominates may respond better than those with a large dermal component. Therefore, the Wood's examination is still a useful adjunct to determine a patient's prognosis in the treatment of melasma.

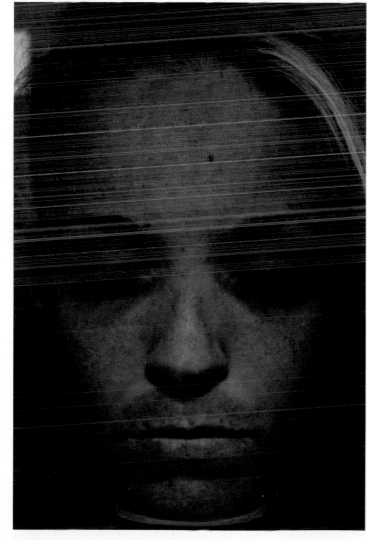

▲ **FIGURE 13-6** Blue light can be used to visualize facial pigment.

Treatment

The therapeutic objective is to retard the proliferation of melanocytes, inhibit the formation of melanosomes, and, further, promote the degradation of melanosomes.[42] Treatment options will be discussed in detail in Chapter 83, but must include a good high-SPF sunscreen with UVA protection and sun avoidance (Box 13-1). The sunscreen must be worn 24 hours a day. Sun avoidance, UVA screens for car and home windows, and protective clothing, such as hats, are a great addition to a topical treatment regimen. Topical treatments may include hydroquinone 2% to 4%, low-potency steroids, kojic acid, arbutin, azelaic acid, hydroxy acids, and retinoids. Topical tretinoin improves epidermal hyperpigmentation by decreasing tyrosinase activity and melanin production as well as enhancing the desquamation of the epidermis.[43] Although tretinoin 0.1% has been studied as a single agent in the treatment of melasma,[44,45] the time to improvement is lengthy (10 months, in one study). Therefore, most physicians use a combination of topical products. The "Kligman formula" is a mixture consisting of 0.1% tretinoin, 5.0% hydroquinone, 0.1% dexamethasone, and hydrophilic ointment.[46] It has been a very popular melasma treatment since its introduction in 1975; however, this formula is currently not commercially available and must be formulated by a pharmacy. A prescription combination preparation similar to the Kligman formula that contains hydroquinone 4%, tretinoin 0.05%, and fluocinolone 0.01% has been approved by the FDA and is a popular treatment for melasma. Most prescription formulas contain 4% hydroquinone; however,

BOX 13-1 Regimen for Patients With Melasma

Morning:

1. Wash with a cleanser that contains an alpha hydroxy acid.
2. Apply a product with hydroquinone, kojic acid, or azelaic acid.
3. Apply a UVA/UVB broad-spectrum sunscreen.
4. Wear a hat and avoid sun and heat when possible.
5. Take an antioxidant supplement such as pycnogenol (see Chapter 34).

Evening:

1. Wash with a cleanser that contains an alpha hydroxy acid.
2. Apply a retinoid such as Retin-A, Renova, Differin or Tazorac, or a product with hydroquinone and a retinoid such as Tri-Luma.

Undergo an in-office peel every 2 weeks (i.e., Jessner's, glycolic, or salicylic acid). Slowly increase the strength of the peel as tolerated. Some physicians use microdermabrasion prior to the peel to increase penetration of the ingredients.

Note: Some patients develop exogenous ochronosis, or increased pigmentation, on exposure to hydroquinone. A good history should be taken and if the patient is sensitive to hydroquinone, it should be avoided. Azelaic acid (Azelex) is another option that is useful in all patients but especially those who cannot tolerate hydroquinone.

there are specialized pharmacies that will prepare formulations with higher concentrations of hydroquinone. The stability of such creams is questionable as retinoids and hydroquinone can work in opposition, thus diminishing overall efficacy if not formulated properly. The author advises using the FDA-approved formulations rather than those compounded by a pharmacy.

Topical steroids have depigmenting effects with an unknown mechanism. It has been proposed that they decrease both production and secretion of melanin in the melanocytes.[46] However, because of potential side effects, such as skin atrophy as well as triggering acne and telangiectasia, the use of steroids is limited to low-potency formulas unless they are combined with a retinoid. Retinoids have been shown to help prevent the atrophy that occurs with topical steroids.[47]

Recent studies have shown that glycolic acid is also beneficial in enhancing the effectiveness of hydroquinone.[48] The addition of glycolic acid facilitates penetration of both agents and hence promotes efficacy. Glycolic acid can be used in a chemical peel formulation or as an additive to home products. Glycolic acid peels and/or Jessner's peels can be used in combination with topical agents to hasten the resolution of melasma (see Chapter 20). Lawrence et al. found that Jessner's solution and 70% glycolic acid (combined with tretinoin and hydroquinone between peels) worked equally well in the treatment of melasma.[41]

The addition of kojic acid may also improve the efficacy of topical agents according to other recent studies. Research performed in Singapore followed 40 Chinese women treated with 2% kojic acid in a gel containing 10% glycolic acid and 2% hydroquinone on one-half of the face.[49] The other half was treated with the same application but without kojic acid. The patients were observed for 12 weeks. All patients showed improvement in melasma on both sides of the face; however, the side treated with the combination containing kojic acid showed more improvement. More than half of the melasma cleared in 24 of the 40 (60%) patients receiving kojic acid compared to 19 of 40 (47.5%) patients receiving the gel without kojic acid.

A tretinoin acid peel is another acceptable option in patients with melasma. In a study of 10 Asian women with melasma, although a 1% tretinoin peel was as effective as a 70% glycolic acid peel, the tretinoin was better tolerated by the patients.[50]

Because there are so many treatment options and compliance is a vital aspect of treating this condition, the regimen should be easy for the patient to understand. Many companies such as La Roche-Posay, Obagi, and Topix package products in an easy-to-follow treatment regimen. Skin care regimens are often combined with microdermabrasion, light treatments, or laser; however, it is the author's opinion that proper skin care and education are paramount for the successful treatment of this disorder.

Intense pulsed light (IPL), a noncoherent broadband light source ranging from 500 to 1200 nm, is another available option for melasma treatment. This procedure is very popular because there is minimal down time and it offers a low risk of side effects. In a study conducted by Wang et al. on 31 Asian women with dermal and mixed melasma, IPL treatment on a monthly basis was compared to 4% topical hydroquinone; 35% of patients in the IPL group showed more than 50% improvement, compared to 14% in the control group.[51] The initial cutoff filter was 570 nm, and 590 to 615 filters were used for the remaining treatments to target deeper components. As expected, epidermal melasma treated with IPL seems to have more promising results as compared to dermal melasma.[52] Although IPL is considered a safe treatment, postinflammatory pigment alteration (PIPA) remains a possibility. Therefore, IPL must be used with caution for individuals with darker skin tones. This treatment will not be successful without a proper skin care regimen and sun avoidance.

The Q-switched Alexandrite laser (755 nm) has also been successfully used to treat melasma.[53] In addition, this laser has been used in conjunction with the UltraPulse CO_2 laser.[54,55] In one study, the combination of the Q-switched Alexandrite laser and UltraPulse CO_2 was associated with more side effects than the Q-switched Alexandrite laser alone, though the combination treatment was more effective.[55]

Fractional photothermolysis is a new option for lightening hyperpigmented areas of the face. In a study performed by Rokhsar et al., 10 patients with refractory melasma and Fitzpatrick skin types III to V received four to six treatments with a Fraxel laser (Reliant Technologies, Palo Alto, CA, USA) at 1- to 2-week intervals; 60% of the patients showed 75% to 100% clearance of their melasma based on the physician evaluation[56] (see Chapter 26).

Patient education is one of the most important aspects of a melasma treatment regimen. Most patients do not realize the important role of UV radiation in this condition, particularly the capacity of UVA rays to penetrate glass. Patients should be instructed to wear, during all daylight hours, a broad-spectrum UVA and UVB sunscreen of the highest SPF that they can tolerate. Patients should also understand that no sunscreen offers complete protection; therefore, sun avoidance should also be practiced. Because patients may have difficulty seeing the improvement in their skin, serial photography with a regular camera and a UV camera can be used to document treatment response.[57]

SOLAR LENTIGOS

Up to 90% of elderly patients have one or more solar lentigos.[58] As the name suggests, the sun is the culprit here, with both acute and chronic exposure linked to engendering these macular brown lesions usually 1 cm in diameter. Solar lentigos are more common in men than

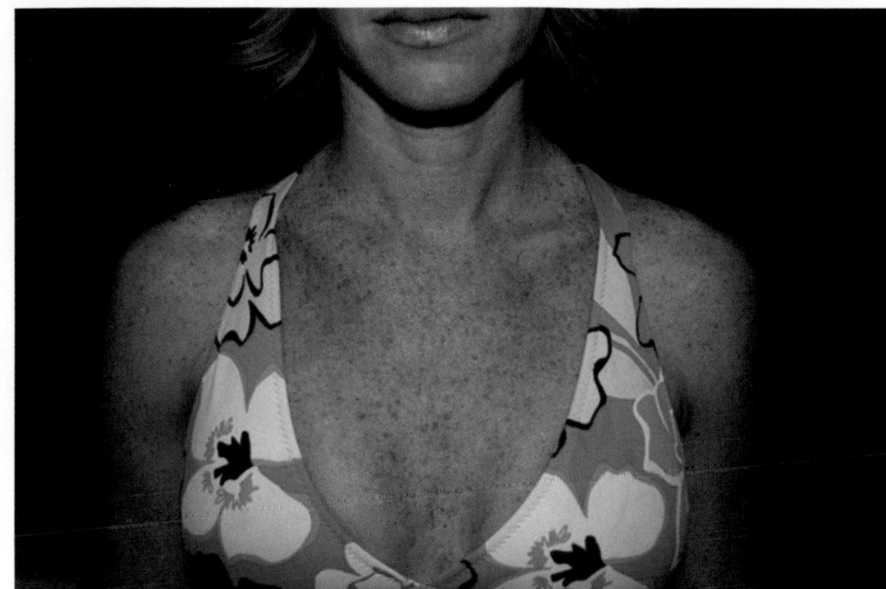

▲ **FIGURE 13-7** Clinical photo of solar lentigos.

women, as opposed to ephelides (freckles), which are reportedly more common in women.[59] The face and backs of hands are the typical areas affected. These lesions are seldom seen among patients younger than 50 years and, therefore, have also been called "senile lentigos." The sun, rather than age, is the causative factor, however. These lesions do not occur on sun-protected skin, even in the elderly (Fig. 13-7). Solar lentigos, ephelides, and lentigos simplex are difficult to distinguish from each other clinically. Taken together, these types of lesions constitute a significant risk factor for melanoma and basal cell carcinoma.[60,61]

Histopathology

Solar lentigos exhibit elongated rete ridges that contain deeply pigmented basaloid cells intermingled with melanocytes. Also, they have an elevated number of melanocytes, which have been shown to have an increased capacity for melanin production.[58] The melanin content of the epidermis in facial solar lentigos has been demonstrated to be 2.2 times higher than that in photodamaged skin.[62] Solar lentigos can be distinguished from freckles histologically because freckles do not have elongated rete ridges and have a normal or lower number of melanocytes (Fig. 13-8).

Prevention of solar lentigos is best achieved through use of sunscreens and sun avoidance. A study in *JAMA* revealed that sunscreen usage helped reduce the occurrence of nevi in white children.[63] Because increased numbers of these nevi are associated with an elevated risk of melanoma, the importance of preventing the onset of such lesions cannot be overstated.

Treatment

Solar lentigos can be treated with various methods depending on convenience for the patient. For example, some patients may want to treat with slower methods that require no down time; other patients want to have the lesions removed in as few office visits as possible and don't mind the down time. All patients should be treated with a home regimen of sunscreen and a combination of topical retinoids, topical bleaching agents, and hydroxy acids. For those patients who want faster and more visible results, TCA peels, lasers (e.g., Q-Switch Ruby, Alexandrite, and Nd:Yag), local dermabrasion, and cryotherapy can be used. When treating a patient with cryotherapy, only a single freeze thaw is recommended, since an aggressive treatment may lead to scarring and hypopigmentation.[64] Chemical peeling agents such as TCA, glycolic acid, and combination peels have been used for many years for the treatment of solar lentigines.[65–67] Although effective, the pain and burning sensation that especially accompanies treatment of a large surface area may be a limiting factor. Several studies have compared the efficacy of these various treatments. An ingenious method developed by Hexsel utilizes a tiny dermabrasion instrument to remove the solar lentigos.[68] She treated 10 female patients who had solar lentigos on the backs of their hands with either localized dermabrasion or cryotherapy. More than 50% of the patients treated with cryotherapy continued to display hypochromia in the treated areas 6 months after treatment, compared with 11% of the patients treated with dermabrasion. The percentage of recurrence of solar lentigos was the same with both treatments (55.55%). In a study comparing liquid nitrogen to 35% TCA in the treatment of solar lentigines of hands in 25 patients, cryotherapy was found to be superior with 71% of subjects showing 50% or more improvement compared to 47% improvement with TCA peel.[69] In this study, although most patients believed that TCA peel has the fastest healing time, liquid nitrogen was rated more efficacious.

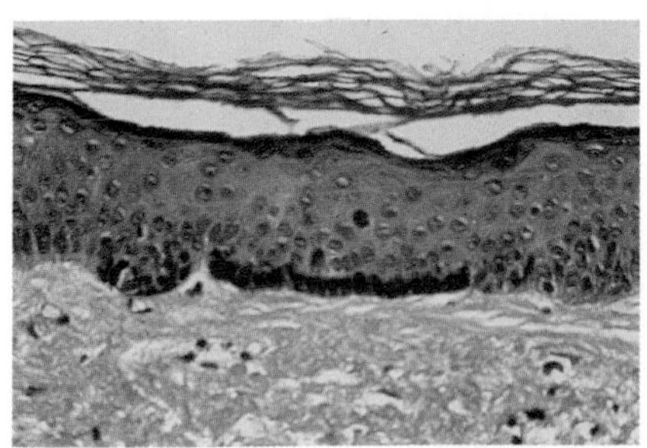

▲ **FIGURE 13-8** Hematoxylin and eosin (H&E) stain of a solar lentigo. *(Photo courtesy of George Ioannides, MD.)*

Laser therapy has also been shown to be effective in treating solar lentigos. One study examining the efficacy of the Q-switched ruby laser in the treatment of solar lentigos demonstrated a response rate of 70% after one or two treatments.[70] The Alexandrite 755 nm,[71] Q-switched Nd:YAG 532 nm, long pulse Nd:YAG 532 nm,[72] 1550 nm diode-pumped erbium fiber laser (Fraxel),[73] and IPL[74] have all been used in the treatment of solar lentigos with success. These methods will be further discussed in Chapter 24. Although lasers are very effective for these lesions, patients should be warned that treated areas will be red or have a scab for approximately 7 to 10 days depending on the type of laser used. The most common side effect of laser treatment is PIPA. A rare side effect worth mentioning is chrysiasis after treatment with Q-switched lasers in patients previously treated with oral or parenteral gold.[75–77] Therefore, it is recommended that all patients get screened for past gold treatment.

Topical creams and bleaching agents are good alternatives for patients who do not wish to undergo aggressive treatments. Topical retinoids (i.e., tretinoin, tazarotene, and adapalene) are effective options and can be used alone or in combination with other bleaching agents such as hydroquinone and azelaic acid. Retinoids have the ability to increase the penetration of bleaching agents and chemical peels in addition to decreasing melanin production. Tretinoin 0.01% in combination with 4-hydroxyanisole (Mequinol) has been shown to be effective in the treatment of solar lentigos.[78,79] Ortonne et al. reported the effect of 4-hydroxyanisole 2%/tretinoin 0.01% solution, and sunscreen in 406 patients with solar lentigines for up to 24 weeks; 325 patients (88%) had an almost complete fading of their facial lesions and 298 (81%) experienced the same in targeted forearm lesions.[80] In another study, Kang et al. treated 90 patients exhibiting solar and actinic lentigines with adapalene gel (0.1% or 0.3%) and compared the results to its vehicle; 1 month following the treatment patients treated with adapalene gel showed significant lightening of their solar lentigines.[81] In addition, the use of tazarotene 0.1% cream once daily in 562 patients with facial photoaging for 24 weeks showed improvement of the lentigines and mottled hyperpigmentation by at least one point using a seven-point scale (0 represented complete response and 6 denoted worsening), when compared to its vehicle.[82] This treatment was followed by an additional 28 weeks of tazarotene 0.1% cream treatment, and continuing improvement was observed with no plateau effect.[83] Accordingly, it is important to inform patients that it may take a few months for topical retinoids to show depigmenting results.

It is also important to remember that patients with multiple solar lentigos are at an increased risk for skin cancer. There is no evidence or reason to believe that successful treatment of these lesions leads to a lower melanoma risk. Therefore, patients with significant numbers of solar lentigos, treated or untreated, should undergo routine skin cancer examinations.

"TANNING-BED" LENTIGINES

The development of unusual melanocytic lesions after exposure to UVA tanning beds has been reported. Clinically, these lesions appear similar to the lentigines that occur after psoralen photochemotherapy.[84] The histologic examination of these lentigos has revealed melanocytic hyperplasia and cytologic atypia.[85] Therefore, patients with these lesions may be at an increased risk of skin cancer. These patients should be cautioned about the hazards of tanning bed use and should have annual skin examinations.

POSTINFLAMMATORY HYPERPIGMENTATION

Postinflammatory hyperpigmentation, also known as postinflammatory pigment alteration (PIPA), can occur as a result of various skin disorders. Occasionally, therapies for skin disease can cause or exacerbate dyschromia. This is most common in patients with darker skin types. A patient's pigmentation risk can be assessed based on historical information by utilizing the Baumann Skin Typing System discussed in Chapter 9 or by having patients take the related self-administered questionnaire, the Baumann Skin Type Indicator (BSTI), which is available online at www.SkinIQ.com. Although postinflammatory hyperpigmentation appears most frequently among patients with darker skin types, it can afflict people of any skin color.[86–88] Those of Asian ancestry tend to be susceptible to PIPA even when their skin tone is light. Minor conditions such as acne, eczema, and allergic reactions can lead to PIPA. Also, more serious cutaneous events (e.g., burns, surgeries, and trauma) or treatments (e.g., chemical peels and laser resurfacing) can precipitate it. Unfortunately, this phenomenon tends to recur in susceptible individuals.[89]

PIPA presents as irregular, darkly pigmented spots arising in areas of previous inflammation.[90] Postinflammatory hyperpigmentation can appear in any part of the skin, but is a particularly significant source of distress to patients when it occurs on the face. In fact, PIPA is one of the most common conditions responsible for spurring patients to visit a dermatologist.

Etiology

Postinflammatory hyperpigmentation is a consequence of increased melanin synthesis in response to a cutaneous insult. It can be diffused or localized and its distribution depends on the location of the original injury.

Histopathology

PIPA is characterized by numerous melanophages in the superficial dermis. An infiltrate of lymphohistiocytes may be seen around superficial blood vessels and in dermal papillae.[91]

Treatment

PIPA is difficult to treat because it occurs in individuals susceptible to hyperpigmentation following inflammation. Further inflammation, as induced by peels or lasers, would therefore worsen the process. Consequently, only nonirritating topical products such as hydroquinone, kojic acid, and retinoids are potentially useful to treat this condition. These agents provide minimal efficacy, though. The best treatment approach is sun avoidance, sunscreen use, and patience because these lesions tend to improve with time.

UNDER EYE CIRCLES

Under eye circles are a common complaint by both men and women. The cause of these dark circles under the eyes is poorly understood. Many believe that the thin skin in this area allows the blood vessels to become more visible. Any inflammation or vasodilation in this area may manifest as darkening. In a Japanese study, it was demonstrated that the lower and lateral parts of the internal canthus have high blood mass and low velocity and therefore contribute to dark circles around eyes.[92] However, there also seems to be a pigmentary component to this process that is poorly understood. There are several anecdotal reports of using pigmented lesion lasers such as the ruby or Nd:Yag to treat these lesions; however, there are no published data evaluating these therapies. Many cosmetic companies claim that their creams erase dark circles. These creams usually contain depigmenting agents; however, it has never been proven that this condition is caused by excessive melanin production. In fact, some physicians have postulated that the circles are caused by hemosiderin deposition. Unfortunately, there is no published research to explain the etiology and best treatment of under eye circles. For now, it seems certain that the best therapeutic approaches are sunscreen and increased rest. There are currently no available treatments proven to be effective.

Recently, prostaglandin analogs such as latanoprost and bimatoprost, used for the treatment of glaucoma, have been reported to cause periocular hyperpigmentation.[93–95] In a study conducted by Doshi et al. on 37 Caucasian patients on bimatoprost who developed periocular hyperpigmentation, this condition was noted in 3 to 6 months after initiation of treatment and resolved within 3 to 12 months following discontinuation of the medication.[95] Eyelid biopsies of patients with hyperpigmentation following bimatoprost treatment revealed increased melanosomes and melanin production,[96] which can be explained by the effects of prostaglandins in the melanin synthesis pathway.

CAMOUFLAGE COSMETICS

In recalcitrant disorders such as melasma, camouflage cosmetics can be used to give the patient a more natural appearance during the treatment process. These products are opaque and do not allow the underlying skin tones to be seen. The product is usually a thick cream that can be made to match a normal skin tone, thus masking the underlying abnormality. Some companies have developed advanced techniques using a spectrophotometer to measure skin color. The data from the spectrophotometer are used to create a pigment-rich foundation that exactly matches the patient's skin tone. Because skin tones are so widely varied, these products provide the best solution for patients with hard-to-match skin tones. Another option is to use a color that is complementary to the unwanted color. For example, green can be used to cover red discolorations, or purple to cover yellow discolorations. Yellow and white camouflage products are the most effective in treating melasma and other brown pigmentation disorders. Patients then apply their normal facial foundation over the color camouflage in order to achieve the most natural look. There are many brands of cover cosmetics available including Cover Blend, Covermark, Christian Dior, Dermablend, Hard Candy, Joe Blasko, MAC, and Neutrogena.

SUMMARY

All skin types are susceptible to pigmentation disorders. Such alterations can be particularly prominent in people with dark skin tones. Therapy is difficult and occasionally frustrating for patients and dermatologists alike as it requires protracted topical application of agents, sun avoidance, and, often, in-office chemical peels. Unfortunately, there is no panacea to treat these intractable disorders and attempts at resolving the particular condition often entail trying many different therapies with varying degrees of success.

REFERENCES

1. Jimbow K, Quevedo WC Jr, Fitzpatrick TB, et al. Some aspects of melanin biology: 1950–1975. *J Invest Dermatol.* 1976;67:72.
2. Bolognia JL, Pawelek JM. Biology of hypopigmentation. *J Am Acad Dermatol.* 1988;19:217.
3. Szabo G, Gerald AB, Pathak MA, et al. Racial differences in the fate of melanosomes in human epidermis. *Nature.* 1969; 222:1081.
4. Mosher D, Fitzpatrick T, Ortonne J, Hori Y. Hypomelanoses and Hypermelanoses. In: Freedberg IM, Eisen AZ, Wolff K, eds. *Fitzpatrick's Dermatology in General Medicine,* 5th ed. New York, NY: McGraw-Hill; 1999:996.
5. Khlgatian MK, Hadshiew IM, Asawanonda P, et al. Tyrosinase gene expression is regulated by p53. *J Invest Dermatol.* 2002; 118:126.
6. Park HY, Russakovsky V, Ohno S, et al. The beta isoform of protein kinase C stimulates human melanogenesis by activating tyrosinase in pigment cells. *J Biol Chem.* 1993;268:11742.
7. Lee JH, Park JG, Lim SH, et al. Localized intradermal microinjection of tranexamic acid for treatment of melasma in Asian patients: a preliminary clinical trial. *Dermatol Surg.* 2006;32:626.
8. Tomita Y, Torinuki W, Tagami H. Stimulation of human melanocytes by vitamin D_3 possibly mediates skin pigmentation after sun exposure. *J Invest Dermatol.* 1988;90:882.
9. Wei Q, Wu X, Hammer JA III. The predominant defect in dilute melanocytes is in melanosome distribution and not cell shape, supporting a role for myosin V in melanosome transport. *J Muscle Res Cell Motil.* 1997;18:517.
10. Ogawa K, Hosoya H, Yokota E, et al. Melanoma dynein: evidence that dynein is a general "motor" for microtubule associated cell motilities. *Eur J Cell Biol.* 1987;43:3.
11. Nordlund JJ. The melanocyte and the epidermal melanin unit: an expanded concept. *Dermatol Clin.* 2007;25:271.
12. Seiberg M, Paine C, Sharlow E, et al. Inhibition of melanosome transfer results in skin lightening. *J Invest Dermatol.* 2000;115:162.
13. Nystedt S, Emilsson K, Larsson AK, et al. Molecular cloning and functional expression of the gene encoding the human proteinase-activated receptor 2. *Eur J Biochem.* 1995;232:84.
14. Seiberg M. Keratinocyte-melanocyte interactions during melanosome transfer. *Pigment Cell Res.* 2001;14:236.
15. Seiberg M, Paine C, Sharlow E, et al. The protease-activated receptor 2 regulates pigmentation via keratinocyte-melanocyte interactions. *Exp Cell Res.* 2000;254:25.
16. Wallo W, Nebus J, Leyden JJ. Efficacy of a soy moisturizer in photoaging: a double-blind, vehicle-controlled, 12-week study. *J Drugs Dermatol.* 2007;6:917.
17. Quast T, Wehner S, Kirfel G, et al. sAPP as a regulator of dendrite motility and melanin release in epidermal melanocytes and melanoma cells. *FASEB J.* 2003;17:1739.
18. Cardinali G, Bolasco G, Aspite N, et al. Melanosome transfer promoted by keratinocyte growth factor in light and dark skin-derived keratinocytes. *J Invest Dermatol.* 2007Sep 20 [Epub ahead of print].
19. Valverde P, Healy E, Jackson I, et al. Variants of the melanocyte-stimulating hormone receptor gene are associated with red hair and fair skin in humans. *Nat Genet.* 1995;11:328.
20. Rees JL. The genetics of sun sensitivity in humans. *Am J Hum Genet.* 2004;75:739.
21. Inoue K, Hosoi J, Ideta R, et al. Stress augmented ultraviolet-irradiation-induced pigmentation. *J Invest Dermatol.* 2003;121:165.
22. Quevedo WC, Fitzpatrick TB, Pathak MA, et al. Role of light in human skin color viariation. *Am J Phys Anthropol.* 1975;43:393.
23. Hermanns J, Petit L, Martalo O, et al. Unraveling the patterns of subclinical pheomelanin-enriched facial hyperpigmentation: effect of depigmenting agents. *Dermatology.* 2000;201:118.
24. Goukassian D, Eller M, Yaar M, et al. Thymidine dinucleotide mimics the effect of solar simulated irradiation on p53 and p53-regulated proteins. *J Invest Dermatol.* 1999;112:25.
25. Gilchrest BA, Eller MS. DNA photodamage stimulates melanogenesis and other photoprotective responses. *J Investig Dermatol Symp Proc.* 1999;4:35.
26. Cui R, Widlund HR, Feige E, et al. Central role of p53 in the suntan response and pathologic hyperpigmentation. *Cell.* 2007; 128:853.
27. Barsh G, Attardi LD. A healthy tan? *N Engl J Med.* 2007;356:2208.
28. Wood JM, Gibbons NC, Schallreuter KU. Melanocortins in human melanocytes. *Cell Mol Biol (Noisy-le-grand).* 2006;52:75.
29. D'Orazio JA, Nobuhisa T, Cui R, et al. Topical drug rescue strategy and skin protection based on the role of Mc1r in UV-induced tanning. *Nature.* 2006;443:340.
30. Mandry Pagán R, Sánchez JL. Mandibular melasma. *P R Health Sci J.* 2000;19:231.
31. Bose SK, Ortonne JP. Pigmentation: dyschromia. In: Baran R, Maibach, HI, eds. *Textbook of Cosmetic Dermatology,* 2nd ed. London, UK: Dunitz Martin, Ltd.; 1998:396-367.
32. In: Arnold HL, Odom RB, James WD, eds. *Andrews' Diseases of the Skin: Clinical Dermatology.* 8th ed. Philadelphia, PA: WB Saunders;1990:991-994.
33. McLeod SD, Ranson M, Mason RS. Effects of estrogens on human melanocytes in vitro. *J Steroid Biochem Mol Biol.* 1994;49:9.
34. Sanchez NP, Pathak MA, Sato S, et al. Melasma: a clinical, light microscopic, ultrastructural, and immunofluorescence study. *J Am Acad Dermatol.* 1981;4:698.
35. Bleehen SS, Ebling FJG, Champion RH. Disorders of the skin colours. In: Champion RH, Burton JH, Ebling FJG, eds. *Textbook of Dermatology.* 5th ed. Oxford, UK: Blackwell Science; 1992:1596- 97.
36. Schauer E, Trautinger F, Kock A, et al. Proopiomelanocortin-derived peptides are synthesized and released by human keratinocytes. *J Clin Invest.* 1994;93:2258.
37. Imokawa G, Yada Y, Morisaki N, et al. Biological characterization of human fibroblast-derived mitogenic factors for human melanocytes. *Biochem J.* 1998; 330:1235.
38. Kang HY, Hwang JS, Lee JY, et al. The dermal stem cell factor and c-kit are overexpressed in melasma. *Br J Dermatol.* 2006;154:1094.
39. Grimes PE, Yamada N, Bhawan J: Light microscopic, immunohistochemical, and ultrastructural alterations in patients with melasma. *Am J Dermatopathol.* 2005;27:96.
40. Gilchrest BA, Fitzpatrick TB, Anderson RR, et al. Localization of melanin pigmentation in the skin with Wood's lamp. *Br J Dermatol.* 1977;96:245.

41. Lawrence N, Cox SE, Brody HJ. Treatment of melasma with Jessner's solution versus glycolic acid: a comparison of clinical efficacy and evaluation of the predictive ability of Wood's light examination. *J Am Acad Dermatol.* 1997;36:589.
42. Pandya AG, Guevara IL. Disorders of hyperpigmentation. *Dermatol Clin.* 2000;18:91.
43. Orlow SJ, Chakraborty AK, Pawelek JM. Retinoic acid is a potent inhibitor of inducible pigmentation in murine and hamster melanoma cell lines. *J Invest Dermatol.* 1990;94:461.
44. Griffiths CE, Finkel LJ, Ditre CM, et al. Topical tretinoin (retinoic acid) improves melasma. A vehicle-controlled, clinical trial. *Br J Dermatol.* 1993;129:415.
45. Kimbrough-Green CK, Griffiths CE, Finkel LJ, et al. Topical retinoic acid (tretinoin) for melasma in black patients. A vehicle-controlled clinical trial. *Arch Dermatol.* 1994;130:727.
46. Kligman AM, Willis I. A new formula for depigmenting human skin. *Arch Dermatol.* 1975;111:40.
47. McMichael AJ, Griffiths CE, Talwar HS, et al. Concurrent application of tretinoin (retinoic acid) partially protects against corticosteroid-induced epidermal atrophy. *Br J Dermatol.* 1996;135:60.
48. Lim JT, Tham SN. Glycolic acid peels in the treatment of melasma among Asian women. *Dermatol Surg.* 1997;23:177.
49. Lim JT. Treatment of melasma using kojic acid in a gel containing hydroquinone and glycolic acid. *Dermatol Surg.* 1999;25:282.
50. Khunger N, Sarkar R, Jain RK. Tretinoin peels versus glycolic acid peels in the treatment of melasma in dark-skinned patients. *Dermatol Surg.* 2004;30:756.
51. Wang CC, Hui CY, Sue YM, et al. Intense pulsed light for the treatment of refractory melasma in Asian persons. *Dermatol Surg.* 2004;30:1196.
52. Moreno Arias GA, Ferrando J. Intense pulsed light for melanocytic lesions. *Dermatol Surg.* 2001;27:397.
53. Rusciani A, Motta A, Rusciani L, et al. Q-switched alexandrite laser-assisted treatment of melasma: 2-year follow-up monitoring. *J Drugs Dermatol.* 2005;4:770.
54. Nouri K, Bowes L, Chartier T, et al. Combination treatment of melasma with pulsed CO_2 laser followed by Q-switched alexandrite laser: a pilot study. *Dermatol Surg.* 1999;25:494.
55. Angsuwarangsee S, Polnikorn N. Combined ultrapulse CO_2 laser and Q-switched alexandrite laser compared with Q-switched alexandrite laser alone for refractory melasma: split-face design. *Dermatol Surg.* 2003;29:59.
56. Rokhsar CK, Fitzpatrick RE. The treatment of melasma with fractional photothermolysis: a pilot study. *Dermatol Surg.* 2005;31:1645.
57. Fulton JE Jr. Utilizing the ultraviolet (UV detect) camera to enhance the appearance of photodamage and other skin conditions. *Dermatol Surg.* 1997;23:163.
58. Hodgson C. Senile lentigo. *Arch Derm.* 1963;87:197.
59. Bastiaens MT, Westendorp RG, Vermeer BJ, et al. Ephelides are more related to pigmentary constitutional host factors than solar lentigines. *Pigment Cell Res.* 1999;12:316.
60. Bliss JM, Ford D, Swerdlow AJ, et al. Risk of cutaneous melanoma associated with pigmentation characteristics and freckling: systematic overview of 10 case-control studies. The International Melanoma Analysis Group (IMAGE). *Int J Cancer.* 1995;62:367.
61. Naldi L, DiLandro A, D'Avanzo B, et al. Host-related and environmental risk factors for cutaneous basal cell carcinoma: evidence from an Italian case-control study. *J Am Acad Dermatol.* 2000;42:446.
62. Andersen WK, Labadie RR, Bhawan J. Histopathology of solar lentigines of the face: a quantitative study. *J Am Acad Dermatol.* 1997;36:444.
63. Gallagher RP, Rivers JK, Lee TK, et al. Broad-spectrum sunscreen use and the development of new nevi in white children: a randomized controlled trial. *JAMA.* 2000;283:2955.
64. Ortonne JP, Pandya AG, Lui H, et al. Treatment of solar lentigines. *J Am Acad Dermatol.* 2006;54:S262.
65. Humphreys TR, Werth V, Dzubow L, et al. Treatment of photodamaged skin with trichloroacetic acid and topical tretinoin. *J Am Acad Dermatol.* 1996;34:638.
66. Collins PS. Trichloroacetic acid peels revisited. *J Dermatol Surg Oncol.* 1989;15:933.
67. Newman N, Newman A, Moy L, et al. Clinical improvement of photoaged skin with 50% glycolic acid. *Dermatol Surg.* 1996;22:455.
68. Hexsel DM, Mazzuco R, Bohn J, et al. Clinical comparative study between cryotherapy and local dermabrasion for the treatment of solar lentigo on the back of the hands. *Dermatol Surg.* 2000;26:457.
69. Lugo-Janer A, Lugo-Somolinos A, Sanchez JL. Comparison of trichloroacetic acid solution and cryosurgery in the treatment of solar lentigines. *Int J Dermatol.* 2003;42:829.
70. Shimbashi T, Kamide R, Hashimoto T. Long-term follow-up in treatment of solar lentigo and cafe-au-lait macules with Q-switched ruby laser. *Aesthetic Plast Surg.* 1997;21:445.
71. Rosenbach A. Treatment of medium-brown solar lentigines using an alexandrite laser designed for hair reduction. *Arch Dermatol.* 2002;138:547.
72. Chan HH, Fung WK, Ying SY, et al. An in vivo trial comparing the use of different types of 532 nm Nd:YAG lasers in the treatment of facial lentigines in Oriental patients. *Dermatol Surg.* 2000;26:743.
73. Jih MH, Goldberg LH, Kimyai-Asadi A. Fractional photothermolysis for photoaging of hands. *Dermatol Surg.* 2008;34:73.
74. Wang CC, Sue YM, Yang CH, et al. A comparison of Q-switched alexandrite laser and intense pulsed light for the treatment of freckles and lentigines in Asian persons: a randomized, physician-blinded, split-face comparative trial. *J Am Acad Dermatol.* 2006;54:804.
75. Trotter MJ, Tron VA, Hollingdale J, et al. Localized chrysiasis induced by laser therapy. *Arch Dermatol.* 1995;131:1411.
76. Yun PL, Arndt KA, Anderson RR. Q-switched laser induced chrysiasis treated with long-pulsed laser. *Arch Dermatol.* 2002;138:1012.
77. Geist DE, Phillips TJ. Development of chrysiasis after Q-switched ruby laser treatment of solar lentigines. *J Am Acad Dermatol.* 2006;55:S59.
78. Fleischer AB Jr, Schwartzel EH, Colby SI, et al. The combination of 2% 4-hydroxyanisole (Mequinol) and 0.01% tretinoin is effective in improving the appearance of solar lentigines and related hyperpigmented lesions in two double-blind multicenter clinical studies. *J Am Acad Dermatol.* 2000;42:459.
79. Colby SI, Schwartzel EH, Huber FJ, et al. A promising new treatment for solar lentigines. *J Drugs Dermatol.* 2003;2:147.
80. Ortonne JP, Camacho F, Wainwright N, et al. Safety and efficacy of combined use of 4-hydroxyanisole (mequinol) 2%/tretinoin 0.01% solution and sunscreen in solar lentigines. *Cutis.* 2004;74:261.
81. Kang S, Goldfarb MT, Weiss JS, et al. Assessment of adapalene gel for the treatment of actinic keratoses and lentigines: a randomized trial. *J Am Acad Dermatol.* 2003;49:83.
82. Phillips TJ, Gottlieb AB, Leyden JJ, et al. Efficacy of 0.1% tazarotene cream for the treatment of photodamage: a 12-month, multicenter, randomized trial. *Arch Dermatol.* 2002;138:1486.
83. Phillips TJ. Tazarotene 0.1% cream for the treatment of photodamage. *Skin Therapy Lett.* 2004;9:1.
84. Salisbury JR, Williams H, du Vivier AW. Tanning-bed lentigines: ultrastructural and histopathologic features. *J Am Acad Dermatol.* 1989;21:689.
85. Roth DE, Hodge SJ, Callen JP. Possible ultraviolet A-induced lentigines: a side effect of chronic tanning salon usage. *J Am Acad Dermatol.* 1989;20:950.
86. Burns RL, Prevost-Blank PL, Lawry MA, et al. Glycolic acid peels for postinflammatory hyperpigmentation in black patients. A comparative study. *Dermatol Surg.* 1997;23:171.
87. Grimes PE, Stockton T. Pigmentary disorders in blacks. *Dermatol Clin.* 1988;6:271.
88. Ruiz-Maldonado R, Orozco-Covarrubias ML. Postinflammatory hypopigmentation and hyperpigmentation. *Semin Cutan Med Surg.* 1997;16:36.
89. Fairley JA. Tretinoin (retinoic acid) revisited. *N Engl J Med.* 1993;328:1486.
90. Bulengo-Ransby SM, Griffiths CE, Kimbrough-Green CK, et al. Topical tretinoin (retinoic acid) therapy for hyperpigmented lesions caused by inflammation of the skin in black patients. *N Engl J Med.* 1993;328:1438.
91. Spielvogel R, Kantor G. Pigmentary disorders of the skin. In: Elenitsas R, ed. *Lever's Histopathology of the Skin.* 8th ed. Philadelphia, PA: Lippincott Williams & Wilkins; 1997:618.
92. Matsumoto M, Kobayashi N, Hoshina O, et al. Study of casual factors of dark circles around the eyes. *IFCC Magazine.* 2001;4:281.
93. Kook MS, Lee K. Increased eyelid pigmentation associated with use of latanoprost. *Am J Ophthalmol.* 2000;129:804.
94. Wand M. Latanoprost and hyperpigmentation of eyelashes. *Arch Ophthalmol.* 1997;115:1206.
95. Doshi M, Edward DP, Osmanovic S. Clinical course of bimatoprost-induced periocular skin changes in Caucasians. *Ophthalmology.* 2006;113:1961.
96. Kapur R, Osmanovic S, Toyran S, et al. Bimatoprost-induced periocular skin hyperpigmentation: histopathological study. *Arch Ophthalmol.* 2005;123:1541.

CHAPTER 14

Skin of Color

Heather Woolery-Lloyd, MD

Skin of color describes individuals with increased epidermal pigment and darker skin. This subset of patients has unique cosmetic concerns and often requires special consideration for cosmetic procedures. Skin of color is typically seen in those of African, Hispanic, Asian, and Southeast Asian descent.

BIOLOGY OF SKIN COLOR

There is little variation in the number of epidermal melanocytes between light- and dark skinned individuals. There are approximately 2000 epidermal melanocytes/mm^2 on the head and forearm and 1000 epidermal melanocytes/mm^2 on the rest of the body. These differences are present at birth.[1] Thus, all persons have the same total number of melanocytes.

Although increased epidermal pigmentation results in a darker skin phenotype, there are actually more distinct ultrastructural characteristics that correlate with skin color. Specifically, the distribution of melanosomes in the keratinocytes correlates with skin color. In white skin, melanosomes are small and aggregated in complexes. In black skin, there are larger melanosomes, which are singly distributed within keratinocytes.[2]

Interestingly, the distribution of melanosomes in darker skin varies with the location on the body. In lighter skin, keratinocytes of both the thigh and volar skin exhibit complexed melanosomes. However, keratinocytes from the thighs of dark-skinned patients display singly dispersed melanosomes, while keratinocytes from the lighter volar skin of these patients have complexed melanosomes.[3] Thus, the melanosomes in the minimally pigmented volar skin of dark-skinned individuals closely resemble the melanosomes of lighter-skinned individuals. This finding further supports the theory that skin color correlates with the distribution of melanosomes. From such studies, one can conclude that melanosome distribution correlates with the color of skin; however, skin color is also determined by other factors.

One study examined the contribution of melanin, oxyhemoglobin, and deoxyhemoglobin on pigmentation observed clinically after ultraviolet B (UVB) exposure. The investigators found that the clinical evaluation of skin complexion was affected both by epidermal melanin concentration and deoxyhemoglobin residing in the superficial venous plexus. Additionally, altering the concentration of deoxyhemoglobin in the skin with pressure or with topical therapies also significantly altered what is visually perceived as skin pigmentation.[4,5]

CATEGORIZING SKIN OF COLOR

Fitzpatrick Skin Typing System

Skin of color is most frequently defined as Fitzpatrick skin phototypes (SPT) IV through VI. These skin types, by definition, tan easily or profusely and burn minimally, rarely, or never. The Fitzpatrick SPT system was originally developed to assess a patient's response to UV exposure for the purpose of treating skin conditions with light.[6] Using this system, patients are assigned a skin type based on the reported ability to tan or burn. The SPT defines a minimum erythema dose (MED) for each skin type, which is then used to guide dosing of UV therapy for various skin diseases. This skin typing system has since evolved into a way to describe a patient's skin color. Dermatologists often assign a patient's SPT based on their clinical assessment of skin color and not necessarily after questioning about a patient's history of sun tanning or burning (Table 14-1).

The Fitzpatrick SPT system originally categorized only white skin and included skin types I to IV. All skin of color (brown or dark brown skin) was identified as SPT V skin. SPT VI skin was later added to further classify skin of color.[7] Although this system is widely accepted and used frequently in dermatology, it does not fully address certain issues related to the darker skin types.

There are two issues that arise when using the Fitzpatrick SPT system. First, some authors have challenged the ability to predict a patient's MED based on the reported ability to tan and burn. In one study involving white patients, there was a poor correlation between SPT (as determined by self-reported tanning history) and MED. This study found a better correlation between MED and skin complexion characteristics such as eye and hair color, freckling tendency, and number of moles.[8] Other studies in Asian and Arab patients have also demonstrated a poor correlation between skin phototype (based on tanning history) and MED.[9–12] These authors have suggested that the SPT system, which was originally developed for white skin, is not applicable in patients of other ethnicities.

The second issue with the SPT system involves the correlation of visually assessed skin color with MED. As mentioned above, most dermatologists often assign a patient's SPT based on their clinical assessment of skin color, and rarely specifically question a patient on skin tanning history. Some authors have proposed that SPT (as determined by observed skin color) does not correlate with the MED in ethnic skin. They suggest that in skin of color, the constitutive pigment does not correlate with MED, as is suggested by the current conventional application of SPT.[4]

For example, most patients of African descent are conventionally labeled as

TABLE 14-1
The Fitzpatrick Skin Phototypes

Skin Type	Appearance	Reaction to Sun Exposure
Type I	Very fair; blond or red hair; light-colored eyes; freckles common	Always burns, never tans
Type II	Fair skinned; light eyes; light hair	Burns easily
Type III	Very common skin type; fair; eye and hair color varies	Sometimes burns, gradually tans
Type IV	Mediterranean Caucasian skin; medium to heavily pigmented	Rarely burns, always tans
Type V	Black skin, Mideastern skin; rarely sun sensitive	Tans
Type VI	Black skin, rarely sun sensitive	Tans easily

Fitzpatrick skin type V (brown) or VI (dark brown). However, upon questioning, some of these patients report that they do frequently burn. This subset of patients likely would be classified as having a skin type of III or IV, if they were truly categorized based on a self-reported tanning history. One study compared skin pigmentation as measured by diffuse reflectance spectroscopy (DRS) of MEDs.[4] This study confirmed that epidermal pigmentation was not an accurate predictor of skin sensitivity to UVB radiation.

Such research highlights the limitation of the SPT, which was originally designed to evaluate lighter skin types. Although the Fitzpatrick SPT continues to be widely used, other systems have been proposed to more clearly define skin of color.

Japanese Skin Type Scale

A Japanese skin type (JST) scale has been used to classify Japanese patients based on personal history of sun-reactivity.[13] This scale, which ranges from JST-I to JST-III, has been correlated with MEDs and minimal melanogenic dose (MMD) in Japanese patients. The MED and the MMD have been shown to increase with increasing JST. The MMD was shown to be greater than corresponding MED for all JST types.[14] These data are in contrast to data in Caucasian skin, revealing that the MED was the same as MMD in SPT II and MMD was less than MED in SPT III and IV.[15] The authors proposed that UVB may elicit more erythema than pigmentation in Japanese patients.

Taylor Hyperpigmentation Scale

The Taylor Hyperpigmentation Scale is a validated scale to describe skin of color and to monitor treatment of hyperpigmentation.[16] It consists of 15 plastic cards representing different hues in skin phototypes IV through VI. Each card also has 10 bands of progressively darker gradations of skin hue. Clinicians can use this system to assess and define skin color in a given patient. The Taylor Hyperpigmentation Scale also provides a simple, convenient tool to measure improvement after treatment of hyperpigmentation (Fig. 14-1).

Lancer Ethnicity Scale

The Lancer Ethnicity Scale (LES) was specifically developed to assess risk and outcome in the cosmetic laser patient.[17] After completing a detailed history of

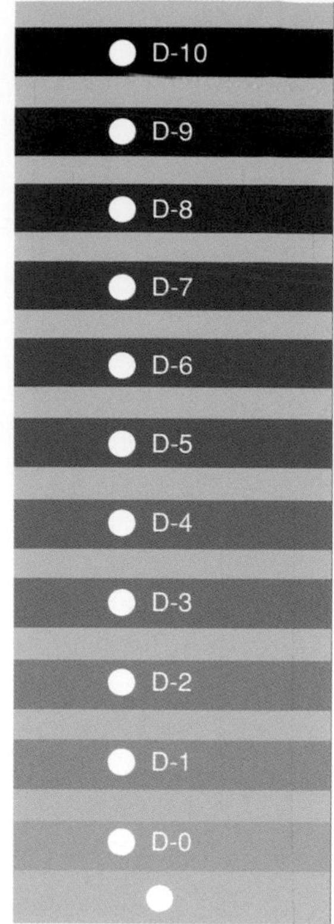

▲ **FIGURE 14-1** An example of one of the cards used to measure color in the Taylor Hyperpigmentation Scale.

the patient's ethnicity, an LES skin type ranging from 1 to 5 is assigned to each grandparent. The LES skin type is based on the geographic origin of the grandparent, ranging from type 5 (African) to type 1 (Nordic). The number is totaled for all four grandparents and then divided by four to determine the LES skin type of the patient. The author suggests that the lower the LES skin type, the lower the risk of scarring and uneven pigmentation after laser and surgical procedures. The LES is a novel approach to treating the cosmetic patient. It places a greater emphasis on ethnicity and country of origin than the patient's actual skin color. This concept is insightful but more studies are needed to validate this novel skin typing system.

Baumann Skin Typing System

Baumann's Skin Typing System addresses a very important cosmetic concern in skin of color, namely, the propensity to develop hyperpigmentation.[18] It does not define ethnicity or skin color. Rather, this questionnaire aids in predicting which patients are most likely to hyperpigment after a given procedure. It also addresses the fact that there are some patients with Fitzpatrick skin types IV to VI who do not have a strong tendency to hyperpigment despite their constitutive pigment. Thus, certain procedures may be less risky in this special group. At the same time, there are some patients with Fitzpatrick skin type III with a strong propensity to develop hyperpigmentation. By determining each individual patient's hyperpigmentation tendencies, this survey provides an excellent tool to the cosmetic dermatologist. It can offer further insight into treatment options for a given patient that transcends the visual assessment of skin complexion (see Chapter 9).

DEFINING STRUCTURE AND FUNCTION IN SKIN OF COLOR

Comparative studies of skin structure and function in skin of color are limited. It is important to note that most studies on this subject involve small numbers of patients. Much of the data are contradictory and can be difficult to interpret. In the following section, these findings will be summarized.

Stratum Corneum: Thickness and Compaction

The stratum corneum (SC) has been extensively studied in black and white skin. Most studies confirm that SC thickness does not differ between black and white individuals.[19–23] However, studies have suggested that the SC of black skin is more compact than white skin.[22,24] Using repeated tape stripping, investigators reported that black skin required an average of 16.6 strips to remove the SC compared to 10.3 strips in white skin.[22] The authors concluded that although SC thickness was equal in both groups, the SC in black skin has more cell layers and increased intracellular adhesion. A subsequent study confirmed these findings. The investigators in this later study also examined recovery time after barrier damage and found that darker skin recovered more quickly after barrier damage from tape stripping.[24] This study included African American, Asian, and Hispanic subjects and found that the skin differences in SC cell layers and barrier function were related to skin color and not related to race. Thus, it appears that although SC thickness is the same between the races, darker skin is more compact (Table 14-2).

Stratum Corneum: Lipid Content, Ceramides, and Barrier Function

Lipids in the SC play an important role in the barrier function of the skin. The

TABLE 14-2
Summary of Findings: Racial Differences in Skin Structure and Function

Structure/Function	Findings	
Stratum corneum: thickness and compaction	Stratum corneum thickness is the same between the races Darker skin is more compact Skin thickness as measured by calipers does not differ between white and black subjects	
Stratum corneum: lipid content, ceramides	Increased lipid content in black subjects Ceramide: Hispanic and Asian>white>black skin Considering the above findings, data are unclear	
Stratum corneum: transepidermal water loss (TEWL)	Contradictory and inconclusive data in black and Asian subjects No difference in TEWL between white and Hispanic subjects demonstrated	
Stratum corneum: corneocyte surface	No difference in corneocyte surface area between black, white, and Asian subjects	
Stratum corneum: spontaneous desquamation	Data are contradictory and inconclusive	
Stratum corneum: water content	Data are contradictory and inconclusive	
Percutaneous absorption	Data are contradictory and inconclusive	
Cutaneous blood vessel reactivity	Five of the nine studies reported no significant difference between the races	
Skin irritancy	No clear difference in skin irritancy in skin of color when compared to white skin	
pH	Data are contradictory and inconclusive	
Elastic recovery/extensibility	Data are contradictory and inconclusive	
Mast cell granules	Electron microscopy of mast cells in black skin demonstrated larger granules, more parallel-linear striations, and less curved lamellae Histologic evaluation showed no difference in mast cell size and number	
Epidermal innervation	No differences in innervation as measured by confocal microscopy were found between European Caucasian, Japanese American, and Chinese American subjects	
Melanosome distribution	Darker skinned subjects have large, singly dispersed melanosomes while lighter-skinned subjects have small grouped melanosomes within keratinocytes Melanosome grouping correlates with the degree of pigmentation in white, black, and Asian subjects Basal cell layer melanosomes correlate with the degree of pigmentation In black skin, melanosomes are not only increased in the basal layer but also distributed throughout all layers of the epidermis, in contrast to white skin where melanosomes are primarily limited to the basal layer Melanosomes greater than 0.35 μm cannot form groups	
Melanin	Total melanin content correlates with the degree of pigmentation	
Protease-activated receptor-2 (PAR-2)	PAR-2 and trypsin have greater expression in darkly pigmented skin when compared to lighter skin	
UV reactivity and photoprotection	*Black*	*White*
Stratum lucidum	Intact and compact	Swollen and cellular
Site of UV filtration	Stratum corneum	Malpighian layer
SPF	13.4	3.4
After solar-simulating radiation	DNA damage in the suprabasal dermis	Epidermal and dermal DNA damage An influx of neutrophils and active proteolytic enzymes Diffuse keratinocyte activation
MED	Darkly pigmented black skin has an MED up to 33 times greater than white skin MED correlated with skin color in Japanese subjects Pigmentation does not always consistently correlate with MED	
Photoaging	*Black-Histology*	*Black-Clinical*
	Flattening of the dermal–epidermal junction	Dark circles and hollowing beneath the eyes
	Elastic fiber degeneration	Lower eyelid bags
	Increase in the superficial vascular plexus	Midface aging
	Asian-Histology	*Asian-Clinical*
	Epidermal atrophy	Hyperpigmentation more prominent than in white subjects
	Cell atypia	Lower wrinkle scores than in white subjects
	Poor polarity	Lower sagging scores than in white subjects
	Disorderly differentiation	Less prominent lower face aging than in white subjects
Dermis	*Black*	
	More numerous and larger fibroblasts	
	Binucleated and multinucleated fibroblasts	
	Binucleated and multinucleated macrophages and giant cells	

(*continued*)

TABLE 14-2 (Continued)
Summary of Findings: Racial Differences in Skin Structure and Function

Eccrine glands	Data are contradictory and unclear
Apocrine glands	May be increased in black patients
Apoeccrine glands	May be increased in black patients
Sebaceous glands	Data are contradictory and unclear
Hair: keratin	No difference identified
Hair: amino acid	Data are contradictory and unclear
Hair:vellus	Vellus follicular hair density was lower in African Americans and Asians when compared to white subjects
Hair: African	Tightly coiled
	Flattened elliptical shape in cross-section
	Naturally shed hairs have a frayed tip
	Spontaneous knotting is often observed
	Longitudinal splitting, fissures, and breaking of hair shaft are also observed
	Fewer elastic fibrils
	Decreased hair density
Hair: Caucasian	Straight or slightly curved
	Elliptical in cross-section
	Smallest cross-sectional area
	Naturally shed hairs usually have original or cut tips
	Spontaneous knotting is rarely observed
Hair: Asian	Straight
	Round in cross-section
	Largest cross-sectional area
	Naturally shed hairs usually have original or cut tips
	No spontaneous knotting is observed

major lipids of the epidermis are ceramides, cholesterol, and free fatty acids. Studies have shown that there is greater lipid content in black SC when compared to white SC.[25,26] Once the lipids are removed from the SC, the weight of delipidized SC is equal in black and white patients.[22]

Although greater overall lipid content has been demonstrated in black SC, a study in the early 1990s showed that ceramide levels were lowest in black skin. In this report, ceramide levels were noted in decreasing order in Hispanic and Asian, white, and black skin. Ceramide levels were inversely correlated with transepidermal water loss (TEWL). Additionally, the ceramide levels directly correlated with water content of the SC.[27]

There is only one study examining lipid content in Asian patients. Scalp lipids in British and Thai subjects were compared, with investigators finding no difference in scalp lipids between the two groups.[28]

Based on the various studies discussed, the data regarding racial differences in lipid content are unclear and inconclusive.

Stratum Corneum: TEWL and Barrier Function

TEWL is one measure of SC barrier function. Five studies of TEWL in black skin indicate that TEWL is greater in black skin than white skin.[27,29–32] There are also six studies that contradict these findings. Five reported no difference in baseline TEWL between the black and white subjects,[33–37] and one reported decreased TEWL in black patients.[38] The variations in the results of the latter study may be explained by the location of the skin examined.[39]

Data on TEWL of Asian skin are inconclusive. Studies have reported that TEWL in Asian skin is greater than, equal to, and less than TEWL in Caucasian skin.[27,31,40] One study comparing Chinese, Malaysian, and Indian subjects demonstrated no differences in TEWL (as measured by skin vapor water loss) among the three groups.[41] There has been no difference demonstrated in TEWL between Hispanic and white skin.[34,42]

From the studies involving black subjects, five out of eleven studies concluded that TEWL was increased in black skin either at baseline or after irritation. The significance of these data is far reaching. If skin color truly does impact barrier function, these data would imply that acquired dyschromias may alter skin barrier properties.[39] It also has implications regarding the ability of people with different skin colors to tolerate environmental insults and to absorb topical agents.

Stratum Corneum: Corneocyte Surface Area and Spontaneous Desquamation

Corneocytes are the nonnucleated cells that comprise the SC. Corneocyte surface area has been demonstrated to influence skin permeabilty.[43] A study examining corneocyte surface area in black, white, and Asian subjects demonstrated no differences in corneocyte surface area among the groups.[44]

In the same study, spontaneous desquamation was measured in black, white, and Asian subjects. The investigators found that spontaneous corneocyte desquamation was equal in white and Asian patients; however, spontaneous corneocyte desquamation was greatest in black patients.[44] The increased desquamation seen in this study may explain the dry "ashy" skin often seen clinically in black patients (Fig. 14-2). Subsequent studies have not confirmed these data. One study reported a greater desquamation index in white subjects.[38] Another study reported no difference in the desquamation index between black and white patients.[45] The data on the differences in spontaneous corneocyte desquamation between these populations remain unclear.

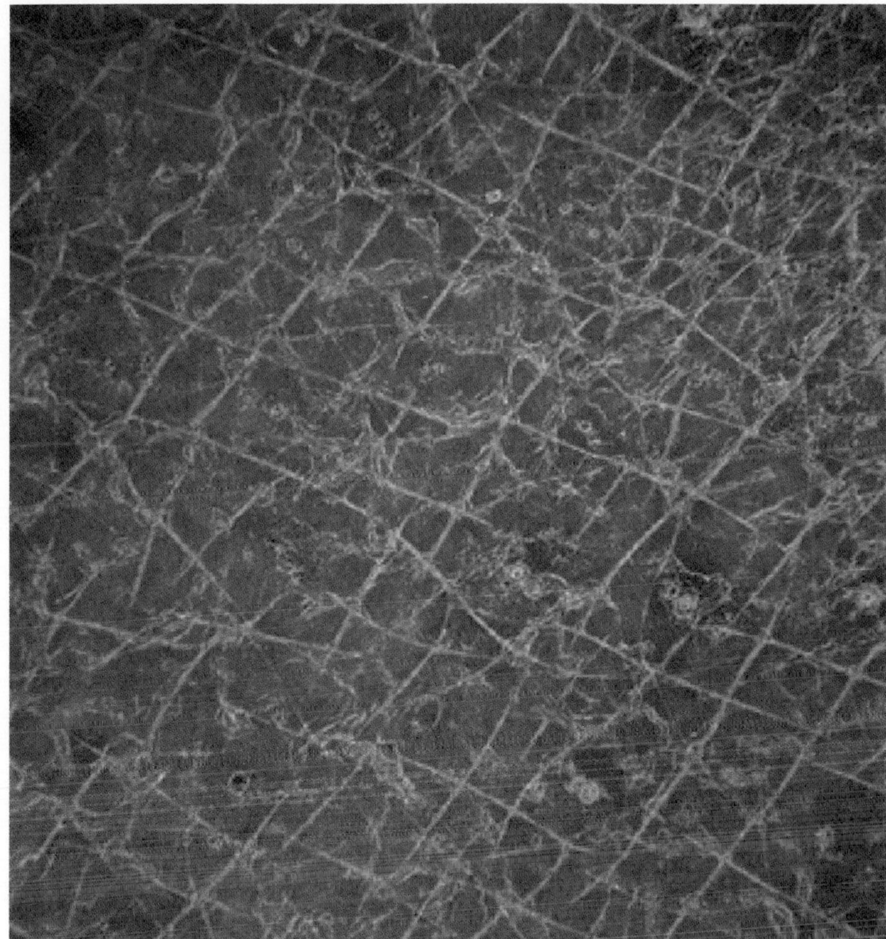

▲ **FIGURE 14-2** Dry skin presents as "ashy skin" in dark-skinned patients.

Stratum Corneum: Water Content

Water content in the skin can be measured by capacitance, conductance, impedance, and resistance. There are seven studies in the literature using these methods to compare water content in the skin of black, white, Hispanic, and Asian subjects.

Five studies examined black and white skin. Three studies showed no significant differences.[30,37,45] In the latter study, skin hydration correlated with scaliness that was seen clinically. One study showed increased water content in black skin while another suggested decreased water content in black skin.[38,46]

One study examined Hispanic and white subjects and found no difference in water content at baseline.[42] Later work contradicts these data. This subsequent study showed racial variability in SC water content among white, black, and Hispanic patients.[34] The water content values also varied by anatomic site. In the only study that included Asian patients, Asian skin was found to have higher water content than white, black, and Hispanic subjects.[27]

Based on a summation of the research, there does not appear to be a clear trend in the difference in water content among various ethnic groups. Indeed, the data on this subject are contradictory and inconclusive.

Percutaneous Absorption

Percutaneous absorption has been studied in black and white patients. Three studies estimated absorption via urinary excretion of a topically applied substance. Two studies saw no difference between black and white patients, while the other showed decreased urinary excretion in black patients.[47–49] All of these studies had a limited sample size. One additional study examined absorption in white and black cadaveric skin.[50] The authors reported decreased absorption in the black cadaveric skin.

Based on a summation of the studies, it is difficult to confirm any differences in percutaneous absorption in skin of color. The studies measuring urinary excretion are limited by other possible variables such as incomplete urine collections, renal function, and metabolism differences. In addition, the study of cadaveric skin may not reflect in vivo absorption. Thus, the data regarding percutaneous absorption in skin of color are inconclusive.

Cutaneous Blood Vessel Reactivity

Cutaneous blood vessel reactivity can be measured via Laser Doppler Velocimetry (LDV) or photoplethysmography (PPG). LDV is a noninvasive method to measure the flow of red blood cells in vasculature. PPG measures the pulsative changes in dermal vasculature and is synchronized with pulse rate.[39] These methods have been used to measure skin irritancy to topical products, absorption of topicals, and efficacy of topical medications. Nine studies compared blood vessel reactivity among ethnic groups via LDV. One of these studies also examined blood vessel reactivity via PPG. In all studies, a topical agent was applied (i.e., vasodilator, vasoconstrictor, or irritant) and then reactivity to the given agent was measured.

In the six studies that included black subjects, two showed no difference,[30,51] three showed decreased blood vessel reactivity in black subjects,[31,52,53] and one showed increased blood vessel reactivity in black subjects when compared to white subjects.[34]

Two studies compared Hispanic and white subjects and found no difference in LDV response to a topical irritant or nicotinate.[42,55]

Three studies included Asian patients. Two studies demonstrated increased blood vessel reactivity in Asian patients,[31,54] and one showed no difference in blood vessel reactivity when compared to white patients.[40]

Much of the data on blood vessel reactivity in skin of color are difficult to interpret because in each study different topical agents were used. However, in five of the nine studies, the authors concluded that there was no significant difference between the subjects studied. Further research is needed to clarify the data on cutaneous blood vessel reactivity in skin of color.

Skin Irritancy

The impact of ethnicity on skin irritancy is controversial. Original studies used visual perception of erythema as a primary endpoint.[56–58] This method of assessing cutaneous irritancy has obvious limitations in darker skin types. The earlier studies suggested that black subjects were less sensitive to irritants than white subjects.[30,42] As described in previous sections, much of this research revealed inconsistent and contradictory data. Subsequent authors have reviewed and reexamined the research on skin irritancy in an effort to determine if definitive conclusions can be made regarding skin irritancy in skin of color.[39,59,60] Most authors agree, from the current data, there does not appear to be a clear increase or decrease in skin irritancy in skin of color.

Stinging, a manifestation of sensory irritation, has also been studied in different skin types. Early reports suggested that stinging was most frequent in fair-skinned persons of Celtic ancestry.[61] A subsequent study showed no skin type propensity for stinging. The authors reported that increased stinging was most related to a history of sensitivity to soaps, cosmetics, and drugs[62] (see Chapter 17).

Most epidemiologic studies of allergic contact dermatitis demonstrate equal incidence among ethnicities.[63–66] Thus, based on current objective data, there does not appear to be any clear difference in skin irritancy in skin of color when compared to white skin (see Chapter 18).

pH, Elastic Recovery/Extensibility, Mast Cell Granules, Epidermal Innervation

Three studies have examined pH in skin of color.[32,37,38] One demonstrated decreased pH in black skin after three tape strips but not at baseline, or after 9, 12, or 15 tape strips.[32] Another showed decreased pH in black skin when compared to white skin on the cheeks but not the legs.[38] The most recent study revealed no difference in pH between black and white subjects.[37] The data from these three studies are insufficient to draw any definitive conclusions on pH in skin of color.

Elastic recovery and extensibility have also been studied in black and white skin.[34,38] The current data are inconsistent and conflicting. Based on the data, no conclusion can be made regarding skin biomechanics in different races.

Mast cell size and characteristics have been studied in black skin. In one study, no histologic differences in the number and size of mast cells were identified.[23] However, electron microscopy of mast cells in black skin demonstrated larger granules, more parallel–linear striations, and less curved lamellae. Tryptase was localized to the parallel-linear striations in black skin and localized to the curved lamellae in white skin. In this small study, significant structural differences were demonstrated in mast cells of black subjects.[67]

Pruritus, atopic dermatitis, and macular amyloid are frequently described in many Asian populations. Epidermal innervation has been studied in Asian and Caucasian patients to investigate differences in skin innervation. No differences in innervation as measured by confocal microscopy were found between European Caucasian, Japanese American, and Chinese American subjects.[68]

Melanin and Melanosome Distribution

As described previously, it is well established that differences in pigmentation are caused by the size and distribution of melanosomes within the keratinocytes.[2] Darker-skinned subjects have large, singly dispersed melanosomes while lighter-skinned subjects have small grouped melanosomes within keratinocytes. Subsequent research confirmed and expanded on the role of melanosomes in skin color. These studies demonstrated that melanosome grouping correlates with the degree of pigmentation in white, black, and Asian subjects.[69,70] Darker-skinned black subjects had large, singly dispersed melanosomes while lighter-skinned black subjects had both large, singly distributed melanosomes and small grouped melanosomes. Similarly, dark-skinned white subjects had singly dispersed melanosomes on sun-exposed skin, while light-skinned white subjects with minimal sun exposure had grouped melanosomes. Melanosome grouping was also correlated with sun exposure. Asian forearm skin primarily had singly distributed melanosomes while unexposed abdominal skin had grouped melanosomes.[69,70]

Further research has determined that the ability of a melanosome to form aggregates is determined by its size. Research suggests that melanosomes greater than 0.35 μm cannot form groups.[69,70]

Basal cell layer melanosomes and total melanin content also correlate with the degree of pigmentation. Darkly pigmented skin has increased melanin as measured by cell culture.[71] Darkly pigmented skin also has increased density of basal cell layer melanosomes.[69] Fewer basal layer melanosomes were observed in fair-skinned Asian patients when compared to darker-skinned individuals.[72] Additional studies have shown that, in black skin, melanosomes are not only increased in the basal layer but also distributed throughout all layers of the epidermis.[23,73] This is in contrast to white skin where melanosomes are primarily limited to the basal layer.

The protease-activated receptor-2 (PAR-2) expressed on the keratinocyte plays a role in melanosome uptake via phagocytosis. Trypsin activates PAR-2 in vivo. Investigators have demonstrated that PAR-2 and trypsin have greater expression in darkly pigmented skin when compared to lighter skin. In addition, PAR-2-induced phagocytosis is more efficient in darker skin types. These data suggest that PAR-2 expression may play a role in darker skin phenotypes[74] (see Chapter 13).

Epidermis: Overall Architecture

It is well established that SC thickness does not differ among ethnicities.[19–23] Overall skin thickness as measured by calipers also does not differ between white and black subjects.[75] Differences in the architecture of the epidermis between the races involve melanin and melanosome distribution as described above. Other differences in epidermal architecture are related to UV damage. These changes are described below.

PHOTOAGING IN SKIN OF COLOR

UV Reactivity and Photoprotection

The photoprotection conferred by melanin in darkly pigmented skin greatly influences the UV-induced differences observed in black and white skin. Epidermal architecture in black and white subjects supports this notion. One study demonstrated an intact, compact stratum lucidum in sun-exposed black skin, in contrast to a swollen, cellular stratum lucidum in sun-exposed white skin. Black skin rarely exhibited atrophy, while white skin had numerous focal areas of atrophy, necrosis, vacuoles, and dyskeratosis.[23]

Melanin clearly offers protection from UV light. It acts as a neutral density filter to reduce penetration of all wavelengths of light equally.[76] In a study using skin samples from blacks and whites, investigators found that 5 times as much UV light reached the upper dermis of white skin when compared to black skin. The authors determined that the main site of UV filtration in white patients was the SC, compared to the malpighian layer in black patients. The average protection offered by melanin in black skin was calculated to be equivalent to a sun protective factor (SPF) of 13.4 compared to 3.4 for white skin. They concluded that the photoprotection observed in black skin was due to both increased melanin content and the unique distribution of melanosomes in dark skin.[76]

Another study examined biopsies in black and white skin before and after solar-simulating radiation (SSR). After SSR, white skin displayed epidermal and dermal DNA damage, an influx of neutrophils, active proteolytic enzymes, and diffuse keratinocyte activation. Black skin only demonstrated DNA damage in the suprabasal dermis. This study of acute changes after SSR confirms the significance of UV protection imparted by melanin.[77]

Racial differences in MED have been described. Darkly pigmented black skin has been determined to have an MED up to 33 times greater than that of individuals with white skin.[70] In Japanese subjects, MED has also been correlated with skin color. In this study, the investigators found that the greater the epidermal melanin content, the less severe the reaction to the sun.[78] It is important to note, however, that darker skin is not always predictive of MED. As mentioned previously, in darker skin, pigmentation does not consistently correlate with MED.[4] Other factors may influence the ability to tan or burn in skin of color.

The process of skin tanning in different racial ethnic groups has been studied. The most significant change noted after 1 MED exposure was an upward shift in the distribution of melanin to the middle layers of the epidermis. This change was most dramatic in darker skin. Such data provide the basis for a better understanding of tanning in the darker skin types.[79]

One study examined skin in Korean subjects and the cumulative response to sun exposure. Investigators compared constitutive and facultative (acquired) pigmentation in different age groups. Facultative pigment of sun-exposed skin in Caucasians appears to reflect cumulative lifetime UV exposure. In this study, constitutive pigment was highest during the first decade of life, decreased during the second decade, and was maintained during the third decade of life in Korean subjects. In contrast to Caucasians, facultative pigmentation did not increase with age.[80]

Histologic Findings

Despite the photoprotection conferred by darker skin, chronologic aging has been observed in black skin. In one study, older black subjects demonstrated flattening of the dermal–epidermal junction when compared to younger subjects.[73] Elastic fiber degeneration and an increase in the superficial vascular plexus were also noted in the aged group. The skin of older black subjects was also characterized by a decrease in the number of melanocytes.[73]

A study in older Thai patients with a history of high sun exposure also showed epidermal atrophy, cell atypia, poor polarity, and disorderly differentiation.[81] In a study of Japanese patients, the relationship between skin phototype and facial wrinkling was examined. As expected, higher scores were recorded for deep wrinkles in individuals with Fitzpatrick SPT I. Interestingly, the same tendency was not demonstrated for fine wrinkle scores.[82]

Clinical Findings

The clinical signs of aging in skin of color have been described. In a study of French Caucasian and Chinese subjects, wrinkle onset was delayed by approximately 10 years in Chinese women. Hyperpigmentation was a much more important sign of aging in Chinese women.[83]

In a study of Japanese and Caucasian patients, young Japanese patients had significantly lower wrinkle scores. The sagging score was also significantly lower in Japanese subjects older than 40 years when compared with Caucasian subjects. Lower face aging was more common in Caucasian subjects.[84]

In African Americans, the clinical signs of aging are less pronounced and tend to be delayed at least a decade when compared to Caucasian skin. Many patients complain of dark circles and hollowing beneath the eyes, while others experience lower eyelid bags. Lower-eyelid signs of aging usually start with midface aging during the 30s. In midface aging, the malar fat pad descends from its location overlying the infraorbital rim and accumulates along the nasolabial fold. This can lead to a hollowed appearance beneath the eyes and an apparent deepening of the nasolablial fold.[85] It is important to note that these changes occur with intrinsic aging and are less related to photodamage. Photoaging in darker skin is manifested primarily by uneven pigmentation, which is one of the most common cosmetic complaints in skin of color. The presence of seborrheic keratosis and dermatosis papulosa nigra is another common clinical sign of aging in patients with skin of color.

Based on these studies, photoaging, although delayed, does occur in skin of color. Despite the significant protection offered by melanin in darker skin types, these data suggest that photoprotection should still be emphasized in patients with skin of color.

ADDITIONAL CONSIDERATIONS REGARDING STRUCTURE AND FUNCTION IN SKIN OF COLOR

Dermis: Overall Architecture

In a comparison of black and white facial skin, dermal differences are evident. Some of these changes are related to UV damage and include decreased elastosis in black skin.[23]

Other differences appear to be primary variations in the fibroblasts, macrophages, and giant cells. In one study, black skin was reported to contain more fiber fragments composed of collagen fibrils and glycoproteins. Fibroblasts were more numerous and larger in size. They were frequently binucleated and multinucleated. Additionally, there were more binucleated and multinucleated macrophages and giant cells.[23]

The changes described in fibroblasts are especially significant in skin of color because of the increased risk of keloids and scarring in these patients. Other differences in dermal structures reported between the races are described below.[23]

ECCRINE GLANDS Research on ethnic differences in eccrine sweat glands is contradictory. Of the four studies measuring sweat production in black and white subjects, two reported decreased sweating in black subjects and two reported no difference.[86–89]

Four other studies have measured resistance to indirectly assess eccrine gland activity. They have shown increased resistance in darker-skinned patients, which suggests increased eccrine gland activity.[46,90–92]

Based on these studies, no conclusion can be made on eccrine gland activity between different ethnic groups.

APOCRINE GLANDS Research on ethnic differences in apocrine glands is limited. Two small nonblinded studies suggest that apocrine glands are larger in black subjects.[93,94] One larger histologic analysis reported that apocrine glands are more numerous in black skin.[90] Based on these data, apocrine glands may be increased in black individuals.

APOCRINE-ECCRINE GLANDS Apocrine-eccrine sweat glands have features of both eccrine and apocrine glands. One study of facial skin reported more numerous apocrine-eccrine glands in black skin when compared to white skin.[23]

SEBACEOUS GLANDS Studies of sebaceous glands and sebaceous gland activity reveal contradictory findings. One study reported increased sebaceous gland size in black patients.[95] Another study reported increased sebum production in black patients.[96] Three studies indicated no difference in sebaceous gland activity between black and white subjects.[37,97,98] Research in Japanese subjects, however, found a correlation between skin surface lipids and increased pigmentation[78] (see Chapter 10).

HAIR Hair composition and structure has been studied between the races. There is no difference in keratin between black and white subjects.[99] One study has shown some differences in amino acid composition; however, a follow-up study demonstrated no difference.[100,101]

Vellus hair follicular density has been studied in African American, Asian, and Caucasian subjects. It has been proposed that vellus hair follicles are a potential reservoir for topically applied substances. Vellus follicular hair density was lower in African Americans and Asians when compared to white subjects. The authors suggested that this difference may impact skin absorption in different ethnic groups.[102]

Differences in terminal hair structure between the races have been well studied and are described below.

AFRICAN HAIR In subjects of African descent, four distinct hair types are recognized: straight, wavy, helical, and spiral. The spiral hair type is the most common subtype.[103] African hair has a flattened elliptical shape in cross-section with a ribbon-like appearance.[104] The hair is typically coiled tightly, and most naturally shed hairs have a frayed tip. Spontaneous knotting is often seen. Longitudinal splitting, fissures, and breaking of the hair shaft are also observed.[105]

Other studies of black hair have revealed that black subjects had fewer elastic fibrils anchoring the hair to the dermis.[23] This has implications in several forms of alopecia frequently seen in black patients, particularly traction alopecia. Additionally, there is decreased hair density in African American subjects when compared to white subjects.[106]

CAUCASIAN HAIR Caucasian hair is typically straight or slightly curved. The hair is elliptical in cross-section. It has the smallest cross-sectional area among ethnic groups and naturally shed hairs usually have the original or cut tip.[104] Spontaneous knotting is rarely observed.[105]

ASIAN HAIR Asian hair is typically straight. The hair is round in cross-section. It has the largest cross-sectional area and naturally shed hairs usually have original or cut tips.[104] No spontaneous knotting is observed.[105]

SUMMARY

Understanding the unique characteristics of skin of color is extremely important in cosmetic dermatology. The most well-defined and distinct differences in skin of color pertain to melanin in the skin. Increased melanin in skin of color offers a significant advantage to these patients, namely, a delay in photoaging.

The disadvantage of melanin also has great impact in cosmetic dermatology, as this constitutive pigment increases the risk of hyperpigmentation from many cosmetic procedures.

Apparent differences in fibroblasts in skin of color also greatly impact the practice of cosmetic dermatology. These fibroblast differences likely place patients with skin of color at increased risk of hypertrophic scars and keloids after invasive surgical and laser procedures.

More than half of the world's population has skin of color. Despite this fact, our understanding of skin structure and function is limited in these patients. Research to date has been quite compelling; however, most research on skin of color is preliminary. Further research and larger population studies are necessary to definitively describe the similarities and differences in skin structure and function among the various ethnic groups.

REFERENCES

1. Jimbow K, Quevedo WC, Prota G, Fitzpatrick TB. Biology of melanocytes. In: Freedberg IM, Eisen AZ, Wolff K, et al., eds. *Fitzpatrick's Dermatology in General Medicine*. 5th ed. New York, NY: McGraw-Hill; 1999:192-200.
2. Szabó G, Gerald AB, Pathak MA, et al. Racial differences in the fate of melanosomes in human epidermis. *Nature*. 1969;222:1081.
3. Milburn PB, Silver DN, Sian CS. The color of the skin of the palms and soles as a possible clue to the pathogenesis of acral-lentiginous melanoma. *Am J Dermatopathol*. 1982;4:429.
4. Smith G, Kollias N, Wallo W. Estimating the ability of melanin to protect skin of color from UV exposure. Program and abstracts of the 64th Annual Meeting of the American Academy of Dermatology; March 3–7, 2006; San Francisco, CA.
5. Stamatas GN, Kollias N. Blood stasis contributions to the perception of skin pigmentation. *J Biomed Opt*. 2004;9:315.
6. Fitzpatrick TB. Soleil et peau. *J Med Esthet*. 1975;2:33.
7. Fitzpatrick TB. The validity and practicality of sun-reactive skin types I through VI. *Arch Dermatol*. 1988; 124:869.
8. Rampen FH, Fleuren BA, de Boo TM, et al. Unreliability of self-reported burning tendency and tanning ability. *Arch Dermatol*. 1988;124:885.
9. Youn JI, Oh JK, Kim BK, et al. Relationship between skin phototype and MED in Korean, brown skin. *Photodermatol Photoimmunol Photomed*. 1997;13:208.
10. Park SB, Suh DH, Youn JI. Reliability of self-assessment in determining skin phototype for Korean brown skin. *Photodermatol Photoimmunol Photomed*. 1998;14:160.
11. Stanford DG, Georgouras KE, Sullivan EA, et al. Skin phototyping in Asian Australians. *Aust J Dermatol*. 1996; 37: S36.
12. Venkataram MN, Haitham AA. Correlating skin phototype and minimum erythema dose in Arab skin. *Int J Dermatol*. 2003;42:191.
13. Satoh Y, Kawada A. Action spectrum for melanin pigmentation to ultraviolet light, and Japanese skin typing. In: Fitzpatrick TB, Toda K, eds. *Brown Melanoderma: Biology and Disease of Epidermal Pigmentation*. Tokyo, Japan: University of Tokyo Press; 1986:87-95.
14. Kawada A. UVB-induced erythema, delayed tanning, and UVA-induced immediate tanning in Japanese skin. *Photodermatol*. 1986;3:327.
15. Pathak MA, Fanselow DL. Photobiology of melanin pigmentation: dose/response of skin to sunlight and its contents. *J Am Acad Dermatol*. 1983;9:724.
16. Taylor SC, Arsonnaud S, Czernielewski J, et al. The Taylor Hyperpigmentation Scale: a new visual assessment tool for the evaluation of skin color and pigmentation. *Cutis*. 2005;76:270.
17. Wolbarsht ML, Urbach F. The Lancer Ethnicity Scale. *Lasers Surg Med*. 1999; 25:105.
18. Baumann L. *The Skin Type Solution*. New York, NY: Bantam Dell; 2006.
19. Thomson ML. Relative efficiency of pigment and horny layer thickness in protecting the skin of Europeans and Africans against solar ultraviolet radiation. *J Physiol*. 1955;127:236.
20. Freeman RG, Cockerell EG, Armstrong J, et al. Sunlight as a factor influencing the thickness of epidermis. *J Invest Dermatol*. 1962;39:295.

21. Mitchell R. The skin of the Australian Aborigines: a light and electron microscopical study. *Australas J Dermatol.* 1968;9:314.
22. Weigand DA, Haygood C, Gaylor JR. Cell layers and density of Negro and Caucasian stratum corneum. *J Invest Dermatol.* 1974;62:563.
23. Montagna W, Carlisle K. The architecture of black and white facial skin. *J Am Acad Dermatol.* 1991;24:929.
24. Reed JT, Ghadially R, Elias PM. Effect of race gender, and skin type of epidermal permeability barrier function [abstract]. *J Invest Dermatol.* 1994;102:537.
25. Rienertson RP, Wheatley VR. Studies on the chemical composition of human epidermal lipids. *J Invest Dermatol.* 1959; 32:49.
26. La Ruche G, Cesarini JP. Histology and physiology of black skin. *Ann Dermatol Venereol.* 1992;119:567.
27. Sugino K, Imokawa G, Maibach H. Ethnic difference of stratum corneum lipid in relation to stratum corneum function [abstract]. *J Invest Dermatol.* 1993;100:597.
28. Harding CR, Moore AE, Rogers JS, et al. Dandruff: a condition characterized by decreased levels of intercellular lipids in scalp stratum corneum and impaired barrier function. *Arch Dermatol Res.* 2002;294:221.
29. Wilson D, Berardesca E, Maibach HI. In vitro transepidermal water loss: differences between black and white human skin. *Br J Dermatol.* 1988;199:647.
30. Berardesca E, Maibach HI. Racial differences in sodium lauryl sulphate induced cutaneous irritation: black and white. *Contact Dermatitis.* 1988;18:65.
31. Kompaore F, Marly JP, Dupont C. In vivo evaluation of the stratum corneum barrier function in blacks, Caucasians, and Asians with two noninvasive methods. *Skin Pharmacol.* 1993;6:200.
32. Berardesca E, Pirot F, Singh M, et al. Differences in stratum corneum pH gradient when comparing white Caucasian and black African-American skin. *Br J Dermatol.* 1998;139:855.
33. Reed JT, Ghadially R, Elias PM. Skin type, but neither race nor gender, influence epidermal permeability barrier function. *Arch Dermatol.* 1995;131: 1134.
34. Berardesca E, de Rigal J, Leveque JL, et al. In vivo biophysical characterization of skin physiological differences in races. *Dermatologica.* 1991;182:89.
35. DeLuca R, Balestrier A, Dinle Y. Measurement of cutaneous evaporation. 6. Cutaneous water loss in the people of Somalia. *Boll Soc Ital Biol Sper.* 1983;59:1499.
36. Pinnagoda J, Tupker RA, Agner T, et al. Guidelines for transepidermal water loss (TEWL) measurement. *Contact Dermatitis.* 1990;22:164.
37. Grimes P, Edison BL, Green BA, et al. Evaluation of inherent differences between African American and white skin surface properties using subjective and objective measures. *Cutis.* 2004; 73:392.
38. Warrier AG, Kligman AM, Harper RA, et al. A comparison of black and white skin using noninvasive methods. *J Soc Cosmet Chem.* 1996;47:229.
39. Wesley NO, Maibach HI. Racial (ethnic) differences in skin properties: the objective data. *Am J Clin Dermatol.* 2003;4:843.
40. Aramaki J, Kawana S, Effendy I, et al. Differences of skin irritation between Japanese and European women. *Br J Dermatol.* 2002;146:1052.
41. Goh CL, Chia SE. Skin irritability to sodium lauryl sulphate–as measured by skin water vapour loss–by sex and race. *Clin Exp Dermatol.* 1988;13:16.
42. Berardesca E, Maibach HI. Sodium-lauryl-sulphate-induced cutaneous irritation. Comparison of white and Hispanic subjects. *Contact Dermatitis.* 1988;18:136.
43. Rougier A, Lotte C, Corcuff P, et al. Relationship between skin permeability and corneocyte size according to anatomic site, age, and sex in man. *J Soc Cosmet Chem.* 1988;39:15.
44. Corcuff P, Lotte C, Rougier A, et al. Racial differences in corneocytes. A comparison between black, white and oriental skin. *Acta Dermatol Venereol.* 1991;71:146.
45. Manuskiatti W, Schwindt DA, Maibach HI. Influence of age, anatomic site and race on skin roughness and scaliness. *Dermatology.* 1998;196:401.
46. Johnson LC, Corah NL. Racial differences in skin resistance. *Science.* 1962;139:766.
47. Wickrema-Sinha WJ, Shaw SR, Weber DJ. Percutaneous absorption and excretion of tritium-labeled diflorasone diacetate: a new topical corticosteroid in the rat, monkey and man. *J Invest Dermatol.* 1978;7:372.
48. Wedig JH, Maibach HI. Percutaneous penetration of dipyrithione in men: effect of skin color (race). *J Am Acad Dermatol.* 1981;5:433.
49. Lotte C, Wester RC, Rougier A, et al. Racial differences in the in vivo percutaneous absorption of some organic compounds: a comparison between black, Caucasian and Asian subjects. *Arch Dermatol Res.* 1993;284:456.
50. Stoughton RB. Bioassay methods for measuring percutaneous absorption. In: Montagna W, Stoughton RB, van Scott EJ, eds. *Pharmacology of the Skin.* New York, NY: Appleton-Century-Crofts; 1969:542-544.
51. Guy RH, Tur E, Bjerke S, et al. Are there age and racial differences to methyl nicotinate-induced vasodilatation in human skin? *J Am Acad Dermatol.* 1985;12:1001.
52. Berardesca E, Maibach HI. Cutaneous reactive hyperemia: racial differences induced by corticoid application. *Br J Dermatol.* 1989;129:787.
53. Berardesca E, Maibach HI. Racial differences in pharmacodynamic responses to nicotinates in vivo in human skin: black and white. *Arch Derm Venereol.* 1990;70:63.
54. Gean CJ, Tur E, Maibach HI, et al. Cutaneous responses to topical methyl bicofinate in black, oriental and caucasian subjects. *Arch Dermatol Res.* 1989;281:95.
55. Berardesca E, Maibach HI. Effect of race on percutaneous penetration of nicotinates in human skin: a comparison of white and Hispanic-Americans. *Bioeng Skin.* 1988;4:31.
56. Marshall EK, Lynch V, Smith HV. Variation in susceptibility of the skin to dichlorethylsulphide. *J Pharmacol Exp Ther.* 1919;12:291.
57. Weigand DA, Mershon GE. The cutaneous irritant reaction to agent O-chlorobenzylidene malonitrile (CS). Quantitation and racial influence in human subjects. Edgewood Arsenal Technical Report 4332, February 1970.
58. Weigand DA, Gaylor JR. Irritant reaction in Negro and Caucasian skin. *South Med J.* 1974;67:548.
59. Taylor SC. Skin of color: biology, structure, function, and implications for dermatologic disease. *J Am Acad Dermatol.* 2002;46:S41.
60. Frosch P, Kligman AM. A method for appraising the stinging capacity of topically applied substances. *J Soc Cosmet Chem.* 1981;28:197.
61. Grove GL, Soschin DM, Kligman AM. Adverse subjective reactions to topical agents. In: Drill VA, Lazar P, eds. *Cutaneous Toxicology.* New York, NY: Raven Press; 1984:200-210.
62. Berardesca E, Maibach H. Ethnic skin: overview of structure and function. *J Am Acad Dermatol.* 2003;48:S139.
63. Kligman AM, Epstein W. Updating the maximization test for identifying contact allergens. *Contact Dermatitis.* 1975;1:231.
64. Fisher AA. Contact dermatitis in black patients. *Cutis.* 1977;20:303.
65. DeLeo VA, Taylor SC, Belsito DV. The effect of race and ethnicity on patch test results. *J Am Acad Dermatol.* 2002;46:S107.
66. North American Contact Dermatitis Group. Epidemiology of contact dermatitis in North America. *Arch Dermatol.* 1973;108:537.
67. Sueki H, Whitaker-Menezes D, Kligman AM. Structural diversity of mast cell granules in black and white skin. *Br J Dermatol.* 2001;144:85.
68. Reilly DM, Ferdinando D, Johnston C, et al. The epidermal nerve fibre network: characterization of nerve fibres in human skin by confocal microscopy and assessment of racial variations. *Br J Dermatol.* 1997;137:163.
69. Toda K, Pathak MA, Parrish JA, et al. Alteration of racial differences in melanosome distribution in human epidermis after exposure to ultraviolet light. *Nat New Biol.* 1972;236:143.
70. Olson RL, Gaylor J, Everett MA. Skin color, melanin, and erythema. *Arch Dermatol.* 1973;108:541.
71. Smit NP, Kolb RM, Lentjes EG, et al. Variations in melanin formation by cultured melanocytes from different skin types. *Arch Dermatol Res.* 1998; 290:342.
72. Goldschmidt H, Raymond JZ. Quantitative analysis of skin color from melanin content of superficial skin cells. *J Forensic Sci.* 1972;17:124.
73. Herzberg AJ, Dinehart SM. Chronologic aging in black skin. *Am J Dermatopathol.* 1989;11:319.
74. Babiarz-Magee L, Chen N, Seiberg M, et al. The expression and activation of protease-activated receptor-2 correlate with skin color. *Pigment Cell Res.* 2004;17:241.
75. Whitmore SE, Sago NJ. Caliper-measured skin thickness is similar in

white and black women. *J Am Acad Dermatol*. 2000;42:76.
76. Kaidbey KH, Agin PP, Sayre RM, et al. Photoprotection by melanin–a comparison of black and Caucasian skin. *J Am Acad Dermatol*. 1979;1:249.
77. Rijken F, Bruijnzeel PL, van Weelden H, et al. Responses of black and white skin to solar-simulating radiation: differences in DNA photodamage, infiltrating neutrophils, proteolytic enzymes induced, keratinocyte activation, and IL-10 expression. *J Invest Dermatol*. 2004;122:1448.
78. Abe T, Arai S, Mimura K, et al. Studies of physiological factors affecting skin susceptibility to ultraviolet light irradiation and irritants. *J Dermatol*. 1983;10:531.
79. Tadokoro T, Yamaguchi Y, Batzer J, et al. Mechanisms of skin tanning in different racial/ethnic groups in response to ultraviolet radiation. *J Invest Dermatol*. 2005;124:1326.
80. Roh K, Kim D, Ha S, et al. Pigmentation in Koreans: study of the differences from Caucasians in age, gender and seasonal variations. *Br J Dermatol*. 2001;144:94.
81. Kotrajaras R, Kligman AM. The effect of topical tretinoin on photodamaged facial skin: the Thai experience. *Br J Dermatol*. 1993;129:302.
82. Nagashima H, Hanada K, Hashimoto I. Correlation of skin phototype with facial wrinkle formation. *Photodermatol Photoimmunol Photomed*. 1999;15:2.
83. Nouveau-Richard S, Yang Z, Mac-Mary S, et al. Skin ageing: a comparison between Chinese and European populations. A pilot study. *J Dermatol Sci*. 2005;40:187.
84. Tsukahara K, Fujimura T, Yoshida Y, et al. Comparison of age-related changes in wrinkling and sagging of the skin in Caucasian females and in Japanese females. *J Cosmet Sci*. 2004;55:351.
85. Harris MO. The aging face in patients of color: minimally invasive surgical facial rejuvenation-a targeted approach. *Dermatol Ther*. 2004;17:206.
86. Robinson S, Dill DB, Wilson JW, et al. Adaptation of white men and Negroes to prolonged work in humid heat. *Am J Trop Med*. 1941;21:261.
87. McCance RA, Purohit G. Ethnic differences in response to the sweat glands to pilocarpine. *Nature*. 1969;221:378.
88. Herrmann F, Prose PH, Sulzberger WB. Studies on sweating v. studies of quantity and distribution of thermogenic sweat delivery to the skin. *J Invest Dermatol*. 1952;18:71.
89. Rebel G, Kirk D. Patterns of eccrine sweating in the human axilla. In: Montagna W, Ellis R, Silver A, eds. *Advances in Biology of Skin*. Vol 3. New York, NY: Pergamon Press; 1962:108-126.
90. Homma H. On apocrine sweat glands in white and negro men and women. *Bull Johns Hopkins Hosp*. 1956;38:365.
91. James CL, Worlana J, Stern JA. Skin potential and vasomotor responsiveness of black and white children. *Psychophysiology*. 1976;13:523.
92. Juniper K Jr, Dykman RA. Skin resistance, sweat-gland counts, salivary flow, and gastric secretion: age, race, and sex differences, and intercorrelations. *Psychophysiology*. 1967;4:216.
93. Schiefferdecker P. Dsaael be (vollkomin. Mitt.). *Zoologica*. 1922;27:1.
94. Hurley HJ, Shelley WB. The physiology and pharmacology of the apocrine sweat gland. In: *The Human Apocrine Sweat Gland in Health and Disease*. Springfield, IL: Charles Thompson; 1960:64.
95. Champion RH, Gillman T, Rood AS, et al. *An Introduction to the Biology of the Skin*. Philadelphia, PA: FA Davis; 1970:418.
96. Kligman AM, Shelley WB. An investigation of the biology of the sebaceous gland. *J Invest Dermatol*. 1958;30:99.
97. Pochi P, Strauss JS. Sebaceous gland activity in black skin. *Dermatol Clin*. 1988;6:349.
98. Abedeen SK, Gonzalez M, Judodihardjo H, et al. Racial variation in sebum excretion rate. Program and abstracts of the 58th Annual Meeting of the American Academy of Dermatology; March 10–15, 2000; San Francisco, CA. Abstract 559.
99. Hardy D, Baden HP. Biochemical variation of hair keratins in man and non-human primates. *Am J Phys Anthropol*. 1973;39:19.
100. Menkart J, Wolfram L, Mao I. Caucasian hair, Negro hair and wool: similarities and differences. *J Soc Cosmetic Chemists*. 1966;17:769.
101. Gold RJM, Schriver CH. The amino acid composition of hair from different racial origins. *Clin Chem Acta*. 1971;33:465.
102. Mangelsdorf S, Otberg N, Maibach HI, et al. Ethnic variation in vellus hair follicle size and distribution. *Skin Pharmacol Physiol*. 2006;19:159.
103. Halder RM. Hair and scalp disorders in blacks. *Cutis*. 1983;32:378.
104. Vernall DG. Study of the size and shape of hair from four races of men. *Am J Phys Anthropol*. 1961;19:345.
105. Khumalo NP, Doe PT, Dawber PR, et al. What is normal black African hair? A light and scanning electron-microscopic study. *J Am Acad Dermatol*. 2000;43:814.
106. Sperling LC. Hair density in African Americans. *Arch Dermatol*. 1999;135:656.

SECTION 3

Specific Skin Problems

CHAPTER 15

Acne (Type 1 Sensitive Skin)

Leslie Baumann, MD
Jonette Keri, MD, PhD

Any discussion of the practice of cosmetic dermatology must include a discussion of acne. Although acne is not typically considered to be a "cosmetic" problem, its highly visible nature makes it a very common complaint among cosmetic patients who are by definition concerned about their appearance. Acne can often have a profound psychological impact on patients. Recently, an evaluation of the psychosocial implications of acne on self-image and quality of life found that it may be equivalent to disorders such as asthma or epilepsy.[1] Acne can be especially troublesome to adults who perceive themselves as too old to have this condition most often associated with adolescence.

Acne vulgaris is a common, multifactorial process involving the pilosebaceous unit. More than 17 million people[2] and 75% to 95% of all teens[3] are affected by some form of acne each year in the United States alone. The majority of patients outside this age range are adult women who typically exhibit a hormonal component to their acne. Approximately 12% of women will have acne until the age of 44, whereas only 3% of men will have acne until the same age.[4] In many cases, adults are more surprised and upset by acne onset than are teenagers. In all cases, though, early and individually tailored treatment is necessary to achieve a satisfactory cosmetic appearance for the patient. This chapter will include a brief survey of the salient aspects of acne pathophysiology as well as suggestions for treatment and prevention. The psychosocial aspects of acne, or the significant psychological distress that this condition provokes, is beyond the scope of this chapter. It is worth noting, however, that many patients seeking treatment only for acne report substantial anxiety associated with this disease. Regardless of acne severity, acne is also one of the chief concerns of patients with body dysmorphic disorder[5] (see Chapter 40).

PATHOPHYSIOLOGY OF ACNE

Comedogenesis and acnegenesis are actually discrete processes, but they are usually associated with one another, with the latter often succeeding the former. Inflammation of the follicular epithelium, which loosens hyperkeratotic material within the follicle creating pustules and papules, characterizes acnegenesis (Fig. 15-1). Comedogenesis is best described as a noninflammatory follicular reaction manifested by a dense compact hyperkeratosis of the follicle, and usually precedes acnegenesis. Because the etiology of such lesions varies from person to person and within individuals also, it is difficult to categorically identify or isolate a basic cause of acne; however, three principal factors have been identified. The primary causal factors in acne work interdependently and are mediated by such important influences as heredity and hormonal activity.

Sebaceous Gland Hyperactivity

Sebum is continuously synthesized by the sebaceous glands and secreted to the skin surface through the hair follicle pore. The excretion of lipids by the sebaceous glands is controlled hormonally. The sebaceous glands are located all over the body but are largest and most numerous in the face, back, chest, and shoulders. These glands become more active during puberty because of the increase in androgens, particularly testosterone, which spurs sebum production. This imbalance between sebum production and the secretion capacity leads to a blockage of sebum in the hair follicle followed by inflammation.

Hormones continue to affect sebaceous gland activity into adulthood. In males, lipid secretion is regulated by the action of testosterone. In females, the immediate increase in luteinizing hormone following ovulation incites acceleration in sebaceous gland activity. The higher sebum secretion then stimulates or exacerbates acne breakouts usually 2 to 7 days prior to menstruation. Women experiencing excessive androgen states, such as those seen in polycystic ovarian disease, frequently suffer from acne as well.

The notion that sebum plays a key role in acnegenesis is buttressed by several facts including its comedogenicity, data showing that it causes inflammation when injected into the skin, and the reportedly higher level of sebum production in people with severe acne.[6] Researchers have also reported that acne patients possess larger sebaceous glands than the general population.[7] Furthermore, drugs that inhibit sebaceous gland activity, such as antiandrogens, estrogens, and oral retinoids, are integral treatment modalities in the successful control of acne.

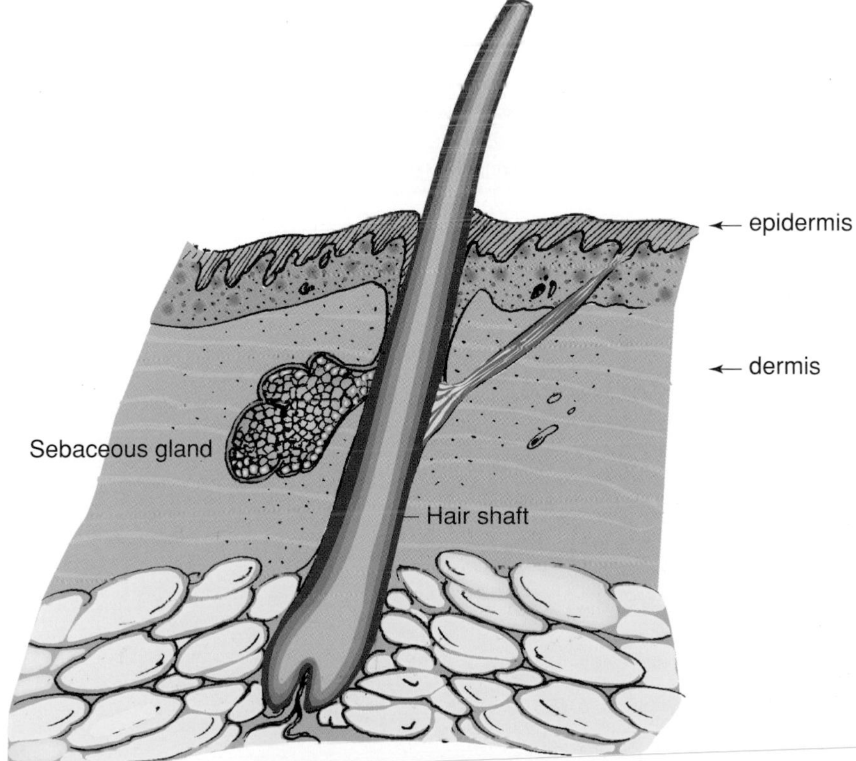

▲ **FIGURE 15-1** The hair follicle or "pore" is the site where acne occurs.

The literature reveals no discernible differences in the sebum composition of acne patients as compared to age-matched controls. Strauss and Thiboutot have noted, though, an inverse relationship between sebum secretion and linoleic acid concentration in the sebum of acne patients—the higher the sebum secretion, the lower the linoleic acid concentration.[7] Downing et al. theorized that the lower concentrations of linoleic acid, which correlated with the high sebum secretion rates of acne patients, leads to a localized deficiency of essential fatty acid of the follicular epithelium.[8] This deficiency then contributes to diminished epithelial barrier function and follicular hyperkeratosis, which aggravates acne.

Changes in Follicular Keratinization

In the lower portion of the follicular infundibulum, the normal process of keratinization occurs in the same way that it occurs on the skin's surface. This maturing of keratinocytes and subsequent exfoliation into the follicle marks the beginning of the formation of comedones. In acne patients, these keratinocytes tend to stick together because of the effects of positive and negative charges, the actions of transglutaminase, and the stickiness of sebum. The clumped keratinocytes block the pore/follicle, creating a blackhead if the pore is open ("open comedone") or a whitehead if it is closed ("closed comedone") (Fig. 15-2). The clogged pore is a great nutritional source for bacteria so *Propionibacterium acnes* gravitate to the blocked pores. The immune system recognizes the presence of bacteria and mounts an immune response resulting in redness, pus, as well as inflammation, and the typical "pimple" results. Most of the inflammation, however, is likely due to inflammatory mediators that are released when bacteria digest sebum (Fig. 15-3).

The Influence of Bacteria

P. acnes has been cited as the cause of acne because it is typically present in teenagers with acne and not those without acne.[7] However, *P. acnes* is commonly found in the facial flora of adults with or without acne. The exact role of bacteria is therefore unclear. It is known that sebum accumulation because of excess lipid secretion and hyperkeratosis at the infundibulum leads to an increase in *P. acnes* around the hair follicles. The presence of the bacteria is likely not a direct cause of acne breakouts, though. It is more likely that the inflammation seen in acne is caused by free fatty acids that result from the breakdown of triglycerides in the sebum owing to bacterial lipases. Other extracellular enzymes, proteases, and hyaluronidases may also play a role in the inflammatory process.[7]

The role of Toll-like receptors (TLRs) has been a recent topic of avid interest regarding the pathogenesis of acne. According to Heymann, these transmembrane proteins, when activated by ligands, modulate the expression of numerous immune response genes.[9] Evidence suggests that *P. acnes*, through its several secreted proinflammatory products, can induce TLR expression with resultant acne inflammation. In vitro work on monocytes has shown that all-*trans*-retinoic acid led to downregulation of TLR2, yielding more details regarding the retinoid mechanism of action[10] (see Chapter 4).

DIFFERENTIAL DIAGNOSIS

There are several acne variants and disorders with similar presentations. A brief survey of these conditions appears near the conclusion of this chapter. In addition, many other dermatologic conditions can be confused with acne (Box 15-1). These are unrelated conditions, but can be mimics.

The Basic Lesion

The fundamental acne lesion is the microcomedo, or microcomedone, an enlarged hair follicle full of sebum and *P. acnes*. Although there is a long list of materials that can cause comedones, the mechanism of spontaneous comedone formation is unknown.[11] The comedo that remains beneath the skin is a whitehead; a comedo that opens to the surface of the skin is labeled a blackhead because it appears black on the epidermis. The diverse array of other acne lesions includes papules (small, inflamed lesions presenting as pink, tender, nonpustular bumps); pustules (small, inflamed, tender, pustular lesions, usually red at the base); nodules (relatively large, spherical, painful lesions located deeper in the dermis); and cysts (even deeper, inflamed, pustular, painful lesions that can cause scarring) (Figs. 15-4 and 15-5).

TREATMENT

There are several therapeutic regimens for acne, most of which focus on prevention of future eruptions rather than treatment of present lesions. This is the reason that the majority of treatments take 8 weeks to work. *Only salicylic acid, benzoyl peroxide, and steroids treat lesions already visible on the skin.* Steroids,

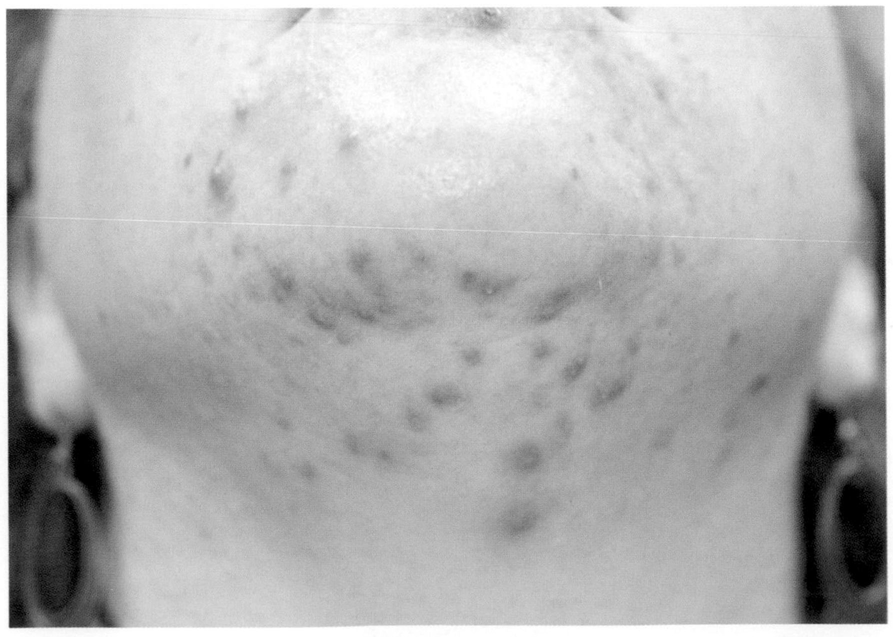

▲ **FIGURE 15-2** Open comedones and inflammatory papules on the neck.

BOX 15-1 Conditions That Can Be Confused with Acne

Adenoma sebaceum
Keratosis pilaris
Perioral dermatitis
Pityrosporum folliculitis
Rosacea
Seborrheic dermatitis
Steroid abuse/use dermatitis
Tinea barbae

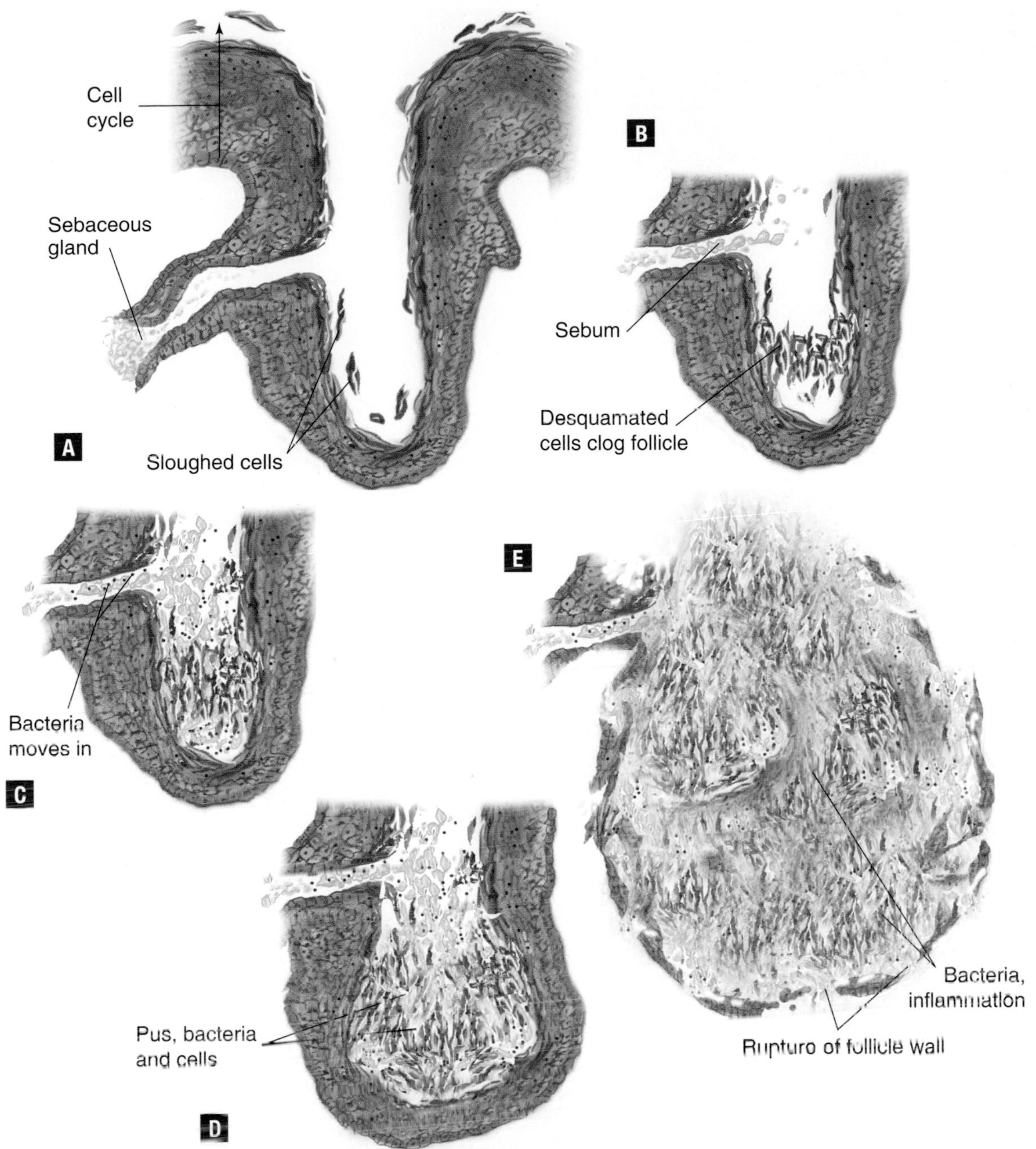

▲ **FIGURE 15-3** A close-up of the hair follicle and sebaceous gland demonstrating the different stages of acne. **A.** Desquamation of keratinocytes occurs in the same way that it does on the skin's surface. However, instead of sloughing into the environment, the keratinocytes slough into the hair follicle. This is a continuous and normal process that represents the culmination of the cell cycle. **B.** The first stage of acne is also known as comedogenesis. The sloughed cells stick together inside the hair follicle, resulting in a clogged pore or comedone. This is caused by several factors including increased amounts of sebum, inflammation of the sides of the hair follicle preventing the release of the desquamated keratinocytes, and inceased cohesion of keratinocytes. **C.** The keratinocyte plug and sebum is an excellent food source for bacteria. The bacteria invade the comedone and release inflammatory factors that lead to the next stage of acne. **D.** Inflammation continues with increased redness and pus. This is clinically detectable as a papule or pustule. **E.** Continued inflammation may lead to so much inflammation that the hair follicle ruptures and the bacteria and debris are released into the dermis. When severe, this can lead to scarring.

although frequently used, are not advised because they can lead to "steroid acne." Five basic principles govern the successful treatment of acne:

The Five Steps

NORMALIZING KERATINIZATION/EXFOLIATION

The first step in controlling acne is to prevent the exfoliated keratinocytes from sticking together (Box 15-2). Retinoids achieve this goal by reducing the positive and negative charges that render the cells sticky and by decreasing the levels of transglutaminase—an enzyme responsible for cross-linking cell membrane proteins of the keratinocytes. In fact, tretinoin has been said to have "superior ability to eradicate existing comedones and prevent the formation of

BOX 15-2 Products That Block Step 1 (Retinoids)

Tretinoin (Avita™, Renova™, Retin-A™, Retin-A Micro™, Atralin™)
Adapalene (Differin™)
Tazarotene (Tazorac™)
Retinol, retinyl linoleate, retinyl palmitate
Oral retinoids: isotretinoin (Accutane™, Claravis, Sotret, Amnesteen)

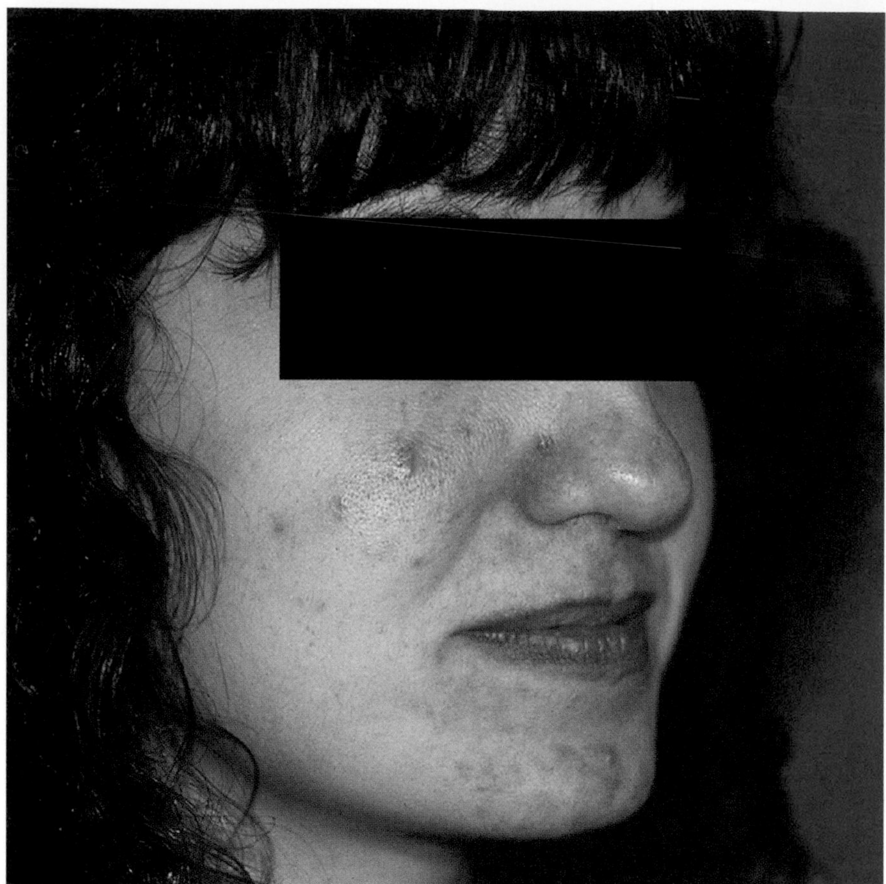

▲ **FIGURE 15-4** Multiple papules and pustules in an acne patient.

new ones."[12] Ultrastructural studies examining tretinoin use have demonstrated the loosening of follicular impactions and loss of cohesiveness within microcomedones.[13] Tretinoin should be considered a first-line therapy for acne because it renders the unplugged follicle more accessible to the penetration of antibiotics.[12]

Patients with cystic acne, or those who are unresponsive to all other regimens, can be treated with oral retinoids such as isotretinoin (Fig. 15-6). This is the only class of drugs that normalize keratinization as well as reduce sebaceous gland function. It has been shown that a marked decrease in sebum production occurs within 2 weeks of the onset of therapy.[14] All oral retinoids have teratogenic effects and patients should be cautioned to avoid pregnancy while taking these medications.

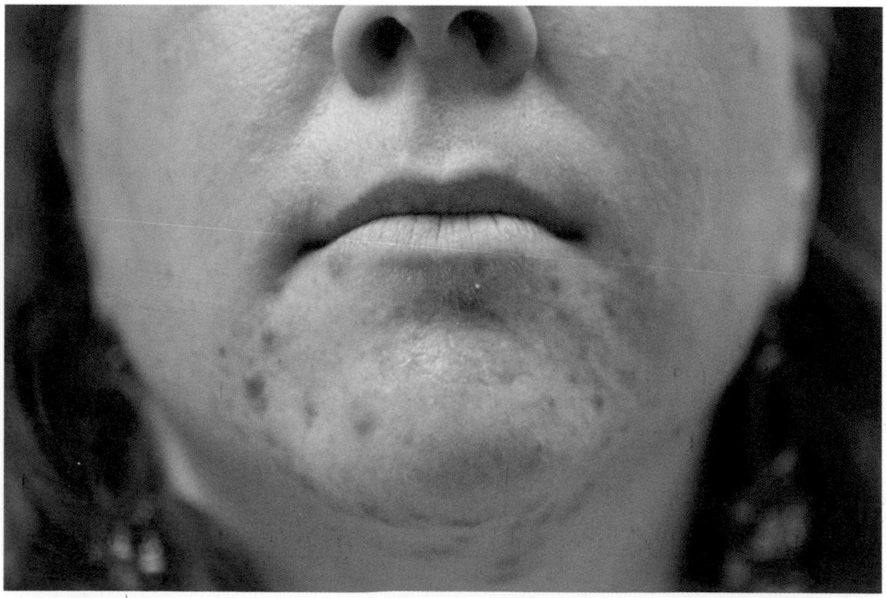

ELIMINATING OR REDUCING *P. ACNES* BACTERIA The use of antibiotics or benzoyl peroxide attacks the bacterial population thereby decreasing the level of inflammatory extracellular products induced by *P. acnes* (Box 15-3). The two antibiotics that are most commonly used in the treatment of acne, and have been shown to be equally effective,[15] are erythromycin and clindamycin. In addition to being antibacterial, these agents exhibit anti-inflammatory activity as they lower the percentage of inflammatory free fatty acids produced by bacterial digestion of surface lipids.[16]

The escalating incidence of antibiotic resistance is also an important consideration when treating the bacterial aspect of acne. Recent research suggests that as many as 60% of acne patients exhibit antibiotic-resistant strains of *P. acnes*.[17] A recent review of 50 controlled trials found that there was a gradual decrease in the efficacy of topical erythromycin, but that the efficacy of topical clindamycin stayed the same.[17] The preponderance of bacteria remain sensitive to medication in most of these patients, but an increasing number of patients have gradually developed less sensitive or more resistant strains. Regardless, the use of two modalities (i.e., benzoyl peroxide and a topical antibiotic) in acne therapies has been shown to decrease the resistance.

Although standard dosing regimens of oral antibiotics remain a mainstay of treatment, newer lower-dose antibiotic formulations represent submicrobial dosing and again are seen as a prudent approach to combating bacterial resistance. With such low-dose antibiotics, the drug works as an anti-inflammatory agent rather than an antimicrobial.

Benzoyl peroxide kills bacteria by generating reactive oxygen species in

BOX 15-3 Products That Affect Step 2

Topical antibiotics: clindamycin, erythromycin solution
Combination products with benzoyl peroxide and either clindamycin or erythromycin
Benzoyl peroxide
Azelaic acid (Azelex™)
Sodium sulfacetamide
Sulfur
Oral antibiotics
Light Therapy

▲ **FIGURE 15-5** Acne on the chin. Patients with this presentation should be asked if they are plucking or waxing hairs on the chin because this distribution mimics folliculitis.

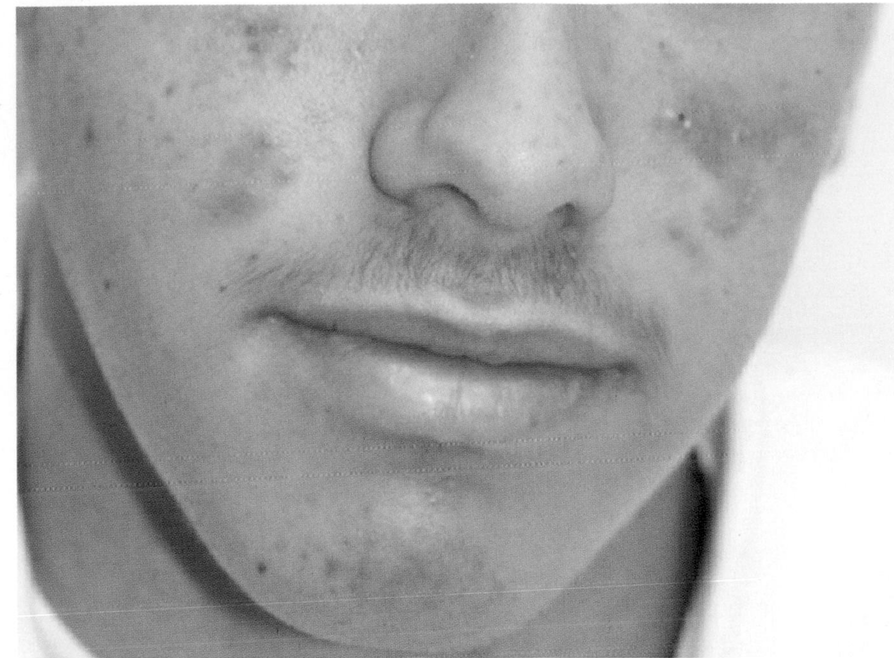

▲ **FIGURE 15-6** Cystic acne on cheeks.

the sebaceous follicle.[18] Because it causes free radical formation, the use of benzoyl peroxide may lead to exaggerated or accelerated aging of the skin and its use should be avoided. When applied at the same time as topical tretinoin, benzoyl peroxide can denature the tretinoin and reduce its effectiveness.[19]

Sodium sulfacetamide and sulfur are present in a variety of combination products. Sodium sulfacetamide is an antibacterial agent, and the mechanism of action of sulfur is also thought to be antibacterial in addition to being keratolytic.

REMOVING THE MATERIAL THAT CLOGS THE PORES Comedolytics, such as salicylic acid (BHA) and AHAs, are used to loosen the keratinocytes and "unclog" the pores (Box 15-4). BHA is more effective in reducing the number of comedones than are AHAs (see "AHAs versus BHA"). Comedone extractions and "acne surgery" can also be performed.

ATTACKING THE INFLAMMATORY RESPONSE The use of anti-inflammatory products, such as salicylic acid, is an effective approach to the most physically troublesome symptom of acne (Box 15-5). Steroid injections and topical corticosteroids, especially potent topical corticosteroids, pose important risks such as steroid atrophy and steroid acne. However, in severe cystic, scarring acne, oral corticosteroids and intralesional steroids may be warranted and necessary to prevent scarring. Finally, in-office BHA peels are effective in reducing the inflammation seen in acne (Table 15-1).

DECREASING THE LEVEL OF SERUM The use of oral and topical retinoids decreases sebaceous gland activity. Hormonal stabilization, using oral contraceptives, is also an effective way for females to reduce sebaceous secretions (Box 15-6). Although there are currently only three oral contraceptive pills approved by the FDA in the United States for the treatment of acne (i.e., Ortho Tri-cyclen, Estrostep, and Yaz), other such pills can be used. Yaz, which was recently approved, is a combination product of ethinyl estradiol and drospirenone. The drospirenone in this product is an antiandrogen and has about the same antiandrogen effect as 25 mg of spironolactone. Yaz and Yasmin, other oral contracep-

AHAs versus BHA

There is a significant chemical distinction between salicylic acid and the alpha hydroxy acids. The AHAs are water soluble, while salicylic acid is lipid soluble. Consequently, the distinct hydroxy acid families enter and function in different areas of the skin; salicylic acid usually effects change only in the upper epidermis while AHAs are believed to penetrate the dermis.[20,21] This difference might account for the longer duration of stinging reported by patients using AHAs as compared to those using BHA.

Because BHA is lipophilic, it is suited, unlike AHAs, to penetrate the sebaceous material in the follicles and thus able to induce exfoliation within the infundibula.[22] The comedolytic properties of BHA were confirmed in a study in which investigators compared the number of microcomedones observed in biopsies of women treated with 2% salicylic acid to those in women treated with 8% glycolic acid.[23] The glycolic formulation did not reduce the density of microcomedones, whereas BHA application resulted in a statistically significant ($p < 0.05$) decrease. Salicylic acid is marketed to patients in a variety of formulations including gels, lotions, masks, and cleansers.

Because of its anti-inflammatory activity, salicylic acid is also widely used in acne peels. A 1995 clinical study by Di Nardo showed that a product containing a combination of glycolic and salicylic acids reduced more inflammatory acne lesions than did benzoyl peroxide.[24] It is noteworthy that this study demonstrated that the combination of the AHA and BHA was more effective against acne lesions than was salicylic acid alone.

Anecdotally, salicylic acid has been reported to work better than AHAs in the treatment of rosacea because the anti-inflammatory properties of BHA induce less erythema. As of the date of this publication, however, there have been no double-blind studies to address this purported benefit.

TABLE 15-1
Anti-inflammatory Agents

Aloe vera
Chamomile
Coenzyme q10
Cucumber extract
Feverfew
Green tea
Licorice extract
Mushrooms
Niacinamide
Pycnogenol
Silymarin

BOX 15-4 Products That Affect Step 3

- Retinoids
- Salicylic acid (BHA)
- Alpha hydroxy acids (primarily glycolic and lactic)
- Azelaic acid

BOX 15-5 Products That Affect Step 4

- Salicylic acid (OTC acne wash, lotion, gel, mask)
- In-office BHA peels
- Oral NSAIDs

BOX 15-6 Products That Affect Step 5

Oral contraceptives
Retinoids (see Step 1)

tives, are similar in that both contain drospirenone, but differ in the amount of estrogen, with Yaz being the lower estrogen pill. (For a more detailed discussion on the effects of hormones on the skin, see Chapter 5.)

MOISTURIZATION AND ACNE

In 1980, Swinyer reported on the differences between treating acne patients in a climate with relatively normal humidity in comparison to treatment in a dry climate. He identified skin dryness as an important factor in exacerbating the pathogenetic cycle of acne, thus hampering its treatment.[25] In a subsequent four-cell study that tested Swinyer's hypothesis, Jackson et al. conducted a 3-month evaluation of the influence of cleansing regimens on the effectiveness of acne therapy using 10% benzoyl peroxide lotion, isolating the type of cleanser as the only variable. An emollient facial wash clearly outperformed pure soap and a benzoyl peroxide wash in decreasing open comedones, papules, and in overall global assessment.[26] (Soap and placebo comprised one cell of the study; in each of the others, the variable—soap, an emollient, or benzoyl peroxide wash—was matched with 10% benzoyl peroxide lotion.)

Washing the skin with a noncomedogenic agent appears to act against acne and serves as a suitable alternative to cleansing with relatively abrasive products while satisfying the acne patient's typical desire to wash one's face. In hydrating while cleansing, use of an emollient facial cleanser will accelerate the pace of acne resolution and contribute to overall response regardless of the patient's treatment regimen.[26]

ACNE PREVENTION REGIMEN

Regimens should contain products that affect each of the five steps of acne formation described above. One such program is the following:

AM

1. Washing with a mild 2% salicylic acid cleanser.
2. Applying a topical antibiotic solution or azelaic acid.
3. Applying a sunscreen SPF 45 with moisturizing cream (unless the skin is very oily, in which case the patient should try a lotion or gel).

PM

1. Washing with the same salicylic acid cleanser.
2. Applying a topical retinoid.

The physician might consider adding in-office salicylic acid peels, oral antibiotics and retinoids, and oral contraceptives in recalcitrant cases. Some make up foundations contain salicylic acid as an additive to aid in the prevention or amelioration of acne.

COMMON ACNE VARIANTS

Acne Cosmetica

Developing acne as a result of cosmetics use is not as common today as it was just a couple of decades ago. Manufacturers test their products for comedogenicity now before putting them on the market. So, if a person chooses nongreasy, nonocclusive products, the cosmetic choice is unlikely to be a source of acne. See Chapter 32 for more information.

Acne Detergicans

The obsessive use of soaps by patients may lead to acne. Many facial cleansers and shampoos contain unsaturated fatty acids that have been shown to be comedogenic.[27] Other components such as bacteriostatic agents and botanical ingredients may irritate the hair follicle and cause acne as well. Therefore, it is important to educate patients that washing does not necessarily improve acne because the detergents used are only capable of removing surface oil and do not affect the sebum in the follicles, where the disease originates. (Of course, one exception to this would be cleansers containing salicylic acid, which has been shown to penetrate into the comedones and improve them.) Acne detergicans is uncommon but should be considered in patients that wash their face or skin more than 4 times daily.[28]

Rosacea

This is an acneiform condition typically presenting in adults between 25 and 60 years of age that is characterized by facial redness, flushing, papules and pustules, and the formation of prominent blood vessels in the face. These patients usually worsen with AHAs and retinoids but do well with antibiotics, BHA, and laser treatment of telangiectasias. The exact cause is unknown, but rosacea is a condition distinct from acne, although a patient may have both conditions at the same time (see Chapter 16).

SUMMARY

The pilosebaceous unit, which comprises the hair follicles, the cells that line them, and nearby sebaceous glands, is the location where acne manifests. This disease is a function of a complex interplay of hereditary, hormonal, and occasional exogenous factors. A change in the inner lining of the hair follicle—cells turn over too quickly and clump together—results in an inhibition of the usual passage of sebum and a blockage at the follicular opening. This sets the stage for the involvement of *P. acnes* and subsequent inflammation.

Just as the etiology is complex and multifactorial, the approach to treatment is variable and requires several steps tailored to the individual patient. There is not, to date, one isolated cause or a panacea—a medication that works for all patients. Early intervention and preventative treatment are largely effective in resolving all but the most recalcitrant cases of this common, cosmetically altering, and distressing condition.

REFERENCES

1. Thomas DR. Psychosocial effects of acne. *J Cutan Med Surg*. 2004;8(suppl 4):3.
2. Health Topics Questions and Answers About Acne: NIDDK. http://www.wrongdiagnosis.com/artic/health_topics_questions_and_answers_about_acne_niddk.htm. Accessed January 25, 2008.
3. Cordain L, Lindeberg S, Hurtado M, et al. Acne vulgaris: a disease of Western civilization. *Arch Dermatol*. 2002;138: 1584.
4. Goulden V, Stables GI, Cunliffe WJ. Prevalence of facial acne in adults. *J Am Acad Dermatol*. 1999;41:577.
5. Bowe WP, Leyden JJ, Crerand CE, et al. Body dysmorphic disorder symptoms among patients with acne vulgaris. *J Am Acad Dermatol*. 2007;57:222.
6. Harris HH, Downing DT, Stewart ME, et al. Sustainable rates of sebum secretion in acne patients and matched normal control subjects. *J Am Acad Dermatol*. 1983;8:200.
7. Strauss JS, Thiboutot DM: Diseases of the sebaceous glands. In: Freeberg I, Eisen A, Wolff K, et al., eds. *Fitzpatrick's Dermatology in General Medicine*. 5th ed. New York, NY: McGraw-Hill; 1999:769.
8. Downing DT, Stewart ME, Wertz PW, et al. Essential fatty acids and acne. *J Am Acad Dermatol*. 1986;14:221.
9. Heymann WR. Toll-like receptors in acne vulgaris. *J Am Acad Dermatol*. 2006;55: 691.

10. Liu PT, Krutzik SR, Kim J, et al. Cutting edge: all-trans retinoic acid down-regulates TLR2 expression and function. *J Immunol.* 2005;174:2467.
11. Webster GF. Acne vulgaris: state of the science. *Arch Dermatol.* 1999;135:1101.
12. Berson DS, Shalita AR. The treatment of acne: the role of combination therapies. *J Am Acad Dermatol.* 1995;32:S31.
13. Lauker RM, Leyden JJ, Thorne EG. An ultrastructural study of the effects of topical tretinoin on microcomedones. *Clin Ther.* 1992;14:773.
14. Farrell LN, Strauss JS, Stranieri AM. The treatment of severe cystic acne with 13 cis-retinoic acid: evaluation of sebum production and the clinical response in a multiple-dose trial. *J Am Acad Dermatol.* 1980;3:602.
15. Thomas DR, Raimer S, Smith EB. Comparison of topical erythromycin 1.5% solution versus topical clindamycin phosphate 1% solution in the treatment of acne. *Cutis.* 1982; 29:624.
16. Esterly NB, Furey NL, Flanagan LE. The effect of antimicrobial agents on leukocyte chemotaxis. *J Invest Dermatol.* 1978;70:51.
17. Simonart T, Dramaix M. Treatment of acne with topical antibiotics: lessons from clinical studies. *Br J Dermatol.* 2005; 153:395.
18. Nacht S, Young D, Beasley JN, et al. Benzoyl peroxide: percutaneous absorption and metabolic disposition. *J Am Acad Dermatol.* 1981;4:31.
19. Martin B, Meunier C, Montels D, et al. Chemical stability of adapalene and tretinoin when combined with benzoyl peroxide in presence and in absence of visible light and ultraviolet radiation. *Br J Dermatol.* 1998;139(suppl 52):8.
20. Draelos Z. Hydroxy acids for the treatment of aging skin. *J Geriatric Dermatol.* 1997;5:236.
21. Brackett W. The chemistry of salicylic acid. *Cosmet Dermatol.* 1997;10(suppl):5.
22. Davies M, Marks R. Studies on the effect of salicylic acid on normal skin. *Br J Dermatol.* 1976;95:187.
23. Kligman A. A comparative evaluation of a novel low-strength salicylic acid cream and glycolic acid. Products on human skin. *Cosmet Dermatol.* 1997;10 (suppl):S11.
24. Di Nardo J. A comparison of salicylic acid, salicylic acid with glycolic acid and benzoyl peroxide in the treatment of acne. *Cosmet Dermatol.* 1995;8:43-44,14.
25. Swinyer LJ, Swinyer TA, Britt MR. Topical agents al one in acne. *JAMA.* 1980;243:1640.
26. Jackson EM. The effects of cleansing in an acne treatment regimen. *Cosmet Dermatol.* 2000;12(suppl):9.
27. Kligman A, Wheatley V, Mills O. Comedogenicity of human sebum. *Arch Dermatol.* 1970;102:267.
28. Mills O, Kligman A. Acne detergicans. *Arch Dermatol.* 1975;111(1):65.

CHAPTER 16

Rosacea (Type 2 Sensitive Skin)

Sogol Saghari, MD
Jonette Keri, MD
Stuart Shanler, MD
Leslie Baumann, MD

Rosacea is a well recognized, chronic, cutaneous condition presenting as central facial erythema, telangiectasia, papules, and pustules. A Swedish study demonstrated a prevalence of approximately 10% in the general population.[1] In the United States, it is believed that there are 13 million people affected with rosacea. It is usually diagnosed between the ages of 30 and 50 years and although both genders can be affected, it is more common in women, with more men experiencing the phymatous changes. Rosacea is also more prevalent in fair-skinned than dark-skinned individuals. Sun damage, a propensity to flush, and genetic predisposition are risk factors in acquiring rosacea.

ETIOLOGY

The precise causal pathway of rosacea still remains unknown. In addition to genetic predisposition, many other factors have been implicated in the pathogenesis of rosacea. These include *Demodex folliculorum* mites, *Helicobacter pylori* infection, vascular lability, response to chemical and ingested agents, and psychogenic factors. Sunlight, heat, alcohol consumption, and spicy food are also very well known for their contributions in aggravating rosacea symptoms. The association of rosacea and digestive tract bacteria is controversial. *Helicobacter pylori* is a very common infection of the digestive tract and there are studies supporting both sides of the argument.[2–4] It has been suggested that intestinal inflammation[5] and bacteria may cause hypersensitization of facial sensory neurons via the plasma kallikrein–kinin pathway and production of bradykinin, a well-known vasodilator[6] (Box 16-1).

BOX 16-1

The kinin-kallikrein system or "kinin system" is a poorly delineated system of blood proteins that plays a role in inflammation, blood pressure control, coagulation, and pain. Its important mediators, bradykinin and kallidin, are vasodilators.

Rosacea is associated with dermal connective tissue damage and pilosebaceous abnormalities. The follicular immune response observed in rosacea has led some authors to suggest that the pilosebaceous inflammation secondary to Demodex mites and bacteria are the key to developing rosacea.[7,8] Although the potential involvement of Demodex mites in rosacea still remains controversial, matrix metalloproteinase-9 (MMP-9), also known as gelatinase, has been implicated with somewhat more confidence in the pathophysiology of this condition. Increased levels of MMP-9, if not controlled by its inhibitors, result in an inflammatory response and the degradation of collagen. Afonso et al. demonstrated that MMP-9 is increased in patients with ocular rosacea.[9] In addition, the expression of MMP-9 has been shown to be increased in the fibroblasts of patients with *Demodex folliculorum* and rosacea when compared to patients with rosacea in the absence of Demodex mites.[10] More research is warranted to study the correlation between Demodex mites and MMPs in the etiology of rosacea.

Another leading theory is based on vascular response. Flushing and telangiectasias are major symptoms in patients affected with rosacea. A combination of superficiality of cutaneous vasculature on the face,[11] higher blood flow of facial skin,[12] and vascular dysregulation via humoral and neural mechanisms[13] may explain the rationale behind this theory.[14] The mechanism of vasodilatation and flushing is believed to be both humoral and neural.[14] Wilkin demonstrated increased blood flow of the cheeks and forearms by both the vasodilator activity of prostaglandins on vascular smooth muscles (nicotinic acid test) and oral thermal challenge mediated by neural mechanisms.[15] In addition to prostaglandins, other neurotransmitters including histamine, serotonin, and substance P may also play a role in the erythema response of rosacea.[16] Vascular endothelial growth factor (VEGF) is known to increase angiogenesis and vascular permeability.[17] A recent study by Smith et al. demonstrated the presence of VEGF receptors on vascular endothelium in addition to the expression of both VEGF and VEGF receptors on inflammatory cells of patients with rosacea.[18] They proposed that VEGF "receptor-ligand binding" may play a role in the pathogenesis of this condition. Topical antiangiogenic growth factors will likely be a focus in future research on rosacea treatments.[19]

In 2007, Richard Gallo and colleagues observed that individuals with rosacea express abnormally high levels of two proteins: cathelicidin (an antimicrobial protein important in mounting an immune response to various bacterial, viral, and fungal pathogens) and stratum corneum tryptic enzyme (SCTE), also called kallikrein 5, a serine protease.[20] They demonstrated that when both of these proteins are present in excess an abnormality in enzymatic processing occurs and yields high levels of *abnormal* cathelicidin, which is proinflammatory, and clinically results in the erythema, inflammation, and vascular dilatation and growth characteristic of rosacea. Cathelicidins have also been implicated in the pathophysiology of psoriasis (increased) and atopic dermatitis (decreased),[21] and therapies designed to modify cathelicidin production are currently being developed.

CLINICAL MANIFESTATION

Diagnostic Criteria

In April 2002, the National Rosacea Society Expert Committee published an article in the *Journal of the American Academy of Dermatology* in which diagnostic criteria were discussed[22] (Table 16-1.) According to the published diagnostic guidelines, the main criteria include "flushing," "nontransient erythema," "papules/pustules," and "telangiectasia," where the presence of one or more on the central face is sufficient for a diagnosis of rosacea. It is important to note that the symptom of flushing alone is enough to diagnose rosacea. Experts have classified rosacea into four subtypes and one variant.[22]

ROSACEA SUBTYPES The characteristics of the four rosacea subtypes are listed in Table 16-2. The condition may progress from the milder subtypes such as flushing to papulopustular and phymatous rosacea. Patients may have more than one subtype. It is important to diagnose and treat rosacea early to try to avoid progression of the disorder. The four subtypes of rosacea are discussed below.

TABLE 16-1
Guidelines for the Diagnosis of Rosacea

One or More of the Following Sufficient for Diagnosis	Additional Symptoms and Signs
Flushing (transient erythema)	Burning/stinging
Persistent erythema	Facial edema
Telangiectasia	Facial dryness
Papules/pustules	Plaques
	Ocular symptoms
	Peripheral involvement (+/− facial roscea)
	Phymatous changes

Adapted from Wilkin J, Dahl M, Detmar M, et al.; National Rosacea Society Expert Committee. Standard grading system for rosacea: report of the National Rosacea Society Expert Committee on the classification and staging of rosacea. *J Am Acad Dermatol.* 2004;50(6):907-912.

Subtype 1: Erythemotelangiectatic Rosacea *(Fig. 16-1.)* This subtype is characterized by erythema (redness) of the central face, in addition to telangiectasias and flushing. The patient may only present with one of the mentioned signs and symptoms. Many patients describe worsening of their symptoms with aggravating factors such as hot beverages, spicy food, sunlight, heat, etc. These patients have a sensitive and irritable skin type. Therefore, complaints of burning and stinging with topical skin regimens are common[28] (see Chapter 17). Many patients in this subtype do not realize that they have rosacea and therefore are not using the proper skin care to avoid progression. Consequently, it is important for dermatologists to screen patients and ask them about facial flushing symptoms.

Subtype 2: Papulopustular Rosacea *(Fig. 16-2.)* Papulopustular rosacea, also called "classic rosacea," presents with papules, pustules, and erythema on the central face. Patients describe the erythema as persistent with episodic breakouts of papules and pustules. This type may be misdiagnosed as acne. Age of onset (older than 30 years of age), absence of comedones, development after precipitating factors, such as spicy food, and the presence of telangiectasias may help the practitioner to distinguish the papulopustular form of rosacea from acne.

Subtype 3: Phymatous Rosacea *(Fig. 16-3.)* Phymatous changes are well recognized by thickened and uneven skin on the nose with an irregular surface and nodularities. This is commonly known as the "WC Field's nose." Although it most commonly affects the nasal area, it also occurs on the malar area and chin. This type is seen more commonly in men and most patients have been affected for many years. Treatment modalities include isotretinoin, laser resurfacing, and surgical intervention.

Subtype 4: Ocular Rosacea *(Fig. 16-4.)* The ocular manifestations of rosacea are usually nonspecific. Most patients with ocular rosacea complain of burning, stinging, itching, and watering of their eyes. Many may go undiagnosed and untreated for several years, since they misinterpret their symptoms as evidence of allergies to different substances. Ocular rosacea should be considered if a patient complains of or

TABLE 16-2
Clinical Subtypes and Variants of Rosacea

Erythemotelangiectatic subtype
Facial flushing
Erythema/edema of central face
Telangiectasias on face
Papulopustular subtype
Persistent erythema of central face
Episodic papules and pustules on face
Phymatous subtype
Thickened skin of nose
Nodularities of nose
Irregular skin surface of nose
Ocular subtype
Burning and stinging of eyes
Foreign body sensation
Photosensitivity
Conjunctivitis/blepharitis/inflamed meibomian glands
Granulomatous variant
Yellow, brown, or red papules and nodules on face
Possible scarring

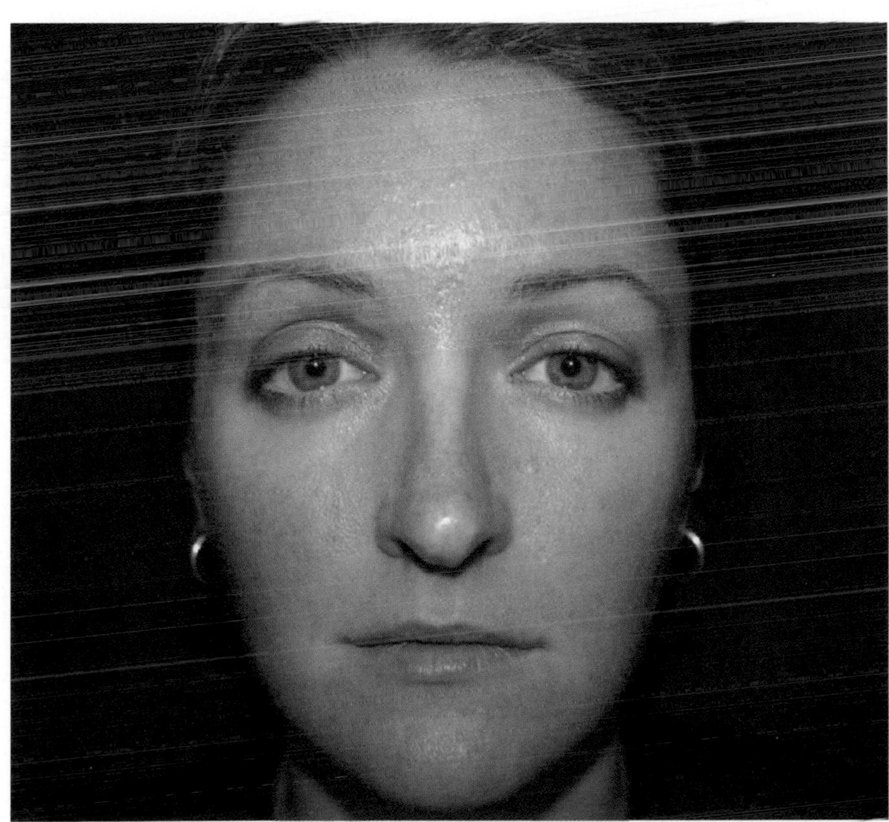

▲ **FIGURE 16-1** Facial flushing is a characteristic of rosacea and its presence alone is enough to diagnose the disorder. Patients with this form of rosacea often do not realize that they have rosacea and do not seek treatment.

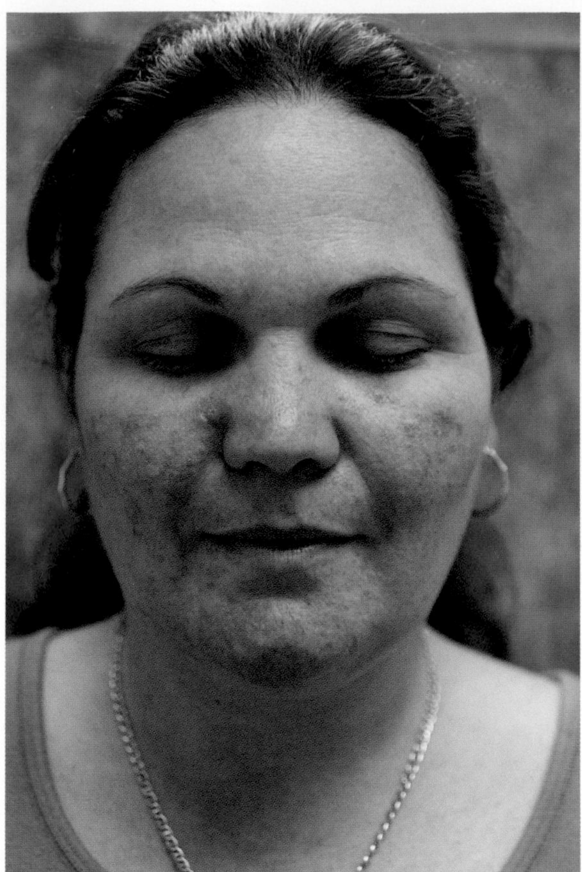

▲ **FIGURE 16-2** Papulopustular rosacea.

exhibits one of the following: interpalpebral conjunctival hyperemia, burning or stinging of the eyes, photosensitivity, telangiectasias of the lid margin, or conjunctiva, and erythema around the eyes.[22] Patients may also present with clinical pictures of conjunctivitis, blepharitis, inflamed meibomian glands (or tarsal glands), or chalazion.[24,25] Notably, the symptoms of ocular rosacea may precede the cutaneous signs, although most patients have some cutaneous manifestation of this condition. Interestingly, children who have styes are more likely to develop rosacea as adults.

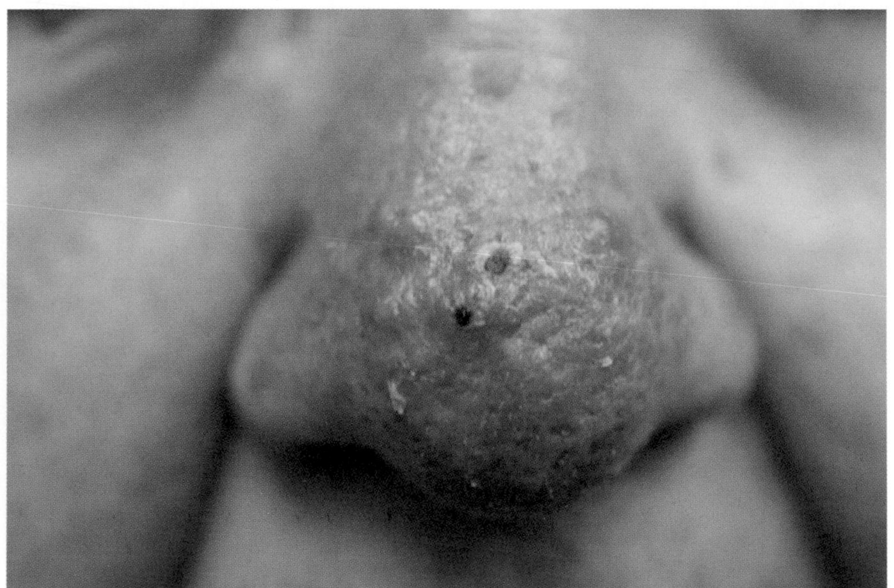

▲ **FIGURE 16-3** Phymatous rosacea. Thickened, irregular skin on the nose. This individual exhibits the papulopustular form of rosacea as well.

VARIANTS OF ROSACEA The National Rosacea Society Expert Committee has only recognized one variant for rosacea, which is the granulomatous form.[22] It is worth noting that pyoderma faciale (also called rosacea fulminans), steroid-induced rosacea, and perioral dermatitis are now considered to be different entities and are no longer classified as subtypes of rosacea.

Granulomatous Rosacea The granulomatous variant of rosacea is characterized by yellow-brown firm papules and nodules usually on the periorificial and malar areas of the face.[22] The papules and nodules appear to be less inflamed than in the papulopustular subtype. The presence of other subtypes is not necessary for diagnosis of this variant.

Differential Diagnosis

Facial erythema and flushing are seen in many dermatologic and systemic disorders. A clinical history and physical examination are very important aspects of the patient evaluation. The Baumann Skin Type Indicator (BSTI) can help determine patients at risk for developing rosacea by asking them historical questions about facial flushing (see Chapter 9). Laboratory tests may be needed to rule out systemic diseases, such as collagen vascular disorders, if these are suspected. Table 16-3 lists the differential diagnosis of rosacea.[26]

TREATMENT

The first step in the treatment of rosacea is to determine the subtype. All subtypes share one common feature—inflammation. Therefore, anti-inflammatory supplements and skin care products can help this condition (see

TABLE 16-3
Differential Diagnosis of Rosacea

Benign cutaneous flushing
Allergic contact dermatitis
Lupus erythematosus
Dermatomyositis
Mixed connective tissue disease
Carcinoid syndrome
Pheochromocytoma
Medullary carcinoma of the thyroid
Pancreatic cell tumor (VIPoma)
Mastocytosis
Photosensitivity from medications
Climacterium/postmenopausal

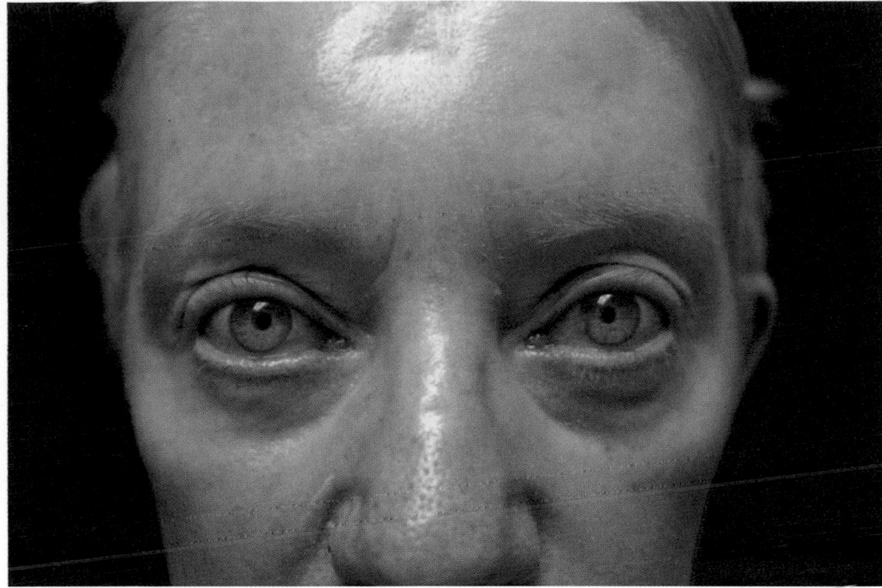

▲ **FIGURE 16-4** Ocular rosacea is characterized by bilateral erythema of the conjunctiva and/or eyelids.

Chapter 35). Sunscreen and sun avoidance are very important aspects of controlling symptoms. Often, because of the facial sensitivity of these patients, selecting the right sunscreen may be challenging. Physical blockers (e.g., zinc oxide and titanium dioxide) are usually tolerated the best by rosacea patients. Green-tinted moisturizers/sunscreens can conceal facial erythema and are therefore favored by many patients with rosacea. Avoidance of aggravating factors also plays an important role in treating this anxiety producing condition (Table 16-4). Based on the severity of symptoms, several topical and oral antibiotics may be used. Although antibiotic therapy controls the inflammatory component of rosacea, and may prevent its exacerbation, antibiotics do not improve the telangiectatic lesions on the face. In recent years, light and laser treatments have been widely and successfully used for this purpose. In a study of 60 patients affected with rosacea who were treated with intense pulsed light (IPL), there was a mean clearance of almost 78% of the telangiectasias. In this study, the mean number of treatments was about four and the wavelength, pulse duration, and energy were adjusted according to patients' skin color.[27] Pulsed dye laser (PDL) is another alternative. It is reasonable to consider an initial treatment plan with IPL and later, treat the resistant telangiectatic areas with PDL. Vascular laser treatments will be discussed in detail in Chapter 24. Table 16-5 summarizes different treatment modalities for rosacea.[28]

TABLE 16-4
Rosacea Aggravating Factors

Food
Hot temperature beverages
Spicy food
Chocolate
Dairy products
Vanilla
Soy sauce
Environmental factors
Heat
UV light
Cold
Humidity
Chemicals
Alcoholic beverages
Medications
Physical exertions
Stress
Chronic cough
Heavy exercise

SUMMARY

The complex etiology and wide spectrum clinical manifestations of rosacea render it a challenging condition for both dermatologists and patients. There is no single and universal approach to treating the patients affected by this condition. However, diagnosing rosacea early in the flushing stage and treating with anti-inflammatory modalities may prevent its progression. Treatment regimens should be individualized and tailored to address patients' concerns.

TABLE 16-5
Rosacea Treatment Modalities

Topical treatments
Antibiotics
Metronidazole
Clindamycin
Erythromycin
Anti-inflammatories
Azelaic acid
Feverfew
Green tea
Licochalcone
Licorice extract
Immunomodulators
Pimecrolimus
Tacrolimus
Sulfur products
Sulfur
Sodium sulfacetamide
Oral antibiotics
Tetracyclines (Tetracycline, doxycycline, minocycline)
Macrolides (Erythromycin, azithromycin, clarithromycin)
Metronidazole
Ampicillin
Trimethoprim/sulfamethoxazole
Other oral treatments
Isotretinoin
Aspirin
Beta-blockers
Selective serotonin reuptake inhibitors (SSRIs)
Clonidine
Hormones (oral contraceptives)
Laser and light treatments
Intense, pulsed-light therapy
Vascular lasers (Pulsed dye laser, Dornier 940 nm, KTP laser)
Carbon dioxide resurfacing laser
Other treatments (for phymatous subtype)
Hot loop electrocoagulation
Dermabrasion

REFERENCES

1. Berg M, Liden S. An epidemiological study of rosacea. *Acta Dermatol Venereol.* 1989;69:419.
2. Rebora A, Drago F, Picciotto A. Helicobacter pylori in patients with rosacea. *Am J Gastroenterol.* 1994;89:1603.
3. Utaş S, Ozbakir O, Turasan A, et al. Helicobacter pylori eradication treatment reduces the severity of rosacea. *J Am Acad Dermatol.* 1999;40:433.
4. Gedik GK, Karaduman A, Sivri B, et al. Has Helicobacter pylori eradication therapy any effect on severity of rosacea symptoms? *J Eur Acad Dermatol Venereol.* 2005;19:398.
5. Sharma JN, Zeitlin IJ, Mackenzie JF, et al. Plasma kinin-precursor levels in clinical intestinal inflammation. *Fundam Clin Pharmacol.* 1988;2:399.
6. Kendall SN. Remission of rosacea induced by reduction of gut transit time. *Clin Exp Dermatol.* 2004;29:297.

7. Rufli T, Büchner SA. T-cell subsets in acne rosacea lesions and the possible role of Demodex folliculorum. *Dermatologica*. 1984;169:1.
8. Powell FC. Rosacea and the pilosebaceous follicle. *Cutis*. 2004;74:9.
9. Afonso AA, Sobrin L, Monroy DC, et al. Tear fluid gelatinase B activity correlates with IL-1alpha concentration and fluorescein clearance in ocular rosacea. *Invest Ophthalmol Vis Sci*. 1999;40:2506.
10. Bonamigo RR, Bakos L, Edelweiss M, et al. Could matrix metalloproteinase-9 be a link between Demodex folliculorum and rosacea? *J Eur Acad Dermatol Venereol*. 2005;19:646.
11. Ryan TJ. The blood vessels of the skin. *J Invest Dermatol*. 1976;67:110.
12. Tur E, Tur M, Maibach HI, et al. Basal perfusion of the cutaneous microcirculation: measurements as a function of anatomic position. *J Invest Dermatol*. 1983;81:442.
13. Wilkin JK: Flushing reactions: consequences and mechanisms. *Ann Intern Med*. 1981;95:468.
14. Crawford GH, Pelle MT, James WD. Rosacea: I. Etiology, pathogenesis, and subtype classification. *J Am Acad Dermatol*. 2004;51:327.
15. Wilkin JK. Why is flushing limited to a mostly facial cutaneous distribution? *J Am Acad Dermatol*. 1988;19:309.
16. Pelwig G, Jansen T. Rosacea. In: Freedberg IM, Eisen AZ, Wolff K, Austen K, Goldsmith L, Katz S, Fitzpatrick T, eds. *Fitzpatrick's Dermatology in General Medicine*. 5th ed. New York, NY: McGraw-Hill; 1999:785.
17. Bates DO, Harper SJ. Regulation of vascular permeability by vascular endothelial growth factors. *Vascul Pharmacol*. 2003;39:225.
18. Smith JR, Lanier VB, Braziel RM, et al. Expression of vascular endothelial growth factor and its receptors in rosacea. *Br J Ophthalmol*. 2007;91:226.
19. Cuevas P, Arrazola JM. Therapeutic response of rosacea to dobesilate. *Eur J Med Res*. 2005;10:454.
20. Yamasaki K, Di Nardo A, Bardan A, et al. Increased serine protease activity and cathelicidin promotes skin inflammation in rosacea. *Nat Med*. 2007;13:975.
21. Ong PY, Ohtake T, Brandt C, et al. Endogenous antimicrobial peptides and skin infections in atopic dermatitis. *N Engl J Med*. 2002;347:1151.
22. Wilkin J, Dahl M, Detmar M, et al. National Rosacea Society Expert Committee. Standard grading system for rosacea: report of the National Rosacea Society Expert Committee on the classification and staging of rosacea. *J Am Acad Dermatol*. 2004;50:907.
23. Lonne-Rahm SB, Fischer T, Berg M. Stinging and rosacea. *Acta Derm Venereol*. 1999;79:460.
24. Quarterman MJ, Johnson DW, Abele DC, et al. Ocular rosacea. Signs, symptoms, and tear studies before and after treatment with doxycycline. *Arch Dermatol*. 1997;133:49.
25. Ghanem VC, Mehra N, Wong S, et al. The prevalence of ocular signs in acne rosacea: comparing patients from ophthalmology and dermatology clinics. *Cornea*. 2003;22:230.
26. Izikson L, English JC III, Zirwas MJ. The flushing patient: differential diagnosis, workup, and treatment. *J Am Acad Dermatol*. 2006;55:193.
27. Schroeter CA, Haaf-von Below S, Neumann HA. Effective treatment of rosacea using intense pulsed light systems. *Dermatol Surg*. 2005;31:1285.
28. Pelle MT, Crawford GH, James WD. Rosacea: II. therapy. *J Am Acad Dermatol*. 2004;51:499.

CHAPTER 17

Burning and Stinging Skin (Type 3 Sensitive Skin)

Leslie Baumann, MD

A subset of people feel stinging and burning when exposed to certain skin care products. These people have traditionally been called "stingers" since Kligman coined the term in 1977. This skin type has also been called reactive skin, hyperreactive skin, intolerant skin, or irritable skin. In the Baumann Skin Typing System, stingers are designated as having Baumann S3 sensitive skin (see Chapter 9); the "3" denotes burners and stingers rather than other types of sensitive skin that develop such as acne (S1), rosacea (S2), or contact dermatitis (S4). One patient can demonstrate one to four different types of sensitive skin. For example, many rosacea (S2) patients are also burners and stingers (S3). Although this skin type is referred to as stingers in the context of applying chemical factors such as skin care ingredients, this skin type also includes those who feel the onset of a prickling, tingling sensation, or slight pain because of physical factors such as ultraviolet radiation, heat, cold, and wind. Psychologic stress or hormonal factors such as menstruation may play a role as well. It is important to know a patient's susceptibility to S3 sensitive skin because this may lead to noncompliance with certain medications and vehicles that cause discomfort to the patient. Finacea is an example of a rosacea medication that causes stinging in a small proportion of users. Retin A Micro contains benzyl alcohol (a derivative of benzoic acid) that can cause stinging in certain people. This chapter will discuss what is known about the mechanisms of burning and stinging, what ingredients are most likely to cause it, and how to identify a potential "stinger."

EPIDEMIOLOGY

Type 3 sensitive skin is common worldwide. In a British study, 57% of women and 31.4% of men reported that they had experienced an adverse reaction to a personal skin care product at some stage in their lives, with 23% of women and 13.8% of men having had a problem in the last 12 months.[1] Another study demonstrated that women showed a greater tendency toward being more sensitive to the subjective effects elicited by lactic acid than males.[2]

MECHANISMS OF BURNING AND STINGING

Stinging is a problem reported to occur primarily on the face, particularly on the nasolabial folds and cheeks. The extreme sensitivity of this region is thought to be caused by a more permeable horny layer, a high density of sweat glands and hair follicles, and an elaborate network of sensory nerves.[3] There is specificity of the stinging response that is not understood. In other words, an individual may be a lactic acid stinger, but not experience such a reaction to other ingredients such as benzoic acid and azelaic acid. One study showed that there was no correlation between patients who stung from lactic acid and those who stung from azelaic acid.[4] This suggests that there is some sort of specificity involved that has not yet been deciphered.

The Role of the Sensory Nervous System

It is likely that the sensory system in the epidermis is involved in this process, rather than the dermal sensory system. In the epidermis, sensory nerves are linked to keratinocytes, melanocytes, Langerhans cells, and Merkel cells (Box 17-1). Sensory nerves are categorized into two groups: the epidermal and the dermal sensory organs. It is the epidermally-located Merkel cells that are thought to play a role in sensory perception; however, the exact role of Merkel cells and their possible involvement in mechanosensation is unclear.[5] Merkel cells consist of neurosecretory granules that contain neurotransmitter-type substances such as metenkephalin, vasoactive intestinal peptide, neuron-specific enolase, and synaptophysin.[6] The Merkel cell-nerve complex has been called by other names including touch domes, hederiform endings, Iggo's capsule, Pinkus corpuscles, and Haarsheibe. Merkel cell-nerve complexes have been found to be associated with hair follicles and eccrine sweat ducts. Little is known about the effects of chemical agents upon the excitability of sensory units such as Merkel cells.

It is believed that those with a predilection toward stinging have an increased nerve response. Capsaicin, the irritant ingredient found in red pepper and used commercially as "pepper spray," causes pain and burning on skin contact on all subjects. Its mechanisms of action have been studied in the pursuit of a better understanding of chemogenic pain. Although it is not known if these same pathways play a role in the skin burning that patients feel when they apply skin care products, it is possible that these follow a similar mechanism; therefore, the actions of capsaicin will be explored here. The C polymodal nociceptor is stimulated by capsaicin and other chemicals. The effects of capsaicin are dependent on concentration. Topical application of 1% capsaicin on intact skin typically produces sensitization to heat.[7] Findings of differential capsaicin effects on heat perception and mechanical stimuli perception have led to the belief in the existence of two categories of functionally different nociceptors in human skin.[8] Much more research needs to be conducted in this area; however, it is plausible that the heat-sensitive nociceptors play a role in this stinging and burning skin type.

VASODILATATION AND ITCHING Type 3 sensitive skin patients complain of abnormal sensations and may or may not exhibit vasodilatation. C nonmyelinated

> **BOX 17-1 Sensory Nerves in the Skin**
>
> The superficial skin layer includes sensory nerve fibers connected to specialized receptors such as Merkel cells.
>
> Three types of fibers are generally recognized in the sensory subclass of fibers:
>
> - Beta fibers, which are the largest fibers and myelinated, mediate the touch, vibration, and pressure sensations (conduction velocity of 2–30 m s^{-1}).
> - Delta fibers, smaller and myelinated, mediate the cold and pain sensations (conduction velocity of >30 m s^{-1}).
> - C fibers, the slowest, smaller and nonmyelinated, mediate the warm and itching sensations (conduction velocity of <2 m s^{-1}). C fibers mediate most of the autonomic peripheral functions.

fibers likely play a role because they are known to mediate warm sensations. Although the stinging and burning that characterize this skin type are not always associated with inflammation, inflammation may occur as well. Neurogenic inflammation may result from neuromediators such as substance P, calcitonin gene-related peptide (CGRP), and vasoactive intestinal peptide, leading to vasodilatation and mast cell degranulation.[9] Nonspecific inflammation may also be associated with the release of IL-1, IL-8, PgE2, PgF2, and TNF.[10] Sorbic acid, a known cause of skin stinging, has been found to release prostaglandin D2 (PGD2) from a cellular source in the skin resulting in cutaneous vasodilatation.[11]

Itching seems to be a different process than burning or stinging; however, there may be some overlap. A detailed explanation of itching is beyond the scope of this chapter but a good recent review can be found in the study by Steinhoff et al.[12] An itch response can be experimentally induced by topical or intradermal injections of various substances such as proteolytic enzymes, mast cell degranulators, and vasoactive agents. Grove compared the cumulative lactic acid sting scores with the histamine itch scores in 32 young subjects; all the subjects who were stingers were also moderate to intense itchers, whereas 50% of the moderate itchers experienced no stinging.[13] Recent studies suggest that a new class of C fibers with an exceptionally lower conduction velocity and insensitivity to mechanical stimuli likely can be considered as afferent units that mediate the itchy sensation.[14]

The Skin Barrier and Stinging

The skin barrier plays an important role in both keeping water from evaporating from the skin as well as keeping out allergens and irritants (see Chapter 11). It has been postulated that an impaired skin barrier allows excessive penetration of applied ingredients, which may lead to stinging. A recent study evaluated 298 women with 5% lactic acid solution and measured transepidermal water loss, skin hydration, sebum content, and pH.[15] A positive correlation between stinging and increased transepidermal water loss was found, suggesting that skin barrier perturbation played a role in the development of stinging. No correlation was observed between stinging responses and other parameters such as skin hydration, sebum content, or pH. However, not all studies show stingers to have impaired barriers. One study examining the relationship between stingers (Baumann S3 type) and those who develop an irritant reaction to a 0.3% sodium dodecyl sulfate patch test (Baumann S4 type) found that stingers were no more likely to develop an irritant response than nonstingers.[3]

Rosacea and Skin Stinging

Patients with rosacea (Baumann S2 type) have a tendency to flush. This flushing is often accompanied by a warm sensation. Many rosacea patients also complain of intolerance to skin care products. One study examined this relationship. Thirty-two patients with rosacea and 32 controls were given the lactic acid stinging test. Twenty-four patients and six controls reacted positively as stingers ($p < 0.001$). This study suggests that patients with rosacea may be more likely to be stingers.[16]

ETHNICITY AND STINGING

Although there is a clinical consensus that blacks are less reactive and Asians are more reactive than whites, the data supporting this hypothesis rarely reach statistical significance.[17] Frosch reported that most common stingers were light-complexioned persons of Celtic ancestry who sunburned easily and tanned poorly.[18] Grove et al. found that stinging was not related to ethnicity, but was associated mainly with a person's history of sensitivity to soaps, cosmetics, and drugs.[19] Aramaki et al. found significant subjective sensory differences between Japanese and German women even though they had significant differences in reactions to sodium lauryl sulfate testing.[20] They concluded that Japanese women might be more likely to report stronger stinging sensations, reflecting a different cultural behavior. Large-scale studies of ethnic differences in this skin type have not been performed.

INGREDIENTS THAT CAUSE STINGING

A list of common stinging ingredients is found in Table 17-1. However, new ingredients are being developed every day so it is impossible to have a complete list. Patients with a proclivity to experience stinging should be advised to make a list of the ingredients found in products that evoke the stinging response. The dermatologist can help the patient identify the responsible ingredient(s) to be avoided in the future. As a general rule, products with a low pH such as any acids (e.g., glycolic, salicylic, lactic) will cause stinging. Vitamin C is formulated with a low pH to enhance absorption, so some forms may cause stinging. In addition, alcohols that are often found in toners and astringents can cause stinging.

TABLE 17-1
Ingredients Known to Cause Stinging in Some People

Alcohol
Avobenzone (Parsol)
Azelaic acid
Benzoic acid
Capsaicin
Eucalyptus oil
Fragrance
Glycolic acid
Lactic acid
Menthol
Peppermint
Salicylic acid
Sorbic acid
Vitamin C
Witch hazel

HOW TO IDENTIFY A POTENTIAL STINGER

The Baumann Skin Type Indicator (BSTI) contains a series of questions that are designed to identify those with the Baumann S3 skin type (see Chapter 9). This questionnaire can be accessed online by registering at www.SkinIQ.com. Using the online version of the questionnaire will allow data to be collected in order to examine issues such as the role of gender, ethnicity, and climate on skin stinging. It is imperative to collect large amounts of worldwide data to identify the factors relevant in this condition.

Objective measures in the research and clinical setting may be used to identify stingers. However, it is important to note that not all stingers react to all known stinging agents. In spite of this, clinical tests can give insight into this distressing condition. The lactic acid stinging test was first described by Kligman in 1977.[18] This method is now used with various stinging agents besides lactic acid. The agent of choice is applied to the cheek using a cotton swab. The stingers experience a moderate to severe sensation within a few minutes. These subjects are then asked to describe the intensity of the sensation using a point scale.[21] It is important to note that substances cannot be simultaneously tested on both cheeks. Strong stinging on one side may enhance the perception of stinging on the opposite cheek. In a laboratory setting, stingers are easy to identify. The problem is that not all people sting in response to the same substance. For example, a lactic acid stinger may sting to lactic acid but not to benzoic acid. For this reason, it is very difficult to predict outside the laboratory setting which ingredients will make a patient sting. The BSTI can help identify susceptible subpopulations who are more likely to develop a stinging response based on historical data.

HOW TO PREVENT STINGING

At this point, identification and avoidance of agents that cause stinging is the most prudent approach. Patients should be instructed to keep a list of ingredients that cause stinging and avoid agents that contain such components. This includes shampoos, conditioners, and shaving products as well as skin care products. It is likely that improving the skin barrier will decrease the incidence of the stinging response. Anti-inflammatory products such as antioxidants, aloe vera, and chamomile can help decrease inflammation that may coincide with the stinging response. It is important to remember that stinging not accompanied by inflammation is not necessarily detrimental to the skin. In fact, chemical peel agents, glycolic acid, and lactic acid agents cause stinging in many because of their low pH. However, these agents have been shown to be very useful in increasing skin hydration and improving the appearance of photodamaged skin.

SUMMARY

Baumann S3 sensitive skin is a poorly understood skin type. Those who exhibit such a skin type find that they are intolerant to some skin care products. This likely affects their brand and product choices. Although stinging skin is usually not accompanied by inflammation, it can be very uncomfortable for the patient and can lead to noncompliance with skin care regimens for other conditions. More research is needed into the mechanisms and associations of this intellectually intriguing skin type so that treatment options can be improved and/or expanded for the patients who suffer symptoms because of this subtype of sensitive skin.

REFERENCES

1. Willis CM, Shaw S, De Lacharrière O, et al. Sensitive skin: an epidemiological study. *Br J Dermatol.* 2001;145:258.
2. Marriott M, Whittle E, Basketter DA. Facial variations in sensory responses. *Contact Dermatitis.* 2003;49:227.
3. Basketter DA, Griffiths HA. A study of the relationship between susceptibility to skin stinging and skin irritation. *Contact Dermatitis.* 1993;29:185.
4. Draelos ZD. Noxious sensory perceptions in patients with mild to moderate rosacea treated with azelaic acid 15% gel. *Cutis.* 2004;74:257.
5. Hitchcock IS, Genever PG, Cahusac PM. Essential components for a glutamatergic synapse between Merkel cell and nerve terminal in rats. *Neurosci Lett.* 2004;362:196.
6. Chu DH. Development and structure of skin. In: Wolff K, Goldsmith LA, Katz SI, Gilchrest BA, Paller AS, Leffell DJ, eds. *Fitzpatrick's Dermatology in General Medicine.* 7th ed. New York, NY: McGraw-Hill; 2007:62.
7. LaMotte RH, Lundberg LE, Torebjörk HE. Pain, hyperalgesia and activity in nociceptive C units in humans after intradermal injection of capsaicin. *J Physiol.* 1992;448:749.
8. Schmelz M, Schmid R, Handwerker HO, et al. Encoding of burning pain from capsaicin-treated human skin in two categories of unmyelinated nerve fibres. *Brain.* 2000;123:560.
9. Misery L, Myon E, Martin N, et al. Sensitive skin: psychological effects and seasonal changes. *J Eur Acad Dermatol Venereol.* 2007;21:620.
10. Reilly DM, Parslew R, Sharpe GR, et al. Inflammatory mediators in normal, sensitive and diseased skin types. *Acta Derm Venereol.* 2000;80:171.
11. Morrow JD, Minton TA, Awad JA. Release of markedly increased quantities of prostaglandin D2 from the skin in vivo in humans following the application of sorbic acid. *Arch Dermatol.* 1994;130:1408.
12. Steinhoff M, Bienenstock J, Schmelz M, et al. Neurophysiological, neuroimmunological, and neuroendocrine basis of pruritus. *J Invest Dermatol.* 2006;126:1705.
13. Grove GL. Age-associated changes in intertegumental reactivity. In: Léveque JL, Agache PG, eds. *Aging Skin: Properties and Functional Changes.* New York, NY:Marcel Dekker; 1993:189-192.
14. Schmelz M, Schmidt R, Bickel A, et al. Specific C-receptors for itch in human skin. *J Neurosci.* 1997;17:8003.
15. An S, Lee E, Kim S, et al. Comparison and correlation between stinging responses to lactic acid and bioengineering parameters. *Contact Dermatitis.* 2007;57:158.
16. Lonne-Rahm SB, Fischer T, Berg M. Stinging and rosacea. *Acta Derm Venereol.* 1999;79:460.
17. Modjtahedi SP, Maibach HI. Ethnicity as a possible endogenous factor in irritant contact dermatitis: comparing the irritant response among Caucasians, blacks and Asians. *Contact Dermatitis.* 2002;47:272.
18. Frosch PJ, Kligman AM. A method for appraising the stinging capacity of topically applied substances. *J Soc Cosmet Chem.* 1981;28:197.
19. Grove GL, Soschin DM, Kligman AM. Adverse subjective reactions to topical agents. In: Drill VA, Lazar P, eds. *Cutaneous Toxicology.* New York, NY: Raven Press; 1984:200-210.
20. Aramaki J, Kawana S, Effendy I, et al. Differences of skin irritation between Japanese and European women. *Br J Dermatol.* 2002;146:1052.
21. Christensen M, Kligman AM. An improved procedure for conducting lactic acid stinging tests on facial skin. *J Soc Cosmet Chem.* 1996;47:1.

CHAPTER 18

Contact Dermatitis (Type 4 Sensitive Skin)

Sharon E. Jacob, MD

OVERVIEW OF CONTACT DERMATITIS

Contact dermatitis is an umbrella expression for a group of dermatoses that are initiated by the pivotal event of the epidermis coming into contact with a triggering chemical. For practical purposes, there are three main clinical forms: (1) irritant contact dermatitis (ICD); (2) contact urticaria (CU); and (3) allergic contact dermatitis (ACD). Approximately 80% of contact dermatitis cases are identified as ICD, because ICD represents a nonspecific inflammatory response to a chemical when the skin barrier function is impaired. Wet work (immersing in detergents, water, or other activities that require frequent hand washing) predisposes an individual to these irritant-type reactions because of disruptions in skin barrier function (see Chapter 11). Irritancy can also occur after chronic exposure to an environment with low humidity,[1] or chronic exposure to saliva (lip smacking), urine, or feces. Another example of an inducible ICD is epidermal keratinocyte damage following a cosmetic peel (Fig. 18-1).

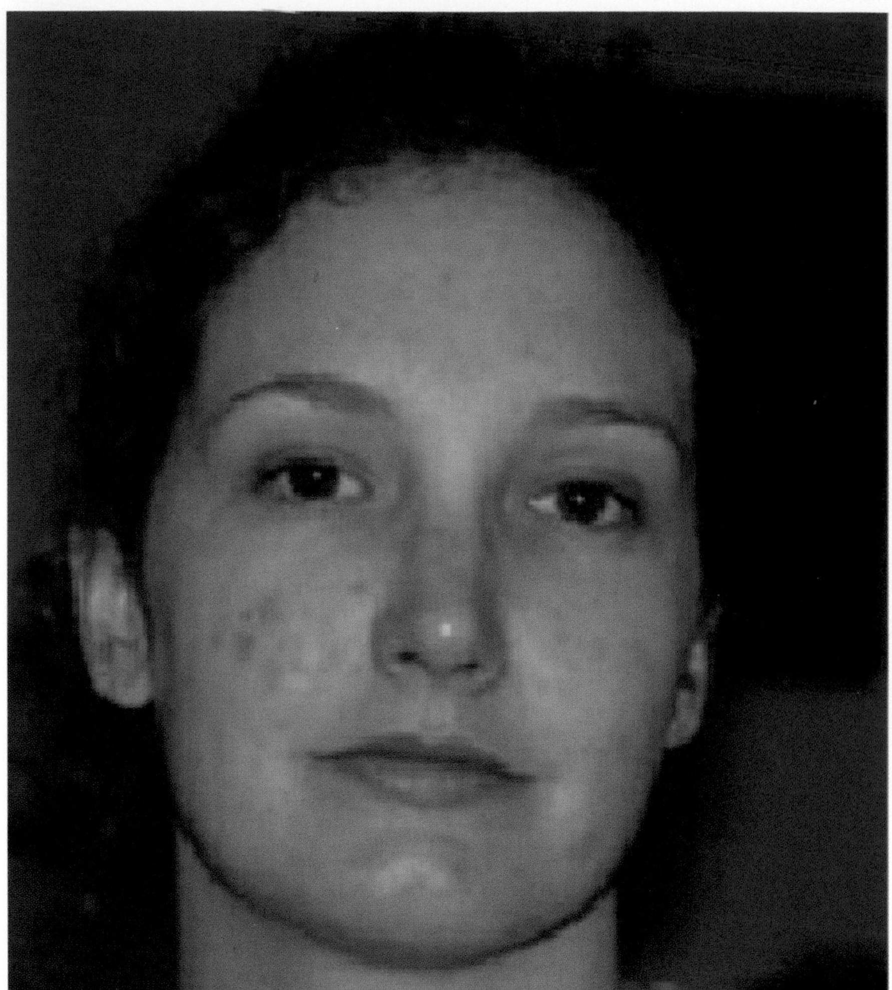

▲ **FIGURE 18-1** Glycolic acid is an irritant that can result in keratinolysis. In this figure, pink tender plaques occurred on the cheeks 1 day after a 30% glycolic acid peel.

At the other end of the spectrum is CU, which accounts for approximately 0.5% of the contact dermatitides. This type of reaction is IgE-mediated and represents an immediate-type hypersensitivity response. Clinically, CU manifests classic wheals and flares (hives); with extreme cases the clinical symptoms may progress to severe respiratory compromise, anaphylaxis, and death. A primary example is latex hypersensitivity.

The pathophysiology of ACD is remarkably different from the other types of contact dermatitis. Like CU, ACD is an immunologic reaction; however, unlike CU, ACD is a consequence of lymphocyte activation (a T-cell mediated Type IV delayed-type hypersensitivity [DTH] reaction). To assist with the visualization of the sensitization process, it can be useful to consider the triggering of ACD as similar to serial vaccination, although scientifically it is important to note that they are different immunologic processes. That is, with each subsequent dose of a chemical the ability to remember that chemical for future interactions becomes more likely. For example, with the hepatitis B vaccine, three shots are required for establishing long-lasting and effective "immunity," or memory of that chemical; conversely, a tetanus vaccine must be "boosted" to guarantee memory. Like the tetanus, the more potent chemicals may only require a single dose, such as poison ivy. In most cases of ACD, however, the "shots" are mini-*doses* that taken sequentially over a given period of time result in the individual being *sensitized* to that chemical.

STEPS LEADING TO ALLERGIC CONTACT DERMATITIS

The chemicals likely to elicit an ACD are generally small lipophilic compounds to which an individual is routinely exposed. These chemicals usually have a molecular weight less than 500 Da allowing them to penetrate the skin or mucous membranes and activate an immunologic cascade.[2,3] Subsequent to entry into the skin these chemicals are taken up by epidermal immunologic cells (Langerhans cells) and further processed for presentation to naïve T lymphocytes. This process of chemical capture and presentation is known as the induction phase of sensitization.

With induction there is clonal expansion of memory T cells, each inheriting the capability to mount an immune response upon reexposure to the allergenic chemical. Upon reexposure, or challenge, the elicitation phase of sensitization ensues, which involves a complex interplay between immune cells (i.e., Langerhans, lymphocytes, and keratinocytes). Each cell releases its respective cytokine repertoire leading to the clinical picture of ACD. It is important to note that while the initial sensitization process may take up to 21 days, subsequent reexposure of the sensitized individual may result in a rechallenge reaction within 48 to 120 hours.[2]

For the most part, primary allergic contact type lesions present in the distribution of allergen—epidermal contact, which ultimately provides a very important diagnostic clue as to the identity of the culprit chemical allergen. There is a notable exception to this rule, however—the "recall reaction." In the recall reaction, sites of previous sensitization may be remotely activated when contact with the chemical is initiated at a distant site. The confounding factors of delay and recall pose a unique challenge in the diagnosis of ACD. For example, one might not suspect the sensitizing role of the hair dye paraphenylenediamine when a patient develops a subsequent reaction to an ester-based topical anesthetic (both are para-aminobenzoic acid derivatives)[4] (Fig. 18-2).

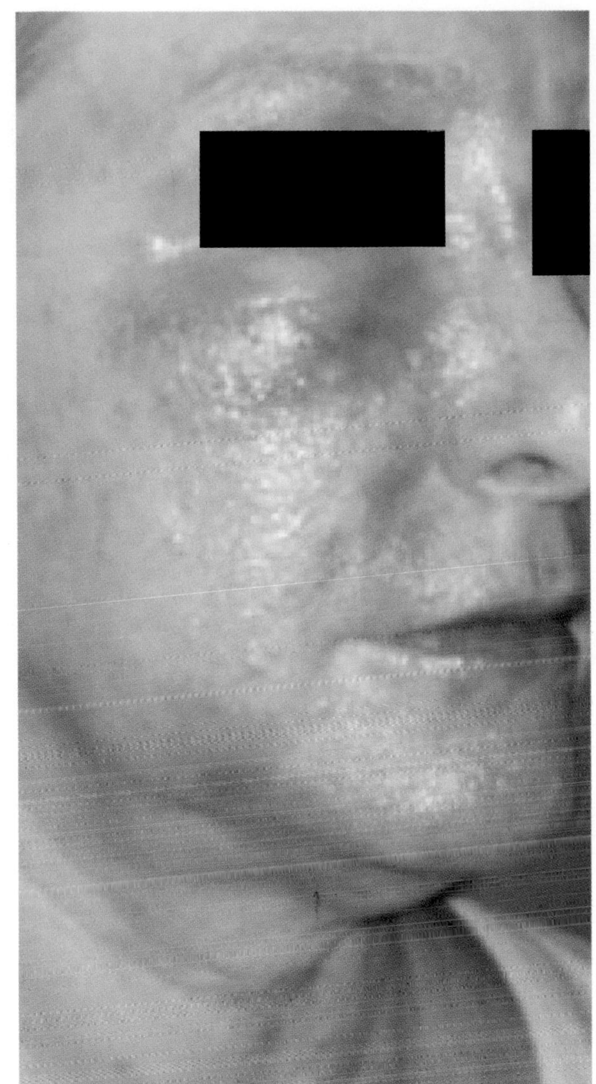

▲ **FIGURE 18-2** Sensitivity to hair dye.

CLINICAL PICTURE OF ALLERGIC CONTACT DERMATITIS

While in ACD the primary clinical dermatitis usually occurs in the distribution of the contact with the instigating allergen, there are inherent differences in the area of the involved epidermis, the potency of the allergen, and the duration of the dermatitis that may alter the presentation.[4] Classic localizations for cosmetic contact allergy are the face, neck, hands, and axillae relating to the use of fragrance-based products in these areas[5] (Fig. 18-3). Flavorings such as peppermint or cinnamon can lead to skin reactions as well and often present as a dermatitis around the mouth known as perioral dermatitis (Fig. 18-4). In some cases, "consort" or "connubial" contact dermatitis occurs when the contact dermatitis is caused by contact with products used by partners or coworkers.

ACD can be classified into three main categories: subacute, acute, and chronic subtypes.[6] In subacute presentations, clinically the skin exhibits macular erythema and scaling. The acute presentation typically displays pruritic erythematous, edematous, and papulovesicular changes in the skin. When the dermatitis is chronic, however, the clinical presentation involves lichenification and fissuring and may not be distinguishable from other chronic dermatoses.

COSMETIC IMPLICATIONS OF CONTACT DERMATITIS

Cosmetic procedure outcomes may be compromised by an ensuing irritant or allergic-based contact dermatitis. Furthermore, failure to effectively detect and avoid subsequent exposures to the allergen may result in unmitigating dermatitis, which may have a seemingly poor correlation with the current personal regimen of the patient. For example, a patient exquisitely sensitized to fragrances containing balsam of Peru,

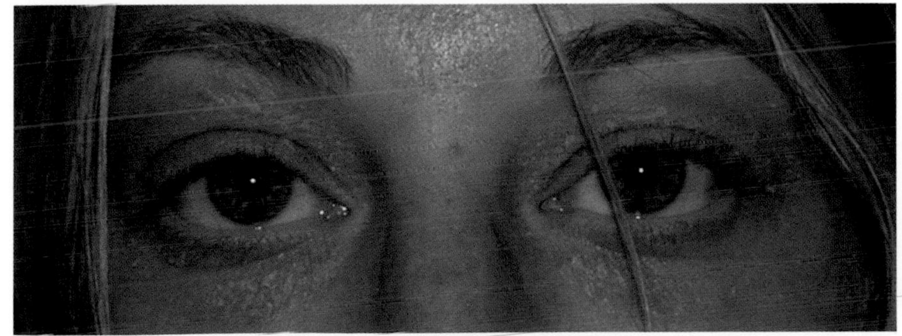

▲ **FIGURE 18-3** Contact dermatitis to fragrance presenting on eyelids.

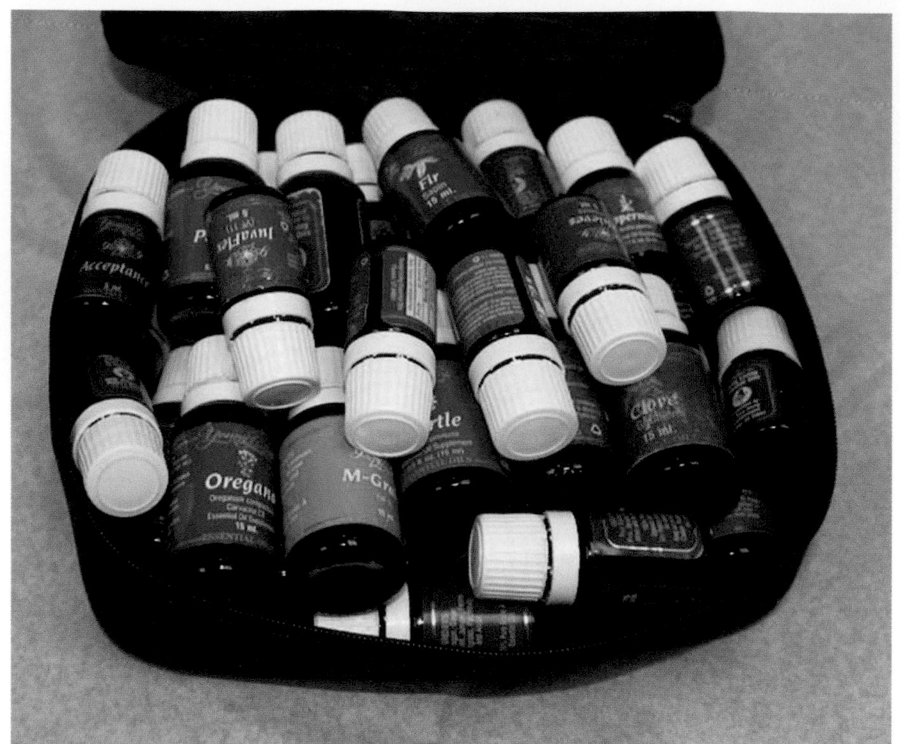

▲ **FIGURE 18-4** Contact dermatitis to flavorings such as peppermint and cinnamon can lead to perioral dermatitis, which is a variant of contact dermatitis. In this figure, the patient's dermatitis was caused by peppermint flavoring in her toothpaste.

such as cinnamic alcohol and aldehyde, may no longer be able to tolerate the fragrance-preservative chemical benzyl alcohol because of cross-reactivity. The "fragrance"-allergic patient may then, in an attempt to avoid fragrances, turn to "fragrance-free" products, which notably may contain the fragrance benzyl alcohol. Indeed, fragrance-based chemicals may be added to products labeled as "fragrance-free" if they are included for an indication other than as a fragrance. Benzyl alcohol has a preservative function as well as a fragrance function and can therefore be found in "fragrance-free" products. In this example, the patient using a benzyl alcohol-containing "fragrance-free" product could end up with recall-type reactions in the distributions of other fragrance sensitivity responses. This may occur in addition to or without a subsequent dermatitis in the area of the new "fragrance-free" product. Obviously, a diagnosis in this case would be difficult to achieve.

As with any ACD, factors to consider in attempting to correlate exposure with reactions and control future outbreaks are (1) the number and duration of exposures to the same chemical (even if it is in a different product composition); (2) status of the skin barrier; (3) occlusion; and (4) the amount (dose) per unit area of skin exposed.[2]

DIAGNOSTIC EVALUATIONS

The epicutaneous patch test is the *gold standard* testing tool in the diagnosis of ACD. There are two commercially available patch test *screening* tools in the United States with Food and Drug Administration (FDA) indications: the Hermal/Trolab 20 allergen standard test and the 24-chamber Thin-layer Rapid Use Epicutaneous (T.R.U.E.) test.[7,8] Beyond these standard assessment tools, comprehensive testing may be performed by tailoring the selection of various fragrances, cosmetics, vehicles, and preservatives for the patient based on the history and clinical distribution of the dermatitis.

In comprehensive testing, suspect chemical substances are, per standard procedure, hand-loaded in chambers and placed in contact with the clinically unaffected epidermis of the back and inner arm for 48 hours (Figs. 18-5 and 18-6). These patches are then removed, marked, and evaluated after the initial 48-hour application period. The patch sites are assessed at both 48 hours and at a delayed reading between 72 and 120 hours postapplication. ACD-type reactions typically will be evolving and worsening at the delayed reading. Reactions are graded per the North American Contact Dermatitis protocol from 0 to 3+ and irritant.

It should be noted that irritant-based reactions may also be seen at the 48-hour reading. However, unlike the ACD-type reactions, these tend to be resolving at the delayed reading. The sodium lauryl sulfate (SLS) test may be a useful adjuvant patch test, especially in the sensitive skin patient, as it may facilitate the differentiation between allergic and irritant reactions.[9] A reaction in the SLS application patch during patch testing indicates that macular erythema in the patch test sample on that patient more likely reflects an irritant etiology. Conversely, if the SLS test fails to demonstrate a reaction upon patch testing, it is more likely that macular erythematous reactions may be allergic in nature. While the SLS testing may be useful, it is important to note that clinical correlation of the presentation and exposure history are crucial for the correct diagnosis of allergic versus irritant contact dermatitis.

TOP SENSITIZERS IN COSMETIC PRODUCTS

A full discussion of the wide range of sensitizing chemicals found in cosmetic-based products is beyond the scope of this chapter, but a list of the most common allergens is found in Table 18-1. Two categories deserve special attention, however, with regard to cosmetic-based contact allergies, most notably fragrances and preservatives.

Fragrances (Table 18-2.)

Since the first report of allergy to fragrance-based chemicals in 1957, fragrances have continued to remain on the top 10 allergen list for contact sensitization.[10] In fact, fragrances are the second most common allergen family identified to cause ACD, and notably **the most frequent cause of contact allergy to cosmetics**. Specifically, cosmetics account for 30% to 45% of these allergic contact reactions, while perfumes and deodorants/antiperspirants account for 4% to 18% and 5% to 17% of cases, respectively.[5] In addition, most likely due to exposure habits, fragrance allergy tends to occur more frequently in women, with a female to male ratio of 3.5:1.[11,12]

Detection of fragrance allergy may be quite complex as, for example, an average of 30 to 50 (and upward of 200) chemicals may be used to create a perfume's fragrance composition![13] Furthermore, there are more than 5000 different synthetic fragrance compounds

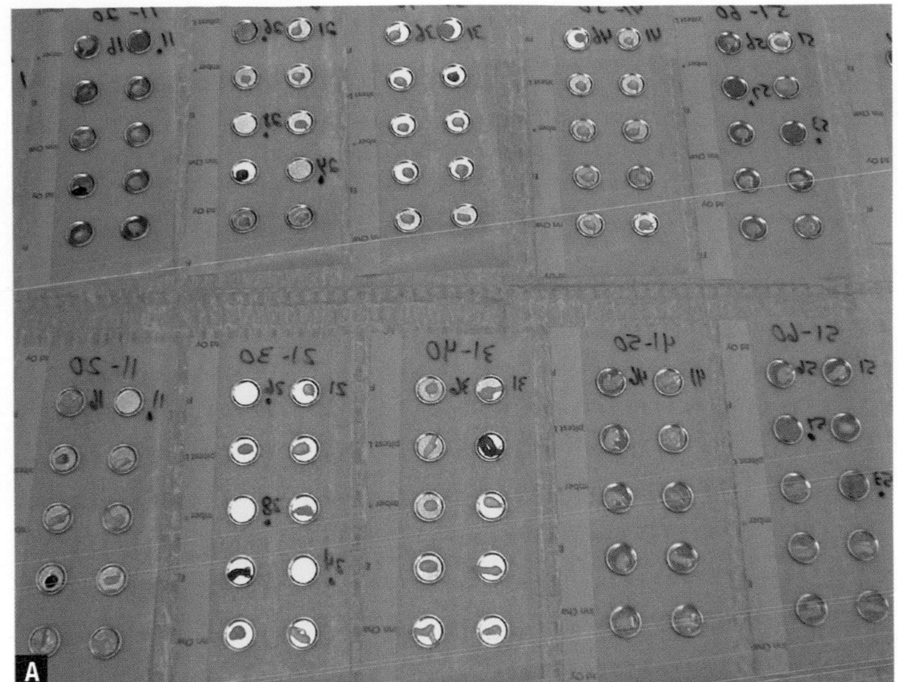

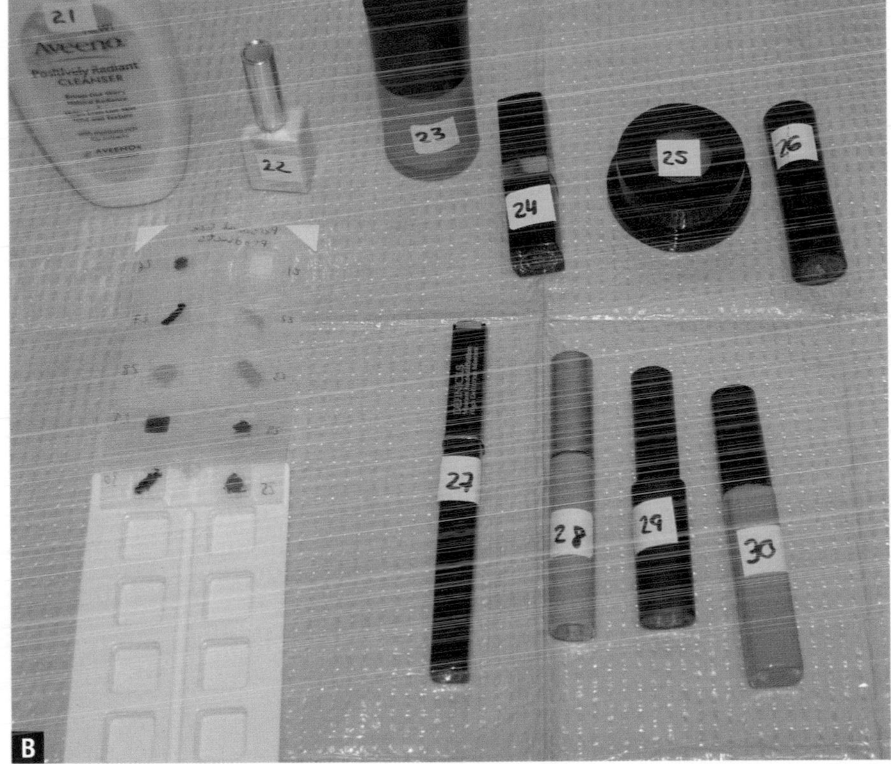

▲ **FIGURE 18-5** Comprehensive chamber preparation. **A.** The standard tray and some cosmetic vehicles. **B.** Preparation of personal products into chambers.

reportedly used in the global fragrance and flavor market (see Chapter 36). This estimated US$12 to 15 billion per year industry provides such chemicals for a wide variety of products from eau de toilettes/colognes and cosmetics to cleaning supplies and medicaments to foods and flavored personal hygiene products.[5,12]

Increasing rates of sensitization, however, have prompted calls for fragrance identification measures to be established. In 1977, Larsen proposed a mixture of eight ingredients (isoeugenol, eugenol, cinnamic aldehyde, cinnamic alcohol [also called cassia oil], geraniol [base substance of the essential oils: geranium, rose, jasmine, lavender, jasmine, citronella], oak moss absolute [tree lichen], hydroxycitronellal [synthetic], and α-amyl cinnamic aldehyde [synthetic]) as a screening tool for fragrance contact allergy.[3,14] This tool, Fragrance Mix 1, is now used in both the commercially available FDA-approved Thin-layer Rapid Use Epicutaneous (T.R.U.E.) screening panel and in comprehensive testing to screen for fragrance allergy and in conjunction with balsam of Peru. Notably, these two components are thought to detect approximately 90% of fragrance allergies.[15]

With regard to the chemicals that comprise the remaining 10%, several fragrance allergens (either essential oils or synthetics) account for the majority of reactions. This underscores the need for awareness of "natural"- or "herbal"-based chemicals as potential sources of ACD. Table 18-2 provides a compilation of estimated sensitization rates from several sources. Of note, patients may be allergic to more than one, and several cross-react.

It is also important to note that the top four sensitizers of the eight ingredients in the Fragrance Mix 1 are also natural cross-sensitizers/components of balsam of Peru.[3] Balsam of Peru is a dark brown, complex viscid fluid harvested from the mature *Myroxylon balsamum* tree primarily found in El Salvador, which was a Peruvian colony when the compound was discovered. The balsam contains the volatile oil cinnamein, a combination of cinnamic acid, benzoyl cinnamate, benzoyl benzoate, benzoic acid, vanillin, and nerodilol, all of which have wide utility in the pharmaceutical, cosmetic, and flavoring industries.[16] In 2005, cinnamic alcohol was found to naturally occur in both tomatoes and balsam of Peru, providing proof to support the common claim that tomatoes were a trigger in patients with a known allergy to balsam of Peru.[17] Because it confers mild bactericidal and capillary-bed stimulant effects, balsam of Peru is widely used in topical medicines for wounds, burns, hemorrhoids, and diaper salves. Furthermore, balsam of Peru components, such as benzyl alcohol, are used widely in cosmetics (i.e., BOTOX™-reconstituted) for its mild anesthetic and preservative properties.

Medical providers should be cognizant of the use of these covert fragrance chemicals. The FDA code of federal regulations, title 21, volume 7, section 700.3 (d), states that the term "fragrance" applies to any natural or synthetic substance or substances used solely to impart an odor to a cosmetic

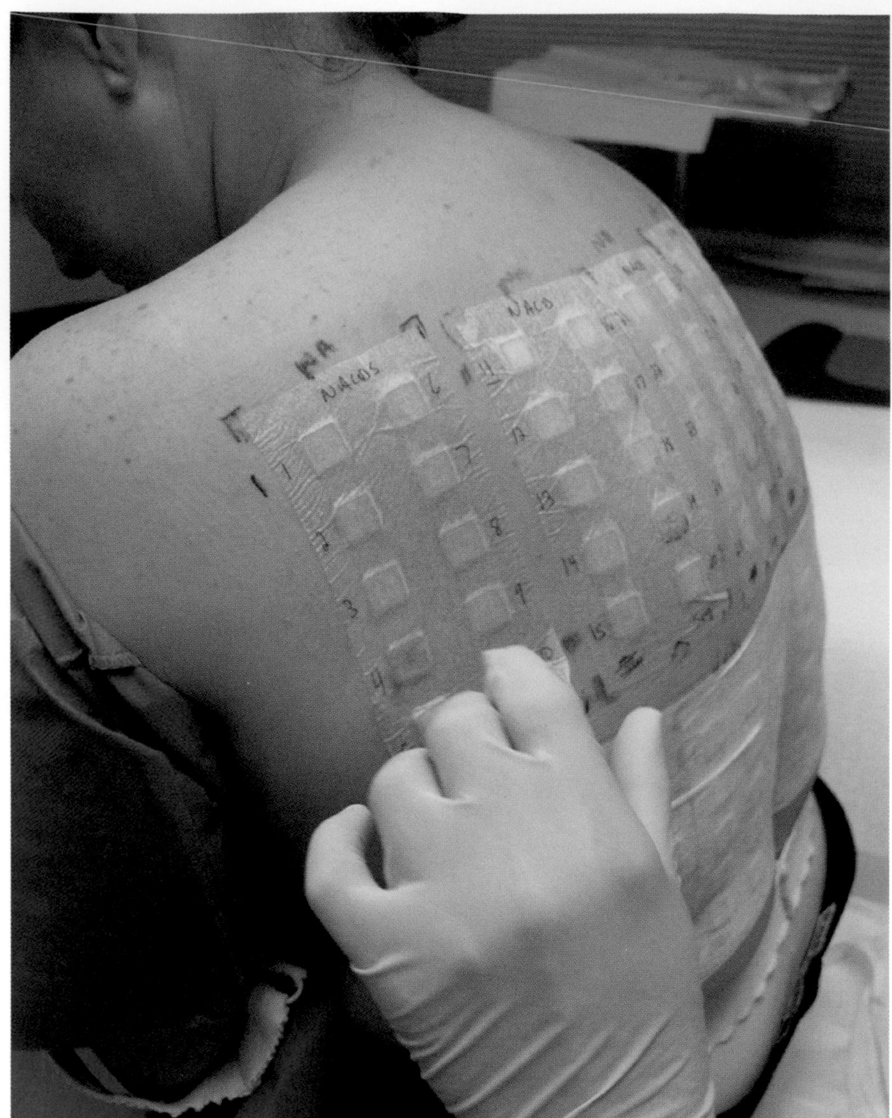

▲ **FIGURE 18-6** Application of the patch to the patient.

product.[18] By this definition, a product can be labeled as "fragrance-free" if fragrance-based ingredients are added to serve a purpose other than affecting the odor of a product, such as for preservation.[19]

Consumers and providers alike should also be aware that "fragrance-free" is not synonymous with "unscented." In general, "fragrance-free" refers to the absence of aroma-enhancing chemicals, whereas unscented may mean that a fragrance-masking chemical has been added.

Preservatives (Tables 18-3 and 18-4.)

FORMALDEHYDE AND FORMALDEHYDE-RELEASING PRESERVATIVES Formaldehyde and formaldehyde-releasing preservatives are second only to fragrances as the most common sources of cosmetic-associated contact dermatitis.[20] In order to decrease sensitization rates and ultimately lower the concentration of formaldehyde in products, it is common for manufacturers to use formaldehyde-releasing-preservatives (FRPs) instead of formaldehyde. Examples of FRPs are listed in Table 18-4. It is important to note, however, that the FRPs are the most sensitizing of the preservative class. Cases of contact dermatitis to formaldehyde/FRPs commonly present as eyelid dermatitis, which is often associated with the use of nail hardeners/lacquers/cosmetics that contain formaldehydes. Several mascaras, blushes, eye shadows, foundations, and shampoos also contain the FRPs that can contribute to the development of eyelid and facial dermatitis in the areas of sensitization. Other important potential sources of exposure to formaldehyde and FRPs include permanent press clothing, cleaning agents, baby wipes, disinfectants, cigarette smoke, and the sweetener aspartame.[21] It is worth noting that formaldehyde is sometimes included in products touted as "natural."

METHYLDIBROMO GLUTARONITRILE AND PHENOXYETHANOL (EUXYL K400) Methyldibromo glutaronitrile (MDGN), first introduced in the cosmeceutical industry in 1985, is a preservative used in a wide variety of toiletry and industrial products. Of note, contact allergy to this chemical is markedly on the rise, with this preservative ranking second only to FRPs (Table 18-3). Initially, the maximum allowable concentration was 0.1% in both leave-on and rinse-off cosmetic products, with one exception—sunscreens, for which the maximum allowable concentration was 0.025%.[22] However, by compounding the MDGN with phenoxylethanol in a ratio of 1:4 (Euxyl K400, Schulke & Mayr Inc., Hamburg, Germany), the manufacturer was able to make a highly effective and stable preservative at even lower concentrations (0.05%–0.02% depending on the product).[3] A higher concentration would be more likely to cause sensitization.

Contact sensitization to Euxyl K400 does occur, however, and is usually due to the MDGN component. Allergy to MDGN has been reported in association with the use of makeup removal wipes, moistened toilet tissue, cucumber eye gel, barrier creams, ultrasonic gel, and makeups.[23,24] High sensitization rates led the European Commission for Cosmetic Products to recommend a ban on the use of MDGN in leave-on products in 2003 and, likewise, in 2005 recommend that MDGN be banned from rinse-off products.[25,26] Products containing these preservatives are still used in the United States and the provider and consumer should be aware of the potential for sensitization.

METHYLCHLOROISOTHIAZOLINONE AND METHYLISOTHIAZOLINONE (EUXYL K100) In 1977, methylchloroisothiazolinone (MCI, 5-chloro-2-methyl-4-isothiazolin-3-one) and methylisothiazolinone (MI, 2-methyl-4-isothiazolin-3-one) were first registered in the United States as Kathon CG and Euxyl K100.[27] These two chemical preservatives are combined in a ratio of 3:1 (MCI:MI) and have been extensively added to bubble bath preparations, cosmetics, and soaps.[28,29] Because of their chemical nature of having polarity (being lipophilic at one end and lipophobic at the other), MCI and MI are compatible with a large number of surfactants and emulsifiers. Furthermore, the isothiazolinones are biocidal, as they interact and oxidize accessible cellular thiols on microbials.[30]

In a multicenter study including 15 different countries, MCI was identified as the culprit contact allergen in 2.9%

TABLE 18-1
Cosmetic Implications of Top Allergens 2001–2002[54]

Order	Substance	Positive Reactions (%)	Potential Cosmetic Implications
1	Nickel sulfate (2.5%)	16.7	Metal: eyelash curlers, razors, tweezers, mineral makeup
2	Neomycin (20%)	11.6	Antibiotic
3	Balsam of Peru (25%)	11.6	Fragrance & Flavorant—perfume, cosmetics, lotions, makeup removers
4	Fragrance mix (8%) (α-amyl cinnamic aldehyde, cinnamic alcohol, cinnamic aldehyde, eugenol, geraniol, hydroxycitronellal, isoeugenol, oak moss absolute)	10.4	Fragrance & Flavorant
5	Thimerosal (0.1%)	10.2	Preservative—mascara
6	Sodium gold thiosulfate (0.5%)	10.2	Metal: Secondary effect, titanium dioxide and zinc oxide abrade gold jewelry during make up application, resulting in gold particle transfer to face
7	Quaternium-15 (2%)	9.3	Preservative—mascara, foundation, eye shadow, blush, cleansers
8	Formaldehyde (1% aqs)	8.4	Preservative—cleansers, cosmetics
9	Bacitracin (20%)	7.9	Antibiotic—Obagi Nuderm step 7
10	Cobalt chloride (1%)	7.4	Metal—eyelash curlers, razors, tweezers, mineral make up

(Finland), 3.6% (United States), 5.7% (Germany), and 8.4% (Italy) of the cases.[31] The rinse off products (i.e., shampoos and soaps) were less likely to provoke dermatitis when compared to leave-on formulations (i.e., moisturizers and cosmetics). Of note, there may be a potential for MCI or MI to cross-react with metronidazole, as the chemicals have similar molecular structures.[32] Thus, the provider may need to be aware of this when prescribing formulations for rosacea, such as Noritate and Metrogel in an MCI- or MI-allergic patient.

Parabens

The **para**-hydroxy**ben**zoic acids (parabens) are a family of five alkyl esters that differ in para-position chemical composition substitutions on the benzene ring (methyl paraben, ethyl paraben, propyl paraben, butyl paraben, and benzyl paraben). These chemical substitutions impart on each paraben ester a different solubility and antimicrobial activity spectrum. Frequently, manufacturers take advantage of this and use the parabens in conjunction with each other to enhance antimicrobial efficacy.[33] In the United States, the average total paraben exposure per individual is estimated to be approximately 76 mg/d (1.3 mg/kg/d for a person weighing 70 kg) with the majority (50 mg/d) derived from cosmetics and personal hygiene product exposure. Notably, food preparations (e.g., mayonnaise, jams, salad dressings, etc.) are thought to account only for approximately 1 mg/d.[33]

The parabens, when absorbed through the skin, are partially metabolized by carboxyl esterases in the skin, liver, and kidney.[34] Recently, it has been demonstrated that a portion of parabens may be retained in human body tissues without hydrolysis by tissue esterases, which has raised concern over the potential for adverse side effects.[35] Special regard has been given to the estrogen-like effects, which were first described by Routledge et al. in 1998 and have been further substantiated by several studies.[36–39]

Since estrogen is a major etiologic factor in the development of human breast tissue and breast cancers, Darbre et al. proposed that parabens and other chemicals that are used in underarm cosmetics may have contributed to what was then, in 2003, the increasing incidence of breast cancer.[40] In an uncontrolled study of 20 patients with breast tumors, parabens were found in 90% of the

TABLE 18-2
Fragrance-Based Allergens[3,54–57]

Allergen Mix	Allergen	Estimated Sensitization Rates
Balsam of Peru[a,d]		11.6%[54]
Fragrance Mix 1[b,d]		11.4%[55]–10.4%[54]
Fragrance Mix 2[c,d]		
	Cinnamic alcohol[a,b]	7.6%[3]
	Eugenol[a,b]	5.4%[3]
	Cinnamic aldehyde[a,b]	4.9%[3]
	Isoeugenol[a,b]	3.1%[3]
	Geraniol[b]	2.8%[3]
	Lyral[c]	2.7%[57]–0.4%[56]
	Ylang-ylang	2.6%[55]
	Hydroxycitronellal[b]	2.1%[3]
	Oak moss absolute[b]	1.8%[3]
	Benzyl Alcohol[a,d]	1.3%[3]
	Narcissus	1.3%[55]
	Jasmine[d]	1.2%[55]–0.4%[56]
	Citral[c]	1.1%[57]
	Sandalwood	0.9%[55]
	Farnesol[c]	0.5%[57]
	Citronellol[c]	0.4%[57]
	Tea tree[d]	0.3%[56]
	a-Hexyl-cinnamic aldehyde[c]	0.3%[57]
	Coumarin[c]	0.3%[57]
	α-amyl cinnamic aldehyde[b]	0.2%[3]

[a]Indicates component/cross-sensitization with balsam of Peru.
[b]Indicates component of Fragrance Mix 1.
[c]Indicates component of Fragrance Mix 2.
[d]Current inclusion on 2007 NACDG screening panel.

TABLE 18-3
Preservatives Found in Cosmetic Products with Estimated Sensitization Rates [3,53,54]

Preservative	Rate
Thimerosal (merthiolate)	10.2%
Quaternium 15 (Dowicil®) (FRP)	9.3%
Bronopol (Bronopol®) (FRP)	3.3%
DiadUrea (Germall 11®) (FRP)	3.2%
Imidurea (Germall 115) (FRP)	3.0%
DMDM Hydantoin (Glydant®) (FRP)	2.8%
Methyldibromo glutaronitrile and phenoxyethanol (Euxyl K 400)	2.7%
Methylchloroisothiazolinone and Methylisothiazolinone (Euxyl K100)	2.3%
Benzyl alcohol	1.3%
Parabens	0.6%
Iodopropynyl butyl carbamate	0.3%

breast tumor samples; however, it has been suggested that there may have been "contamination" of the glassware that the samples were processed in from the detergents used by the technicians.[37,41]

The close proximity of the axilla and the breast has further fueled queries as to the possibility of an association of parabens with breast cancer.[42] This led the Cosmetic Ingredient Review Board to reevaluate the safety of parabens in 2005.[43] The panel determined that the original conclusion on the safety of parabens in cosmetics withstood, and that parabens were shown to have much less estrogenic activity than the body's naturally-occurring estrogen.[44] Nevertheless, lack of information on the effects of long-term exposure to low levels of parabens and subsequent accumulation in the body tissues suggests the need for prospective longitudinal studies.[37]

With regard to topical adverse effects from cosmetic preparations, the parabens have caused both irritant and allergic type contact dermatitis.[45–48] For example, paraben allergy has been described in association with facial cosmetics, ultrasound gels, topical steroid creams, and food additives.[49–52] A recent meta-analysis by Krob et al. revealed that despite widespread use of this preservative class, the overall prevalence and relevance of paraben allergy was remarkably low (0.5%), when compared to other preservative chemicals.[53]

IODOPROPYNYL BUTYL CARBAMATE In 1996, iodopropynyl butyl carbamate (IPBC) was approved for use in the United States by the Cosmetic Ingredient Review at an allowable level of up to 0.1% in topical formulations.[3] Testing for this allergen began in Denmark in 1996 and in the United States in 1998, with current data suggesting that the sensitization potential is relatively low when compared to the other preservative allergens.[54] (See Chapter 37 for further discussion of preservatives.)

OTHER ALLERGENS IN SKIN, HAIR, AND NAIL CARE PRODUCTS (TABLES 18-5 TO 18-8) Skin reactions have been described with hair care products as well as hair processing and coloring chemicals. Toluene sulfonamide formaldehyde resin in nail polish is such a common cause of contact dermatitis that companies such as Sally Hansen and Revlon have developed "formaldehyde- and toluene-free" nail polish. In fact, in some countries such as Switzerland, "formaldehyde resins" are banned in nail care products. Sunscreen ingredients

TABLE 18-4
Preservatives That Can Cause Contact Dermatitis

- Benzoic acid
- Benzyl alcohol
- Euxyl K 400 (Methyldibromo glutaronitrile and phenoxyethanol)
- Formaldehyde
- Formaldehyde-releasing-preservatives (FRPs):
  - Quaternium 15
  - Imidazolidinyl urea (Germall)
  - Diazolidinyl urea (Germall II)
  - Bromonitropropane diol (Bronopol)
  - DMDM hydantoin
- Methylchloroisothiazolinone (MCI)
- P-tert-Butylphenol formaldehyde resin
- Parabens
- Propylene glycol
- Sodium benzoate
- Toluenesulphonamide Formaldehyde Resin (tosylamide)

TABLE 18-5
Other Sensitizers Found in Skin and Hair Care Products

- 2,6-Ditert-butyl-4-cresol (BHT)
- 2-tert-Butyl-4-methoxyphenol (BHA)
- 4-Chloro-3-cresol (PCMC)
- Benzyl alcohol
- Benzyl salicylate
- Cetyl alcohol
- Chloracetamide
- Chlorhexidine digluconate
- Isopropyl myristate
- Lanolin alcohol
- Propyl gallate
- Sorbic acid
- Sorbitan monooleate (Span 80)
- Sorbitan sesquioleate
- Stearyl alcohol
- tert-Butylhydroquinone
- Triclosan (Irgasan DP 300)
- Triethanolamine
- Benzoyl peroxide
- Cocamide DEA
- Cocamidopropyl Betaine
- Di-alpha-tocopherol acetate (vitamin E)
- Methyl methacrylate
- Potassium dichromate

TABLE 18-6
Botanicals That Can Cause Allergy in Skin and Hair Care Products

- Aloe vera
- Angelica
- Arnica
- Balsam of Peru (*Myroxylon pereirae*)
- Beeswax
- Bladderwrack
- Catnip
- Chamomile
- Colophony (rosin)
- Compositae Mix
- Coriander
- Cucumber
- Dog rose hips
- Echinacea
- Ginkgo
- Goldenseal
- Gotu kola (*Centella asiatica*)
- Green tea
- Hops
- Kelp
- Lavender
- Licorice
- Marigold
- Propolis (bee's glue)
- Rosemary
- Sage
- Sesquiterpene lactone
- St. John's wort
- Tea tree oil
- Witch hazel
- Ylang-ylang oil

TABLE 18-7
Products in Hair Coloring and Processing that Can Cause Skin Sensitization

- 2,5 Diaminotoluene sulfate
- 2-Nitro-P-phenylenediamine
- 3-Aminophenol
- 4-Aminophenol
- Ammonium persulfate
- Ammonium thioglycolate
- Glyceryl thioglycolate
- Hydrogen peroxide
- Hydroquinone
- Paraphenylenediamine (PPD)$^{+}$
- Resorcinol

TABLE 18-8
Sunscreen Ingredients that Can Cause Sensitization

Sunscreen Ingredients
2-Ethylhexyl-4-dimethylaminobenzoate (Eusolex 6007) (Padimate O) (Octyl Dimethyl paba)
2-Ethylhexyl-4-methoxycinnamate (Parsol MCX)
2-Hydroxy-4-methoxy-4-methylbenzophenone (Mexenone)
2-Hydroxy-4-methoxy-benzophenon-5-sulfonic acid (Sulisobenzone)
2-Hydroxy-4-methoxybenzophenone (Eusolex 4360)
3-(4-Methylbenzyliden)camphor (Eusolex 6300)
4-Aminobenzoic acid (PABA)
4-tert-Butyl-4'-methoxydibenzoylmethane (Parsol 1789) (Avobenzone)
Benzophenone-3 (oxybenzone)
Homomenthylsalicylate (Homosalate)
Isoamyl-p-methoxycinnamate
Octyl salicylate (Octisalate)
Phenylbenzimidazol-5-sulfonic acid (Eusolex 232)

have also been reported to cause skin allergy. In order to elucidate the cause of contact dermatitis in most patients, a thorough history is crucial. Having the patients bring in the offending skin care products, when known, is also necessary.

TREATMENT

The first step in the treatment of any contact dermatitis is to identify the offending agent, whether an allergen or a caustic irritating chemical. Once identification has been made, the subsequent step is avoidance of the culprit compound and, in the case of ACD, all cross-reactive substances. Alternative product substitution is imperative for the well-being of the patient. Furthermore, measures should be taken to ensure barrier integrity (i.e., decreased hand washing with soaps and increased emollient use) for both allergic- and irritant-based dermatoses. The use of emollients to help heal the skin is important, especially with regard to reactions that are irritant in nature (see Chapter 31).

In the interim, while the avoidance regimen is being instituted and the immune system is being given a chance to "forget" the sensitization, symptomatic treatment in ACD and CU may consist of topical corticosteroids or topical immunomodulators. At times, with severe acute or chronic extensive involvement, the use of systemic agents such as prednisone, cyclosporine, or ultraviolet light treatments may be indicated. The use of ICD corticosteroids is controversial, but seems to be advantageous if applied early.

REFERENCES

1. Rietschel RL. Clues to an accurate diagnosis of contact dermatitis. *Dermatol Ther.* 2004;7:224.
2. Jacob SE, Amado A, Cohen DE. Dermatologic surgical implications of allergic contact dermatitis. *Dermatol Surg.* 2005;31:1116.
3. Fisher's. In: Rietschel RL, Fowler JF Jr, eds. *Contact Dermatitis.* 5th ed. Philadelphia, PA: Lippincott Wiliams & Wilkins; 2001.
4. Camarasa JG, Lluch M, Serra-Baldrich E, et al. Allergic contact dermatitis from 3-(aminomethyl)-pyridyl salicylate. *Contact Dermatitis.* 1989;20:347.
5. de Groot AC, Frosch PJ. Adverse reactions to fragrances. A clinical review. *Contact Dermatitis.* 1997;36:57.
6. de Groot A. Allergic contact dermatitis. In: Marks R, ed. Eczema. London, UK: Martin Dunitz; 1992:104-125.
7. Mekos Laboratories Web site. http://www.mekos.dk/page.asp?sideid=2& zcs=27. Accessed November 8, 2005.
8. Fischer T, Maibach HI. The thin layer rapid use epicutaneous test (TRUE-test), a new patch test method with high accuracy. *Br J Dermatol.* 1985;113:63.
9. Uter W, Geier J, Becker D, et al. The MOAHLFA index of irritant sodium lauryl sulfate reactions: first results of a multicentre study on routine sodium lauryl sulfate patch testing. *Contact Dermatitis.* 2004;51:259.
10. Chatard H. Case of sensitization to perfumes with cutaneous and general reactions. *Bull Soc Fr Dermatol Syphiligr.* 1957;64:323.
11. Scheinman PL. Allergic contact dermatitis to fragrance: a review. *Am J Contact Dermat.* 1996;7:65.
12. Johansen JD. Fragrance contact allergy: a clinical review. *Am J Clin Dermatol.* 2003;4:789.
13. International Fragrance Association (IFRA) Web site. http://www.ifraorg.org. Accessed January 1, 2007.
14. Larsen WG. Perfume dermatitis. A study of 20 patients. *Arch Dermatol.* 1977;113:623.
15. Militello G, James W. Lyral: a fragrance allergen. *Dermatitis.* 2005;16:41.
16. Hjorth N. Eczematous allergy to balsams, allied perfumes and flavouring agents, with special reference to balsam of Peru. *Acta Derm Venereol Suppl (Stockh).* 1961;41:1.
17. Srivastava D, Chang YT, Kumar S, et al. Identification of the constituents of balsam of Peru in tomatoes. Poster presentations. *Dermatitis.* 2005;16:101.
18. Food and Drug Administration Department of Health and Human Services. Code of Federal Regulations. Food and Drugs. http://www.accessdata.fda.gov/scripts/cdrh/cfdocs/cfcfr/CFRSearch.cfm?CFRPart=700 &showFR=1. Accessed January 2, 2007.
19. Scheinman PL. The foul side of fragrance-free products: what every clinician should know about managing patients with fragrance allergy. *J Am Acad Dermatol.* 1999;41:1020.
20. Adams RM, Maibach HI. A five-year study of cosmetic reactions. *J Am Acad Dermatol.* 1985;13:1062.
21. Hill AM, Belsito DV. Systemic contact dermatitis of the eyelids caused by formaldehyde derived from aspartame? *Contact Dermatitis.* 2003;49:258.
22. Jensen CD, Johansen JD, Menne T, et al. MDGN in rinse-off products causes allergic contact dermatitis: an experimental study. *Br J Dermatol.* 2004;150:90.
23. De Groot AC, van Ginkel CJ, Weijland JW. Methyldibromoglutaronitrile (Euxyl K 400): an important "new" allergen in cosmetics. *J Am Acad Dermatol.* 1996;35:743.
24. Sánchez-Pérez J, Del Rio MJ, Jiménez YD, et al. Allergic contact dermatitis due to methyldibromo glutaronitrile in make-up removal wipes. *Contact Dermatitis.* 2005;53:357.
25. Schnuch A, Kelterer D, Bauer A, et al. Quantitative patch and repeated open application testing in methyldibromo glutaronitrile-sensitive patients. *Contact Dermatitis.* 2005;52:197.
26. Jong CT, Statham BN. Methyldibromoglutaronitrile contact allergy—the beginning of the end? *Contact Dermatitis.* 2006;54:229.
27. U.S. Environmental Protection Agency Web site. http://www.epa.gov/oppsrrd1/REDs/factsheets/3092fact.pdf. Accessed January 2, 2007.
28. Mowad CM. Methylchloro-isothiazolinone revisited. *Am J Contact Dermat.* 2000;11:115.
29. Isaksson M, Gruvberger B, Bruze M. Occupational contact allergy and dermatitis from methylisothiazolinone after contact with wallcovering glue and after a chemical burn from a biocide. *Dermatitis.* 2004;15:201.
30. Collier PJ, Ramsey A, Waigh RD, et al. Chemical reactivity of some isothiazolone biocides. *J Appl Bacteriol.* 1990;69:578.
31. Dermatitis linked to preservative in moisturizers (Kathon CG found to be cause of cosmetic allergy.) *Nutrition Health Review.* 9/22/1990.
32. Wolf R, Orion E, Matz H. Co-existing sensitivity to metronidazole and isothiazolinone. *Clin Exp Dermatol.* 2003; 28:506.
33. Cashman AL, Warshaw EM. Parabens: a review of epidemiology, structure, allergenicity, and hormonal properties. *Dermatitis.* 17(1). http://medscape.com/parabens. Accessed August 30, 2007.
34. Lee CH, Kim HJ. A study on the absorption mechanisms of drug through membranes. *Arch Pharm Res.* 1994;17:182.
35. Oishi S. Lack of spermatotoxic effects of methyl and ethyl esters of p-hydroxybenzoic acid in rats. *Food Chem Toxicol.* 2004;42:1845.
36. Endocrine disruption. http://envirocancer.cornell.edu/Bibliography/cENDOCRINE.cfm. Accessed September 3, 2006.
37. Routledge EJ, Parker J, Odum J, et al. Some alkyl hydroxyl benzoate preservatives (parabens) are estrogenic. *Toxicol Appl Pharmacol.* 1998;153:12.
38. Blair RM, Fang H, Branham WS, et al. The estrogen receptor relative binding affinities of 188 natural and xenochemi-

cals: structural diversity of ligands. *Toxicol Sci*. 2000;54:138.
39. Darbre PD, Byford JR, Shaw LE, et al. Oestrogenic activity of benzylparaben. *J Appl Toxicol*. 2003;23:43.
40. Darbre PD. Underarm cosmetics and breast cancer. *J Appl Toxicol*. 2003;23:89.
41. Darbre PD, Aljarrah A, Miller WR, et al. Concentrations of parabens in human breast tumours. *J Appl Toxicol*. 2004;24:5.
42. Darbre PD., Environmental oestrogens, cosmetics and breast cancer. *Best Pract Res Clin Endocrinol Metab*. 20;121:206.
43. CTFA Response Statement, April 17, 2003; RSPT 03–12. http://www.nuskin.com/corp/science/hottopics/parabens. Accessed September 3, 2006.
44. Parabens. http://www.cfsan.fda.gov/~dms/cos-para.html. Accessed August 13, 2006.
45. Menne T, Hjorth N. Routine patch testing with paraben esters. Contact Dermatitis. 1988;19:189.
46. Verhaeghe I, Dooms-Goossens A. Multiple sources of allergic contact dermatitis from parabens. *Contact Dermatitis*. 1997;36:269.
47. Scanberg IL. Allergic contact dermatitis to methyl and propyl paraben. *Arch Dermatol*. 1967;95:626.
48. Wiepper KD. Paraben contact dermatitis. *JAMA*. 1967;202:579.
49. Simpson JR. Dermatitis due to parabens in cosmetic creams. *Contact Dermatitis*. 1978;5:311.
50. Eguino P, Sánchez A, Agesta N, et al. Allergic contact dermatitis due to propylene glycol and parabens in an ultrasonic gel. *Contact Dermatitis*. 2003; 48:290.
51. Fisher AA. Allergic paraben and benzyl alcohol hypersensitivity relationship of the “delayed” and “immediate” varieties. *Contact Dermatitis*. 1975;1:281.
52. Fisher AA. Dermatitis of the hands from food additives. *Cutis*. 1982;30:21.
53. Krob HA, Fleischer AB Jr, D’Agostino R Jr, et al. Prevalence and relevance of contact dermatitis allergens: a meta-analysis of 15 years of published T.R.U.E. test data. *J Am Acad Dermatol*. 2004; 51:349.
54. Pratt MD, Belsito DV, DeLeo VA, et al. North American Contact Dermatitis Group patch-test results, 2001–2002 study period. *Dermatitis*. 2004;15:176.
55. Frosch PJ, Johansen JD, Menne T, et al. Further important sensitizers in patients sensitive to fragrances. *Contact Dermatitis*. 2002;47(5):279.
56. Belsito DV, Fowler JF Jr, Sasseville D, et al. Delayed-type hypersensitivity to fragrance materials in a select North American population. *Dermatitis*. 2006; 17:23.
57. Frosch PJ, Johansen JD, Menne T, et al. Further important sensitizers in patients sensitive to fragrances. *Contact Dermatitis*. 2002;47(2):78.

CHAPTER 19

Wrinkled Skin

Sogol Saghari, MD
Leslie Baumann, MD

The desire to maintain or restore a youthful appearance has become a significant concern for many people in today's world. Evidently, "wrinkles" are considered one of the major obstacles in this arena. In 2004, Botox Cosmetic™ injections were shown to be the most often performed cosmetic procedure in the United States.[1] Cutaneous wrinkles, defined as furrows or ridges on the skin surface, appear to be multifactorial in etiology and a consequence of intrinsic and extrinsic aging (discussed in Chapter 6). While genetic predisposition is an important factor in developing wrinkles, engaging in particular life style behaviors such as excessive sun exposure and smoking are also known causes of cutaneous aging (see Chapter 6). This chapter will concentrate on wrinkles not caused by sun exposure but, rather, by intrinsic aging. Treatment approaches focus more on the condition itself, but also address behavioral elements pertaining to extrinsic aging.

AGING

Aging is a process that occurs in all organs, but is most visible in the skin. The skin may very well reflect or act as an outward sign of processes occurring in the internal organs. In fact, the amount of facial wrinkling has been shown to correlate with the extent of lung disease in COPD.[2] The naturally-occurring functional decline of organs with age can be exacerbated by environmental factors, but there is certainly a genetic component that influences the aging process. Little is known at this point about the genetics of skin aging except for the genes that have been implicated in premature aging syndromes such as Werner's syndrome[3] (Table 19-1). Mammalian cells can undergo only a certain number of cell divisions before replicative senescence occurs and they are no longer able to divide.[6] This may be nature's way of preventing these cells from becoming cancerous; however, this process plays a role in aging as well.

TABLE 19-1
Premature Aging Syndromes[a]

SYNDROME	DEFECT
Werner's syndrome[3]	DNA helicase
Cockayne syndrome[4]	DNA helicase
Progeria[5]	Lamin A

[a]These premature aging syndromes suggest that DNA repair capacity is very important to mitigate aging.

Pathology and Etiology

The histopathology of wrinkles is a combination of interesting findings. Epidermal thinning is an outstanding microscopic feature, where the atrophy is more prominent in the deepest area of the wrinkle (Fig. 6-8). Other changes include flattening of the dermal-epidermal junction, atrophy of the subcutaneous adipose tissue of the hypodermis, as well as the loss of collagen, glycosaminoglycans, and elastin tissue.

COLLAGEN LOSS Abnormal and reduced collagen is a major finding in the pathology of wrinkles, both in sun-exposed and non-sun-exposed skin.[7] Collagen modification in wrinkled skin can be explained with a combination of different concepts. It is well known that collagen synthesis is decreased in aging skin. In addition, because of higher levels of matrix metalloproteinases (MMPs), collagen degradation also appears to increase with aging. Another explanation for abnormal dermal collagen in cutaneous aging is collagen glycation.[8] As discussed in Chapter 2, glycation of collagen is a nonenzymatic process that involves the addition of a reducing sugar molecule to extracellular matrix collagen and proteins. Following an oxidative reaction, the end products of glycated collagen and proteins, known as advanced glycation end products (AGEs), are formed. The AGEs are then deposited on the collagen and elastin tissue, rendering them stiffer and less susceptible to contracture and remodeling. In addition, glycated collagen modifies the actin cytoskeleton of fibroblasts and inhibits their contracture effect on the collagen.[9] AGEs can interact with certain receptors to induce intracellular signaling that leads to enhanced oxidative stress and elaboration of key proinflammatory cytokines. The resulting free radicals and cytokines lead to a breakdown of collagen.[10]

Decorin, a small leucine-rich proteoglycans (SLRPs) found in the extracelluar matrix protein, is involved in "decorating" the collagen (see Chapter 2). It is shaped in a "horseshoe" pattern and holds collagen fibers in the proper arrangement.[11] Interestingly, a fragment of decorin also known as "decorunt" has been shown to be higher in adult versus fetal skin.[12] Since decorunt has a lower affinity for collagen fibers, the breakdown of decorin to decorunt may play a role in the disorganization of the dermal collagen network seen in aged skin.

ELASTIN DEGRADATION Wrinkled skin is known to exhibit decreased resilience because of abnormal elastic tissue. In the setting of UV exposure, the quantity of elastase, the enzyme responsible for degrading elastin, increases and leads to "elastosis," a hallmark of photoaged skin. However, studies have demonstrated that nonexposed aged skin also displays less elastin tissue.[13,14]

TELOMERE SHORTENING Telomeres are the terminal portions of mammalian chromosomes that are composed of hundreds of short sequences of repeats of the base pairs TTAGGG. They cap the ends of chromosomes preventing fusion.[15] During cell division, when the chromosomes divide, the enzyme DNA polymerase cannot replicate the final base pairs of the chromosome. Therefore, these terminal sequences are continuously lost on replication, resulting in shortening of the chromosome. When telomeres get "too short," apoptosis of the cells is triggered. For this reason, telomeres are thought to play a role in aging. Telomerase is a reverse transcriptase enzyme found in stem cells that can replicate the terminal base pairs but this enzyme is not found in most cells. Many studies are ongoing that are looking at the role of telomerase in aging and cancer.

UV exposure may contribute to telomere shortening. Telomeres normally exist in a loop configuration, with the loop held in place by the final 150 to 200 bases on the 3 strand that forms a single-stranded overhang (Figs. 19-1A and B). It is believed that when the loop is disrupted and the overhang becomes exposed, p53 (a tumor suppressor protein) and other DNA damage response proteins are induced,[16] resulting in apoptosis or senescence. UV light leads to the

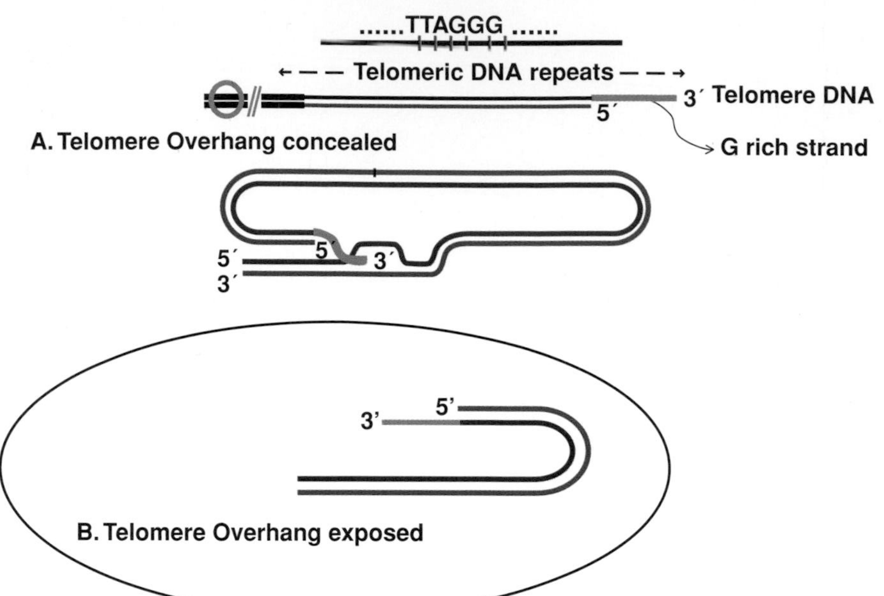

▲ **FIGURE 19-1** **A.** Telomeres in normal loop configuration. The 3-prime end is held in place by the last 150 to 200 base pairs on the 3-prime strand. **B.** Once damaged, the loop structure opens and the 3-prime end is exposed. (Adapted from page 965 Fitzpatrick's 7th edition.)

bonding together of thymine dimers, which may lead to disruption of the telomere loop (Fig. 19-2). This is one way to explain the overlap seen in intrinsic and extrinsic aging.

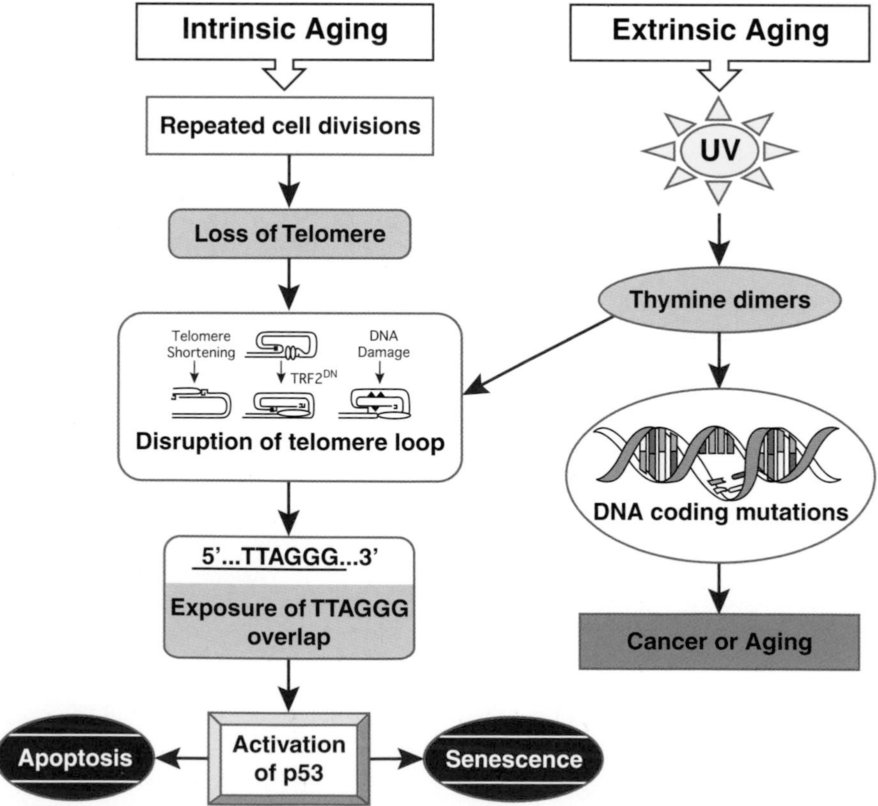

▲ **FIGURE 19-2** Extrinsic aging and intrinsic aging can both result in the same outcome—cellular apoptosis or senescence. This diagram shows the proposed mechanisms in which these two processes overlap to lead to aging. Repeated cell division, thymine dimers, and other causes of telomere damage lead to disruption of the telomere loop. This leads to exposure of the TTAGGG overlap and activation of p53. (*Yaar M, Gilchrest BA. Photoaging: mechanism, prevention and therapy. Br J Derm. 2007;157:877.*)

Immune System

Aging is associated with an increase in proinflammatory cytokines (see Chapter 4). These cytokines result in inflammation, which plays a role in degrading collagen and elastin as well as other vital skin components. The role of cytokines in aging has not been completely elucidated, but this will likely be an area of extreme interest in upcoming research. The function of antigen-presenting cells, T cells, and B cells declines with age. These changes are thought to contribute to the higher risk of infections and cancer observed in older patients.[17]

Other Factors

The endocrine system may contribute to aging. It is likely that insulin, vitamin D, and thyroid hormone levels influence skin aging in ways that have not yet been elucidated. Hormones, especially estrogen and androgens, are significant factors in the aging of skin (see Chapter 5).

PREVENTION AND TREATMENT

Identifying skin types predisposed to wrinkling is the first step in patient management. The Baumann Skin Typing System (Chapter 9) is a useful classification approach, aiding physicians and patients to understand and manage their skin needs to prevent and treat wrinkles. Other classification systems, such as those by Lemprele and Glogau (see Chapter 40), also help physicians quantify the amount of wrinkling. After assessing the degree of wrinkling, patient education is the next essential step. Patients must understand that prevention of additional wrinkling is the mainstay of managing wrinkled skin. Effects of certain behaviors such as excessive sun exposure and smoking should be discussed, and treatment plans with expected and realistic results should be explained in detail with patients. It is well known that sunscreen and sun avoidance are key elements in preventing extrinsic photoaging. Although UVA is more often implicated in cutaneous aging, coverage for both UVA and UVB is recommended when selecting a sunscreen. A routine skin regimen containing retinoid application is also valuable in both the prevention and treatment of aging skin. Topical retinoids have been shown to both increase collagen synthesis[18] and decrease the MMPs involved in collagen and elastin degradation.[19] Since oxidative stress resulting from UV irradiation and free radicals are implicated in skin aging, antioxidants have an important role in the prevention and treatment of wrinkles (see Chapter 34). Of antioxidants, vitamin C (ascorbic acid) deserves special attention. Vitamin C is well recognized for its role in the collagen synthesis pathway via the prolyl hydroxylase enzyme. Studies have revealed a reduction of wrinkles following topical application of ascorbic acid,[20–22] correlating with increased collagen on histology of the treated areas.[21] Other antioxidants such as coenzyme Q10 (ubiquinone), green tea, and vitamin E are also believed to be of value in the prevention and treatment of aging.

Recently, photorejuvenation has become a popular approach to wrinkle reduction. Procedures with intensed pulsed light (IPL) and light emitting diodes (LEDs) have also shown promising results in the treatment of wrinkled skin and photoaging[23–26] (see Chapter 24).

SUMMARY

Much remains to be learned regarding the science or biomechanics of aging. However, the field is rapidly progressing with increased knowledge about the roles of genetics, stem cells, telomeres, the immune system, and hormones. Advances in these theoretical realms and in the laboratory will certainly lead to novel therapies in the future. Specific preventive measures and treatment modalities are well recognized and discussed at length in various chapters of this book, including the roles of diet and cigarette smoking. Sunscreen and topical retinoids are the basic treatment options, proven to be valuable in treating wrinkled skin. New data show that retinoids improve skin texture in intrinsically aged skin as well as photodamaged skin.[27] Patient education and compliance, which are crucial in this matter, may be achieved by providing thorough information, including illustrations of the benefits of treatments and behavioral changes and the disadvantages of noncompliance.

REFERENCES

1. PR Newswire. 11.9 Million Cosmetic Procedures in 2004; American Society for Aesthetic Plastic Surgery Reports 44 Percent Increase. Publication date: 17 February, 2005. http://goliath.ecnext.com/coms2/summary_0199-3691791_ITM. Accessed February 24, 2008.
2. Patel BD, Loo WJ, Tasker AD, et al. Smoking related COPD and facial wrinkling: is there a common susceptibility? *Thorax*. 2006;61:568.
3. Yu CE, Oshima J, Fu YH, et al. Positional cloning of the Werner's syndrome gene. *Science*. 1996;272:258.
4. Troelstra C, van Gool A, de Wit J, et al. ERCC6, a member of a subfamily of putative helicases, is involved in Cockayne's syndrome and preferential repair of active genes. *Cell*. 1992;71:939.
5. De Sandre-Giovannoli A, Bernard R, Cau P, et al. Lamin a truncation in Hutchinson-Gilford progeria. *Science*. 2003;300:2055.
6. Campisi J. Replicative senescence: an old live's tale? *Cell*. 1996;84;497.
7. Varani J, Fisher GJ, Kang S, et al. Molecular mechanisms of intrinsic skin aging and retinoid-induced repair and reversal. *J Investig Dermatol Symp Proc*. 1998;3:57.
8. Dyer DG, Dunn JA, Thorpe SR, et al. Accumulation of Maillard reaction products in skin collagen in diabetes and aging. *J Clin Invest*. 1993;91:2463.
9. Howard EW, Benton R, Ahern-Moore J, et al. Cellular contraction of collagen lattices is inhibited by nonenzymatic glycation. *Exp Cell Res*. 1996;228:132.
10. Goh SY, Cooper ME. REVIEW: the role of advanced glycation end products in progression and complications of diabetes. *J Clin Endocrinol Metab*. 2008 Jan 8 [Epub ahead of print].
11. Scott JE. Proteodermatan and proteokeratan sulfate (decorin, lumican/fibromodulin) proteins are horseshoe shaped. Implications for their interactions with collagen. *Biochemistry*. 1996;35:8795.
12. Carrino DA, Onnerfjord P, Sandy JD, et al. Age-related changes in the proteoglycans of human skin. Specific cleavage of decorin to yield a major catabolic fragment in adult skin. *J Biol Chem*. 2003;278:17566.
13. El-Domyati M, Attia S, Saleh F, et al. Intrinsic aging vs. photoaging: a comparative histopathological, immunohistochemical, and ultrastructural study of skin. *Exp Dermatol*. 2002;11:398.
14. Seite S, Zucchi H, Septier D, et al. Elastin changes during chronological and photo-ageing: the important role of lysozyme. *J Eur Acad Dermatol Venereol*. 2006;20:980.
15. Blackburn EH. Switching and signaling at the telomere. *Cell*. 2001;106:661.
16. Eller MS, Puri N, Hadshiew IM, et al. Induction of apoptosis by telomere 3' overhang-specific DNA. *Exp Cell Res*. 2002;276:185.
17. Yaar M, Gilchrest BA. Aging of skin. In: Wolff K, Goldsmith LA, Katz SI, Gilchrest BA, Paller AS, Leffell DJ, eds. *Fitzpatrick's Dermatology in General Medicine*. 7th ed. New York, NY: McGraw-Hill; 2007:963.
18. Woodley DT, Zelickson AS, Briggaman RA, et al. Treatment of photoaged skin with topical tretinoin increases epidermal-dermal anchoring fibrils. A preliminary report. *JAMA*. 1990;263:3057.
19. Fisher GJ, Datta SC, Talwar HS, et al. Molecular basis of sun-induced premature skin ageing and retinoid antagonism. *Nature*. 1996;379:335.
20. Humbert PG, Haftek M, Creidi P, et al. Topical ascorbic acid on photoaged skin. Clinical, topographical and ultrastructural evaluation: double-blind study vs. placebo. *Exp Dermatol*. 2003;12:237.
21. Fitzpatrick RE, Rostan EF. Double-blind, half-face study comparing topical vitamin C and vehicle for rejuvenation of photodamage. *Dermatol Surg*. 2002;28:231.
22. Traikovich SS. Use of topical ascorbic acid and its effects on photodamaged skin topography. *Arch Otolaryngol Head Neck Surg*. 1999;125:1091.
23. Sadick NS, Weiss R, Kilmer S, et al. Photorejuvenation with intense pulsed light: results of a multi-center study. *J Drugs Dermatol*. 2004;3:41.
24. Brazil J, Owens P. Long-term clinical results of IPL photorejuvenation. *J Cosmet Laser Ther*. 2003;5:168.
25. Trelles MA, Allones I, Velez M. Non-ablative facial skin photorejuvenation with an intense pulsed light system and adjunctive epidermal care. *Lasers Med Sci*. 2003;18:104.
26. Trelles MA. Phototherapy in anti-aging and its photobiologic basics: a new approach to skin rejuvenation. *J Cosmet Dermatol*. 2006;5:87.
27. Kafi R, Kwak HS, Schumacher WE, et al. Improvement of naturally aged skin with vitamin A (retinol). *Arch Dermatol*. 2007;143:606.

CHAPTER 20

Chemical Peels

Leslie Baumann, MD
Sogol Saghari, MD

The use of chemical peels to treat the aging face is well established and poses minimal risk when performed by educated practitioners. In addition to improving the texture of the skin and reducing hyperpigmentation and mild wrinkling, peels are also useful in the treatment of acne, rosacea, and melasma. In 1999, chemical peels were so popular that they were found to be the most common cosmetic procedure performed in the United States.[1] In 2006, chemical peels were second only to Botox among the top five minimally invasive cosmetic procedures performed by board-certified members of the American Society of Plastic Surgeons, with 1.1 million procedures performed.[2] The introduction of lasers in skin rejuvenation may have some impact on the frequency of chemical peel treatments. Although the claims of what chemical peels can do have been frequently overstated, there is actually an abundance of research on the utility of these products, which are used in physicians' offices and salons worldwide.

Chemical peels are categorized based on the depth of the procedure: superficial, medium or deep. Superficial peels induce necrosis of all or parts of the epidermis, from the stratum granulosum to the basal cell layer (Figs. 20-1 and 20-2). Medium-depth peels create necrosis of the epidermis and part or all of the papillary dermis in the treatment area. The necrosis extends into the reticular dermis following deep peels.[3] Currently, superficial peels are the most frequently performed peels, as intense pulsed light, laser resurfacing and dermabrasion have essentially supplanted medium and deeper-depth peels. Superficial- and medium-depth peels do not significantly ameliorate deep wrinkles or sagging skin, but can improve the color and texture of the skin thereby yielding a more youthful appearance. This chapter will focus on and differentiate between the most frequently used in-office types of superficial and medium-depth peels, including mechanisms of action, side effects and results obtained with the various acids used in peels. Many of the ingredients in these peels are also found in home products; therefore, some skin care products will be mentioned in this chapter as well.

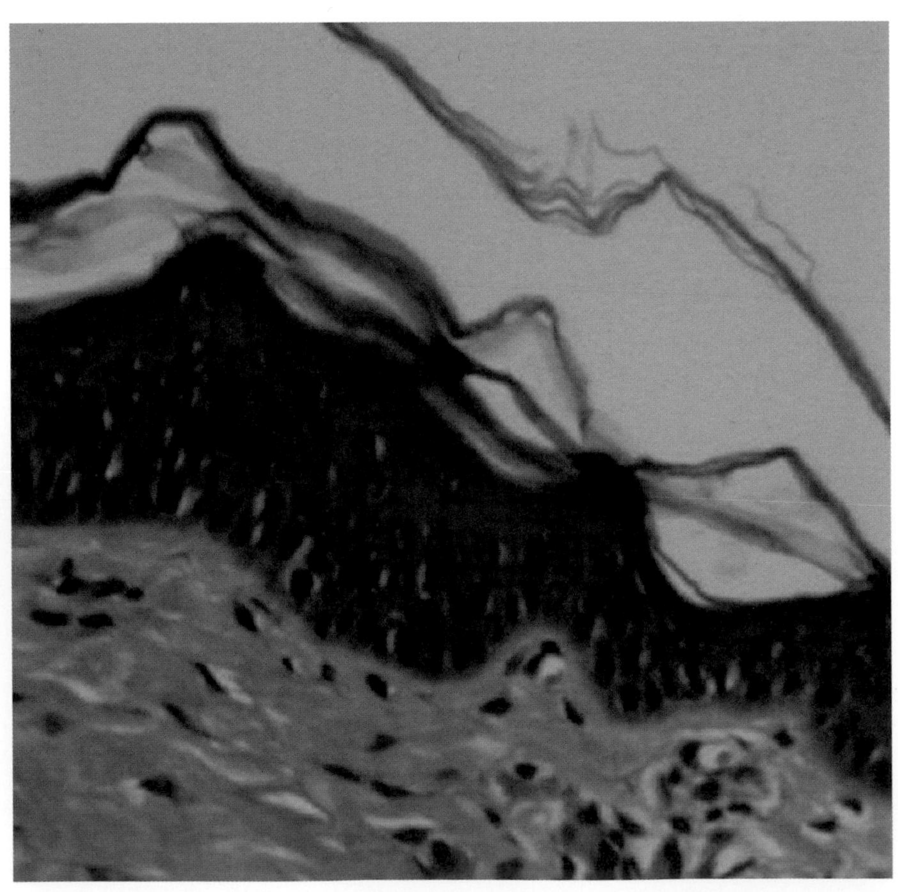

▲ **FIGURE 20-1** A hematoxylin and eosin (H&E) stain of untreated normal bovine skin.

SUPERFICIAL PEELS

Although a wide variety of agents have been shown to be effective for superficial peeling, alpha hydroxy acids (AHAs), beta hydroxy acid (BHA), Jessner's solution, modified Jessner's solution, resorcinol, and trichloroacetic acid (TCA) are the most commonly used in-office peel compounds. All of these compounds produce effects on the skin by inducing desquamation with resultant hastening of the cell cycle. These solutions remove the superficial layer of the stratum corneum (SC), yielding skin that is smoother in texture and more evenly pigmented. The individual ingredients of these peels will be discussed but, notably, these ingredients are often used in combination. Many of these ingredients are found in home products as well.

AHAs AND BHA

AHAs and BHA are naturally-occurring organic acids that contribute to inducing exfoliation and accelerating the cell cycle. Clearly there are myriad uses for AHAs and BHA in the practice of cosmetic dermatology. Authors have reported success using such products in the treatment of photoaging by improving mottled pigmentation, fine lines, surface roughness, freckles, and lentigines. AHAs and BHA have also been used with success to treat actinic and seborrheic keratoses.[4]

Research in the 1970s demonstrated that topical preparations that contain AHAs exert profound influence on epidermal keratinization.[5] AHAs and BHA affect corneocyte cohesiveness at the lower levels of the SC,[6] where they alter its pH, thereby acting on the skin.[7] When AHAs and BHA are applied to the skin in high concentrations, the result is detachment of keratinocytes and epidermolysis; application at lower concentrations reduces intercorneocyte cohesion directly above the granular layer, advancing desquamation and thinning of the SC.[7] This has two major effects: quickening of the cell cycle (which is slowed in aged skin) and increased desquamation, which results in improvement of hyperpigmentation and a smoother skin surface.

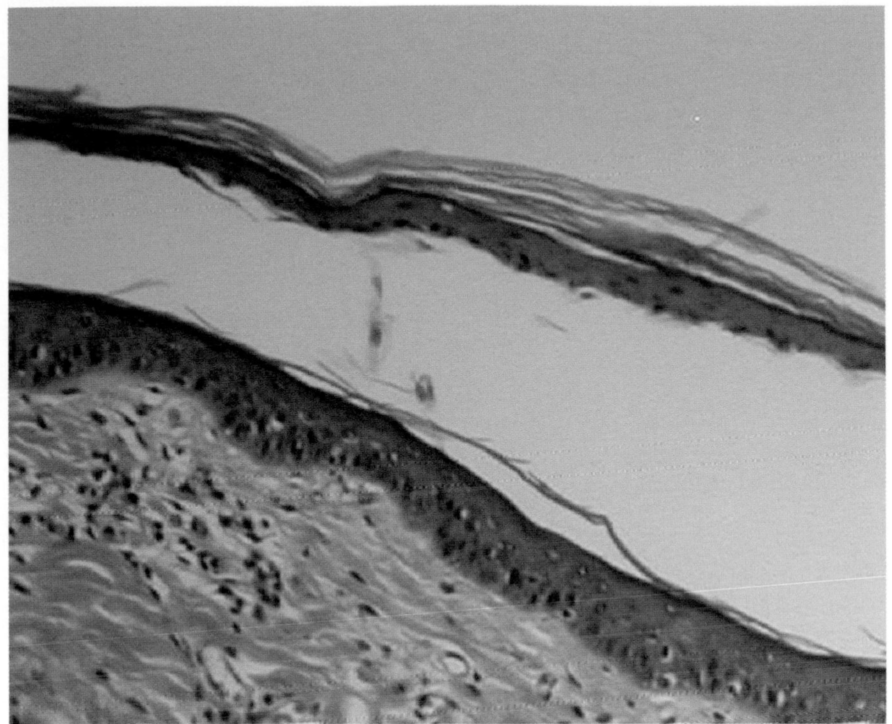

▲ **FIGURE 20-2** A hematoxylin and eosin (H&E) stain of bovine skin treated with a superficial chemical peel (two coats of the Pigment Peel Plus). This biopsy demonstrates a split in the spinous layer of the epidermis.

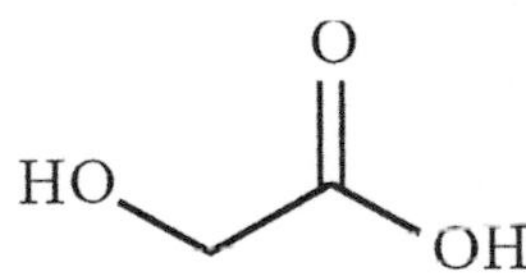

Glycolic Acid
(2-Hydroxyethanoic acid)

▲ **FIGURE 20-3** Chemical structure of glycolic acid. The OH group is in the alpha position; therefore, this is in the alpha hydroxy acid family.

AHAs

AHAs are a group of naturally-occurring compounds that contain the hydroxy group in the alpha position. This versatile group of acids includes glycolic acid, which is derived from sugar cane, lactic acid, from sour milk, citric acid, from citrus fruits, and phytic acid, which is derived from rice. The use of hydroxy acids in skin care products dates back to ancient Egypt and Cleopatra, who was said to have applied sour milk to her face to enhance its youthfulness.

GLYCOLIC ACID Glycolic acid (Fig. 20-3) is the AHA most commonly used in chemical peels in the offices of dermatologists and aestheticians. It is popularly known as "the lunchtime peel" because it can be completed during the patient's lunch hour and the patient can return to work without any telltale signs. The glycolic peel was one of the first superficial chemical peels to become popular because of its effectiveness and ease of use.

Well-designed studies have demonstrated the efficacy of AHA peels as a treatment for photoaging. In 1996, Ditre showed that application of AHAs resulted histologically in a 25% increase in skin thickness, increased acid mucopolysaccharides in the dermis, improved quality of the elastic fibers, and increased collagen density.[8] These findings are desirable because they imply that AHAs reverse some of the histologic signs of aging. This was again illustrated in a mouse model by Moon et al., who reported that mice treated with glycolic acid showed a significant decrease in wrinkle score and an increase in the amount of collagen synthesized.[9] It has been well established that collagen synthesis decreases with aging (see Chapter 6); therefore, increased synthesis of collagen may help retard the aging process. This increase of collagen production after treatment with AHAs has been demonstrated both in vivo and in vitro by using fibroblast cultures. In fact, in a study by Kim et al., glycolic acid treatments increased fibroblast proliferation in vitro as well as collagen production.[10] Glycolic acid peels are sometimes used in patients with acne; however, in a study by Lee et al., application of two glycolic acid peels (30%) or Jessner's solution with a 2-week interval failed to display any effect on sebum production.[11] Table 20-1

TABLE 20-1
Commonly Used Glycolic Acid Peel Brands[a]

Product name	Company	Percent Glycolic Acid	Percent Free Acid	pH	Neutralized	Buffered	Additives
Refinity Skin Solution	Cosmederm Technologies	70%	70%	>1	No	No	Strontium Nitrate
M.D. Forté Glycolic Chemical Peel Kit I	Allergan	70% peel	48% glycolic and ammonium glycolate	2.75	Partially	Yes	
M.D. Forté Glycolic Chemical Peel Kit II	Allergan	99% peel	68% glycolic and ammonium glycolate	2.25	Partially	Yes	
Glyderm—50% GA swab	ICN	50%	Free acid is esterified; . as such it probably is not active				Citric alcohol<5%
MicroPeel 20	BioMedic	20	20	1.3	No	No	Glycerin
MicroPeel 30	BioMedic	30	30	1.3	No	No	Glycerin
MicroPeel 50	BioMedic	50	50	0.8	No	No	Glycerin

[a]The amount of free acid determines the strength of the peel. Esterified free fatty acid must be hydrolyzed to the free acid by the skin's natural esterases to be active.

provides a list of the most commonly used glycolic acid peel brands.

Glycolic acid peels are inexpensive and easy to use. However, unlike many other peels, glycolic acid must be neutralized after use so as to prevent burning. For this reason, it is difficult to use on large areas of the body. It is best used in a small area on which application can be quickly applied and quickly neutralized.

LACTIC ACID Lactic acid (Fig. 20-4) is a popular AHA that is found in many at-home products and prescription moisturizers. It is usually not used as an in-office peel. Lactic acid is hypothesized to be part of the skin's natural moisturizing factor which plays a role in hydration[12] (see Chapter 11). Several studies on the activity of buffered 12% ammonium lactate lotion (LacHydrin™) have documented its moisturizing ability.[13] Lactic acid also has been shown to impart antiaging benefits similar to those seen with glycolic acid. One study demonstrated an increase in skin firmness and thickness and improvement in skin texture and moisturization using 5% and 12% lactic acid. These effects were limited to the epidermis as no effect on dermal firmness or thickness was seen.[14]

OTHER EFFECTS OF AHAs Aged skin, in addition to manifesting wrinkles and pigmentation abnormalities, is generally dryer than younger skin. Most cosmetic dermatologists forget that AHAs are also effective moisturizing agents because they have humectant properties (see Chapter 32). Interestingly, lactic acid is one of the few ingredients in the United States that is available in the same strength over the counter (OTC) and in prescription form. LacHydrin™ is actually an FDA-approved drug for use in dry skin, but not for photoaged skin. AHAs are beneficial in dry skin because they function as humectants, causing the skin to hold onto water. They also

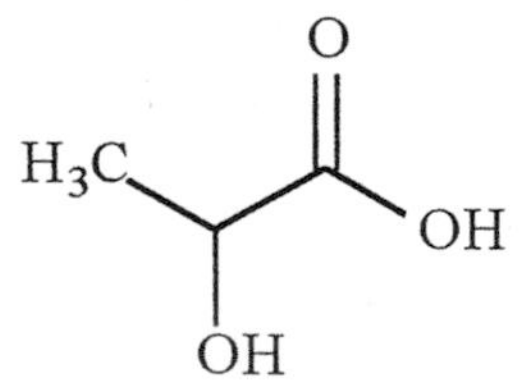

Lactic Acid
(2-Hydroxypropanoic acid)

▲ **FIGURE 20-4** Chemical structure of lactic acid.

enhance desquamation thereby normalizing the SC by getting rid of the clinging keratinocytes that make the skin look rough and scaled. Once the desquamation is enhanced, the skin is more flexible and better able to reflect light. Although many patients with sensitive skin are afraid to try AHAs, the irritation induced by some of these acids has been shown to be related to the formulation rather than the AHA itself.[15] In fact, AHAs have actually been demonstrated to reduce the irritation experienced when known irritants are placed on the skin. It is thought, but not proven, that AHAs can actually increase skin barrier function. In one study, glycolic acid, lactic acid, tartaric acid, and gluconolactone were compared in a double-blind, vehicle- and negative-controlled randomized trial. It was found that all of these AHAs protected the skin from irritation caused by a 5% sodium lauryl sulfate challenge patch test as measured by resulting erythema and changes in transepidermal water loss (TEWL). In fact, this study showed that TEWL is not altered by application of AHAs. It is interesting that AHAs are able to cause a sheet-like separation of the SC that is not associated with compromise of the barrier function.[7] The exact mechanism of action of how AHAs impart this protection is currently unknown; however, these agents may prove useful in the management of skin diseases associated with diminished barrier function and a susceptibility to irritant contact dermatitis.

BHA

Also known as salicylic acid (SA), BHA is another commonly used type of in-office chemical peel used by aestheticians and cosmetic dermatologists. These formulations are also available in OTC home products that have lower concentrations of acids (usually 0.5%–2%) than those used in the office (usually 20%–30%). Derived from willow bark, wintergreen leaves, and sweet birch, SA is the only member of the BHA family, so named because the aromatic carboxylic acid has a hydroxy group in the beta position (Fig. 20-5). This is actually a misnomer because the carbons of aromatic compounds are traditionally given Arabic numerals (1, 2, etc.) rather than the Greek letter designations typical for the nonaromatic structures. It is likely that SA was labeled as a BHA at the time BHA peels were introduced in order to market the products and benefit from the popularity of AHAs. Although BHA is a newer category of chemical peels, SA is hardly a

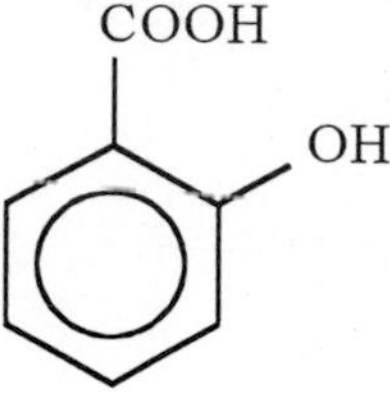

Salicylic Acid

▲ **FIGURE 20-5** Chemical structure of salicylic acid.

new agent—it had a long history of effectiveness before it was labeled as a BHA.

Most physicians use preparations of 20% or 30% SA for in-office peels. Such peels have been shown to fade pigment spots, decrease surface roughness, and reduce fine lines,[16] with similar results to those seen with AHAs. In the early 1990s, Swinehart reported satisfactory results using 50% SA on the hands and forearms of patients exhibiting actinically induced pigmentary changes in those areas.[4] These effects are likely caused by increased exfoliation and an accelerated cell cycle, as seen with AHAs. However, unlike AHAs, BHA affects the arachidonic acid cascade and, therefore, exhibits anti-inflammatory capabilities. These properties may allow SA peels to be effective while inducing less irritation than AHA peels. A 1997 double-blind consumer-perception study of neurosensory discomforts after 3 weeks of use confirmed that SA is perceived by patients as being milder than glycolic acid. Of subjects treated with glycolic acid, 20% reported subjective adverse reactions, while 4% to 7% of the SA group reported such reactions.[17] The lower incidence of perceived irritation caused by SA has contributed to the great popularity of in-office peels and home products that contain BHA. The anti-inflammatory effects of BHA make it a very useful peel in patients with acne and rosacea (Fig. 20-6). It can be combined with traditional acne therapy to speed the resolution of comedones and red inflamed papules (see Chapter 15). SA peels may have a whitening effect in patients with darker skin types. In a study of 24 Asian women who were treated with bi-weekly facial peeling with 30% SA in absolute ethanol for 3 months, some lightening of skin color was seen.[18] These peels can also lead to postinflammatory hyperpigmentation. The risks of skin lightening or darkening should be explained to patients with darker skin types prior to their use. The trick is to use a strong enough peel to be

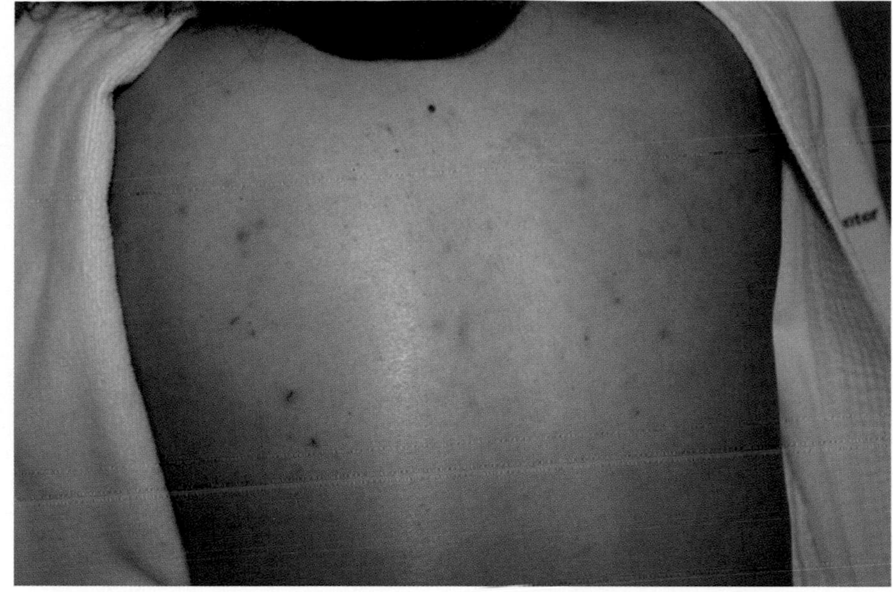

▲ **FIGURE 20-6** Beta hydroxy acid peels can be used to treat acne and photoaging on any part of the body. This patient was treated with BHA for acne and postinflammatory hyperpigmentation on the back.

effective but not strong enough to induce inflammation. If in doubt use a lower strength peel and titrate to stronger peels in future sequential treatments.

Another difference between AHAs and BHA is that BHA is lipophilic, which enables it to penetrate the sebaceous material in the hair follicle and exfoliate the pores.[18] AHAs, which are water-soluble, do not exhibit this comedolytic characteristic[19] (Table 20-2). Kligman evaluated this phenomenon in a study that compared the number of microcomedones seen in biopsies of women treated with 2% SA to those from women treated with 8% glycolic acid. The glycolic formulation did not decrease the density of microcomedones, whereas a statistically significant ($p < 0.05$) decrease was seen after BHA application.[17] Therefore, because of its lipophilic nature, BHA confers a stronger comedolytic effect than do AHAs.

BOX 20-1

It is important to note that the frost seen in a BHA peel represents precipitated SA, while the frost in a TCA peel represents precipitated skin proteins. These "skipped" areas seen in a TCA peel should not be touched up as they can be with a BHA peel, because the TCA peel frosting time depends on the concentration used. Lower concentrations take longer to frost. BHA peels frost in 2 minutes. Retouching the unfrosted areas of a TCA peel could result in burning the patient and should be strongly discouraged.

Although there is a wealth of evidence that suggests that AHAs stimulate collagen production, there are no published data examining the effects of BHA on collagen synthesis. Many authors postulate, however, that the increased collagen synthesis seen with AHAs and retinoids may be due in part to the resulting inflammation, which may stimulate collagen synthesis. If this is true, one would expect that SA would also increase collagen synthesis.

BHA also differs from the AHAs insofar as it does not need to be neutralized and the frost is visible once the peel is complete (Box 20-1). The practitioner can readily observe the uniformity of application of a BHA peel because of the white precipitate of SA that forms (Fig. 20-7).

TABLE 20-2
Comparison of AHAs and BHA

	AHAs	BHA
Useful in photoaging	Yes	Yes
Useful in acne	Yes	Yes
Useful in melasma	Yes	Yes
Useful for dry skin	Yes	Yes
Speeds cell cycle	Yes	Yes
Enhances exfoliation	Yes	Yes
Lipophilic	No	Yes
Inhibits arachidonic acid	No	Yes
Anesthetic properties	No	Yes
Anti-inflammatory properties	Maybe	Yes
Must be neutralized	Yes	No
Visible frost	No	Yes
Risk of salicylism	No	Yes (low)
Variety of available concentrations	Yes	A few
FDA-approved for prescription use	Yes (dry skin)	No
Shown to increase collagen synthesis	Yes	No
Useful in pregnancy/ breast feeding	Yes	No

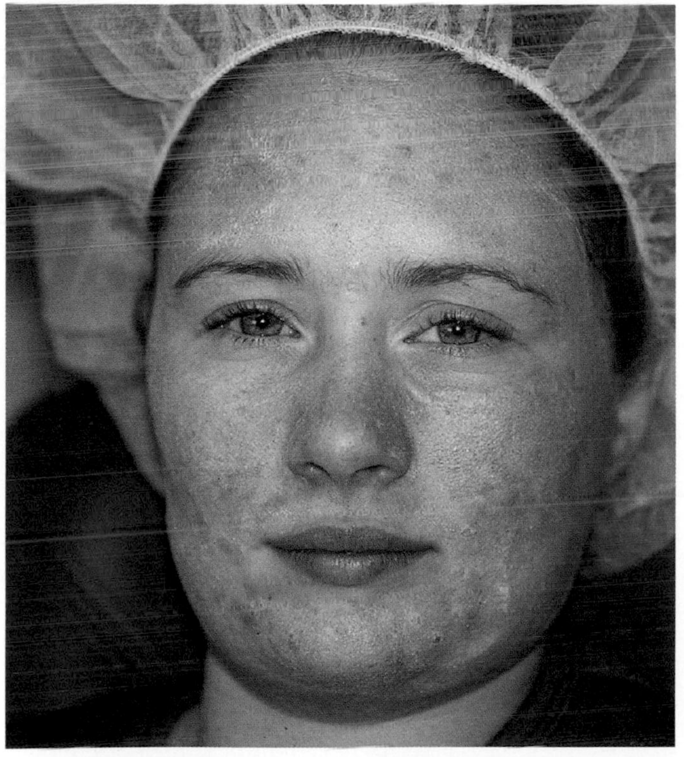

▲ **FIGURE 20-7** The white frost appears 2 minutes after application of the salicylic acid peel and signals that the peel is complete.

effective moisturizer in combination with BHA products to prevent this problem.

SA is currently a popular component of many in-office peels using a combination of ingredients. Examples include the Jessner's Peel, the PCA Peel™ by Physician's Choice, and the Pigment Plus Peel™ by Biomedic.

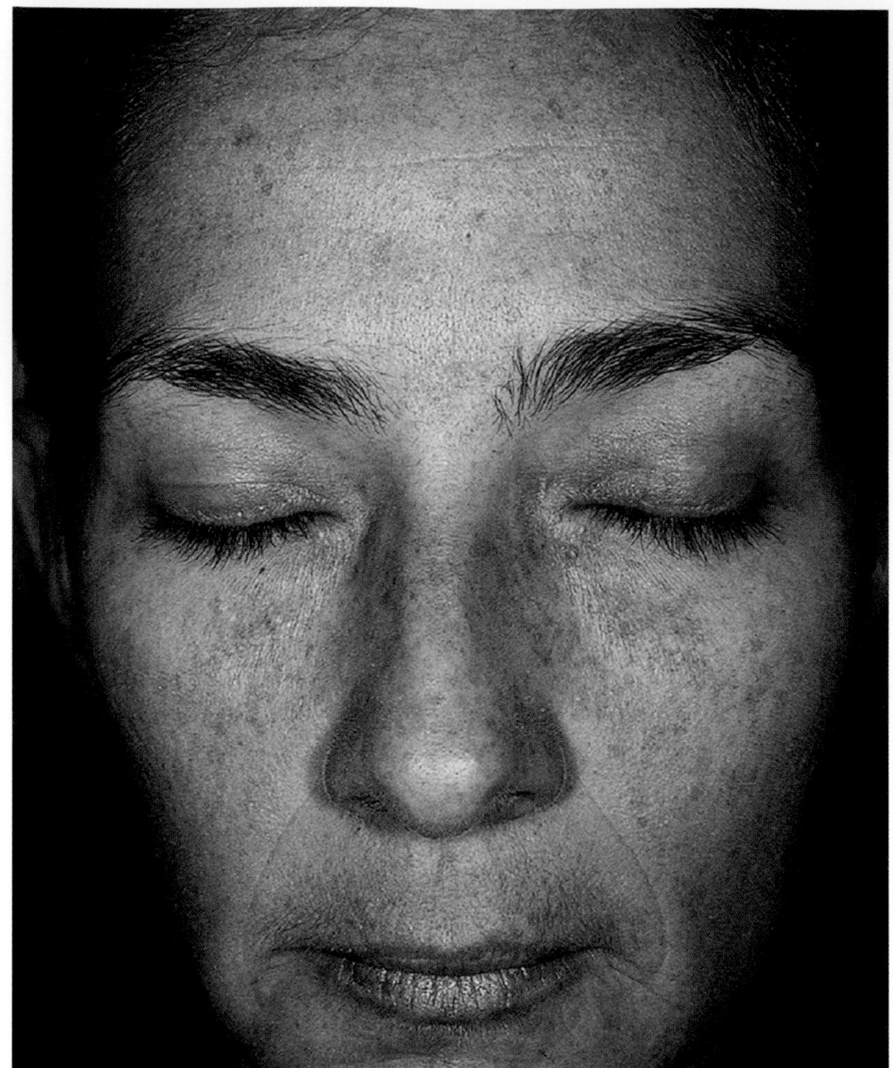

▲ **FIGURE 20-8** Prior to a superficial modified Jessner's peel. Note the solar lentigos.

Any areas that have been inadequately peeled can be easily identified and then treated by reapplying the BHA solution. Also, timing of the peel is unnecessary, and the risk of overpeeling is remote because once the vehicle becomes volatile, which occurs in approximately 2 minutes, there is very little penetration of the active agent. It is important to immediately use the chemical peel liquid once the cap has been taken off the bottle, otherwise it will evaporate and change the efficacy. In addition, do not use a fan when you use this peel because it will increase the rate at which the vehicle becomes volatile and will lessen the effect of the peel. Because neutralization of the BHA peel is unnecessary, it is easier to apply to larger areas of the body such as the back and chest that are difficult to adequately neutralize. However, it is unwise to peel large surface areas of the body with SA in one office visit. Although toxic levels of salicylates have not been reported in association with the concentrations currently used for SA peels,[3] there have been case reports of children with multiple excoriations and elderly patients with ichthyosis treated with topicals containing SA that developed salicylism.[20] Therefore, large body surfaces should be treated with care and the physician should watch for the signs of salicylism, which include nausea, disorientation, and tinnitus. Of course, BHA, whether in concentrations developed for in-office peels or in at-home products, is contraindicated in patients who are pregnant, breast-feeding, or allergic to aspirin.

Many home care product formulations contain SA. Typically, they are labeled as "acne washes" and contain 0.5% to 2% SA. These products are an excellent addition to a home care regimen for acne, rosacea, photoaging, and pigmentation disorders. Notably, irritation and skin dryness can result from such products, especially since patients tend to use higher and higher concentrations of home products to maintain exfoliation. Patients should use an

DISADVANTAGES OF HYDROXY ACIDS AHAs are a significant set of options in an antiaging armamentarium; however, it is important for patients to have realistic expectations. Superficial chemical peels are only able to produce subtle changes in the skin with each peel. It is the cumulative benefits of the peels that yield the most noticeable changes in the skin. At least four superficial peels are usually necessary before patients can begin to see amelioration of photodamage, solar lentigos, and melasma. Those with more severe damage may require eight or more. If this is not explained to patients, they will become discouraged after one or two chemical peels and will not be compliant with the prescribed regimen. Patients must also be told that superficial peels are unable to correct moderate to severe wrinkles and scars even though many OTC cosmetic products promise these unrealistic changes. If patients' expectations are realistic, they will be pleased with the results that superficial peels can provide (Figs. 20-8 and 20-9).

Although AHAs are very popular as ingredients in daily cleansers and moisturizers, some experts have suggested that continued use of hydroxy acids may lead to a decrease in efficacy with continued use because of accommodation of the skin. It is postulated that this occurs because the skin becomes a better acid buffer and is able to more efficiently neutralize the effects of the acids.[14] At this time there is no published evidence to support this claim, but this possibility should be kept in mind. It may be beneficial to have patients stop their hydroxy acid preparations periodically to enhance the efficacy of these products when used long term.

Although AHAs are well known to make the SC appear more compact, this effect has not been associated with the use of SA in the literature. However, it is likely that BHA has the same effect. AHAs, but surprisingly not BHA, were under scrutiny in the past because of the fear that AHAs "thinned" the skin. This has not been proven. There is concern that the thinner SC will provide less of a barrier to harmful environmental factors

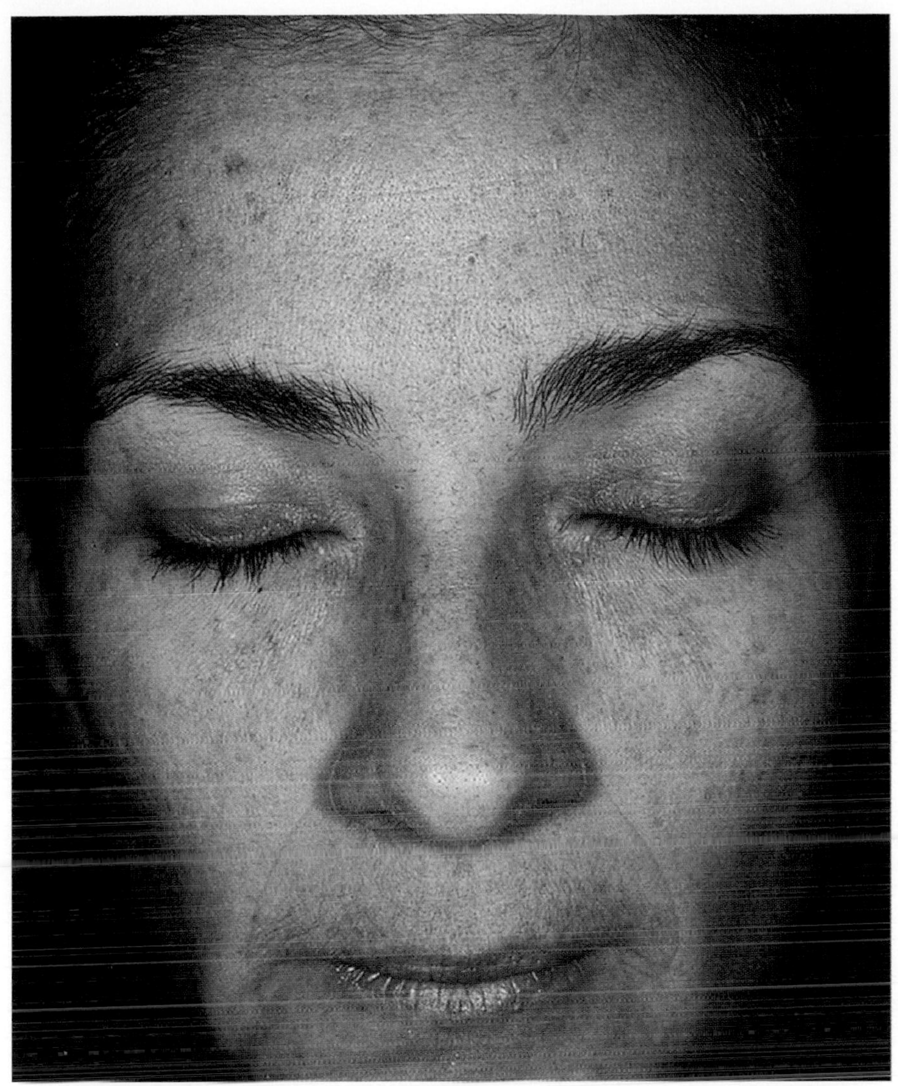

▲ **FIGURE 20-9** After one modified Jessner's peel. The solar lentigos are mildly improved, but it will take at least three more peels for the patient to note a significant difference in these pigmented lesions.

such as ultraviolet (UV) light and toxins in the environment. Although studies have shown that TEWL is not affected by the use of AHAs, there was still concern that the barrier would be disturbed in skin treated with AHAs. In 1999, a study evaluated the barrier integrity of hairless guinea pigs after treatment with 5% and 10% glycolic acid at pH 3.0. Investigators found no increase in skin penetration of exogenously applied hydroquinone, musk xylol, and 3H water when compared to controls. However, they did find that the guinea pigs treated with the glycolic preparations had approximately a two-fold *increase* in epidermal thickness and almost double the number of nucleated cell layers as compared with the control group.[21] This suggests that although the SC is thinned by AHAs, the overall epidermis is thicker. Another concern with AHAs is that they may increase photosensitivity. A study by Tsai et al. demonstrated that pretreatment of human skin with 10% glycolic acid caused an increase in UVB-induced skin tanning in Caucasian and Asian subjects and an increase in UVA tanning in Asian subjects (but not Caucasians).[22] Many cosmetic companies have also noted that increased numbers of sunburn cells have been seen in patients treated with AHA preparations. The FDA is now requiring that all AHA preparations be labeled to inform patients about photosensitivity and to advise using sunscreens.

EVALUATING AND COMPARING HYDROXY ACID PREPARATIONS The most important aspect of chemical peel strength is the amount of available free acid. The amount of free acid itself is affected by the following: concentration of the peel (% hydroxy acid), the pK_a of the acid preparation, the pH of the solution (which is also affected by the type of vehicle used), and whether or not the peel is buffered. Because of this complex interplay of factors, it is difficult to compare one brand of chemical peel to another. For example, a 30% glycolic acid peel from one company is not necessarily the same strength as a 30% glycolic peel from another company. The acid percentage is only a small part of the story. It is necessary to consider the pH, the amount of free acid, the additive ingredients, and whether or not the peel is buffered before comparing different peeling brands.

The Significance of the pK$_a$ In order to use AHAs and BHA properly, one must understand the pK$_a$ and how the pH of a peel affects its efficacy. The pK$_a$ of a substance measures its capacity to donate protons. The pK$_a$ is the pH at which the level of free acid is the same as the level of the salt form of the acid. When the pH is less than the pK$_a$, the free acid form, the one responsible for exfoliation of the skin, predominates; when the pH is greater than the pK$_a$, the salt form predominates. The acid form is the "active form" in the peel because it causes exfoliation. It is necessary to have the proper balance of the salt and acid forms to have an efficacious peel with minimal irritation. The pK$_a$ for salicylic acid is 2.97 while 3.83 is the pK$_a$ for the AHAs.[23,24] Because the pK$_a$ of BHA differs from that of the AHA family, it is difficult to formulate a combination product containing both that reaches an optimal pH. For example, in a combination AHA–BHA product with a pH of 3.5, the AHA acid form would predominate but the BHA salt form would predominate. The effects of BHA would be rendered suboptimal then

Significance of the pH The higher the pH, the more basic the solution is; the lower the pH, the more acidic the solution is. The irritation induced by a product is often directly related to how low the pH is. Lower pH equates to increased irritation, as well as efficacy.

Buffered solutions Some chemical peel formulations are "buffered." Many companies claim that this increases the tolerability of these agents. A product is buffered when a base such as sodium bicarbonate or sodium hydroxide is added to the solution. This produces an increased amount of the salt form, which results in less free acid and a higher pH. Buffered solutions are resistant to pH changes when a salt or an acid is added to the preparation. Because these solutions have a lower pH and less free acid, there is a decrease in side effects; however, there may also be a decrease in efficacy. These formulations are safer for use by beginners and nonphysicians, which may account for their popularity.

Vehicle It is important to remember that the vehicle can also cause irritation to the patient. In fact, studies indicate that irritation associated with AHA products is usually related to the formulation of the product and not to the AHA itself.[7] Also, the difference in vehicles can contribute to variations in the clinical response. Some companies add strontium nitrate (e.g., Cosmederm-7™) to decrease the sensory irritation of AHA solutions. In one study, when strontium nitrate and 70% glycolic acid were applied to the volar arm, patients exhibited less burning and stinging than when 70% glycolic acid was applied alone to the other arm.[25] There is no evidence that the strontium nitrate decreases redness or epidermolysis, but there is good evidence that it decreases the itching and burning sensations without affecting the efficacy of the glycolic preparations. Other agents that increase penetration, such as urea, may affect the efficacy of these topical products; therefore, it is important to know all the ingredients in each topical preparation.

RESORCINOL Resorcinol has been used as a chemical peeling agent since Unna described its use in 1882.[26] A phenol derivative, resorcinol (m-dihydroxybenzene) exhibits antipruritic, keratolytic, antimycotic, and antiseptic properties. It is mainly used as a treatment for pigmentary disorders and acne, but is also a lone peeling agent and a common component of combination chemical peels, including the Jessner's peel (Fig. 20-10). In a study of nine patients treated with a 53% concentration of resorcinol once weekly for 10 weeks, all subjects showed an average of 0.03 mm improvement in thickness of their epidermis and five patients exhibited enhanced elastosis. Verhoeff's stain showed an improvement of elastic fibers in all cases.[27]

Care must be taken to limit the surface area treated because systemic toxicity similar to that seen with phenol has been reported. Prolonged use has been associated with myxedema because the drug has an antithyroid action and methemoglobinemia in children. Resorcinol is a primary irritant and a moderately strong sensitizer that seldom produces allergic contact dermatitis. However, contact allergy to resorcinol in topical acne products and in Castellani's paint have been reported.[28] Although resorcinol is very useful in the treatment of hyperpigmentation disorders, it can cause hyperpigmentation in patients with a Fitzpatrick skin type greater than IV and should be used with great care in these patients. The possibility of deeper penetration and achieving a medium-depth peel with resorsinol is also worth consideration.[29] This can be achieved by pretreatment with tretinoin, increasing the absorption of the peeling agent.

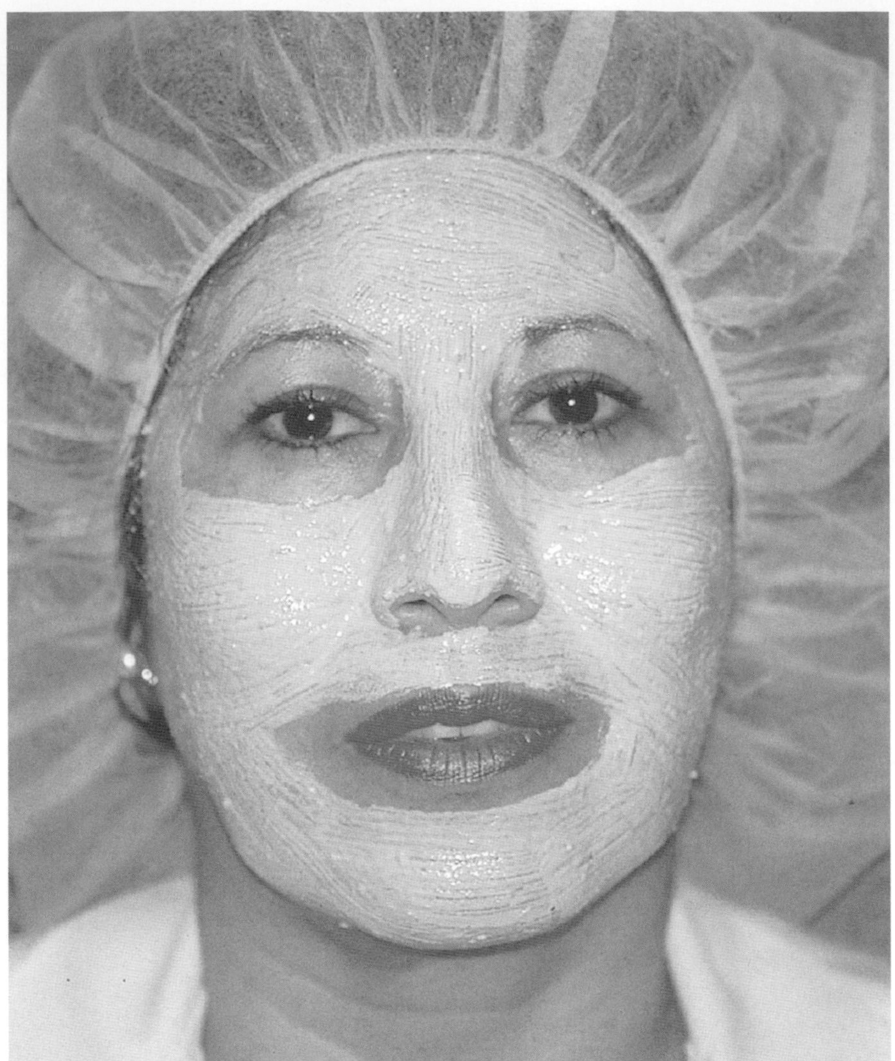

▲ **FIGURE 20-10** Resorcinal paste mask.

Other Peels

Several popular peels consist of a combination of active ingredients. The first combination peel to gain wide usage was Jessner's peel. It is still commonly used today. Many peels such as the PCA Peel by Physician's Choice use a formula known as a "modified Jessner's peel." These peels contain many of the same ingredients as the classic Jessner's peel but employ different combinations. They will not be discussed in this chapter but are listed in Table 20-3.

JESSNER'S SOLUTION This popular peel is a combination of resorcinol 14 g, salicylic acid 14 g, and lactic acid 14 g in a sufficient quantity of ethanol (95%) to make 100 cc of solution. It can be purchased already made from many companies. Dr. Max Jessner originally formulated this peel to reduce the concentration and toxicity of each of the individual ingredients while increasing efficacy.[30] The strength of the peel is determined by how many layers are applied and if it is used in combination with other peeling formulas. Jessner's peel is popularly used with other peels because it does not have to be neutralized. Once the peel frosts, a second type of peel such as TCA can be applied on top of the Jessner's peel to increase the depth of the overall peel. Although this peel is very safe, it should be used with caution on patients with darker skin types because resorcinol is associated with an increased risk of postinflammatory hyperpigmentation in those with Fitzpatrick skin type IV and

TABLE 20-3
Examples of Superficial Peels Currently on the Market

Biomedic LHA Peel sold by La Roche-Posay contains 5% or 10% LHA lipohydroxy acid.
The Biomedic Pigment Peel Plus™ contains 20% salicylic acid and 30% TCA in a glycerin base. It is sold by La Roche-Posay.
Esthetique Peel is sold by Physician's Choice™. It contains L-lactic acid, L-retinol, polyphenols, and antioxidants.
Jessner's Peel—contains resorcinol 14 g, salicylic acid 14 g and lactic acid 14 g in a sufficient quantity of ethanol (95%) to make 100 cc of solution. It is sold by many companies including Delasco.
Miami Peel S-30 is sold by Quintessence Skin Care. It contains salicylic acid 30%, ascorbic acid (vitamin C), green tea extract, and other antioxidants.
The PCA Peel is sold in 4 oz bottles by Physician's Choice. This peel comes in three forms (each is formulated at a pH of 2.2):
PCA Peel® with hydroquinone and resorcinol: contains ethanol 52%, lactic acid 14%, resorcinol 14%, salicylic acid 14%, kojic acid 3%, hydroquinone 2%, and citric acid 1%.
PCA Peel with hydroquinone: contains ethanol 55%, salicylic acid 15%, lactic acid 15%, citric acid 10%, kojic acid 3%, and hydroquinone 2%.
PCA Peel without hydroquinone: contains ethanol 57%, salicylic acid 15%, lactic acid 15%, citric acid 10%, and kojic acid 3%.
Sensi Peel™ contains 6% TCA, 12% lactic acid, kojic acid, l-arbutin, meadowfoam oil, l-ascorbic acid, azelaic acid, chaste tree extract, and plant and marine polysaccharides. It is sold by Physician's Choice.
Ultra Peel I ™ contains10% TCA, 20% lactic acid, l-ascorbic acid, kojic acid, plant and marine polysaccharides, and chaste tree extract. It is sold by Physician's Choice.
Ultra Peel® II Exfoliating Treatment contains retinol and vitamin C. It can be layered over other peels to increase exfoliation. It is sold by Physician's Choice.
Ultra Peel Forte™ contains 20% TCA, 5% l-lactic acid, l-ascorbic acid, kojic acid, compound Z, and chaste tree extract (plant sourced progesterone). It is sold by Physician's Choice.

greater. Patients may also develop a contact dermatitis to resorcinol that manifests as redness and swelling. Topical or oral steroids may be used to treat this uncommon side effect.

Use of the Jessner's peel The solution can be used in conjunction with other agents like glycolic acid, 5-fluouracil, and TCA as it enhances the effects of each. When used alone, a thin coat of the solution is applied to all areas to be treated. Prior to treatment, a thin layer of Vaseline or Aquaphor is applied to the areas not intended for treatment, such as the nasoalar grooves, where the solution tends to pool, and the lips. The practitioner should take precautions to avoid dripping the solution into undesired areas. The first coat is complete once frosting occurs (usually in 3 to 5 minutes). The patient usually experiences noticeable flaking for approximately 7 days. If a deeper peel is desired, two or three coats may be applied with a resulting elevation in peeling, efficacy and, of course, side effects. When using this peel on patients with a tendency to develop dyschromias, such as patients with melasma, postinflammatory hyperpigmentation, etc., it is a good idea to proceed slowly with one coat of the solution every 2 to 3 weeks to avoid exacerbating the hyperpigmentation. This peel is excellent for use in acne patients because resorcinol is a well-known treatment for acne. It is also effective in rosacea patients because it contains salicylic acid. Modified Jessner's peel combinations containing added ingredients such as hydroquinone and kojic acid (see Chapter 38), or ones that omit resorcinol for individuals that are sensitive to this component, are available. In order to avoid systemic absorption and the combined effects of the resorcinol and salicylic acid, this peel should not be used on large body areas at once.[31]

TRETINOIN PEEL For several years, topical tretinoin has been successfully used in various preparations for the treatment of melasma, acne, and photoaging. Topical tretinoin is known to induce increased collagen deposition,[32] and inhibit the metalloproteinases responsible for degrading collagen.[33] The tretinoin peel is not available in the United States; however, it is used in many countries such as Brazil off-label for the treatment of photoaging, melasma, acne, and keratosis pilaris. The peeling solution is orange in color, preserved in brown containers, and painted on the desired treatment site. The patient is advised to wash off the solution after 4 to 6 hours of treatment. The peeling may be variable and usually begins after 2 days. Kligman et al. studied tretinoin 0.25% in a solution of 50% ethanol and 50% polyethylene glycol 400 in 50 women between 30 and 60 years of age with diagnoses of photoaging, rosacea, and acne. The solution was applied to the face by the patients every other night for 2 weeks and later, on a nightly basis. Patients showed clinical improvements as manifested by a smoother appearance of the epidermis, reduction of fine lines, and improvement of hyperpigmentation. Histologic examination of the skin revealed increased thickness of the basal layer and fibroblasts in the papillary dermis, decreased numbers of melanosomes, diminished SC thickness, and better organized rete ridges. Kligman and colleagues proposed that the effects of using low-strength tretinoin for 6 to 12 months may be achieved by higher strengths in 4 to 6 weeks.[34]

Cucé et al. conducted a study on 15 women between 23 and 40 years old with Fitzpatrick skin types I to IV to assess the clinical and histologic effects of a 1% tretinoin peel. A pretreatment biopsy was done. The chemical peel was performed with an interval of 2 to 3 days and patients had the peel on for 6 to 8 hours. Fifteen days following the last application a second biopsy was performed, which showed increasing of the epidermal thickness and thinning of the SC.[35] These findings also correlated with clinically better looking skin. The histologic and clinical evaluation of patients' skin in this study indicated that to achieve the same effect of a tretinoin peel after 2.5 weeks one must use topical tretinoin for approximately 4 to 6 months. In another study of 10 patients with Fitzpatrick skin types III to V and moderate to severe melasma, a 1% tretinoin peel was compared to a 70% glycolic acid peel. The tretinoin peel was left on the treated area for 4 hours while the glycolic peel was placed for a maximum of 3 minutes. Both peels were found to be equally effective at 3 months posttreatment, though less erythema and desquamation were associated with the tretinoin peel, which was therefore better tolerated by the patients.[36]

Side Effects of All Types of Superficial Peels

Although superficial chemical peels are very safe when used properly they can all cause erythema, itching, peeling, increased skin sensitivity, and even epidermolysis. Allergic contact dermatitis has been reported to occur with resorcinol, salicylic acid, kojic acid, lactic acid, and hydroquinone. Irritant contact dermatitis has been linked to glycolic acid. Any peel can cause an irritant dermatitis when used with excessive frequency, inappropriately high concentrations, or with a vigorous skin preparation using acetone or another "degreasing" solution. Patients with a recent insult to the SC, such as beginning a regimen with tretinoin, facial shaving, use of "exfoliating" scrubs and Buff-Puffs™, or kissing a person with a heavy beard for prolonged periods, are more susceptible to chemical peels extending deeper than intended. Consequently, it is necessary to closely examine the condition of the skin and get a good history from the patient prior to performing a peel (Box 20-2).

BOX 20-2 How to Use Chemical Peels—Dr. Baumann's Perspective

There are several brands of superficial chemical peels available on the market. In the case of AHAs, one must know the pH and concentration of free acid in the individual products in order to compare strength and efficacy across products. The practitioner must exercise extra caution when treating patients with darker skin types, regardless of the chemical peel selected, to avoid hyperpigmentation. For such patients, the practitioner should start with the lowest concentration of free acid and slowly increase the concentration.

1. At the first visit, assess the patient's skin using a UV or Wood's light to determine the extent of pigmentation abnormalities. This will help convince the patient of the necessity of sunscreen use. Take regular pictures and UV camera photographs if possible. Determine the patient's Baumann Skin Type (see Chapter 9). Discuss skin care, sunscreen use and the importance of topical retinoid treatments (Chapter 30) and offer product recommendations based on the patient's skin type. Also at this juncture, it is imperative to caution patients to refrain from using at-home topical AHAs, BHA, and other irritating ingredients such as vitamin C in order to avoid excessive skin irritation. In addition, the physician should make sure that the patient is not using another form of exfoliation such as facial scrubs or Buff-Puffs™. The practitioner should treat each patient, even those with type I skin, with the lowest strength peel of the chosen brand (or the one requiring the shortest duration on the face) on the first visit to ascertain the patient's level of sensitivity. Explain to patients that they will not notice much difference in their skin after the first peel because it is only a low-strength solution used to determine their ability to tolerate the peel. It is important at each visit, but particularly so at the first visit, to find out if the patient has any significant forthcoming social obligations that might be compromised or made embarrassing owing to erythema or conspicuous skin flaking. There is a low incidence of hypersensitivity reactions (most commonly seen with the Jessner's peel) that, according to Murphy's law, occur preferentially in those patients with an important party or lecture coming up. Patients should return within 10 to 14 days for a follow-up and to receive the next peel.

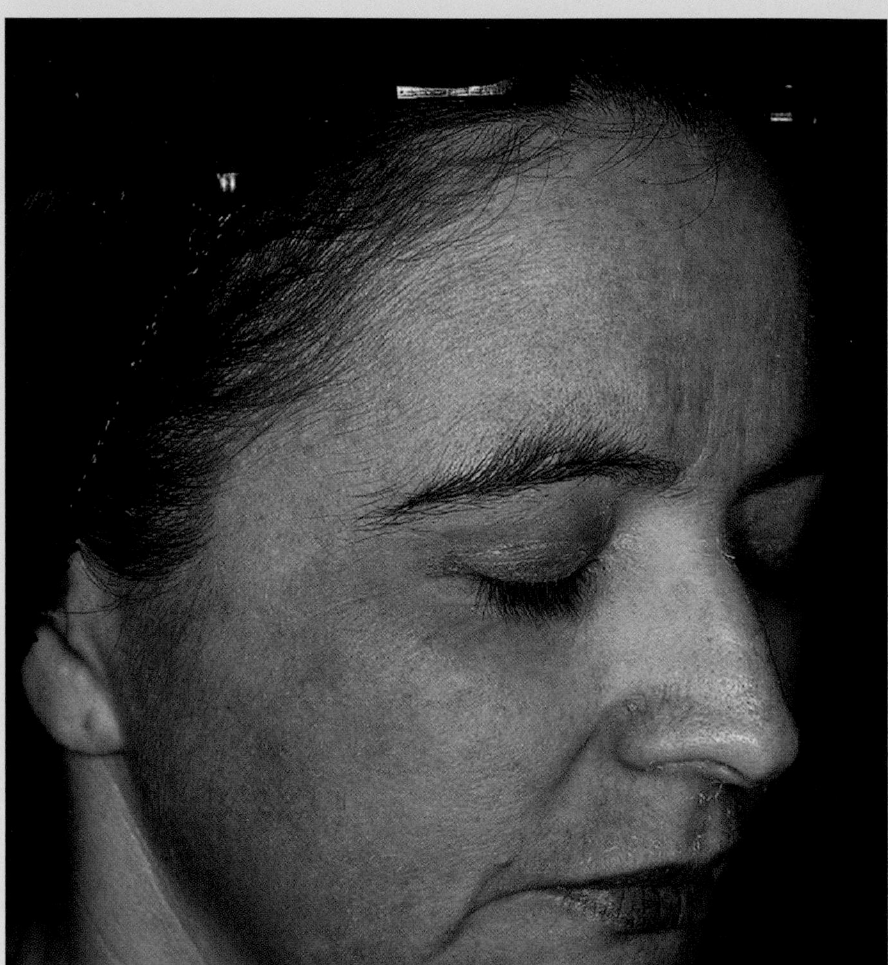

▲ **FIGURE 20-11** Patient on Retin A with retinoid dermatitis. Peeling this patient will result in excessive redness and scaling. It is best to wait 1 week prior to proceeding with chemical peeling.

2. At the second visit, the practitioner can go to the next level in peel strength if the patient experienced minimal or no peeling after the initial peel. Most patients are started on a topical retinoid on the first visit so care must be taken to avoid peeling skin that exhibits "retinoid dermatitis" (Fig. 20-11). In such a case, the practitioner should refrain from performing a peel until the retinoid dermatitis resolves. On this visit, it is also important to assess how well the patient tolerates the social/psychological impact of peeling. If the patient complains about flaking skin or erythema, the physician should titrate the peels more slowly. If the patient feels that significant erythema and/or flaking are the sine qua non of an adequate peel, the physician may want to proceed more rapidly.
3. Visit Three and Beyond—Manufacturers of most superficial chemical peel brands recommend treatments at 10- to 14-day intervals. One may continue the peelings until the initial presenting symptoms have resolved and, thereafter, perform peels at 4-week intervals for maintenance. One should occasionally inquire about retinoid and sunscreen use to ensure patient compliance. After the third peel, patients should be consistently using the retinoids with no skin irritation. If this is the case, it is a good time to add an at-home AHA or BHA preparation. There are many brands to choose from and skin care product ingredients are discussed at length throughout this text to help you decide which products to recommend.

Postinflammatory hyperpigmentation is a rare complication in superficial chemical peels that are started at low strengths and titrated up very slowly. Grimes followed 25 patients with Fitzpatrick skin types V and VI who were treated with 20% and 30% salicylic acid peels.[37] These patients were pretreated with hydroquinone 4% for 2 weeks prior to peeling. Only three patients developed temporary postinflammatory hyperpigmentation. No residual hyperpigmentation was seen. Several studies have shown that superficial peels can also be used safely in Asian patients.[38,39] However, most dermatologists agree that these patients should be pretreated with a depigmenting agent and tretinoin and should be advised to use effective sun protection offering broad UVA and UVB coverage.

MEDIUM-DEPTH PEELS

Trichloroacetic Acid 10% to 40%

TCA became popular in the 1960s through the work of Ayres.[40] Low-strength TCA (10%–15%) is used to ameliorate fine wrinkles and dyschromias and to provide the skin with a smooth, healthy appearance. TCA, at these strengths, does not improve deeper wrinkles or scars.[41,42] Higher-strength TCA (35%–40%) produces epidermal and dermal necrosis without serious systemic toxicity. It must be used with extreme caution, however, because hyperpigmentation and scarring can result. Practitioners should carefully select patients, noting that patients with darker skin types should not be treated with TCA as they have an increased risk for postinflammatory hyperpigmentation.

TCA at 35% to 40% is the standard solution for medium-depth peels for the face and hands. When discussing the strength of TCA peels, it is imperative to discuss the strength in weight per volume (wt/vol) measurements. Unfortunately, not all authors use this form of measuring so one must take care when reading and basing a peel on the literature to know how the strength was calculated in order to avoid underestimating the strength of the peel. This precaution reduces the risk of inducing scarring.[43] For instance, 25% TCA cannot be formed by diluting 50% TCA with an equal volume of water because this type of dilution is vol/vol and actually yields a solution stronger than 25% wt/vol TCA. When following a protocol from the literature, the practitioner should calculate the TCA percentage by wt/vol measurements to avoid mistakes. TCA can be purchased according to the desired wt/vol strength.

Following application of a TCA peel, denatured protein causes a "frosting" of the skin, signaling the completion of the peel. The time lag between the application and the appearance of the frost varies according to the acid concentration. The delay might last 5 to 7 seconds after application of 40% TCA, but can last as long as 15 to 20 minutes after application of a more dilute acid. This is crucial for the practitioner to remember in order to avoid overtreatment.

TCA can be applied alone or after use of Jessner's solution or glycolic acid to achieve a deeper peel. Healing time is usually between 5 and 7 days for patients treated only with TCA and between 7 and 10 days for patients treated with a combination of TCA and either Jessner's solution or glycolic acid.[41,42]

Available Brands of TCA Peels

Many physicians use the Delasco brand of liquid TCA, which is available in various concentrations (Fig. 20-12). Other physicians prefer to use chemical peel kits that combine TCA with an indicator that reveals when the peel has frosted. Because there are legal concerns associated with the shipping of TCA, most of the companies that sell these kits require that the practitioner purchase the TCA solution separately. Table 20-4 lists the more commonly used TCA peels on the market. Biomedic developed a combination of TCA and SA called "The Pigment Peel Plus," which is used for dyschromias and photoaging in addition to acne. Although one coat of these peels produces a superficial peel, several coats can be applied to increase the peel to one of medium depth. Other peels, such as the Obagi Blue Peel™, contain only TCA (Figs. 20-13 and 20-14). This peel is also applied in coats. One or two coats produce a superficial peel while three to four coats produce a medium-depth peel.

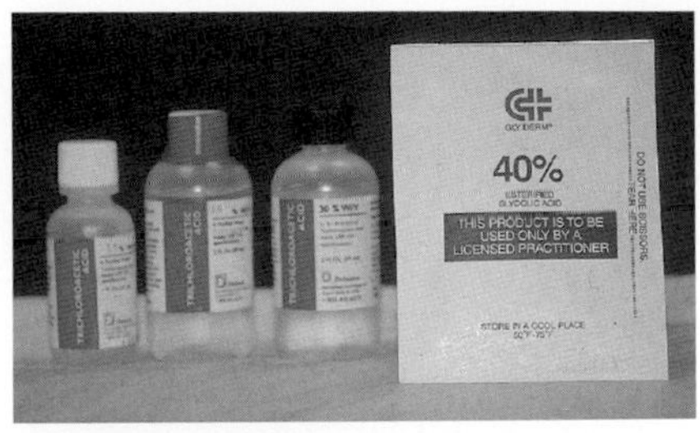

▲ **FIGURE 20-12** Delasco brand trichloroacetic acid in varying strengths. These TCA peels may be used with a prep of glycolic acid (40% shown here) or Jessner's solution.

Pyruvic Acid

Pyruvic acid is an alpha ketoacid that is physiologically converted to lactic acid, thereby rendering it a chemical peeling agent while providing hydration to the skin. Pyruvic acid penetrates down to the papillary dermis and results in increased production of collagen and elastic tissue.[44] It is important to note that pyruvic acid must not be used in high- or full strength concentration since there is the potential for scarring.[45] The pyruvic acid peel has been used

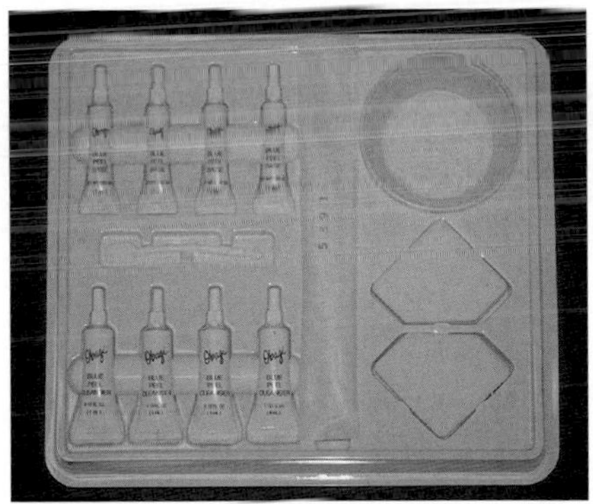
▲ **FIGURE 20-13** Obagi Blue Peel kit contains cleanser and blue base. TCA must be purchased separately.

TABLE 20-4
Comparison of Costs and Properties of Available TCA Peels

Name	Company	Strength	TCA Included	How Supplied	Cost	Cost per Patient	Ease of Use	Other
TCA 30% liquid	Delasco	30% wt/vol	Yes	2 oz bottle	$28.00	$1.00	Fast	Clear, so can drip
TCA 40% liquid	Delasco	40% wt/vol	Yes	2 oz bottle	$31.75	$1.00	Fast	Clear, so can drip
Obagi Blue Peel	Obagi	4 coats	No	Box of 6 kits	$475.00	$80.00	Time-consuming	Blue, very hard to wash off

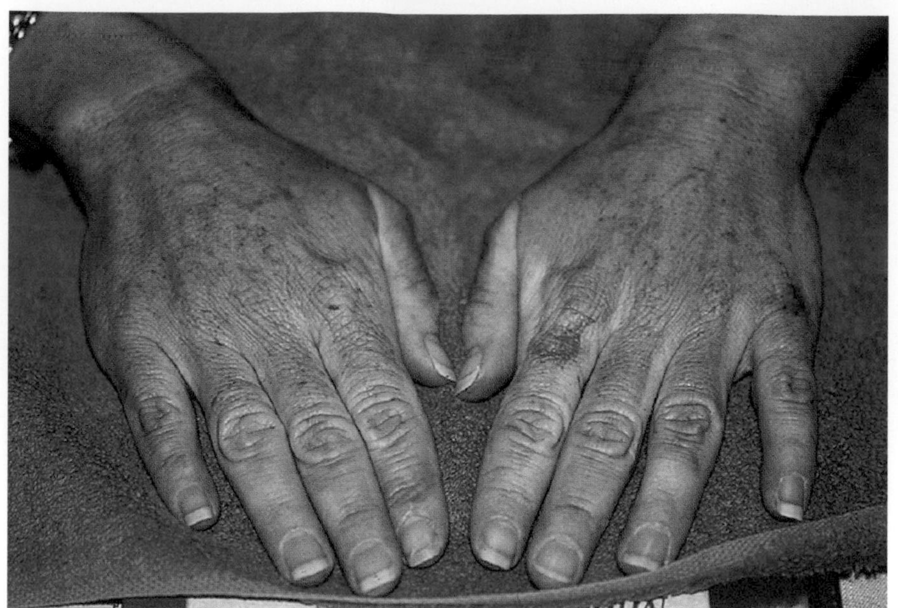

▲ **FIGURE 20-14** Obagi Blue Peel applied to hands.

with success in the treatment of moderate acne, photoaging, and melasma.[46–48] Given the fact that pyruvic acid is converted into CO_2 and acetaldehyde, the CO_2 buildup in the bottle may lead to explosion if the container is left in place for a while.[49]

This chemical peel is usually used at 40% to 60% concentrations on facial skin, previously prepared with topical retinoids. At such concentrations, it is considered a medium-depth peel and therefore must be used with caution in darker skin types or patients with sensitive or irritated skin. After 2 to 5 minutes, or when adequate frosting is observed, the face is soaked in water, which is more for the patient's comfort rather than neutralizing the peel.[50] Some authors recommend neutralizing a pyruvic acid peel with 10% sodium bicarbonate and water.[48] Since the vapors from the chemical peel may be strong and irritating to the upper respiratory tract, the procedure is best done in a well-ventilated room and with use of an electrical fan. Reepithelialization is observed in 1 to 2 weeks, while erythema may last for up to 2 months.[50] Pyruvic acid has also been used successfully in combination with 5-fluouracil for the treatment of actinic keratoses and warts.[51,52]

Side Effects and Precautions

Patients should be warned that they will look terrible for at least 10 days following a medium-depth peel. During the first 2 days, the skin appears slightly pink. On days 3 and 4 the skin darkens. By day 5 the skin begins to peel off in sheets. The peeling should be complete by day 10; however, the erythema may last until day 14. Patients should be shown pictures of how they will look so that there will be no surprises (Fig. 20-15). Many authors advise against using TCA at greater than 50% concentration. Contraindications for medium-depth peels include patients with darker skin types and those who have been recently treated with isotretinoin or topical radiation.[53] Because reepithelialization occurs from adnexal structures, some authors have theorized that patients recently treated for hair removal with lasers may have trouble healing after medium- or deep-depth peels. However, at this point, this complication has not been reported. One should be extra cautious when using medium-depth peels on the mandible, neck, and chest because these areas are more likely to get scars.

Patients should be warned that lesions such as solar lentigos may initially disap-

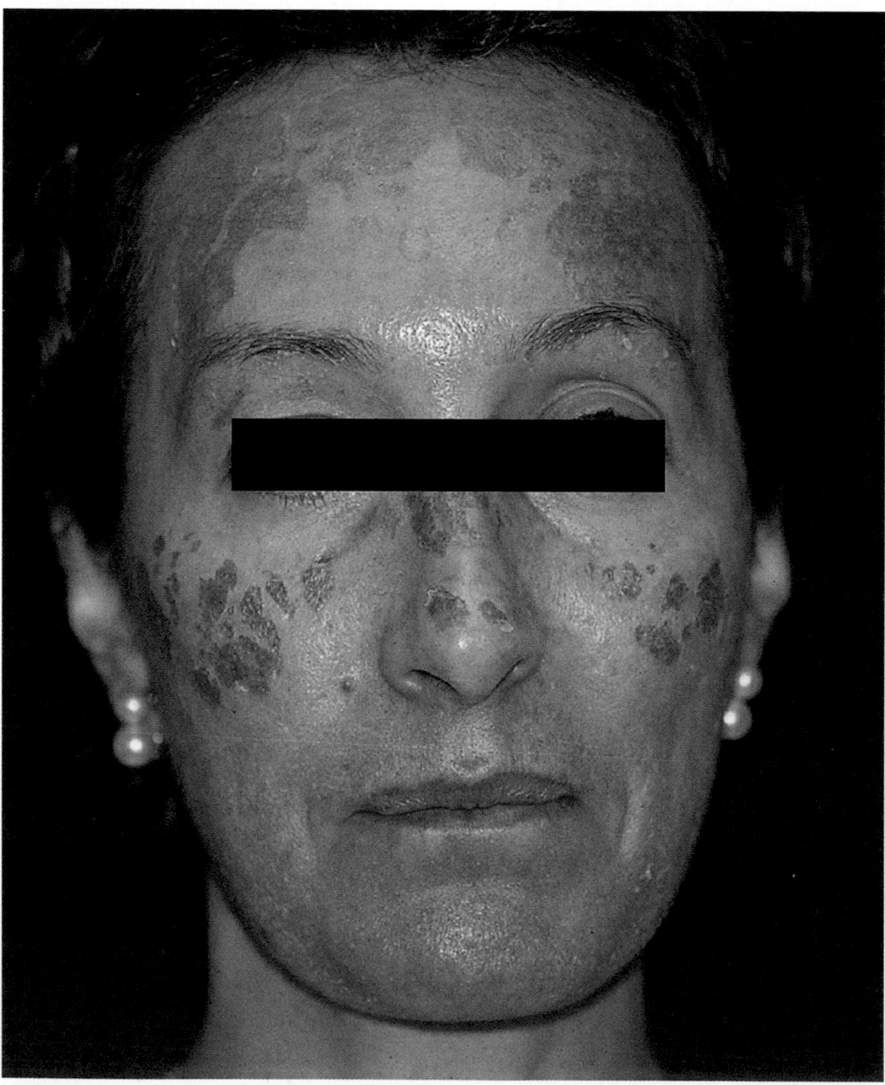

▲ **FIGURE 20-15** Patient 4 days after four coats of the Obagi Blue Peel. Patient should be told not to peel off the dark skin, but to let it peel naturally.

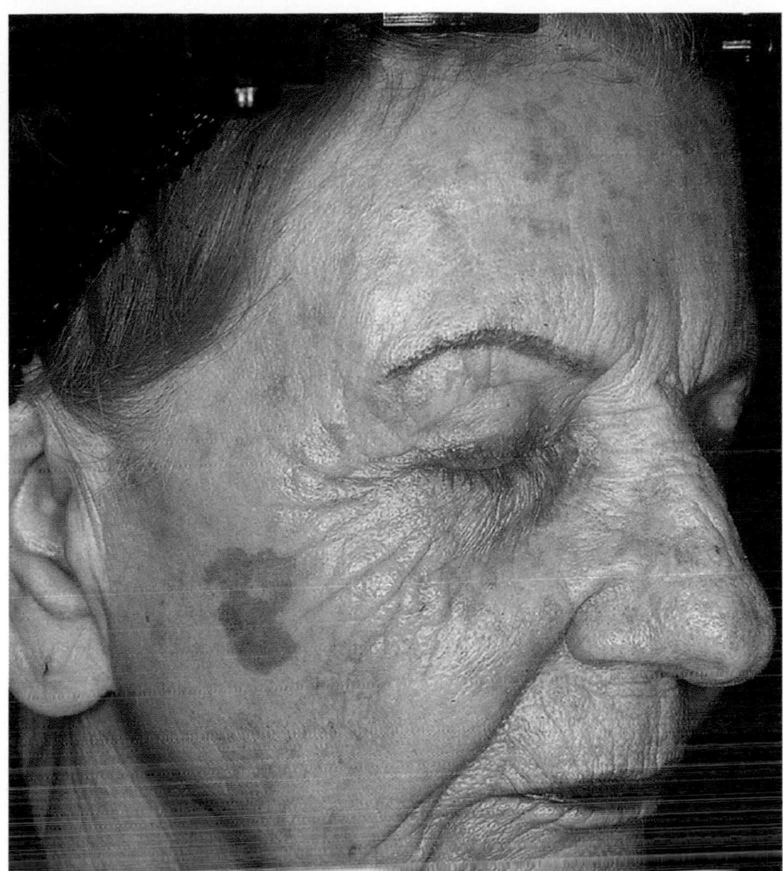

▲ **FIGURE 20-16** Patient with photodamage prior to one coat of a Jessner's peel followed immediately by the Accupeel 16%.

pear and then return after the chemical peel. This occurs because the melanocytes that are responsible for pigmentation reside below the level of the chemical peel (see Chapter 13). The results will be improved if patients use retinoids, sunscreen, and hydroquinone or other bleaching agents (Figs. 20-16 to 20-18).

Following medium peels, as with superficial ones, it is important for patients to use sunscreen and to practice sun avoidance. Patients with darker skin types should use hydroquinone after the peel to lower the incidence of hyperpigmentation. Practitioners should administer antiviral medication to patients with a history of herpes simplex infection. Also, it is important for the practitioner to avoid overzealously applying TCA, which can cause scarring. Patients recently treated with isotretinoin are also particularly vulnerable to scarring from medium peels.

COMBINATION OF SUPERFICIAL AND MEDIUM-DEPTH PEELS

Many physicians use a superficial peeling method to decrease and even out the SC and follow that up with the application of TCA. Various combinations have been used including glycolic acid followed by TCA ("Coleman peel")[54] and Jessner's peel followed by TCA ("Monheit peel"). The initial application of Jessner's solution results in reducing the cohesion of the epidermal cells, allowing better and more even penetration of the 35% TCA solution. This combination is effective in mild to moderate photoaging, including lentigines, pigmentary changes, and rhytides[55] (Box 20-3). Patients may need mild sedation and would benefit from the anti inflammatory effects of NSAIDs prior to this procedure. Dr. Harold Brody popularized the use of solid CO_2 (dry ice) followed by 35% TCA. The application of solid CO_2 also causes interruption in the epidermal consistency and deep penetration of TCA.[56] There are several excellent texts on chemical peeling that further discuss these combination methods.

DEEP-DEPTH PEELS

Laser surgery and dermabrasion have largely supplanted deep-depth peels, having shown superior results with fewer complications. Currently, there

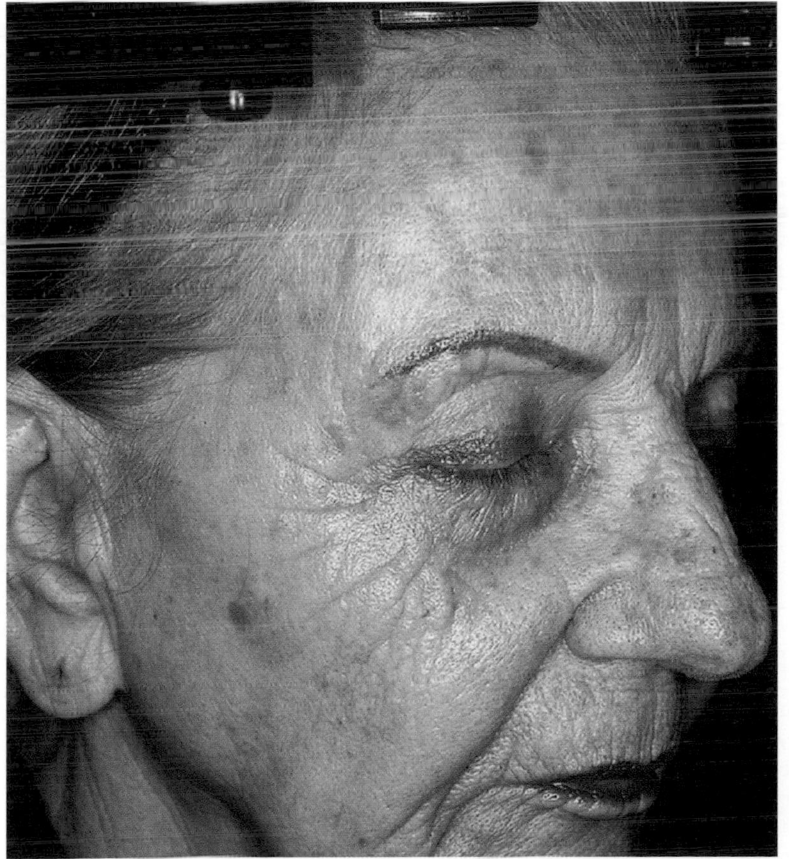

▲ **FIGURE 20-17** Same patient 4 days later. The peeling has begun. The solar lentigo on the right cheek is much inproved.

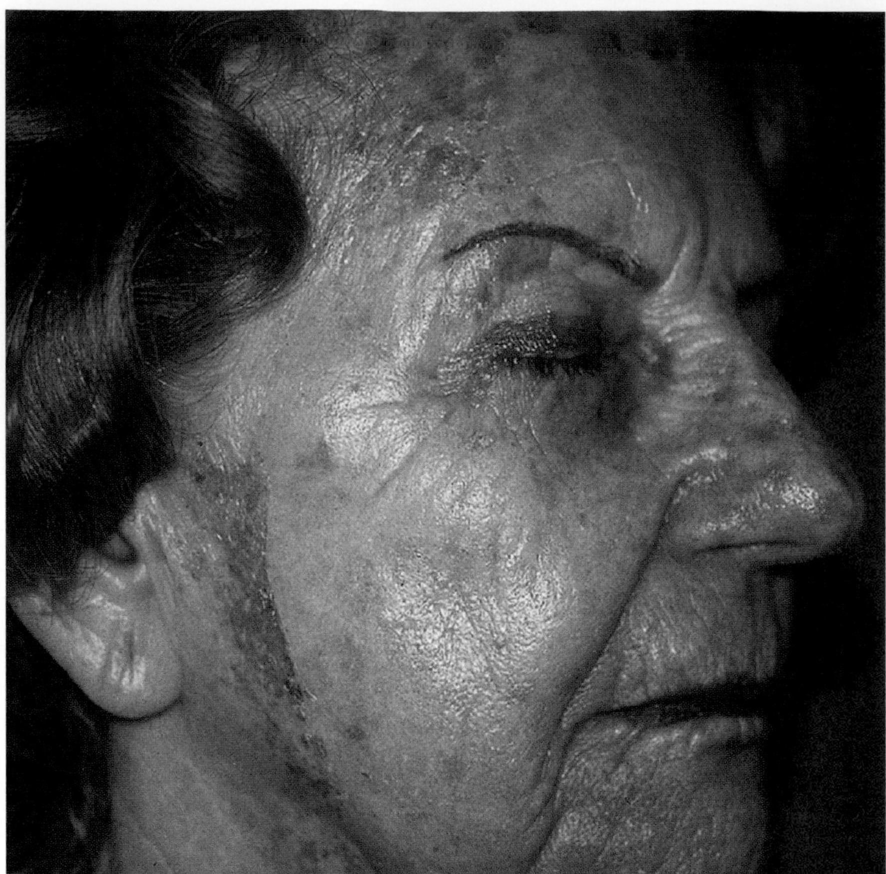

▲ **FIGURE 20-18** Eight days later. The solar lentigo on the right cheek is beginning to reappear, which is often the case with larger lesions.

BOX 20-3 Superficial Peel Indications

- *Acne and Rosacea*—BHA peels can be used in all skin types. Resorcinol can be used in Fitzpatrick skin types I and II and light type III skin. Do not treat rosacea patients with AHAs and retinoids because it worsens the erythema.
- *Melasma*—Jessner's peels, modified Jessner's peels and resorcinol are first-line choices here. Resorcinol can be used in Fitzpatrick skin types I and II and light type III skin. AHAs and BHA are also effective.
- *Photoaging and mild wrinkles*—All of the mentioned chemical peels have been shown to be useful for treatment of photoaging. The choice of which to use should be based on patient history, other concurrent pathology, and the downtime that the patient can tolerate.
- *Pretreatment for a medium-depth peel*—One can "condition" the skin for a medium peel by pretreating with any of the superficial peels. The likely method of action is the quickening of the cell cycle pace. Most physicians pretreat with topical retinoids, bleaching agents, and three to four superficial peels prior to a medium-depth peel for patients with Fitzpatrick skin type III.

Medium-depth peel indications—The indications are the same as those for superficial peels. The pathology is more significant, though. Therefore, severe acne and photoaging would respond better to medium-depth peels. Patients with a history of hyperpigmentation disorders or with Fitzpatrick skin type III or greater skin should be treated very cautiously with medium-depth peels.

are modified phenol peels such as the Stone Venner-Kellson peel (composed of phenol, croton oil, water, olive oil, and septisol solution) available, but they are rarely used by physicians in the United States. The Stone Venner-Kellson peel can be ordered from Delasco and the ordering physician must specify the ingredients. Since deep-depth peels are no longer popular and have been replaced by laser surgery, phenol peels and other deep-depth peels will not be discussed here.

AT-HOME CHEMICAL PEELS

Chemical peels used to be offered by dermatologists or trained professionals at beauty salons. Recently, many companies have developed at-home skin peel kits mostly using AHA as their main ingredient. Considering the potential side effects, especially increased photosensitivity, the FDA's AHA Review Committee and the Cosmetic, Toiletry, and Fragrance Association's (CTFA) Cosmetic Ingredient Review (CIR) Expert Panel reviewed the use of AHAs in cosmetic products.[57] In 1998, the CIR Expert Panel came to the following conclusion:

"Based on the available information included in this report, the CIR Expert Panel concludes that glycolic and lactic acid, their common salts and their simple esters, are safe for use in cosmetic products at concentrations ≤10%, at final formulation pH ≥ 3.5, when formulated to avoid increasing sun sensitivity or when directions for use include the daily use of sun protection. These ingredients are safe for use in salon products at concentrations ≤30%, at final formulation pH ≥3.0, in products designed for brief, discontinuous use followed by thorough rinsing from the skin, when applied by trained professionals, and when application is accompanied by directions for the daily use of sun protection."[58]

There are several AHA products available as at-home peel kits. Resurface Peel by Lancôme (8% glycolic acid and 5% Physio-Peel enhancer), Glytone Boost Mini Peel Gel (10.8% glycolic acid), and Dermo-Expertise ReNoviste Antiaging Glycolic Peel Kit by L'Oréal (10% glycolic acid with a patented Biosaccharide Complex) are examples of at-home glycolic acid products. Olay Regenerist Microdermabrasion & Peel System is another AHA-containing at-home peel agent in which dermacrystals are applied and gently massaged through the face for approximately 1 minute, followed by application of the activator serum. Advanced Solutions™ Facial Peel by Neutrogena is an at-home chemical peel using CelluZyme™ technology, which is touted for delivering an effect equal to 20% glycolic acid.[59]

At-home chemical peels intended for acne treatment currently on the market primarily contain SA as their main ingredient. L'Oréal's Acne Response Intensive Adult Acne Peel, which is a 2% salicylic acid-based product, and Neutrogena's Advanced Solutions Mask Eliminating

Peel, which also contains 2% SA, in addition to CelluZyme are examples of these products. Also available are peels that combine AHA and BHA, such as the Swiss Formula Peel-Off Hydroxy Masque by St. Ives, which contains both lactic acid and salicylic acid.

SUMMARY

Superficial and medium-depth peels are dynamic tools when used as part of office procedures for the treatment of acne, pigmentation disorders, and photoaging. They should be used in combination with sun avoidance, sunscreen, retinoids, and home care products to achieve maximum efficacy.

REFERENCES

1. American Society of Aesthetic Plastic Surgery 1999 statistics found at http://www.surgery.org/download/2007stats.pdf. Accessed January 17, 2008.
2. American Society of Plastic Surgeons Web site. http://www.plasticsurgery.org/media/statistics/2006-Statistics.cfm. Accessed January 15, 2008.
3. Rubin MG. What are skin peels? In: *Manual of Chemical Peels: Superficial and Medium Depth*. Philadelphia, PA: Lippincott Williams & Wilkins; 1995:19-20.
4. Swinehart JM. Salicylic acid ointment peeling of the hands and forearms. Effective nonsurgical removal of pigmented lesions and actinic damage. *J Dermatol Surg Oncol.* 1992;18:495.
5. Van Scott EJ, Yu RJ. Control of keratinization with alpha-hydroxy acids and related compounds. I. Topical treatment of ichthyotic disorders. *Arch Dermatol.* 1974;110:586.
6. Van Scott EJ, Yu RJ. Hyperkeratinization, corneocyte cohesion, and alpha hydroxy acids. *J Am Acad Dermatol.* 1984;11:867.
7. Berardesca E, Distante F, Vignoli GP, et al. Alpha hydroxyacids modulate stratum corneum barrier function. *Br J Dermatol.* 1997;137:934.
8. Ditre CM, Griffin TD, Murphy GF, et al. Effects of alpha-hydroxy acids on photoaged skin: a pilot clinical, histologic, and ultrastructural study. *J Am Acad Dermatol.* 1996;34:187.
9. Moon SE, Park SB, Ahn HT, et al. The effect of glycolic acid on photoaged albino hairless mouse skin. *Dermatol Surg.* 1999;25:179.
10. Kim SJ, Park JH, Kim DH, et al. Increased in vivo collagen synthesis and in vitro cell proliferative effect of glycolic acid. *Dermatol Surg.* 1998;24:1054.
11. Lee SH, Huh CH, Park KC, et al. Effects of repetitive superficial chemical peels on facial sebum secretion in acne patients. *J Eur Acad Dermatol Venereol.* 2006;20:964.
12. Middleton J. Sodium lactate as a moisturizer. *Cosmet Toiletries.* 1978;93:85.
13. Wehr R, Krochmal L, Bagatell F, et al. Controlled two-center study of lactate 12 percent lotion and a petrolatum-based cream in patients with xerosis. *Cutis.* 1986;37:205.
14. Smith WP. Epidermal and dermal effects of topical lactic acid. *J Am Acad Dermatol.* 1996;35:388.
15. Yu R, Van Scott E. Bioavailability of alpha-hydroxyacids in topical formulations *Cosmet Dermatol.* 1996;9:54.
16. Kligman D, Kligman AM. Salicylic acid peels for the treatment of photoaging. *Dermatol Surg.* 1998;24:325.
17. Kligman A. A comparative evaluation of a novel low-strength salicylic acid cream and glycolic acid. Products on human skin. *Cosmet Dermatol.* 1997; 10(suppl):11S.
18. Ahn HH, Kim IH. Whitening effect of salicylic acid peels in Asian patients. *Dermatol Surg.* 2006;32:372.
19. Davies M, Marks R. Studies on the effect of salicylic acid on normal skin. *Br J Dermatol.* 1976;95:187.
20. Brubacher JR, Hoffman RS. Salicylism from topical salicylates: review of the literature. *J Toxicol Clin Toxicol.* 1996;34:431.
21. Hood H, Kraeling M, Robl M, et al. The effects of an alpha hydroxy acid (glycolic acid) on hairless guinea pig skin permeability. *Food Chem Toxicol.* 1999; 37:1105.
22. Tsai T, Paul B, Jee S, et al. Effects of glycolic acid on light-induced skin pigmentation in Asian and Caucasian subjects. *J Am Acad Dermatol.* 2000;43:238.
23. Clark CP III. Alpha hydroxy acids in skin care. *Clin Plast Surg.* 1996;23:49.
24. Draelos Z. Hydroxy acids for the treatment of aging skin. *J Geriatric Dermatol,* 1997;5:336.
25. Zhai H, Hannon W, Hahn GS, et al. Strontium nitrate suppresses chemically-induced sensory irritation in humans. *Contact Dermatitis.* 2000;42:98.
26. Unna PG. Therapeutiques generales des maladies de la peau. 1882.
27. Hernández-Pérez E, Carpio E. Resorcinol peels: gross and microscopic study. *Am J Cosm Surg.* 1995;12:337.
28. Serrano G, Fortea J, Millan F, et al. Contact allergy to resorcinol in acne medications: report of three cases. *J Am Acad Dermatol.* 1992;26:502.
29. Karam PG. 50% resorcinol peel. *Int J Dermatol.* 1993;32:569.
30. Brody HJ. *Chemical Peeling and Resurfacing.* 2nd ed. New York, NY: Mosby-Year Book; 1996:82.
31. Rubin MG. Jessner's peels. In: *Manual of Chemical Peels: Superficial and Medium Depth.* Philadelphia, PA: Lippincott Williams & Wilkins; 1995:88.
32. Griffiths CE, Russman AN, Majmudar G, et al. Restoration of collagen formation in photodamaged human skin by tretinoin (retinoic acid). *N Engl J Med.* 1993;329:530.
33. Fisher GJ, Datta SC, Tawlar HS, et al. Molecular basis of sun-induced premature skin aging and retinoid antagonism. *Nature.* 1996;379:335.
34. Kligman DE, Sadiq I, Pagnoni A, et al. High-strength tretinoin: a method for rapid retinization of facial skin. *J Am Acad Dermatol.* 1998;39:S93.
35. Cucé LC, Bertino MC, Scattone L, et al. Tretinoin peeling. *Dermatol Surg.* 2001; 27:12.
36. Khunger N, Sarkar R, Jain RK. Tretinoin peels versus glycolic acid peels in the treatment of Melasma in dark-skinned patients. *Dermatol Surg* 2004;30.756.
37. Grimes PE. The safety and efficacy of salicylic acid chemical peels in darker racial-ethnic groups. *Dermatol Surg.* 1999;25:18.
38. Lim J, Tham S. Glycolic acid peels in the treatment of melasma among Asian women. *Dermatol Surg.* 1997;20:27.
39. Wang C, Huang C, Hu C, et al. The effects of glycolic acid on the treatment of melasma amoung Asian skin. *Dermatol Surg.* 1997;23:23.
40. Ayres S III. Superficial chemosurgery in treating aging skin. *Arch Dermatol.* 1962;85:385.
41. Chiarello SE, Resnik BI, Resnik SS. The TCA Masque. A new cream formulation used alone and in combination with Jessner's solution. *Dermatol Surg.* 1996;22:687.
42. Brody HJ. Chemical peels in skin resurfacing. In: Freedberg IM, Eisen AZ, Wolff K, Austen KF, Goldsmith LA, Katz SI, eds. *Fitzpatrick's General Dermatology.* 5th ed. New York, NY: McGraw-Hill; 1999:2937-2947.
43. Bridenstine JB, Dolezal JF. Standardizing chemical peel solution formulations to avoid mishaps. Great fluctuations in actual concentrations of trichloroacetic acid. *J Dermatol Surg Oncol.* 1994;20:813.
44. Moy LS, Peace S, Moy RL. Comparison of the effect of various chemical peeling agents in a mini pig model. *Dermatol Surg.* 1996;22:429.
45. Brody HJ. *Chemical Peeling and Resurfacing.* 2nd ed. New York, NY: Mosby-Year Book; 1996:130.
46. Cotellessa C, Manunta T, Ghersetich I, et al. The use of pyruvic acid in the treatment of acne. *J Eur Acad Dermatol Venereol.* 2004;18:275.
47. Ghersetich I, Brazzini B, Peris K, et al. Pyruvic acid peels for the treatment of photoaging. *Dermatol Surg.* 2004;30: 32.
48. Berardesca E, Cameli N, Primavera G, et al. Clinical and instrumental evaluation of skin improvement after treatment with a new 50% pyruvic acid peel. *Dermatol Surg.* 2006;32:526.
49. Milstein E. Is pyruvic acid potentially explosive? *Schoch Lett.* 1990;40:41.
50. Brody HJ. *Chemical Peeling and Resurfacing.* 2nd ed. New York, NY: Mosby-Year Book; 1996:131.
51. Griffin TD, Van Scott EJ. Use of pyruvic acid in the treatment of actinic keratoses: a clinical and histopathologic study. *Cutis.* 1991;47:325.
52. Halasz CL. Treatment of warts with topical pyruvic acid: with and without added 5-fluorouracil. *Cutis.* 1998;62: 283.
53. Dinner MI, Artz JS. The art of the trichloroacetic acid chemical peel. *Clin Plast Surg.* 1998;25:53.
54. Coleman WP III, Futrell JM. The glycolic acid trichloroacetic acid peel. *J Dermatol Surg Oncol.* 1994;20:76.
55. Monheit GD. Medium-depth chemical peels. *Dermatol Clin.* 2001;19:413.
56. Brody HJ. *Chemical Peeling and Resurfacing.* St. Louis, MO: Mosby; 1997:109-110.

57. Guidance for Industry. Labeling for Topically Applied Cosmetic Products Containing Alpha Hydroxy Acids as Ingredients. January 20, 2005. http://www.cfsan.fda.gov/~dms/ahaguid2.html. Accessed January 14, 2008.
58. Andersen FA. Final report on the safety assessment of glycolic acid, ammonium, calcium, potassium, and sodium glycolates, methyl, ethyl, propyl, and butyl glycolates, and lactic acid, ammonium, calcium, potassium, sodium, and TEA-lactates, methyl, ethyl, isopropyl, and butyl lactates, and lauryl, myristyl, and cetyl lactates. *Int J Toxicol*. 1998; 17:S1.
59. Neutrogena Corp. http://www.neutrogena.com/. Accessed February 25, 2008.

CHAPTER 21

Prevention and Treatment of Bruising

Susan Schaffer, RN
Sogol Saghari, MD
Leslie Baumann, MD

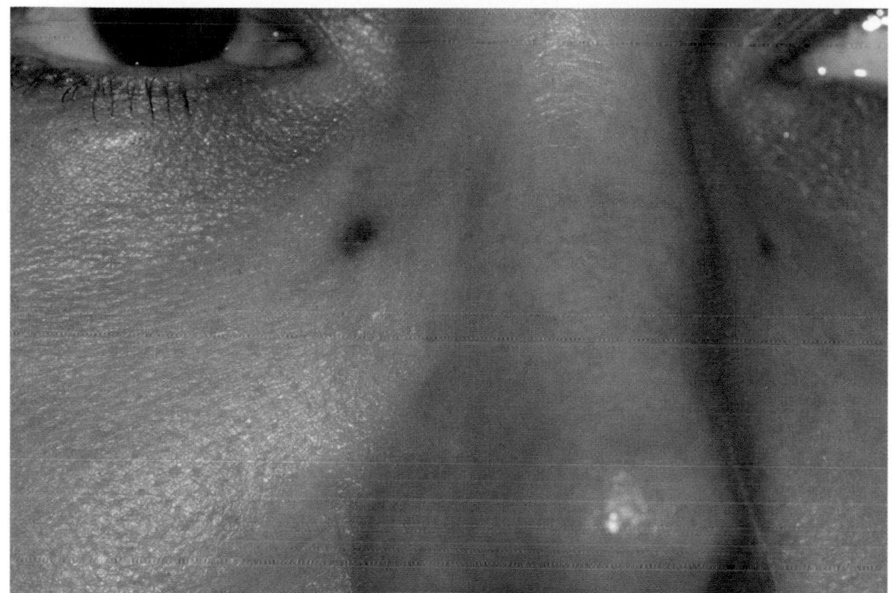

▲ **FIGURE 21-2** Bruising 2 days after treatment with Botox to bunny lines in a patient on ibuprofen.

Ecchymoses, also known as bruises, occur as a result of an injury to the capillaries, allowing blood to leak into the underlying tissue (Figs. 21-1 and 21-2). This is a benign process that resolves within a few days. Hematoma is a more serious entity, when an injury to a blood vessel results in the collection of blood in the surrounding tissue. The enlarging size of the hematoma may push on vital organs or lead to tissue necrosis; therefore, they should be avoided. Hematomas may be treated conservatively with pressure dressings, if active bleeding is not present, or by drainage, if there is active bleeding or the hematoma is enlarging in size.

In a healthy individual with a small injury to a capillary, the coagulation process results in a fibrin clot in the damaged area and eventually healing of the vessel. Platelets are an essential component in the coagulation process. They become activated via exposure to the endothelial lining of the damaged blood vessel, and produce coagulation factors in addition to adhering to the damaged tissue and forming a platelet clog. The process of hemostasis also involves the coagulation pathway, a complicated cascade involving two routes: the *contact activation pathway*, also known as the *intrinsic pathway*, and the *tissue factor pathway*, also known as the *extrinsic pathway* (Fig. 21-3). Several cofactors are required for the proper functioning of the coagulation pathway. Vitamin K is an essential factor for a hepatic enzyme known as gamma glutamyl carboxylase, which is involved in the synthesis of factors II, VII, IX, and X. Calcium is also required in several steps of the coagulation pathway. In addition, there are natural anticoagulants present, such as proteins C and S, which are beyond the scope of our discussion.

Following coagulation and clot formation, the fibrinolysis process, which is necessary for breaking down the clot, occurs. This pathway starts with the activation of plasminogen, a protein synthesized in the liver that is converted to plasmin via tissue plasminogen activator (tPA) and other factors (Fig. 21-4). Plasmin degrades fibrin into fibrin degradation products (FDPs), which are the end result of this cascade.

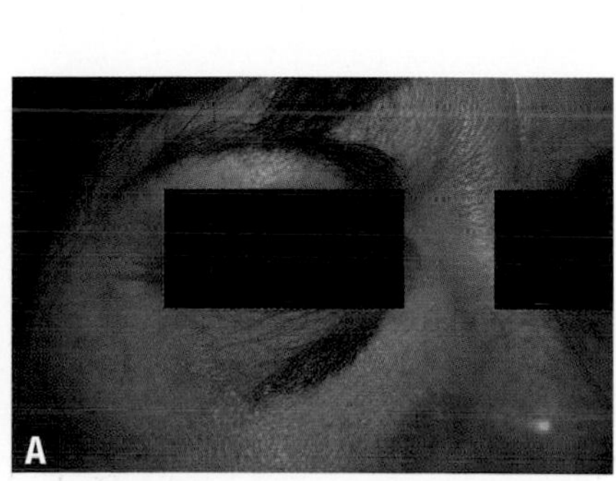

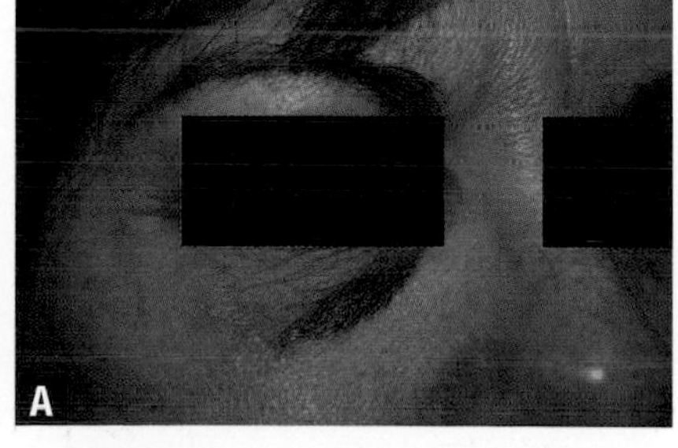

▲ **FIGURE 21-1** **A.** Bruising after Juvéderm to the under eye area. **B.** Bruising after Hylaform to the under eye area.

RATING BRUISE SEVERITY

At this time there are no published scales rating bruise severity. Rating bruise severity is important if one wants to evaluate treatments aimed at preventing bruising or accelerating the healing of bruises. The authors have developed the Baumann-Castanedo scale to rate bruises. This scale is displayed in Tables 21-1 and 21-2. The Baumann-Castanedo scale will allow the user to track the color and size of the bruise in order to gauge severity and improvement.

PREVENTION AND TREATMENT

The initial bruised area is purplish-red in color, later changing to green and yellow before the discoloration eventually disappears. Hemoglobin in the red blood cells is responsible for the red-purple color of the bruise. The two natural

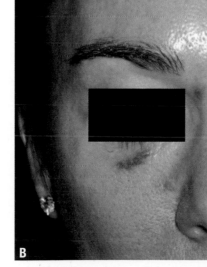

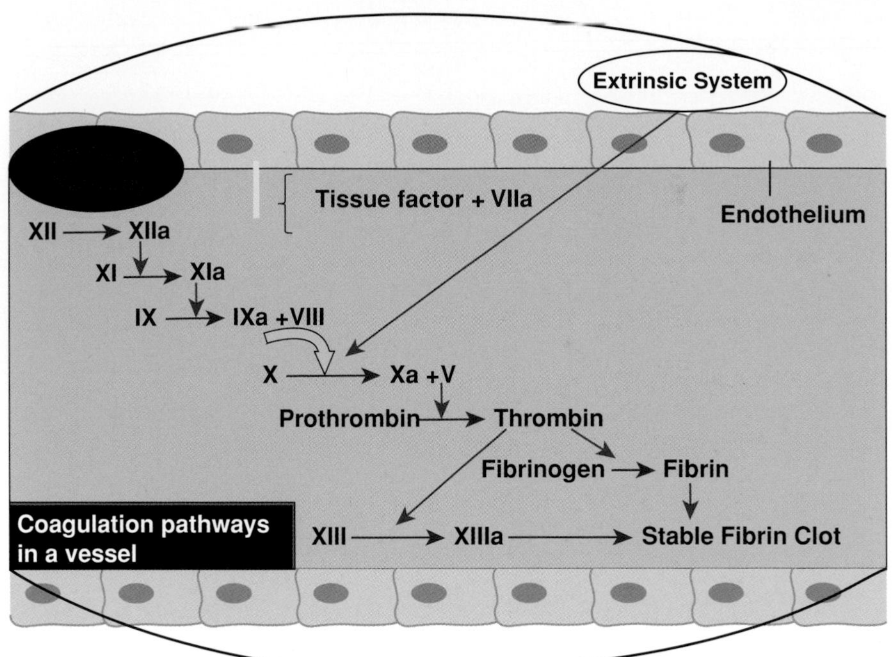

▲ **FIGURE 21-3** Coagulation pathway.

breakdown products of hemoglobin cause the color alteration in a bruise. Hemoglobin breaks down to biliverdin (green), which in turn is metabolized to bilirubin (yellow) (Fig. 21-5).

When performing a cosmetic procedure with possible bleeding, it is helpful to ask patients about any history of bleeding disorders or usage of anticoagulant medications. It is also important to advise patients to avoid certain medications 10 days prior to the procedure (Table 21-3). A list of these medications and supplements should be reviewed over the phone and faxed or mailed to the patient at the time the appointment is made so that when they arrive at their appointment, they will not have taken any of these products. This practice will greatly decrease the amount of bruising that occurs if the staff is methodical about this warning. NSAIDs including ASA are well recognized for their antiplatelet effects. Other supplements such as garlic and ginkgo are also known for inhibitory effects on platelets.[1] In addition, green tea enhances the tendency to bleed by antiplatelet activity.[2] Vitamin E appears to exert its bleeding effect by inhibition of the intrinsic coagulation pathway.[3]

Bruising may also be prevented or treated by using certain herbal supplements such as bromelain and arnica, which will be discussed briefly.

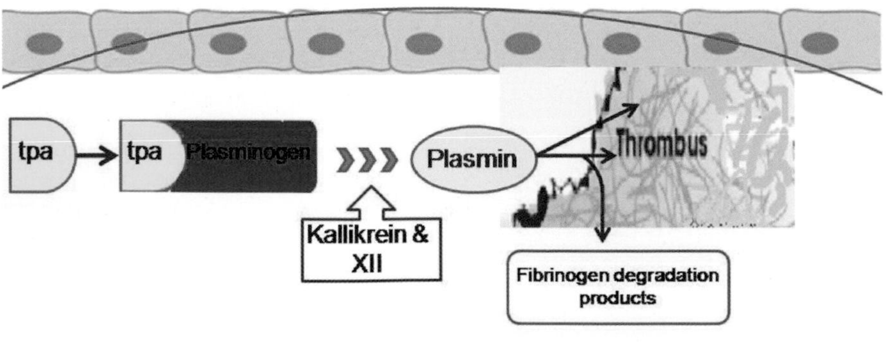

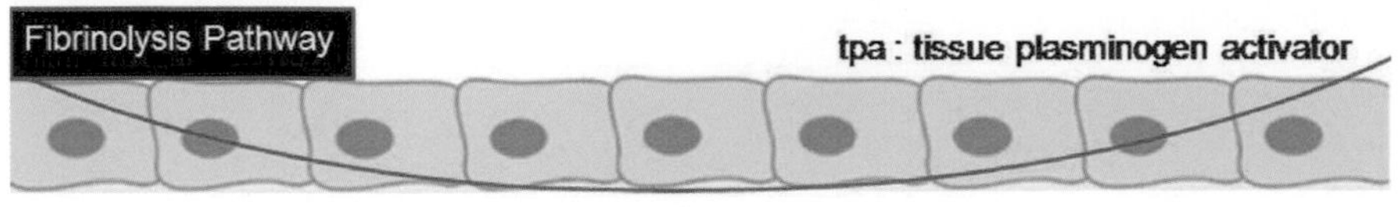

▲ **FIGURE 21-4** Fibrinolysis pathway.

TABLE 21-1
Bruise Dimension Scale

0 = no bruise
1 = 0.1 cm–0.4 cm
2 = 0.5–1.0 cm
3 = 1.1–2.0 cm
4 = 2.1–3.0 cm
5 = 3.1 cm or larger

Bromelain

Bromelain is a substance naturally present in mature pineapple stem (*Ananas comosus*) and contains proteolytic enzymes.[4,5] Over the years it has been used in medical settings for its antithrombotic, fibrinolytic, and anti-inflammatory effects.[6] It is believed that bromelain exerts its anticoagulant activity via inhibition of platelet aggregation.[7] Pirotta and De Guili-Morghen explained the fibrinolytic activity of bromelain in rats by activating plasminogen conversion to plasmin.[8] Bromelain has also been shown to decrease vascular permeability by lowering the levels of bradykinin, resulting in decreased edema, pain, and inflammation.[9] There is no standard recommended dose for bromelain consumption. Bromelain has been used in different doses ranging from 200 to 2000 mg.[6] In treating human osteoarthritis, bromelain has been used in doses anywhere from 540 to 1890 mg/d with successful results.[10–12] Bromelain is considered safe; however, a higher incidence of adverse events (e.g., headache, gastrointestinal symptoms, and cutaneous rash) have been observed with higher doses.[13] Notably, bromelain should not be recommended to patients on anticoagulant medications, such as warfarin and aspirin, prior to consulting their primary care physicians. Most cosmetic dermatology practices recommend bromelain 500 mg twice a day for 1 day following a procedure to prevent bruising, or if bruising occurs, 500 mg twice a day until the bruising has cleared. Bromlelain should not be taken *prior* to the procedure because in the author's experience it seems to increase bruising rather than prevent it.

TABLE 21-2
Bruise Progression Scale (According to Changes in Color)

1 = Pink/Red
2 = Purple/Dark Blue
3 = Green/Dark Yellow
4 = Pale Yellow/Brown
5 = Hint of color

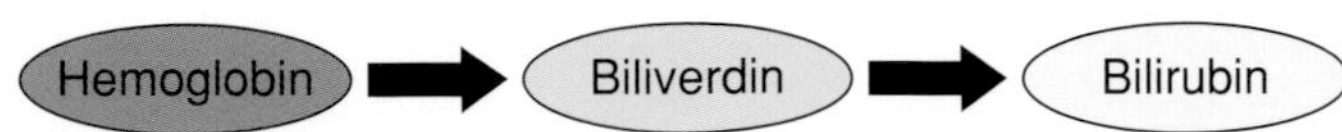

▲ **FIGURE 21-5** Color change in bruising.

Arnica

Arnica, also known as leopard's bane or mountain tobacco, is an extract derived from several mountain plants, including *Arnica montana, Arnica chamissonis, Arnica fulgens, Arnica cordifolia,* and *Arnica sororia.* It is widely used in homeopathic practice because arnica contains helenalin, a sesquiterpene lactone that is the major active ingredient conferring anti-inflammatory effects.[14] Helenalin has been shown to inhibit the activation of NF-κB in T cells, B cells, and epithelial cells;[14] NF-κB is considered a transcription factor of several cytokines.[15] The exact mechanism of action of arnica in the treatment of bruises remains unknown; however, it has been proposed that arnica affects platelet function in vitro.[16] The clinical trials for treatment of ecchymoses with arnica are conflicting. In a study of 200 patients who underwent a wisdom tooth removal or apicoectomy, subjects received arnica 3 days prior to the procedure and twice daily after the procedure in case of edema. A 90% success rate with no swelling or ecchymoses was reported. However, this study lacked a blinded control group. Alonso et al. evaluated 19 patients with facial telangiectasia in a double-blinded, placebo-controlled laser study.[17] Subjects were divided into pre and posttreatment groups for treatment with pulsed dye laser. The pretreatment group received topical arnica gel with vehicle on one side and vehicle only on the other side of the face for 2 weeks prior to laser treatment. The posttreatment group followed the same regimen after the laser procedure. No statistically significant differences were noted in the prevention or accelerated clearing of the ecchymoses.[18] However, this study used a homeopathic formulation of arnica that contained very low amounts of arnica. It is possible that a formulation with a higher amount of arnica would have showed success. Another multicenter, randomized, double-blind, placebo-controlled study of 130 patients with phlebectomy also failed to show a difference among patients treated with arnica (pre- and postprocedure) compared to the control group.[19] However, in the author's experience, bruising seems to be prevented when the patient is advised to take four homeopathic arnica pills labeled "with 30x dilution" 4 to 6 hours prior to a cosmetic procedure. High doses of oral arnica can be harmful, so patients should be warned not to exceed this dose. Some people are sensitive to the compound helenalin found in arnica. If they as develop a mild rash, they are likely helenalin sensitive and should stop using arnica. In the author's practice, arnica gel is applied to the treated area after every cosmetic procedure. It is used to massage patients after Sculptra treatments (see Chapter 23). Patients are instructed to apply the arnica creams 3 times a day at home until bruises clear. Donell Super Skin K-Derm Gel and Boiron Arnica Cream are popular brands of topical arnica that are easily found in pharmacies and mass market outlets.

TABLE 21-3
Medications and Supplements to Avoid at Least 10 Days Prior to Undergoing Cosmetic Procedures

NSAIDs (Aspirin, Advil, Motrin, Ibuprofen)
Vitamin E
Green tea
Garlic
Ginkgo
Ginseng
St. John's Wort

SUMMARY

Although bruising may be prevented by certain techniques in dermatologic practice, bruises are considered an inevitable side effect of injectable procedures. Therefore, it is incumbent upon the practitioner to inform the patient of this minor side effect. Patients need to be aware that bruises may take approximately 7 to 14 days to clear, so they can make appropriate adjustments to their schedules.

REFERENCES

1. Ang-Lee MK, Moss J, Yuan CS. Herbal medicines and perioperative care. *JAMA.* 2001;286:208.
2. Kang WS, Lim IH, Yuk DY, et al. Antithrombotic activities of green tea catechins and (−)-epigallocatechin gallate. *Thromb Res.* 1999;96:229.
3. Marsh SA, Coombes JS. Vitamin E and alpha-lipoic acid supplementation increase bleeding tendency via an intrinsic coagulation pathway. *Clin Appl Thromb Hemost.* 2006;12:169.
4. Rowan AD, Buttle DJ, Barrett AJ. The cysteine proteinases of the pineapple plant. *Biochem J.* 1990;266:869.
5. Rowan AD, Buttle DJ. Pineapple cysteine endopeptidases. *Methods Enzymol.* 1994;244:555.
6. Maurer HR. Bromelain: biochemistry, pharmacology and medical use. *Cell Mol Life Sci.* 2001;58:1234.
7. Glaser D, Hilberg T. The influence of bromelain on platelet count and platelet activity *in vitro. Platelets.* 2006;17:37.
8. Pirotta F, De Giuli-Morghen C. Bromelain—A deeper pharmacological study. I. Anti-inflammatory and serum fibrinolytic activity after administration of bromelain in the rat. *Drugs Exptl Clin Res.* 1978;4:1.
9. Kumakura S, Yamashita M, Tsurufuji S. Effect of bromelain on kaolin-induced inflammation in rats. *Eur J Pharmacol.* 1988;150:295.
10. Singer F, Singer C, Oberleitner H. Phlogenzyme versus diclofenac in the treatment of activated osteoarthritis of the knee. *Int J Immunother.* 2001;17:135.
11. Singer F, Oberleitner H. Drug therapy of activated arthrosis. On the effectiveness of an enzyme mixture versus diclofenac. *Wien Med Wochenschr.* 1996;146:55.
12. Tilwe GH, Beria S, Turakhia NH, et al. Efficacy and tolerability of oral enzyme therapy as compared to diclofenac in active osteoarthritis of knee joint: an open randomized controlled clinical trial. *J Assoc Physicians India.* 2001;49:617.
13. Brien S, Lewith G, Walker A, et al. Bromelain as a treatment for osteoarthritis: a review of clinical studies. *Evid Based Complement Alternat Med.* 2004;1:251.
14. Lyss G, Schmidt TJ, Merfort I, et al. Helenalin, an anti-inflammatory sesquiterpene lactone from *Arnica,* selectively inhibits transcription factor NF-κB. *Biol Chem.* 1997;378:951.
15. Baeuerle PA, Henkel T. Function and activation of NF-κB in the immune system. *Annu Rev Immunol.* 1994;12:141.
16. Schroder H, Losche W, Strobach H, et al. Helenalin and 11α, 13-dihydrohelenalin, two constituents from *Arnica montana* L., inhibit human platelet function via thiol-dependent pathways. *Thromb Res.* 1990;57:839.
17. McIvor EG. Arnica montana: a clinical trial following surgery or trauma. *J Am Inst Homeopath.* 1973;66:81.
18. Alonso D, Lazarus MC, Baumann L. Effects of topical arnica gel on post-laser treatment bruises. *Dermatol Surg.* 2002;28:686.
19. Ramelet AA, Buchheim G, Lorenz P, et al. Homeopathic arnica in postoperative haematomas: a double-blind study. *Dermatology.* 2000;201:347.

SECTION 4

Cosmetic Procedures

CHAPTER 22

Botulinum Toxin

Leslie Baumann, MD
Mohamed L. Elsaie, MD
Lisa Grunebaum, MD

Botulinum toxin (BTX), an exotoxin produced by the bacteria *Clostridium botulinum,* occurs naturally in nature. BTX induces a bilaterally symmetric descending neuroparalytic condition called botulism. The word "botulinum" is derived from the Latin word for sausage, "botulus." Botulism was so named during the Napoleonic Empire in the early 1800s when it was noted to be triggered by the ingestion of spoiled sausages. Later, German physician Justinus Kerner described food-borne botulism and its clinical symptoms during the period between 1817 and 1822. In 1946, Schantz reported isolating BTX type A in its crystalline form, and nearly a quarter of a century later, Alan Scott became the first to harness the effects of BTX for medicinal use in monkey strabismus.[1]

The use of *C. botulinum* A exotoxin, commonly known as botulinum toxin type A (BTX-A), has emerged over the last decade as one of the most popular methods of combating cutaneous signs of aging, particularly the dynamic wrinkles of the face. The therapeutic application of this potent neurotoxin has carved a comfortable niche in the cosmetic realm of dermatology practice for practical reasons: Results appear within several days of administration, the procedure itself is short in duration and relatively uncomplicated, and side effects are minimal.

Although medicinal use of BTX by physicians is widespread, professional opinions vary as to the best ways to administer the treatment. For instance, the ideal dilution of the toxin, the number of units to inject, and the longevity of prepared and refrigerated BTX remain debated issues (Box 22-1). The methods described in this chapter are those used most frequently by the primary author. The novice injector should try the various methods espoused by experienced specialists to determine which yields the best results in his/her own practice.

BOX 22-1 Units of Botulinum Toxin

One unit (U) of BTX is the dose that would be lethal to 50% (LD_{50}) of the specific mouse species tested. For a 70-kg person, the LD_{50} of Botox is 2500 to 3000 U. However, manufacturers use different mouse models, so a unit of one brand is not equivalent to a unit of another brand. Because of these variations, it is important to know which type of BTX was used when evaluating dosing information in the literature. For cosmetic indications, injection of approximately 20 to 75 U doses of Botox is typical. Practitioners have used doses as high as 1000 Botox units to treat cerebral palsy and other neurologic conditions.

MECHANISMS OF ACTION

Acetylcholine (ACh) is the neurotransmitter associated with induction of muscle movement. BTX achieves chemical denervation of striated muscles by cleaving one or more of the proteins required for the release of ACh (Fig. 22-1). The target protein depends on the serotype of toxin used (Table 22-1). The result is temporary flaccid paralysis of the injected muscles, which persists approximately 3 to 5 months. As new neuromuscular junctions form, muscle function returns. There are seven BTX serotypes (A–G). Serotype A is the most potent and was the first to be made available in the United States for medical use. Botox Cosmetic™ (Allergan Inc., Irvine, CA) and Dysport™ (Ipsen Products, Maidenhead, Berkshire, UK) are both formed from serotype A, which functions by cleaving the SNAP-25 protein, a component of the SNARE (Soluble *N*-ethylmaleamide-sensitive factor Attachment protein Receptor) complex (Box 22-2). The presence of an intact SNARE complex, composed of synaptobrevin, SNAP-25, and syntaxin, is necessary for vesicles containing ACh to fuse with the cell membrane and to release ACh into the neuromuscular junction (Fig. 22-1). BTX B, now available in the United States as Myobloc™ (known as Neurobloc in Europe), cleaves synaptobrevin, thus preventing the release of ACh.

TABLE 22-1
Binding Sites of Various Toxin Serotypes

Toxin Serotype	Binding Site
BTX-A	SNAP-25
BTX-B	Synaptobrevin
BTX-C1	SNAP-25 and syntaxin
BTX-D	Synaptobrevin
BTX-E	SNAP-25
BTX-F	Synaptobrevin
BTX-G	Synaptobrevin

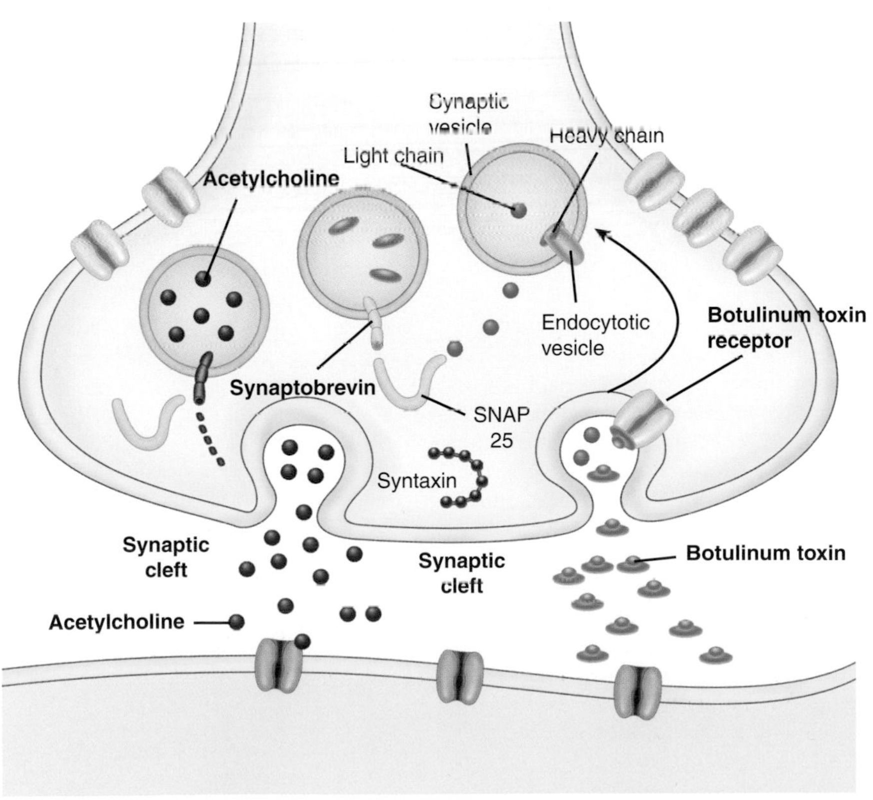

▲ **FIGURE 22-1** Botulinum toxins inhibit the release of acetylcholine into the neuromuscular junction.

BOX 22-2 Composition of Botulinum Toxin

BTX is composed of three domains: the binding domain, the translocation domain, and the enzymatic domain. The binding domain is responsible for attaching to the presynaptic nerve terminal. (These receptors are specific to each BTX serotype and the serotypes do not bind to each other's acceptors.) Binding of the toxin initiates endocytosis and internalization of the molecule. Once inside the endosome, the acidic environment is believed to create a change in the conformation of the translocation domain of the toxin that allows the light chain to cross the membrane of the endosome and enter the cytosol.[2] Once released into the cytosol, the enzymatic domain residing in the light chain cleaves a protein in the SNARE complex that inactivates this complex, preventing the fusion of ACh vesicles and blocking release of ACh into the synaptic cleft. The specific cleaved SNARE complex protein depends on the BTX serotype. BTX-A cleaves the SNAP-25 molecule at the peptide bond between glutamine 197 and arginine 198 and BTX-B cleaves synaptobrevin between the amino acid residues glutamine 76 and phenylalanine 77.[3] Interestingly, tetanus toxin also cleaves synaptobrevin, but uses a different enzyme.

CLINICAL INDICATIONS

In the 1970s, Dr. Alan Scott became the first scientist to use BTX to treat strabismus in monkeys. Within 7 years, he had performed the first human trials.[4] Subsequently, ophthalmologists began using BTX to treat strabismus, nystagmus, and blepharospasm.[5,6] In 1990, the first paper reporting the use of BTX for cosmetic purposes was published.[7] Since that time, the use of BTX has become increasingly widespread and is currently the most popular nonsurgical cosmetic procedure, with 2.78 million injections performed in 2007.[8] The use of Botox Cosmetic in the United States grew by 4159.2% from 1997 to 2007 despite the fact that the FDA had yet to approve of its use for cosmetic purposes until halfway through this period![7,8]

The cosmetic indications for BTX currently include the prevention and treatment of dynamic wrinkles (wrinkles "in motion") and amelioration of excessive sweating (hyperhidrosis). BTX is also used to ameliorate platysmal banding in the neck, which leads to a condition commonly known as "turkey neck." Some practitioners have also obtained satisfactory results in treating the signs of aging in the lower face.[9,10] New indications are frequently reported.

BOTULINUM TOXIN TYPE A

Botox Cosmetic

Initially introduced as Botox™, this product was first used for cosmetic purposes in 1981. Botox Cosmetic, still usually referred to as Botox, was approved by the FDA in 2002 for treatment of (glabellar) frown lines. Botox is formed from fermented cultures of *C. botulinum*. The cultures are subjected to autolysis, releasing a 900 kD toxic complex. Prior to placement in storage vials, the compound is diluted with human serum albumin. The manufacturers then freeze dry and seal the toxin. One vial of Botox contains 100 U of BTX-A.

DILUTION AND STORAGE Physicians do not agree on the optimal dilution ratio for the toxin or on how long the toxin retains its potency after dilution. However, Klein published a survey of expert Botox users and found that most of them use a dilution of 2.5 cc per 100-U vial.[11] This dilution was used in the Allergan FDA trials as well. Reports in the literature support the use of 1 cc to 10 cc dilutions.[11] See Table 22-2 for dilution guidelines.

The 100-U bottle of Botox is diluted with 0.9% saline. Preservative-free saline was recommended initially until studies showed that pain perception was decreased when preservative-containing saline was used.[12] When diluting the bottle, care must be taken to gently inject the saline into the bottle to prevent foaming and bubbles, which may denature the toxin and decrease its potency. Many physicians remove the rubber stopper before adding the saline, which prevents the rapid addition of saline to the bottle because of the vacuum of the bottle and helps avoid leaving a few expensive drops of BTX-A in the vial. Novice practitioners should be advised to never insert the needle of the syringe that is to be used for injection into the rubber stopper. This would make it dull and increase the pain on injection. In addition, it is important not to shake the bottle or "flick" the syringe to eliminate air bubbles as agitation of the toxin may lead to loss of potency.

Once the BTX-A has been diluted with saline, it begins to lose potency, but the point at which the potency losses become clinically significant is unknown. Many authors suggest that BTX-A should be used within 48 hours; however, a few authors state that Botox may remain in the refrigerator up to 4 weeks.[13] If one plans to keep Botox for an extended period of time, preservative-containing saline should be used and the reconstituted Botox should be kept in a refrigerator. In the primary author's experience, the best Botox is "fresh" Botox and should be used within 24 hours of dilution. Botox should not be refrozen once prepared as this also causes a definite loss of potency, due to the formation of ice crystals.

TABLE 22-2
The Amount of Saline Used to Dilute Botox Determines the Number of Units in Each 0.1 cc

Dilution Table for Botox

Volume of Diluent Added (cc)	Number of Units per 0.1 cc
1.0	10
2.0	5
2.5	4
3.0	3.3

Reloxin/Dysport

Dysport is sold in bottles containing 500 U of BTX-A. Dysport will be marketed in the United States as Reloxin™. Medicis Pharmaceutical Corporation, which will manufacture and distribute Reloxin in the United States, was awaiting FDA approval for this product at the time of publication. Because Reloxin is simply the American brand name for Dysport, which is produced in the United Kingdom, the terms are interchangeable. Reloxin will be the term used for the remainder of this portion of the discussion. Similar to Botox, the neurotoxin is produced from *C. botulinum*. One unit of Botox is equivalent to 2.5 to 4 U of Reloxin.[14,15] The units and dilution must be adjusted accordingly. Reloxin is manufactured as freeze-dried 500-U vials and preserved as a powder. One bottle of Botox contains 5 ng of protein while a vial of Reloxin contains 4.35 ng.[16]

DILUTION AND STORAGE The shelf life of the packaged Reloxin vial is approximately 1 year, if refrigerated at 2 to 8°C.[17] The vial should be used within 24 hours of reconstitution, for the same reasons that this is recommended with Botox. Reloxin can be diluted with 0.9% preservative-free or preservative-containing saline as suggested in Table 22-3. Using a dilution with 2.5 mL provides 20 U of Reloxin per 0.1 mL. Reconstituted Reloxin should not be frozen.

A series of separate studies on glabellar lines were carried out at major cosmetic centers across the United States in order to assess the efficacy, tolerability, and safety of Reloxin prior to FDA approval. In two parallel groups of placebo-controlled double-blinded studies including 300 and 158 patients, respectively, subjects were randomized to either Reloxin (50 U) or placebo. The study durations were respectively 150 and 180 days. Based on visual response scales assessed by investigators and patients, both studies concluded that at 30 days postinjection, Reloxin significantly reached study-designed improvement endpoints in 90% of patients and reduced the severity of glabellar lines significantly better than placebo ($p < 0.001$). The median time of onset was either 2 or 3 days for both studies. The median duration of effect was 85 days, with significant efficacy through day 120.[18]

A larger multicenter open-label study was carried out in 21 centers across the United States and enrolled 1200 patients over a 13-month duration. Reloxin (50 U) was used for glabellar lines to assess effectiveness and duration. Results suggested an onset of action within 3 days and a median duration of 88 days for effect. In all series, Reloxin was deemed safe with negligible adverse effects.[19] Reloxin performs similarly to Botox and is injected in the same sites and manner as Botox. It is important to remember that the dose of Reloxin is different than the dose of Botox; otherwise, these are virtually identical products.

XEOMIN Xeomin® (Merz Pharmaceuticals, Frankfurt, Germany) is also a BTX-A product containing only the 150 kDa neurotoxin component. The smaller size of this compound may increase its diffusion rates; however, this has not been clearly established. Xeomin was introduced in Germany in 2005 and is not currently available in other European countries or the United States. It is manufactured as 100-U vials. Merz Pharmaceuticals claims that the product is highly purified and contains only 600 pg of bacterial proteins,[20] which may result in lower immune response. In addition, Xeomin differs from Botox and Reloxin in one of its constituent elements. While Botox and Reloxin contain sodium chloride and lactose, respectively, Xeomin contains saccharose. The clinical conversion rate of Botox to Xeomin is reported as 1:1.[21] A number of major studies conducted and reported by Jost et al. demonstrated equal efficacy and safety profiles of Xeomin in the treatment of focal dystonias as compared to Botox. The five clinical trials involved 862 patients and found no difference between the two BTX-A toxins in terms of onset of action, duration, or waning of effect.[22] Further research is needed to evaluate efficacy in cosmetic dermatology and antigenic response of this product.

TABLE 22-3
Reloxin Dilution Table[a]

DILUENT: 0.9% SALINE	300 U VIAL	125 U VIAL
1.0 mL	30 U	12.5 U
2.0 mL	15 U	6.25 U
2.5 mL	12 U	5 U
3.0 mL	10 U	4.1 U

[a]Units per 0.1 mL.

NEURONOX Neuronox® is a BTX-A complex manufactured by Medy-Tox, Inc. (Seoul, South Korea). Neuronox was introduced in South Korea and is currently available in Asia, the Middle East, and Africa. It is manufactured as 100-U vials of neurotoxin along with 0.5 mg of human serum albumin and 0.9 mg of sodium chloride. The conversion rate of Neuronox to Botox is reported to be 1:1. The manufacturers of Neuronox claim that their product is safe and effective; however, efficacy, tolerability, and safety needs to be evaluated by further well-designed research investigations.[23]

PROSIGNE Prosigne® (Lanzhou Institute of Biological Products, Lanzhou, China) is a BTX-A product available in China, Southeast Asia, and certain parts of South America. The product is manufactured as 50- and 100-U vials. There is a lack of evidence regarding the clinical efficacy and safety of Prosigne for the treatment of focal dystonias and hemifacial spasm. Evidence is also lacking in terms of ascertaining the precise role of Prosigne in the cosmetic realm. To date, only two studies have evaluated this product. Tang et al. retrospectively studied 785 patients with hemifacial spasm and various types of focal dystonias, including blepharospasm to compare Prosigne with Botox. They found no significant differences between the two preparations and found an equivalence ratio of 1:1.5 between Botox and Prosigne.[24] In the other study, Rieder et al. evaluated 28 patients using equivalent units of Botox and Prosigne. They demonstrated similar results with both drugs, suggesting a direct bioequivalence. Because of the discrepancy between the two studies, which could be due to heterogeneity of patients and methods of sampling, further research is needed in this area to accurately establish the bioequivalence of Prosigne in comparison to other BTX-A preparations.[25]

BOTULINUM TOXIN TYPE B

Myobloc

Myobloc™ (Solstice Neurosciences, South San Francisco, CA) received FDA approval for use in the United States in December 2000. Myobloc is composed of BTX-B, which acts by cleaving the protein synaptobrevin preventing ACh release in the synaptic cleft. The drug is available in a ready-to-use formula that does not require reconstitution, but it should be kept refrigerated. Myobloc is stable for up to 21 months in refrigerator storage. This product is available in three-vial configurations of 2500, 5000, and 10,000 U, with a composition of 5000 U BTX-B/mL. Once the bottle has been opened, Myobloc begins to lose its potency. A physician who performs few Myobloc injections per week can opt to use a smaller size bottle to avoid wasting the residual toxin, thus ensuring that the toxin is as potent as possible.

The FDA has approved Myobloc for the treatment of cervical dystonia; however, its use in cosmetics has not yet been approved. Phase III clinical trials of the drug for the treatment of cervical dystonia reported a 12- to 16-week duration of effect. In a study by Baumann et al., 20 patients were treated for crow's feet with Myobloc and the maximum efficacy was determined to be at day 30, with the effect beginning to dissipate at a mean of 67.5 days.[26]

Approximately 50 U of Myobloc are equivalent to 1 U of Botox. Although Myobloc is shipped in a reconstituted form, preservative-free saline may be added to change the amount of units in 0.1 cc. When diluting a bottle of Myobloc, it is important to recognize that the bottles are overfilled and actually contain slightly more Myobloc than the label states in order to compensate for the volume that may be lost in the needle tip and on the edges of the bottle (Table 22-4).

DIFFUSION CHARACTERISTICS OF BOTULINUM TOXINS

With the emergence of different brands of botulinum toxins, differences in preparations and effects need to be assessed for optimal patient benefit with minimal complications. Although the various BTX preparations have very similar results, there are a few differences to take into account. Diffusion rates may result in different "fields of effects" or surface area affected by the toxin.

The diffusion potential of botulinum neurotoxins and their migration is dependent on a number of factors such as the size and structure of the molecule,[27] the subtype of the toxin,[28,29] the volume of injections,[30] the protein load and the formulation's excipient content,[31] and finally on the muscle and site of injection.[19] The field of effects or diffusion of BTX-A and BTX-B have been characterized and targeted in a few studies concerned with their extent of diffusion and potential complications.

Myobloc appears to have a greater field of effect than Botox. One study compared the radius of diffusion of Myobloc to Botox in eight patients with moderate to severe forehead wrinkles. Patients were injected with 5 U of Botox on one side of their frontalis muscle and with 500 U of Myobloc to the other side (1:100 Botox:Myobloc conversion rate). The field of effect of Myobloc was assessed using a digital micrometer on traced scanned images and demonstrated a higher diffusion.[32] In another comparative study of Botox and Myobloc, Matarasso showed that treating crow's feet with Myobloc produces more sensation of tightness and freezing in comparison to Botox and he speculated that the observation is caused by increased Myobloc diffusion.[33] An increased field of effect may be advantageous in that it would allow fewer injection points to produce the same effect. This is particularly beneficial when treating hyperhidrosis of the palms, where the pain of injection is significant. In fact, in the primary author's experience, Myobloc is the most efficacious toxin in the treatment of hyperhidrosis because of the greater amount of diffusion.[34]

Reloxin/Dysport may also have a greater field of effect than Botox. In a recent study, the diffusions of Botox and Dysport were compared in 20 patients with forehead hyperhidrosis.[35] Patients were randomly injected with 3 U of Botox or Dysport (conversion rate of 1:2.5, 1:3, and 1:4 correlating to 7.5, 9, or 12 U) in four areas of the forehead. The injection volume was consistent in all treatments. The anhidrotic area was assessed by using the starch-iodine test. Subjects who received Dysport had a significantly higher mean area of anhidrosis on their forehead as compared to patients treated with Botox. Another study compared 12 healthy volunteers who were randomly assigned to receive three 0.1 mL intradermal injections in their forehead: 4 U Botox on one side, 12 U Dysport (conversion rate of 1:3) on the contralateral side, and saline in the center. The anhidrotic area was assessed by using the starch-iodine test. A higher mean area of anhidrosis was observed in 11 of the 12 subjects who received Dysport and the authors concluded that Dysport has a higher migration potential than Botox.[36] A higher migration potential would likely result in fewer injections required in a treated area. (Box 22-3 for a brief discussion related to the number of injections and the business aspects of these treatments.) This would be beneficial in areas such as the crow's feet, where bruising from the needle is common. More studies need to be performed to determine if an increased field of effect provides an advantage. Xeomin is the smallest of the BTX-A preparations because it is composed of the neurotoxin component alone and not the surrounding complexing proteins.[20] For this reason, it may diffuse more than the other BTX-A preparations. More research is necessary to determine how much diffusion is preferred for cosmetic indications.

BOX 22-3 The Business Side of Botulinum Toxin

The amount of BTX needed per site depends on the musculature of the individual patient. Therefore, BTX should be priced by the number of units used and not by the area treated. When using a consistent dilution technique, one can charge by the number of units used. The price per unit varies geographically. The patient should understand that additional injections (and charges) may occur at the next visit because individual musculature varies. In other words, if you charge by the number of units, you will likely need to charge for touch-ups as well.

CLINICAL USES

Dynamic Wrinkles

BTX can be injected into specific muscles to induce temporary paralysis resulting in an inability to move and wrinkle the skin overlying the treated muscle. BTX is only beneficial for dynamic wrinkles, also known as "wrinkles in motion." It is not as effective for static wrinkles ("wrinkles at rest"), although prolonged use of BTX may help prevent wrinkles in motion from becoming wrinkles at rest. BTX can be combined with dermal fillers (Chapter 23) and resurfacing techniques (Chapter 24) to optimize patient satisfaction. The upper part of the face contains distinct muscle groups that can be selectively paralyzed by a knowledgeable injector. In the lower part of the face, the muscle groups are less distinct and thus more difficult to inject accurately (Fig. 22-2). The paralytic effects of BTX appear approximately 3 to 7 days after injection. However, the effects may increase for up to 2 weeks.

TABLE 22-4
Saline Can be Added to Myobloc to Change the Number of Units in 0.1 cc

Dilution Needed to Change the Amount of Myobloc in 0.1 cc		
	2500-Unit Vial	
Target Concentration (units-mL)	mL of Saline Added to Vial	Units per 0.1 cc
2500	0.8 cc	250
2000	1.2 cc	200
	5000-Unit Vial	
2500	1.4 cc	250
2000	2.1 cc	200

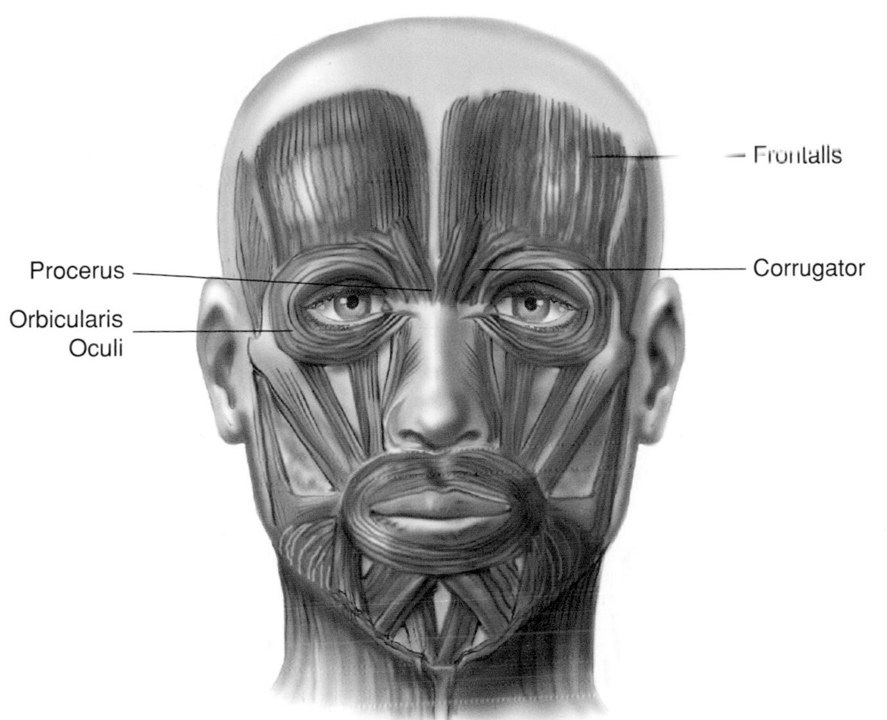

▲ **FIGURE 22-2** The muscles of the face. Each can be deliberately relaxed with an injection of botulinum toxin. Note that the muscles of the upper face are more distinct and separate from each other than the muscles in the lower face.

To use Botox, dilute the 100-U vial with 2.5 cc of preservative-free saline. This yields 4 U per 0.1 cc. To use Reloxin/Dysport, dilute the 500-U vial with 2.5 mL of 0.9% preservative-free saline. This provides 20 U per 0.1 mL. To use Myobloc, dilute a 2500-U vial with 1.2 cc of saline. This yields 200 U per 0.1 cc. Inject with a 1-cc syringe and a 30-gauge needle.

GLABELLAR REGION To treat the glabellar region, inject 0.1 cc (4 U of Botox or 200 U Myobloc) into each corrugator muscle along with 0.1 cc into the procerus muscle (Figs. 22-3 to 22-5). Glabellar injections are currently the only injections approved by the FDA for cosmetic use. The glabellar indication is also the only one under consideration by the FDA for Reloxin. Rzany et al. studied the effect of Dysport in a double-blinded placebo-controlled study of 221 subjects with glabellar lines. Participants were injected with 30 U, 50 U, or placebo in the glabellar area and followed for 16 weeks. After 4 weeks, there was little statistical difference between the treatment groups. The response rate among the 30- and 50-U receivers compared to placebo was 86.1% versus 18.9% and 86.3% versus 7.9%, respectively.[37]

The injection sites for female and male patients are shown in Fig. 22-6. In men or patients with stronger musculature, two sites superior to the corrugator muscle may need to be injected (Fig. 22-7A and B). The primary author has found that doses of 20 U in the glabella work for most men while retaining a natural look; one study showed that 40 to 60 U in the glabellar area was more effective in males.[38] The injector should avoid the periosteum as this can induce postinjection headache. After injecting the procerus muscle, massage the area laterally across the bridge of the nose to ensure that the toxin enters the depressor supercilii portion of the corrugator muscle (Fig. 22-8), which will subtly lift the patient's medial brow, resulting in a more youthful appearance. Proper treatment of the glabellar area or "brow furrow" prevents the patient from frowning, leading to a more relaxed, less angry look (Fig. 22-9A and B). In addition, relaxation of these muscles for long periods of time may prevent or reduce wrinkle formation in the brow area.

FOREHEAD REGION BTX-A is clinically used more broadly than its FDA indication of glabellar treatment. Expanded use is permissible for licensed physicians and is referred to as "off label" use. To treat wrinkles of the forehead, inject 0.1 cc (4 U Botox, 200 U Myobloc) across the forehead as demonstrated in Figs. 22-10 and 22-11. Injection of the forehead is an art as well as a science as it can dramatically affect eyebrow shape. Therefore, prior to injecting the

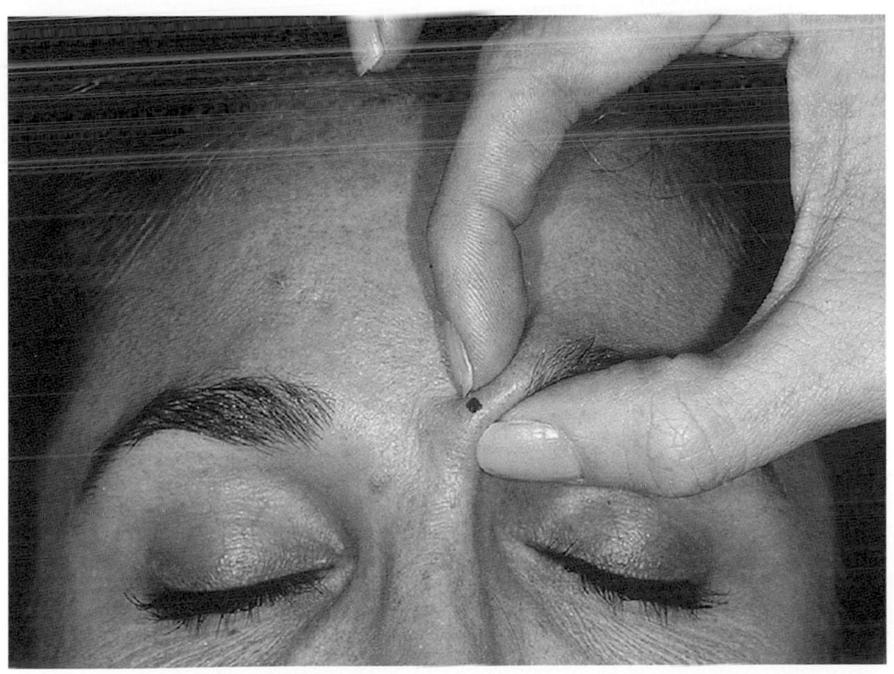

▲ **FIGURE 22-3** Corrugator injection site.

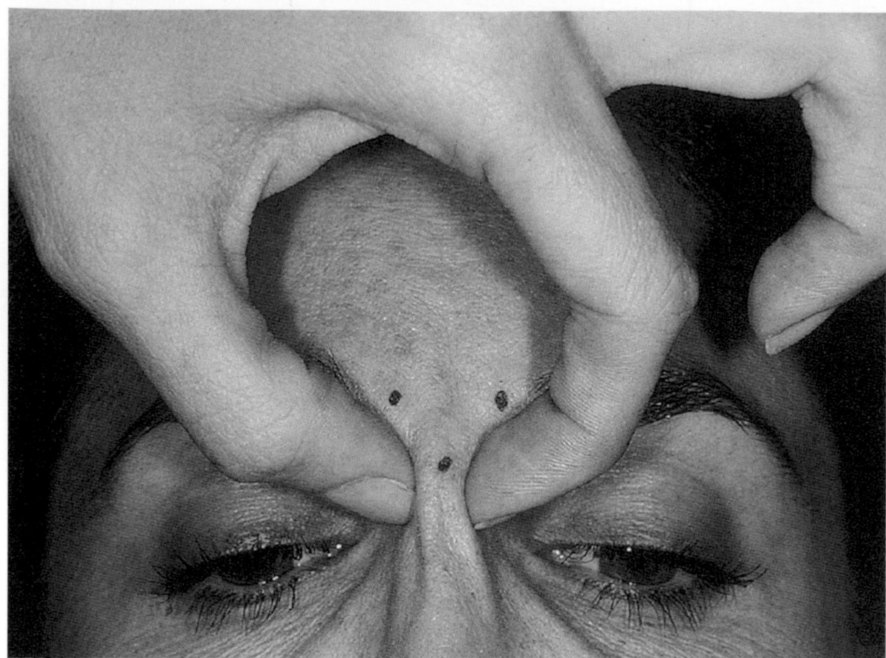

▲ **FIGURE 22-4** Procerus injection site.

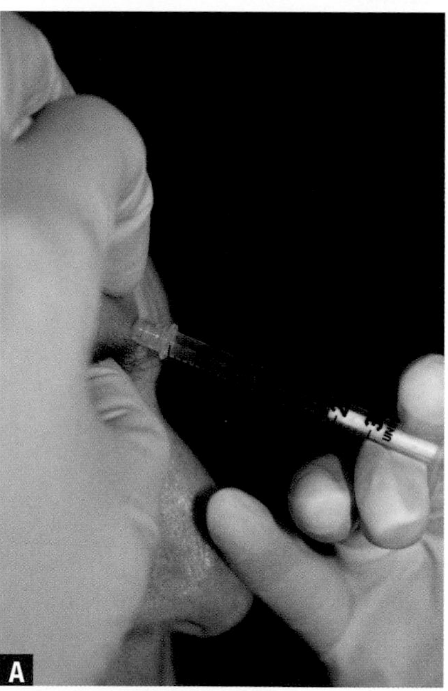

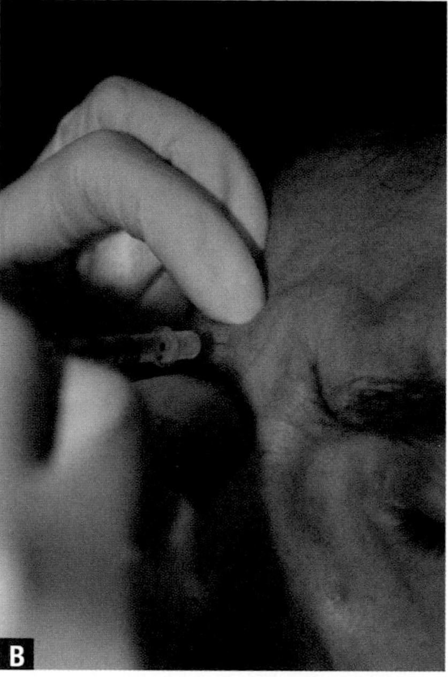

▲ **FIGURE 22-5** Angle of injection of the corrugator muscle. **A.** Use one hand to isolate the corrugator muscle. **B.** Rest the finger of the other hand on the nose as shown in **A** to stabilize the hand.

▲ **FIGURE 22-6** Each 4 represents 0.1 cc of medication that contains either 4 units of Botox or 500 units of Myobloc. Women with increased musculature and men often need two extra injection sites as depicted,because they have increased muscle mass. (Younger women age 18 to 25 usually need only the three depicted injection sites.)

forehead, the physician should consider whether she/he wants to enhance the arch of the eyebrow to create a more horizontal eyebrow shape. Generally, women prefer a more arched brow because it imparts a more feminine look, while men prefer a more horizontal brow (Table 22-5). The forehead should be injected about every two square centimeters where movement of the muscles is seen on eyebrow elevation. It is important not to inject all patients in the same way. Forehead injections should be tailored or customized to the patient's forehead size and shape. In addition, one must take into consideration the placement of the eyebrow over the superior orbital rim. Low brows will become even lower after injections of BTX to the forehead; therefore, forehead injections should be avoided in some patients. Alternately, injections can be performed in the higher regions of the forehead in patients with low brows. Use the recommendations in this chapter as rough guidelines and vary injection technique to suit the needs of each individual patient's anatomy. The major pitfalls with forehead injections are the following: (1) unwanted eyebrow shape (Fig. 22-12), (2) brow ptosis, (3) missed areas (Figs. 22-13 and 22-14), and (4) drooping eyelids. It is important not to overinject the forehead area as this may lead to brow ptosis. Additionally, one must take care to avoid the area 1 cm above the eyebrows to reduce the chances of brow ptosis (Fig. 22-15). The physician should warn the patient with low forehead wrinkles within this 1-cm area that these wrinkles cannot be treated with BTX, and will remain after treatment as demonstrated in Figs. 22-16 and 22-17. Care must be taken to avoid forehead injections in individuals with low-set brows and/or excessive eyelid skin. In older patients and patients with excess eyelid skin, overtreatment of the forehead area may result in drooping eyelids. Hooding of the upper eyelids by the descending eyebrow tissue results in a neural reflex

TABLE 22-5
Masculine and Feminine Characteristics of Brow Shape

FEMININE BROWS	MASCULINE BROWS
Arched	Horizontal
Longer lid to brow distance	Lower lid to brow distance
Thinner brow	Thicker brow

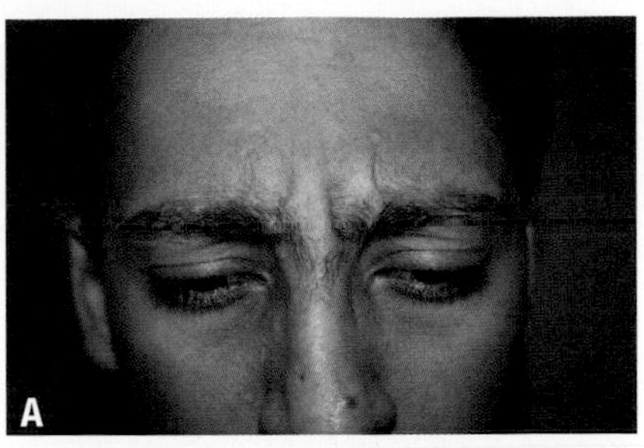

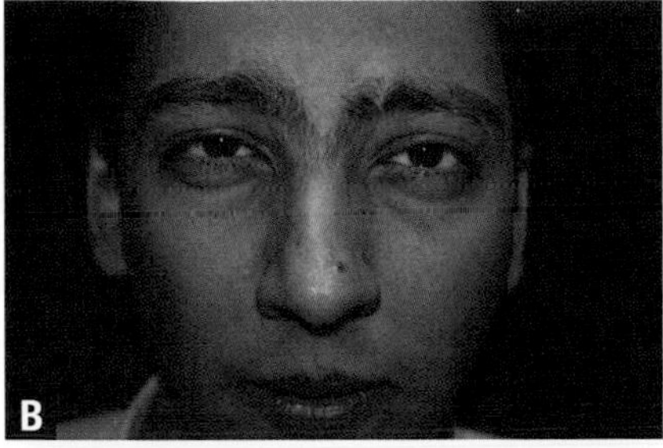

▲ **FIGURE 22-7** Male patient before and after injection of 20 units of Botox.

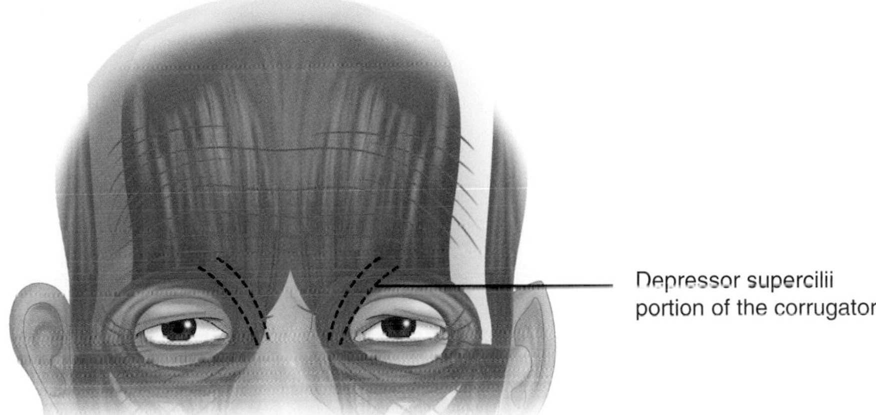

▲ **FIGURE 22-8** The depressor supercilii is a branch of the corrugator muscle responsible for depressing the medial eyebrow. Massaging the toxin into this area usually causes elevation of the medial brow.

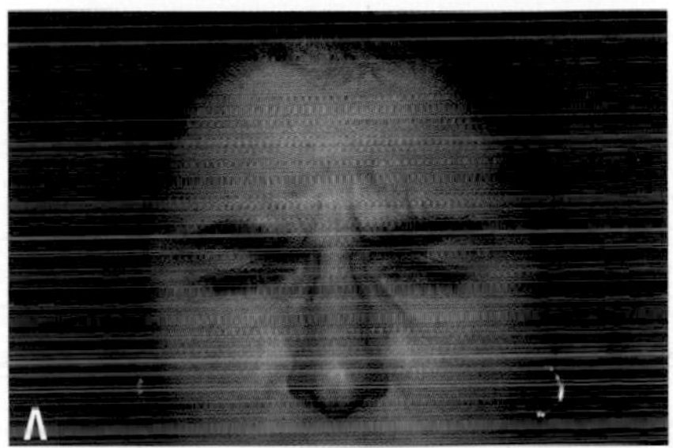

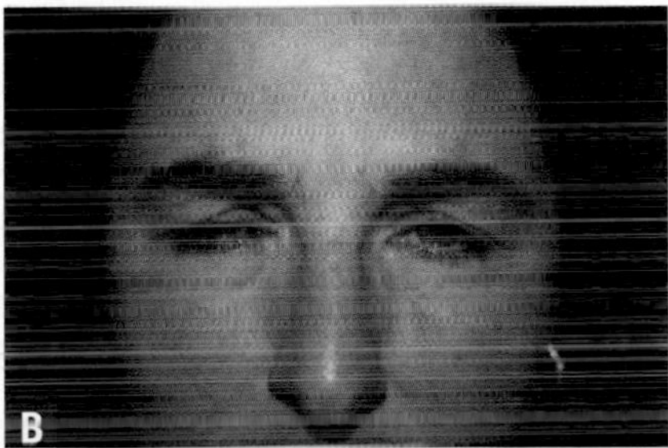

▲ **FIGURE 22-9** Female patient. **A.** before and **B.** after 12 units to the glabella. Note that she is recruiting facial muscles in the center of the brow in order to frown.

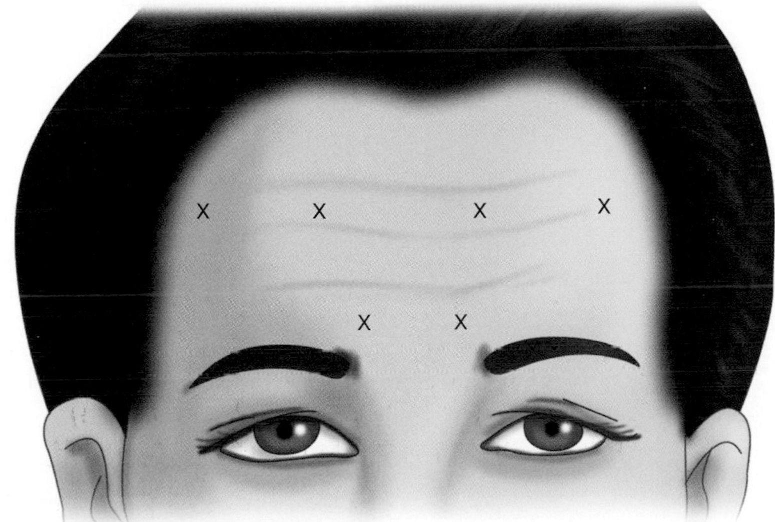

▲ **FIGURE 22-10** The pattern of injection to encourage arched brows.This pattern is used to promote a more feminine brow shape. Each x denotes 4 Botox units or 500 Myobloc units.

that increases the activity of the frontalis muscle in an effort to keep the vision clear of the descending tissue that would otherwise obstruct vision or interfere with eyelid function.[39] In this population the upward pulling of the frontalis muscle is needed to raise the baggy upper eye skin. These patients are better treated with blepharoplasty first, then with BTX. The ideal patient for BTX treatment in the forehead is a young patient (20s–40s) with no excess upper eyelid skin (Figs. 22-18 and 22-19).

CROW'S FEET To treat crow's feet with Botox, inject 0.1 cc 1 cm lateral to the lateral canthus. Then inject 0.05 cc 1 cm above the first injection and 0.1 cc 1 cm below as shown in Figs. 22-20 and 22-21. If wrinkles progress medially, one can inject 0.05 cc approximately 1 cm apart along the orbital rim to the midpupillary line. When using Dysport, fewer injection sites may be required because of increased diffusion. Injecting medial to the midpupillary line does not correct medial wrinkles and can lead to an ectropion; therefore, this area should be avoided. Most patients do not notice these wrinkles prior to BTX injections and sometimes mistakenly believe that BTX "caused" these previously unobserved wrinkles. When used properly, BTX can temporarily erase the lateral crow's feet lines (Fig. 22-22).

BROW LIFT AND THE MICRODROPLET TECHNIQUE

BTX has been used to elevate the eyebrow position by treating between the eyebrows as well as the lateral eyebrow with relatively few injection sites,[23] and with relatively large quantities of BTX (1.5–2.5 U BTX-A).[40] This technique is limited by the possibility of inducing the undesired side effect of upper eyelid ptosis caused by the unwanted diffusion of BTX into the levator palpebrae superioris muscle, which is responsible for eyelid elevation.[41]

The position and appearance of the eyebrows is determined at rest and dynamically by the opposing action of several groups of muscles that act on the eyebrow. The frontalis muscle primarily performs eyebrow elevation. Brow elevation is opposed by the septal and orbital portions of the orbicularis oculi muscle, including the depressor supercilii component of the orbicularis oculi muscle, and the procerus muscle.[42] The medial position of the eyebrow is also influenced by the activity of the corrugator

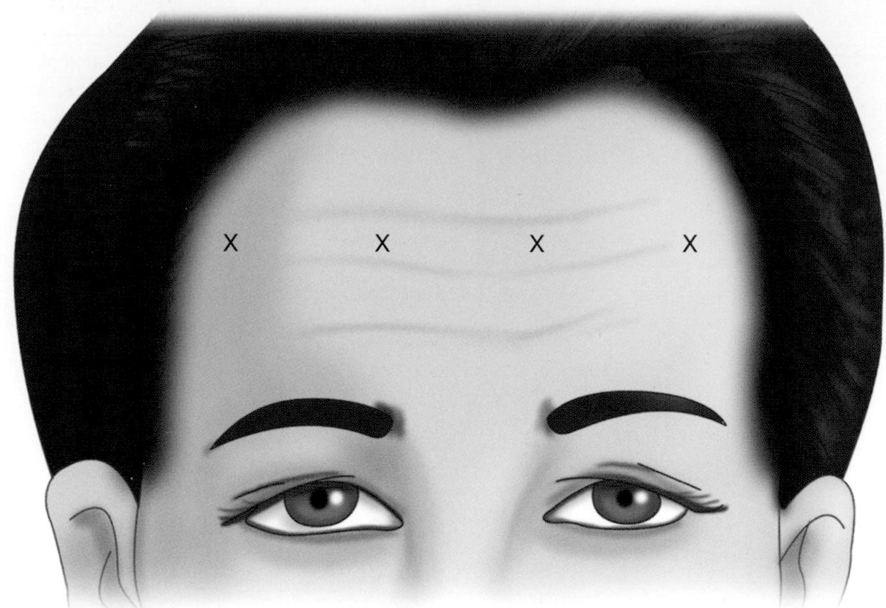

▲ **FIGURE 22-11** The pattern of injection to encourage horizontal brows. This pattern is used to cause a more masculine brow shape. Each x denotes 4 Botox units or 500 Myobloc units.

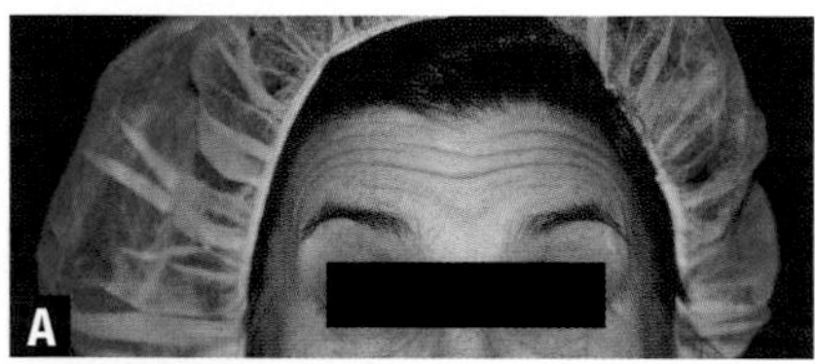

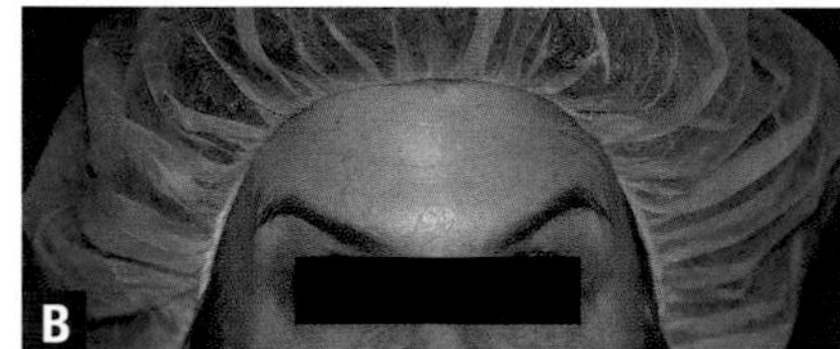

▲ **FIGURE 22-12** Before (**A**) and after (**B**) injection of Botox in the V-shaped pattern taught by many BTX experts. However, in this patient, significant use of the lateral forehead muscles is seen in **A.** Using the V-shaped injection technique in a patient with this forehead muscle function results in an unpopular "Diablo eyebrow" as seen in **B**. This can be avoided or corrected by injecting 4 units of Botox 2 cm above the lateral brow in the area of muscle movement.

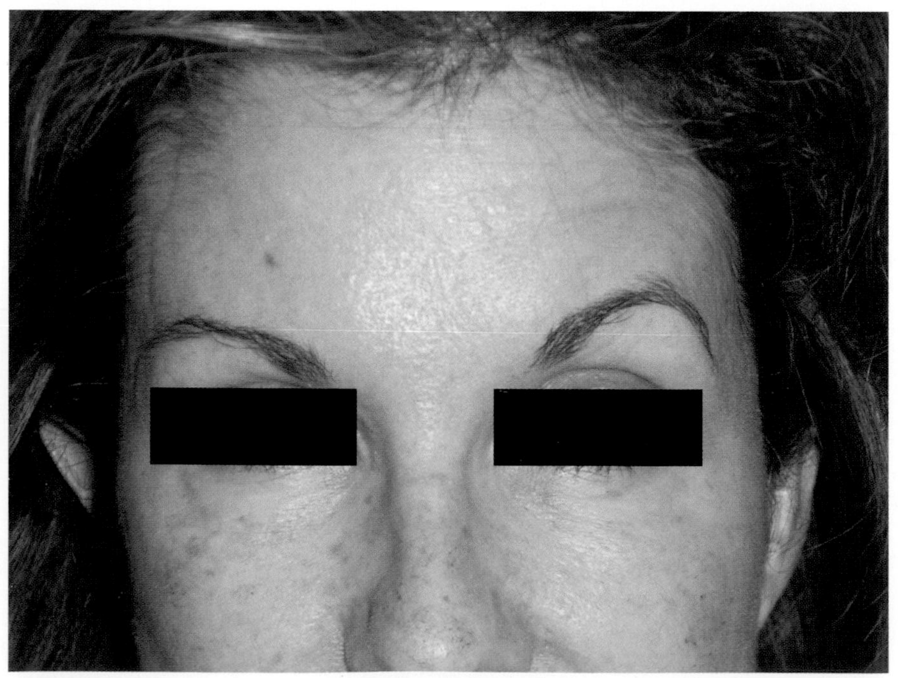

▲ **FIGURE 22-13** This patient was treated with Botox in the forehead by a beginning BTX injector. On her right side the lateral forehead was treated. On the left side it was not. It is crucial to inject the forehead equally on both sides to prevent asymmetry.

supercilii muscle. Additionally, the shape of the brows is affected by the activities of the eyebrow elevators and the eyebrow depressor muscles where they interdigitate along the eyebrow to create facial expression.[43] With age there is a gradual fall in the position of the eyebrows, which is known as brow ptosis, resulting in smaller appearing eyes that is not aesthetically desirable.

BTX can also be used to elevate the brows, resulting in a more youthful appearance. This has been referred to in the literature as a chemical brow lift. The technique of lifting the brow includes injection of the glabellar area as described above. After injecting the procerus muscle with 0.1 cc of Botox the nasal bridge should be massaged in order to ensure that the toxin enters the depressor supercilii portion of the corrugator muscle as shown in Fig. 22-8. This can be used to try and correct an asymmetry of the medial brow. Injecting 0.05 cc of Botox into the lateral brow depressor muscles as shown in Fig. 22-23 can raise the lateral aspect of the eyebrow.[44] Ahn et al. showed that treatment of the lateral depressors of the brow results in an average brow elevation of 4.83 mm when measured from the lateral canthus.[45] Injections of Botox into the glabellar area and lateral brow have also been shown to yield brow elevations of 1 to 3 mm when measured from the eyebrow to the midpupillary point.[44] However, it is the primary author's experience that the lateral brow lift with Botox provides inconsistent results and leads to lateral brow lowering in some patients. (The procerus injection consistently raises the brows.) Therefore, the lead author prefers using a dermal filler injected into the lateral brow to achieve a brow lift (Chapter 23).

A novel technique introduced by Steinsapir is intended to temporarily elevate the eyebrows without provoking any undesirable side effects. This "microdroplet technique" uses small quantities of BTX dissolved in microdroplets of injectable saline carrier to treat the septal and orbital orbicularis muscles, on each side of the patient's face. He treats the frontalis at and below the brow by injecting very small volumes of fluid in multiple locations.[46] These microdroplets have volumes of 10 to 50 μL of injectable saline containing as small as 0.001 to 1 U Botox. Treatment is based on 100 U Botox and 3 mL of injectable saline, which equals approximately 0.33 U of Botox per 10 μL. A typical treatment involves a total of approximately 100 microdroplets placed in double or triple rows just above, in, and

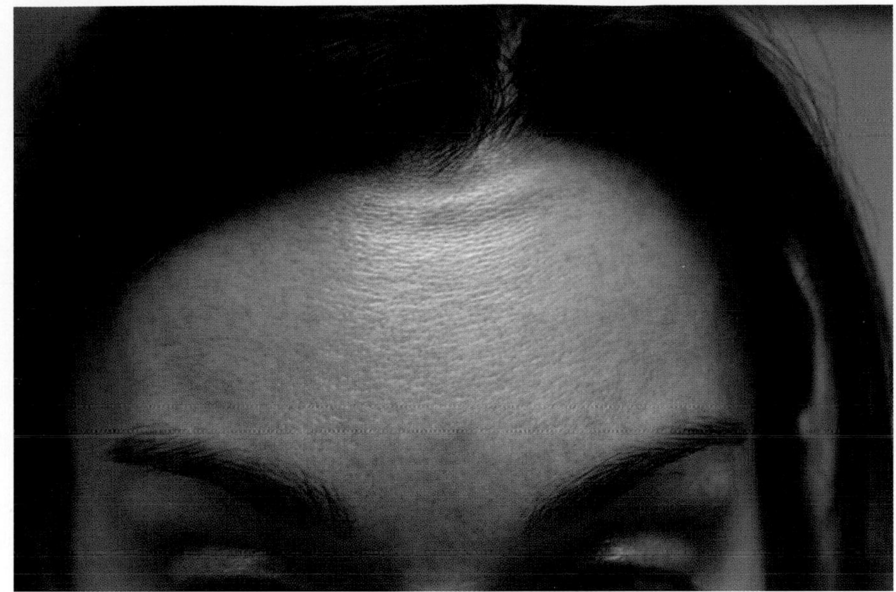

▲ **FIGURE 22-14** The physician who injected this female missed the area just below the hairline. In men, this can often occur laterally in areas of hair loss, so men may need to be injected in the upper lateral regions just below the receding hairline.

below the brow, stopping around the level of the lowest brow cilia. The microdroplet injections are placed superficially approximately 1 mm into the skin to trap the Botox at the interface between the orbicularis oculi and the skin. For crow's feet, the needle is inserted before the midline of the lateral palpebral raphe. The glabellar area is also treated. The combination of these treatments produces a uniform brow-lift effect.[14]

Bunny Lines

The upper nasalis muscle across the bony dorsum of the nose causes fanning wrinkles ("bunny lines") at the radix of the nose[47] and can lead to medial wrinkling around the eyes. Two to four units of Botox can be injected into the nasalis muscle as shown to reduce or eliminate these lines. Many physicians inject into the wrinkles rather than into the nasalis muscle resulting in an incomplete correction. The correct injection points are in the belly of the muscle, inferior to the angular vein as shown in Figs. 22-24 to 22-26. If the injection is too low, the levator labii superioris will be relaxed, which leads to an unwanted upper lip ptosis.

Treating Nasal Tip Ptosis/Nasal Tip Lift

BTX has been used for lifting the nasal tip. More than one technique exists but there is no consensus on an optimal method. The main muscles that influence the nasal tip are the nasalis, the depressor septi nasi, the levator labii superioris, and the alaeque nasi muscle. Atamoros in 2003 described the injection of 4 U of Botox into each of the alar portions of the nasalis and 4 U into the depressor septi.[48] Dayan and Kempiners later described the injection of 5 U of Botox into each depressor septi nasi and 3 U into each levator labii superioris.[49] Ghavami et al. demonstrated similar results as Dayan and Kempiners with only 1 to 2 U injected to each of the depressor septi nasi and further stressed that proper studies excluding confounding variables, such as concomitant rhinoplasty or chemodenervation of synergistic muscles, are required before Botox injection alone can be recommended as a treatment for dynamic nasal tip ptosis.[50] The primary author uses 2 to 3 U injected at the base of the columella.[51] This procedure is most effective for those with a short- or normal-sized upper lip. Those with a long length between the top of the columella and the top of the lip, that is, long upper lip, do not receive good results from this procedure (Fig. 22-27). Those with a long upper lip will benefit from a dermal filler to raise the nasal tip (Chapter 23).

COSMETIC USE OF BOTULINUM TOXIN TYPE A IN THE LOWER FACE

Cosmetic treatments with BTX-A have focused mainly on the upper face, particularly the glabellar, forehead, and periocular areas. With the huge increase in the number of cosmetic Botox injections delivered each year and its clinical effectiveness, a variety of off-label interventions using BTX-A for the lower face have emerged.[52] However, this area has an increased incidence of side effects and should only be treated by experienced BTX users.

As such, BTX-A is now more widely used in lower face and neck rejuvenation, in treating the chin and corners of the mouth as well as in recontouring of the jawline. Yet another area where BTX-A has shown promise cosmetically is in the treatment of facial and chest wall flushing. The response of the

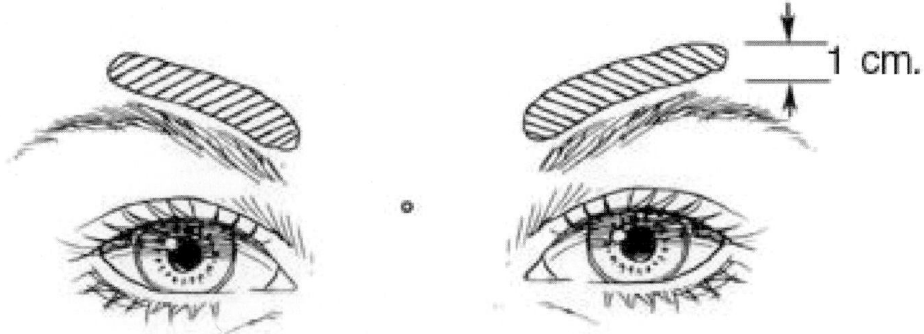

▲ **FIGURE 22-15** The 1-cm area above the medial portion of the eyebrow is a "danger zone" and, to avoid ptosis, should not be injected.

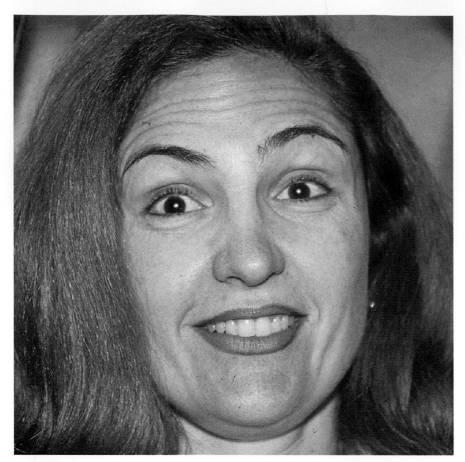

▲ **FIGURE 22-16** Forehead with eyebrows elevated prior to injection of botulinum toxin.

lower facial muscles to BTX-A is greater than upper facial muscles. Moreover, it has been established that the lower facial muscles will have a longer-lasting response to BTX-A than upper facial musculature. The dose for the lower muscles therefore needs to be adjusted to the muscle size and patient gender to be approximately half or one-third the dose injected in the upper facial muscles.

Upper Gum Show—The levator labii superioris alaeque nasi muscle retracts the upper lip. In some individuals, this muscle is overactive and pulls the lip back excessively, allowing visualization of the upper gums and upper incisors. Injecting 1 to 2 U into the levator labii superioris alaeque nasi muscle on each side of the bony nasal prominence will slightly drop the lip, preventing the upper gum show. This procedure works better in young patients because it causes vertical elongation of the lip. This can be used in combination with fillers such as CosmoPlast in the vermilion border to prevent the elongated lip (Fig. 22-28).

Melomental Folds

The melomental folds are also called marionette lines. They extend from the downturned corner of the mouth to the lateral chin. The depressor anguli oris pulls down the corner of the mouth in opposition to the zygomaticus major and minor contributing to these folds. Marionette lines are often corrected by dermal fillers; however, some physicians prefer to combine dermal fillers with BTX injections. BTX can be injected into the depressor anguli oris to weaken it, allowing the zygomaticus to elevate the corners of the mouth and return them to a horizontal position.[10] For reducing the melomental folds, a dose of 2 to 4 U should be injected at the depressor anguli oris immediately above the angle of the mandible and 1 cm lateral to the lateral oral commissure.[53] Care must be taken not to use too high of a dose as this can lead to drooping of the lateral lower lip, flaccid cheeks, an incompetent mouth, or an asymmetric smile.

Perioral Lines

Many factors are implicated in the formation of perioral lines. Smoking, photoaging, loss of subcutaneous tissue in the lower face, and the purse string-like action of the orbicularis oris muscles are the most important causes. BTX-A injection is usually reserved for deep perioral lines worsened with muscular

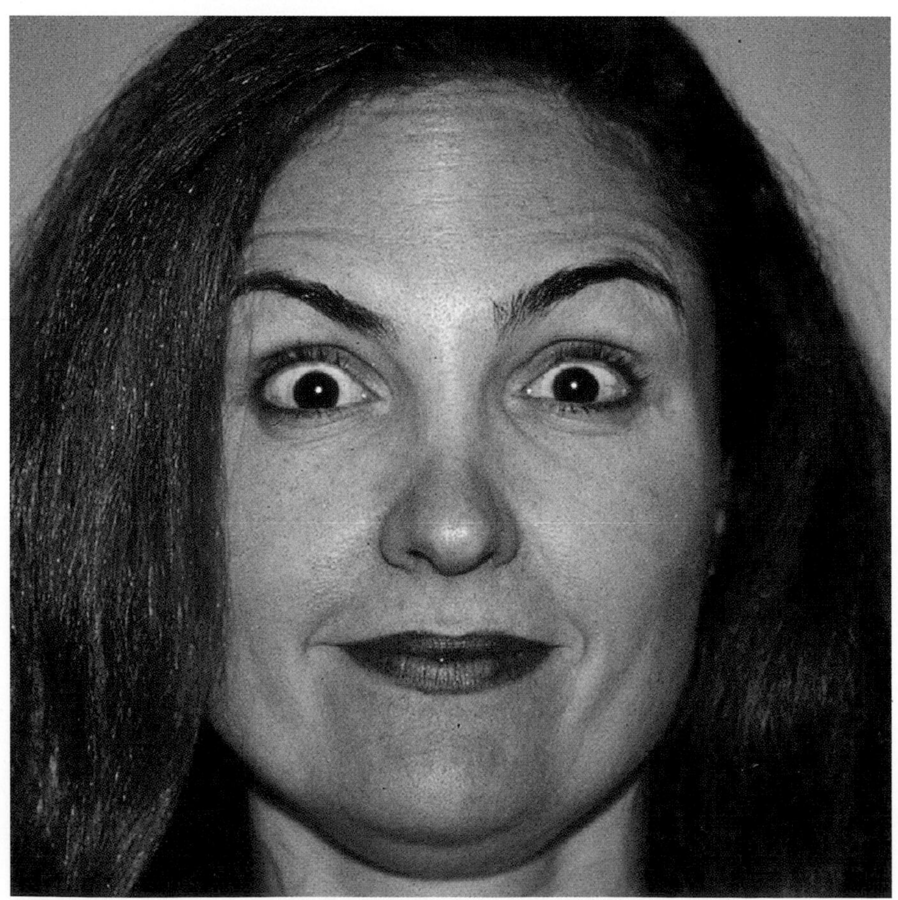

▲ **FIGURE 22-17** Forehead with eyebrow elevated after injection of botulinum toxin. Note that lower forehead wrinkles are still present. However, they are not apparent when eyebrows are not elevated.

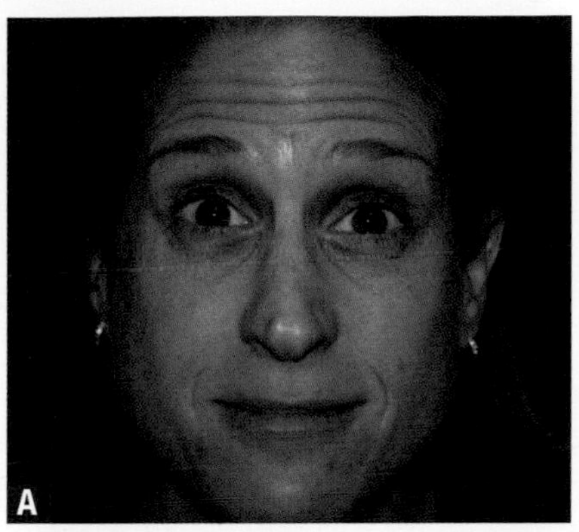

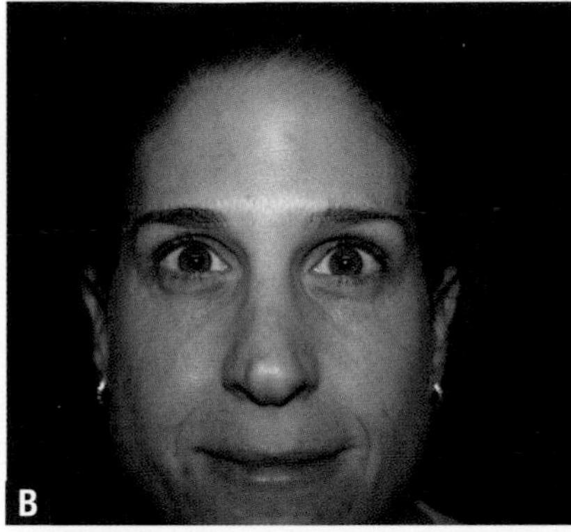

▲ **FIGURE 22-18** Before (**A**) and after (**B**) Botox injections.

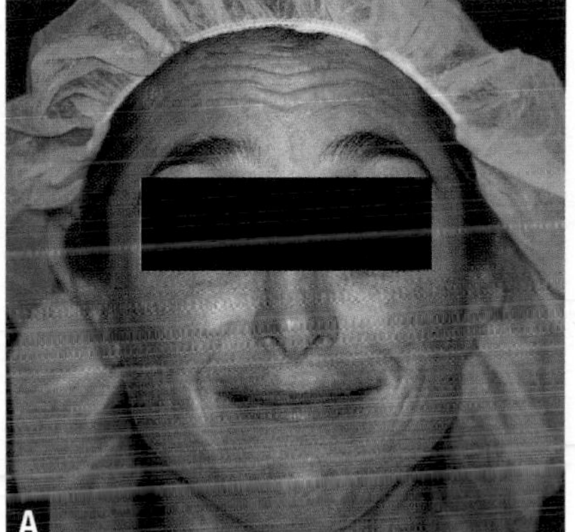

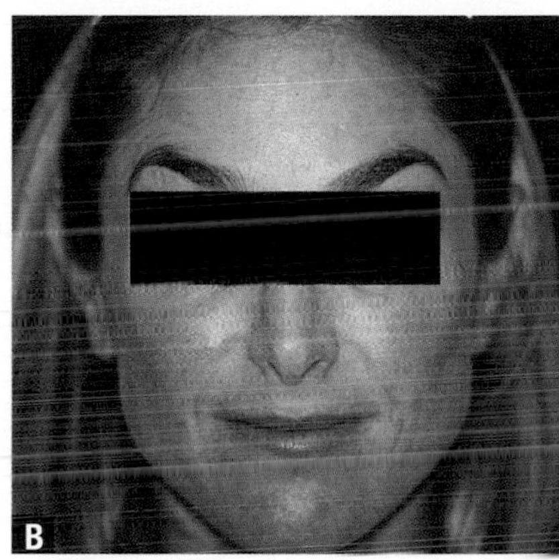

▲ **FIGURE 22-19** Before (**A**) and after (**B**) Botox injections to the forehead, glabella, and crow's feet.

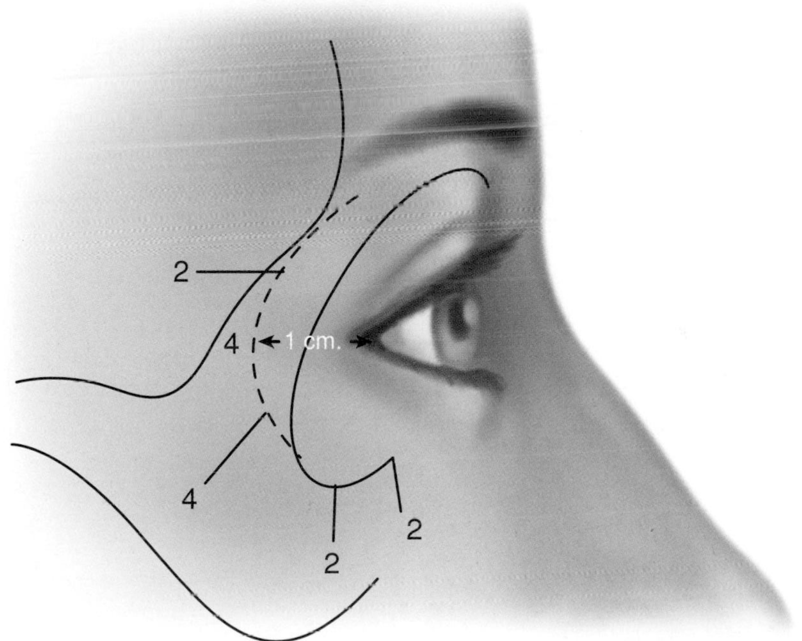

▲ **FIGURE 22-20** Injection points in the crow's feet area. The injection technique depends on the field of effect of the substances used. If Reloxin is used, fewer injection sites (two) may be required because of an increased field of effect. Botox should be injected as shown in this diagram. The exact placement of injection is determined by the patient's facial anatomy but this is a rough guide of placement.

pursing of the lips. The dosage is dependent on the depth of lines but generally 1 U of BTX-A injected into each site with a total of 2 U per half of the upper lips. The middle upper lip should be avoided in patients wanting to retain their cupid bow. It is critical to measure the placement on the upper lips first so that the sides are treated in exactly the same spot to preserve symmetry (Fig. 22-29). The best results occur when BTX is combined with laser resurfacing or lip fillers to enhance the vermillion border and smooth the surface of the skin.

Mentalis Muscle and Chin Puckering

Relaxing the hyperkinetic muscle fibers of the chin and the mentalis muscle with BTX-A can reduce and eliminate chin puckering (Fig. 22-30). A single dose of 4 to 6 U of BTX-A placed in the exact center of the point of the chin is effective.[51] An overdose in this area can result in the inability to approximate the lower lips tightly against the teeth, ultimately leading to involuntary dribbling from the lip when drinking or drooling from the corners of the mouth.[54]

Neck Lines and Platysma

Brandt and Bellman were the first to report using BTX to treat aging of the neck.[55] Platysmal bands and neck vertical lines represent an accurate gauge of chronological age specifically for those people with exaggerated outdoor sun exposure. Separation of the platysma anteriorly occurs with aging, resulting in banding or "turkey neck." Vertical platysmal bands may be successfully treated with BTX-A. The extended or marked platysmal bands are grasped between the thumb and index fingers and the needle is vertically inserted into the muscle band. The dose is usually 2 to 4 U spaced 4 cm apart with an overall cumulative dose of 8 to 12 U per band and a total maximum in the neck of 25 to 30 U. Because of the nature of the muscle and the site of injection, complications such as dysphagia and dysphonia can be encountered.[56] Patients should be warned about the possibility of such untoward effects.

NEFERTITI LIFT The platysma muscle pulls downward with age, leading to jowl formation and frequent rhytides. Jawline redefinition with neurotoxin has not been widely exposed in the literature and there exists a discrepancy in the exact dosing and techniques to best define this area. A technique described

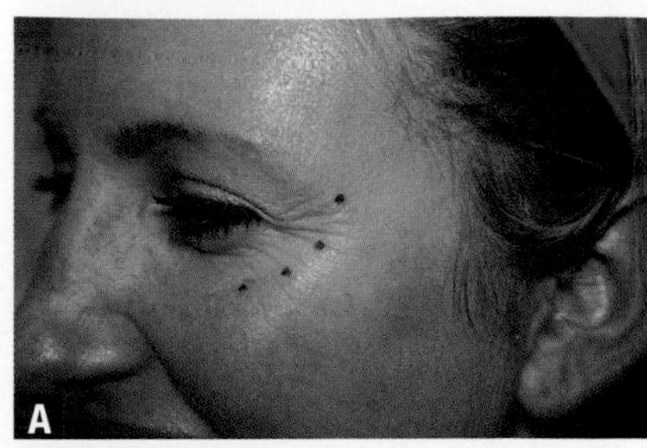

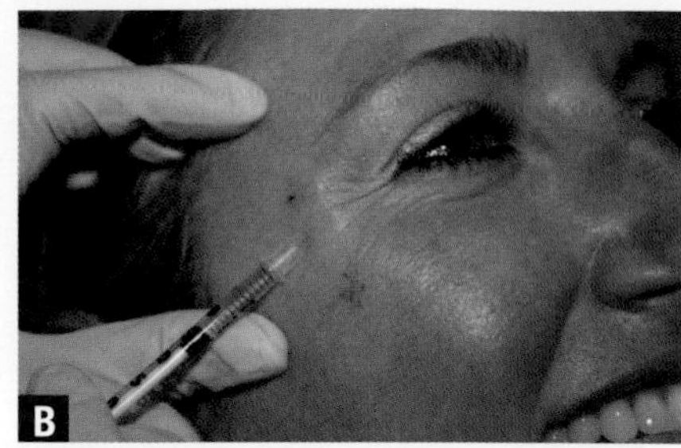

▲ **FIGURE 22-21** To inject Botox in crow's feet, have the patients gently smile. Inject at sites of maximal muscle contraction, which will be about 1.0 to 1.5 cm lateral to the corner of the eye.

recently by Levy was named the "Nefertiti Lift" (after the perfect jawline of the ancient queen).[57] This technique releases the downward tension of the depressor effect of the aging platysma and releases the skin to the elevator muscles for lifting action. The "mini-lift" technique requires an injection of 2 to 3 U of BTX-A along and under each mandible and to the upper part of the posterior platysmal band for a total of 15 to 20 U per side.[57]

CHEST The upper area of the chest is a site of predilection for photodamage. Textural, pigmented, and photodamage changes are frequently seen in the V-shaped area of the chest. Static and dynamic wrinkles are caused by both photodamage and muscular sagging of the upper chest. Anatomically, the platysma is known to originate at the second rib; however, it can still present as far down as the fourth rib after which it traverses the pectoralis major and inserts in the mandible.[58] To date there is no consensus or indication for upper chest injection of BTX-A; however, there are various ways to inject BTX in the upper chest. The techniques used are the curved, the "V," and the triangular approaches, during which BTX is injected over a curved, V-shaped area, or a triangular area with "5 to 10" sites identified within, each targeted with 2 to 8 U of BTX.[48]

BOTOX AND GENDER

Interest among men seeking cosmetic procedures is increasing every day. Men had nearly 1.1 million cosmetic procedures performed in 2007, accounting for 9% of the total cosmetic procedures carried out in the United States. The number of cosmetic procedures for men increased 17% from 2006.[8] The BTX injection technique in men and women is similar; however, it is important to appreciate that higher doses are often required by men in comparison to women.[59] One study compared the muscle mass differences among 468 men and women aged 18 to 88 years and demonstrated a significantly higher amount of skeletal muscle in men than women in the muscles of the face, potentially because of the hypertrophic effect of testosterone.[60] Moreover, Monks et al. found androgen receptors to be abundant in the vicinity of the neuromuscular junction.[61] They speculated that androgens may even increase the number of junctions. The primary author's recommendation is to use a total of 20 U of BTX for glabellar injection in men as a starting dose. Five injection sites of 4 U each is the preferred method to preserve a more natural look. Significant care must be taken when injecting brows in men so as to avoid cosmetically undesired effects such as feminization of the brow or arching. With temporalis and masseter injections, men likely need an additional 25% to 100% as compared to women. Furthermore, men need higher doses for orbicularis oculi paralysis owing to its broader circumference.

ETHNIC DIFFERENCES IN BOTULINUM TOXIN RESPONSES

Very little information is available regarding the possible ethnic differences in the clinical effects of BTX or for dosing considerations. To date there is a lack of consensus on dosing considerations for different skin types and there exists a discrepancy regarding which skin type requires higher or lesser doses for an optimal response.[62] Several variables must be taken into consideration, such as skin thickness, skin musculature, and circumference of bony prominences. Skin thickness and texture contribute to dosing decisions. Although the injections are generally muscular, the thickness of the dermis might influence the delivery technique. For instance, some studies have suggested that the skin of Asians tends to be thicker than that of Caucasians with more collagen fibers, which might demand a higher dose of injection.[63] However, other studies in Asians have found that lower doses may be needed than in Caucasians.[64] Arimura et al. evaluated the differences in the muscle-relaxing effect of BTX-B using electrophysiologic measurements in 48 Asian and Caucasian volunteers. They concluded that the muscle-relaxing effects of BTX-B were similar in both Asian and Caucasian study populations.[65] Racial differences in BTX responses remain unclear. More studies are required to determine any potential variations in the response of different skin types to botulinum toxins. The primary author has not noted any consistent differences among the various ethnicities treated in her practice.

HYPERHIDROSIS

Hyperhidrosis is a troublesome problem leading to awkward social situations for those affected. Unfortunately, topical and oral medications, iontophoresis, and surgery have not proven efficacious in the majority of patients. The eccrine glands are innervated by sympathetic nerves that use ACh as the neurotransmitter. Therefore, BTX is effective in temporarily reducing or abolishing sweat production. Botox is the only BTX that is approved by the FDA for axillary hyperhidrosis.

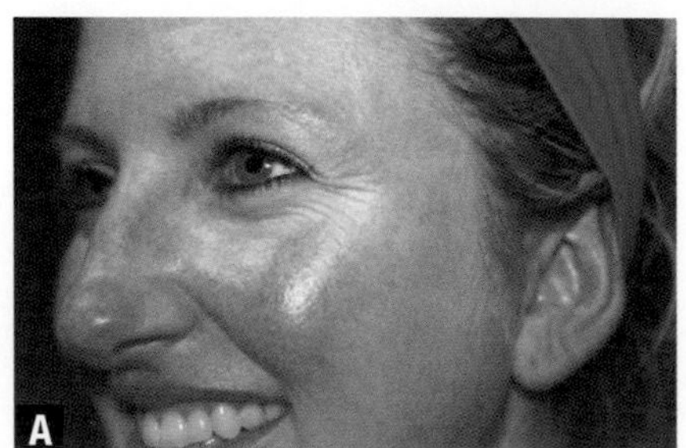

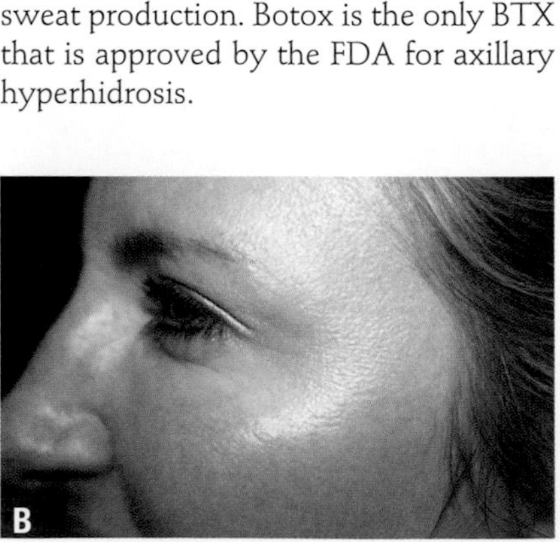

▲ **FIGURE 22-22** Before (**A**) and after (**B**) Botox injections.

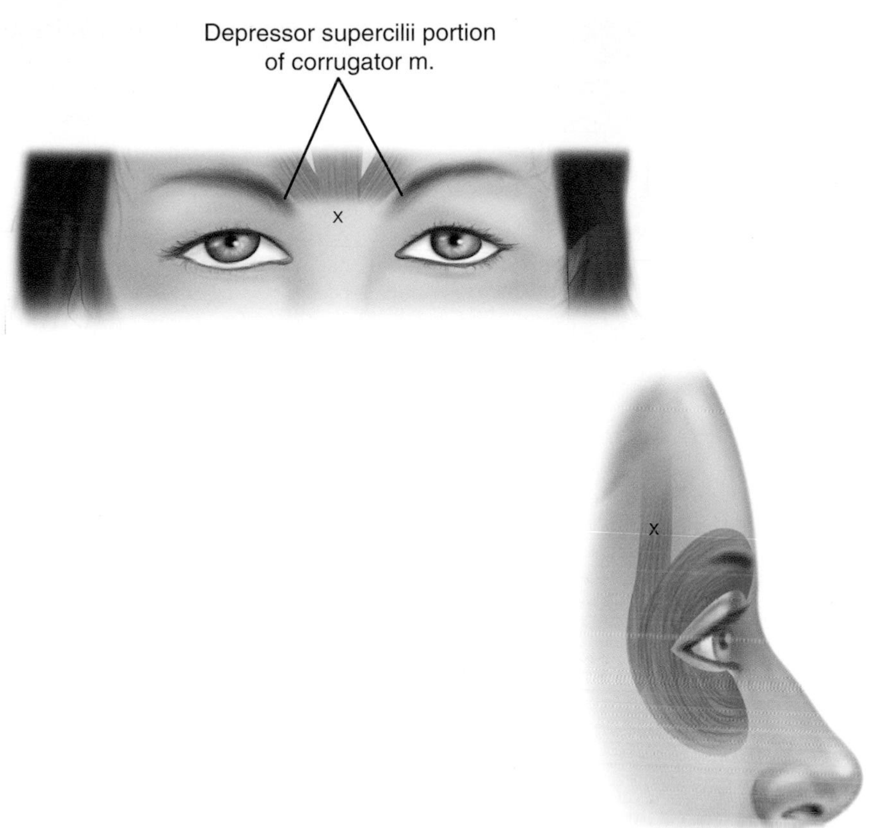

▲ **FIGURE 22-23** Injection points to elevate the brow. Four units of Botox are placed in the procerus muscle and massaged laterally. Two units of Botox are then placed in the upper lateral brow as shown.

Botox for hyperhidrosis is diluted with 5.0 cc of preservative-free saline, yielding 2 U per 0.1 cc. Reloxin/Dysport can also be diluted with 5.0 cc of preservative-free saline, providing 10 U per 0.1 cc. To use Myobloc, dilute a 5000-U vial with 2.1 cc of saline. This yields 200 U per 0.1 cc. Using a 1-cc tuberculin syringe with a 30-gauge needle, subcutaneously inject 0.05 cc with an approximate depth of 3 mm with care to avoid intramuscular injections. The palm or sole, including the webs of the hands and feet, should be injected every square centimeter. When treating the axilla, ask patients which areas bother them to determine how far beyond the hair-bearing area to inject. A starch-iodine test may be performed prior to injections to ascertain which areas need to be injected. The iodine solution is applied to the affected area and then covered with starch. The areas that produce sweat will turn black, indicating which areas to inject (Fig. 22-31A–E). Although this test is messy, it is a useful technique for evaluating the efficacy of the injections and for determining which areas to inject. The primary author injects the tips of the fingers and toes as well to avoid compensatory sweating in these areas (Figs. 22-32 and 22-33). It is usually necessary to inject 100 U Botox or 5000 U Myobloc per palm or sole and 50 U Botox or 2500 U Myobloc per axilla. The effects last approximately 4 months although there are reports in the literature of longer lasting results.[66] Lowe et al. studied 322 patients with axillary hyperhidrosis in a multicenter, double-blind trial for 52 weeks.[67] Subjects received 50 or 75 U of Botox and were compared to a control group of placebo injection. Seventy-five percent of the patients who received Botox noticed a reduction of hyperhidrosis, while only 25% of the placebo group noticed a difference. The median duration of effect was also significantly higher in patients who received Botox when compared to the placebo group. There was no statistically significant difference between the two groups receiving toxin. Following the first treatment, the median duration of effect was 205 days for the patients receiving 50 U and 197 days in patients injected with 75 U of Botox.

Baumann et al. studied Myobloc in the treatment of 20 patients with axillary hyperhidrosis in a double-blind, randomized, placebo-controlled trial. Subjects received either Myobloc (2500 U, or 0.5 mL, per axilla) or 0.5 mL vehicle (100 mmol NaCl, 10 mmol succinate, and 0.5 mg/mL human albumin) into the bilateral axillae. The onset and duration of action were determined to be 5 to 7 days and 2.2 to 8.1 months (mean of 5 months), respectively.[68] In another study conducted by Baumann et al., Myobloc was used to treat 20 patients with palmar hyperhidrosis. Participants were injected with either Myobloc (5000 U per palm) or a 1.0 mL vehicle (100 mM NaCl, 10 mM succinate, and 0.5 mg/mL human albumin) into bilateral palms. The duration of action of Myobloc in these patients ranged from 2.3 to 4.9 months, with a mean of 3.8 months.[34]

INGUINAL HYPERHIDROSIS

Inguinal hyperhidrosis (IH) is a focal and primary form of hyperhidrosis in which the individual has intense sweating in

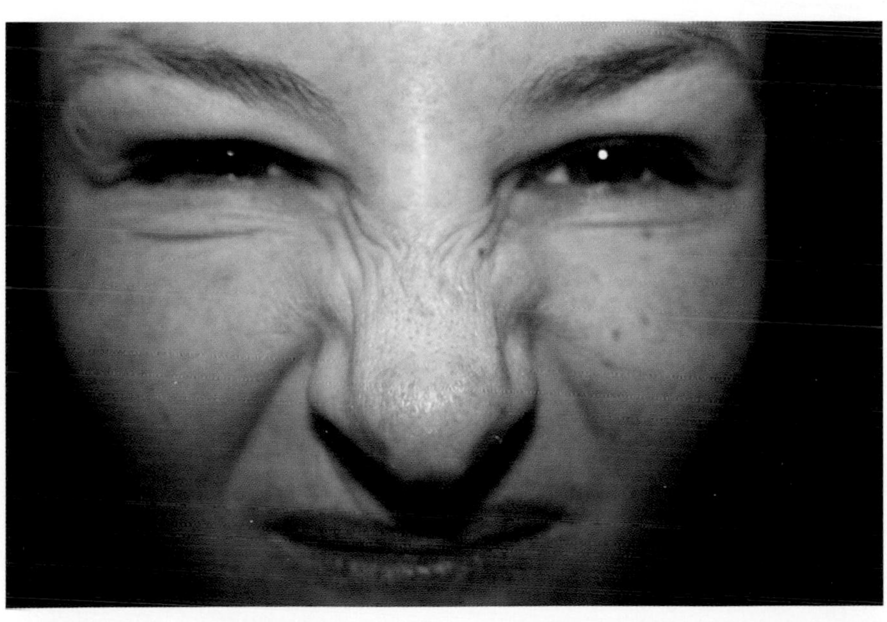

▲ **FIGURE 22-24** Wrinkling of the nasalis muscle or "bunny lines" leads to medical wrinkling under the eyes.

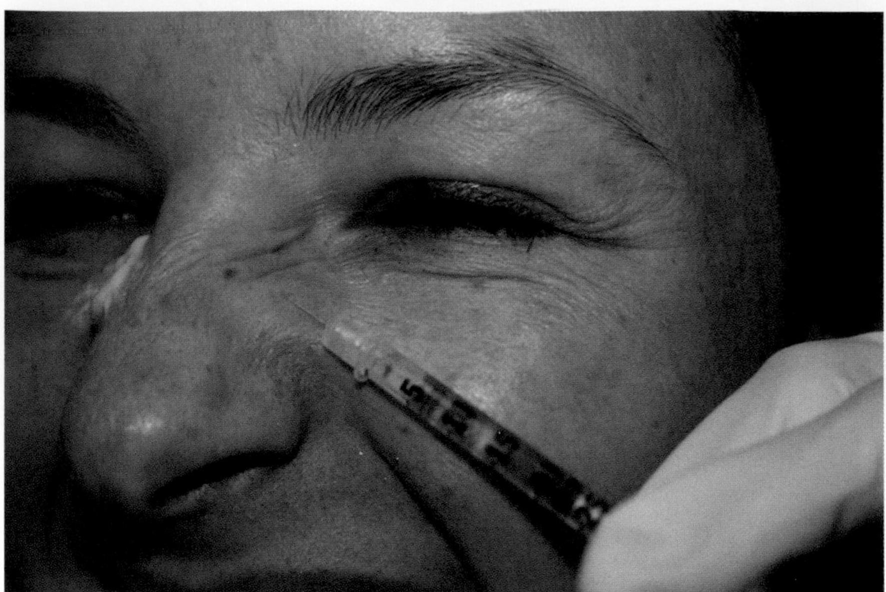

▲ **FIGURE 22-25** Injection site to treat bunny lines.

the inguinal region. Appearing in adolescence, usually not later than the age of 25, the condition continues into adulthood. IH is characterized by chronic, intense sweating in the inguinal region, a situation that is potentially embarrassing for the patient. IH symmetrically affects the groin region, including the suprapubic area, the shallow depression that lies immediately below the fold of the groin (corresponding to the femoral triangle), the medial surfaces of the upper inner thighs, and the genital area. It may also include the lower part of the gluteus maximus, gluteal fold, and natal cleft.[69] No study to date has described the ideal doses of BTX for the treatment of IH. The threshold doses of BTX-A for the treatment of hyperhidrosis depend on the severity of the condition.[70] Two or three units of BTX-A per square centimeter can be used to treat the hyperhidrotic area in the inguinal region. The only side effects reported in the sparse literature are those related to the injections, such as rare small hematomas and temporary edema.[71]

OTHER NEUROGLANDULAR DISORDERS

The effects of BTX-A at the neuroglandular junction have not been explored as extensively as those occurring at the neuromuscular junction. Clinical studies examining the effect of intracutaneous BTX for focal hyperhidrosis found complete abolition of sweating in the injected area within 3 to 7 days. No adverse effects were reported, and in a 5-month follow-up there were no clinical recurrences of the hyperhidrosis.[72] Gustatory sweating is another area of neuroglandular dysfunction in which BTX-A has proven effective. Gustatory sweating (or Frey's syndrome) is a disabling disorder in which the cheek skin sweats profusely during eating. The syndrome may occur after parotidectomy, and is likely due to the misdirection of regenerating parasympathetic fibers that innervate the sweat glands of the face. Intracutaneous BTX-A has been reported to significantly decrease or prevent sweating for more than 6 months, with no clinical evidence of facial weakness in any patients.[73] BTX-A injected into the submandibular glands has been reported to significantly decrease salivation resulting from stimulation of the lingual nerves. The decreased salivation was temporary, and did not appear to be directly toxic to the acinar cells of the gland.[74] Canine studies have also shown that vasomotor rhinorrhea, a parasympathetically controlled phenomenon, responds favorably to topical BTX-A. While the duration of action of BTX-A at the neuromuscular junction appears to be approximately 3 months, a longer-lasting effect may occur at the glandular level. BTX-A has produced anhydrosis for more than 12 months in patients with gustatory sweating. The reason for the difference in duration of action is uncertain; hypotheses include a higher rate of resynthesis of SNAP-25 (the protein cleaved by BTX) in neuromuscular synapses, and a higher area of axonal sprouting and consecutive reinnervation of muscle fibers as compared to that in glandular tissue.[75,76]

PAIN CONTROL

With the expanding use of botulinum toxins in cosmetic practice, pain alleviation remains an important aspect of the injection. Pain sensation is dependent on many factors, most importantly the concentration of the neuropeptides (substance P) at the site of injection, the tissue density (higher tissue density implies more pain), and the density of the nociceptor distribution at the site of injection. Other factors include the volume injected, the bore of the needle used, the layer of skin within which the toxin is injected, the rate of the fluid injection, and, of course, the physician's level of experience.[77]

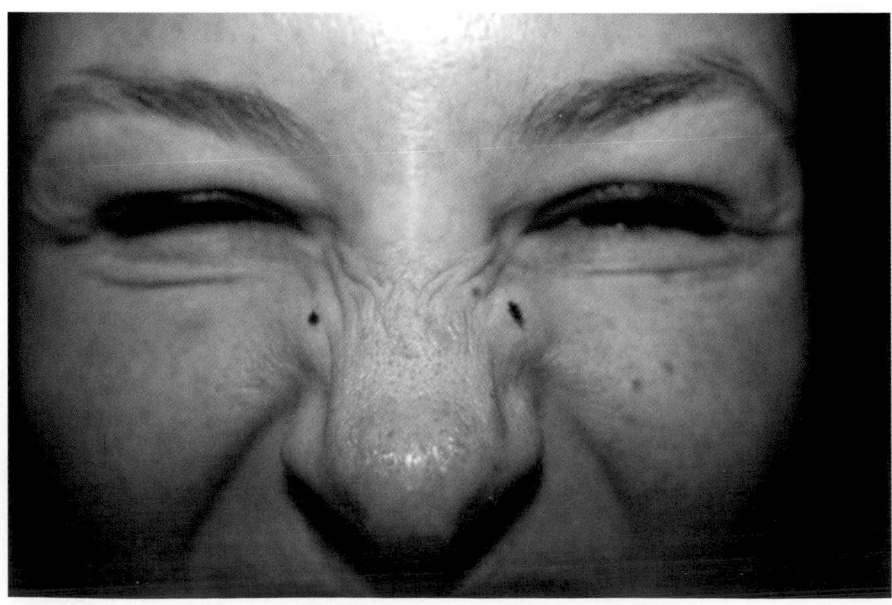

▲ **FIGURE 22-26** Injection sites to treat nasal bunny lines.

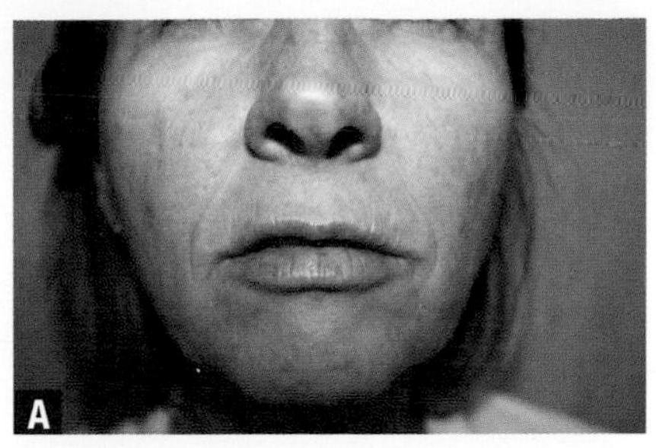
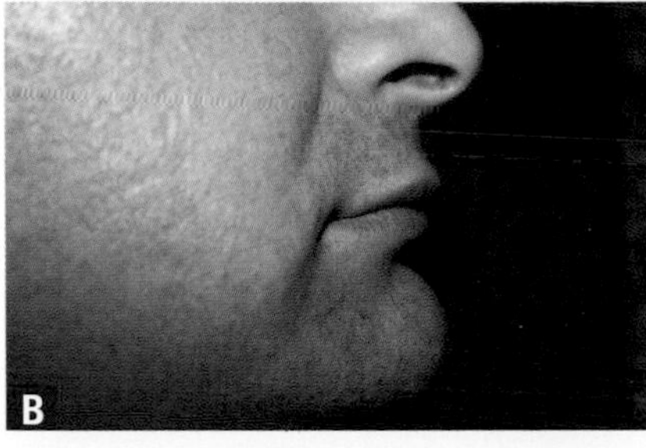

▲ **FIGURE 22-27** **A.** Patient with a long upper lip. **B.** Patient with a short upper lip. This patient is a better candidate for Botox injection to raise the tip.

Differences in pain perception among patients treated with the commercially available toxin preparations have not been studied extensively; however, results from the only comparative study of three available preparations of the toxin showed that the pain induced by Neurobloc (BTX-B) was found to be significantly higher than that induced by Botox and Dysport (BTX-A), between which no significant difference was found. The study concluded that the different chemical properties and pharmaceutical adjuvants in toxins A and B likely affect the pain sensation and speculated that the pH difference of Neurobloc (pH 5.6) and Botox/Dysport (pH 6.8) influences pain perception.

Pain sensation during toxin injections is usually fleeting, and simple measures can improve patient comfort.[78] For facial wrinkles, anesthesia is not necessary unless the patient prefers it. The 30-gauge needles that are used to inject the medication are the same size as acupuncture needles and cause minimal pain in a calm patient. Allowing the BTX to come to room temperature may decrease the level of pain otherwise felt by the patient. When the physician approaches the patient in a calm and reassuring manner, not allowing the patient see the needles prior to and during the injections, the patient's anxiety is significantly reduced as is the perception of pain.

Topical anesthetic creams such as EMLA™ or LMX™ can be applied prior to injection to decrease the sensation of pain. BTX should not be mixed with local anesthetics because they can alter the pH of the preparation and cause the toxin to lose potency. Ice packs can be applied prior to injections, which may decrease the pain and encourage vasoconstriction, resulting in less bruising (see Chapter 21).

For hyperhidrosis, pain control is a necessity, especially for the palms and soles. Although some physicians perform nerve blocks, the primary author uses the following method: at least 1 hour prior to treating for hyperhidrosis, the topical anesthetic Ela-Max™ or EMLA (eutectic mixture of local anesthetic) is applied to the area to be treated. Next, these areas are occluded with plastic bags or gloves when treating hands and feet or with tape when treating axillae. Many attempts have been made to decrease the pain associated with the use of BTX for palmar hyperhidrosis. These have included topical anesthetics, intravenous regional anesthesia, nerve blocks, ice, Frigiderm spray,[79] and others. The use of nitrous oxide ("laughing gas") requires office training and can induce an anxiolytic rather than a pain-diminishing effect.[79] Ongoing trials to assess the effects of different anesthetics for an optimal injection with minimal pain are needed to establish the full potential of the different approaches of pain reduction with BTX injections.

POTENTIAL ADVANTAGE OF BOTULINUM TOXIN TYPE A IN HEADACHES

Migraine headaches occur in approximately 18% of women and 6% of men, resulting in a significant disability and decreased quality of life.[80] A subset of patients who have undergone BTX therapy for cosmetic indications have also reported improvement in migraine and chronic headache symptoms. Studies of the effects of BTX on headaches are controversial. While a few investigations failed to show a positive effect of Botox in the prevention of migraine or chronic headaches,[81–83] BTX may have a role in reducing the severity of headaches experienced by some patients.[83] Some recent studies specifically designed to target headaches and chronic migraines demonstrated efficacy of botulinum toxins in patients with chronic migraines and suggested further trials to reach an ideal optimal consensus on the safety and efficacy of this toxin in migraine/headache therapy.[84]

BOTULINUM TOXIN IN PERSISTENT FACIAL FLUSHING

Facial flushing is not an uncommon problem in fair-skinned individuals of Celtic and northern European descent. A vasomotor phenomenon that results in increased erythema, persistent facial flushing can be accompanied by facial telangiectasias and gustatory sweating. Facial flushing is categorized as either autonomic neural-mediated (wet) or direct vasodilator-mediated (dry). The method by which BTX-A works to affect vasodilation is unknown, and the results regarding its efficacy for this indication are inconclusive. One theory is that BTX might work through reduction of local subclinical inflammation, which contributes to persistent erythema. Moreover, the anti-inflammatory role of BTX-A in blocking substance P, vanilloid receptor 1 (TRPV-1), and calcitonin gene-related peptide (CGRP) is important in decreasing the subclinical inflammation that might present as erythema.[85] Only Yuraitis et al. have described an improvement related to facial flushing in limited case reports.[86] Alexandroff as well as Kranendonk et al. failed to show an effective response to BTX-A for facial flushing in three published cases.[87,88] Further studies are required to better assess the safety and efficacy of this procedure.

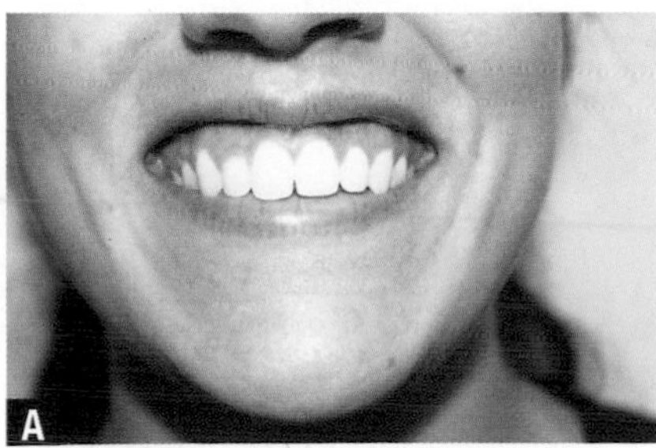
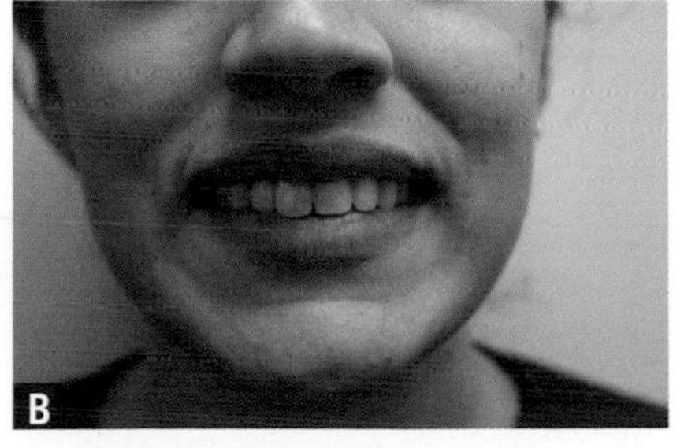

▲ **FIGURE 22-28** Upper gum shown (**A**) prior to Botox injections and (**B**) after Botox injections.

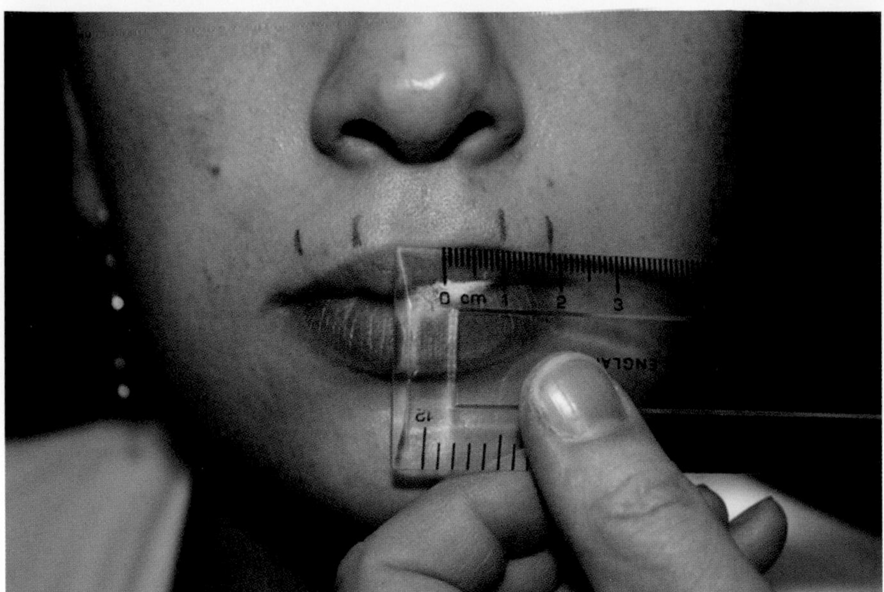

▲ **FIGURE 22-29** Placement of Botox on the upper lip to treat smoker's lines. Only 1 unit should be used in each injection site for a total of 4 units for the entire upper lip.

BOTULINUM TOXINS AND ACNE VULGARIS

Acne, which most commonly occurs during adolescence, is influenced by several factors (see Chapter 15). The pathology centers on the pilosebaceous follicle (comprising the sebaceous gland), the follicle (pore), and vellus hair. Factors that promote the formation of comedones (whiteheads or blackheads) include the following: (1) increased sebum production; (2) inflammation of the dermis and follicles by inflammatory mediators; (3) hyperkeratinization and obstruction of the upper region of the follicle; and (4) colonization of the follicle by the bacterium *Propionibacterium acnes*. Adolescence is marked by an increase in levels of circulating androgens, particularly dehydroepiandrosterone sulfate (DHEAS). The increased androgen levels are thought to cause sebaceous glands to enlarge and increase sebum production. While most acne patients have normal hormone levels, increased sebum production plays an important role in acne. A correlation exists between the rate of sebum production and the severity of acne. In addition, acne patients typically produce sebum that is deficient in linoleic acid, which is a potential cause of abnormal keratinization and follicular obstruction. Increased sebum levels can also irritate keratinocytes, causing the release of interleukin-1, which in turn can cause follicular hyperkeratinization. The final common pathway in each of these acne-causing routes, which are not mutually exclusive, is follicular obstruction.[89]

BTX may inhibit the cascade of events leading to acne. This is likely achieved through parasympathetic effects, inhibiting sweat gland activity, and sebaceous gland secretion as well as stimulating keratinocyte locomotion. Associated anti-inflammatory and antiandrogenic effects may also contribute. We hypothesize that BTX-A toxin inhibits the formation of acne through at least three different pathways. First, BTX inhibits sebum production by sebaceous glands through cholinergic inhibition and sebocyte differentiation. Cholinergic secretions normally attributed to increased sebum production are inhibited by BTX resulting in a lowered sebum potential across the ducts and skin.[90] Moreover, decreased sebocyte promoter differentiation and lower sebum levels may clinically improve acne by decreasing the growth of *P. acnes*. Thus, the ability to decrease sebum production decreases *P. acnes* growth and acne development. Additionally, BTX inhibits sweat production by sweat glands. Decreased perspiration may clinically improve acne by reducing the growth of *P. acnes*.[91] Furthermore, follicular occlusion by keratinocytes is the final common pathway in each of the various routes leading to acne. Keratinocyte migration is inhibited by the high-dose stimulation of nicotinic ACh receptors. By inhibiting the release of ACh, BTX may indirectly increase the migration of keratinocytes, thus reducing follicular occlusion.[92] The androgen surge during puberty is a known instigator of acne, and studies have shown that androgens increase the number of ACh receptors. Interestingly, androgen receptors are found on pilosebaceous duct keratinocytes, which are important in follicular occlusion. It is postulated that during puberty androgens increase the number of ACh receptors on the pilosebaceous keratinocytes, leading to further inhibition of keratinocyte locomotion through increased ACh stimulation. By inhibiting the release of ACh, BTX decreases the number of ACh receptors on the pilosebaceous keratinocytes, thereby increasing keratinocyte locomotion through decreased ACh stimulation.[93]

Finally, surprising results from recent research have shown that holocrine

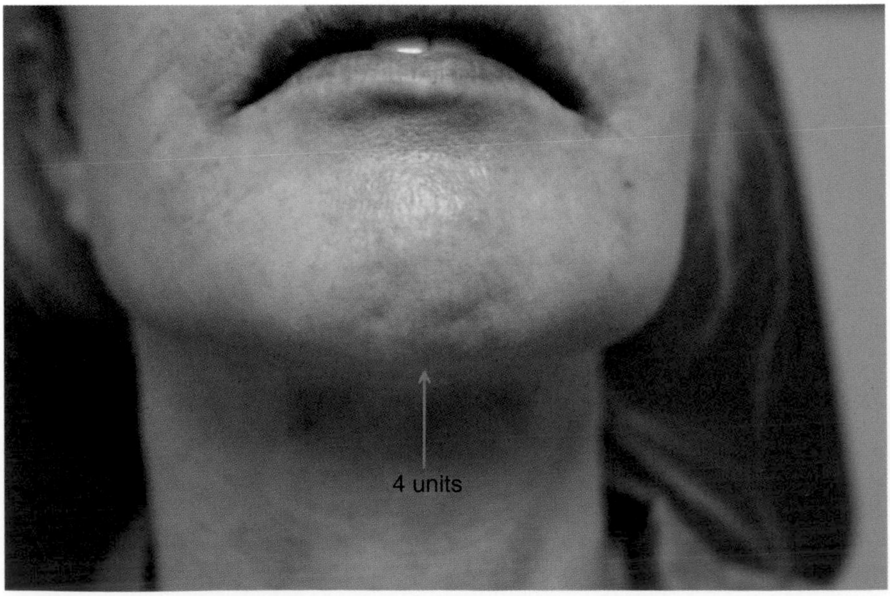

▲ **FIGURE 22-30** Chin puckering or Peau d' orange can be treated with BTX.

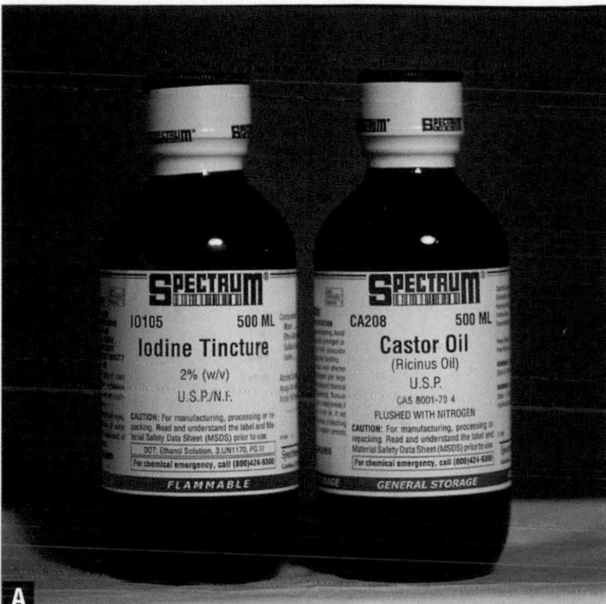

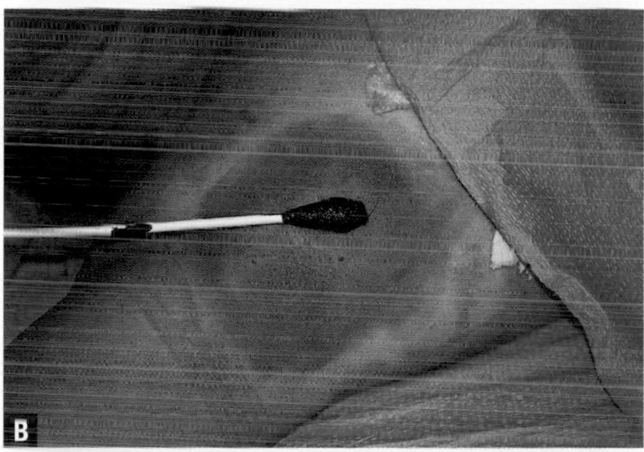

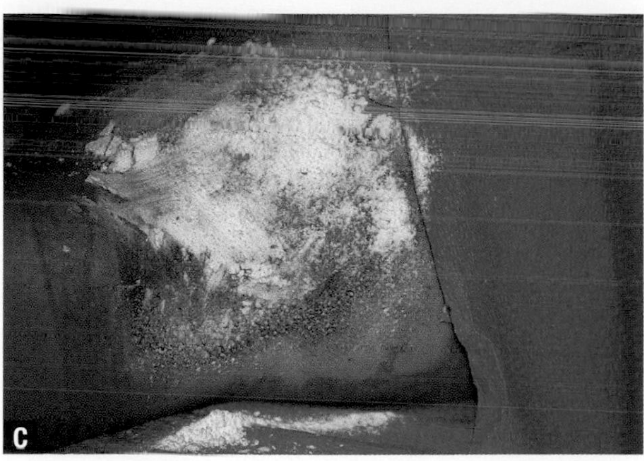

▲ **FIGURE 22-31** **A.** The iodine starch test solution is made by combining 9 parts of iodine with 1 part of castor oil. **B.** The iodine solution is then applied to the affected area using a swab. **C.** Potato starch is sprinkled over the iodine solution. (continued)

gland secretions are controlled by various neuropeptides, with substance P playing a significant role.[94] BTX-A blocks substance P, TRPV-1, and CGRP, which are important mediators in inflammation, and therefore helps decrease the inflammatory aspect of acne development.

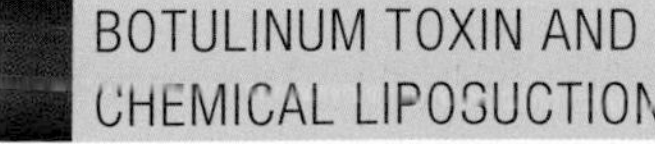

BOTULINUM TOXIN AND CHEMICAL LIPOSUCTION

Obesity is a medical problem with obvious cosmetic implications. Liposuction, gastric volume reduction, laparoscopic banding, lipase inhibitors, and mesotherapy are all methods employed in the treatment of obesity. Fat distribution and its physiology are partly known to be under the control of the autonomic nervous system. Multiple research studies have revealed that lipoatrophy and degradation of adipocytes was noticed after denervation.[95] There is disagreement regarding whether or not nervous system innervation plays a role in fat accumulation. Bilbao et al. showed that vagotomy reduced fat accumulation in rats and postulated that vagotonia plays a role in the development of obesity.[96] On the other hand, Jones et al. showed that muscle action-related sympathetic activity is associated with advancing age and increased abdominal adiposity.[97] This disparity was linked to a high sympathetic to parasympathetic ratio.[98] Following observations of coincidental lipoatrophy after BTX injections, it has been postulated that BTX injected in subcutaneous fat might achieve fat loss for cosmesis.[99] Lim et al. suggested a scheme by which subcutaneous fat denervation and hence focal lipoatrophy could be achieved. They recommended a maximum injectable total dose of 200 U for the intended area of fat reduction with an even distribution of each injection.[95] Further research in this area is required to establish a better risk–benefit ratio of this potential Botox use and to provide a guided consensus for its optimal use.

BOTULINUM AND HAIR GROWTH CONTROL

Focal hair loss following BTX-A treatment for blepharospasm and oromandibular dystonia has been reported, but remains controversial.[100,101] Several theories have been suggested to explain this observation, specifically the fact that hair follicles contain cholinergic receptors, which are essential signaling elements for nerve transmission that send growth signals to hair follicles.[102] When inhibited by BTX, those receptors may lead to hair loss.[103] Hair loss has also been described in conditions related to peripheral nerve dysfunction such as diabetic peripheral neuropathy, myxoma of the nerve sheath, and after occipital nerve block with corticosteroid. BTX could have the same effect through chemodenervation. These observations need to be studied before arriving at a conclusion or establishing a new indication for BTX. Cutrer and Pittelkow have actually reported regrowth of hair rather than loss after Botox was administered for alopecia areata, extending the debate over whether Botox actually causes hair regrowth or loss.[104]

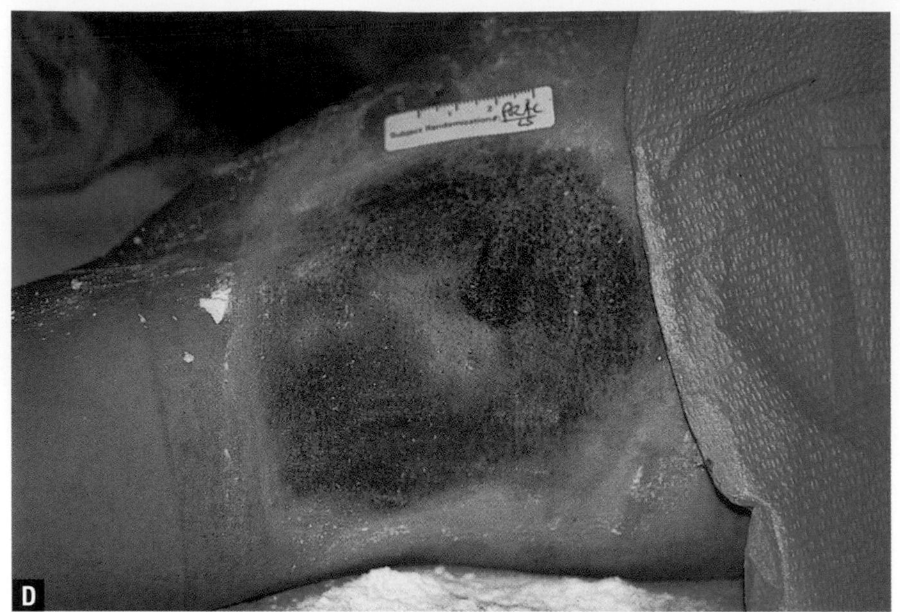

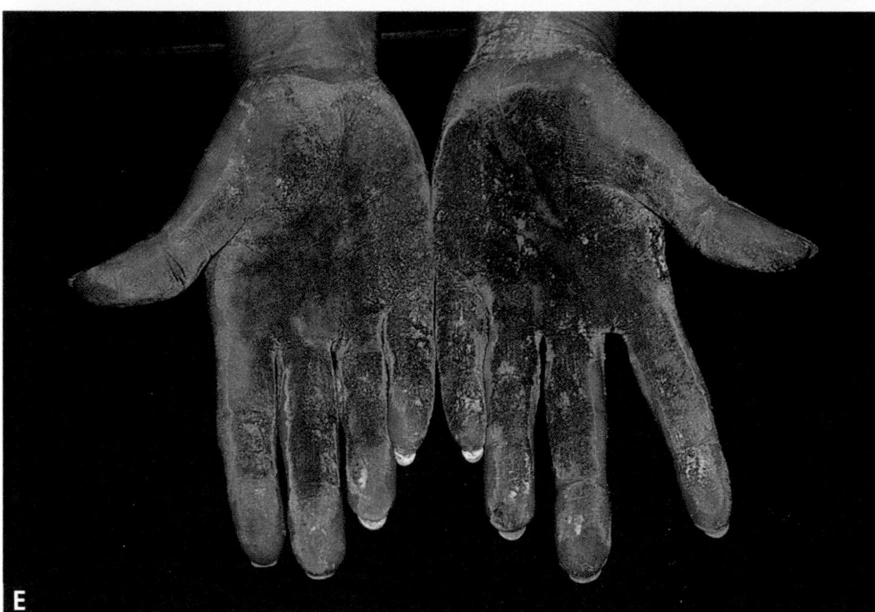

▲ **FIGURE 22-31** (continued). **D.** Sweat turns the starch black, delineating the affected areas. **E.** This test is useful to determine which areas to inject. In this patient, the fingertips can be avoided because the starch iodine test indicates that there is no sweating on the fingertips.

BTX-A AND COSMETIC SURGERY

BTX-A can be used before or after the surgical manipulation to either enhance or sustain benefits. If injected in the preoperative period, the toxin may allow improved tissue manipulation and reduced incisional tension leading to improved healing. Prior to endoscopic brow lift or a face lift using endoscopy, BTX-A injections help in raising the position of the brow and can reduce the amount of surgical manipulations necessary. Finally, when used after surgery, BTX-A weakens the musculature, prolonging the anticipated effect.[105]

COMBINED THERAPIES: BTX-A AND OTHER REJUVENATION MODALITIES

The superiority of BTX-A when used with other cosmetic procedures has been documented in a number of studies. When administered 1 week prior to the treatment with filling agents, BTX-A prevents the distortion of the fillers and prolongs the effects of augmentation by reducing the muscular activity associated with rhytide formation.[106]

BTX-A therapy works synergistically with resurfacing techniques to provide an optimal improvement of dynamic rhytides and in some cases enhance overall skin tone and texture. One study indicated that CO_2 ablative laser resurfacing combined with BTX-A provided a stronger and longer-lasting effect.[107] Within many cosmetic practices, BTX-A is now a part of the standard resurfacing protocol.

The synergistic effects of BTX-A and other rejuvenation procedures can extend to intense pulsed light protocols. In one study, the combined effect of intense pulsed light and BTX-A produced a more pronounced global aesthetic improvement in reducing crow's feet, telangiectasia, pore size, and lentigines, as well as ameliorating facial skin texture as compared with the use of intense pulsed light alone.[108]

RESISTANCE TO BOTULINUM TOXIN

Development of Antibodies

Botulinum neurotoxins may be immunogenic, and antibodies may inactivate the molecule. The BTX molecule is composed of a light chain and a heavy chain. The toxin is embedded in a protein complex that protects the toxin's binding site until the desired pH is reached and the toxin is released. Antibodies to this critical binding site on the heavy chain of the BTX molecule will prevent binding of the toxin to its receptor, thereby crippling the actions of the toxin. "Neutralizing antibodies" have been reported in patients treated with high doses of BTX for neurologic disorders such as cerebral palsy. It is important to understand that there are many types of antibodies that can interact with BTX; however, the only antibodies that can affect the efficacy of the toxin are neutralizing antibodies. Antibodies may develop to BTX that are inconsequential to the patient, yet the antibodies that are capable of neutralizing the toxin are a concern as they have the potential to decrease the efficacy of the toxin. By definition, antibodies that neutralize BTX-A would not neutralize BTX-B and vice versa. Patients who develop antibodies to BTX-A can still enjoy the benefits of BTX-B. For this reason, it is recommended that practitioners have several different BTX serotypes available on the market.

The incidence of antibody-mediated resistance to BTX, as determined by the mouse lethality assay, is reported between 3% and 9.5% and is accepted generally to be approximately 5%. The only apparent symptom of the development of antibodies is lack of response to

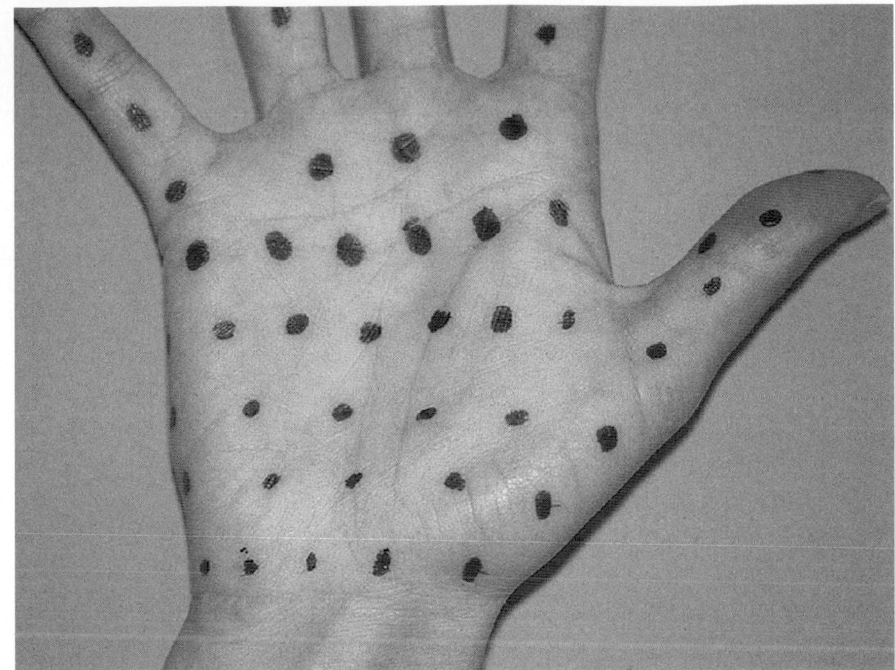

▲ **FIGURE 22-32** Injection sites on hands are approximately 1.5 cm apart.

TABLE 22-6
Factors of Proteins That Increase Immunogenicity

Foreign instead of endogenous
Large rather than small size
Denatured rather than native
Presence of adjuvants
Aggregated rather than unaggregated
Quantity present
Frequency encountered

These properties of toxin preparations make them more likely to cause an antibody response. Of course, other factors such as the age and genetics of a patient are also important.

further injections. The use of other serotypes (F or B) may benefit those who have developed antibody resistance. There are two types of therapy resistance to BTX, primary and secondary. A patient who does not respond to the first injection of BTX-A is referred to as a "primary nonresponder," but reasons for nonresponse can include inappropriate site of injection, poor technique, and/or insufficient dose.[109,110]

Immunogenicity should be suspected in a patient who no longer responds to BTX-A ("secondary nonresponder") following a successful course of earlier injections. Antibody formation could be targeted against the neurotoxin component of BTX or against its nontoxic protein component. The recommended approach is to inject 20 U BTX into the hypothenar or forehead muscles. If the patient responds to BTX, then transient weakness will develop in the muscle 1 to 2 weeks after injection. An alternative is to take blood for an antibody assay that is rarely used. In secondary nonresponders, the problem can be further overcome by using a different BTX serotype, for example, BTX-B if resistance develops to BTX-A.

Risk factors for the development of antibodies include higher doses, shorter intervals between injections, booster doses, and young age. Recommendations to help prevent development of antibodies include the following: (1) use of the smallest possible dose to achieve relief, (2) an interval between injections of at least 1 month (the preferred interval is 3 months), and (3) "touch-up injection" avoidance.

Many researchers have postulated that the risk of antibody formation is due in part to the quantity of protein or the "protein load" of the toxin, the type of protein present in the toxin, and to other factors listed in Table 22-6. Manufacturers of BTX have attempted to minimize each of these factors in order to create a less immunogenic product. For example, the original Botox that was used until December 1997 contained a higher level of protein than the Botox currently in use; therefore, it should lead to a lower incidence of antibody formation. As previously discussed, Merz Pharmaceuticals, the manufacturer of the new BTX product Xeomin, claims that its product contains a negligible amount of bacterial proteins (0.6 ng) with lower immune response. In spite of the concerns regarding immunogenicity, there are no known or published reports of antibody production in patients treated with doses of any of the available BTX products for cosmetic indications, which may be explained by the lower doses used in comparison with neurologic and cervical dystonia indications where reports of resistance are centered.[111]

SIDE EFFECTS

Complications from the use of BTX injections occur infrequently and are transient and reversible. Bruising at the

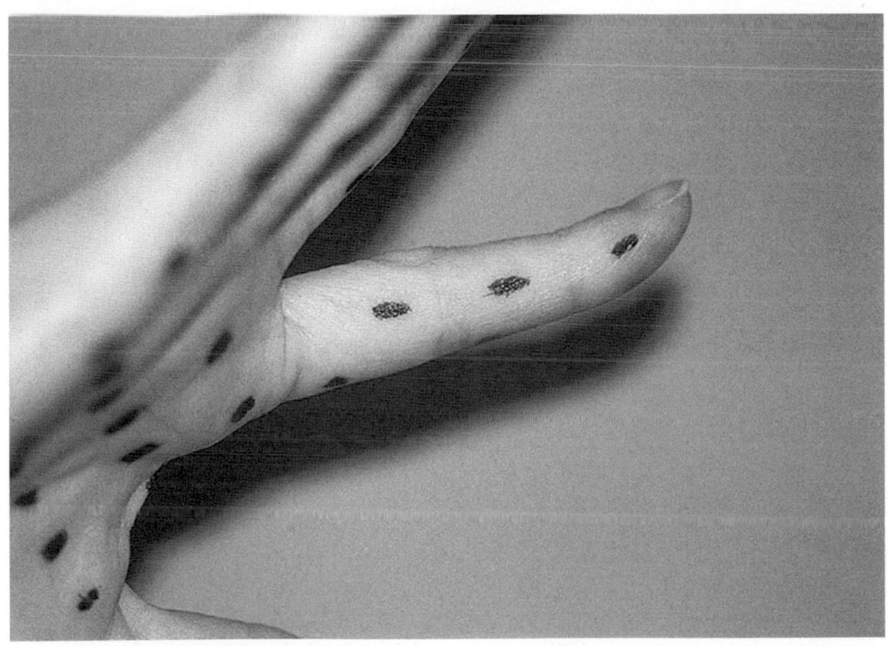

▲ **FIGURE 22-33** Injection sites on fingers.

injection site(s) is one of the most common adverse events and the incidence can be lessened by avoiding aspirin, NSAIDs, green tea, vitamin E, and other anticoagulants for 10 days prior to treatment. Anecdotal reports reveal that application of ice packs to the area prior to injection reduces the pain of the procedure and the incidence of bruising. Some studies have shown an association with flu-like symptoms (Botox and Myobloc) and dry mouth (Myobloc) after injection of these products in larger doses used for neurologic indications.

The most serious side effects of BTX treatment in the upper face are ptosis and, very rarely, diplopia or ectropion.[112] Proper placement of the toxin with good injection technique will drastically reduce the incidence of these temporary side effects. In fact, many experts anecdotally state that physicians just learning to perform BTX injections in the upper face have approximately a 4% incidence of inducing ptosis, which, with practice, falls to 0.5%.

Adverse effects from injection into the platysma can include bruising, drooling, downturning of the corner of the mouth, weakness in the neck muscles, and dysphagia. Lip ptosis or mouth asymmetry may result from injections in this area.

Treatment of the palms and soles for hyperhidrosis can induce temporary muscle weakness. One should exercise caution when treating patients that require a strong grip (e.g., tennis players) and manual dexterity (e.g., piano players) and these patients should be aware of the risks of treatment of the palms. One other cautionary note: the use of Botox has been reported, in one patient, to have unmasked underlying myasthenia gravis;[113] therefore, its use is contraindicated in patients with myasthenia gravis, systemic lupus, and other autoimmune disorders associated with a preexisting neuromuscular condition. Dysport is the only brand of BTX that contains lactose. Its use has been blamed for a fixed drug eruption in one patient.[114] Care should be taken to label all syringes containing BTX to avoid inadvertent administration of the toxin.

SUMMARY

The injection of the *C. botulinum* A exotoxin is a safe; fast, and nontraumatic approach to correcting wrinkles, raising eyebrows, and improving hyperhidrosis. A significant number of physicians worldwide perform this procedure for cosmetic purposes. There are many new forms and brands of BTX entering the market. It is certain that we will see much more research examining this interesting agent in the near future.

REFERENCES

1. Savardekar P. Botulinum toxin. *Indian J Dermatol Venereol Leprol.* 2008;74:77.
2. Finkelstein A. Channels formed in phospholipid bilayer membranes by diphtheria, tetanus, botulinum and anthrax toxin. *J Physiol.* 1990;84:188.
3. Setler P. The biochemistry of botulism toxin type B. *Neurology.* 2000;55:S22.
4. Scott A. Clostridial toxins as therapeutic agents. In: Simpson LL, ed. *Botulinum Neurotoxin and Tetanus Toxin.* New York, NY: Academic Press; 1989:399-412.
5. Blitzer A, Binder WJ, Aviv JE, et al. The management of hyperfunctional facial lines with botulinum toxin. A collaborative study of 210 injection sites in 162 patients. *Arch Otolaryngol Head Neck Surg.* 1997;123:389.
6. Carruthers JD, Carruthers JA. Treatment of glabellar frown lines with C. botulinum-A exotoxin. *J Dermatol Surg Oncol.* 1992;18:17.
7. Carruthers A, Carruthers J. History of the cosmetic use of Botulinum A exotoxin. *Dermatol Surg.* 1998;24:1168.
8. The American Society for Aesthetic Plastic Surgery. Cosmetic surgery national data bank statistics 2007. http://www.surgery.org/download/2007stats.pdf. Accessed March 21, 2008.
9. Ocampo J. Indicaciones cosm'eticas de la toxina botulinica. *Piel.* 1997;12:434.
10. Carruthers A, Carruthers J. Clinical indications and injection technique for the cosmetic use of botulinum A exotoxin. *Dermatol Surg.* 1998;24:1189.
11. Klein AW. Dilution and storage of botulinum toxin. *Dermatol Surg.* 1998;24:1179.
12. Sarifakioglu N, Sarifakioglu E. Evaluating effects of preservative-containing saline solution on pain perception during botulinum toxin type-a injections at different locations: a prospective, single-blinded, randomized controlled trial. *Aesthetic Plast Surg.* 2005;29:113.
13. Hui JI, Lee WW. Efficacy of fresh versus refrigerated botulinum toxin in the treatment of lateral periorbital rhytids. *Ophthal Plast Reconstr Surg.* 2007;23:433.
14. Sampaio C, Ferreira JJ, Simoes F, et al. DYSBOT: a single-blind, randomized parallel study to determine whether any differences can be detected in the efficacy and tolerability of two formulations of botulinum toxin type A—Dysport and Botox—assuming a ratio of 4:1. *Mov Disord.* 1997;12:1013.
15. Odergren T, Hjaltason H, Kaakkola S, et al. A double blind, randomised, parallel group study to investigate the dose equivalence of Dysport and Botox in the treatment of cervical dystonia. *J Neurol Neurosurg Psychiatry.* 1998;64:6.
16. Pickett A, O'Keeffe R, Panjwani N. The protein load of therapeutic botulinum toxins. *Eur J Neurol.* 2007;14:e11.
17. Package insert on Dysport. Berkshire, UK. Ipsen Ltd., 2001.
18. Brandt F, Swanson N, Baumann L: A phase III randomized double-blind, placebo-controlled study to assess the efficacy and safety of Reloxin in the treatment of glabellar lines. Poster presented at Winter Clinical Dermatology Conference-Hawaii®, March 14-18, 2008, The Ritz Carlton, Kapalua, Maui, Hawaii.
19. Data on file, Medicis Corporation.
20. Wohlfarth K, Müller C, Sassin I, et al. Neurophysiological double-blind trial of a botulinum neurotoxin type a free of complexing proteins. *Clin Neuropharmacol.* 2007;30:86.
21. Dressler D. Pharmacological aspects of therapeutic botulinum toxin preparations. *Nervenarzt.* 2006;77:912.
22. Jost WH, Blümel J, Grafe S. Botulinum Neurotoxin type A free of complexing proteins (XEOMIN) in focal dystonia. *Drugs.* 2007;67:669.
23. Package insert. Neuronox®. Medy-Tox Inc. South Korea, 2006.
24. Tang X, Wan X. Comparison of Botox with a Chinese type A botulinum toxin. *Chin Med J (Engl).* 2000;113:794.
25. Rieder CR, Schestasky P, Socal MP, et al. A double-blind, randomized, crossover study of prosigne versus botox in patients with blepharospasm and hemifacial spasm. *Clin Neuropharmacol.* 2007;30:39.
26. Baumann L, Slezinger A, Vujevich J, et al. A double-blinded, randomized, placebo-controlled pilot study of the safety and efficacy of Myobloc (botulinum toxin type B)-purified neurotoxin complex for the treatment of crow's feet: a double-blinded, placebo-controlled trial. *Dermatol Surg.* 2003;29:508.
27. Aoki KR, Ranoux D, Wissel J. Using translational medicine to understand clinical differences between botulinum toxin formulations. *Eur J Neurol.* 2006;13(suppl 4):10.
28. Dolly JO, Black J, Williams RS, et al. Acceptors for botulinum neurotoxin reside on motor nerve terminals and mediate its internalization. *Nature.* 1984;307:457.
29. Black JD, Dolly JO. Interaction of 125I-labeled botulinum neurotoxins with nerve terminals. I. Ultrastructural autoradiographic localization and quantitation of distinct membrane acceptors for types A and B on motor nerves. *J Cell Biol.* 1986;103:521.
30. Gracies JM, Weisz DJ, Yang BY, et al. Impact of botulinum toxin A (BTX-A) dilution and end plate targeting technique in upper limb spasticity. *Ann Neurol.* 2000;52:S87.
31. Wohlfarth K, Göschel H, Frevert J, et al. Botulinum A toxins: units versus units. *Naunyn Schmiedebergs Arch Pharmacol.* 1997;355:335.
32. De Almeida AT, De Boulle K. Diffusion characteristics of botulinum neurotoxin products and their clinical significance in cosmetic applications. *J Cosmet Laser Ther.* 2007;9(suppl 1):17.
33. Matarasso SL. Comparison of botulinum toxin types A and B: a bilateral and double-blind randomized evaluation in the treatment of canthal rhytides. *Dermatol Surg.* 2003;29:7.
34. Baumann L, Slezinger A, Halem M, et al. Double-blind, randomized, placebo-controlled pilot study of the safety and

efficacy of Myobloc (botulinum toxin type B) for the treatment of palmar hyperhidrosis. *Dermatol Surg.* 2005;31:263.
35. Trinidade de Almeida AR, Marques E, de Almeida J, et al. Pilot study comparing the diffusion of two formulations of botulinum toxin type A in patients with forehead hyperhidrosis. *Dermatol Surg.* 2007;33:S37.
36. Cliff SH, Judodihardjo H, Eltringham E. Different formulations of botulinum toxin type A have different migration characteristics: a double-blind, randomized study. *J Cosmet Dermatol.* 2008;7:50.
37. Rzany B, Ascher B, Fratila A, et al. Efficacy and safety of 3- and 5-injection patterns (30 and 50 U) of botulinum toxin A (Dysport) for the treatment of wrinkles in the glabella and the central forehead region. *Arch Dermatol.* 2006;142:320.
38. Carruthers A, Carruthers J. Prospective, double-blind, randomized, parallel-group, dose-ranging study of botulinum toxin type A in men with glabellar rhytids. *Dermatol Surg.* 2005;31:1297.
39. Teske SA, Kersten RC, Devoto MH, et al. Hering's law and eyebrow position. *Ophthal Plast Reconstr Surg.* 1998;14:105.
40. Huang W, Rogachefsky AS, Foster JA. Browlift with botulinum toxin. *Dermatol Surg.* 2000;26:55.
41. de Almeida AR, Cernea SS. Regarding browlift with botulinum toxin. *Dermatol Surg.* 2001;27:848.
42. Knize DM. Limited-incision forehead lift for eyebrow elevation to enhance upper blepharoplasty. *Plast Reconstr Surg.* 1996;97:1334.
43. Karacalar A, Korkmaz A, Kale A, et al. Compensatory brow asymmetry: anatomic study and clinical experience. *Aesthetic Plast Surg.* 2005;29:119.
44. Huilgol SC, Carruthers A, Carruthers JD. Raising eyebrows with botulinum toxin. *Dermatol Surg.* 1999;25:373.
45. Ahn MS, Catten M, Maas CS. Temporal brow lift using botulinum toxin A. *Plast Reconstr Surg.* 2000;105:1129.
46. Evans J. Microdroplets provide less aggressive brow lift. *Skin and Allergy News.* 2007;3:42.
47. Carruthers J, Carruthers A. The adjunctive usage of botulinum toxin. *Dermatol Surg.* 1998;24:1244.
48. Atamoros FP. Botulinum toxin in the lower one third of the face. *Clin Dermatol.* 2003;21:505.
49. Dayan S, Kempiners J. Treatment of the lower third of the nose and dynamic nasal tip ptosis with botox. *Plast Reconstr Surg.* 2005;115:1784.
50. Ghavami A, Janis JE, Guyuron B. Regarding the treatment of dynamic nasal tip ptosis with botulinum toxin A. *Plast Reconstr Surg.* 2006;118:263.
51. Carruthers J, Carruthers A. Aesthetic botulinum A toxin in the mid and lower face and neck. *Dermatol Surg.* 2003;29:468.
52. Wise JB, Greco T. Injectable treatments for the aging face. *Facial Plast Surg.* 2006;22:140.
53. Foster JA, Wulc AE. Cosmetic use of botulinum toxin. *Facial Plast Surg Clin North Am.* 1998;6:79.
54. Benedetto AV. Cosmetic uses of botulinum toxin A in the lower face, neck and upper chest. In: Benedetto AV, ed. *Botulinum Toxin in Clinical Dermatology.* Boca Raton, FL: Taylor & Francis Group; 2005;3-12.
55. Brandt FS, Bellman B. Cosmetic use of botulinum A exotoxin for the aging neck. *Dermatol Surg.* 1998;24:1232.
56. Lowe NJ. Botulinum toxin:combination treatments for the face and neck. In: Lowe NJ, ed. *Textbook of Facial Rejuvenation.* London, England: Martin Dunitz/Taylor and Francis; 2002:158-170.
57. Levy PM. The 'Nefertiti Lift': a new technique for specific re-contouring of the jawline. *J Cosm Laser Ther.* 2007;9:249.
58. Becker-Wegerich PM, Rauch L, Ruzicka T. Botulinum toxin A: successful décolleté rejuvenation. *Dermatol Surg.* 2002;28:168.
59. Flynn TC. Botox in men. *Dermatol Ther.* 2007;20:407.
60. Flynn TC. Update on botulinum toxin. *Semin Cutan Med Surg.* 2006;25:115.
61. Monks DA, O'Bryant EL, Jordan CL. Androgen receptor immunoreactivity in skeletal muscle : enrichment at the neuromuscular junction. *J Comp Neurol.* 2004;473.59.
62. Carruthers J, Fagien S, Matarasso L, et al. Consensus recommendations on the use of botulinum toxin type a in facial aesthetics. *Plast Reconstr Surg.* 2004;114:1S.
63. Ahn KY, Park MY, Park DH, et al. Botulinum toxin A for the treatment of facial hyperkinetic wrinkle lines in Koreans. *Plast Reconstr Surg.* 2005;105:778.
64. Kim J. Cosmetic treatments for ethnic skin. Papers presented at: 65th Annual summer meeting of American Academy of Dermatology, focus session 872; February 2007; Washington, DC.
65. Arimura K, Arimura Y, Takata Y, et al. Comparative electrophysiological study of response to botulinum toxin type B in Japanese and Caucasians. *Mov Disord.* 2008;23:240.
66. Heckmann M, Ceballos-Baumann AO, Plewig G. Botulinum toxin A for axillary hyperhidrosis (excessive sweating). *N Engl J Med.* 2001;344:488.
67. Lowe NJ, Glaser DA, Eadie N, et al. Botulinum toxin type A in the treatment of primary axillary hyperhidrosis: a 52-week multicenter double-blind, randomized, placebo-controlled study of efficacy and safety. *J Am Acad Dermatol.* 2007;56:604.
68. Baumann LS, Halem ML. Botulinum toxin-B and the management of hyperhidrosis. *Clin Dermatol.* 2004;22:60.
69. Barankin B, Wasel N. Treatment of inguinal hyperhidrosis with botulinum toxin type A. *Int J Dermatol.* 2006;45:985.
70. Goldman A. Treatment of axillary and palmar hyperhidrosis with botulinum toxin. *Aesthetic Plast Surg.* 2000;24:280.
71. Moraru E, Voller B, Auff E, et al. Dose thresholds and local anhidrotic effect of botulinum A toxin injections (Dysport). *Br J Dermatol.* 2001;145:368.
72. Kinkelin I, Hund M, Naumann M, et al. Effective treatment of frontal hyperhidrosis with botulinum toxin A. *Br J Dermatol.* 2000;143:824.
73. Pomprasit M, Chintrakarn C. Treatment of Frey's syndrome with botulinum toxin. *J Med Assoc Thai.* 2007;90:2397.
74. Suskind DL, Tilton A. Clinical study of botulinum-A toxin in the treatment of sialorrhea in children with cerebral palsy. *Laryngoscope.* 2002;112:73.
75. Manchese RR, Blotta P, Pastore A, et al. Management of parotid sialocele with botulinum toxin. *Laryngoscope.* 1999;109:1344.
76. Laskawi R, Drobik C, Schönebeck C. Up-to-date report of botulinum toxin type A treatment in patients with gustatory sweating (Frey's syndrome). *Laryngoscope.* 1998;108:381.
77. Kranz G, Sycha T, Voller B, et al. Pain sensation during intradermal injections of three different botulinum toxin preparations in different doses and dilutions. *Derm Surg.* 2006;32:886.
78. Carruthers A, Carruthers J, Said S. Dose-ranging study of botulinum toxin type A in the treatment of glabellar rythides in females. *Derm Surg.* 2005;31:414.
79. Baumann L, Frankel S, Welsh E, et al. Cryoanalgesia with dichlorotetrafluoroethane lessens the pain of botulinum toxin injections for the treatment of palmar hyperhidrosis. *Dermatol Surg.* 2003;29:1057.
80. Lipton RB, Bigal ME. Migraine: epidemiology, impact and risk factors for progression. *Headache.* 2005;45:S3.
81. Aurora SK, Gawel M, Brandes JL, et al. Botulinum toxin type a prophylactic treatment of episodic migraine: a randomized, double-blind, placebo-controlled exploratory study. *Headache.* 2007;47:486.
82. Silberstein SD, Stark SR, Lucas SM, et al. Botulinum toxin type A for the prophylactic treatment of chronic daily headache: a randomized, double-blind, placebo-controlled trial. *Mayo Clin Proc.* 2005;80:1126.
83. Vo AH, Satori R, Jabbari B, et al. Botulinum toxin type-a in the prevention of migraine: a double-blind controlled trial. *Aviat Space Environ Med.* 2007;78:B113.
84. Freitag FG, Diamond S, Diamond M, et al. Botulinum toxin type a in the treatment of chronic migraine without medication overuse. *Headache.* 2008;48:201.
85. Bansal C, Omlin KJ, Hayes CM, et al. Novel cutaneous uses for botulinum toxin type A. *J Cosmet Dermatol.* 2006;5:268.
86. Yuraitis M, Jacob CI. Botulinum toxin for the treatment of facial flushing. *Dermatol Surg.* 2004;30:102.
87. Alexandroff AB, Sinclair SA, Langtry JA. Successful use of botulinum toxin a for the treatment of neck and anterior chest wall flushing. *Dermatol Surg.* 2006;32:1536.
88. Kranendonk SK, Ferris LK, Obagi S. Re: Botulinum toxin for the treatment of facial flushing. *Dermatol Surg.* 2005;31:491.
89. Simonart T, Dramaix M, De Maertelaer V. Efficacy of tetracyclines in the treatment of acne vulgaris: a review. *Br J Dermatol.* 2008;158:208.
90. Yosipovitch G, Reis J, Tur E, et al. Sweat secretion, stratum corneum hydration, small nerve function and pruritus in patients with advanced chronic renal failure. *Br J Dermatol.* 1995;133:561.

91. Kurzen H, Kari U. Novel aspects in cutaneous biology of acetylcholine synthesis and acetylcholine receptors. *Exp Dermatol*. 2004;13:27.
92. Chernyavsky AI, Arredondo J, Wess J, et al. Novel signaling pathways mediating reciprocal control of keratinocyte migration and wound epithelialzation through M_3 and M_4 muscarinic receptors. *J Cell Biol*. 2004;166:261.
93. Shapiro E, Miller AR, Lepor H. Down regulation of the muscarinic cholinergic receptor of the rat prostate following castration. *J Urol*. 1985;1:179.
94. Toyoda M, Morohashi M. Pathogenesis of acne. *Med Electron Microsc*. 2001;34:29.
95. Lim EC, Raymond CS. Botulinum toxin injections to reduce adiposity: possibility, or fat chance? *Med Hypotheses*. 2006;67:1086.
96. Balbo SL, Mathias PC, Bonfleur ML, et al. Vagotomy reduces obesity in MSG-treated rats. *Res Commun Mol Pathol Pharmacol*. 2000;108:291.
97. Jones PP, Davy KP, Alexander S. Age-related increase in muscle sympathetic nerve activity is associated with abdominal adiposity. *Am J Physiol*. 1997;272:E976.
98. Lindmark S, Lönn L, Wiklund U, et al. Dysregulation of the autonomic nervous system can be a link between visceral adiposity and insulin resistance. *Obes Res*. 2005;13:717.
99. Lim EC, Seet RC. Botulinum toxin, Quo Vadis? *Med Hypotheses*. 2007;69:718.
100. Rubegni P, Fimiani M, Tosi GM, et al. Conjunctival edema and alopecia of the external third of the eyebrows in a patient with Meige syndrome. *Graefes Arch Clin Exp Ophthalmol*. 2000;238:98.
101. Kowing D. Madarosis and facial alopecia presumed secondary to botlinum a toxin injections. *Optom Vis Sci*. 2005;82:579.
102. Hasse S, Chernyavsky AI, Grando SA, et al. The M_4 muscarinic acetylcholine receptor plays a key role in the control of murine hair follicle cycling and pigmentation. *Life Sci*. 2007;80;2248.
103. Kurzen H, Berger H, Jager C, et al. Phenotypical and molecular profiling of the extraneuronal cholinergic system of the skin. *J Invest Dermatol*. 2004;123: 937.
104. Cutrer FM, Pittelkow MR. Cephalalgic alopecia areata: a syndrome of neuralgiform head pain and hair loss responsive to botulinum A toxin injection. *Cephalalgia*. 2006;26:747.
105. Carruthers A, Carruthers JD. Botulinum toxin type A in facial aesthetics—an update. *US Dermatology Review*. 2006; 1-5.
106. Patel MP, Talmor M, Nolan WB. Botox and collagen for glabellar furrows: advantages of combination therapy. *Ann Plast Surg*. 2004;52:442.
107. Carruthers J, Carruthers A, Zelichowska A. The power of combined therapies: Botox and ablative facial laser resurfacing. *Am J Cosm Surg*. 2000;17:129.
108. Carruthers J, Carruthers A. The effect of full-face broadband light treatments alone and in combination with bilateral crow's feet botulinum toxin type A chemodenervation. *Dermatol Surg*. 2004;30:355.
109. Lee SK. Antibody-induced failure of botulinum toxin type A therapy in a patient with masseteric hypertrophy. *Dermatol Surg*. 2007;33:S105.
110. Pellett S, Tepp WH, Clancy CM, et al. A neuronal cell-based neurotoxin assay for highly sensitive and specific detection of neutralizing serum antibodies. *FEBS Lett*. 2007;581:4803.
111. Dressler D. Clinical presentation and management of antibody-induced failure of botulinum toxin therapy. *Mov Disord*. 2004;19(suppl 8):S92.
112. Guyuron B, Huddleston SW. Aesthetic indications for botulinum toxin injection. *Plast Reconstr Surg*. 194;93:913.
113. Borodic G. Myasthenic crisis after botulinum toxin. *Lancet*. 1998;352:1832.
114. Cox NH, Duffey P, Royle J. Fixed drug eruption caused by lactose in an injected botulinum toxin preparation. *J Am Acad Dermatol*. 1999;40:263.

CHAPTER 23

Dermal Fillers

Leslie Baumann, MD
Marianna Blyumin, MD
Sogol Saghari, MD

The dermal filler market is rapidly growing worldwide. According to the American Academy of Aesthetic Plastic Surgeons, 1,448,716 people received hyaluronic acid (HA) injections by plastic surgeons in 2007 (Table 23-1). The actual number is likely much higher when factoring in procedures performed by dermatologists and other aesthetically oriented physicians and physician extenders. Although collagen products (Zyplast and Zyderm) were the first dermal fillers to become widely available, collagen fillers have largely been replaced by HA fillers.

The ultimate goal of dermal fillers is to smooth out wrinkles and folds, even out scars, volumize furrows and sunken valleys, contour unevenness and laxity, and sculpt skin into a 360-degree, rejuvenated look. Over the last quarter century, several kinds of products suitable for soft tissue augmentation have become available, with intense industry research yielding more and more filler options with increasing regularity. Different regulatory mechanisms usually leave the US a few months or years behind other developed countries in making the latest products available to patients.

TABLE 23-1
Soft Tissue Augmentation Procedures Performed in 2007 by Members of the Academy of Aesthetic Plastic Surgeons

PROCEDURES	NUMBER PERFORMED IN 2007
Fat injections	44,547
Calcium hydroxylapatite (Radiesse/Radiance)	119,397
Collagen	63,769
Hyaluronic acid	1,448,716
Sculptra (not yet FDA approved)	34,972
Polymethyl methacrylate (Artecoll, Artefill)	12,075

Data obtained from www.surgery.org.

HISTORY

In 1893, by transplanting fat from the arms into facial defects, Neuber became the first physician to practice soft tissue augmentation.[1] In the middle of the 20th century, soft tissue augmentation could best be characterized by the use of silicone. Although popular in the 1940s and 1950s, silicone use was associated with the development of foreign body granulomas, which ultimately prompted the banning of silicone in 1992 until a new form of the substance (intended for ophthalmologic use) was approved by the United States Food and Drug Administration (FDA) in the late 1990s. In the meantime, though, the field of soft tissue augmentation had come into its own, in the 1970s, with the introduction by Stanford University researchers of animal-derived collagen implants.[2] By the 1980s, the use of collagen injections for wrinkles had entered the mainstream. While Americans were enjoying the benefits of bovine collagen fillers (i.e., Zyderm and Zyplast), other countries began to experiment with dermal HA fillers such as Hylaform and later Restylane in the mid to late 1990s. The beginning of the 21st century ushered in the introduction of newer nonbovine collagen fillers, CosmoDerm and CosmoPlast, and HA fillers, such as Captique and Juvéderm, as well as other synthetic fillers, Sculptra, Radiesse, and Artefill into the United States market. With different forms of soft tissue augmentation agents currently available in the United States and others in the pipeline, selecting the appropriate filler is challenging for physicians and patients alike. In order to achieve optimal cosmetically-pleasing results, it is incumbent upon dermatologists to obtain thorough comprehension of the characteristics of available fillers, their indications, contraindications, benefits and drawbacks, and ways to resolve potential complications. In this chapter, we will review the basics behind the art and science of the broad array of dermal fillers on the market in the United States. This will be preceded by a brief discussion of regulatory issues and the patient evaluation and consultation.

REGULATION

In the US, dermal fillers are regulated as medical devices. In order to obtain FDA approval, the company applying for approval for a dermal filler must satisfy the intense safety and efficacy criteria including nonteratogenicity, nonmigration, noncarcinogenesis, biocompatibility, and optimal purity, as well as reproducible and durable efficacy in correcting skin defects. Unfortunately, some physicians and physician extenders choose to use dermal filling substances that have not yet received FDA approval for any indication. This is not advisable for several reasons including the fact that it is illegal and that the safety of these products has not been established. With the multitude of safe, efficacious, and durable fillers on the market, there is no need or justifiable reason to use unapproved dermal fillers in the US.

PATIENT EVALUATION AND CONSULTATION

When embarking on soft tissue augmentation, proper preparations are essential. An initial consultation should include distant and close evaluation of the patient's facial structure and discussion of the cosmetic treatment options. The patient's history is taken to assess contraindications including allergy to filler components, herpes facialis, pregnancy/lactation, keloid predisposition, and autoimmune diseases. In addition, use of medications that inhibit clotting such as aspirin and ibuprofen should be examined. The ideal cosmetic outcome is achieved through a combination of various cosmetic procedures in order to attain an even tone, smooth texture, and adequate facial volume and shape. The discussion of the sequence and description of each proposed procedure, alternatives, risks and benefits, financial cost, and recovery period prepares the patient for realistic expectations and informed decision-making. After the treatment procedures are selected and informed consent is signed and witnessed, the patient should undergo pretreatment photography for the purpose of documentation; posttreatment photography is scheduled immediately after and on the follow-up visits. For novice patients, it is better to start the soft tissue intervention with the temporary and predictable fillers (e.g., collagen and HA), and then gradually advance with more lasting fillers (e.g., Sculptra and Radiesse) based on their comfort level and desire.

The best approach to minimizing the side effects of soft tissue augmentation is, first, to prevent them. To reduce bruising, patients should avoid anticoagulant medications or supplements (e.g., aspirin, vitamin E, etc.) for 10 days prior and several days after the procedure (see Chapter 21). The utility of *Arnica montana* oral tablets or topical gel or postprocedure oral bromelain supplements to decrease ecchymoses is anecdotal but these are often used in the primary author's practice. The pain associated with injection can be diminished with topical (e.g., lidocaine cream, ice), regional (e.g., infraorbital, dental nerve block), or intraprocedural anesthesia (e.g., fillers that contain lidocaine). Patients prone to regional herpes outbreaks should obtain antiviral prophylaxis with systemic medications (e.g., valcyclovir 1 g twice daily for 3 days, starting a day before the procedure). The procedure should be conducted in a clean, safe, well-lit, and soothing environment that is prepared to address any potential complications. Vasovagal responses are not uncommon; therefore, orange juice should be available in the event that the patient feels dizzy or faint. Topical steroids may be needed in case of a contact allergy to lidocaine cream. Most importantly, nitropaste should be immediately available in case a purple duskiness is seen on injection, warning of a possible arterial occlusion. Some physicians suggest keeping hyaluronidase on hand in case an arterial occlusion occurs with HA.[3]

TYPES OF FILLERS

Dermal fillers can be classified based on various criteria: depth of implantation (superficial upper and middermis, deep dermis, and subcutaneous levels); longevity of correction (temporary, semipermanent, and permanent); allergenicity (whether preprocedure allergic testing is required); composition of the agent (xenografts, allografts, or autologous, semi/fully synthetic); and stimulatory behavior (capacity to drive physiologic processes of endogenous tissue proliferation) versus replacement fillers (space-replacing effect). Safety and efficacy studies of the available fillers are required by the FDA; however, studies looking at the durability of the filler are not required and, therefore, subject to disagreement and frequent citing of anecdotal evidence. The lasting effect of the filler is dependent on the composition, amount used, depth injected, and carrier of the agent. Our discussion of fillers will proceed by dividing them according to composition: collagen fillers will be discussed first, followed by HA fillers, and then other agents.

TEMPORARY FILLERS

Injectable fillers such as collagen and HA are biodegradable and last from 4 to 9 months. These fillers commonly serve an important role as the initial step for new patients interested in soft tissue augmentation. Because of their transient effect, the potential patient dissatisfaction and side effects are also short-lived. Therefore, temporary fillers should always be the first line of therapy, saving the longer-lasting fillers for future patient visits.

Collagen

The major structural component of the dermis, collagen is the most abundant protein in the human organism as well as the skin, in particular, and confers strength and support to the skin. Collagen is also one of the strongest natural proteins, imparting durability and resilience to the skin, and comprising 70% of dry skin mass[4] (see Chapter 2). What is known as "collagen" is actually a meshwork of scaffolding-like structures composed of a complex family of over 18 types, 11 of which are found in the dermis. Type I collagen (80%–85%) and type III collagen (10%–15%) are the primary collagen constituents in the dermal matrix of adult human skin. Dermal fibroblasts produce a precursor form of collagen, α procollagens, which in turn produce both collagen types I and III, each of which is composed of three collagen chains.

Skin fragility and wrinkles result from the loss of collagen, which occurs with aging as well as solar exposure and other insults. UV light, free radicals, and other factors cause the body to produce collagenase, an enzyme that breaks down collagen. The injection of various forms of collagen into the skin helps it regain a youthful appearance, but such results are temporary. The range of collagen products has increased in recent years as manufacturers have worked to extend the duration of product effects.

BOVINE COLLAGEN

Overview With a record of safety and efficacy spanning over two decades, bovine collagen was the traditional dermal filler agent used to ameliorate undesirable signs of cutaneous facial aging.[5] In 1977, Zyderm I was introduced as the first injectable bovine collagen implant; it was approved by the FDA in 1981 for fine lines and shallow acne scars. Zyderm II and Zyplast were introduced and approved, respectively, in 1983 for moderate lines and deeper acne scars and 1985 for deep dermal folds and lines. Although these products were the standard for years to which newer implants were compared, because of better safety profiles, human-derived collagen and HA products have become more widely used. Zyderm I is 96% type I collagen and 4% type III collagen derived from the bovine skin of US enclosed cattle herds. Zyderm I and II differ only by collagen concentration. Zyderm I contains 35 mg/cc, while Zyderm II contains 65 mg/cc. The difference in concentration is significant insofar as it renders Zyderm II thicker and stiffer than Zyderm I. Like Zyderm I, Zyplast contains 35 mg/cc of collagen, but this collagen is cross-linked with glutaraldehyde, which makes it last longer via resistance to degradation (Table 23-2). Consequently, Zyplast is more viscous and less immunogenic than Zyderm.[6]

Zyderm and Zyplast are white substances prepackaged in 0.5-, 1-, and 2-mL syringes and injected with a 30-gauge 0.5-inch needle. The product should be stored in the refrigerator ideally at 4°C. While Zyderm I is properly injected into superficial dermis at 20- to 30-degree angles with the expectation of temporary skin blanching, Zyderm II can be injected slightly deeper at 35- to 45-degree angles with less anticipated blanching and minimal overcorrection.

TABLE 23-2
Collagen Concentration Comparison

Collagen from Cow Hide	Collagen from Bioengineered Skin	Concentration
Zyderm I	CosmoDerm I	35 mg collagen/cc
Zyderm II	CosmoDerm II	65 mg collagen/cc
Zyplast	CosmoPlast	35 mg collagen/cc cross-linked with glutaraldehyde

Since Zyderm is diluted with phosphate-buffered sterile saline, which is rapidly reabsorbed in skin, to achieve the optimal effect, overcorrecting implantation is necessary. Zyplast is implanted into even deeper dermis at 45- to 90-degree angles with minimal delayed blanching and without overcorrection.

Benefits Bovine-derived collagen dermal filling agents effectively reduce wrinkles and scars. Zyplast is appropriate for shaping the vermilion border of the lips and treating moderate and deep wrinkles, such as nasolabial folds and atrophic scars. Zyderm I is well suited for treating superficial rhytides (e.g., horizontal forehead wrinkles, crow's feet, fine perioral wrinkles, and scars) or for use over Zyplast in deeper wrinkles. The higher concentration of collagen in Zyderm II renders this product more appropriate for acne scar revision (see Chapter 26), but Zyplast lasts longer because it is cross-linked. Collagenase ultimately succeeds in degrading these products, returning the skin to its appearance prior to injection. Zyplast is the most commonly used bovine collagen product and lasts approximately 4 months, just slightly longer than Zyderm I and II. Bovine collagen can be safely reinjected 3 to 4 times per year if needed. Zyderm and Zyplast are the least expensive dermal fillers on the market and typically engender less bruising than products that contain HA. All the bovine collagen products contain 0.3% lidocaine to reduce the pain associated with the procedure.

Drawbacks Two skin tests, 6 and 2 weeks before the scheduled treatment, are required before the use of bovine collagen agents to reduce the risk of inducing hypersensitive or allergic reactions. Such responses can occur as early as 6 hours after the test, but are more likely to emerge 48 hours or 4 weeks after the test. A positive skin test disqualifies a patient for treatment with bovine collagen.

Approximately 3% of the general population is thought to be sensitive to bovine collagen.[7] Although a patient is unlikely to react to bovine collagen implants after two negative skin tests, the risk is never completely eliminated. The risk of hypersensitive reaction is 1.3% to 6.2% after one negative test[8,9] and 0.5% after two negative tests (Fig. 23-1). Patients should be advised that should such a reaction occur, it can be expected to spontaneously resolve within 4 to 24 months.[8,9] Allergic reactions also arise, albeit rarely, following multiple treatments. Topical, intralesional, or a brief course of systemic corticosteroids can be effective to treat these reactions. Oral cyclosporine[10] (Figs. 23-2 and 23-3) and topical tacrolimus[11] have also reportedly been used for the successful treatment of recalcitrant hypersensitive reactions to bovine collagen. Patients with lidocaine hypersensitivity are contraindicated for obtaining these injections because the fillers contain lidocaine.

Nonhypersensitive reactions to bovine collagen fillers can also infrequently occur (e.g., abscesses, bacterial infections, beading, cyst and granuloma formation, ecchymoses, and local necrosis). Several previously discussed preventative steps can be taken to reduce the likelihood of such outcomes. Because of its viscosity, Zyplast should not be injected into the glabellar region, as there have been reports of local necrosis and retinal artery occlusion leading to visual loss.[12] However, Zyderm I or II can be injected into the glabellar area very slowly and with extreme caution. Vascular occlusion or compression manifests as prominent

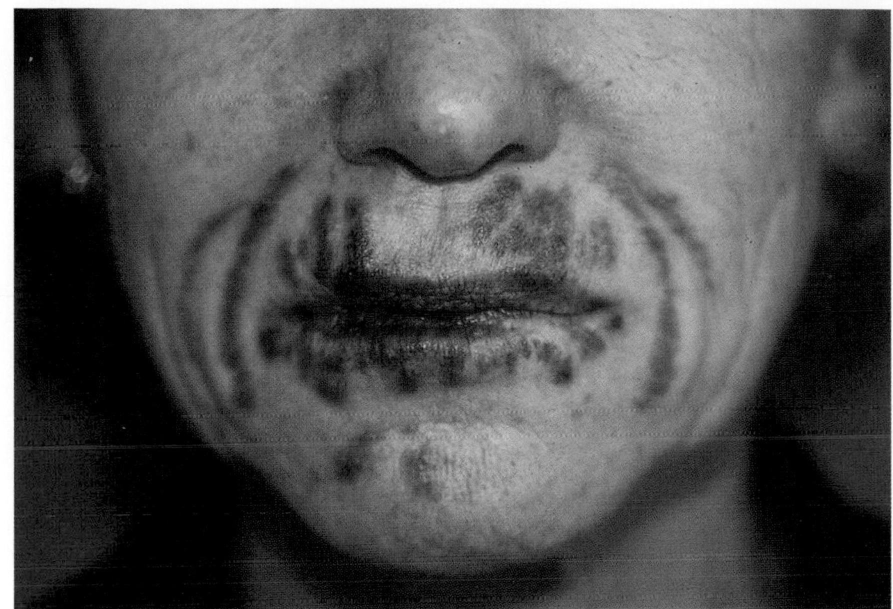

▲ **FIGURE 23-1** Collagen hypersensitivity reaction in a patient treated by another physician after only one skin test.

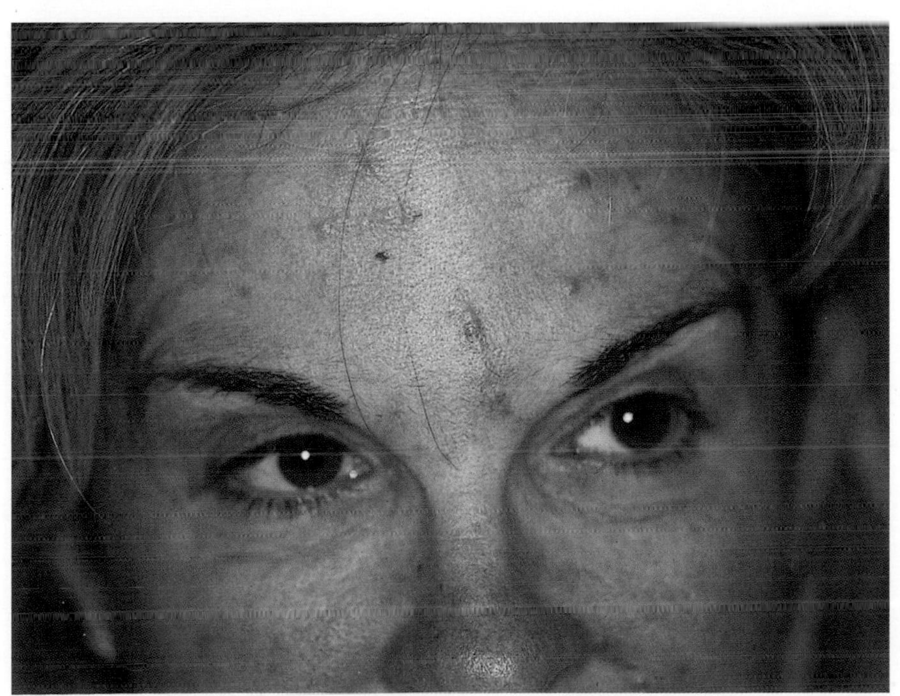

▲ **FIGURE 23-2** Collagen hypersensitivity reaction prior to treatment with cyclosporine. Note the indicated lesions in the forehead and glabellar area.

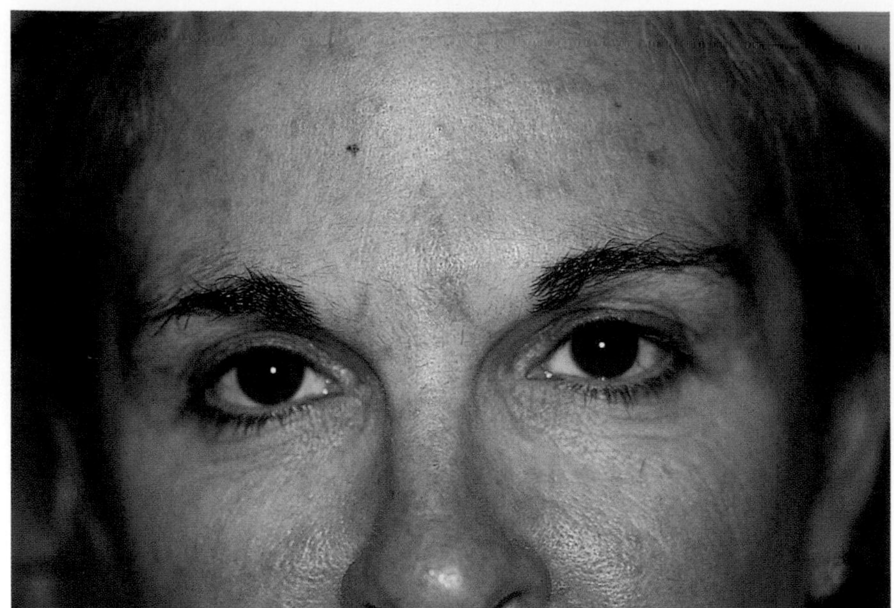

▲ **FIGURE 23-3** Collagen hypersensitivity reaction after 11 days of treatment with cyclosporine 5 mg/kg/d. The lesions flattened and had decreased redness. Only hyperpigmentation remained and resolved after a week.

immediate blanching and pain. Warm compresses, topical nitroglycerin, and meticulous wound care are necessary treatments. Prior to 1990, beads and cysts were reported at the injection site in 0.04% of patients treated with Zyderm or Zyplast, most likely caused by injections that were too superficial.[12] Injections should be made only into the dermis to avoid such reactions.[13] Abscesses should be treated with incision and drainage and a combination of antibiotics and corticosteroids to reduce secondary scarring. More than a decade ago, there was some speculation that autoimmune diseases, namely, polymyositis and dermatomyositis, might be induced by the injection of bovine collagen,[14] but studies have demonstrated that antibodies to bovine collagen do not cross-react with human collagen.[15,16] Therefore, the FDA has agreed that it is unlikely that bovine collagen causes connective tissue disease in humans.[9,17] Further, a study by Hanke et al. showed that the incident rate of polymyositis/dermatomyositis in patients receiving bovine collagen was not higher than the control-matched population.[18] However, the authors recommend avoiding the use of bovine collagen-containing fillers in patients with a history of autoimmune disease. Another major downside to using bovine collagen is the minimal durability of about 3 to 4 months.

BIOENGINEERED HUMAN COLLAGEN

Overview Over the last 10 years, several companies, motivated by the drawbacks of bovine-derived collagen, have developed human-derived soft tissue fillers. Unlike earlier cadaver-derived collagen (i.e., Cymetra) and, more recently, autologous collagen (i.e., Isolagen), bioengineered human collagen is pregenerated to ensure ease of accessibility. The manufacturing process begins with the harvesting of dermal fibroblasts from bioengineered human skin and placement into a three-dimensional mesh. The fibroblasts are then cultured in a bioreactor that simulates the conditions of the human body. Then, the fibroblasts synthesize collagen and extracellular matrix proteins. The derived collagen is purified to enhance safety. Human-bioengineered collagen implants include CosmoDerm I, CosmoDerm II, and CosmoPlast (Allergan Corporation, Irvine, CA), which contain human collagen types I and III, and were approved by the FDA in March 2003. CosmoDerm I is composed of 35 mg/cc human-bioengineered collagen distributed in a phosphate-based saline solution and 0.3% lidocaine. CosmoDerm II contains twice the collagen concentration of CosmoDerm I. CosmoPlast contains the same ingredients as CosmoDerm I, but is cross-linked by glutaraldehyde, yielding a product more resistant to degradation, thus lasting longer, and more appropriate for use in treating deeper furrows. While CosmoDerm is indicated for superficial wrinkles and shallow scars, CosmoPlast, which exhibits a stiff consistency (even more so than products containing HA), is well suited to treating the vermilion border of the lips (Fig. 23-4), as well as raising the corners of the mouth. In addition, it is a good choice to correct deformities of the bridge of the nose or to raise the nasal tip (Fig. 23-5). CosmoPlast is typically used in combination, usually with an HA agent, to treat medium and deep wrinkles, with the collagen product injected first to create a volume-filling base and the HA filler injected more superficially into the same location.

Similar to bovine collagens, CosmoDerm and CosmoPlast are white substances prepackaged in 1-mL syringes and injected via 30-gauge 0.5-inch needles. Although some anecdotal reports indicate better rheology of human collagen fillers, their technique of injection, cosmetic outcome, and durability are

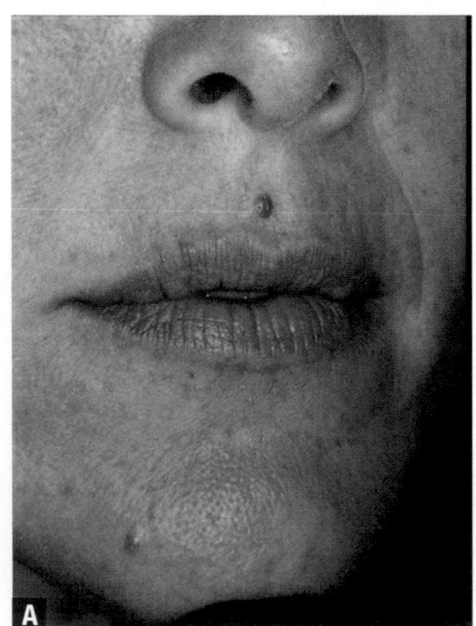

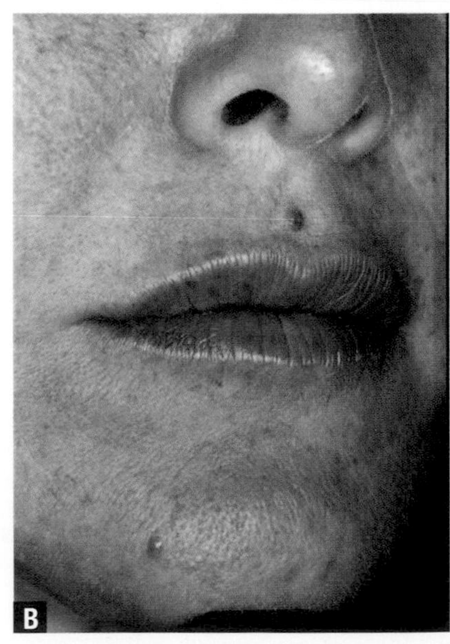

▲ **FIGURE 23-4** **A.** Before CosmoPlast to vermilion border. **B.** Immediately after CosmoPlast.

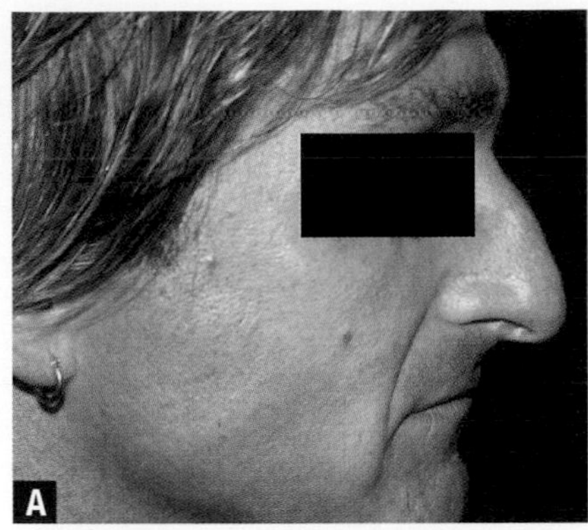
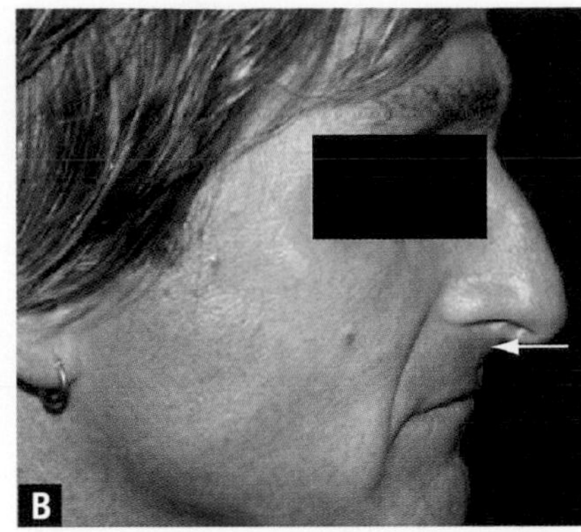
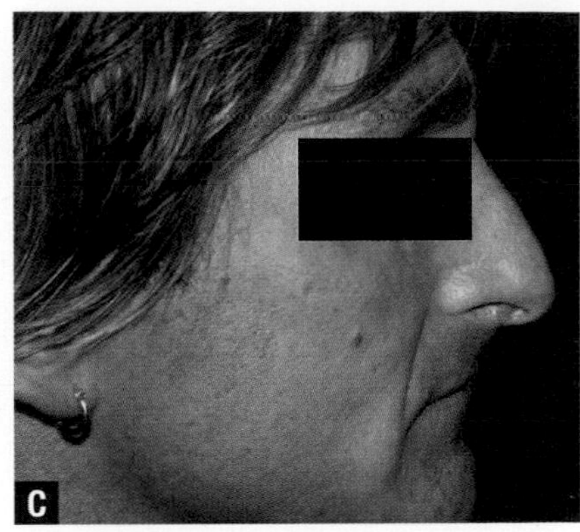

▲ **FIGURE 23-5** **A.** This patient has a dropped nasal tip. Options to raise the tip include a dermal filler or a botulinum toxin. **B.** CosmoPlast or Restylane is placed just below the cartilage of the central nose as shown with the white arrow. **C.** After CosmoPlast or Restylane is injected, the tip of the nose rises immediately. Note that it is now parallel to the ground rather than curling down.

comparable to bovine collagen fillers. Furthermore, like bovine collagen, CosmoDerm and CosmoPlast must be kept refrigerated when stored. For human-derived collagen devices, on average, one syringe is used for patients in their twenties, two syringes for patients in their thirties, three syringes for patients in their forties, and as needed for older patients in order to correct age related lines and folds.

Benefits Given the absence of allergy risk associated with these agents, no skin testing is required. This allows for patients to be treated in their initial visit to the physician. The cosmetic effects of CosmoDerm and CosmoPlast are immediate, lasting about 3 months for the former and about 4 months for the latter,[19] and are typically associated with less bruising than the effects of procedures using agents containing HA. Also similar to the bovine-derived fillers, CosmoDerm and CosmoPlast contain lidocaine to mitigate the pain of injection and lower the risk of edema and ecchymoses by inhibiting the activation of eosinophils.[20] CosmoPlast can create the beautiful "Snow White line" and "Cupid's bow" shape of the lip borders as well as upturn the tip of the nose to create a poised appearance. Although HA fillers are favored because they last longer and are softer, CosmoDerm I can be used to plump the body of the lip. CosmoDerm I can be layered over CosmoPlast for the purpose of ideal contouring of deep lines, such as nasolabial folds and marionette lines. In addition, to treat medium and deep wrinkles, HA fillers can be superimposed on top of CosmoPlast or injected in the same plane as CosmoPlast. Although fillers should be used rarely and with great caution in the glabellar rhytides because of the potential risk of tissue necrosis, CosmoDerm I can be used with great care in this region. At the time of publication of this text, there were no HA fillers geared for superficial placement, although Prevelle, Juvéderm, and Restylane may have superficial fillers soon. Therefore, CosmoDerm I, although it lasts only about 3 months, is the filler of choice for periorbital wrinkles and smoker's lines above the top lip. CosmoDerm II is most often used for acne scars.

Drawbacks Bioengineered human-derived collagen is expensive to produce, rendering these agents somewhat costly. Further, the cosmetic effects from these products do not last, on average, any longer than the bovine-derived products. The duration is thought to be around 4 months. However, these products are associated with less bruising, erythema, and pain than other filling agents and, consequently, remain desirable options for those who cannot afford to have downtime. Excluding the reduction in immunogenic potential, human collagen fillers have similar side effect profiles to bovine collagen fillers. Likewise, patients with lidocaine allergies should avoid these agents.

CADAVERIC COLLAGEN

Overview Approved by the FDA in 2000 for soft tissue augmentation, Cymetra® (LifeCell Corp., Palo Alto, CA) is a micronized collagen derived from processed human cadaver skin. A similar product, Fascian (Fascia Biosystems, Beverly Hills, CA), is obtained from cadaver fascia, and has a heavier consistency. Cymetra is packaged as a 330 mg white powder in a 5-cc syringe, stored at room temperature and reconstituted with 1 mL of 1% lidocaine to create a thick paste.[6] Tunneling and threading injection methods are accomplished through a 26-gauge syringe into a subcutaneous plane, avoiding overcorrection.

Benefits This acellular and purified filler negates a potential sensitivity reaction and pretesting is, therefore, unnecessary. The cadaver collagen has somewhat longer durability versus other collagen products, lasting from 3 to 9 months, although durability is controversial.[6] Cymetra is indicated for use in deep rhytides (i.e., nasolabial folds), depressed scars, and volumizing of the lips. Reconstitution with lidocaine yields reduction in intraprocedural pain.

Drawbacks Based on the composition of the product, Cymetra is contraindicated in patients with gentamicin allergies. The product is very viscous, which makes it difficult to operate, generating more local tissue discomfort and trauma as well as leading to longer recovery time for patients. Fascian is an even thicker and stiffer product, which translates to more side effects and difficulty in administration. The implantation of cadaver products into superficial and mobile wrinkles can induce migration and, therefore, is discouraged. The major issues with employing these agents are the cumbersome preparations and deficit of adequate clinical trials demonstrating their long-term efficacy and safety.

Hyaluronic Acid

In the last few years, HA filler substances have become the new gold standard, far outpacing in usage the other soft tissue augmentation agents.[21] HA, or hyaluronan, is a nonsulfated glycosaminoglycan (GAG) that occurs naturally in the skin and other tissues (specifically, connective, epithelial, and neural tissues) as space-occupiers of the extracellular matrix. HA is also ubiquitous across animal species, which makes it nonimmunogenic. This polysaccharide has the capacity to bind water up to 1000 times its mass. The biologic behavior of HA is predictable; it creates lubrication and volume with an aqueous and pliable framework that suspends and adheres to collagen, elastin, and cells. With age, the concentration of HA in skin decreases, translating to more lax, sallow, and dull skin. The viscoelastic qualities of HA serve to plump up the skin, yielding a more youthful appearance. Naturally-occurring, unmodified, or uncross-linked HA has a half-life of about 24 hours. For this reason, HA is cross-linked when formulated into a dermal filler product. Higher concentrations and moderate cross-linking of the HA in a product impart greater longevity. There exists a certain threshold where beyond that value additional cross-linking can cause biocompatibility issues. In effect, cross-linking has to be in the right balance to maintain duration and biocompatibility of the HA filler. HA is readily metabolized by the liver into by-products, water, and carbon dioxide. In the skin, HA is broken down by hyaluronidase, mechanical degradation caused by facial movement, and by free radicals. Supplementation with oral antioxidants theoretically will increase the duration of HA fillers, but this has not been proven (see Chapter 34).

There are two main categories of HA fillers: animal derived (e.g., Hylaform) and bacteria derived (e.g., Restylane, Captique, Juvéderm, etc). Medicis, the company that sells Restylane, trademarked the name "nonanimal derived synthetic hyaluronic acid (NASHA)" to show that their products, Restylane and Perlane, are not animal based. Because of the expense of animal-derived products, the vast majority of HA products are bacterial derived. At the time this chapter was written, no HA products on the market contained lidocaine and, therefore, were more painful than fillers that contain lidocaine. However, lidocaine-containing injectables, such as Prevelle Silk, have recently entered the market. Because of their nonallergenic nature and manufacturing, HA fillers do not require prior testing and can be stored at room temperature. Their advantages over collagen products are longer duration (6–12 months), better pliability, and less immunogenic and allergic side effects. On the whole, side effects of various HA fillers are similar, mild, and rare; these include bruising (Fig. 23-6), temporary swelling, lumps, acneiform eruptions, and, rarely, acute hypersensitivity.[22] In addition, arterial occlusion, thought to be due to swelling of the HA implant, causing vascular compromise, can rarely occur. (Fig. 23-7).

A major advantage of HA fillers is that if skin nodules do arise, these reactions can be easily dissolved with intralesional hyaluronidase (Fig. 23-8). The disadvantages of the currently available HA fillers are increased pain on injection and postprocedure edema, erythema, and ecchymoses as compared to CosmoPlast injections.

CONSIDERATIONS IN CHOOSING AN HA FILLER HA fillers do not require skin testing and the risk of allergy with all products that are FDA approved is minimal. Cost, availability, duration of correction, and size of the required needle for injection all play a role in product selection and manufacturers all strive to create an affordable, long-lasting product that can be injected with a 30-gauge or smaller needle. However, there are other, less obvious, scientific considerations to be taken into account when choosing a filler (Table 23-3). The stiffness or G′ (G prime) of a product is one of the most important considerations. G′ is a measurement of gel hardness. It is obtained when a gel is placed on a plate. A second plate is placed over the

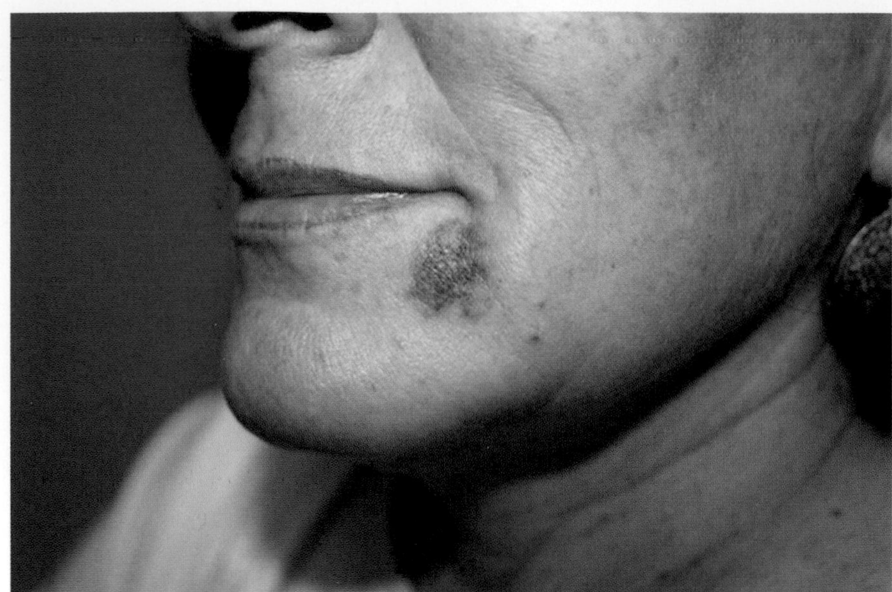

▲ **FIGURE 23-6** This is a common site at which bruises occur after a dermal filler is injected.

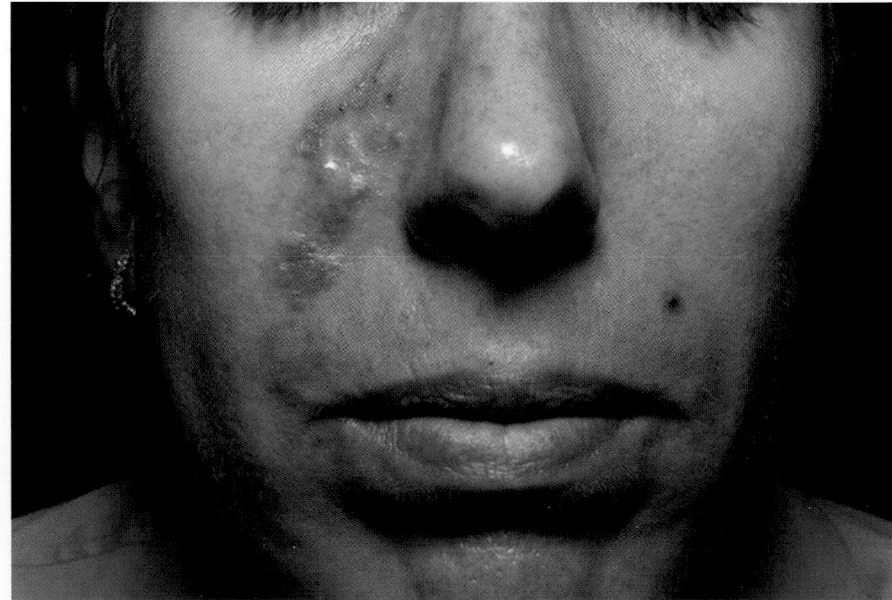

▲ **FIGURE 23-7** This patient developed redness, blisters, and lumps after receiving an HA injection. The most likely cause was vascular compromise due to swelling of the implant. All cultures were negative, other treated sites were normal and the lesions resolved without scarring.

TABLE 23-3
Factors to Consider When Choosing a Hyaluronic Acid Filler

Concentration of HA
Cost
Cross-linking
  Degree of cross-linking
  Quantity of HA cross-linked versus uncross-linked
  Type of cross-linking technology used
Duration of correction
G′ (elastic modulus)
Hydration level of product in the syringe
Presence of lidocaine
Required needle size for injection
Sizing technology
Syringe
  Design of syringe
  Size

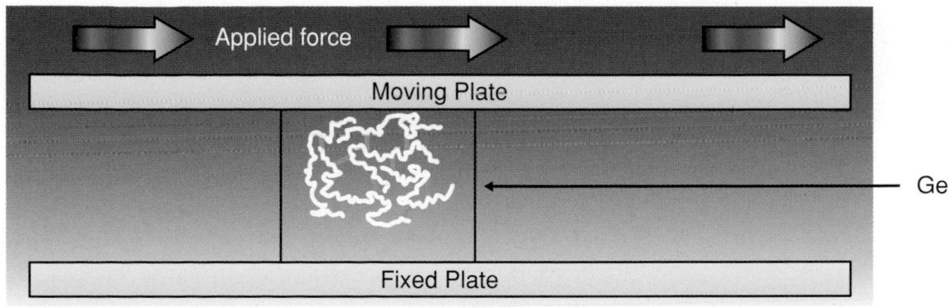

▲ **FIGURE 23-9** Measurement of G′. A force is applied laterally on the top plate. The more the gel resists the movement, the harder the gel, the higher the G′.

gel and a lateral force is applied. The measurement of resistance to deformation is known as the elastic modulus or the G′ (Fig. 23-9). Together with the cohesivity of the product, G′ values could be used to determine the appropriate placement of an HA dermal filler. For example, more robust products (higher G′ values and higher cohesivities) such as Juvéderm Ultra Plus and Perlane, in the primary author's opinion, should be used in deeper lines, such as nasolabial folds and marionette lines, as well as to lift the lateral brow, to correct the nasal bridge, to give the ear lobe youthful volume, to evert the nipples, and to raise the nasal tip. More fluid products such as Juvéderm Ultra and Restylane are better suited to be used over large areas such as the cheekbones and cheeks. Low G′ products such as Hylaform and Juvéderm Ultra are necessary in areas that require a softer agent, such as the body of the lip or the tear trough. As new products reach the market, knowing the G′ will help practitioners match fillers with indications.

The concentration of HA in a product is important to consider as well (Table 23-4). Many authorities believe that the higher the concentration of HA, the stiffer the product and the longer its duration. This is true in general when comparing products within a brand, for example, when comparing Juvéderm 18 to Juvéderm 24. However, this does not hold true across brands because not all of the HA in the dermal fillers is cross-linked. Many HA fillers contain uncross-linked HA and lightly cross-linked chains and fragments. The uncross-linked HA, fragments of HA, and lightly cross-linked HA are included in the overall concentration measurement but only remain in the skin for a limited time and should minimally contribute to the longevity of the filler. The uncross-linked HA does help decrease extrusion force and make injection easier, which is the main reason it is included. Therefore, the fact that Restylane contains 20 mg of HA/cc and Juvéderm contains 24 mg of HA/cc does not give a physician enough information to decide which filler will have longer duration. It is actually the amount of modified HA that plays the primary role in duration.

The type of modification (cross-linking) and the cross-linking agent used is also important. Cross-linking can be best visualized by imagining a ladder (Fig. 23-10). Each side of the ladder is an HA chain. The rungs of the ladder are the cross-links. When the "rungs" of the ladder attach to both sides of the ladder, the agent is considered completely modified. However, the cross-linking agent used may incompletely cross-link the chains of HA, leaving the sides of the rungs unattached and resulting in incomplete modification. Such a product might not be as durable as a completely modified product. In addition, there are two types of rungs in the HA ladder. One is called an ether linkage and the other is called an ester linkage. Ether linkages are formed by 1,4-butanediol diglycidyl ether (BDDE, the cross-linking agent in Restylane and Juvéderm) and divinyl sulfone (DVS, the agent used in Prevelle Silk, Captique, and Hylaform). The cross-linking agent used in Prevelle Dura, 1,2,7,8 diepoxyoctane (DEO), forms both ether and ester linkages (known as "double cross-linking"). It is

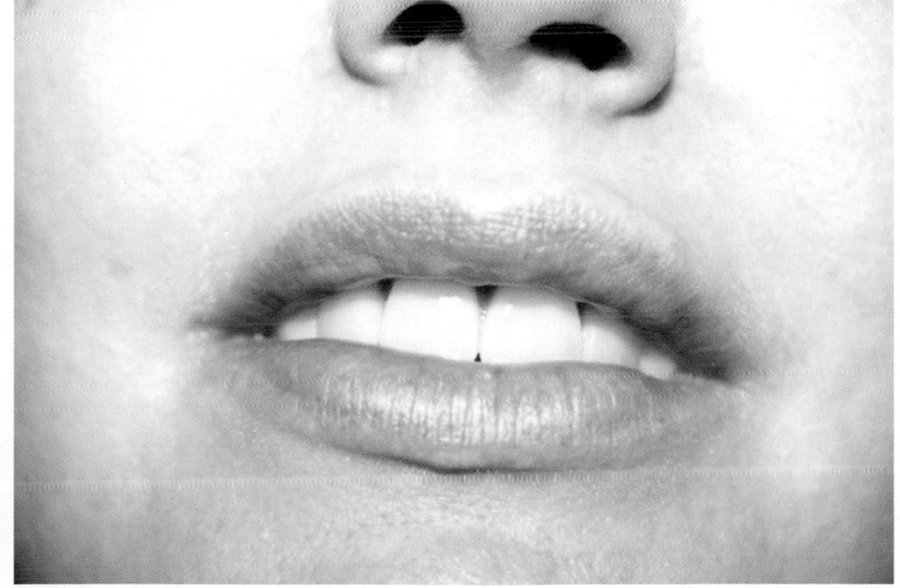

▲ **FIGURE 23-8** Visible lumps of Hylaform in the upper lip.

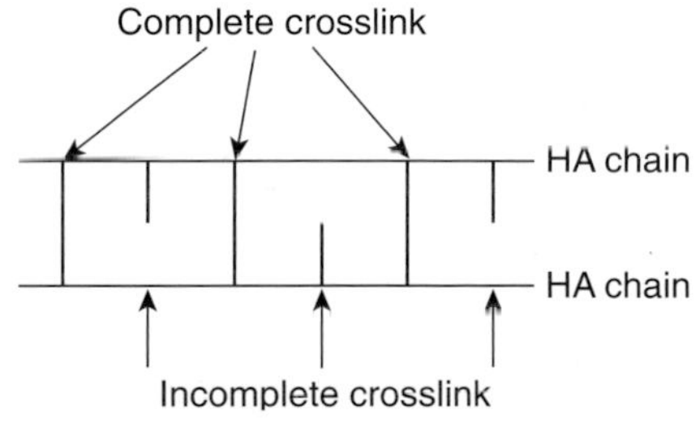

▲ **FIGURE 23-10** Cross-links that occur during the cross-linking process may be complete or incomplete.

TABLE 23-4
Hyaluronic Acid Fillers: Cross-Linking Agents and Concentration of HA

Product	Cross-linking Agent	Concentration (mg/mL)
Captique	DVS	4.5–6.5
Hylaform	DVS	4.5–6.5
Juvéderm Ultra and Ultra Plus	BDDE	24
Prevelle Dura	DEO	20
Prevelle Silk	DVS	4.5–6.5
Restylane and Perlane	BDDE	20

unknown at this time what advantages, if any, ether linkages impart to a dermal filler.

The hydration status of the filler once it is packaged in the syringe also affects filler performance. HA is well known to bind up to 1000 times its weight in water. The amount of water bound to the HA prior to its packaging in the syringe determines how much more water the filler can absorb once it is injected into the skin. In other words, fillers that are completely hydrated in the syringe will bind less water on injection and the volume will expand less upon injection as compared to fillers that are not completely hydrated in the syringe. Fillers that are not completely hydrated in the syringe will swell somewhat within 24 hours after correction; therefore, it is prudent to slightly undercorrect with these substances. In addition, patients can be told that they will "look even better" 24 hours after the injection. Restylane and Juvéderm are not completely hydrated in the syringe while Captique and Hylaform are close to being fully hydrated (Table 23-5).

Another process that may affect the performance of the filler is referred to as "sizing technology." This term is used by Allergan to differentiate Juvéderm from the other HA fillers. When an HA filler is cross-linked, the chains of modified sugars form a gel. In the process of manufacturing Restylane, Restylane Fine Line, Restylane Lip, Restylane Touch, Perlane, and Restylane Sub-Q, this gel is extruded through a screen. This produces various sizes of the gel that are considered "sized." The large pieces become Perlane or Restylane Sub-Q, while the small pieces are marketed as Restylane Fine Line or Restylane Lip. The medium-sized pieces are Restylane. The larger pieces yield products that are best used in the mid to lower dermis while the small pieces such as Restylane Fine Line can be used more superficially. The Juvéderm family of products is not sized. In other words, Juvéderm is not pushed through a screen and broken into sized pieces and, therefore, it consists of randomly sized and shaped pieces.[23] It is unknown at this time what role sizing technology plays, if any, in the performance of a filler.

There are many factors that must be understood in order to make the most suitable choice of HA filler. There are no peer-reviewed publications that review the above mentioned properties so it is difficult at this point to know how important these various characteristics are in choosing a filler. More data need to be collected to properly ascertain if, for example, sizing technology makes a difference or if ester bonds last longer than ether bonds. These distinctions will become clearer and more important as more HA fillers are introduced onto the market and more data are collected. A discussion of the individual HA brands follows.

TABLE 23-5
Hyaluronic Acid Filler Hydration in the Syringe

Almost Completely Hydrated in the Syringe[a]	Not Completely Hydrated in the Syringe[b]
Captique	Restylane
Hylaform	Juvéderm
Prevelle Silk	Prevelle Dura

[a]No need to undercorrect.
[b]Slightly undercorrect.

HYLAFORM (NO LONGER ON THE MARKET)

Overview Although Hylaform is no longer on the market, it will be discussed because it was the first product on the market that used the DVS cross-linking system. The knowledge gleaned from this revolutionary agent has led to many spin-off products using similar technology such as Captique and Prevelle. Hylaform is an animal-based HA product derived from rooster combs. It is produced by cross-linking the hydroxyl groups of HA with DVS to yield a gel-like substance that is sized by extruding the gel through a sieve in the production process discussed above.[24] The smallest pieces of the gel are packaged as Hylaform Fine Line, which is indicated for superficial wrinkles, but has never been approved for the US market. Hylaform, composed of medium-sized (average size 400 μm) particles, is indicated for injection into the middermis for medium facial wrinkles and fine lines. Hylaform Plus is composed of larger particles (average size 700 μm) and is used for deeper furrows. In 2004, the FDA approved two products in this family, Hylaform and Hylaform Plus (Allergan, Irvine, CA), the latter of which remains on the US market. The moderate density of cross-linking renders the Hylaform fillers biocompatible, soft, and pliable. The G′ of this filler is low compared to other HA products on the market; therefore, this is the softest HA filler currently on the market. This softness makes it an ideal filler for use in the lips. The Hylaform products contain 5.5 mg/mL of cross-linked HA.

Benefits Hylaform has a low G′, which means that it is not very stiff and has a very natural feel in the skin. It is soft and malleable making it ideal for use in the body of the lip, smoker's lines, and the periorbital tear-trough as well as in large areas such as the cheekbones and jowls. Hylaform is very easy to inject with a low extrusion force through a 30-gauge needle. The side effects of Hylaform are rare, mild, and temporary.

Drawbacks Side effects, which are rare and relatively mild, typically include bruising, erythema, induration, and pruritus.[25] The contraindications for Hylaform products are similar to those for most fillers (e.g., autoimmune and inflammatory disorders, allergic background, history of anaphylactic reactions, immunosuppressant therapy, and pregnancy or breastfeeding). In addition, patients allergic to products of avian origin (e.g., eggs) cannot use these agents.[25,26] Hylaform is close to being fully saturated with water in the syringe;[27] therefore, there is no volume expansion of the filler after injection. Additionally, the injection of Hylaform, as with other fillers that do not contain an anesthetic, could be painful. However, the softness of Hylaform renders it less painful than other HA fillers to inject. The use of topical anesthetics reduces the pain on injection. The cosmetic effects of Hylaform and Hylaform Plus are believed to last only about 3 to 4 months, most likely because of their cross-linking properties and lower concentration of HA than the newer HA fillers (e.g., Restylane and Juvéderm).

CAPTIQUE (NO LONGER ON THE MARKET)

Overview Captique (Allergan, Irving, CA) differs from Hylaform only insofar as the former is derived from bacterial fermentation rather than rooster combs; otherwise, it is also composed of 5.5 mg/mL of HA. In 2004, it was approved by the FDA for moderate to severe wrinkles. The bacterial origin of Captique renders it slightly stiffer than Hylaform, but not as firm as Restylane. Captique is packaged as a clear gel in a 0.75-mL syringe and injected dermally with a 30-gauge needle via the serial puncture method. Like Hylaform, Captique is no longer available.

Benefits This product is suitable for treating similar periorbital and perioral wrinkles as Hylaform as well as enhancing lip fullness and shallow scars. No testing or refrigeration is required and the agent can be injected in the initial physician's visit. As an HA filler, it has a low side effect profile because of its immunogenic inertness and low likelihood of allergic reactions. The equilibrium hydration of Captique is also comparable to Hylaform, meaning that it is fully hydrated with water in the syringe. In the primary author's experience, patients complained of less stinging after injection with Captique as compared with Juvéderm.

Drawbacks The longevity of Captique is questionable but believed to be about 4 to 6 months. Few duration studies were performed, however. It has a high extrusion force when injected through a 30-gauge needle, which renders injection more difficult than that for Hylaform or Restylane. Captique does not contain lidocaine, thus it is similar to other HA fillers in the capacity to cause moderate pain, bruising, edema, and redness on injection. Captique has been taken off the market because its parent company, Allergan, is focusing on promoting Juvéderm.

RESTYLANE

Overview Restylane (Medicis, Scottsdale, AZ) was the first nonanimal HA product approved in the US. It is a NASHA gel formulated through fermentation, with sugar present, in bacterial cultures of equine streptococci. Restylane has a higher concentration of HA compared to Hylaform and Captique and the highest G′ of the fillers currently on the market, denoting that it is a slightly stiffer product. It is the most popular of the HA fillers in the US because of its safety profile, brand recognition, and ease of injection. Restylane is composed of approximately 100,000 particles/mL (approximately 250 μm on average)[28] and contains 20 mg/mL of HA. Restylane is indicated for middermal wrinkle reduction and was the first HA filler approved in the US in 2003.[29] Perlane, another product in the Restylane family, was more recently approved by the FDA for significantly deeper folds and furrows. Restylane is made of medium-sized particles of HA gel, while Perlane is composed of larger HA gel particles (approximately 1000 μm),[28] but with the same HA concentration. The Restylane family of products also includes Restylane Fine Line, Restylane Touch, Restylane Lip, and Restylane Sub-Q, which are not currently approved for use in the US. These products have the same formulation as Restylane and differ only in their particle size. Restylane and Perlane are packaged as transparent gels, with a shelf life of 18 months, and stored at room temperature. Restylane is enclosed in 0.4- and 1-mL syringes while Perlane is packaged in a 0.7-mL syringe; both are injected via a 27-gauge needle. Restylane is implanted using linear threading anterograde or retrograde techniques. It is important to avoid injecting at withdrawal of the needle, which can result in superficial injection, creating blue colored nodules. A fanning threading technique can also be employed with Restylane at the nasolabial fold or lip commissures.

Benefits The stiffness of Restylane renders it well suited for moderate to deep wrinkles and it is this quality among other factors that is thought to impart greater longevity in human tissue as compared to Hylaform and Captique. The cosmetic effects of Restylane are thought to last over 6 months; Perlane delivers a durability of 6 to 9 months. Product stiffness makes Restylane and Perlane more suitable for moderate and deep wrinkles than for use in the body of the lips or the tear trough. Restylane is ideal to fill nasolabial and marionette lines, chin and jowl depressions, nasal deformities, and for nasal tip-lift as well as acne scars and other defects.

Drawbacks Bruising is associated with all HA fillers. However, the stiffness is a downside if the product is used by a poorly skilled physician, with bumps and blue blebs possibly arising from improper injection technique. Injection into the tear trough may result in visible blebs. Slower injection of any HA filler will limit the risk of inflammation. Restylane can be used in the vermilion border to augment the shape of the lip. In the primary author's opinion, Restylane and Perlane are a poor choice for the body of the lips. However, outside the US, Restylane Lip is available and is a better choice for use in this area. As with other fillers that do not contain an anesthetic, the injection of Restylane can be painful. The use of topical anesthetics and/or dental nerve blocks is recommended to reduce the pain on injection. Restylane tends to sting less after injection when compared to Juvéderm. It is unknown why this occurs as they are both the same pH of approximately 7.0.

JUVÉDERM™

Overview Juvéderm (Allergan, Irvine, CA), is manufactured by a bacterial fermentation process similar to that used for other stabilized bacterial-based HA fillers and was approved by the FDA in late 2006. There are many products in the Juvéderm line (Juvéderm 18, Juvéderm 24, Juvéderm 24 HV, Juvéderm 30, and Juvéderm 30 HV), but only Juvéderm 24 HV (also known as Juvéderm Ultra) and Juvéderm 30 HV (also known as Juvéderm Ultra Plus) are currently approved by the FDA and sold in the US. All the products in the line vary by the amount of HA concentration, the amount of cross-linking, and the regularity of the cross-linking. Both Juvéderm Ultra and Ultra Plus consist of 24 mg/cc of HA, but Juvéderm Ultra Plus has a higher degree of cross-linking than Juvéderm Ultra, which makes Ultra Plus more suitable for the deepest facial grooves and furrows. Unlike Restylane, which consists of stiff and a fairly narrow range of particle sizes, Juvéderm is a smooth consistency gel composed of a broad range of particles of various sizes and shapes[30] (referred to as "Hyalacross technology").

Juvéderm products are packaged as a clear gel in 0.8-mL syringes. They are stored at room temperature. Juvéderm Ultra is injected into the middermis via a 30-gauge needle while Juvéderm Ultra Plus is implanted deeper via a 27-gauge needle.[27] The needles must be tightly attached to the Luer-lock syringe to prevent detachment during injections. Various techniques of injection can be used with Juvéderm, including serial puncture and tunneling.

Benefits Juvéderm Ultra and Ultra Plus are in the medium range of stiffness; therefore, they can be used in any wrinkles, moderate or deep, and to correct scars. Juvéderm Ultra is easily placed in the vermilion border or the body of the lips. The high concentration of HA in Juvéderm Ultra and Ultra Plus and the high degree of cross-linking results in longer-lasting aesthetic effects as compared to products such as Hylaform. As other HA products, these agents have an overall low, mild, and transient adverse-event profile. Juvéderm is not completely hydrated in the syringe,[27] so it will slightly expand after injection as it absorbs more water. This is important to remember when injecting the body of the lips, which should be slightly undercorrected to allow for the expansion. Similar to Restylane, the longevity of Juvéderm Ultra is about 6 to 9 months and Ultra Plus may last up to 12 months.

Drawbacks All HA products can cause erythema, swelling, and bruising after implantation (see Chapter 21). Pain during injection caused by lack of anesthetic can be alleviated with the use of topical or regional anesthesia. Juvéderm can be placed with care in the tear trough area, but the proximity to the eye is unnerving with the risk of the needle popping off, so injections should be very slow with only moderate extrusion force. The needle is more likely to pop off when the syringe is almost empty; therefore, the tear trough area should be injected with a new syringe and the last part of the syringe can be saved for less dangerous areas such as the nasolabial folds. As with all fillers, the skill and experience of the physician is crucial for optimal outcome. If Juvéderm is injected too superficially, it can create a bluish hue. Caution should be taken in overinjecting the vermilion border and creating an unnatural "duck-bill" appearance. In addition, superficial placement of Juvéderm in the tear trough defects can result in blue nodules. Blue nodules and unwanted bulges can be corrected with the use of hyaluronidase.

PREVELLE SILK

Overview Prevelle Silk is sold by the Mentor Corp. (Santa Barbara, CA). This bacterial-derived product is similar to the Captique formulation with moderate softness illustrated by its G′ in the middle of the spectrum. This product is softer than Restylane and is similar in softness to Juvéderm. Prevelle Silk has a higher degree of cross-linking density than Hylaform and therefore is slightly stiffer than Hylaform. The gel contains 5.5 mg/mL of cross-linked HA with an average particle size of 300 μm. Prevelle is suitable for treating shallow to moderate wrinkles, lips, and scars. The longevity of the product is unknown but reported to be about 4 months. Prevelle Silk contains 0.3% lidocaine. It was approved in the United States in 2008. This product is suitable for use in the lips since it generates less pain during injections. Side effects, which are rare and relatively mild, include redness, swelling, and pruritus.

Benefits This product is softer than other products on the market since Hylaform and Captique were discontinued. It can be used in any moderate to deep facial wrinkles, the body of the lip, and periorbital areas. Prevelle Silk is the first lidocaine-containing HA in the United States.

Drawbacks Longevity of the correction is not known but thought to be 4-6 months.

PREVELLE DURA

Overview Prevelle Dura (Mentor Corp.) is another bacterial-derived filler approved for the US market in 2008. It is composed of 220-μm HA particles cross-linked with DEO. As mentioned previously, DEO cross-linking results in both ether bonds and ester bonds, known as double cross-linking. These ester bonds may confer better stability and longer duration but this has not yet been proven.[31] Prevelle Dura is touted for suitability in any dermal layer to correct middermal and deep rhytides. The G′ (stiffness) of this product is 900 Da, which renders it slightly stiffer than Restylane.

Benefits Preliminary studies demonstrate the safety of this product;[31] however, more trials need to be performed to establish its strengths and weaknesses. Based on double cross-linking technology, the company claims that this device may last longer than previous HA fillers; however, this has not been proven. The role of the double cross-linking technology in terms of duration of the filler has not been ascertained.

Drawbacks Prevelle Dura is slightly more viscous and, therefore, requires more pressure on injection.

Hyaluronidase

Hyaluronidase is a soluble enzyme that hydrolyzes HA, other GAGs, and other connective tissue components in the skin and vitreous humor of the eye.[32] It has been approved by the FDA, as Vitrase and Amphadase, for enhancement of injectable drug absorption and resorption of radiopaque agents. However, effective off-label uses include wound care and postsurgical flap care among other uses.

Several reports have indicated the usefulness of hyaluronidase to dissolve HA filler overcorrection for symmetric contouring, as well as to manage impending tissue necrosis because of HA skin injections.[33–35] Specifically, Hirsch et al. published two cases of imminent tissue necrosis caused by intra-arterial injection of HA and surrounding tissue compression of vital vessel, which resolved with employment of hyaluronidase. After using other appropriate techniques to manage impending tissue necrosis including systemic aspirin, Nitro BID under occlusion, and hot compresses with massage without significant response, the authors injected 30 units of hyaluronidase into deep dermal tissue and subcutis using a serial puncture method along the distribution of affected arteries, which led to the resolution of symptoms within a day.[32,33] Although early reports have recommended the utility of hyaluronidase only within 16 minutes of the critical event, Hirsch et al. reported successful responses after several days.[32] Furthermore, the effectiveness of hyaluronidase for bluish (Tyndall) manifestations and asymmetric lumpiness from HA overcorrection has also been reported at various concentrations.[34–36]

Because of the described benefits of hyaluronidase for the treatment of complications of the popular HA fillers, it has been recommended as a necessary agent to keep in an aesthetic physician's office.[37] Hyaluronidase is a clear liquid that is stored in the refrigerator and reconstituted with 1 mL of normal saline to generate 150 units. Very rare adverse acute and delayed-type hypersensitivity reactions to hyaluronidase have been reported, so it may be prudent to perform a skin test prior to the use of this agent. Injection of hyaluronidase into patients with an allergy to hymenoptera stings and thimerosal is contraindicated.[33,38]

Semipermanent Fillers

Fat, Radiesse, and Sculptra are considered semitransitory because they are partly biostimulatory and partially biodegradable; this balance allows them to last approximately 1 to 3 years.[39] The adverse events associated with semipermanent fillers include rare granuloma formations. The aesthetic effects of these fillers are best preserved with annual touch-up sessions.

AUTOLOGOUS FAT

Overview Originating in the 1890s, transplantation of fat from a patient's excess adipose areas to other skin defects is the oldest soft tissue augmentation method.[1] Fat injection filling has gained recognition for several reasons. Naturally, the patient's own cells are unlikely to cause sensitivity or inflammation and are therefore considered supremely biocompatible. Furthermore, the technique of fat implantation has undergone remarkable polishing over many years, especially with the advent of harvesting subcutis through liposuction. The procedure is a multistep process, whereby the fat cells are obtained from the buttock, thigh, and abdominal regions, then segregated, stored (refrigerated up to 18 months), and injected back into the patient's subcutis on the face, hands, and any other areas requiring volume enhancement. As anticipated, this process is more invasive, time-consuming, both for the clinician to prepare and perform as well as the patient to recover from, as well as more costly. In effect, the optimal efficacy with minimal adverse effects is mainly achieved in the hands of a qualified dermasurgeon. Approximately 0.1 cc aliquots of fat are inserted into subcutis through a 17- to 18-gauge needle via a tunneling technique, without overcorrection.[40] Postprocedure massage is recommended for proper shaping of contours.

Benefits Because of its autologous character, lipotransfer is unlikely to cause sensitivity and reactivity of the tissue, minimizing potential long-term side effects and obviating prior testing. Nasolabial folds, sunken cheeks, tear troughs, marionette lines, scars, and lips are the most appropriate areas of correction with fat. Furthermore, fat transfer provides a reported duration of about 12 months; although the concrete duration is controversial.[41] Because the injectable material used is the patient's own tissue, its use decreases the amount of money spent on the actual filler. The procedure also has an attractive double-gain, where two cosmetic areas can be simultaneously addressed, lipoexcess and lipodystrophy. Stem cells have been isolated from fat cells. It is believed that the stem cells found in fat lead to increased skin rejuvenation (see Chapter 3). When performed by a skilled physician, the results of lipotransfer are remarkable.[42]

Drawbacks Fat injections require prophylactic local or regional anesthesia. Because of the fact that the procedure is more surgically invasive, more complex preparations and settings are required with longer and more frequent office visits. Although the harvesting portion can cause a longer recovery time and an increased risk of side effects (e.g., infection, scarring), the actual injection has a similar adverse event profile to the other fillers (e.g., edema, redness, bruising, and discomfort lasting a few days).[34] Another variable to consider when selecting candidates for this procedure is to ensure that the patient has a sufficient graft supply. In some patients, the fat injections last several years and in other patients the injections last merely months. Many tricks are employed to try and increase longevity, but at this time there are no guarantees.[32]

RADIESSE

Overview Radiesse (BioForm Medical, San Mateo, CA) was approved by the FDA in 2006 for the correction of moderate to severe folds and wrinkles along with HIV-associated lipoatrophy. It is composed of 30% calcium hydroxylapatite (CaHA) microspheres (25–45 μm) suspended in an aqueous gel carrier (1.3% sodium carboxymethyl cellulose, 6.4% glycerin, and 36.6% sterile water). As the gel carrier of this filler dissipates in several months, the microspheres stimulate cutaneous cells to generate focal foreign body reaction and neocollagenesis.[32,33] This leads to envelopment of the microspheres by fibrin, collagen, and fibroblasts, and slows the degradation by macrophages and metabolism into calcium and phosphate ions. Because of a similar mineral constitution as human bones, and no foreign antigenic properties, CaHA is particularly biocompatible. It is critical for patients to be aware that Radiesse is a radiopaque material that can be visualized and misinterpreted on facial radiographs, but importantly, it does not radiographically mask surrounding tissues.

Radiesse is a white material packaged in a 1-mL syringe and injected via a 25- to 27-gauge and 11/4-inch needle into the deep dermis or subcutis without overcorrection.[33] The product should be stored at room temperature. A reasonable injection method for Radiesse is tunneling or crisscross threading techniques.[32] A placement of Radiesse in the supraperiosteal plane yields better control and ability to contour skin with this stiffer filler.[43]

Benefits Since Radiesse is immunologically inert, it does not require skin testing. With more than 20 years of use as implantable devices for otolaryngology and orthopedic specialties, CaHA possesses an excellent safety record. The average duration of Radiesse is 9 to 18 months. The proper locations of injection include the nasolabial folds, marionette lines, prejowl sulcus, and cheek depressions. Unlike Sculptra, where time is necessary to build up new collagen, Radiesse offers the advantage of immediate wrinkle ablation. Interestingly, although Radiesse induces foreign body reaction, it is not known to cause granuloma formation.[36] In its gel form, the device is also quite pliable, permitting timely manipulation and appropriate modification. In addition, it can be combined with other fillers, such as Sculptra, HA, and collagen.

Drawbacks The main drawback of Radiesse is that it is not reversible like HAs. Radiesse also does not contain an anesthetic and because of its high viscosity, requires administration through a high-bore needle. However, Radiesse can be combined with lidocaine in the syringe to decrease pain on injection. Hence, the use of topical or regional anesthesia is recommended. Minimal side effects such as ecchymoses, edema, and erythema appear soon after Radiesse injection and are transitory. Rare nodules have also been associated with Radiesse and can be managed with intralesional steroids or excision. Similar to Sculptra, an implantation of Radiesse in the superficial and mobile wrinkles (e.g., lips and periorbital area) and the body of the lips is discouraged because of the palpable and visible white papules that can develop (also known as "popcorn lips"). Radiesse should not be performed in the nose of a patient anticipating rhinoplasty. Several facial plastic surgeons have given anecdotal reports in lectures suggesting that this complicates rhinoplasty surgery. An HA or collagen filler would be a more appropriate choice in preoperative rhinoplasty patients.

SCULPTRA

Overview. Sculptra is a synthetic, biodegradable, biocompatible, immunologically inert peptide polymer (also known as NewFill).[44–46] Sculptra (Dermik Laboratories, Sanofi-Aventis, Bridgewater, NJ) is composed of poly-L-lactic acid (PLLA) microspheres, sodium carboxymethylcellulose, and nonpyrogenic mannitol and is manufactured from powdered, absorbable suture material (e.g., Vycryl). This agent is not a true dermal filler because it does not fill the dermis the way collagen and HA do but, rather, it promotes the production of new and organized collagen in the dermis. Many physicians refer to it as a "dermal stimulator." Sculptra is thought to foster neocollagenesis by stimulating fibroblasts and gradually restoring facial volume.[47–49] However, Sculptra is eventually cleared from the skin via phagocytic digestion. In the US, Sculptra was approved by the FDA in 2004 for the treatment of HIV-associated facial lipoatrophy, but it has been used off-label for cosmesis, and Dermik is currently applying for approval for its use in facial rejuvenation. NewFill has been used in Europe and Asia for many years. When it was first introduced, NewFill was diluted with a lower amount of saline and many granules and nodules were reported. This led to new recommendations to dilute one bottle with 5 to 10 cc of sterile water and massage after application. With the new recommendations, adverse events have been minimal.

Freeze-dried Sculptra powder is stored at room temperature and reconstituted approximately 2 to 4 hours prior to injection. The package label states that the product should be used within 72 hours. In our practice, we prefer using Sculptra that has been reconstituted for at least 2 days because the solution is easy to work with and results in less needle clogging. Sculptra is reconstituted and kept in the refrigerator for 2 days to 2 weeks. Although the package label recommends that the formulation be reconstituted with 5 cc of sterile water, many physicians reconstitute with 4 mL of sterile water and 1 mL of 2% lidocaine with epinephrine. The lidocaine decreases pain while the epinephrine reduces bruising. Strong agitation of the filed syringes is recommended directly before injection to homogenize the white suspension. (Sculptra tends to settle in the bottom of the syringe.) By means of tunneling and threading techniques, a 25- or 26-gauge needle is utilized to implant Sculptra into overlapping deep dermal and subcutaneous layers of the skin.

The mechanism of action and proper technique of injecting Sculptra require practitioners to restore volume to a selected treatment plane rather than a specific wrinkle.[50] Indeed, injecting Sculptra is more similar to fat injection procedures than collagen or HA injections, because it serves to sculpt the prominent hollows and deep grooves associated with loss of deep soft tissue. In addition, specialized training to use Sculptra is required prior to injections. Small and exact aliquots of Sculptra are injected in the correct tissue plane without overcorrection. In general, 2 to 3 cc of the product are used for patients in their thirties, 4 cc for patients in their forties, and 5 cc or more for older patients. The cost is approximately $230 per syringe.

Once Sculptra is injected, there is a transient period lasting about 1 hour during which the patient can see a slight effect because of the volume of fluid injected. Once this resolves, results are not seen until about 4 weeks after treatment when results *may* begin to appear. Injections are performed on a monthly basis until desired results have been obtained. The number of injection sessions required varies greatly from person to person and it is difficult to predict the total number of sessions needed. Injections are performed 3 to 6 weeks apart. Anecdotal reports state that premenopausal women and postmenopausal women on hormone replacement therapy (HRT) require fewer sessions than postmenopausal women not on HRT. Postmenopausal women not on HRT may require up to eight sessions. Men tend to correct more quickly than women for unknown reasons. After the procedure, the patient's skin is strenuously massaged with topical arnica (for its anticoagulant properties) for about 5 minutes to reduce bruising, pain, and nodule formation. Patients should be told to massage the treated area for 5 minutes every night for five nights.

Sculptra treatments can be combined with other fillers for instant gratification. In this case, Sculptra is injected first, the massage with arnica is performed, and then the HA or collagen filler is applied in the treatment area. Sculptra is often used in the cheeks and cheekbone area while an HA filler is used in the nasolabial folds, marionette lines, and the lips. Alternatively, a course of three to four Sculptra treatments is used and then an HA filler is used after Sculptra at the last visit. Sculptra should always be used first, then massaged, before the HA is injected so that the lidocaine and epinephrine in the Sculptra will reduce the pain and bruising of the HA injection, and the massaging will not affect the placement of the HA filler.

Benefits Sculptra does not require prior skin testing. It is ideal for treating volume loss in the cheeks, nasolabial folds, and the malar area. Once the desired result is achieved, results last about 18 to 24 months.[42,44,51,52] The correction is very natural looking. Having been used successfully in various medical devices for more than 30 years, PLLA has an established safety record.[53] Moreover, new product guidelines and injection techniques (e.g., using a more dilute product, avoiding overcorrection, not injecting too superficially, and postinjection massage) have reduced the incidence of side effects (i.e., formation of granulomas and nodules) as compared to when the product was originally packaged as NewFill.[54]

Drawbacks Sculptra injection results are not immediate and multiple courses are required to achieve the optimal cosmetic effect, with the number of treatments depending on volume of the defect being treated.[45] Preinjection reconstitution can contribute to scheduling limitations because it must be made at least 2 hours in advance. Injecting suspension can be slightly difficult because of recurrent clogging of the needles, which leads to frequent needle changes. Adverse events are rare, but PLLA can cause postinjection site pain, bruising, and swelling, as compared to other products, partly because of the larger needle used. Adding lidocaine to the diluent mitigates injection pain. Ecchymoses can be reduced by mixing epinephrine into the PLLA suspension and taking bromelain supplements (500 mg twice daily) *after* injection (see Chapter 21). Hyperkinetic areas (e.g., crow's feet and the corner of the mouth) and regions with thin skin (e.g., around the eyes, smoker's lines above the lips) should not be treated with Sculptra because of irregular papules that can emerge. Most lumps that do arise are from superficial administration of Sculptra and are not visible, although they are palpable by the patient. Reassuring patients that these lumps are transient in nature is important. Nodule and hematoma formation are the other rare adverse effects that have been reported, but are less likely if the new injection guidelines are followed.[55,56] Sculptra injection technique is very different than that of HA fillers and the learning curve is higher. In addition, there is lack of reversibility as with HA fillers. Specialized training is required by the manufacturers of Sculptra before they will sell the product to a physician.

Permanent Fillers

Although the current momentum in the cosmetic market is toward the less invasive procedures, which are safer, permanent fillers are very popular outside the US because of the lower cost. Many of these products are used by unskilled practitioners and lead to disfiguring results. If practitioners are to use a permanent filler, they should be skilled in the technique and certain of the patient's expectations. In the primary author's opinion, it is best to use a temporary filler first, to make sure that a patient is pleased, before proceeding to a permanent or semipermanent option. Newer fillers (e.g., Artefill) as well as older fillers (e.g., silicone) are being used for this purpose. These nonbiodegradable fillers stay enclosed by the skin for an indeterminate and lasting period of time. However, these fillers are not to be used for and by the lighthearted. They are associated with rare, significant side effects such as granulomas, migration, and asymmetry and are best implanted into a patient experienced with prior soft tissue augmentations and by a proficient physician. Remember, as with anything enduring, if one is not pleased with the results, one has to live with long-term consequences.

ARTEFILL

Overview In October 2006, the FDA approved the novel permanent filler Artefill (Artes Medical, Inc., San Diego, CA) for the correction of nasolabial folds.[57] Artefill is constituted with 20% homogenous polymethylmethacrylate (PMMA) suspended in equilibrium with partly denatured 3.5% bovine collagen (from enclosed US cattle herds) and 0.3% lidocaine. As opposed to the original European product, Artecoll, which contained different size microspheres of PMMA that potentially contributed to a higher risk of granulomas, Artefill is composed of uniform size PMMA microspheres (30–50 μm) that are less likely to result in the formation of granulomas. Small size, uniformity, and smoothness are refined characteristics of Artefill that promote biocompatibility and resistance to phagocytic degradation and migration as well as ensure encapsulation by patients' collagen leading to lasting nonimmunogenic results.

Artefill is packaged in a kit of three 0.8-mL and two 0.4-mL syringes that are injected through a 26-gauge needle into subdermal and subcutaneous space via a tunneling technique without overcorrection.[33] After injection, gentle massage is recommended to evenly distribute material in the skin and prevent clumping. Artefill must be stored via refrigeration (2°C–10°C) and warmed before use. In order to achieve optimal correction of rhytides, two to three treatment sessions, a few months apart, are suggested.[51] Like Sculptra, specific injection training for Artefill is required.

Benefits Artefill offers the dual action of immediate wrinkle correction from collagen (lasting about 1–3 months) and permanent deep-fold ablation from PMMA (lasting for more than 5 years).[51] The long-term efficacy is believed to be because of the stimulatory influence of PMMA on the surrounding skin, causing fibroblast and collagen proliferation around the material starting at 1 month.[33] Although approved only for nasolabial folds, PMMA has also been successfully used in other deeper defects (e.g., the cheek and malar regions). Lidocaine content eliminates the necessity for alternative anesthesia and alleviates intrainjection discomfort. As compared to the standard of bovine collagen, PMMA filler has been found to be superior in efficacy with a comparable safety profile.[51] Widely used in implantable medical devices for more than 50 years, PMMA has a long safety record.[32]

Drawbacks Artefill contains bovine collagen; therefore, skin testing prior to injections is strongly advised to reduce the incidence of hypersensitivity. This means that patients cannot be treated on the initial office visit. Furthermore, because of Artefill's higher viscosity, more administration pressure is required by the clinician, and the product is more difficult to inject than collagen and HA fillers. Although the majority of side effects caused by Artefill are mild and transient (e.g., swelling, redness, hypersensitivity, and temporary lumpiness, which is amenable to massage), rare moderate-to-severe effects have been reported (e.g., granuloma and inflamed nodule formation, manageable with intralesional steroids or excision).[51] Because of the reported lumpiness with this product, it is currently discouraged for lip augmentation or any superficial wrinkle correction. Having to inject through a larger bore needle may induce more posttreatment edema and ecchymoses, which require slightly longer downtime. The disadvantage of implanting permanent fillers such as Artefill is the inability to foretell the long-term appearance of the patient; since the skin changes with age, the natural look may be altered. Time will tell the exact risk-to-benefit ratio of this filler.

SILICONE

Overview Silicone is composed of dimethylsiloxane chains linked by oxygen with varied viscosity based on the length of the polymer. Used in patients since the 1940s, the liquid form of this product is one of the oldest soft tissue augmentation materials.[58] The use of this injectable filler is fraught with controversy because the initial unpurified product was associated with long-term disfiguring side effects, including migration and granuloma formation. It was illegal to perform silicone injections in the US in some states until recently. However, because of the purification of liquid silicone and honing of the injection technique, this soft tissue filler has returned and is very popular in Brazil. At the turn of the 21st century, the FDA approved two forms of medical-grade silicone oils: ADATO (or Sil-ol 5000, Bausch & Lomb Surgical, Inc., San Dimas, CA) with 5000 centistoke (cs) viscosity and Silikon 1000 (Alcon Laboratories, Inc., Fort Worth, TX) with 1000 cs viscosity. These are both indicated for the ophthalmologic uses of retinal temponade and detachment.[32,33] Although neither of these products have been approved by the FDA as skin injectables, they are used off-label. Furthermore, there are ongoing studies in the US assessing the safety and efficacy of SilSkin (a 1000 cs, highly purified polydimethylsiloxane, OFAS-Therapeutic Silicone Technologies, Inc., New York, NY) for the correction of nasolabial folds and HIV-associated lipoatrophy. Pilot studies in patients with HIV-lipoatrophy have revealed satisfactory results with minimal side effects.[59]

Similar to PMMA and PLLA, silicone oil biostimulates the surrounding skin to slowly generate a focal fibro-granulomatous reaction that leads to a permanent volumizing. Zappi et al. analyzed the microscopic biologic behavior of liquid silicone and concluded that it was an effective, durable (up to 23 years), and immunologically compatible filler.[60]

Silikon 1000 is the preferred injectable filler over ADATO because of its lower viscosity and therefore easier injectability. It is stored at room temperature and packaged as clear oil. The proficiency in the injection technique is the crucial variable in achieving successful soft tissue augmentation with silicone. The favored technique is a serial puncture of microdroplets and subdermal implantation of 0.01 to 0.02 mL silicone aliquots at 2- to 4-mm intervals using a glass syringe with a 30-mL needle.[32,52] The key is not to overcorrect. Instead, patients should anticipate steady changes with multiple treatment sessions, 1 to 2 months apart, in order to achieve the most natural and safe outcome in several months.

Benefits Since it is immunologically inert, no prior skin testing is required. Practitioners with experience in using Silikon have reported its value in correcting wrinkles and scars, augmenting lips, and panfacial contouring of deeper folds and valleys.[61] Its low cost and longevity are obvious benefits.

Drawbacks As with any temporary filler, potential long-term consequences should be broached when discussing this treatment option with patients. Most side effects associated with medical-grade silicone injectables are minimal and include anticipated temporary pain, edema, bruising, and redness.[53] The pain is likely because of the absence of anesthetic as part of the product formulation, so appropriate preprocedure anesthesia should be provided. However, it is important to keep in mind that rare reports of appropriately-injected, purified silicone causing significant nodules, granulomas, cellulitis, and ulceration also exist.[53] The skill of the physician is crucial as this is a permanent filler. The primary author has seen myriad unhappy patients who have lumps and asymmetry after treatment by other physicians (Figs. 23-11 and 23-12). In addition, many patients who are treated by nonphysicians are treated with impure silicone. This results in disfiguring edema and long-term complications. In our clinic, we have tried to treat complications of silicone injections by nonphysicians with injectable steroids, tacrolimus, cyclosporine, and Aldara with minimal and short-term improvement. Surgical excision has remained the only effective long-term treatment.

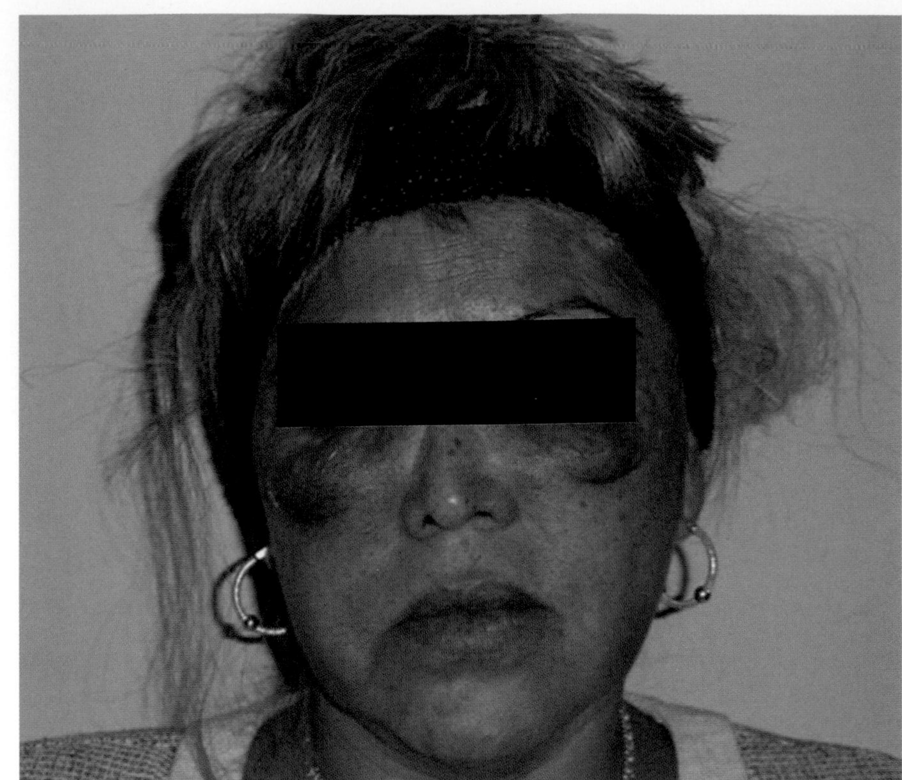

▲ **FIGURE 23-11** Patient who had an unknown substance injected by an aesthetician in a hotel room in Miami. Analysis of biopsy material showed silicone. No treatments have been effective long-term in this patient.

POLYTETRAFLUOROETHYLENE

Overview. Approved by the FDA in the 1990s for the purpose of soft tissue augmentation, several forms of expanded polytetrafluoroethylene (PTFE) are currently on the market: Gore-Tex strings or strands (Gore Advanced Technologies Worldwide, Newark, DE); Soft-Form and UltraSoft tubes (Tissue Technologies, Inc., San Francisco, CA); and newer dual-porous, soft, varied-shape Advanta (Atrium Medical Corporation, Hudson, NH).[62,63] PTFE is a synthetic material used in medical devices since the 1970s with a good safety record. These are spongy products that provide significant volume enhancement and stimulate local tissue fibrosis and integration, which relays permanence and stability. PTFE is

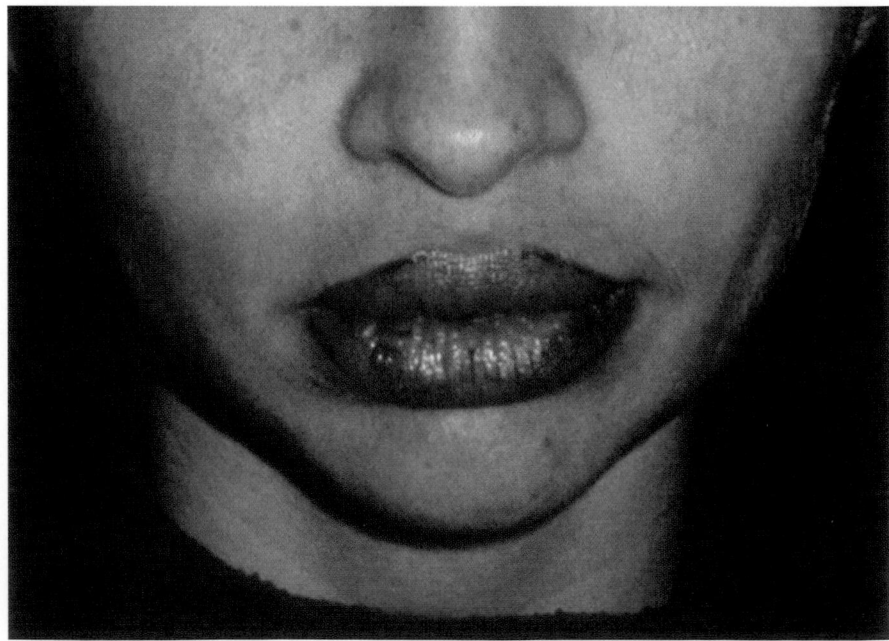

▲ **FIGURE 23-12** Patient who had silicone injections to the lips. She is unhappy with the large size of her lips.

biocompatible with rare instances of inflammatory reactions.

The extended PTFE subdermal implants require a more invasive procedure via surgical implantation, which translates to higher procedural risks and the necessity for a more specialized setting and training. Because of these complex features and generally lower physician satisfaction, the use of these devices by cosmetic dermatologists is not popular.[57]

Benefits PTFE fillers have been shown to impart an enduring correction of the nasolabial folds, marionette lines, malar and mandibular deficits, and enhancement of the lips.[56] Additionally, these products do not require prior testing because of immunologic inertness. Although the implants are considered permanent, if patients are dissatisfied with their image alterations, the products can be removed in bulk within 3 months.

Drawbacks The side effects of bleeding, bruising, redness, postoperative pain, scarring, palpability, and secondary infection occur more frequently with PTFE fillers as compared to HA fillers and the recovery time is longer.[64] These products have high displacement and extrusion rates and an unnaturally stiff appearance.[58] In addition, they can shrink with time leading to an asymmetric correction.

Fillers on the Horizon

As noninvasive cosmetic interventions have become more prominent, the manufacturing market has responded by developing newer products. In fact, there are so many products to consider, it has become ever more challenging for regulatory organizations, physicians, and patients to discern their differences. While some clinicians opt to jump on the bandwagon and use novel filling agents by interpreting newer as better, others await satisfactory clinical evidence before integrating these fillers into their practices. It is crucial to appreciate the fact that the products once proclaimed innovative have either stood the test of time, with manufacturers reaping the rewards, or they have been superseded. This section provides an overview of the up and coming soft tissue augmentation devices.

EVOLENCE

Overview Evolence (Colbar LifeScience Ltd., Herzliya, Israel) is cross-linked porcine-derived collagen (30 mg/mL concentration). Because of the greater biologic similarity between pig and human skin versus bovine and human skin, this filler has potentially lower immunogenicity than bovine collagen fillers, with no preprocedure sensitivity testing required.[65] It is currently only approved in Europe and Israel as two products, Evolence and Evolence Breeze (finer version), for soft tissue augmentation.

Evolence is injected through a 25- to 27-gauge 1.25- to 1.5-inch needle into mid-depth dermal space using tunneling and cross-hatching techniques, while Evolence Breeze is injected in 0.1-mL aliquots via a 31-gauge needle using a serial puncture technique into the superficial dermis; overcorrection is to be avoided.[66] Postimplantation massage is advised to enhance molding.

Benefits Without prior allergy testing needed, these products can be injected on the first visit. Special cross-linking technology, Glymatrix, yields a more stable collagen product that creates immediate effects potentially lasting for up to 1 year. Evolence products may be used in combination with other agents such as HA fillers. This collagen filler is stored at room temperature. A recent study comparing the safety and efficacy of Evolence and Restylane showed that Evolence performed similarly to Restylane.[67]

Drawbacks Evolence does not contain lidocaine as other collagen fillers do. It is more difficult to inject than Restylane and Juvéderm. Needle jamming has been noted on occasion, which makes injections a bit awkward.[60] Religious beliefs have to be considered prior to implantation because this product contains porcine collagen, which may be rejected on religious grounds by Jewish and Muslim patients. This product had not yet been approved by the FDA at the time of publication, but approval is expected shortly. Although postprocedure side effects of porcine collagen fillers are comparable to HA fillers (e.g., transient edema, erythema, pain, ecchymoses), the development of infrequent lumps and nodules that last several months has also been noted.[60] These papules can be treated with massage and intralesional corticosteroids. Because of these side effects, injecting Evolence into thin skin areas should be avoided.[60] This filler is new and does not have the years of experience associated with other collagen and HA fillers. Its use should be approached with caution.

ISOLAGEN

Overview Although presently approved in the UK, Isolagen (Isolagen Inc., Exton, PA) is undergoing clinical studies in the US to obtain FDA approval. Utilizing the patient's skin, fibroblasts are cultured and stimulated to generate injectable material for aesthetic augmentation. The appeal of Isolagen is that it uses a minimally invasive harvesting technique, employing very little tissue (a 3-mm skin punch biopsy from a noncosmetic area), to produce an individual, immunologically inert supply of volume-enhancing product.[68] About 2 months after harvesting, a 1 to 2 cm^3 amount of product is created and injected at about 2-week intervals in several sessions to provide longer-lasting results. This product may contain fibroblasts that could confer long-term benefits not found with other fillers.

Benefits The crucial benefits of Isolagen are biocompatibility and safety. This product contains the donor's own fibroblasts, which may provide ameliorative effects by increasing the production of desired cytokines and growth factors, stimulating collagen and elastin production. Correction is believed, but not proven, to last about 6 to 12 months. As other collagen fillers, it is injected at superficial and moderate dermal depth to treat rhytides and nasolabial folds as well as the lips.

Drawbacks This product is particularly expensive because of the specific engineering technique of cultured autologous fibroblasts and collagen. There is a waiting period of 2 months and the product derived from the biopsy is relatively sparse. However, this product can be used in conjunction with other fillers to make up the volume difference. Special product shipping, handling and storage, as well as a narrow time-frame of implantation (within 24 h of Isolagen delivery) are limitations. The side effects of the product have not been clarified, but are likely similar to other fillers on the market.

LARESSE

Overview Laresse is a novel dermal filler composed of two polymers in solution, carboxymethyl cellulose (CMC) and polyethylene oxide (PEO), both of which are hydrophilic. The product is a viscoelastic gel that is injected into the dermis as a space-filling substance. Although the clinical data are limited, it has been available in the UK since mid-2006 and has become a competitor to cross-linked HA products. Since Laresse is not cross-linked, it is smoother to inject than HA fillers and imparts a soft contour to the dermis.

Benefits Skin testing is not required with this product. The components have been used in numerous injectable therapeutics and medical devices and are known to be immunologically inert. Laresse is easily injected and is reported to produce less pain on injection than other fillers. The product is particularly smooth and natural feeling in the skin and it has been used in nasolabial folds and other superficial wrinkles. Because of its ability to stabilize and compact in higher concentrations without a need for cross-linking, it is hypothesized that Laresse will have longer durability than HA fillers.[69] However, no studies have been published in the US to support these claims.

Drawbacks Although studies have shown that Laresse lasts 6 months in some patients, limited clinical studies have been performed so its duration will become evident as it becomes available in the marketplace. The extent of its potential applications in facial augmentation is unclear as the product has been used clinically only since 2007 and its use in the hands of practitioners is still being evaluated. Laresse does not contain lidocaine and, therefore, preprocedure anesthesia is usually topical or a nerve block, similar to HA fillers. Side effects are analogous to the HA fillers and consist mainly of transient swelling, bruising, and redness. Other adverse events are yet to be revealed as Laresse is being investigated by the FDA.

AQUAMID

Overview A novel permanent filler, Aquamid (Ferrosan A/S-Contura International SA, Cophenhagen, Denmark) has been approved and used in Europe, South America, and the Middle East for the past few years.[33] Aquamid is composed of 97.5% pyrogenic water linked to 2.5% cross-linked polyacrylamide polymer. When it is introduced into skin tissue, acrylamide stimulates fibrotic and localized foreign-body reactions. The gel is packaged in a 1-mL syringe and stored at room temperature. It is injected through a 27-gauge needle using a threading technique without overcorrection.

Benefits The material is inert, obviating prior sensitivity testing. Aquamid is biocompatible and nonabsorbable, which yields an inert and durable device that can last indefinitely. Aquamid has shown efficacy in lip augmentation, correction of nasolabial folds, depressed mouth commissures, as well as glabellar and perioral rhytides.[33]

Drawbacks Lacking lidocaine content, Aquamid requires local or regional anesthesia prior to the procedure. Although postimplantation side effects are similar to those of HA fillers (e.g., temporary erythema, edema, redness), rare long-term and more severe adverse effects are more prominent with Aquamid. The primary author has seen several patients treated in South America with prolonged swelling and edema (Fig. 23-13). The exact duration of Aquamid in the skin is still unclear,

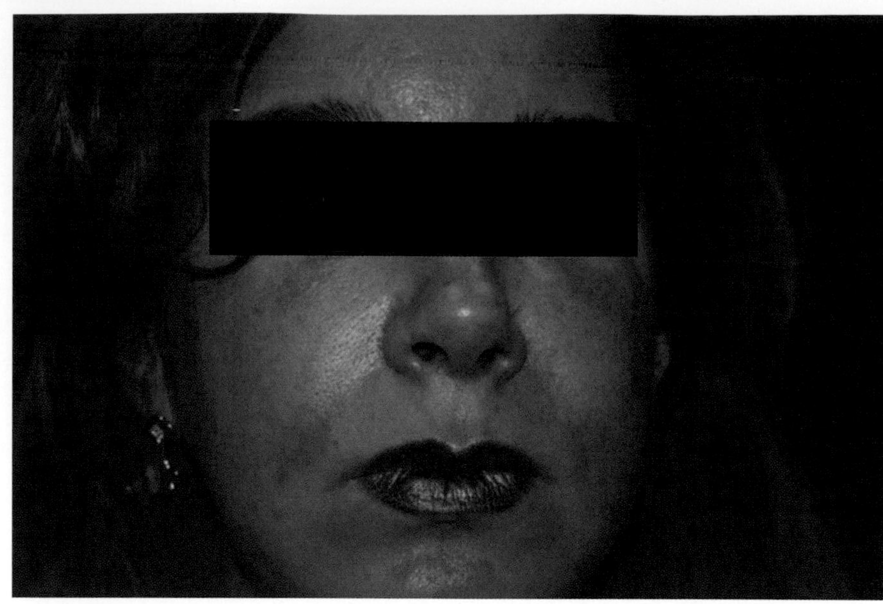

▲ **FIGURE 23-13** Patient with prolonged facial swelling one month after Aquamid injections.

TABLE 23-6
The A, B, C, D Approach to Choosing the Appropriate Filler

A—Assess the patient
- a. Which areas show aging or asymmetry?
- b. Which areas can be easily corrected?
- c. Imagine how the patient will look if various areas are corrected.
- d. Determine the best areas of injection and proceed to next step.

B—Budget
- a. Determine the patient's financial budget.
- b. Determine the patient's time budget.
- c. Refine plan in your mind about which areas are most important to treat.

C—Considerations
- a. Learn more about the patient.
- b. What bothers the patient most?
- c. Ask about prior experience with fillers.
- d. Are there any religious restrictions?
- e. Can the patient return for future treatments?
- f. Does the patient have an event coming up?
- g. Is the patient on anticoagulants?
- h. Are there any concerns about outcome?
- i. Are there any product promotions going on?

D—Device
- a. Assess pros and cons of available fillers.
- b. Match attributes of fillers to what was learned in steps A, B, and C.
- c. Choose the appropriate device.
- d. Discuss the plan with the patient.

with most recent studies demonstrating about 2-year durability.[70] Rare hematomas, lumps, granulomas, and indurations do occur with the use of Aquamid.[33] Use of this filler should be discouraged until more safety data are gathered.

HOW TO SELECT A FILLER

There are many filler options available, so deciding on which filler to use is difficult. The A, B, C, D approach can help (Table 23-6). "A" stands for *assess* the patient. Determine which areas can be treated with the greatest potential for improvement. Look at the entire face and decide where to get the "best bang for the buck." For example, if the patient has prominent nasolabial folds, there are two main options: treating the nasolabial folds, or treating the cheek or cheekbone area to add volume that will improve the fold by pulling the skin back. A patient with large round cheeks would do better to have the nasolabial fold treated (Fig. 23-14), while a patient with thin cheeks and facial volume loss would have a better result if the cheeks were treated (Figs. 23-15 and 23-16). As a practitioner, it is important to form your own impression first before the patient tells you their thoughts. In some cases you may notice factors that the patient does not even realize are contributing to an aged appearance (Figs. 23-17 and 23-18). These observational skills are developed with experience. Table 23-7 provides an overview of which fillers are best suited for each facial area. Once you have an idea of what areas would make the most significant impact if treated, then move to the "B" section, which is ***budget***. It is crucial to determine how much money the patient is willing to spend. It is often the case that the budget is lower than what is necessary, so the physician must determine what areas to treat to achieve the best cosmetic effect possible within the patient's budget. In addition, the practitioner must consider the patient's time budget or schedule. For example, if a patient is visiting from another country and planning to leave the following day, a course of Sculptra injections is not an option. Once the time and financial budget have been determined, the practitioner should talk to the patient about other ***considerations***. The most important question is what bothers them about their face. It is often different than what the physician sees.

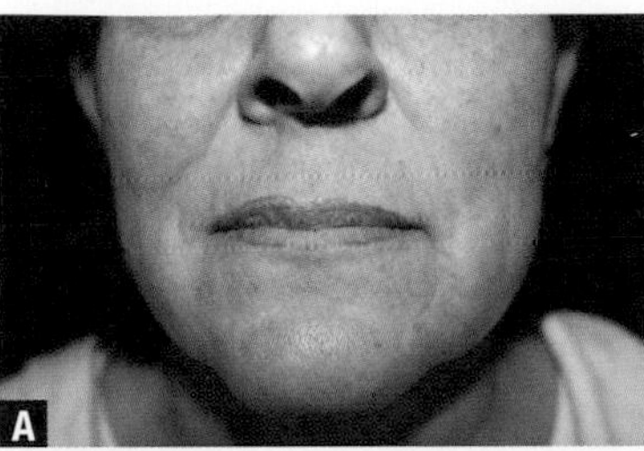

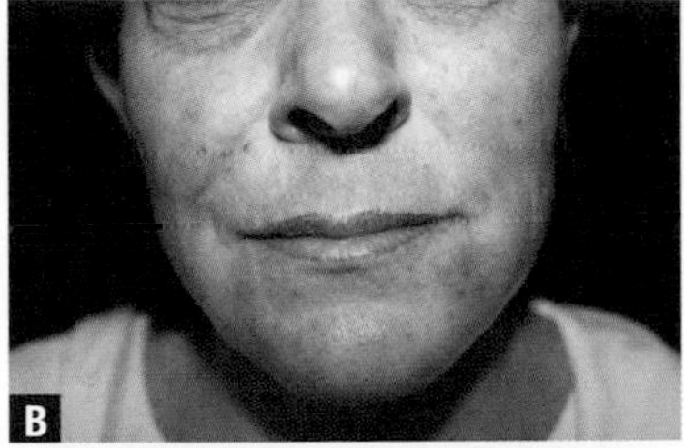

▲ **FIGURE 23-14 A.** Those with a normal to large buccal fat pad are best treated with injections directly into the nasolabial folds and marionette lines. **B.** Immediately after treatment of nasolabial folds and marionette lines.

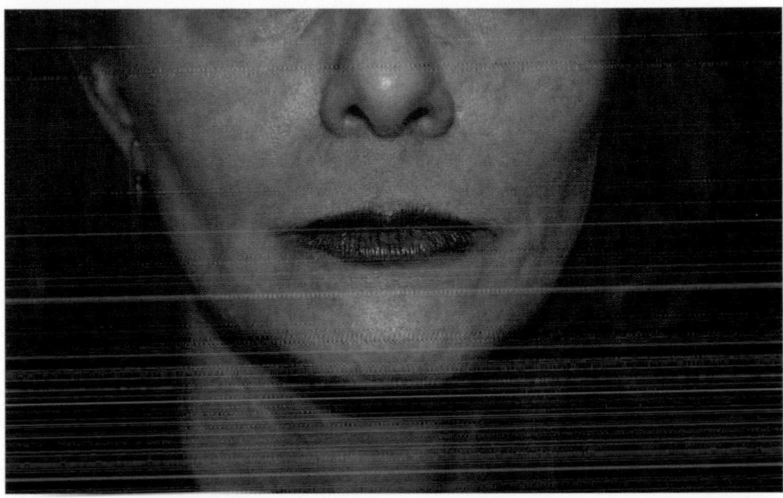

▲ **FIGURE 23-15** This patient has thin cheeks from buccal fat pad wasting; therefore, she is a good candidate for a filler such as Sculptra, Juvéderm Ultra, or Restylane to the cheek area below the cheekbones.

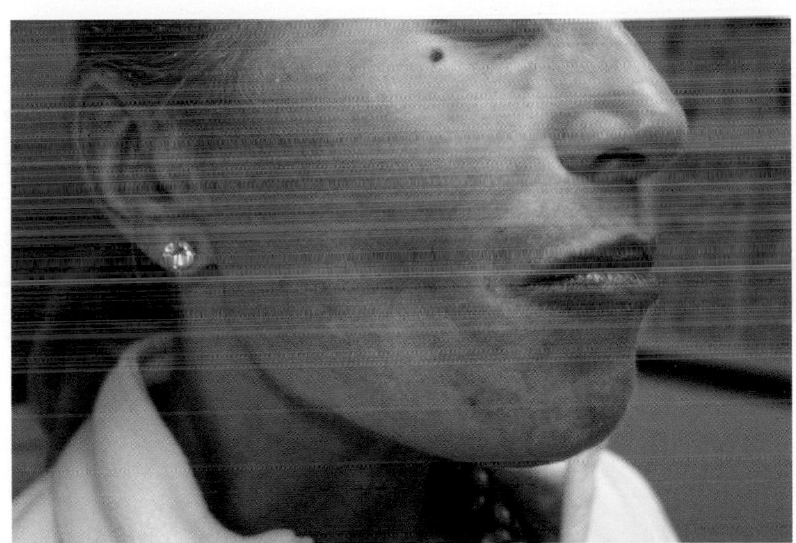

▲ **FIGURE 23-16** This patient appears to have buccal fat pad wasting, but actually is missing a tooth on this side, leading to the defect. A dental consult is more appropriate for this patient rather than a dermal filler.

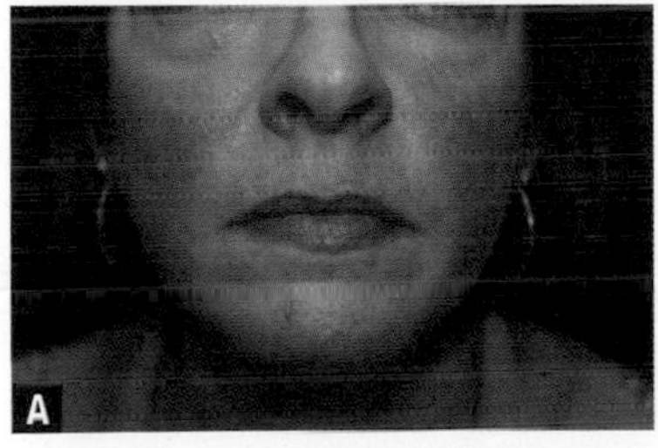

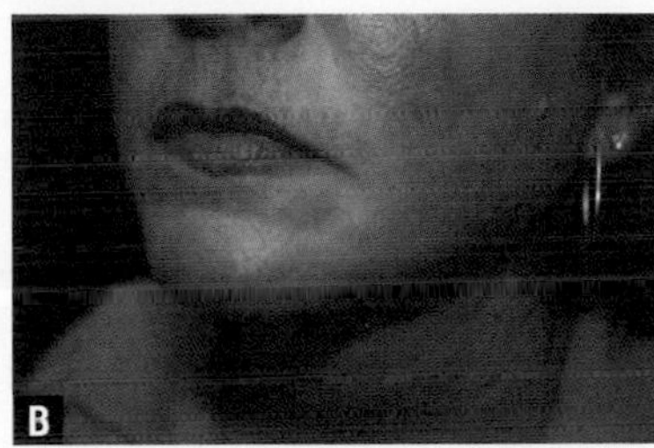

▲ **FIGURE 23-17** (**A** and **B**) Soft tissue loss around the mental area is often one of the first signs of facial aging. It is hard to capture on film and patients do not really notice it until it is pointed out to them.

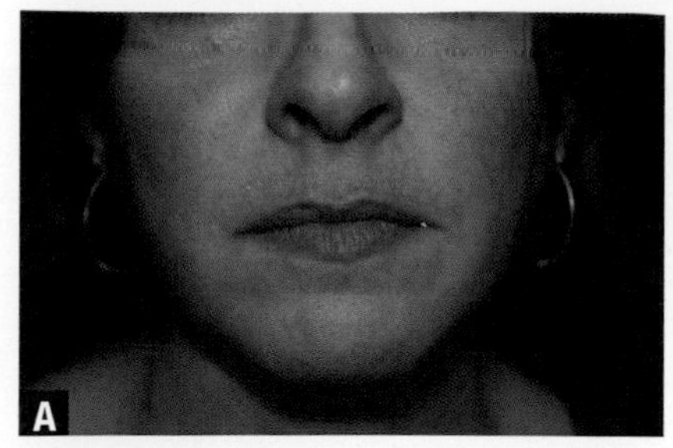

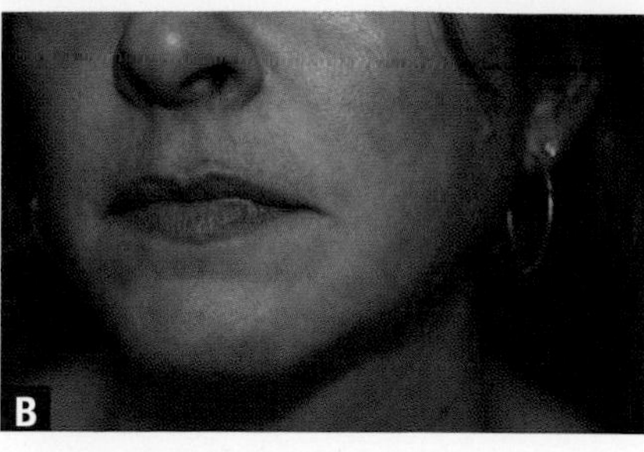

▲ **FIGURE 23-18** (**A** and **B**) Once the soft tissue around the mental bone has been filled, the face looks more youthful. An HA filler was used in this patient.

TABLE 23-7
Fillers by Region (Listed from the Top of the Face Down)

- Forehead lines
  - Cosmoderm I
  - Restylane Fine Lines, Juvéderm[18], or Prevelle Silk
  - Zyderm I
- Raising lateral brows (almost any will work)
  - CosmoPlast
  - Evolence
  - Juvéderm Ultra
  - Juvéderm Ultra Plus
  - Perlane
  - Prevelle Silk
  - Prevelle Dura
  - Radiesse
  - Restylane
  - Zyplast
- Glabella (use with caution)
  - CosmoDerm I
  - Zyderm I
- Tear trough (soft fillers preferred)
  - Hylaform
  - Juvéderm 18
  - Prevelle Silk
  - Restylane Touch
- Crow's feet
  - CosmoDerm I
  - Juvéderm 18
  - Prevelle Silk
  - Restylane Touch
  - Zyderm I
- Cheek bones
  - Juvéderm Ultra
  - Juvéderm Ultra Plus
  - Perlane
  - Prevelle Dura
  - Prevelle Silk
  - Radiesse
  - Restylane
  - Sculptra
- Nasolabial folds
  - CosmoPlast
  - Evolence
  - Juvéderm Ultra
  - Juvéderm Ultra Plus
  - Perlane
  - Prevelle Silk
  - Prevelle Dura
  - Radiesse
  - Restylane
  - Sculptra
  - Zyplast
- Vermilion border of the lip
  - CosmoPlast
  - Evolence
  - Juvéderm Ultra
  - Prevelle Silk
  - Restylane
  - Zyplast
- Body of the lip
  - Hylaform
  - Prevelle Silk
  - Restylane Lip
- Marionnette lines
  - CosmoPlast
  - Evolence
  - Juvéderm Ultra
  - Juvéderm Ultra Plus
  - Perlane
  - Prevelle Silk
  - Prevelle Dura
  - Radiesse
  - Restylane
  - Zyplast
- Pre-jowl sulcus
  - CosmoPlast
  - Evolence
  - Juvéderm Ultra
  - Juvéderm Ultra Plus
  - Perlane
  - Prevelle Silk
  - Prevelle Dura
  - Radiesse
  - Restylane
  - Sculptra
  - Zyplast

Patient happiness is contingent on improving what they see as the problems on their face, not what bothers the physician. The following or similar questions may be appropriate to frame such a discussion, then, in the attempt to identify the most suitable filler for a patient: What have you tried before? Were you satisfied with the results? Why or why not? What concerns do you have? Are you a frequent bruiser? Are you worried that your lips will look too big? Do you hate it when your lipstick bleeds up into the lines on the top lip? Do you have any religious restrictions? Do you have any events coming up? What amount of downtime can you tolerate? These are all critical issues in determining the most appropriate filler. Once all this information has been gathered, the physician must choose a filling *device* that meets all the criteria. It is a relatively easy choice after the preceding questions have been answered. In addition, the physician should have many filler choices on hand to give the patient the best result.

Injection Technique

Injection technique varies from filler to filler. Most physicians use either an anterograde, retrograde, or serial puncture technique. Most collagen and HA fillers are injected at a 45-degree angle (Fig. 23-19). It is important to be individually trained on the injection techniques of each filler. Fillers can be used in combination with botulinum toxins and other cosmetic procedures (Fig. 23-20). Although this chapter focused on facial use, fillers can also be injected in other areas of the body such as the hands (Fig. 23-21). Many injection techniques can be used. However, it is difficult to teach various techniques without video and live demonstrations. In the future, instructional videos will be available at www.derm.net and training courses will be offered at the University of Miami. In addition, the American Academy of Dermatology and the American Society of Dermatologic Surgeons offer training courses for dermatologists.

SUMMARY

Filling agents for soft issue augmentation procedures are now widely available, based on the long-standing successful track records of the earliest products. Most agents in the soft tissue augmentation armamentarium can be safely used alone or in combination. The

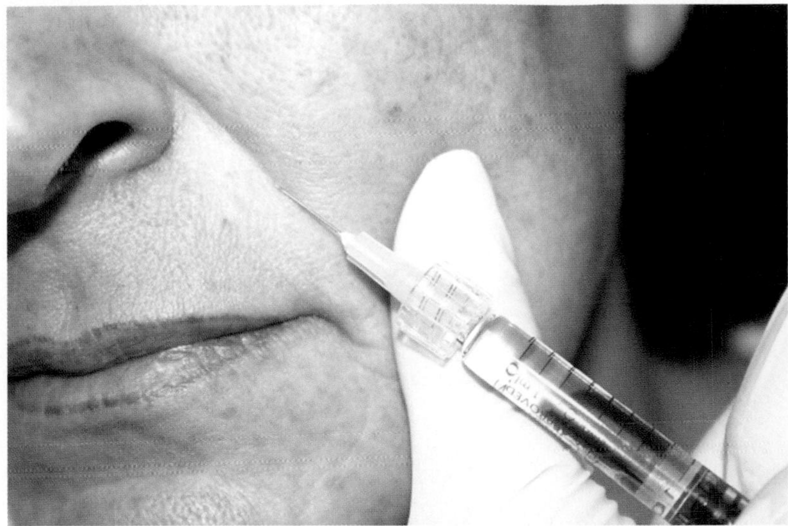

▲ **FIGURE 23-19** Most collagen and HA fillers are injected using a 45-degree angle. Injecting over the thumb can help ensure this angle.

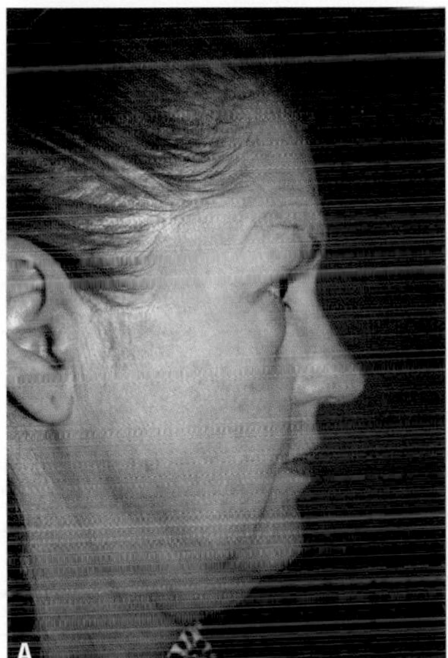

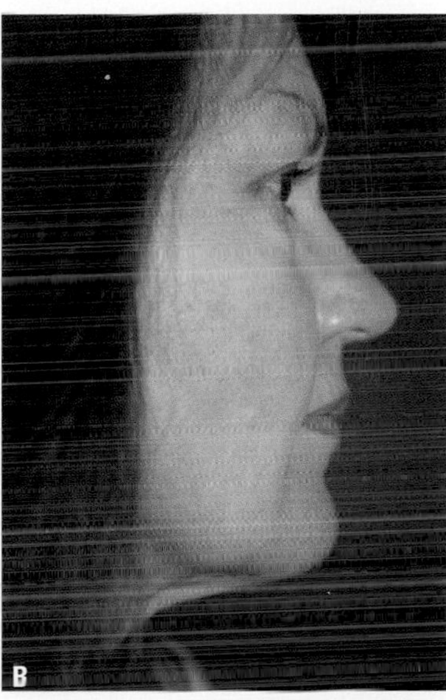

▲ **FIGURE 23-20** (**A** and **B**) A patient treated with Radiesse to several facial areas and with Botox to the platysma. (Photos courtesy of Lisa Grunebaum, MD.)

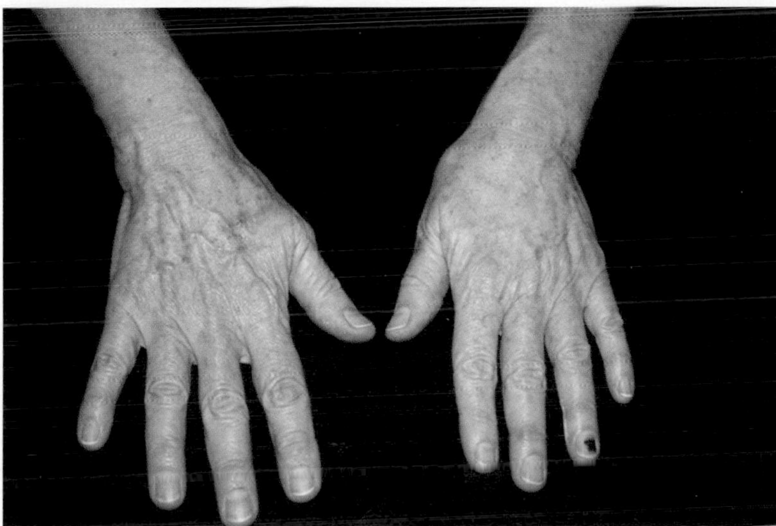

▲ **FIGURE 23-21** The hand on the left is before Radiesse treatment. The image with the dark nail is after Radiesse. (Photos courtesy of Lisa Grunebaum, MD.)

most frequently used agents are those that contain HA. Given the widespread popularity of soft tissue augmentation and the ever-present need to develop safer fillers that last longer than the current products, new fillers frequently enter the market. Soon to be made available in the US is an HA filler that contains lidocaine as well as more durable and safer synthetic agents. In short, the demand for soft tissue augmentation procedures has steadily increased since their inception and research is ongoing to develop products that address the shortcomings of the earlier products while incorporating and expanding on their advantages. Moreover, the "coupling" of fillers with other cosmetic interventions (e.g., Botox injections) enhances their longevity and efficacy, and creates an overall realistically aesthetic appearance.[71] To keep astride with the rapidly changing cosmetic dermatology arena, it behooves the aesthetic practitioner to be aware of the current availability, application, and future potential of dermal fillers.

REFERENCES

1. Neuber F. Fettransplantation. *Chir Kongr Verhandl Dsch Gesellch Chir.* 1893;22:66.
2. Klein A, Elson M. The history of substances for soft tissue augmentation. *Dermatol Surg.* 2000;26:1096
3. Glaich AS, Cohen JL, Goldberg LH. Injection necrosis of the glabella: protocol for prevention and treatment after use of dermal fillers. *Dermatol Surg.* 2006;32:276.
4. Gniadecka M, Nielsen OF, Wessel S, et al. Water and protein structure in photoaged and chronically aged skin. *J Invest Dermatol.* 1998;111:1129.
5. Baumann L. Soft tissue augmentation. In: Baumann L, ed. *Cosmetic Dermatology: Principles and Practice*. New York, NY: McGraw-Hill; 2002:155-172.
6. Eppley BL, Dadvand B. Injectable soft-tissue fillers: clinical overview. *Plast Reconstr Surg.* 2006;118:98e.
7. Stegman SJ, Chu S, Armstrong RC. Adverse reactions to bovine collagen implant: clinical and histologic features. *J Dermatol Surg Oncol.* 1988;14:39.
8. Castrow FF II, Krull EA. Injectable collagen implant-Update. *J Am Acad Dermatol.* 1983;9:889.
9. Siegle RJ, McCoy JP Jr, Schade W, et al. Intradermal implantation of bovine collagen. Humoral immune responses associated with clinical reactions. *Arch Dermatol.* 1984;120:183.
10. Baumann LS, Kerdel F. The treatment of bovine collagen allergy with cyclosporin. *Dermatol Surg.* 1999;25:247.
11. Moody BR, Sengelmann RD. Topical tacrolimus in the treatment of bovine collagen hypersensitivity. *Dermatol Surg.* 2001;27:789.
12. Hanke CW, Higley HR, Jolivette DM, et al. Abscess formation and local necro-

sis after treatment with Zyderm or Zyplast collagen implant. *J Am Acad Dermatol.* 1991;25:319.
13. Cooperman LS, Mackinnon V, Bechler G, et al. Injectable collagen: a six-year clinical investigation. *Aesthetic Plast Surg.* 1985;9:145.
14. Cukier J, Beauchamp RA, Spindler JS, et al. Association between bovine collagen dermal implants and a dermatomyositis or a polymyositis-like syndrome. *Ann Intern Med.* 1993;118:920.
15. Rosenberg MJ, Reichlin M. Is there an association between injectable collagen and polymyositis/dermatomyositis? *Arthritis Rheum.* 1994;37:747.
16. Elson ML. Injectable collagen and autoimmune disease. *J Dermatol Surg Oncol.* 1993; 19:165.
17. Klein AW. Bonfire of the wrinkles. *J Dermatol Surg Oncol.* 1991;17:543.
18. Hanke CW, Thomas JA, Lee WT, et al. Risk assessment of polymyositis/dermatomyositis after treatment with injectable bovine collagen implants. *J Am Acad Dermatol.* 1996;34:450.
19. Baumann L. CosmoDerm/CosmoPlast (human bioengineered collagen) for the aging face. *Facial Plast Surg.* 2004;20:125.
20. Okada S, Hagan JB, Kato M, et al. Lidocaine and its analogues inhibit IL-5-mediated survival and activation of human eosinophils. *J Immunol.* 1998; 160:4010.
21. Cosmetic Surgery National Data Bank 2005 Statistics (American Society of Aesthetic Plastic Surgery website). http://www.surgery.org/download/2005stats.pdf. Accessed June 7, 2006.
22. Lemperle G, Rullan PP, Gauthier-Hazan N. Avoiding and treating dermal filler complications. *Plast Reconstr Surg.* 2006;118:92S.
23. Baumann LS, Shamban AT, Lupo MP, et al. Comparison of smooth-gel hyaluronic acid dermal fillers with cross-linked bovine collagen: a multicenter, double-masked, randomized, within-subject study. *Dermatol Surg.* 2007;33:S128.
24. Balazs EA, Bland PA, Denlinger JL, et al. Matrix engineering. *Blood Coagul Fibrinolysis.* 1991;2:173.
25. Hylaform® [package insert]. Genzyme Biosurgery, Ridgefield, NJ. 2004.
26. Bergeret-Galley C. Comparison of resorbable soft tissue fillers. *Aesthetic Surg J.* 2004;24:33.
27. Monheit GD, Prather CL. Juvéderm: a hyaluronic acid dermal filler. *J Drugs Dermatol.* 2007;6:1091.
28. McCracken MS, Khan JA, Wulc AE, et al. Hyaluronic acid gel (Restylane) filler for facial rhytids: lessons learned from American Society of Ophthalmic Plastic and Reconstructive Surgery member treatment of 286 patients. *Ophthal Plast Reconstr Surg.* 2006;22:188.
29. Narins RS, Brandt F, Leyden J, et al. A randomized, double-blind multicenter comparison of the efficacy and tolerability of Restylane versus Zyplast for the correction of nasolabial folds. *Dermatol Surg.* 2003;29:588.
30. Tezel A, Walker P. P2906. The influence of formulations on persistence with hyaluronic acid dermal fillers. [Abstract] *J Am Acad Dermatol.* 2007;56(2):AB198.
31. Kinney BM. Injecting Puragen Plus into nasolabial folds: preliminary observations of FDA trial. *Aesthetic Surg J.* 2006;26:741.
32. Hirsch RJ, Lupo M, Cohen JL, et al. Delayed presentation of impending necrosis following soft tissue augmentation with hyaluronic acid and successful management with hyaluronidase. *J Drugs Dermatol.* 2007;6:325.
33. Hirsch RJ, Cohen JL, Carruthers JD. Successful management of an unusual presentation of impending necrosis following a hyaluronic acid injection embolus and a proposed algorithm for management with hyaluronidase. *Dermatol Surg.* 2007;33:357.
34. Goldberg RA, Fiaschetti D. Filling the periorbital hollows with hyaluronic acid gel: initial experience with 244 injections. *Ophthal Plast Reconstr Surg.* 2006;22:335.
35. Lambros V. The use of hyaluronidase to reverse the effects of hyaluronic acid filler. *Plast Reconstr Surg.* 2004;114:277.
36. Pierre A, Levy PM. Hyaluronidase offers an efficacious treatment for inaesthetic hyaluronic acid overcorrection. *J Cosmet Dermatol.* 2007;6:159.
37. Hirsch RJ, Brody HJ, Carruthers JD. Hyaluronidase in the office: a necessity for every dermasurgeon that injects hyaluronic acid. *J Cosmet Laser Ther.* 2007;9:182.
38. Amphastar. com. http://www.amphastar.com/amphadasewhatis.htm. Accessed, February 29, 2008. .
39. Goldman MP. Optimizing the use of fillers for facial rejuvenation: the right tools for the right job. *Cosmetic Dermatology.* 2007;20(7S):14.
40. Broder KW, Cohen SR. An overview of permanent and semipermanent fillers. *Plast Reconstr Surg.* 2007;118:7S.
41. Bucky LP, Kanchwala SK. The role of autologous fat and alternative fillers in the aging face. *Plast Reconstr Surg.* 2007; 120:89S.
42. Stashower M, Smith K, Williams J, et al. Stromal progenitor cells present within liposuction and reduction abdominoplasty fat for autologous transfer to aged skin. *Dermatol Surg.* 1999;25: 945.
43. Baumann L, Narins R, Werschler P. Dermal filling agents: evaluating more choices for your patients. Part 2. *Skin Aging.* 2007;15(6):50.
44. Majola A, Vainionpää S, Vihtonen K, et al. Absorption, biocompatibility, and fixation properties of polylactic acid in bone tissue: an experimental study in rats. *Clin Orthop Relat Res.* 1991; 268:260.
45. Gogolewski S, Jovanovic M, Perren SM, et al. Tissue response and in vivo degradation of selected polyhydroxyacids: polylactides (PLA), poly(3-hydroxybutyrate) (PHB), and poly(3-hydroxybutyrate-co-3-hydroxyvalerate) (PHB/VA). *J Biomed Mater Res.* 1993;27:1135.
46. Viljanen JT, Pihlajamäki HK, Törmälä PO, et al. Comparison of the tissue response to absorbable self-reinforced polylactide screws and metallic screws in the fixation of cancellous bone osteotomies: an experimental study on the rabbit distal femur. *J Orthop Res.* 1997;15:398.
47. Burgess CM, Lowe NJ. NewFill for skin augmentation: a new filler or failure? *Dermatol Surg.* 2006;32:1530.
48. Sherman RN. Sculptra: the new three-dimensional filler. *Clin Past Surg.* 2006;33:539.
49. Thioly-Bensoussan D. A new option for volumetric restoration: poly-L-lactic acid. *J Eur Acad Dermatol Venereol.* 2006;20(Suppl 1):12.
50. Vleggaar D, Bauer U. Facial enhancement and the European experience with poly-L-lactic acid. *J Drugs Dermatol.* 2004;3:526.
51. Keni Sp, Sidle DM. Sculptra (injectable poly-L-lactic acid). *Facial Plast Surg Clin North Am.* 2007;15:91.
52. Vleggaar D. Facial volumetric correction with injectable poly-L-lactic acid. *Dermatol Surg.* 2005;31:1511.
53. Lowe NJ. Dispelling the myth: appropriate use of poly-L-lactic acid and clinical considerations. *J Eur Acad Dermatol Venereol.* 2006;20(Suppl 1):2.
54. Vleggaar D. Poly-L-lactic acid: consultation on the injection techniques. *J Eur Acad Dermatol Venereol.* 2006;20(Suppl 1):17.
55. Borelli C, Kunte C, Weisenseel P, et al. Deep subcutaneous application of poly-L-lactic acid as a filler for facial lipoatrophy in HIV-infected patients. *Skin Pharmacol Physiol.* 2005;18:273.
56. El-Beyrouty C, Huang V, Darnold CJ, et al. Poly-L-lactic acid for facial lipoatrophy in HIV. *Ann Pharmacother.* 2006;40:1602.
57. Cohen SR, Berner CF, Busso M, et al. Five-year safety and efficacy of a novel polymethylmethacrylate aesthetic soft tissue filler for the correction of nasolabial folds. *Dermatol Surg.* 2007;33:S222.
58. Narins RS, Beer K. Liquid injectable silicone: a review of its history, immunology, technical considerations, complications, and potential. *Plast Reconstr Surg.* 2006;118:77S.
59. Jones DH, Carruthers A, Orentreich D, et al. Highly purified 1000-cSt silicone oil for treatment of human immunodeficiency virus-associated facial lipoatrophy: an open pilot trial. *Dermatol Surg.* 2004;30:1279.
60. Zappi E, Barnett JG, Zappi M, et al. The long-term host response to liquid silicone injected during soft tissue augmentation procedures: a microscopic appraisal. *Dermatol Surg.* 2007;33:S186.
61. Hevia O, Cazzaniga A, Brandt F, et al. Liquid injectable silicone (polydimethylsiloxane): four years of clinical experience. [Abstract] *J Am Acad Dermatol.* 2007;56(2):AB1.
62. Hanke W. A new ePTFE soft tissue implant for natural-looking augmentation of lips and wrinkles. *Dermatol Surg.* 2002;28:901.
63. Cox SE. Who is still using expanded polytetrafluoroethylene? *Dermatol Surg.* 2005;31:1613.
64. Duffy DM. Complications of fillers: overview. *Dermatol Surg.* 2005;31:1626.
65. Beer K. Evolence: the thing of shapes to come. *Skin Aging.* 2007;15:22.
66. Smith KC. New fillers for the new man. *Dermatol Ther.* 2007;20:388.
67. Narins RS, Brandt FS, Lorenc ZP, et al. A randomized, multicenter study of the

safety and efficacy of Dermicol-P35 and non-animal-stabilized hyaluronic acid gel for the correction of nasolabial folds. *Dermatol Surg.* 2007;33:S213.

68. Homicz MR, Watson D. Review of injectable materials for soft tissue augmentation. *Facial Plast Surg.* 2004; 20:21.
69. Falcone SJ, Doerfler AM, Berg RA. Novel synthetic dermal fillers based on sodium carboxymethylcellulose: comparison with crosslinked hyaluronic acid-based dermal fillers. *Dermatol Surg.* 2007;33:S136.
70. Von Buelow S, Pallua N. Efficacy and safety of polyacrylamide hydrogel for facial soft-tissue augmentation in a 2-year follow-up: a prospective multicenter study for evaluation of safety and aesthetic results in 101 patients. *Plast Reconstr Surg.* 2006;118:85S.
71. Michaels J, Michaels B. Coupling advanced injection techniques for cosmetic enhancement. *Cosmetic Journal.* 2008;21:31.

CHAPTER 24

Lasers and Light Devices

Joely Kaufman, MD

Since 1960, when the first laser was invented by T.H. Maiman at the Hughes Research Laboratory, the research arm of the Hughes Aircraft Company in Malibu, CA, research into and development of lasers has blossomed into a multibillion dollar industry. People have been especially fascinated by the capabilities and possibilities of "laser light." Beginning with the ruby laser, these instruments have quickly become an integral part of many medical specialties, including dermatology. Lasers and light devices are now used in almost every area of medicine and our daily lives, including DVD and CD players, grocery store scanners, holograms, and even traffic lights.

LASER BASICS

To realize their usefulness in medicine and aesthetic medicine in particular, it is important to understand the basics of laser terminology (Box 24-1). Understanding the interactions of light with the skin helps make clinical treatments more successful. The word "laser" is actually an acronym for light amplification by stimulated emission of radiation. A laser amplifies light by stimulating photons, storing them, and releasing them as a beam of light. In order to accomplish this, the laser must have a source of energy referred to as the "pump." This energy gets absorbed by atoms in the form of photons. When the atom emits its photons, it releases its energy in the form of light. All of this occurs in the lasing medium. Many lasers are named based on the type of lasing medium that they contain. Lasing mediums can be liquid (dyes such as rhodamine), solid [e.g., ruby, alexandrite, Nd:YAG, diode (semiconductor)], or gas (e.g., helium-neon, argon, CO_2).

BOX 24-1 A device is not deemed a true laser unless it fulfills three criteria:

- Monochromicity: the device emits light of a single wavelength.
- Collimation: all waves travel in a single direction.
- Coherence: all waves are in phase with each other.

BOX 24-2 The three main chromophores in the skin include:

- Water
- Hemoglobin
- Melanin

Several of the instruments in the cosmetic armamentarium that will be discussed here are not "true" lasers. This fact does not render them any less useful in treating patients, but it is an important distinction to make. The importance lies in the nature of the interaction between light and skin. In 1983, Anderson and Parish introduced the theory of selective photothermolysis.[1] This theory states that the selectivity of a laser for its target relies on the fact that different wavelengths of light will be absorbed by different chromophores in the skin (Box 24-2). This allows us to "selectively" destroy these targets without damaging the surrounding tissues. In order to accomplish this, the pulse width should be sufficiently long to heat the tissue to the level of destruction, but not long enough for that heat to transfer out of the target to the surrounding normal skin. The duration of active lasing is termed the "pulse width" or "pulse duration." The ideal pulse duration for selective destruction of a target is determined by the size of the target. The time it takes for the target to dissipate two-thirds of its heat to the surrounding tissue is directly proportional to its size. This is termed the thermal relaxation time (Trt). The pulse width should be equal to or shorter than this Trt in order to selectively destroy the target and not the normal surrounding tissue. If the laser pulse is longer than the Trt, then there is more risk of unwanted damage to other tissues. Lasers can emit light in a continuous fashion, or in spurts, or pulses. The theory of selective photothermolysis really only applies to pulsed laser systems, as continuous lasing results in bulk heating of tissue, and hence little "selectivity."

When light of any wavelength or intensity hits the skin four possible results ensue. The light can be directly *reflected from the skin*. This usually takes place at the stratum corneum, and this is the reason that practitioners wear protective eyewear even when not lasing near the eye. Light that passes through the stratum corneum can be *scattered by collagen in the dermis* or *transmitted through the dermis to the subcutaneous tissues*. The light that results in actual work being done on the tissues is the light that is *absorbed*. Absorption in the skin is by three main chromophores.

Each of these target chromophores absorbs light at a different wavelength (Fig. 24-1). Using these absorption spectra, we can select a laser with a wavelength that will be absorbed by the chromophore. This allows us to treat the target and not the normal skin. When the target tissue is beneath the epidermis, treatment of the target without damage to the epidermis is difficult to achieve without protection of the epidermis. This protection is achieved via cooling systems. Cooling systems are critical in several laser procedures including vessel destruction and laser hair removal. There are several modes of cooling used in lasers today, including cryogen cooling, contact, ice, and direct cold air. Employing these devices reduces injury to the epidermis. Conversely, employing too much cooling when the target is in the epidermis results in an ineffective treatment. Cooling systems are essential in laser

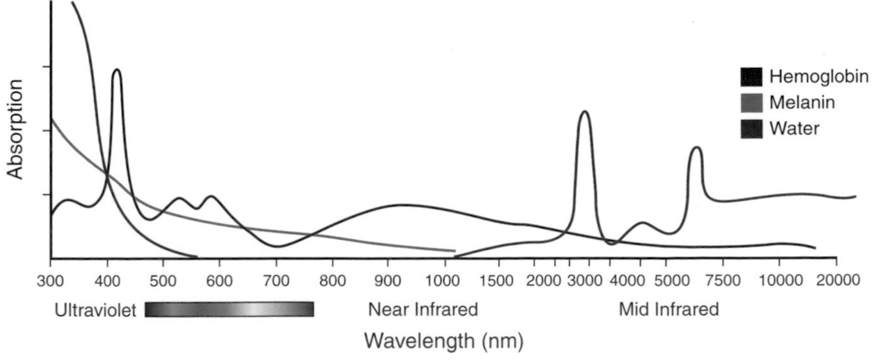

▲ **FIGURE 24-1** Absorption spectrum for the three primary skin chromophores.

hair removal, as high energies are needed to produce damage to the follicle. Applying this much energy to the skin without cooling the epidermis would result in catastrophic epidermal damage. Even with cooling, in some instances epidermal protection may still be unattainable, as is sometimes the case with darker skin types.

The energy of lasers is expressed in joules. Fluence is the energy per area, expressed in joules per centimeter squared (J/cm^2). The power of a laser is expressed in watts. When using lasers in clinical applications, it is important to remember all aspects of the laser, including wavelength, pulse duration, fluence, and cooling. Lasers are just machines; it is up to the operator to adjust and use them correctly.

In the next sections, the use of lasers by clinical diagnosis will be reviewed. Several lasers can be used for each type of lesion, some more effectively than others. The most effective lasers for each condition will be discussed.

TABLE 24-1
Vascular Laser and Light Devices

LASER TYPE	WAVELENGTH (nm)	LASER DEVICES
Pulsed dye lasers	585, 595 +1064	Candela Vbeam Cynosure Cynergy
Intense pulsed light	500–1200	Lumenis One, Lumenis IPL Quantum, Palomar StarLux, Palomar MediLux
Diodes	940	Dornier
KTP	532 (for cutaneous and endovenous)	
Long-pulsed Nd:YAG	1064	Cutera Xeo, Cutera Coolglide, Candela Gentle Yag, Laserscope Lyra, Wavelight Mydon, Cynosure Acclaim
Nd:YAG for endovenous	1320	Cooltouch CTEV

A 1064 nm handpiece for vascular lesions is also available on several IPL devices.

VASCULAR LASERS

There are many different vascular lesions that can be treated with lasers. Treating vascular lesions with the laser became popular with the advent of the argon laser in the 1970s. Since that time several laser systems targeting vascular lesions have been developed. The chromophore for vascular lesions is oxyhemoglobin. The peak absorption by oxyhemoglobin lies somewhere between 500 and 600 nm. It is for this reason that most of the lasers used for vascular lesions emit light with wavelengths within this range. Because longer wavelengths penetrate deeper owing to less scattering by collagen, wavelengths outside of this range are also used for deeper vascular lesions. Lesions amenable to laser treatment with a vascular wavelength include hemangiomas, nevus flammeus (port wine stains), lymphangiomas, venous lakes, angiomas, telangiectasias, spider veins, poikiloderma of Civatte, scars, and erythema from rosacea. Additional reports have emerged of successful treatment with vascular lasers for conditions such as verruca vulgaris, hypertropic scars, striae, sebaceous gland hyperplasia, granuloma faciale, and lupus erythematosus.

Because of the location of the vessel in the dermis, the need for epidermal cooling with the treatment of vascular lesions is critical when using wavelengths that are also within the melanin absorption spectrum. The longer wavelength vascular lasers can be operated with care without epidermal cooling. Selective photothermolysis plays a critical role in the treatment of vascular lesions. The oxyhemoglobin target must absorb the light, generating heat, and coagulating the vessel, all without damaging the surrounding tissue. The early vascular lasers were associated with a high incidence of hypopigmentation and scarring. The realization of the importance of photothermolysis and pulse widths ultimately allowed for the safe and effective treatment of vascular lesions without scarring.

The pulsed dye laser (PDL) was introduced in 1989 and remains the gold standard in laser treatment for hemangiomas. The original pulsed dye operated at a wavelength of 577 nm. Subsequent generations of PDLs have slightly longer wavelengths, corresponding to deeper penetration. Longer-wavelength lasers, however, operate further outside the peak absorption of oxyhemoglobin, and therefore require more fluence for comparable results. PDLs come equipped with dynamic cooling systems in the form of a cryogen burst. Today, the most popular systems used for vascular lesions are the PDL (585 nm), long-pulsed dye laser (595 nm), the potassium titanyl phosphate (532 nm), and the 1064 nm neodymium-doped yttrium aluminum garnet (Nd:YAG). There are also a few diode systems that are very effective for vascular lesions, including a 940 nm diode that functions very well for telangiectasias on the face, spider veins on the body, and angiomas (Table 24-1).

PDL devices are effective for telangiectasias on the face, neck, and chest, but perform less well on the body (Fig. 24-2). This is related to the short wavelength and superficial penetration of the laser. PDLs are also used for

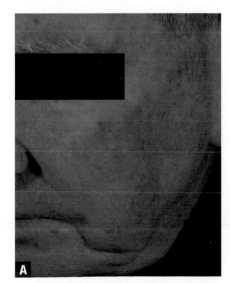

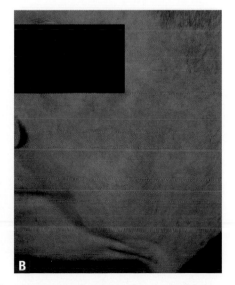

▲ **FIGURE 24-2** **A.** Before treatment with PDL for telangiectasia. **B.** After treatment with PDL for telangiectasia.

vascular malformations in adults and children, including hemangiomas, port wine stains, and lymphangiomas. The PDLs available today come equipped with cryogen cooling, various spot sizes, and adjustable pulse durations. The desired pulse duration should be adjusted to the vessel diameter and its thermal relaxation time. The larger the vessel diameter, the longer the optimal pulse width should be. Very short pulse widths lead to rupture of the vessel and resultant purpura. This common side effect made the PDLs very unpopular with cosmetic patients in the past. The recent use of longer pulse widths and double passes with these lasers results in comparable efficacy for telangiectasias, with little purpura. Still, with the treatment of hemangiomas and port wine stains, purpuric settings are often needed for adequate clearing of the lesion. Side effects in addition to purpura include blistering, postinflammatory pigment alteration (PIPA) caused by the cryogen spray, as well as scarring from overly aggressive fluences. Lesions on the chest and neck should always be treated with lower energies than those on the face.

The potassiumtitanylphosphate (KTP) laser, with a wavelength of 532 nm, is also highly absorbed by oxyhemoglobin. It has proven to be at least as effective for facial telangiectasias as the PDLs.[2] The KTP laser can operate in a range of longer pulse widths, resulting in no purpura. Its shortcomings are related to its short wavelength and lack of penetration. Treatment with the KTP is most effective for very superficial vessels. In addition, treatment of tanned or darker skin types should be performed with caution if at all, as the 532 nm wavelength is well absorbed by melanin.

Longer-wavelength lasers can also be used effectively for vascular lesions. The longer wavelengths allow for deeper penetration and hence are excellent choices for the lower extremities. In addition, they are particularly useful for high flow vessels on the face. Examples of lasers used for spider veins include the 940-nm diode laser and the 1064-nm Nd:YAG.

LASERS FOR PIGMENTED LESIONS

The first laser invented was also the first to be used for removal of pigment. The ruby laser emits a wavelength that is very well absorbed by melanin. This superior absorption by melanin has been the source of both the ruby's rise and fall. The ruby is excellent at removing any pigment. Unfortunately, it cannot distinguish between normal pigment and unwanted pigment, and quickly fell out of favor for pigment and hair removal because of the high incidence of hypopigmentation. The Q-switched ruby is still used for tattoo removal in light-skinned patients. Longer-wavelength lasers have displaced the ruby for pigment removal.

Melanosomes are very small, and hence have a very short thermal relaxation time, around 1 millisecond. In order to selectively target melanin, without harming the surrounding tissue, pulse durations equal to or shorter than the thermal relaxation time of melanin are used. Q-switched lasers are devices outfitted with a mechanism, a Q-switch, that stores the generated energy and releases it as very short, intense pulses. The pulse width on a Q-switched laser is in the nanosecond range. This extremely short pulse duration makes Q-switched lasers ideal for selective destruction of melanin. The most common Q-switched lasers used today are the Q-switched ruby (694 nm), Q-switched alexandrite (755 nm), Q-switched Nd:YAG (1064 nm), and the frequency-doubled Nd:YAG (532 nm). Choosing which Q-switched laser to use largely depends on the color and depth of the lesion to be treated. Longer wavelengths are better for deeper pigment and pigment in dark-skinned patients, whereas shorter wavelengths are used in fair-skinned patients with superficial lesions. Recently, longer-pulsed systems were shown to be effective for removal of lentigos, but the Q-switched lasers remain the gold standard. Q-switched lasers are also ideal for removal of nevi of Ito and Ota, lentigines, as well as café-au-lait macules (Fig. 24-3). When using any laser with a wavelength that is absorbed by melanin, it is important to remember that the laser does not distinguish between normal melanin in the skin and abnormal unwanted melanin. The most common and significant complication with these lasers is pigment alterations. Hypopigmentation can occur from the laser ablating normal melanin. PIPA can occur as a direct result of the inflammation caused by high-peak energies attained with Q-switching. Both of these complications are more common in darker skin types.

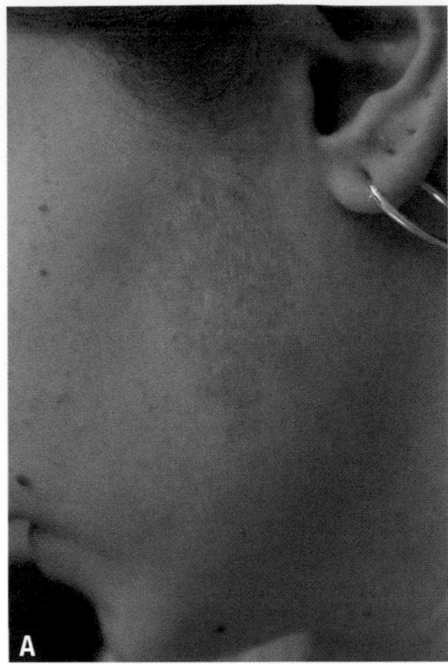

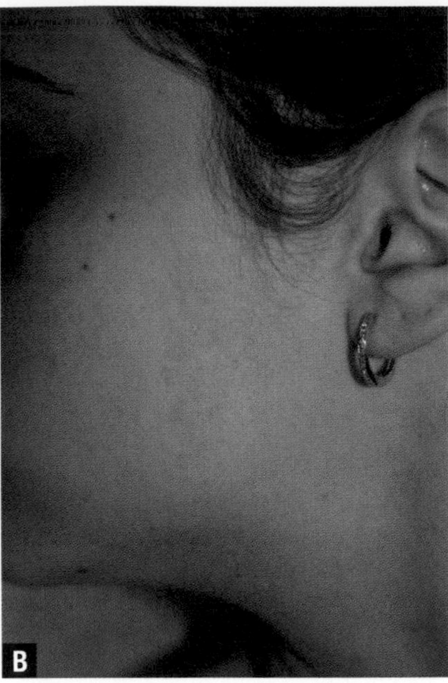

▲ **FIGURE 24-3** Café-au-lait macules before and after treatment with Q-switched laser.

LASERS FOR TATTOOS

The prevalence of tattoos has increased dramatically over the past several years. With continued improvement in colors, including fluorescent and glowing inks, this trend should be expected to continue. The more tattoos placed, the more that will need to be removed. In the past, laser tattoo removal involved the nonspecific ablation of the skin overlying the tattoo, resulting in removal, but also pigment alterations, and even scarring. Nonselective removal devices/procedures include the CO_2 laser, the argon laser, and dermabrasion. Currently, tattoo removal is performed primarily via selective photothermolysis, using the tattoo ink as the target chromophore for the laser. Each color of ink is absorbed by a different wavelength of light, and hence the more ink colors in the tattoo, the more difficult it is to remove. With the recent introduction of new inks and new colors, complete removal of modern tattoos is becoming more and more difficult. Cosmetic tattoos are usually a blend of several different inks, rendering them extremely challenging to remove with laser. Professional tattoos typically place ink in the mid-dermis, requiring a device that can penetrate to this depth in order to achieve adequate treatment. Amateur tattoos typically use less ink and placement is more superficial, making them easier to remove.

Just as in removal of melanosomes from the skin, removal of tattoo ink must be achieved with a very short pulse-width system, in the nanosecond range. These systems are the Q-switched laser devices, of which three are currently available on the market: the Q-switched ruby, the Q-switched alexandrite, and the Q-switched Nd:YAG. The ruby was the first Q-switched system available, and at a wavelength of 694 nm, it is good for removing blue and black pigments.[3] The alexandrite (755 nm) is also very effective at removing blue and black tattoo pigments.[4] In addition, it has the unique ability to remove green, which is historically one of the most difficult colors to eliminate. The alexandrite is the gold standard for removal of green tattoos, in fact, as the other two Q-switched lasers tend to perform inadequately in this area.[5]

The Nd:YAG (1064 nm) is the workhorse for professional tattoo removal because of its capacity for deep penetration. It is used for the basic black ink seen in both amateur and professional tattoos. The frequency-doubled Nd:YAG (532 nm) can be used for red pigments. Generally a combination of these lasers is needed for successful removal of a tattoo. Even then, residual ink or a shadow of the tattoo may persist despite numerous treatment sessions.

The most important aspect of tattoo removal is setting realistic expectations for the patient from the beginning. Laser tattoo removal is not an eraser, as many tattoos will not be completely removed no matter how many treatments are performed. In addition, there are reports of some tattoo inks actually darkening because of oxidation of the tattoo particles. This may result in an ink that is unremovable. Test spots are important especially in cosmetic tattoos. For the removal of professional tattoos, six to ten treatments, spaced at least 6 weeks apart, may be required. For amateur tattoos, three to five treatments are generally effective.[6] In patients with darker skin types, tattoo removal may result in scarring or dyspigmentation. Many authors advocate the use of topical bleaching agents prior to sunscreen to reduce the competing chromophores (skin melanosomes). With every patient, regular use of sunscreen in the treatment area is essential. Any patient with a tan in the area of treatment should not be treated.

Wound healing and postoperative care are also essential parts of laser tattoo removal. Moist wound healing via topical emollient creams and a dressing are recommended for all patients for 1 to 2 weeks after laser treatment. Straying from this regimen will increase the risk of postinflammatory changes and scarring, and delay additional treatments.

The future of tattoo removal may be represented by Q-switched devices that emit picosecond pulses, which would be even shorter than the currently used nanosecond devices. In addition, the introduction of dissolvable inks or more easily removed inks may improve the treatment of tattoos.

LASERS FOR EPILATION

Hair removal is one of the most popular cosmetic procedures performed today. It seems that every salon, spa, and medical office offers this service to their patients, all using different devices. Several methods of hair removal with light devices have been explored. The most common of these is via selective photothermolysis, with melanin as the chromophore. This melanin lies in the hair shaft itself and in the bulge region of the follicle. In order to permanently remove hair, one must eradicate not only the hair itself but the reproducing cells of the follicle. The energy, in the form of heat, must travel from the hair to the bulge area where the reproducing cells reside (1.5 mm below the epidermis). Although the Trt of melanin is very short, simply destroying the melanin would only result in fragmentation of the hair, with subsequent regrowth. Use of the Q-switched Nd:YAG (1064 nm) results in fragmentation of the hair, and temporary hair removal. Although an appropriate laser was readily available, it was not until Anderson and Dierickx lengthened the pulse width of the ruby that this device could be used for hair removal. Since that discovery, many other systems have come to the market, rendering the ruby essentially obsolete for hair removal.

The choice of which laser to use for epilation should be based on two overarching factors: (1) the hair color and texture and (2) the patient's skin color. Both of these factors must be considered for successful and semipermanent removal. Darker and coarser hair absorbs more light energy from the laser device, and hence can be removed at even longer wavelengths, which are traditionally less absorbed by melanin. The strongest absorption of light by melanin is at the shorter wavelengths (Fig. 24-4). Therefore, light or fine hairs are better treated at these wavelengths. However, melanin in the skin competes with the melanin in the hair for laser absorption. Hence the darker the skin color, the more difficultly the laser has in distinguishing the hair melanin from the skin melanin, and the more difficult the treatment. Cooling is critical in hair removal for protection of the epidermis. Without cooling of the epidermis, the melanin in

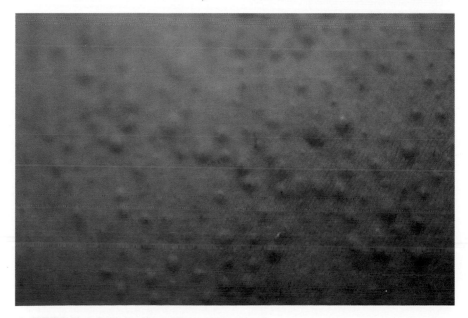

▲ **FIGURE 24-4** Follicular edema with laser hair removal.

the skin would first absorb the laser light and burn the skin, as opposed to removing the hair. Many of the wavelengths used for hair removal can also be used for epidermal pigment removal when used without cooling. Hair without or with very little pigment (white or light blonde) cannot be permanently removed by any device available at the time of this writing. Also, as discussed previously, the shorter wavelengths penetrate less deeply; therefore, some do not effectively reach the hair bulb. The ruby laser (694 nm) is no longer used for hair removal for this reason. The alexandrite laser (755 nm) is the shortest wavelength hair removal system used. Because of the high absorption of light by melanin at this wavelength, the alexandrite is able to remove lightly pigmented hairs from light skin.

One drawback of using a laser with a wavelength that is highly absorbed by melanin is that it needs to be used with extreme caution in darker skin types. Treatment of darker skin types with the alexandrite can result in hypopigmentation or postinflammatory hyperpigmentation.

The alexandrite laser is my laser of choice for patients with Fitzpatrick skin types I to III. It is also the best choice for light or very fine hairs. There are reports of it being used safely in types IV and V, but it should be used with caution. Reports of dyspigmentation in darker skin types are frequently seen with the alexandrite. In addition, use on recently tanned skin can also result in pigment abnormalities, though typically transient. There are also reports of paradoxical hypertrichosis after laser hair removal with the alexandrite.[7] This is even more common on darker skin types.

The diode is the workhorse of all the hair removal systems, as it can be used on all skin types. Optimal results are achieved with coarse, dark hair. There are two wavelengths of diode lasers for hair removal currently on the market, 800 nm and 810 nm. There is very little difference between the two wavelengths as far as clinical results are concerned. One would expect deeper penetration of the light with the longer 810 nm, but slightly less absorption by melanin would occur.

The Nd:YAG (1064 nm) systems operate at a wavelength that is minimally absorbed by melanin. Consequently, this laser is effective for removal primarily of dark, coarse hairs. The introduction of this laser made laser hair removal available to darker-skinned patients.

Comparisons of laser systems for hair removal have considered the clinical efficacy of the alexandrite, diode, and Nd:YAG. The alexandrite and the diode are comparable in efficacy and pain tolerability. The Nd:YAG was rated more painful and less efficacious in one study.[8] This laser, however, is the safest system in dark-skinned patients with dark hair, because of the longer wavelength and less absorption by melanin in the skin. Other studies have shown comparable efficacy among all three laser systems.[9] See Table 24-2 for a list of lasers used for hair removal.

TABLE 24-2
Hair Removal Light Devices

Wavelength	Light Device
694-nm ruby	Not currently used for hair removal
755-nm alexandrite	Candela GentleLASE, Cynosure Apogee
800–810-nm diode	Lumenis LightSheer, Opusmed F1 Diode, Syneron eLaser
1064-nm Nd:YAG	Candela GentleYag, Cutera Coolglide, Cynosure Apogee Elite

Prior to full treatment each patient should be evaluated by a physician trained in laser hair removal practices. Skin should not be tanned, damaged, or show any signs of infection. In many cases, in darker-skinned patients, pretreatment with bleaching agents is needed. For adequate removal, hair should have at least some pigment, as melanin is the chromophore for laser epilation. Patients must understand that white, fine, or very blonde hairs will not be removed by these devices. Prior to full treatment, test spots are generally performed. Full treatment can be carried out 2 weeks after the test spot, if there is a good response without adverse effects. Immediately after treatment, the area should exhibit follicular edema and erythema. This is the normal response to laser heating of the follicle (Fig. 24-5). Postprocedure application of a class 5 or 6 topical steroid for 5 days is often used in darker skin types to avoid postinflammatory changes. Depending on the hair, the treatment area, and the patient's skin type, complete removal can take anywhere from three to twelve sessions. These should be spaced 1 month apart, longer for the slower growing areas such as the legs and back. Sun protection is critical both before and after laser hair removal.

Laser hair removal is an effective method of epilation that can yield long-lasting effects. Choosing the right system for each patient depending on skin color, hair color, and hair caliber is essential. Patient compliance with a regimen including sun protection is also a critical part of any successful laser procedure.

RESURFACING LASERS

Ablative resurfacing has historically been performed using the CO_2 laser. Since its introduction in 1968, the CO_2 laser has been used for the treatment of acne scars, rhytides, actinic chelitis, and

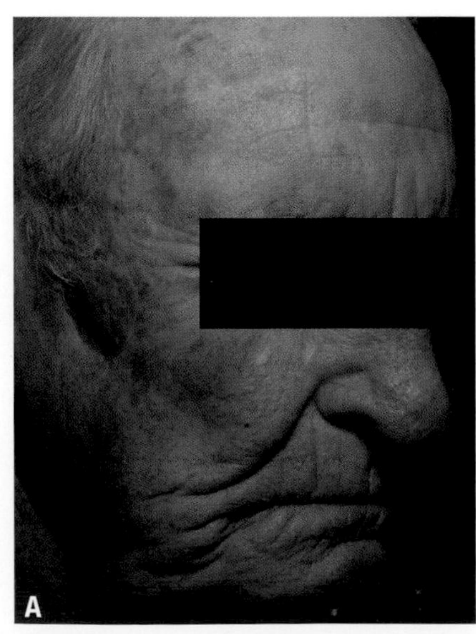

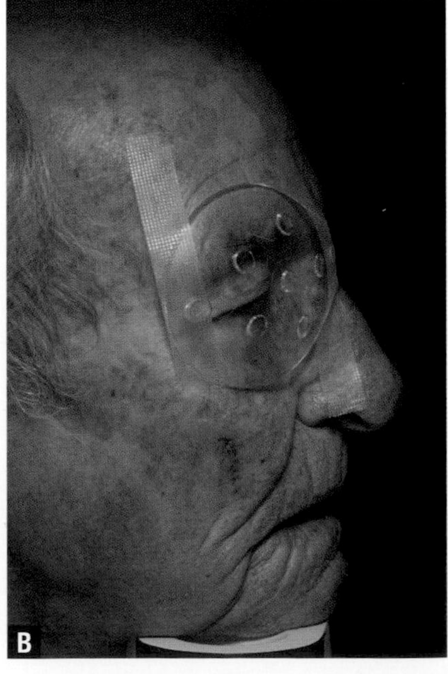

▲ **FIGURE 24-5 A.** Surgical scar before fractional resurfacing with Fraxel. **B.** Surgical scar after fractional resurfacing with Fraxel.

other symptoms of photoaging. At a wavelength of 10,600 nm, high water absorption results in rapid ablation of the epidermis. The erbium:YAG (Er:YAG) emits a wavelength of 2940 nm and is even more highly absorbed by water. This intense absorption by water results in a more superficial depth with the Er:YAG when compared to the CO_2 laser. With the rapid vaporization of tissue with any ablative laser comes tissue tightening and smoothing of the skin, which is not achieved with most other nonablative laser systems. Of the ablative devices, the tightening is most dramatic with the CO_2 lasers. However, the complication rates, and the downtime, have resulted in a decrease in the use of these systems for rejuvenation. Proper patient selection is critical, and even then, side effects can be high, including permanent scarring. In the hands of an experienced user, the CO_2 still remains an excellent instrument for facial rejuvenation in the right patient. These devices are currently being modified into fractional ablative devices that should achieve some of the tightening effects seen with ablation, yet with a lower risk of side effects.[10]

Fractional Resurfacing

The search for laser rejuvenation alternatives was prompted by the high complication rates associated with traditional ablative resurfacing. Nonablative lasers became popular for the treatment of rhytides and acne scarring as they were established as safe. These devices did stand up to their safety profile, but efficacy was questionable in many cases. In fact, before and after photographs demonstrated minimal changes and these devices are used primarily for acne treatment. Laser rejuvenation in a manner that could produce good clinical results with a high safety profile was the next step. The novel concept of fractional resurfacing was introduced in 2004 by Manstein et al.[11] The term "fractional" refers to treating a portion or fraction of the skin. Unfortunately, the definition does not specify laser type, spot size requirements, or wavelength; it just describes the manner of distribution of the treatment spots. These parameters will be determined in the future with more research in this area. By only treating microscopic areas in one session, healing time is greatly reduced. Each treated area is surrounded by normal viable skin from which migration of keratinocytes occurs, increasing the time to healing. Each treatment spot is termed a microscopic treatment zone (MTZ). The MTZs heal via migration of the normal surrounding epidermis, as opposed to healing via differentiation. Because of this unusual manner of spot placement, very high energies can be tolerated without bulk heating. Epidermal healing with a true microspot fractional device has been shown to be complete within 36 hours. This rapid healing time reduces the incidence of infections, pigment alterations, and scarring.

Spot size is a critical part of fractional resurfacing. Exactly how small the spot size needs to be is still being debated at this time. It is important to clarify that there are currently many different lasers that use the term fractional. Most of these are merely lasers with a scanner that distributes small spots, resulting in treatment of a portion of the face. It is unclear at this point how small the treatment spots must be to still obey the concept of "fractional resurfacing." Fractional devices have energy adjustments just as with any other laser system. In addition, they feature density adjustments, which is also a critical part of treatment efficacy. The higher the density, the closer together the MTZs will be, and the more aggressive the treatment. "Ablative" results can be obtained with very high energies at very high densities with any device.

Fractional devices come in two varieties: ablative and nonablative. The first fractional nonablative device, Fraxel (Reliant), was introduced in 2004. At the time of publication there were three fractional nonablative devices on the market. The Fraxel laser is a 1550 nm nonablative erbium-doped fiber laser. The fractional handpiece from Palomar is a 1540 nm wavelength fiber laser powered by the Palomar StarLux Intense Pulsed Light system. The Affirm (Cynosure) system offers a device with a wavelength of 1440 nm. The wavelength for these lasers lies within the water absorption spectrum, and hence water is the chromophore. These lasers are termed nonablative as they do not result in ablation, but rather coagulation of the epidermis. MTZs can be placed in a random or stamped pattern. Different devices use various methods of MTZ placement, and it is not clear at this time which one is best. The untreated skin surrounding each MTZ serves as a reservoir for epidermal cells, which migrate to rapidly heal the treated area. Higher energies translate to deeper penetration by the laser. Penetration well into the dermis results in better collagen production. MTZ diameters also increase as the energy is increased, so ideally each device should have density adjustments that would account for this change. To avoid bulk heating, at very high energies, the density of the treatment should be reduced, with wider spacing of the MTZs. These devices are currently approved for treatment of periorbital rhytides, acne and surgical scars, and melasma. They have also been reported to be effective for striae, photoaging, and lentigines. Fractional nonablative lasers are safe for use off the face as well. Studies in darker-skin types indicate that the fractional nonablative lasers (1440 nm, 1540 nm, and 1550 nm) are safe to use in all skin types at adjusted energy and density settings.

The fractional ablative devices were still in their infancy at the time of publication (Table 24-3). The gold standard for ablative resurfacing was once the CO_2 laser, but its use has plunged because of the high associated risks seen with full-face resurfacings. The reintroduction of the CO_2 with a fractional delivery system (Reliant) is sure to change the recent conventional thought about the CO_2 laser. A fractional CO_2 device (ActiveFX, Lumenis) is also currently available. This laser uses a scanning delivery of millimeter spots at an ablative 10,600-nm wavelength. The fractional CO_2 is equipped with a millimeter spot size with a new micron spot delivery just released. This random placement of lesions results in better cooling of surrounding tissues and less chance of bulk tissue heating. Healing times average several days. There is currently a fractional ablative Er:YAG (2940 nm) device on the market that is powered by an intense pulsed light system (IPL) (Pixel, Alma). This laser delivers energy to the skin in a small spot stamp pattern. Several treatments are recommended. With the high absorption of light by water at this wavelength, penetration is approximately 50 μm per pass. A fractional yttrium scandium gallium garnet (YSGG) (Cutera) at a wavelength of 2790 nm was also recently introduced. With a wave-length less

TABLE 24-3
Devices for Fractional Resurfacing

NONABLATIVE	ABLATIVE
1440 nm, Cynosure affirm	CO_2 10,600 nm, Reliant re:pair, Lumenis ActiveFX
1540 nm, Palomar fractional	YSGG 2790 nm, Cutera Pearl
1550 nm, Reliant restore Fraxel	Er:YAG 2940 nm, Alma Pixel

absorbed by water than a traditional Er:YAG, this device should theoretically allow for deeper penetration with concurrent ablation of the epidermis. Though this wavelength is relatively new to the aesthetic market, the results are promising.

NONLASER SYSTEMS

Intense Pulsed Light

IPL devices are light instruments that look and act like lasers, but do not qualify as true lasers because of their lack of coherent, monochromatic light. Newer IPL systems are able to pump true laser devices in a separate handpiece, allowing for the purchase of one system for many indications. This has made these systems very popular since their introduction in 1995. The first system introduced, the Photoderm (ESC/Sharplan, now Lumenis), was touted as the best modality for treating leg veins. It was only after early use of the system that its true capabilities of removing lentigines and telangiectasias were recognized.[11] There are many IPLs on the market today, with new ones introduced every year. IPLs have been used in several of the above conditions, including acne, facial telangiectasias, photodamage, lentigines, poikiloderma, nevus flammeus, venous malformations, spider veins, keratosis pilaris, and hair removal.

IPL devices emit noncoherent light with wavelengths between 500 and 1200 nm. These are flashlamp-based systems that contain an internal filter and several external "cut-off filters." These filters are used to block the emission of light lower than the desired wavelengths. Many cutoff filters are available for each system and generally come in a handpiece that can be changed on the unit body. By using these filters, one can employ the theory of selective photothermolysis with noncoherent, polychromatic light.

IPL devices also benefit from multiple adjustable pulse durations. Depending on the target and the patient's skin type, pulse widths can be manipulated accordingly. For treatment of targets with short thermal relaxation times, the pulse widths can be shortened. For larger vessels with longer Trts, pulse widths can be lengthened. This is important in the treatment of telangiectasias, as when the vessels seem to be resistant to treatment, simply changing the pulse width can result in an effective clinical response. Sequential pulsing, which allows time for cooling in between pulses, reduces the risk of bulk heating of tissues; therefore, the risk of scarring is also decreased. Sequential pulsing is also thought to aid in the treatment of telangiectasias by generating deoxygenated hemoglobin with the first pulse, and using this as the target for the second pulse.[12]

IPLs have also been favored over some of the lasers for treating telangiectasias and dyspigmentations because of the large spot sizes available with these devices. This renders treatment of larger areas more feasible. Another important component of IPL instruments is the cooling apparatus. With cooling of the epidermis, complications such as blistering and dyspigmentation are kept to a minimum. Most IPL devices are now outfitted with a cooling device, whether contact or cool air.

IPLs are one of the primary treatments for facial telangiectasias, lentigines, poikiloderma, and photorejuvenation. Several IPLs also have interchangeable filter handpieces for hair removal, nonablative skin tightening, and even fractional resurfacing. Preparation of a patient for IPL involves determining skin type and sun protection. Treating a patient who is recently tanned may result in hypopigmentation caused by the absorption of melanin by the laser. Patients should be instructed to use proper photoprotection both before and after treatments. Special care should be taken when using these devices to treat patients with darker skin types (IV and V).[13,14] Pulse widths and delays between pulses should be lengthened when treating this population. A thin layer of cool ultrasound gel is placed on the skin surface and the laser is placed directly against the gel. (Some of the newer systems do not require gel.) Care should be taken to place pulses close together, and far spacing can result in striping in patients with severe photodamage (Fig. 24-6). Striping can also occur in any patient when higher fluences are used and pulses are not placed closely together. This complication is easily remedied by further treatment of the untreated areas. After the treatment, the areas are cleansed of all gel, and sun protection is applied. A full-face treatment generally takes approximately 15 minutes. No topical anesthesia is required for most types of IPL treatment. With high fluences used for port wine stains, some patients may require topical anesthesia. Three to five treatments at 1-month intervals are recommended for clearing of photodamage.[15] More are generally needed for port wine stains and other vascular malformations. Downtime is minimal, if there is any at all, with mild darkening of treated lentigines, and erythema of treated areas. Patients can generally return to work immediately following the procedure, which makes IPLs very popular with patients. The ability to treat vascular and pigmented lesions with one instrument, as well as the rapid treatment times, and consistent, reproducible results achieved when these device are used properly have catapulted the IPL systems to the forefront of the industry (Fig. 24-7).

Light Emitting Diodes

Light emitting diodes (LEDs) have garnered recent attention because of their ease of use and popularity as activation sources for aminolevulinic acid (i.e., photodynamic therapy). These devices emit noncoherent light of either one primary wavelength or of a short range of wavelengths. Unlike the previously mentioned instruments, LEDs do not operate by the theory of selective photothermolysis. LEDs operate on the

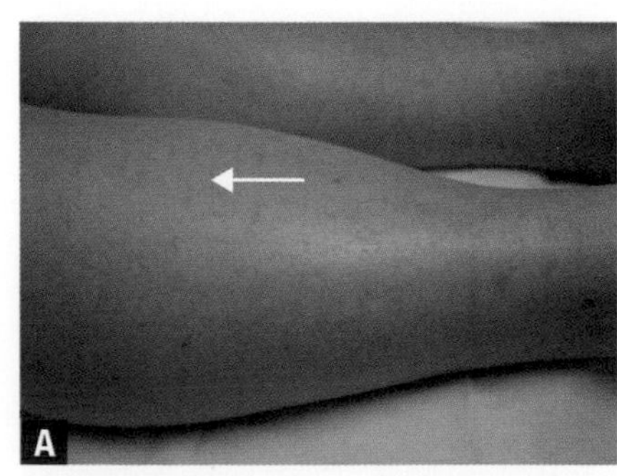

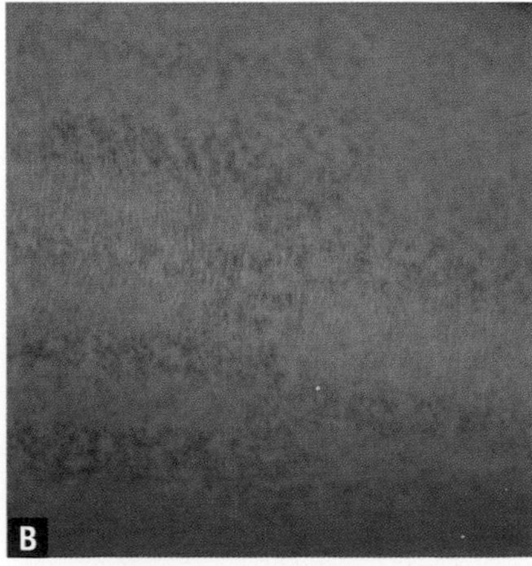

▲ **FIGURE 24-6 A.** The IPL device can result in rectangular-shaped "striped" areas. These are treated by turning the handpiece 90 degrees for the next treatment. **B.** Closer view of striping from the IPL. This occurs most commonly on the legs and chest.

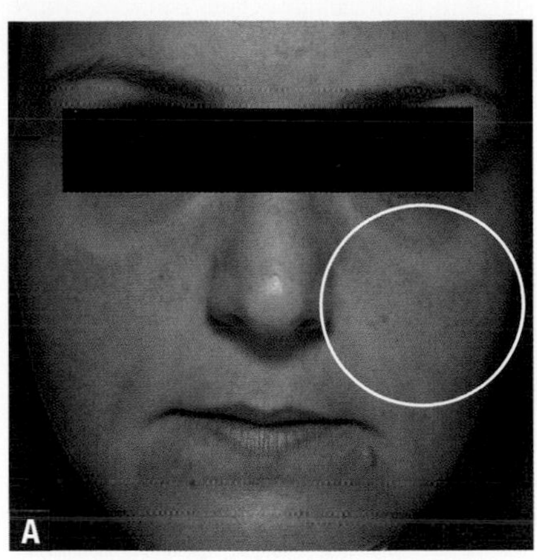

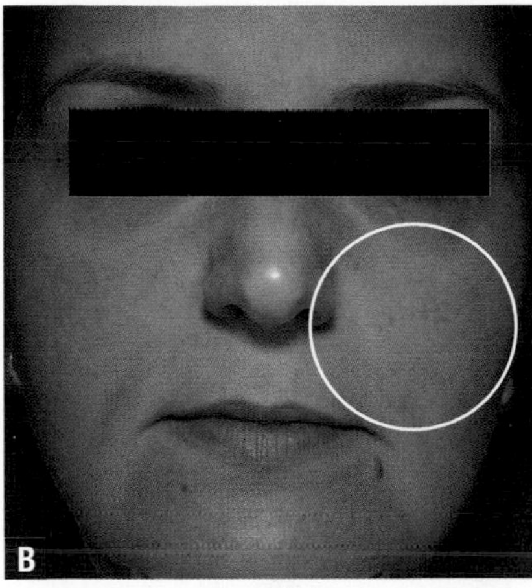

▲ **FIGURE 24-7 A.** Rosacea before IPL treatment. **B.** Rosacea after one IPL treatment. 2–3 more will be needed for maximum results.

theory of photobiomodulation, or photomodulation, which is the ability of light to alter cellular activity. This capacity to change the cellular metabolism via light energy has been demonstrated in the laboratory.[16] It is an essentially nonthermal manner of treating the skin, and has been shown to be effective for several conditions when used as low level laser therapy (LLLT).[17,18] LLLT uses small spot sizes, rendering full-face treatments difficult. The advent of LED systems introduced a method by which large areas could be easily and painlessly treated. These systems consist of panels of lights of a particular wavelength or range of wavelengths. Currently available LEDs include blue, yellow, red, near infrared, and infrared. LEDs are most commonly used for acne and photorejuvenation. Case reports for use in wound healing, psoriasis, and rhytides also appear in the literature. The advantage of LEDs over other lasers is the ease of treatment, including a painless, rapid, and safe manner of treating all skin types. The disadvantage is that the clinical results may not be as dramatic as some of the other laser and light procedures.

In 2003, a visible red light device was approved by the FDA for skin rejuvenation (Omnilux Revive). A novel yellow LED has also been approved for photorejuvenation in the US. These instruments not only differ in the wavelength of light emitted, but also in the mode of delivery. Some systems pulse the light in sequences and some have nonpulsed, constant delivery systems. Which manner is the most effective has not yet been determined.

LEDs have been shown in vivo to alter cell activity, including that of fibroblasts and immune cells. Takezaki et al. reported an increase in vimentin filaments and mitochondria in the fibroblasts from skin irradiated with a 633 nm LED.[19] In vivo studies have demonstrated an increase in collagen production postradiation with 633-nm LED.[20]

Several LEDs are currently available on the market in a range of wavelengths and pulse sequencing. To date no one has demonstrated that one particular pulsing sequence is superior to another. Such studies, along with comparisons of the different wavelengths, are warranted to hone the use of these devices and perhaps expand the range of indications. The need for additional studies notwithstanding, the use of LEDs to activate aminolevulinic acid has become an important component in photodynamic therapy.

PHOTODYNAMIC THERAPY

The notion of photodynamic therapy (PDT) has been around since the early 1900s, but it was not until Kennedy introduced PDT that its true advantages could be discovered in dermatology.[21] PDT represents the use of a photosensitizer activated by light to selectively treat the skin. The currently approved use for PDT in the United States is for nonhyperkeratotic actinic keratoses of the face using 5-aminolevulinic acid (ALA) (Levulan® Kerastick, DUSA Pharmaceuticals) activated by blue light. However, several off-label indications have received attention in the literature and are now commonly used in cosmetic practice. These conditions include photoaging[22] and sebaceous hyperplasia.[23]

5-ALA is a prodrug that is applied to target areas and selectively absorbed by proliferating cells and pilosebaceous units. Then, 5-ALA is metabolized into protoporphyrin IX (PpIX), which is innately photosensitizing. PpIX is activated by several different wavelengths of light, resulting in the production of free radicals and selective destruction of target cells. The currently approved drugs for PDT include 5-ALA and the methyl ester of ALA (mALA) (Metvix, Galderma). Commonly used activation sources include LEDs (red and blue), pulsed dye laser (585 nm, 595 nm), and IPL devices.

PDT has recently been used to enhance the effectiveness of commonly used photorejuvenation procedures. Split-face studies have shown that the addition of ALA to traditional IPL treatments results in better clinical amelioration of the signs of photoaging than IPL alone.[22,24] One group even demonstrated a greater increase in collagen production on the PDT/IPL side when compared with IPL alone.[25] The addition of ALA to an IPL photorejuvenation procedure is useful in patients looking for treatment of precancerous lesions in addition to the aesthetic aspects of photodamage.

TIGHTENING DEVICES

The newest wave in light devices is directed at the problem of achieving skin tightening. Although nonablative fractional resurfacing has been quite successful at rejuvenation, it has proven insufficient in actual tightening. Evaluation of the action of "tightening" is difficult in itself, as there is no standardized, quantitative measure. Photographic assessments are generally inadequate, as even a slight change in position will alter the result. In addition, it is almost impossible to measure the slight tightening that occurs, especially if it occurs over many months. Nevertheless, many of the practitioners who use these devices do believe in their efficacy in a percentage of patients.

The practice of tightening the skin is based on the notion that collagen will contract when heat is applied. Several light-based devices have been introduced with the goal of delivering heat to the dermis while leaving the epidermis unharmed. This heat presumably causes collagen contraction and hence lifting. The epidermis

TABLE 24-4
Skin Tightening Devices

Device	Technology
Titan (Cutera)	Infrared light
Aluma (Lumenis)	Radiofrequency: Bipolar
Accent (Alma)	Radiofrequency: Bipolar, unipolar
ReFirme (Syneron)	Radiofrequency
Lux Deep IR (Palomar)	Infrared light (850–1350 nm)
ThermaCool (Thermage)	Radiofrequency: Monopolar

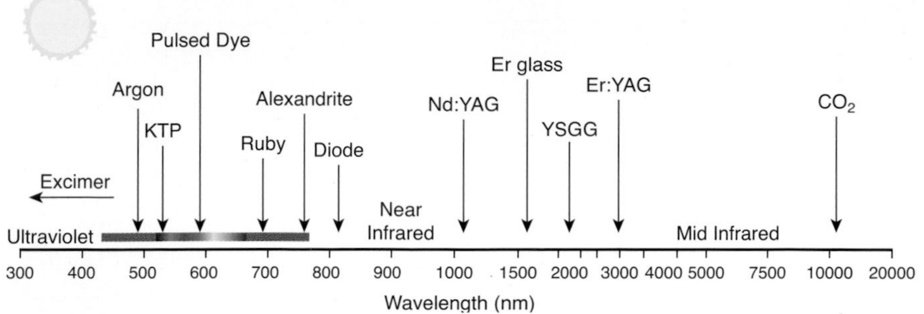

▲ **FIGURE 24-8** Wavelength diagram of available devices. KTP: potassiumtitanylphosphate; Nd:YAG: neodymium-doped yttrium aluminium garnet; YSGG: Yttrium Scandium Gallium Garnet; CO_2: Carbon dioxide.

remains protected as a result of dynamic cooling during the application of the infrared light. One of the most popular skin-tightening instruments is the Titan (Cutera). The Titan emits a long pulse of infrared light with wavelengths ranging from 1200 to 1500 nm. The procedure is completely painless with resultant mild erythema that resolves in a few minutes to hours. Collagen contraction is immediate, but in addition to this contraction collagen synthesis is also induced. Many patients see results with these devices, yet some do not respond to the treatment. Patient selection, energies used, and overall skin quality may play a role in determining if a treatment will be successful.

Other "tightening" products include monopolar, bipolar, and combination unipolar and bipolar radiofrequency devices (Table 24-4). The theory is the same, in that nonselective heat is applied to the dermis via direct contact with the skin. The epidermis must be protected with a cooling system. The radiofrequency devices tend to be somewhat more painful than the infrared devices. Some radiofrequency instruments require application of topical anesthesia prior to the procedure. Side effects are limited and include erythema (lasting up to 1 week), depressions, and superficial burns. No cases of permanent scarring have been reported.

The literature contains very few studies measuring the effectiveness of these tightening devices. Most reports are anecdotal and demonstrate high safety, but not efficacy. Clearances for these devices are for the face and neck, but many are using them in areas such as the arms, buttocks, and abdomen. Both the infrared and radiofrequency systems can be used in all skin types, as long as the cooling systems are functional.

SUMMARY

Since their introduction in 1960, lasers have continued to expand in popularity and availability. Laser science was changed forever with the introduction of the theory of selective photothermolysis by Anderson and Parrish. Based on this theory, our understanding of how lasers can be used to treat numerous conditions has flourished. Paired with our continued understanding of wound healing, new developments in the laser industry have significantly increased the safety of these procedures while managing to improve efficacy. With each year comes the introduction of newer technologies with the goal of developing even safer and more effective devices for various dermatologic conditions (Fig. 24-8). Of course, it is recommended that with any new device or new user, start slow. Overaggressiveness with any laser or light device can cause severe complications, sometimes permanent. Additional research in this area is ongoing and warranted, as are increased regulations in laser training and operation. This will ensure the safe and effective treatment of all laser patients.

REFERENCES

1. Anderson RR, Parrish JA. Selective photothermolysis: precise microsurgery by selective absorption of pulsed radiation. *Science*. 1983;220:524.
2. Uebelhoer NS, Bogle MA, Stewart B, et al. A split-face comparison study of pulsed 532-nm KTP laser and 595-nm pulsed dye laser in the treatment of facial telangiectasias and diffuse telangiectatic facial erythema. *Dermatol Surg*. 2007;33:441.
3. Taylor CR, Gange RW, Dover JS, et al. Treatment of tattoos by Q-switched ruby laser. A dose-response study. *Arch Dermatol*. 1990;126:893.
4. Alster TS. Q-switched alexandrite laser treatment (755 nm) of professional and amateur tattoos. *J Am Acad Dermatol*. 1995;33:69.
5. Fitzpatrick RE, Goldman MP. Tattoo removal using the alexandrite laser. *Arch Dermatol*. 1994;130:1508.
6. Bernstein EF. Laser treatment of tattoos. *Clin Dermatol*. 2006;24:43.
7. Alajlan A, Shapiro J, Rivers JK, et al. Paradoxical hypertrichosis after laser epilation. *J Am Acad Dermatol*. 2005;53:85.
8. Rao J, Goldman MP. Prospective, comparative evaluation of three laser systems used individually and in combination for axillary hair removal. *Dermatol Surg*. 2005;31:1671.
9. Amin SP, Goldberg, DJ. Clinical comparison of four hair removal lasers and light sources. *J Cosmet Laser Ther*. 2006;8:65.
10. Hantash BM, Bedi VP, Chan KF, et al. Ex vivo histological characterization of a novel ablative fractional resurfacing device. *Lasers Surg Med*. 2007;39:87.
11. Manstein D, Herron GS, Sink RK, et al. Fractional photothermolysis: a new concept for cutaneous remodeling using microscopic patterns of thermal injury. *Lasers Surg Med*. 2004;34:426.
12. Goldman MP, Weiss RA, Weiss MA. Intense pulsed light as a nonablative approach to photoaging. *Dermatol Surg*. 2005;31:1179.
13. Negishi K, Tezuka Y, Kushikata N, et al. Photorejuvenation for Asian skin by intense pulsed light. *Dermatol Surg*. 2001;27:627.
14. Kawada A, Shiraishi H, Asai M, et al. Clinical improvement of solar lentigines and ephelides with an intense pulsed light source. *Dermatol Surg*. 2002;28:504.
15. Bitter PH. Noninvasive rejuvenation of photodamaged skin using serial, full-face intense pulsed light treatments. *Dermatol Surg*. 2000;26:835.
16. Whelan HT, Buchmann EV, Dhokalia A, et al. Effect of NASA light-emitting diode irradiation on molecular changes for wound healing in diabetic mice. *J Clin Laser Med Surg*. 2003;21:67.
17. Baxter GD. *Therapeutic Lasers: Theory and Practice*. Oxford, UK: Churchill Livingstone; 1994.
18. Enwemeka CS, Parker JC, Dowdy DS, et al. The efficacy of low-power lasers in tissue repair and pain control: a meta-analysis study. *Photomed Laser Surg*. 2004;22:323.
19. Takezaki S, Omi T, Sato S, et al. Light-emitting diode phototherapy at 630 +/− 3 nm increases local levels of skin-homing T-cells in human subjects. *J Nippon Med Sch*. 2006;73:75.
20. Rigau J, Trelles MA, Calderhead RG, et al. Changes in fibroblast proliferation and metabolism following in vitro helium-neon laser irradiation. *Laser Therapy*. 1991;3:25.
21. Kennedy JC, Pottier RH, Pross DC. Photodynamic therapy with endogenous protoporphyrin IX: basic principles and present clinical experience. *J Photochem Photobiol B*. 1990;6:143.
22. Dover JS, Bhatia AC, Stewart B, et al. Topical 5-aminolevulinic acid combined with intense pulsed light in the treatment of photoaging. *Arch Dermatol*. 2005;141:1247.
23. Alster TS, Tanzi EL. Photodynamic therapy with topical aminolevulinic acid and pulsed dye laser irradiation for sebaceous hyperplasia. *J Drugs Dermatol*. 2003;2:501.
24. Alster TS, Tanzi EL, Welsh E. Photorejuvenation of facial skin with topical 20% 5-aminolevulinic acid and intense pulsed light treatment: a split-face comparison study. *J Drugs Dermatol*. 2005;4:35.
25. Marmur ES, Phelps R, Goldberg DJ. Ultrastructural changes seen after ALA-IPL photorejuvenation: a pilot study. *J Cosmet Laser Surg*. 2005;7:21.

CHAPTER 25

Sclerotherapy

Larissa Zaulyanov-Scanlan, MD

In addition to the face, neck, chest, and hands, the aesthetic appearance of the legs is a significant area of concern to patients. In 2005, according to statistics gathered by the American Society for Aesthetic Plastic Surgery, sclerotherapy ranked as the sixth most common nonsurgical cosmetic procedure.[1] In order to maximize the successful treatment of leg veins with sclerotherapy, a thorough understanding of venous pathology, specifically venous hypertension and chronic venous insufficiency, is crucial for practitioners.

The aim of this chapter is to familiarize the reader with the underlying pathology, the diagnosis, and the treatment of venous hypertension, and to help the reader differentiate between the medical and the cosmetic sclerotherapy patient. In keeping with the theme of this textbook, the treatment section of this chapter will focus on sclerotherapy as it pertains to the cosmetic patient, specifically regarding the treatment of leg telangiectasias, venulectasias, and reticular veins. Treatment options for patients with clinically relevant venous disease will be briefly mentioned.

THE VENOUS SYSTEM AND VARICOSE VEINS

The venous system is a low-pressure system and a blood reservoir. Unlike arteries, which carry oxygenated blood and have a thick elastic muscular lining designed to withstand high pressures, veins carry deoxygenated blood, are thin-walled, and easily distend with increased pressure. The map of venous circulation is more variable than that of arterial circulation, and anastomoses between veins commonly occur. This multiplicity allows for surgical repair of the venous system as there are several routes for deoxygenated blood to return to the heart. Veins rely on the heart as well as skeletal muscle contraction for circulation. Contraction of skeletal muscle compresses the veins within them and helps to propel blood back to the heart. This is particularly important in the lower extremities where the force of gravity must be overcome to maintain proper circulation. The contractile action of the skeletal muscles, primarily the calf muscles, helps to transport blood upward.

The Venous System of the Leg

The venous system of the leg consists of both a superficial and a deep component. The superficial component is located above the fascia, and the deep component is located below the fascia. The principal superficial veins are the lesser saphenous vein, which runs from the ankle to the knee, and the greater saphenous vein, which runs from the ankle to the groin. The superficial veins of the leg connect and empty into the deep veins via perforating veins, which pierce through the fascia separating the compartments of the leg. The skin surface of the leg may consist of superficial pink telangiectasias found in the papillary dermis that empty into blue-appearing reticular veins found in the reticular dermis, which empty into the superficial venous system located above the fascia. These superficial veins drain into the deep venous system that is located below the fascia and within the muscle. Besides being identified according to their location, veins can also be categorized by size. Telangiectasias are flat red vessels that are up to 1 mm in diameter, venulectasias are bluish vessels that may distend above the skin surface and are usually 1 to 2 mm in diameter, and reticular veins are those that have a cyanotic hue and are 2 to 4 mm in diameter. Nonsaphenous varicose veins are 3 to 8 mm in diameter, and saphenous varicose trunks are usually greater than 5 mm in diameter. These larger vessels typically lie deep below the skin surface and are better visualized with duplex ultrasound.

Varicose Veins

Veins have one-way valves that occur every few inches along their course and are positioned to oppose back flow so deoxygenated blood can continue to flow in the direction of the heart. A varicose vein is a vein that has lost its elasticity. While any vein in the body may be affected, the superficial veins of the legs are by far the most frequently involved. These weakened veins dilate under the pressure of supporting a column of blood against the force of gravity. Varicose veins have a caliber greater than normal, and their valve cusps no longer meet. They are incompetent and result in reflux. Varicose veins impede proper circulation by permitting blood to flow away from the heart, decreasing the efficiency of the entire venous system, and leading to venous hypertension. The severity of venous hypertension is directly related to the skin changes seen in chronic venous insufficiency. The progression to chronic venous insufficiency follows the leaking of fluids out of the veins into the perivascular tissue, engendering symptoms of leg swelling, aching, and eventually dermatologic manifestations such as increased vascular markings, skin discoloration (hyper- or hypopigmentation and hemosiderin deposition), dermatitis, fibrosis, and ulceration.

The etiology of varicose vein formation is multifactorial. There is a familial tendency to develop varicose veins, usually in patients who present with this disease early in life. Its relation to gender appears to be a more significant factor, as it is seen in approximately 26% of women versus 5% of men. In addition, advancing age appears to be involved, as those older than age 35 almost triple their risk compared to those aged 24 to 35 years.[2] Physical states that increase the pressure on the venous system by physically compromising venous return, such as pregnancy, obesity, decreased mobility, and frequent constipation, are also associated with an increased risk of varicose vein formation.[2–4] Other factors, such as the presence of estrogen, have been shown to have an impact on the vascular system. While estrogen appears to protect against the formation of venous ulcers of the lower limbs,[5] it has been implicated in raising telangiectatic matting (the appearance of tiny vessels less than 0.2 mm in diameter), which occurs in women after undergoing sclerotherapy for the treatment of leg veins.[6]

Current research on the etiology and pathology of varicose veins and chronic venous insufficiency suggests that the underlying pathologic mechanism is an inflammatory response that is hypothesized to be initiated by an increase in shear stress on the venous endothelium. Several studies suggest that an increase in venous pressure induces leukocyte accumulation and subsequent free radical production that leads to degradation of valve leaflets by metalloproteinases,[7–9] which are enzymes that degrade collagen, elastin, and other components of the extracellular matrix. Based on this free radical-driven model of venous damage, flavonoids (plant-derived free radical scavengers) have been shown to ameliorate the symptoms and progression of chronic venous insufficiency.[10–13]

EXAMINATION OF THE SCLEROTHERAPY PATIENT AND DIAGNOSIS OF CHRONIC VENOUS INSUFFICIENCY

The current test of choice to investigate blood flow in the superficial and deep venous system is the duplex ultrasound. This test is indicated for symptomatic patients and for patients who have clinical evidence of chronic venous insufficiency (see below). Duplex ultrasound is more reliable than Doppler ultrasound because it provides actual visualization of veins. It is recommended that duplex ultrasound be performed on the upper and lower leg (superficial and deep veins, and venous perforators) in order to accurately locate points of reflux that should be targeted for treatment.[14]

Most patients with chronic venous insufficiency have specific symptoms and clinical signs that reveal their disease state. A detailed clinical examination is adequate to diagnose most patients suffering from primary varicose veins,[15] and Doppler vascular studies have been shown to be useful in patients presenting with recurrent varicose veins or obese patients with signs and symptoms of chronic venous insufficiency with no clinically clear varicosity.[16] Not all patients with venous reflux have symptoms of chronic venous insufficiency, but patients with symptoms of chronic venous insufficiency are more likely to have venous reflux. Moreover, the degree of symptoms correlates with the degree of venous disease.[17,18] Pain and a sensation of heaviness are the most common symptoms of chronic venous insufficiency,[16,19] while edema is the most frequent and the first objective sign.[19–21] Vessel diameter greater than approximately 4 mm is directly related to the likelihood of venous incompetence,[22] and patients with corona phlebectatica (fan-shaped intradermal telangiectasias in the medial and sometimes lateral portions of the ankle and foot; Fig. 25-1) have a 4.4 times greater risk of incompetent leg or calf perforators by duplex ultrasound than patients without this clinical finding.[23]

Based on these current research findings, the recommended approach to the sclerotherapy patient is as follows: if the patient is symptomatic (reports symptoms of leg pain, heaviness, swelling, aching, cramping, itching, or any other symptoms attributable to venous dysfunction), vascular testing is indicated. Likewise, if the patient is asymptomatic, but upon physical examination has two or more of the following symptoms, vascular testing is indicated: signs of edema, vessel diameter greater than 4 mm, corona of the lower extremities, hyper- or hypopigmentation, dermatitis, fibrosis, and/or current or healed ulcer. In addition, if there is a history of previous sclerotherapy with poor results, such as recurrence of vessels or appearance of new vessels in the previous treatment area after sclerotherapy, then vascular testing is indicated. Otherwise, patients who present with leg telangiectasias with or without reticular veins and without the previously listed features may be presumed to be cosmetic treatment candidates. In this case, the treating physician may decide that these patients do not need to undergo initial vascular studies.

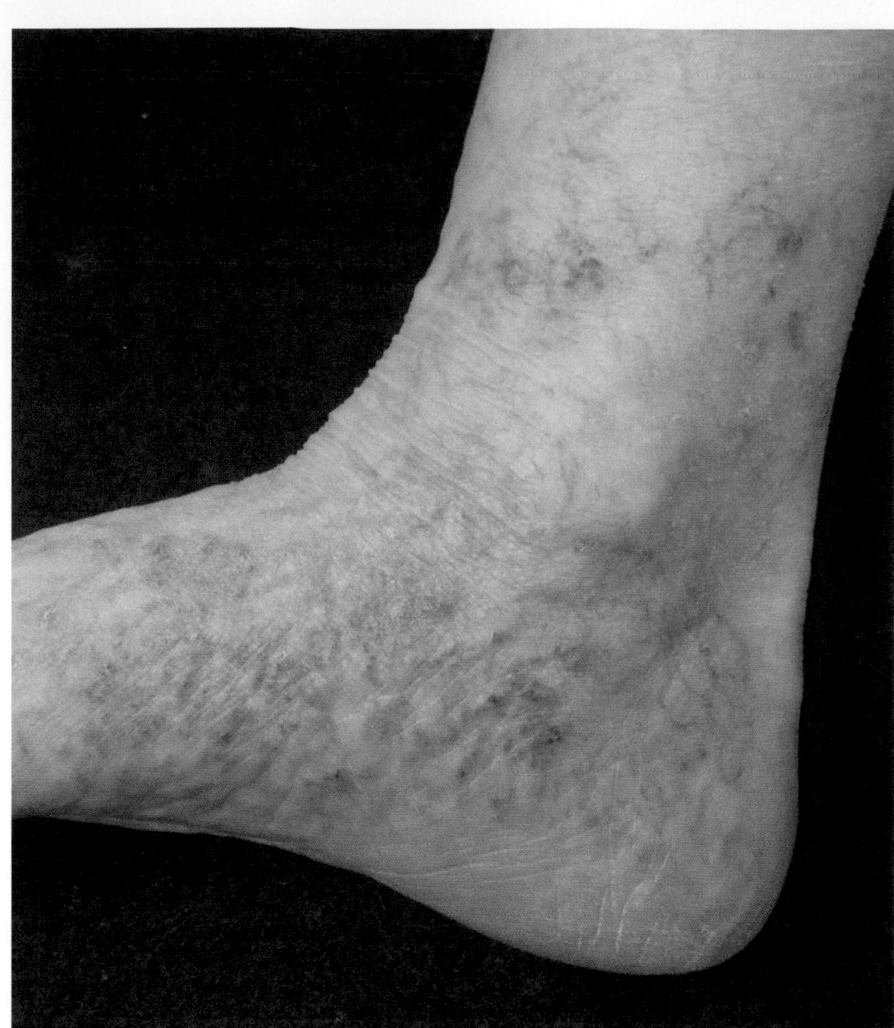

▲ **FIGURE 25-1** Corona phlebectatica around the medial malleolus. Presence of these fan-shaped vessels around the ankle is a clinical sign of underlying venous reflux. Patients with this finding should be examined by duplex ultrasound.

SCLEROSING AGENTS

There are several studies in the literature reporting that sclerotherapy has been successfully used to treat both functional and cosmetic vein disorders. When it performs as expected, the sclerosant significantly damages the endothelial lining of the vessel wall being treated and results in inflammation, fibrosis, and in the eventual obliteration of the vessel.

There are three classes of sclerosants based on their mechanism of action: hyperosmotic agents, detergents, and chemical irritants. Hyperosmotic agents, such as hypertonic saline, produce endothelial damage through dehydration. Detergents, such as sodium tetradecyl sulfate, sodium morrhuate, ethanolamine oleate, and polidocanol, cause vascular injury by altering the surface tension around endothelial cells, diminishing their ability to adhere to one another. Chemical irritants, such as chromated glycerin, injure cells by acting as a corrosive secondary to the metal component.

Current practice includes the use of sclerosants in solution or those that are manually foamed. Foamed sclerosants (either sodium tetradecyl sulfate or polidocanol mixed with air) are mainly used to treat functional vein disorders, such as chronic venous insufficiency and venous ulceration under duplex-guided ultrasound.[24,25] This approach has been very successful for the medical sclerotherapy patient. However, a known risk of foam sclerotherapy includes transient vision disturbances.[26]

In the United States, the only agents approved by the FDA for sclerotherapy are sodium tetradecyl sulfate (Sotradecol®), sodium morrhuate (Scleromate®), and ethanolamine oleate; the latter two have an extensive side effect profile and are used primarily for esophageal varices. The most common sclerosing agent used in dermatology is hypertonic saline, although it is approved as an abortifacient rather than a sclerotherapy agent. Chromated glycerin (72% glycerin with 8% chromium potassium alum, Scleremo®) is an agent recognized for superior treatment of leg telangiectasias. In the treatment of telangiectatic leg veins, chromated glycerin has been shown to clear vessels significantly better than polidocanol in solution or polidocanol foam.[27] Chromated glycerin is not FDA approved for sclerotherapy and is not available in the United States; however, sterile glycerin is available on hospital formulary for use in cerebral edema and acute glaucoma. A solution of 72% glycerin has been shown to clear leg telangiectasias significantly better and with fewer complications (such as formation of microthrombi, telangiectatic matting, or hyperpigmentation) than sodium tetradecyl sulfate in solution.[28] Used in this nonchromated form, 72% of sterile glycerin solution is mixed in a ratio of 2:1 with 1% lidocaine and epinephrine (ratio 1:100,000) for injection into leg telangiectasias.[28] Glycerin alone is a hyperosmotic agent and it is likely that its mechanism of action in sclerotherapy is dehydration of the vessel wall, similar to hypertonic saline. Other sclerosing solutions that are not FDA approved include polidocanol and polyiodinated iodine.

It is important to know the risk profiles of commonly used sclerosants (Table 25-1). Hypertonic saline is associated with burning and cramping upon injection and an increased risk of ulcerative necrosis secondary to extravasation. Sodium tetradecyl sulfate has also been associated with hyperpigmentation, pain upon extravasation, and skin necrosis. Rarely, sodium tetradecyl sulfate and, even more rarely, polidocanol have been associated with allergic hypersensitivity reactions. While it has been suggested that allergic reactions to detergent sclerosants are often caused by solubilized latex products from the rubber plunger in the syringe into the sclerosant solution, this has not been substantiated and remains a subject of controversy. Overall, the estimated incidence of allergic reactions is 0.3% and may occur with the use of any sclerosing agent,[29] as allergic reactions to components found in gloves, syringes, and other supplies that come in contact with a patient through treatment can arise. As such, it may be prudent to take at least 20 minutes for in-office observation postprocedure after every sclerotherapy session, especially in patients with a history of asthma or a history of allergies. Likewise, it is imperative to have basic life support skills as well as subcutaneous epinephrine, intravenous corticosteroids, intravenous antihistamines, oxygen, and other resuscitative equipment readily available to treat this potentially life-threatening complication if it arises.

The optimal concentration of sclerosant may vary with the diameter of the vessel being treated, with a greater concentration of sclerosant being required for vessels of larger diameter.[30] If the sclerosant is too weak, insufficient damage to the endothelium results and a thrombus may form that eventually recanalizes. If the sclerosant is too strong, then ulceration and hyperpigmentation can occur because of extravasation of the sclerosant.

Management of side effects can be a challenge. While pain and cramping are acute and quickly resolve, hyperpigmentation, telangiectatic matting, and ulceration are more chronic.

TABLE 25-1
Characteristics of Common Sclerosing Solutions

Solution	FDA Approval	Advantages	Risks/Disadvantages	Recommended Dose Limitations Per Treatment Session
Hypertonic saline (23.4%)[a]	Yes, as abortifacient	Nonallergenic	Off-label Pain and cramping Skin necrosis Hyperpigmentation Microthrombi formation	10 mL
Sodium tetradecyl sulfate (Sotradecol) (0.25%)[a]	Yes	Can be foamed to treat varicose veins under ultrasound guidance	Pain upon extravasation Skin necrosis Hyperpigmentation Microthrombi formation Rare anaphylaxis	10 mL of 3%
Polidocanol (0.25%)[a]	No	Painless Can be foamed to treat varicose veins under ultrasound guidance	Hyperpigmentation Microthrombi formation Allergic reactions Rare anaphylaxis	10 mL of 3%
Glycerin (72% glycerin mixed with 1% lidocaine and 1:100,000 epinephrine, combined 2:1)[b]	No	Rare hyperpigmentation	Pain and cramping Rare allergy Too weak for large veins	10 mL

[a]Average reported concentration used to treat veins from 1 to 4 mm in diameter.
[b]Best used for the treatment of fine telangiectasias (vessels up to 1 mm in diameter).

Hyperpigmentation after sclerotherapy is delayed and can take several months to a year to resolve. It has been associated with high total body iron stores.[31] This type of hyperpigmentation is caused by hemosiderin deposition and is not melanocytic; therefore, it does not respond to topical bleaching agents as much as to tincture of time. Telangiectatic matting is usually permanent and more common in hyperestrogenemic states.[6,32] It may also be a sign of underlying venous reflux and should be investigated by duplex ultrasound. Both hyperpigmentation and telangiectatic matting may benefit from treatment with intense pulsed light as this modality has shown some success in treating vascular lesions, including telangiectasias,[33,34] as well as treatment of dyspigmentation.[34,35] It is important to emphasize that necrosis with subsequent ulceration can potentially occur with extravasation of any of the sclerosants into the skin or by inadvertent intra-arterial or periarterial injection of sclerosants. The sclerosant with the least risk of inducing necrosis seems to be glycerin, effective only for the treatment of leg telangiectasias. When extravasation of sclerosant occurs in the skin it is generally secondary to the treatment of small vessels, such as telangiectasias or reticular veins. This complication presents as a small and painful slow-to-heal blister, erosion, or ulceration. Healing typically resolves with a skin-colored scar. In contrast, reports of intra-arterial injection occur when treating larger, deeper vessels. This risk is increased when targeting veins around the ankle or when treating deeper veins, both cases where veins and their accompanying arteries are in close proximity to one another. When arteries are accidentally injected, the entire area supplied by the artery quickly becomes ischemic and pale, and is usually painful. In this situation, affected areas are large, involving a segment of the leg or foot. Fortunately, intra-arterial injection is a very rare event, but the risk is not completely avoidable and can still occur even under ultrasound guidance.[36] Management in this case is emergent, and may result in possible amputation. To minimize the incidence of most complications, use of proper injection technique is critical. Using the minimal concentration of sclerosant for the vessel size, small volumes, and slow injection to maintain low pressure in the vessel will assure the best results. Cosmetic treatment of veins around the ankle with sclerotherapy should be avoided and, in this specific group of patients, the possibility of reflux should be explored.

SCLEROTHERAPY FOR THE COSMETIC PATIENT

When treating leg veins, it is important to treat proximal sites and larger vessels first, as treatment of these vessels may obliterate those vessels that are smaller and distally located. As previously mentioned, cosmetic treatment is undertaken only if the patient does not have any clinical signs or symptoms of chronic venous insufficiency or has had all sources of reflux already treated. Preoperative photographs and fully informed consent outlining all possible risks and complications should be obtained prior to therapy. A discussion of postprocedure care is also essential.

A body map with segmental divisions of the legs is helpful in documenting each session (Fig. 25-2). Treatment is repeated at 6-week intervals to allow for complete resolution of previously treated sites. The number of treatment sessions may vary, usually from one to six, based on the aggressiveness of the physician as well as the clinical presentation and expectations of the patient.

There are four injection techniques commonly used in the treatment of cosmetic leg veins: the puncture-fill technique, the aspiration technique, the empty vein technique, and the air-bolus technique. The puncture-fill technique relies on the feeling associated with perforating a vessel wall. It is probably the most common, but also the most difficult to grasp for beginners and better mastered over time while using the other listed approaches. The aspiration technique is most useful for the treatment of reticular veins, with the observation of the aspirated dark blood into the hub of the syringe or the tubing of a butterfly needle confirming correct needle placement. The empty vein technique involves leg elevation and kneading the vessel to remove as much blood as possible prior to injecting the sclerosant. The air-bolus technique uses the injection of a small amount of air (0.2 cc or less) prior to the introduction of sclerosant. The air in the tip of the syringe displaces the blood in the vessel confirming correct needle placement.

Alcohol is used to clean the skin as well as increase the refractile index of the skin, rendering vessels more visible upon the skin surface. A common approach by the author is to use a combination of the aspiration and empty vein techniques for reticular veins, and puncture-fill for venulectasias and telangiectasias. It is also helpful when using the puncture-fill technique to target the most superficial portion of the vessel. For telangiectasias less than 1 mm in size, where cannulating the vessel is a challenge, it is necessary to start injecting with the tip of the needle just barely underneath the skin surface, bevel side facing up (Fig. 25-3). When treating reticular veins, the use of a butterfly needle helps to secure venous access; however, prior to injecting these vessels it is essential to pull back on the plunger to visualize dark blue blood in the tubing and ensure location inside the lumen of the vein (Fig. 25-4). Injection can then proceed slowly. In all cases, when resistance is encountered,

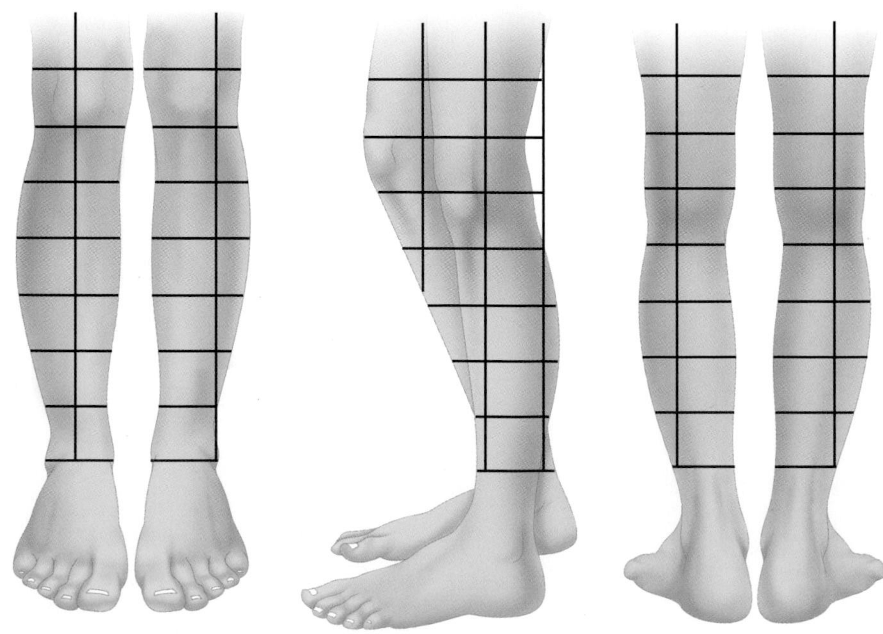

▲ **FIGURE 25-2** Sample flow sheet or map for recording sclerotherapy sessions.

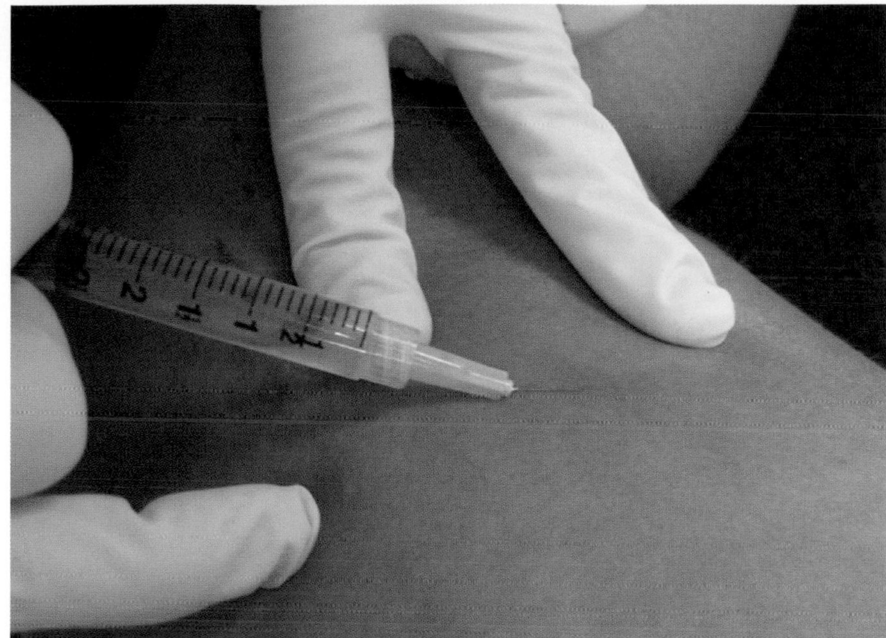

▲ **FIGURE 25-3** Injection of leg telangiectasias. Hand traction is employed to keep the skin taut. The needle is bent at a 30-degree angle and inserted just below the skin surface, bevel side up. Injections are performed slowly to maintain low pressure on the vessel wall to minimize extravasation of sclerosant.

BOX 25-1 Materials Used for Sclerotherapy for Cosmetic Patients

1. Cotton balls or swabs soaked with 70% isopropyl alcohol
2. Protective gloves
3. Protective eyewear
4. 3-cc disposable syringes
5. 32-gauge needles
6. Light source
7. 25- or 27-gauge butterfly needle
8. Dental rolls (or dry cotton balls)
9. Paper tape
10. Coban® or elastic bandage

injection should be stopped or extravasation can occur.

Prior to injecting, the needle may be bent at an angle of 20 degrees to 45 degrees. Upward hand traction is employed by the sclerotherapist using the nondominant hand or by an assistant to keep the skin taut. Sclerosant is injected slowly to allow adequate time for contact with the endothelium as well as to prevent vascular distention and rupture. A small amount of sclerosant is used at each puncture site (approximately 0.1 to 0.3 cc for telangiectasias and 0.5 to 1 cc for reticular veins) in order to minimize side effects such as ulceration caused by extravasation. Reticular veins are treated at intervals of approximately 3 cm along the length of the vessel, proximal to distal. Larger vessels, such as reticular veins, are injected before smaller vessels, such as venulectasias and telangiectasias, and areas of arborization are treated before isolated linear areas.

Immediately upon withdrawal of the needle, the treatment areas should be compressed manually. Then each area is taped with either dry cotton balls or dental rolls, and wrapped with Coban or an elastic wrap (Box 25-1). The patient is instructed to keep this in place for a minimum of 4 hours, after which time graduated compression stockings are substituted for an average of 1 to 3 weeks. The garment should have a pressure of at least 15 mm Hg. Compression therapy is known to tighten the paracellular barrier by elevating expression of specific tight junctions, inhibiting permeability of fluid into the perivascular tissue, and thereby preventing progression of chronic venous insufficiency.[37] It also decreases symptoms of chronic venous insufficiency,[38] such as pain and discomfort,[39] as well as edema.[40] While graduated compression garments are not favorably accepted by most patients, especially cosmetic patients in warm climates, it should be emphasized that the use of these garments is associated with greater clinical resolution and decreased risk of hyperpigmentation.[40]

Lasers for Cosmetic Leg Veins

Laser leg vein treatment has been explored with a variety of wavelengths, and the long-pulsed 1064-nm Nd:YAG laser has shown the most promising results.[41,42] However, when compared with sclerotherapy in the treatment of lower extremity telangiectasias, sclerotherapy continues to offer superior clinical results.[41] Notably, laser therapy should only be an option for patients who have avoided sun exposure to the intended treatment areas for several weeks prior to the procedure and who have Fitzpatrick skin type I to III. Primary indications for laser or intense pulsed light treatment of leg veins include ankle telangiectasias, needle phobia, and telangiectatic matting or vessels too small to cannulate. As with sclerotherapy, optimal results are achieved with lasers when larger feeding vessels are treated first.

Treatment of Varicose Veins

Varicose veins, an eventual complication of venous hypertension and chronic venous insufficiency, may be managed in several ways. Daily graduated

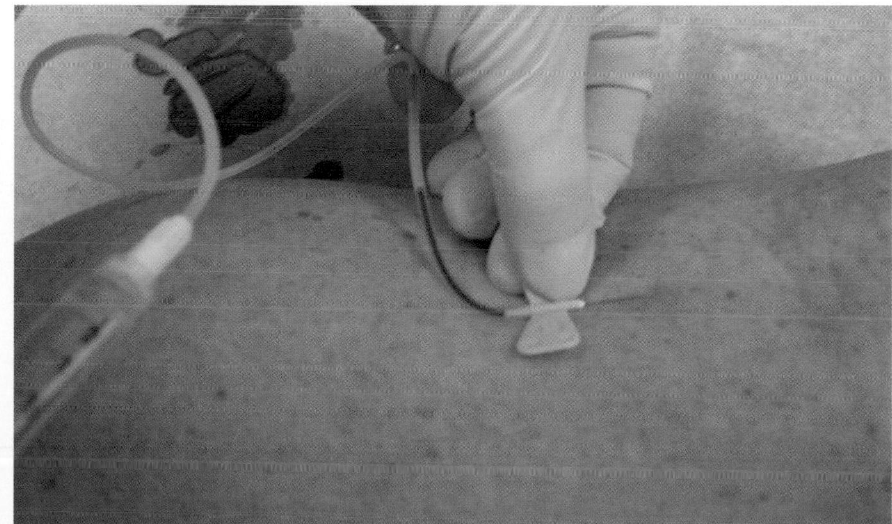

▲ **FIGURE 25-4** Injection of reticular veins. A 25-gauge butterfly needle is attached to a 3-cc syringe. Intraluminal vein placement is confirmed by pulling back on the plunger of the syringe prior to injection. Sclerosant is then slowly injected.

compression is of paramount importance in slowing its progression and controlling the associated symptoms. Oral agents, like flavonoids (found in such foods as citrus fruits, berries, green tea, red wine, and dark chocolate with cocoa content of at least 70%), have also proven to be beneficial. Similarly, daily intake of vitamin C, while not directly investigated, may also be helpful. Maintaining an active lifestyle and avoiding obesity are additional recommended measures.

Treatment options are best explored after duplex ultrasound examination once all points of reflux have been determined. Besides sclerotherapy, mainly using the foamed method,[24,25,43,44] other types of procedures that can be used to treat leg varicosities include ambulatory phlebectomy, vein stripping and/or ligation, or endovascular closure.

SUMMARY

Sclerotherapy remains the gold standard for treatment of cosmetic leg veins. Optimal results occur when individual patient characteristics are evaluated, thus separating the cosmetic sclerotherapy patient from the medical sclerotherapy patient. Sclerotherapy is a technique that is mastered with practice. By understanding venous pathology and etiology, and by being able to choose the right sclerosant and right technique for the vein in question, a successful outcome will surely be achieved.

REFERENCES

1. The American Society for Aesthetic Plastic Surgery. http//www.plasticsurgery.org. Accessed January 25, 2008.
2. Ahumada M, Vioque J. Prevalence and risk factors of varicose veins in adults. *Med Clin (Barc)*. 2004;123:647.
3. Fowkes FG, Lee AJ, Evans CJ, et al. Lifestyle risk factors for lower limb venous reflux in the general population: Edinburgh Vein Study. *Int J Epidemiol*. 2001;30:846.
4. Jawien A. The influence of environmental factors in chronic venous insufficiency. *Angiology*. 2003;54(suppl 1):S19.
5. Bérard A, Kahn SR, Abenhaim L. Is hormone replacement therapy protective for venous ulcer of the lower limbs? *Pharmacoepidemiol Drug Saf*. 2001;10:245.
6. Davis LT, Duffy DM. Determination of incidence and risk factors for postsclerotherapy telangiectatic matting of the lower extremity: a retrospective analysis. *J Dermatol Surg Oncol*. 1990;16:327.
7. Pascarella L, Penn A, Schmid-Schonbein GW. Venous hypertension and the inflammatory cascade: major manifestations and trigger mechanisms. *Angiology*. 2005;56(suppl 1):S3.
8. Kosugi I, Urayama H, Kasashima F, et al. Matrix metalloproteinase-9 and urokinase-type plasminogen activator in varicose veins. *Ann Vasc Surg*. 2003;17:234.
9. Fileta B, Chang A, Barnes S, et al. Varicose veins possess greater quantities of MMP-1 than normal veins and demonstrate regional variation in MMP-1 and MMP-13. *J Surg Res*. 2002;106:233.
10. Bergan JJ. Chronic venous insufficiency and the therapeutic effects of Daflon 500 mg. *Angiology*. 2005;56(suppl 1):S21.
11. Cesarone MR, Belcaro G, Rohdewald P, et al. Comparison of Pycnogenol and Daflon in treating chronic venous insufficiency: a prospective, controlled study. *Clin Appl Thromb Hemost*. 2006;12:205.
12. Smith PC. Daflon 500 mg and venous leg ulcer: new results from a meta-analysis. *Angiology*. 2005;56(suppl 1):S33.
13. Cesarone MR, Belcaro G, Pellegrini L, et al. Venoruton vs Daflon: evaluation of effects on quality of life in chronic venous insufficiency. *Angiology*. 2006;57:131.
14. Wong JK, Duncan JL, Nichols DM. Whole-leg duplex mapping for varicose veins: observations on patterns of reflux in recurrent and primary legs, with clinical correlation. *Eur J Vasc Endovasc Surg*. 2003;25:267.
15. Ad Hoc Committee, American Venous Forum. Classification and grading of chronic venous disease in the lower limbs. A consensus statement. *J Cardiovasc Surg (Torino)*. 1997;38:437.
16. Safar H, Shawa N, Al-Ali J, et al. Is there a need for Doppler vascular examination for the diagnosis of varicose vein? A prospective study. *Med Princ Pract*. 2004;13:43.
17. Jantet G. Chronic venous insufficiency: worldwide results of the RELIEF study. Reflux assessment and quality of life improvement with micronized Flavonoids. *Angiology*. 2002;53:245.
18. Ruckley CV, Evans CJ, Allan PL, et al. Chronic venous insufficiency: clinical and duplex correlations. The Edinburgh Vein Study of venous disorders in the general population. *J Vasc Surg*. 2002;36:520.
19. Callejas JM, Manasanch J; for ETIC Group. Epidemiology of chronic venous insufficiency of the lower limbs in the primary care setting. *Int Angiol*. 2004;23:154.
20. Boccalon H, Janbon C, Saumet JL, et al. Characteristics of chronic venous insufficiency in 895 patients followed in general practice. *Int Angiol*. 1997;16:226.
21. Langer RD, Ho E, Denenberg JO, et al. Relationships between symptoms and venous disease: the San Diego population study. *Arch Intern Med*. 2005;165:1420.
22. Kurt A, Unlu UL, Ipek A, et al. Short saphenous vein incompetence and chronic lower extremity venous disease. *J Ultrasound Med*. 2007;26:163.
23. Uhl JF, Cornu-Thenard A, Carpentier PH, et al. Clinical and hemodynamic significance of corona phlebectatica in chronic venous disorders. *J Vasc Surg*. 2005;42:1163.
24. Pascarella L, Bergan JJ, Menkenas LV. Severe chronic venous insufficiency treated by foamed sclerosant. *Ann Vasc Surg*. 2006;20:83.
25. Barrett JM, Allen B, Ockelford A, et al. Microfoam ultrasound-guided sclerotherapy of varicose veins in 100 legs. *Dermatol Surg*. 2004;30:6.
26. Coleridge SP. Saphenous ablation: sclerosant or sclerofoam? *Semin Vasc Surg*. 2005;18:19.
27. Kern P, Ramelet AA, Wutschert R, et al. Single-blind, randomized study comparing chromated glycerin, polidocanol solution, and polidocanol foam for treatment of telangiectatic leg veins. *Dermatol Surg*. 2004;30:367.
28. Leach BC, Goldman MP. Comparative trial between sodium tetradecyl sulfate and glycerin in the treatment of telangiectatic leg veins. *Dermatol Surg*. 2003; 29:612.
29. Ramelet AA, Monti M. *Phlebology: The Guide*. Paris, France: Elsevier; 1999.
30. Sadick NS. Sclerotherapy of varicose and telangiectatic leg veins. Minimal sclerosant concentration of hypertonic saline and its relationship to vessel diameter. *J Dermatol Surg Oncol*. 1991;17:65.
31. Thibault PK, Wlodarczyk J. Correlation of serum ferritin levels and postsclerotherapy pigmentation. A prospective study. *J Dermatol Surg Oncol*. 1994;20:684.
32. Sadick NS. Predisposing factors of varicose and telangiectatic leg veins. *J Dermatol Surg Oncol*. 1992;18:883.
33. Fodor L, Ramon Y, Fodor A, et al. A side-by-side prospective study of intense pulsed light and Nd:YAG laser treatment for vascular lesions. *Ann Plast Surg*. 2006;56:164.
34. Ross EV, Smirnov M, Pankratov M, et al. Intense pulsed light and laser treatment of facial telangiectasias and dyspigmentation: some theoretical and practical comparisons. *Dermatol Surg*. 2005;31:1188.
35. Gupta AK, Gover MD, Nouri K, et al. The treatment of melasma: a review of clinical trials. *J Am Acad Dermatol*. 2006; 55:1048.
36. Trinh-Khac JP, Roux A, Djandji A, et al. Nicolau livedoid dermatitis after sclerotherapy of varicose veins. *Ann Dermatol Venereol*. 2004;131:481.
37. Herouy Y, Kahle B, Idzko M, et al. Tight junctions and compression therapy in chronic venous insufficiency. *Int J Mol Med*. 2006;18:215.
38. Vayssairat M, Ziani E, Houot B. Placebo controlled efficacy of class 1 elastic stockings in chronic venous insufficiency of the lower limbs. *J Mal Vasc*. 2000;25:256.
39. Weiss RA, Weiss MA. Resolution of pain associated with varicose and telangiectatic leg veins after compression sclerotherapy. *J Dermatol Surg Oncol*. 1990;16:333.
40. Goldman MP, Beaudoing D, Marley W, et al. Compression in the treatment of leg telangiectasia: a preliminary report. *J Dermatol Surg Oncol*. 1990;16:322.
41. Lupton JR, Alster TS, Romero P. Clinical comparison of sclerotherapy versus long-pulsed Nd:YAG laser treatment for lower extremity telangiectasias. *Dermatol Surg*. 2002;28:694.
42. Eremia S, Li C, Umar SH. A side-by-side comparative study of 1064 nm Nd:YAG, 810 nm diode and 755 nm alexandrite lasers for treatment of 0.3–3 mm leg veins. *Dermatol Surg*. 2002;28:224.
43. Kakkos SK, Bountouroglou DG, Azzam M, et al. Effectiveness and safety of ultrasound-guided foam sclerotherapy for recurrent varicose veins: immediate results. *J Endovasc Ther*. 2006;13:357.
44. Darke SG, Baker SJ. Ultrasound-guided foam sclerotherapy for the treatment of varicose veins. *Br J Surg*. 2006;93:969.

CHAPTER 26

Facial Scar Revision

Suzan Obagi, MD
Angela S. Casey, MD

Facial scarring is a common complaint among patients seen by cosmetic dermatologic surgeons. Several etiologies, including inflammatory acne, trauma, previous surgical procedures, and viral infections such as varicella or herpes simplex, can lead to permanent scarring. Treatment of scarring remains an evolving subject among dermatologic surgeons. In order to better understand the optimal treatments for facial scarring, we first explore the different morphologies of facial scars. This is followed by a review of treatments grouped according to each distinct type of scar. We conclude with a discussion of combination treatments and how to apply these modalities to the patient with acne scarring to achieve the maximum results.

MORPHOLOGY OF ATROPHIC SCARS

There are two broad classifications of facial scarring: atrophic and hypertrophic. This review focuses on atrophic facial scarring. We expand upon the classification previously proposed by Jacob et al.[1] by dividing atrophic facial scarring into four main types: ice pick, boxcar, shallow/atrophic, and valley/rolling scars (Fig. 26-1). Ice pick scars are typically small (1–2 mm) and have a wide aperture with steep edges that taper to a single point at the base, as if the skin has been pierced by an ice pick. An epithelial tract forms along the sides of the opening within the scar. These scars may be shallow or deep, and may extend as far as the dermal–subcutaneous junction. Boxcar scars are round to oval in shape with well-defined vertical edges and a flat base, as if the scar has been punched out of the skin. They typically range from 0.1 to 0.5 mm in depth and are usually widely spaced out on the skin surface, occurring as solitary scars. Unlike ice pick scars, this type of scar does not converge to a single point. Shallow/atrophic scars present as a cluster of miniaturized boxcar scars. They usually emerge in groups of four or more and occur mainly on the cheeks. Valley scars ("rolling" scars) are deeper and have an undulating appearance that is best appreciated in indirect lighting (Fig. 26-2). Valley-shaped scars arise from a variable loss of dermis and/or subcutaneous tissue. Because acne and varicella scars are dermal defects, they require a treatment modality that reaches the dermis in order to achieve clinical improvement.

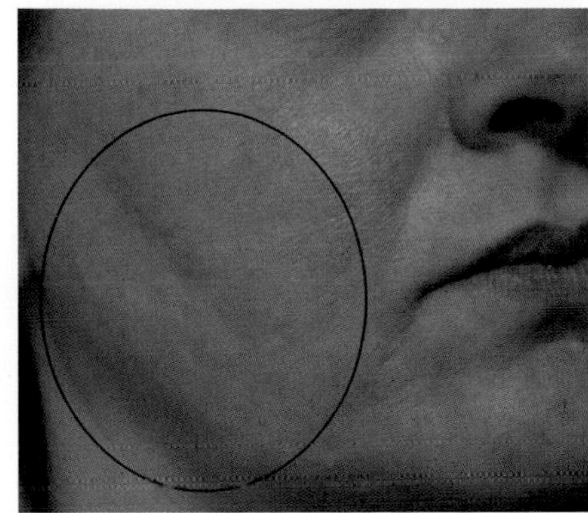
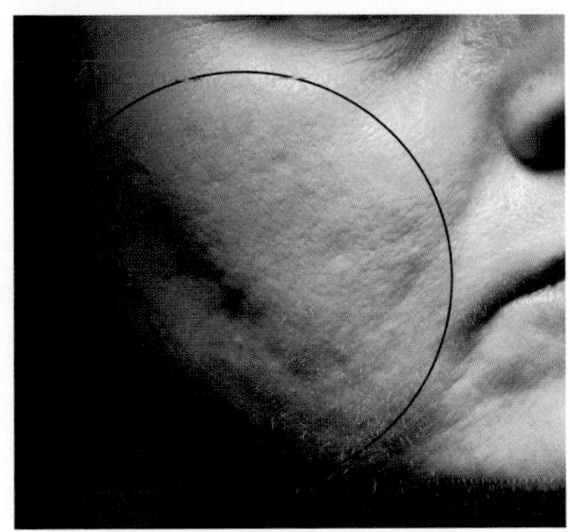

▲ **FIGURE 26-2** Valley scars viewed in direct light (left) and indirect light (right).

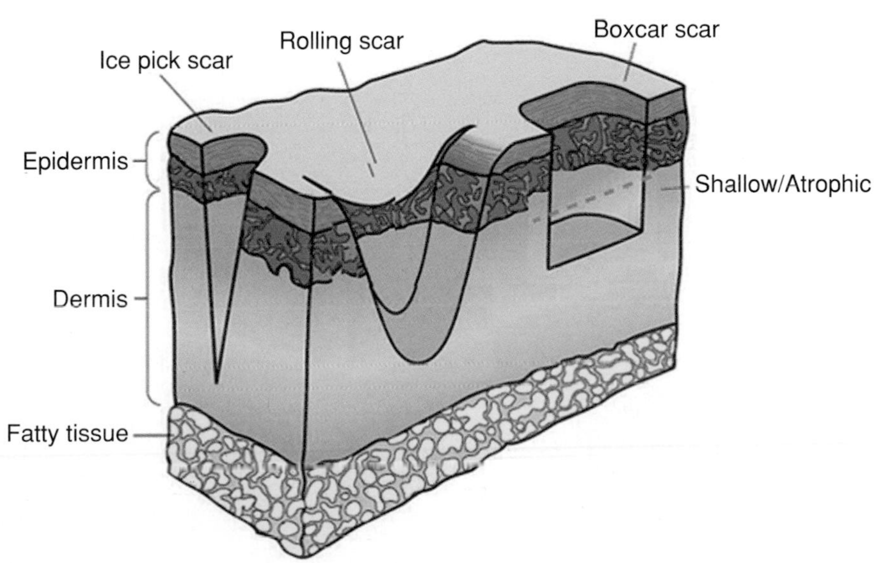

▲ **FIGURE 26-1** Schematic illustrating the different types of acne scars.

Pretreatment Considerations

Open communication and good rapport with the patient cannot be emphasized enough. Patients paying for cosmetic procedures tend to have high expectations of the results; therefore, realistic outcomes of the various treatment modalities must be discussed in detail with the patient prior to the procedure. Potential side effects and adverse outcomes must also be revealed to the patient prior to the procedures. Additionally, it is important to discuss expected "downtime" and possible discomfort during the recovery period. Furthermore, pre- and postoperative skin conditioning regimens as well as necessary time and monetary investment should be covered in detail during the patient consultation. Finally, assessment of the patient's pain threshold and discussion of topical, local, or oral analgesia should be initiated.

Pre- and postoperative photographs are mandatory as these photographs serve as an important source of documentation. Patients should remove their makeup prior to having the photographs taken, and all photography should be performed in a standardized manner with constant lighting, settings, and views.

A complete and thorough discussion of these issues, while important, is beyond the scope of this chapter; therefore, we direct readers to several references by the senior author.[2–6]

ALGORITHM FOR ATROPHIC SCARS

Ice Pick Scars

Because of the deep and steeply sloped morphology of ice pick scars, fillers do not typically produce significant cosmetic improvement.[7] Likewise, resurfacing is not optimal since the depth of the scar usually far exceeds that which can be safely reached with resurfacing procedures. Therefore, the treatment choices include punch excisions, punch grafts, and spot trichloroacetic acid (TCA) peels (Fig. 26-3).

PUNCH EXCISION Punch excision and punch grafting are best suited for ice pick scars that are less than 2 mm in diameter (including the walls of the scar); scars larger than 2 mm should be excised in an elliptical fashion and closed in a layered manner. Punch excision describes a technique of eliminating the scar through the use of a trephine. After infiltration of local anesthesia, the smallest possible trephine that will completely remove the scar is used to punch-excise down to subcutaneous fat. Excisions of 1 mm in size are left to heal by secondary intention. Excisions that are 1 to 2 mm in size are closed with 5-0 nylon (Ethilon, Ethicon, Inc., Somerville, NJ), with gentle eversion of the wound edges. Aquaphor Healing Ointment (Beiersdorf, Inc., Wilton, CT) and a bandage are then placed over the site. Sutures are removed at 1 to 2 weeks (depending on skin thickness) following the procedure to prevent track-mark deformities.

PUNCH GRAFTING Punch grafts have been used for many years as an option for treating pitted scars of the face,[8,9] as well as scars from previous surgical procedures.[10] After local anesthesia, the scar is removed using a 1-, 1.5-, or 2-mm trephine. The donor grafts are typically obtained from the postauricular skin. Donor grafts are taken 0.5 mm larger than the excision, which allows for optimal alignment after healing and scar contraction take place. The graft is placed so that it is level with the surrounding skin, and it may be held in place with Steri-Strips (3M, St. Paul, MN). The donor site is bandaged as described earlier. Approximately 6 weeks following graft placement, the area can be leveled with dermabrasion, if necessary.

SPOT TRICHLOROACETIC ACID Another effective treatment for ice pick scar revision is spot treatment with TCA. TCA causes precipitation of proteins and coagulative necrosis of cells in the epidermis and collagen necrosis in the papillary and upper reticular dermis. Dermal collagen production and remodeling occurs over several months and results in dermal thickening. Lee et al. described the technique of using a sharpened wooden applicator to firmly and directly apply 65% to 100% TCA into the ice pick scar. They found that the application of a higher TCA concentration was more effective in treating atrophic acne scars.[11] Based on our experience with this method, extreme caution must be used since the application of such a strong concentration of TCA can actually cause deepening and widening of scars. We prefer using 30% to 50% TCA. These treatments can be repeated at 6-week intervals until satisfactory results are achieved.

Boxcar Scars

Boxcar scars are round or oval in shape with well-defined vertical edges. Varicella and herpes simplex scars are good examples. The difference in elevation requires that the base of the scar be raised to the level of the surrounding skin or that the surrounding skin be planed down to the level of the scar base. Options for treating this type of scarring include punch elevation or resurfacing with dermabrasion, laser, or modified phenol peels (Fig. 26-4). These scars do not respond well to superficial or medium-depth peels because of the depth of the scar when compared to the surrounding skin. Additionally, the underlying fibrosis of the dermis in these scars prevents the scar from stretching and smoothing out with peels.

PUNCH ELEVATION Punch elevation describes the technique of elevating tissue within a depressed scar so that it is level with the normal skin surface surrounding it. When choosing a site to be punch elevated, it is essential that the scar have a smooth, normal base and sharp vertical edges. Using a trephine that is equal in size to the inner diameter of the scar, the inner aspect of the scar is excised down to subcutaneous fat. The tissue is then elevated to sit slightly above the surface level of the skin to overcome the retraction that occurs during the healing phase. The tissue may be held in place with Steri-Strips (3M, St. Paul, MN) or 5-0 or 6-0 polypropylene (Prolene, Ethicon, Inc.). The area is bandaged as discussed previously, and the patient is seen in follow-up 1 week later for suture removal/evaluation.

DEEP PEELS/PHENOL PEELS Phenol peels are deep peels that quickly penetrate the skin to the level of the reticular dermis[12]; the efficacy of the phenol is due to the resulting protein denaturation and coagulation as well as induction of new collagen synthesis.[13] Phenol requires hepatic metabolism followed by renal excretion. Systemic absorption of phenol can directly cause arrhythmias, so patients must be on a cardiac monitor throughout the procedure.

One of the significant risks of phenol peels is permanent hypopigmentation [14]; therefore, careful patient selection is essential. The original formulation of phenol and croton oil has been modified to prevent the peel from penetrating as deeply as the Baker-Gordon formulation. Both Hetter and Stone independently described a modification of phenol peels that yields better control over depth of penetration.[14,15] This has allowed patients with various skin types to be treated with favorable results.[16] While laser resurfacing with CO_2 and Er:YAG (erbium:yttrium-aluminum-garnet) has largely replaced

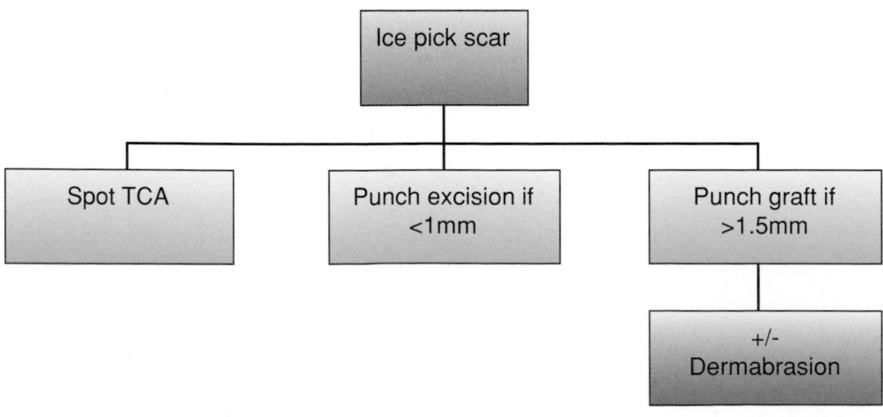

▲ **FIGURE 26-3** Treatment algorithm for ice pick scars.

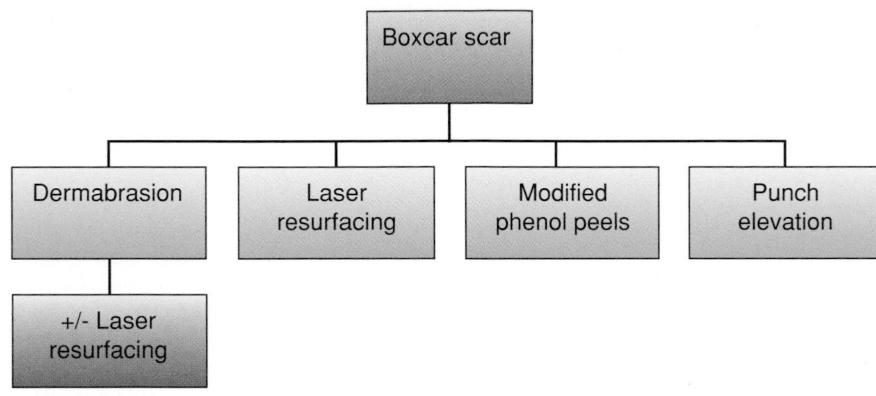

▲ **FIGURE 26-4** Treatment algorithm for boxcar scars.

peels for the treatment of scars, the modified phenol peels are making a comeback.

DERMABRASION Dermabrasion attempts to level down normal skin so that it is brought close to the depth of the scar; this method is very effective in creating a new contour plane. However, the depth of the plane that can be achieved with dermabrasion is limited as extensively deep abrading can cause additional scarring. Wounding to the depth of papillary dermis produces "tightening" while a wound in the upper reticular dermis results in "leveling." The presence of pinpoint bleeding indicates abrasion to the level of the papillary dermis while continued abrasion reveals the parallel lines of the superficial reticular dermis. When frayed white strands of collagen are evident, the mid-reticular dermis is visible and this should be an absolute endpoint as further invasion may lead to additional scarring. For a detailed description on the technique of dermabrasion, we refer the reader to articles by Bradley and Park[17] as well as Orentreich and Orentreich.[18]

LASERS Both ablative and nonablative laser resurfacing have been effective in treating facial scarring, and these are discussed in detail below.[19–24]

Ablative lasers Ablative laser resurfacing targets and vaporizes water-containing tissue, thereby allowing epidermal renewal as well as the reorientation and regeneration of collagen fibers in the superficial dermis.[25–27] The CO_2 laser has a wavelength of 10,600 nm and primarily targets water in the epidermis and superficial dermis. The Er:YAG laser has a wavelength of 2940 nm, which corresponds to the peak absorption coefficient of water. This laser produces minimal thermal injury, thereby resulting in faster reepithelialization and an improved side-effect profile, but less vascular coagulation as well as reduced collagen contraction and remodeling.[28,29]

Combined CO_2/Er:YAG is a commonly used treatment modality because it avoids many of the side effects encountered with pure CO_2 laser treatment while still producing a satisfying result.[30] Following the procedure, an occlusive dressing is applied for 2 days; for a comprehensive review of occlusive dressings, we refer the reader to a review article by Newman et al.[31] A postprocedure wound care regimen consists of Domeboro compresses (Bayer Corp., Morristown, NJ) every 4 hours and Aquaphor Healing Ointment or Biafine (OrthoNeutrogena, Skillman, NJ). Re-epithelialization typically occurs in 7 to 10 days. If an occlusive dressing is used for more than 48 hours, prophylaxis with a first-generation cephalosporin and fluconazole is recommended for 4 days, starting the day of the procedure.[3]

Fractional photothermolysis To date, there have been few controlled studies regarding the impact of fractional photothermolysis (Fraxel Laser, Reliant Technologies, Inc., Mountain View, CA) for treatment of scars; however, this relatively new modality has had reported success in the treatment of hypertrophic scars[32] and atrophic scars.[33–35] Fractional photothermolysis creates hundreds to thousands of microthermal zones (MTZ), or microscopic columns of thermal injury, sparing the tissue surrounding each zone.[35–37] Fractional photothermolysis has a 1550-nm wavelength and targets tissue water but not melanin, allowing its use in patients with all skin types; the depth of penetration is approximately 1500 μm. The fractional heating of the chromophore avoids bulk heating of the skin and reduces the risk of thermal injury to the dermis thereby minimizing the chance of worsening scarring. Reepithelialization takes place at approximately 24 hours posttreatment. The stratum corneum remains intact as it contains less water and therefore is not targeted.

In our experience, results with fractional photothermolysis are still not as dramatic as laser resurfacing plus dermabrasion. In order to get more dramatic clinical results with fractional photothermolysis high energies must be used, which cause a recovery time that approaches that of traditional resurfacing procedures. However, newer fractionated *carbon dioxide* lasers are on the market and comparative studies will be very helpful.

Nonablative lasers Nonablative lasers such as the pulsed dye laser (585–600 nm), long wavelength Nd:YAG (1320 nm), and the long wavelength diode (1450 nm) can produce improvement in boxcar and shallow atrophic scars. The pulsed dye lasers target hemoglobin and are useful for pink scars that are still exhibiting collagen remodeling and inflammation, likely through elimination of blood vessels within the scar.[38] Purpura is the main side effect of pulsed dye laser treatment and can last up to 14 days; however, the risk of hyperpigmentation should also be discussed with the patient prior to treatment.

For more mature scars that are no longer exhibiting collagen remodeling, the depth of the scarring process must be taken into account when choosing a laser. The energy from the laser causes partial denaturing of the collagen fibers; in response, there is an increase in collagen synthesis by fibroblasts. Synchronization of surface cooling and heating allows control of the depth of dermal injury.[39] Improvement in acne scarring following treatment with the 1320-nm Nd:YAG laser (CoolTouch CT3 Laser, CoolTouch, Inc., Roseville, CA) has been demonstrated in numerous studies.[40–42] The 1450-nm midinfrared diode laser (SmoothBeam, Candela Corporation, Wayland, MA) affects the dermis between 100 and 500 μm of depth. Improvements in atrophic acne scars,[43] as well as other atrophic scars,[44] have been reported with this laser.

Shallow Atrophic Scars

Shallow atrophic scars are most easily thought of as mini-boxcar scars that occur in clusters. They are most commonly located on the cheeks. Many of the same treatment modalities that are used to treat boxcar scars are also effective in treating

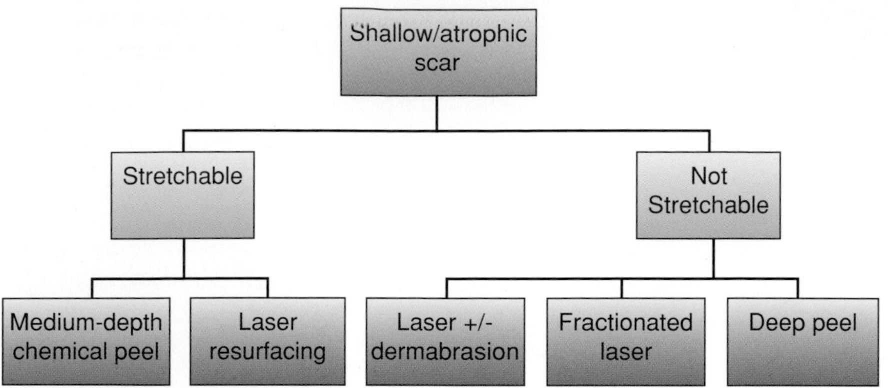

▲ **FIGURE 26-5** Treatment algorithm for shallow atrophic scars.

shallow atrophic scars. These scars respond well to both ablative and nonablative laser resurfacing, fractionated lasers, and dermabrasion just as boxcar scars do (Fig. 26-5). Additionally, chemical peels may be used to improve the appearance of shallow atrophic scars, especially scars that are "stretchable," meaning that the scar appearance is improved with lateral traction. Chemical peel options are discussed in greater detail below.

MEDIUM AND DEEP CHEMICAL PEELS Peel depth is affected by acid concentration, number of coats applied or "passes," skin thickness, skin preconditioning, body surface being treated, and in some instances, the duration of contact of the acid on the skin. Keratolytics are used for superficial exfoliation and are not discussed in this chapter as they do not significantly impact the deeper scarring of atrophic facial scars. Medium-depth chemical peels destroy the stratum corneum as well as epidermis and penetrate into the papillary dermis causing destruction, protein denaturation, and inflammation at a deeper level. This, in turn, results in collagen remodeling and, therefore, scar improvement and skin tightening (Fig. 26-6). Examples of medium-depth chemical peels include TCA, and variations of TCA peels such as the Obagi Blue Peel (Obagi Medical Products, Long Beach, CA), TCA and Jessner's solution (Monheit peel), or TCA combined with glycolic acid (Coleman peel). See the "Deep Peels/Phenol Peels" section.

Valley Scars

Valley scars result from a defect in volume in the area of the scar. This loss of volume may be at the level of the dermis or of the subcutaneous tissue. Correction of this volume loss can be achieved in two ways: fillers may be injected into the area of volume loss or a reaction may be induced in the patient that will result in collagen remodeling and an increase in collagen volume as wound healing takes place (Fig. 26-7).

FILLERS Soft tissue fillers have been used for decades in the correction of surface deformities. Several factors must be taken into consideration when choosing a filling agent, including: duration of filler, anatomic location, depth of scar to be filled, risk of allergic or granulomatous reaction, and risk of infection. Also, any history of keloid scar formation, known allergy to any components of the filler, active infection in the treatment site, or history of autoimmune disease are contraindications to using fillers. There is a higher risk of skin necrosis within the glabellar area in these procedures; therefore, extra care in this region is advocated. The most important predictor of filler success may be the actual texture and degree of fibrosis in the scar being filled. When more fibrosis is present, less correction is achieved with fillers.

Biologic Fillers

AUTOLOGOUS FAT Perhaps the most permanent of all filling substances, autologous fat transfer offers many advantages including the fact that it is nonimmunogenic, abundant in supply, and is a living tissue with potential for permanent augmentation. There is debate over the fragility of the adipocyte that predisposes it to damage during harvesting, preparation, and implantation. Atraumatic harvesting of the fat is essential. Blunt cannulae or a 20-gauge needle may then be used to place the fat into the desired area. Special care must be taken to avoid causing an embolism with a sharp needle.

COLLAGEN Collagen may be human-derived (CosmoDerm-I®/CosmoPlast®, Allergan, Irvine, CA) from human foreskin fibroblast culture or bovine-derived (Zyderm®/Zyplast®, Allergan, Irvine, CA). CosmoDerm-I received approval by the US Food and Drug Administration (FDA) in March 2003 for the treatment of acne scars. It is placed into the superficial dermis with a slight degree of overcorrection, while CosmoPlast is placed in the upper to middle dermis.

Zyplast and Zyderm are similar in concentration to CosmoPlast and CosmoDerm®. Two skin tests must be performed prior to placing bovine collagen in a patient as the risk of an allergic reaction to bovine collagen despite one negative skin test is 1.3% to 6.2%. Placement is similar to that of CosmoDerm and CosmoPlast.

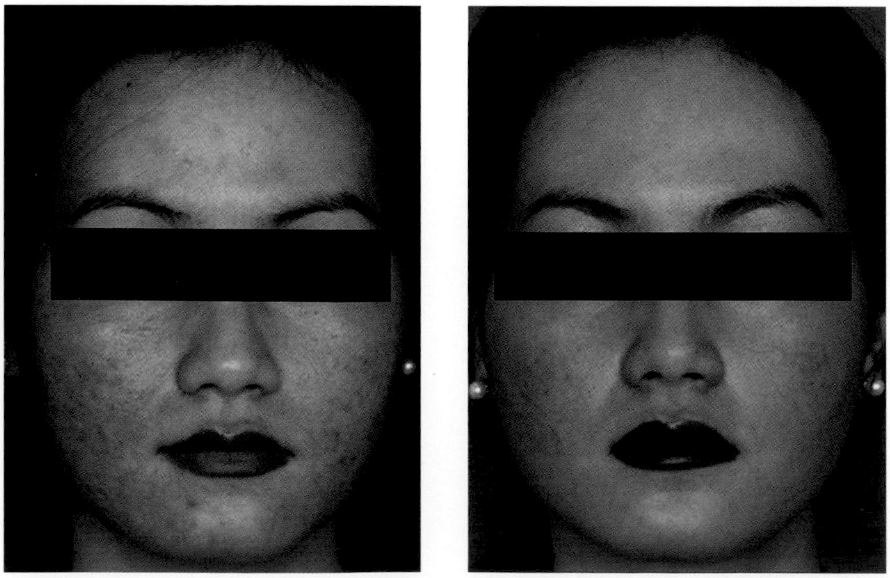

▲ **FIGURE 26-6** Shallow atrophic scars before (left) and after (right) treatment with the Obagi® TCA blue peel. (*Photograph courtesy of Dr. Zein E. Obagi.*)

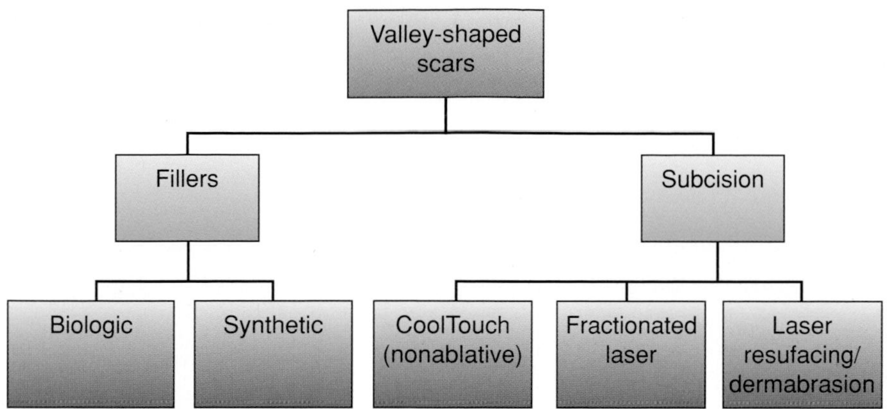

▲ **FIGURE 26-7** Treatment algorithm for valley-shaped scars.

Synthetic Fillers

HYALURONIC ACID Hyaluronic acid consists of alternating residues of D-glucuronic acid and N-acetyl-D-glycosamine that can bind up to 10,000 times its weight in water. It is found throughout the body in connective tissue as well as in synovial tissue and fluid. Hyaluronic acid is marketed as Restylane®, Restylane Fine Lines®, and Perlane® (Medicis Aesthetics, Scottsdale, AZ), Hylaform®, and Juvederm Ultra Plus® (Allergan, Irvine, CA), all of which have been approved by the FDA for superficial rhytides. All these formulations are composed of stabilized hyaluronic acid at 20 mg/mL but have varying sizes of injected particles.

Hyaluronic acid is popular because of its ease of injection, excellent safety profile, low rate of hypersensitivity reactions (1 in 2000), and superior longevity when compared with collagen. Complications include mild bruising, edema, arterial embolization, and visible papules.[3]

POLY-L-LACTIC ACID Poly-L-lactic acid (Sculptra, Dermik Laboratories, Bridgewater, NJ) belongs to the alpha hydroxy acid family and Sculptra is composed of crystalline, irregularly sized microparticles of poly-L-lactic acid that are 40 to 60 μm in diameter. This synthetic polymer has been approved for HIV-related facial lipoatrophy by the FDA. Sculptra is packaged as a sterile freeze-dried preparation that is reconstituted with sterile water 48 hours before injection. After injection of the poly-L-lactic acid, a foreign body reaction occurs over several weeks to months, presenting as a volumetric expansion.[45] It is important to note that there is no visual endpoint at the time of injection, and a waiting period of at least 4 to 6 weeks after initial product placement is recommended before subsequent injections.

Complications of poly-L-lactic acid include nodules (typically arising several weeks after injection) and granulomas (emerging months to years after injection); incidence rates range from 6% to 52%.[46] Early nodules may be broken up with needle fragmentation or further diluted with sterile saline. Late nodules and granulomas typically require treatment with excision; steroid injections may also be effective. Metabolism occurs via bioabsorption and gradual degradation.

CALCIUM HYDROXYLAPATITE Calcium hydroxylapatite (CaHA) (Radiesse®, Bioform Medical, San Mateo, CA) is a synthetic filler that typically lasts 12 to 18 months before subsequent injections are needed.[47] Radiesse was recently approved by the FDA for the correction of moderate to severe facial folds, such as nasolabial folds, as well as treatment of HIV lipoatrophy. There is no need for a skin test prior to use, and the correction that is obtained is close to 1:1, meaning that no expansion of the implant will occur after injection. CaHA has been used for superficial depressed scars[48] and acne scars.[49]

Side effects are generally mild; occasionally, nodules may form following treatment. This is especially more common when CaHA is used in the lips. Additionally, CaHA is radiopaque, so patients should be aware that it may appear on X-ray films or other imaging.

ARTEFILL Polymethylmethacrylate (PMMA) (ArteFill®, Artes Medical, San Diego, CA) is a permanent dermal filler that has been recently approved by the FDA for the correction of nasolabial folds. To our knowledge, there are no studies examining the effectiveness of ArteFill in treating facial scarring. The concern with this filler agent is the risk of nodule formation. The formulation approved for use in the United States has undergone changes so that the PMMA beads are of a more uniform size and therefore do not undergo phagocytosis.

Subcision

Subcutaneous incision, or subcision, for the treatment of depressed scars was first described in 1995.[50] After outlining, anesthetizing, and sterilizing the affected areas, a 22-gauge needle or a tribeveled 18-gauge hypodermic needle (Nokor, Becton Dickinson, Franklin Lakes, NJ) is inserted into the superficial fat with the bevel up just adjacent to the scarred area. The needle is turned so that the bevel is perpendicular to the skin surface, and the needle is moved back and forth in a fanning motion to break up the fibrous tissue that is depressing the scar. Audible rasping and popping is observed as the underside of the dermis is released from its subcutaneous attachment.[51] Following the procedure, patients can expect bruising for up to 1 week.

The exact mechanism of action of subcision is not fully understood. Orentreich and Orentreich described two mechanisms including release of tethers that bind down the scar and reactive formation of new connective tissue.[50] Alam et al. studied the effectiveness of subcision on acne scarring in 40 patients and noted that the investigators as well as the patients found that subcision improved the appearance of rolling acne scars.[51]

COMBINATION THERAPIES

Any individual patient may have several different morphologies of facial scars and therefore may require a combination of treatments that targets each specific scar type. It is important to understand the timeline of these combination therapies and which treatments may be employed simultaneously versus those that are spaced out several months apart; timing of combination treatments depends on the modalities and mechanisms of action. Each patient is unique, and clinical improvement may vary significantly among patients. We recommend reassessment of the patient 3 to 6 months following treatment to determine if further procedures would be beneficial. In the following section, we present a general guideline of combination treatment options that may be considered in approaching the patient with facial scarring.

Chemical Peels and Laser Resurfacing

A combination of chemical peels and laser resurfacing at the same visit is ideal for patients with numerous shallow atrophic scars intermixed with deeper boxcar scars. In these patients, chemical peeling is performed first, as this works at a more superficial level compared to laser resurfacing and improves the contour of the shallow atrophic scars. We use 24% to 26% TCA as a peeling agent. The chemical peel is applied to regions of the entire face with emphasis on the areas with shallow atrophic scarring. The endpoint is a peel into the papillary dermis or just into the reticular dermis. In patients who also have ice pick scars (in addition to shallow atrophic and boxcar scars), straight 30% TCA is used to spot treat the ice pick scars. At the conclusion of the peel, the skin is cleansed to remove excess peel solution. We then use the CO_2/Er:YAG laser over the entire scarred area in order to smooth out the contour of the skin, focusing on areas that have deeper boxcar-type scars. The combination treatment allows blending of the treated areas while optimizing the improvement of each distinct scar type.

Fractional photothermolysis may also be used in combination with chemical peeling for patients with shallow atrophic and boxcar scars. In this scenario, the chemical peel is applied during the first treatment session to the entire scarred area. Approximately 3 months after the peel, the patient returns to the office for reevaluation. At that point, fractional photothermolysis may be used to correct any deeper boxcar scars or shallow atrophic scars that have not responded to the chemical peeling. Alternatively, the patient may undergo fractionated laser treatments over the areas of deeper acne scarring followed immediately by the performance of a chemical peel. If this approach is employed, care must be taken so that the chemical peel does not penetrate more deeply than intended.

Laser Resurfacing and Dermabrasion

Laser resurfacing plus dermabrasion is another option for patients with a combination of shallow atrophic scars and deeper boxcar scars (Fig. 26-8). The laser is used over the entire scarred area or on the entire face (if clinically beneficial to reduce photodamage as well) to both ablate and tighten the skin. At the same visit, following laser resurfacing, dermabrasion is then used to plane down the skin that is elevated relative to any remaining atrophic areas and smooth out the contours of the entire skin surface; this achieves a more level surface topography.[52]

Subcision and Fractional Photothermolysis

Subcision may be combined with fractional photothermolysis to treat patients who have a combination of valley-shaped scars and boxcar or shallow atrophic scars. Subcision targets the valley-shaped scars while fractional photothermolysis may be used to treat any residual boxcar or shallow atrophic scars. These two treatments can be employed on the same day as long as they are not performed on the same scars. Alternatively, the subcision treatments may be performed at 3-month intervals until a satisfactory degree of filling is achieved. At that point in time, fractional photothermolysis may be performed.

Subcision and Laser Resurfacing with the 1320-nm Nd:YAG Laser

As previously mentioned, subcision alone is effective in the treatment of valley-shaped scars but can be associated with a fairly common risk of dermal nodule formation. To reduce this risk, we have found that nonablative laser therapy with the 1320-nm Nd:YAG laser (CoolTouch-CT3) is effective if started 1 week after subcision.[53] The laser treatments are performed at 2-week intervals for a total of six treatments.

Laser Resurfacing/Dermabrasion/Subcision/Fillers/Chemical Peel

Patients with a combination of shallow atrophic scars and boxcar scars may also have coexistent deeper valley-shaped scars at a depth that does not maximally respond to dermabrasion and laser resurfacing alone. After completion of dermabrasion and laser resurfacing, a series of two to three subcision treatments may be required to address the valley scars. If the patient still has atrophic areas following the above treatments, dermal fillers are ideal for evening out

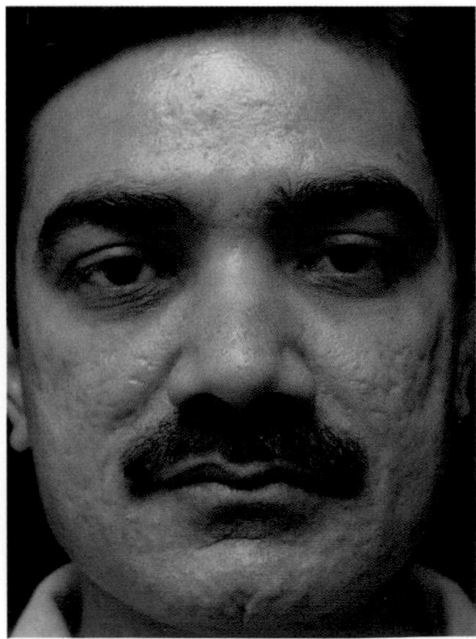
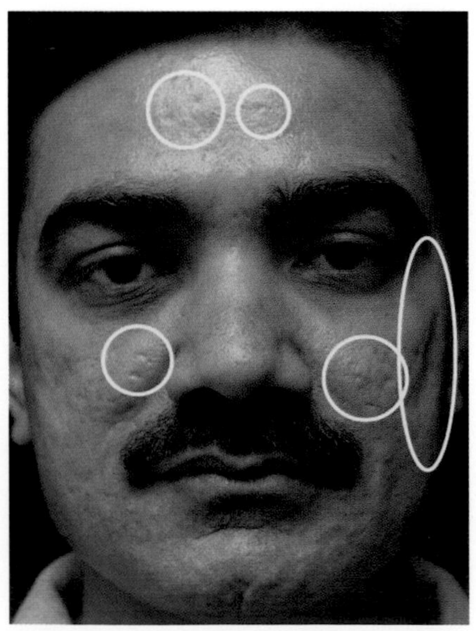
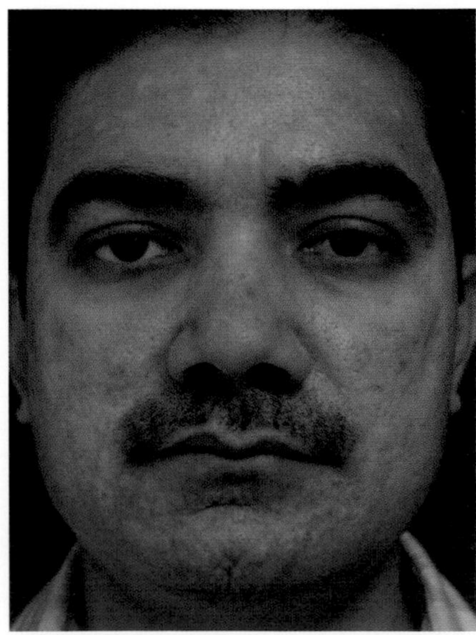

▲ **FIGURE 26-8** Combination of shallow atrophic scars, boxcar scars, and valley-shaped scars before (left). The middle photo shows the scars that were treated with subcision. The patient underwent subcision and spot TCA peels followed several months later by full-face laser resurfacing and dermabrasion of the cheeks (right).

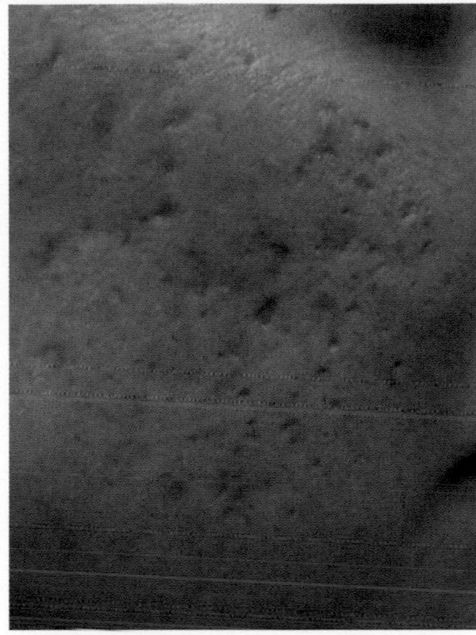
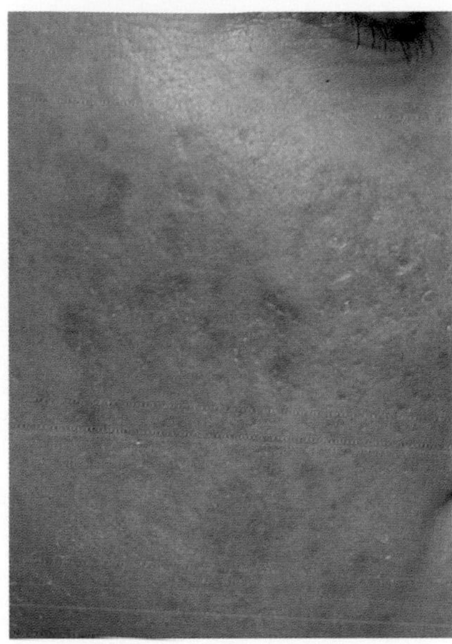

▲ **FIGURE 26-9** Boxcar and ice pick scars before (left) and after (right) punch grafts followed 6 weeks later by resurfacing with laser and dermabrasion as well as punch excisions of any remaining small scars.

any remaining discrepancies in contour. We do not advocate using fillers immediately prior to laser resurfacing as the effects of laser energy on various fillers have not been well studied.

Fulton and Silverton described a comprehensive and aggressive resurfacing of the acne-scarred face employing these treatments. They started with a Jessner's/TCA peel on the chest and neck regions (and other areas that are not resurfaced by the CO_2 laser). Atrophic valley scars were then filled with adipose tissue. After adipose tissue infiltration, CO_2 laser resurfacing and then dermabrasion were performed. This was followed by laser touch-up with the CO_2 laser. Then excision and/or grafting were performed, and finally manual dermabrasion was applied to any transition zones or residual irregularities. Postoperative semiocclusive wound dressings were placed after the above procedures were completed. The authors found a 75% to 80% improvement of acne scars.[52]

Punch Excision and Laser or Dermabrasion

Punch excision may be used at the same time as skin resurfacing (Fig. 26-9). Upon completion of the skin resurfacing procedure with laser or dermabrasion, any remaining ice pick scars up to 2 mm in size can be punch excised as discussed earlier. The advantages of performing the punch excision at the same time as the skin resurfacing are to combine procedures (thus reducing recovery time) and to allow the sutures to heal with less noticeable marks on the skin since the entire surface has to undergo reepithelialization.

SUMMARY

There are many treatment options available for facial scars. Proper patient assessment, determination of scar morphology, and selection of the appropriate treatment modality are essential when addressing facial scarring. It is also necessary to bring patients back for regular follow-up 3 to 6 months after treatment (in addition to routine postprocedure follow up) to properly assess efficacy of any given treatment. Finally, use of a pre- and posttreatment skin-conditioning regimen will optimize patient outcomes. Recent technologies in skin resurfacing enhance more traditional therapies and allow us further options in selecting the best treatments for our patients.

REFERENCES

1. Jacob CI, Dover JS, Kaminer MS. Acne scarring: a classification system and review of treatment options. *J Am Acad Dermatol.* 2001;45:109.
2. Obagi S. Correction of surface deformities: botox, soft-tissue fillers, lasers and intense pulsed light, and radiofrequency. *Atlas Oral Maxillofac Surg Clin North Am.* 2004;12:271.
3. Obagi S. Pre- and postlaser skin care. *Oral Maxillofac Surg Clin North Am.* 2004;16:181.
4. Obagi S, Bridenstine JB. Skin resurfacing. *Oral Maxillofacial Surg Knowledge Update.* 2001;3:5.
5. Obagi S, Bridenstine JB. Lifetime skin care. *Oral Maxillofac Surg Clin North Am.* 2000;12:531.
6. Obagi S, Chaudhary-Patel M. Overview of skin resurfacing modalities. In: Guthoff RF, Katowitz JA, eds. *Essentials in Ophthalmology: Oculoplastics and Orbit.* New York, NY: Springer; 2007:259-275.
7. Goldberg DJ, Amin S, Hussain M. Acne scar correction using calcium hydroxyapatite in a carrier-based gel. *J Cosmet Laser Ther.* 2006;8:134.
8. Johnson WC. Treatment of pitted scars: punch transplant technique. *J Dermatol Surg Oncol.* 1986;12:260.
9. Mancuso A, Farber GA. The abraded punch graft for pitted facial scars. *J Dermatol Surg Oncol.* 1991;17:32.
10. Dzubow LM. Scar revision by punch-graft transplants. *J Dermatol Surg Oncol.* 1985;11:1200.
11. Lee JB, Chung WG, Kwahck H, et al. Focal treatment of acne scars with trichloroacetic acid: chemical reconstruction of skin scars method. *Dermatol Surg.* 2002;28:1017.
12. Brody HJ. Deep peeling. In: Brody HJ, ed. *Chemical Peeling and Resurfacing.* 2nd ed. St. Louis, MO: Mosby; 1997:137-160.
13. Stegman SJ. A comparative histologic study of the effects of three peeling agents and dermabrasion on normal and sun-damaged skin. *Aesthetic Plast Surg.* 1982;6:123.
14. Hetter GP. An examination of the phenol-croton oil peel: part I. Dissecting the formula. *Plast Reconstr Surg.* 2000;105:227.
15. Stone P. Modified phenol peels—role of the application technique. *Clin Plast Surg.* 1998;25:21.
16. Rullan PP, Lemon J, Rullan J. The 2-day light phenol chemabrasion for deep wrinkles and acne scars: a presentation of face and neck peels. *Am J Cosm Surg.* 2004;21:15.
17. Bradley DT, Park SS. Scar revision via resurfacing. *Facial Plast Surg.* 2001;17:253.
18. Orentreich N, Orentreich DS. Dermabrasion. As a complement to dermatology. *Clin Plast Surg.* 1998;25:63.
19. Kwon SD, Kye YC. Treatment of scars with a pulsed Er:YAG laser. *J Cutan Laser Ther.* 2000;2:27.
20. Jeong JT, Park JH, Kye YC. Resurfacing of pitted acne scars using Er:YAG laser with ablation and coagulation mode. *Aesthetic Plast Surg.* 2003;27:130.
21. Tanzi EL, Alster TS. Treatment of atrophic facial acne scars with a dual-mode Er:YAG laser. *Dermatol Surg.* 2002;28:551.
22. Sawcer D, Lee HR, Lowe NJ. Lasers and adjunctive treatments for facial scars: a review. *J Cutan Laser Ther.* 1999;1:77.
23. Lent WM, David LM. Laser resurfacing: a safe and predictable method of skin resurfacing. *J Cutan Laser Ther.* 1999;1:87.
24. Koo SH, Yoon ES, Ahn DS, et al. Laser punch-out for acne scars. *Aesthetic Plast Surg.* 2001;25:46.
25. Alster TS. Cutaneous resurfacing with CO_2 and erbium:YAG lasers: preoperative, intraoperative, and postoperative considerations. *Plast Reconstr Surg.* 1999;103:619.
26. Ross EV, McKinlay JR, Anderson RR. Why does carbon dioxide resurfacing work? A review. *Arch Dermatol.* 1999;135:444.

27. Smith KS, Skelton HG, Graham JS, et al. Depth of morphologic skin damage and viability after one, two, and three passes of a high-energy, short-pulse CO_2 laser (TruPulse) in pig skin. *J Am Acad Dermatol*. 1997;37:204.
28. Alster TS. Clinical and histological evaluation of six erbium:YAG lasers for cutaneous resurfacing. *Laser Surg Med*. 1999;24:87.
29. Sapijaszko MJ, Zachary CB. Er:YAG laser skin resurfacing. *Dermatol Clin*. 2002;20:87.
30. Weinstein C. Modulated dual mode erbium/CO_2 lasers for the treatment of acne scars. *J Cutan Laser Ther*. 1999;1: 204.
31. Newman JP, Fitzgerald P, Koch RJ. Review of closed dressings after laser resurfacing. *Dermatol Surg*. 2000;26:562.
32. Behroozan DS, Goldberg LH, Tianhong D, et al. Fractional photothermolysis for the treatment of surgical scars: a case report. *J Cosmet Laser Ther*. 2006;8:35.
33. Manstein D, Herron GS, Sink RK, et al. Fractional photothermolysis: a new concept for cutaneous remodeling using microscopic patterns of thermal injury. *Laser Surg Med*. 2004;34:426.
34. Hasegawa T, Matsukura T, Mizuno Y, et al. Clinical trial of a laser device called fractional photothermolysis system for acne scars. *J Dermatol*. 2006;33:623.
35. Alster TS, Tanzi EL, Lazarus M. The use of fractional laser photothermolysis for the treatment of atrophic scars. *Dermatol Surg*. 2007;33:295.
36. Khan MH, Sink RK, Manstein D, et al. Intradermally focused laser pulses: thermal effects at defined tissue depths. *Laser Surg Med*. 2005;36:270.
37. Fisher GH, Geronemus RG. Short-term side effects of fractional photothermolysis. *Dermatol Surg*. 2005;31:1245.
38. Alster TS. Improvement of erythematous and hypertrophic scars by the 585-nm flashlamp-pumped pulsed dye laser. *Ann Plast Surg*. 1994;32:186.
39. Levy JL, Besson R, Mordon S. Determination of optimal parameters for laser for nonablative remodeling with a 1.54 μm Er:glass laser: a dose-response study. *Dermatol Surg*. 2002;28:405.
40. Sadick NS, Schecter AK. A preliminary study of utilization of the 1320-nm Nd:YAG laser for the treatment of acne scarring. *Dermatol Surg*. 2004;30:995.
41. Rogachefsky AS, Hussain M, Goldberg J. Atrophic and mixed pattern of acne scars improved with a 1320-nm Nd:YAG laser. *Dermatol Surg*. 2003;29:904.
42. Tanzi EL, Alster TS. Comparison of a 1450-nm diode laser and a 1320-nm Nd:YAG laser in the treatment of atrophic facial scars: a prospective clinical and histologic study. *Dermatol Surg*. 2004;30:152.
43. Chua SH, Ang P, Khoo L, et al. Nonablative 1450-nm diode laser in the treatment of facial atrophic acne scars in type IV to V Asian skin: a prospective clinical study. *Dermatol Surg*. 2004;30:1287.
44. Jih MH, Friedman PM, Kimyai-Asadi A, et al. Successful treatment of a chronic atrophic dog-bite scar with the 1450-nm diode laser. *Dermatol Surg*. 2004;30:1161.
45. Hamilton MM, Hobgood T. Emerging trends and techniques in male aesthetic surgery. *Facial Plast Surg*. 2005;21:324.
46. Humble G, Mest D. Soft tissue augmentation using Sculptra. *Facial Plast Surg*. 2004;20:157.
47. Silvers SL, Eviatar JA, Echavez MI, et al. Prospective, open-label, 18-month trial of calcium hydroxylapatite (Radiesse) for facial soft-tissue augmentation in patients with human immunodeficiency virus-associated lipoatrophy: one-year durability. *Plast Reconstr Surg*. 2006;118:34S.
48. Roy D, Sadick N, Mangat D. Clinical trial of a novel filler material for soft tissue augmentation of the face containing synthetic calcium hydroxylapatite microspheres. *Dermatol Surg*. 2006;32: 1134.
49. Tzikas TL. Evaluation of the Radiance FN soft tissue filler for facial soft tissue augmentation. *Arch Facial Plast Surg*. 2004;6:234.
50. Orentreich DS, Orentreich N. Subcutaneous incisionless (subcision) surgery for the correction of depressed scars and wrinkles. *Dermatol Surg*. 1995;21:543.
51. Alam M, Omura N, Kaminer MS. Subcision for acne scarring: technique and outcomes in 40 patients. *Dermatol Surg*. 2005;31:310.
52. Fulton JE, Silverton K. Resurfacing the acne-scarred face. *Dermatol Surg*. 1999;25:353.
53. Fulchiero GJ Jr, Parham-Vetter PC, Obagi S. Subcision and 1320-nm Nd:YAG nonablative laser resurfacing for the treatment of acne scars: a simultaneous split-face single patient trial. *Dermatol Surg*. 2004;30:1356.

SECTION 5

Skin Care

CHAPTER 27

Starting a Skin Care Product Line

Leslie Baumann, MD

The notion of developing one's own line of skin care products to offer patients and, possibly, the general public, may be inspired by the sight of infomercials for very popular formulations designed by dermatologists, or hearing about practitioners who sell their own product lines, or even the realization that such a step just seems to be the logical way to expand a successful cosmetic dermatology practice. Regardless of its origins, the prospect of starting one's own line of products is pondered by an increasing number of cosmetic dermatologists.

On the surface it may appear that the act of developing one's own line of skin care products is a scientific enterprise; however, the bottom line is that designing one's own product line is very much a business. The process may include science (although, unfortunately, it often does not include enough), as it certainly includes chemistry. However, designing a line of skin care products involves much more than just scientific knowledge. Business experience, which many cosmetic dermatologists may lack, is required. This chapter will discuss the challenges inherent in starting one's own line of skin care products.

QUESTIONS TO CONSIDER BEFORE DRAWING UP THE BUSINESS PLAN

Before embarking on the arduous journey of initiating one's own line of skin care products, it is advisable to explore the motivating factors. Specifically, it is incumbent upon the professional who is weighing such a business decision to consider the following questions: Why are you thinking about starting your own line of skin care products? Are your patients consistently dissatisfied with what they find on their own or with formulations for which you offer either a ringing endorsement or, maybe, just a tepid nod? Is your chemistry background sufficient? Do you have an innovative approach to product development? Are you simply trying to take the next step in the evolution of your thriving cosmetic dermatology practice? The practitioner who asks such questions might find that the answers stop them in their tracks or lead them to getting their feet and hands a little dirty in a challenging new business.

THE BUSINESS (AND COSTS) OF DEVELOPING SKIN CARE PRODUCTS

Few, if any, cosmetic dermatologists who contemplate this venture are chemists. Therefore, it is unlikely that physicians preparing to launch a product line would be able to create the formulas necessary to develop new products. In this scenario, thousands of dollars in investment would be needed to accompany the creation of new formulas. In most cases, however, the physician is striving to rebrand quality products already on the market. Essentially, this means going to manufacturers and paying them to tweak current formulas with signature ingredients so as to differentiate their brand and package them under the physician's name for limited distribution. In a few cases, the dermatologist may pay to test a new formula before generating the new line.

In either of the main scenarios, payment is not a simple matter. There are costs associated with each step of the process. First, the physician must decide on the volume of the order, the time frame or launch date, and, of course, the ingredients.

Volume

The volume of the order is always the first item on the agenda. Deciding on the initial supply can be tricky because it is difficult to predict demand. Practitioners must factor into this decision the understanding that the minimum quantities required range across manufacturers, and companies adjust minimum quantity requirements based on the type of packaging selected. A survey of companies conducted by the author revealed that if you are planning to change an existing formula or packaging, most manufacturers would consider this your "run" (or requested supply) and require a minimum of 2500 to 5000 units per product in the line. One small company requires minimums as low as 12 to 36 pieces, depending on the item, for products that they already carry and simply need to relabel. (However, this company requires a minimum order of 5000 to 10,000 units per product for a practitioner's own unique formulation—the range is related to the complexity of the project and/or custom packaging, with a higher minimum required for more complex work.) Most stipulated a minimum of 10,000 pieces. One company requires 25,000 units when the practitioner requests that the formulation be packaged in tubes. Packaging is the next major decision.

Packaging

Deciding on the type of packaging for each item in the product line is part and parcel of placing a product order. Products are typically packaged in tubes, bottles, jars, and airless pump containers. Jars tend to be more expensive, particularly if gold tops are used. Companies generally try to match products with the appropriate packaging—sunscreens in tubes, liquids in bottles, creams in jars, and serums in airless pump bottles. Some companies use only plastic containers, which confer several advantages such as reduced breakage, lighter shipping weight, and ease of labeling. However, the wrong grade of plastic, regardless of the packaging, can adversely affect the stability of a product. Also, it is important to note that in the case of products with active ingredients (i.e., sunscreens, acne products, etc.), changing even one ingredient or any part of the packaging requires 90-day stability testing in order to achieve 2-year expiration dating.

Labeling is another important aspect of product packaging, as costs and aesthetics must be considered. Setting up printing plates for labeling and using multiple colors can be quite expensive. Some companies employ one or more in-house graphic artists whose services do not result in any extra charges. When this service is not available, or when a physician wants more input, a $300 plate fee per color is typical for this more elaborate but still downscale labeling approach. For example, if a dermatologist chooses to create a logo in red and green, along with the copy in black, the cost would be for the one-time setup charge of three color plates or $900. If multiple products are to be included in the line, all colors on the labels, as well as the size of the labels, might be kept the same, with only a slight change in copy made to distinguish the different products. In this case, only one additional plate (at $300) would be needed. This is an unrealistic scenario, however, simply to illustrate the cost structure of printing. A more realistic scenario is a line that includes products for different uses, necessitating various container sizes. In turn, various label sizes would be needed for suitable fit and presentation (e.g., an 8-oz bottle for a cleanser, a 1–2-oz jar for a facial moisturizer, a 4-oz tube for sunscreen, and a 1-oz bottle with pump dispenser for a skin lightener). In this scenario, initial printing plate charges would be multiplied by the number of different size containers in the product line. It is important to note that with the rising popularity of digital technology, plate charges are slowly waning. Of course, technology still varies among label companies.

Labels themselves are inexpensive (usually ranging from $0.10 to $0.50 per label depending on colors and finish), but may influence the volume order because some companies may require at least 5000 labels per product. Label material is another cost variable. Regular paper labels that include some minimal protective coating, neither waterproof nor sufficient to prevent creasing if the bottle is squeezed, are the least expensive. Polylaminate or vinyl labels that are water- and weatherproof as well as slightly elastic, thus retaining form upon being squeezed, are superior and slightly more expensive (Table 27-1). Although additional design costs are not uncommon, the physician is really getting scant more than her/his name and address on the product. In order to achieve an upscale look for a finished product it is often recommended that the packaging be "screened" (in other words, getting the product labels silkscreened onto the package as opposed to having them painted). This usually involves a one-time setup charge with the screener, running between $500 and $1000 per product with a lead time ranging from 3 to 4 weeks. Once the manufacturer receives the screened product, they will process the order. Physicians marketing only through their offices need not screen products but it is often recommended for those who are marketing products through upscale department stores or on a home shopping network, such as QVC or HSN, or on an infomercial. Pricing for screening varies based on quantity to be screened and the number of colors used. In most cases, the use of silkscreening would be considered for runs of 5000 units or more. Manufacturers typically have relationships with screening companies. The benefit of having labels silkscreened is that such labels do not peel off or scuff and, therefore, are ideally suited for imparting an upscale appearance.

Usually available in the United States, ordinary packaging is associated with lead times of 6 to 8 weeks and minimum orders of 2500 to 10,000 pieces. High-end or upscale packaging minimums tend to range from 25,000 to 50,000 pieces, accompanied by a lead time of anywhere from 8 to 15 weeks. Most upscale packaging is obtained from Italy, Spain, South Korea, and China, with little available in the United States. Most physicians naïvely begin the ordering process with a plan to custom design their product packages, but quickly revise their expectations when confronted with the prospect of exorbitant packaging and labeling costs. Physicians also have to cover shipping costs to the point of delivery, usually the clinical practice. When feasible, costs can be reduced by shrewd, frugal manipulation of package minimums (e.g., packaging products together, netting two or three products per 30,000-piece minimum versus one product per 30,000-piece minimum).

Overall costs per unit are especially important for a would-be product designer to consider. A low-end simple cleanser or lotion might range from $2 to $2.50 per unit; medium-range products, $3 to $6 per unit. Sophisticated products, which might include advanced liposome delivery systems or bio- or nanotechnology, could be as high as $7 at the low end and as high as $20 or $30 per unit for the most advanced products. Such products can usually be purchased in smaller minimum quantity sizes, so it is reasonable to expect to pay from $20,000 to $25,000 per product.

TABLE 27-1
Product Label Quote Range[a]

	Polylaminate		Paper w/Coating	
	5000 Labels	10,000 Labels	5000 Labels	10,000 Labels
1-Color	$0.143 ea.	$0.106 ea.	$0.075 ea.	$0.058 ea.
2-Color	$0.152 ea.	$0.111 ea.	$0.085 ea.	$0.064 ea.
3-Color	$0.162 ea.	$0.116 ea.	$0.094 ea.	$0.069 ea.
4-Color	$0.183 ea.	$0.122 ea.	$0.173 ea.	$0.113 ea.

[a]This is a representative quote range for an 8-oz body lotion label, listed by label material and number of colors used. Note: The larger the volume, the less significant the additional charge for added colors. Polylaminate labels are generally 35% to 40% more expensive than paper labels.

Product Choices: Rebranding, Timing, and Starting from Scratch

A typical range of products in a dermatologist's own line includes basic cleansers; bleaching agents; shampoos; AHAs; sunscreens; topical antioxidants such as green tea, grape seed extract, and stable vitamin C; growth factors; retinols; and even new AHA and sunscreen formulations that incorporate antioxidants and liposomal delivery systems. Companies that provide such OTC and private-label products cite ease of manufacture, high patient and physician satisfaction, and stability of products. Stable, efficacious skin care products are not easy to formulate, however.

The easiest, lowest-risk approach to starting one's own line is to work with one of the smaller companies that already carries the type of product(s) of interest and requires low minimums in the initial order volume. If this rebranding is successful, new products can be easily added to the line. At that point, the physician might want to branch out with a unique formula or two.

From conception of the plan to release of a new line of products, developing a new cosmetics or cosmeceutical line can take anywhere from 6 months to a year. If a practitioner is able to quickly identify a company to work with and that company already provides the desired products for rebranding, the business could take off in a few months. If a practitioner hopes to peddle a unique formula, there are additional associated financial and time costs. Developmental laboratory fees can range from $15,000 to $50,000 per product. (Simple formulations produced at smaller laboratories more likely incur research and development charges of $1000 to $5000.) In addition, the FDA requires a 90-day stability assessment for an established product that is to be tweaked with the addition of a new ingredient or two according to a physician's specifications. If a physician decides to change the packaging on an established product, retesting is required. The same is true if anything is changed in the formulation (e.g., adding or removing a fragrance or an antioxidant). It is recommended that more than one variation of the formulation be submitted simultaneously in case one separates.

It is best to order packaging at least 2 months into the stability-testing process. Although a product may be perfectly stable, some types of packaging might not be ideally suited to it. Experienced formulators should know which resins have the best track records in terms of maintaining stability when exposed to certain elements or compounds (e.g., light exposure causes decomposition of antioxidant products). It takes 2 to 4 months for packaging to arrive, and typically another 3 weeks or more for inclusion in the manufacturing schedule (once all components, including packaging, have arrived at the manufacturer's plant).

Formulating new products from scratch, rather than relabeling, is an easier enterprise if the product is a nondrug, which contains no active ingredient as defined by the FDA. Examples include antioxidant products, cleansers, shampoos, and AHAs. Stability does not have to be established in these cases. Some companies will still perform such testing, though, as they prefer to manufacture under pharmaceutical guidelines. As stated previously, prescription or OTC drugs (defined as containing an active ingredient and listed on the back label) must undergo stability testing. Examples of these products include sunscreens, prescription and OTC acne products, and antifungals.

Testing, Promotional Considerations and Costs in Dollars and Time

Implicit in the timeline cited above is a substantial amount of personal (and, possibly, personnel—depending on how many people a physician has employed to devote to the start-up) time consumed in the development and product launch process. If the practitioner is not taking a half-year sabbatical, a significant commitment of staff time will be required from those with strong critical thinking and executive decision-making skills to orchestrate and supervise a process that involves a wide array of diverse professionals—manufacturers, formulating chemists, packaging companies, graphic artists, printers, trucking and logistics companies, and, ultimately, banks and finance companies, if the physician does not plan to pay for everything out of pocket. Once the product line has been manufactured, marketing and promotion costs come into play. Promotional pamphlets and brochures must be designed and printed to coincide with the introduction of the product line, which is best accompanied by an advertising and public relations campaign. Such necessary business adjuncts comprise some of the additional, arguably hidden or initially ignored, associated costs of launching a product line that a physician must consider before deciding to embark on this challenging venture.

At this point, it should be clear that the cost stream involved in creating a product line is quite extensive. As mentioned above, additional costs are incurred from stability testing. For example, the FDA requires in vivo studies (with a minimum of five patients) to validate SPF claims for sunscreen products or formulations with SPF claims. Costs depend on the complexity of the study and the number of study subjects, but typically range from $5000 to $25,000. Practitioners opting simply to relabel an existing product with their own name are usually given permission by the sunscreen's manufacturer to use their validation data. New validation studies are mandatory for new formulations. If a practitioner chooses to include three products that have SPF (e.g., sunscreen, a skin lightener with SPF, and an AHA body lotion with SPF), three SPF validation studies would be required. It is important to note that the FDA requires two forms of stability testing on prescription and OTC drugs. The 90 day accelerated program allows for a product launch with a 2-year shelf life. This is followed by ongoing 2-year real-time stability testing. It is important to note that the FDA's final monograph on sunscreen, issued and debated since 1999 but not yet enforced, recommends a minimum of 20 SPF test subjects as well as a UVA test requirement (only UVB testing is conducted currently).[1] Such policies, once implemented, would lead to higher costs for sunscreen developers that, in turn, would be borne by physicians starting their own product lines.

FINAL MARKETING QUESTIONS TO CONSIDER

To start a successful product line, a well-organized business plan is necessary. If you plan to create (not just label with your name) and market your line beyond the scope of your practice, remember that you are competing with professionals, people backed with significant funding, purchasing teams, and strong business plans. It is worth noting that not even all of their projects succeed. For every success, such as Rodan and Field's Proactiv, there are several flashes in the pan—lines that last a few weeks and then fizzle.

Although infomercials represent an obvious marketing route, given the example of Proactiv, they are hardly the best first approach to marketing. This leads to fundamental sales questions that are important to ask oneself as part of an initial business plan when mulling over starting a product line: Where and how will you sell your products? Will you mass market, through companies such as Wal-Mart, K-Mart, or Target? Will you focus on pharmacy chains such as CVS, Walgreens, or Eckerd? Do you have the contacts there to facilitate sales? A sound business plan will address these questions. Mass marketers want to know the practitioners' plans for "moving" or selling their product line. Accordingly, they will want to know the advertising schedule and public relations program. The Internet, of course, is another popular sales option. Cursory consideration of this approach is appealing because the overhead appears to be low. In addition, most practitioners probably know someone who can create an attractive Web site. However, it takes money to pay for advertising links to steer people to a Web site. An advertising budget and public relations campaign will still be necessary. It should be noted that, anecdotally, online sales by most practitioners selling private-label lines are dwarfed by in-office sales.

Some practitioners hoping to sell their own products may rely on sales to colleagues (via exhibit hall booths at conferences) or vending the private-label products in their colleagues' offices. However, only Obagi has been successful at this. Besides offering something innovative, Obagi had public relations support and educational seminars. It is not easy to sell to physicians, particularly when peddling a variation of something already widely available. An expansive, expensive sales force and support staff would likely be necessary to even have a chance at selling a private line this way. For physicians choosing to limit sales to their own offices, the best bet is to arrange to sell an established product line relabeled under one's own name. Convinced that their idea is a surefire hit, some physicians ask manufacturers to fund their start-up. When companies can own the project and simply hire a spokesperson, though, there is scant incentive for them to fund a speculative start-up.

Whether you sell products in your office, online, or in a store, a significant concern is how to make sure that the customers who buy your products are using the right products? Using the Baumann Skin Typing System (BSTS) discussed in Chapter 9 can greatly simplify this. The BSTS divides people into 16 skin types based on skin hydration, sensitivity, pigmentation tendency, and extent of photoaging. This allows the user to accurately determine what ingredients are most efficacious for each of the 16 skin types. The system can be used by registering at www.SkinIQ.com. Once you are accepted and given a password, you can invite consumers to complete the online quiz to determine their skin type. Once you and they know their skin type, you can easily suggest which products are right for them. If you would like to label your products with the various Baumann Skin Type Designations, contact info@skintypesolutions.com to learn how to proceed. In addition, you may choose to set up an online store to sell your products and use the BSTS to help the customers know which products are right for their skin as is done at www.Baumannstore.com. For information about using the questionnaire, online store or the BSTS contact info@skintypesolutions.com.

SUMMARY

For the cosmetic dermatologist or other practitioner thinking about starting one's own line of products to offer to her/his patients, it is essential to understand that this is a business, not medical, matter. It is also a big business decision at that, insofar as significant work is required on the physician's part upon committing to such a risk. As a practitioner, the first questions you should ask yourself are "Why start a new line of products? Would my patients be more likely to adhere to therapeutic regimens if my name is on the label?"

Upon deciding to initiate a line of products, it is important to be aware that start-up costs vary by company. Some are especially adept at facilitating and streamlining the process. Shopping around among the different cosmetic manufacturing and packaging companies and conducting one's own cost–benefit analysis, factoring in time and ultimate benefits to one's patients as important variables, is advisable. As a practitioner considering this business venture, one must be prepared with an initial desired volume of product, the ideal launch date, and ingredients/product types. It is important to remember, though, that while manufacturers will usually reassure customers regarding the ease of concocting products, the reality is that they are quite difficult to formulate. The bottom line in this business, nonmedical, decision is that significant research is necessary—"look before you leap"—before entering into this difficult, competitive enterprise.

REFERENCE

1. U.S. Food and Drug Administration Center for Drug Evaluation and Research: Rulemaking History for OTC Sunscreen Drug Products. http://www.fda.gov/cder/otcmonographs/Sunscreen/new_sunscreen.htm. Accessed March 18, 2008.

CHAPTER 28

Cosmetic and Drug Regulation

Edmund Weisberg, MS
Leslie Baumann, MD

COSMECEUTICALS: DRUGS VERSUS COSMETICS

According to the United States Food and Drug Administration (FDA), a personal care product can be classified as a drug, a cosmetic, or both. Moisturizers with skin protection factor (SPF) and antidandruff shampoos are examples of dermatologic products classified as both a drug and a cosmetic. The term "cosmeceutical" was introduced approximately 25 years ago by Albert Kligman, MD, at a meeting of the Society of Cosmetic Chemists because he felt that a new category of regulation should exist.[1] Although this topic has been debated for decades, the category "cosmeceuticals" has still not been codified or officially recognized. In other words, it has no legal meaning. The term, however, is increasingly a part of the mainstream vernacular and frequently used to describe products that are known to have a biologic action but are regulated as cosmetics (e.g., products containing retinol). Although it is well known that retinol stimulates retinoic acid receptors resulting in biologic activity, retinol is a popular ingredient contained in numerous cosmetics. Companies often list retinol as an inactive ingredient on product labels to avoid regulatory action by the FDA.

The stage for this unforeseen regulatory loophole in which cosmeceuticals reside was set in 1938 when the US Congress passed a statute known as The Federal Food, Drug, and Cosmetic Act (FD&C Act), which outlined formal criteria for classification of drugs and cosmetics. In this document, cosmetics were defined as: "*... articles intended to be rubbed, poured, sprinkled, or sprayed on, introduced into, or otherwise applied to the human body or any part thereof for cleansing, beautifying, promoting attractiveness, or altering the appearance.*" In contrast, a drug is defined as a substance "*intended to affect the structure and function of the body.*" Based on this definition, the actual *intent* of the product and not its actions govern how it is classified. This allows for the classification of retinol as a cosmetic because it is listed as an inactive ingredient on product labels; therefore, retinol is not *intended* to serve a biologic purpose.

As in several other realms of society during our era of rapidly propagating technology, numerous legal implications fail to anticipate future developments. In terms of the debate over classifying products as drugs, cosmetics, or cosmeceuticals, there are some salient points to consider. The first is that the current regulations discourage companies from publishing supportive scientific clinical trials to evaluate the efficacy of their products. For example, if a manufacturer establishes in a study that an ingredient increases collagen synthesis, the company is proving that its product affects the "function of the body." If they were then to market or sell that product as a cosmetic intended to increase collagen synthesis, as would be desirable in an antiaging product or a wrinkle cream, they would be violating the 1938 statute. The only legal option for the manufacturer would be, instead, to market its product as a drug.

Before approval for marketing in the United States, every new drug must be clinically tested in accordance with FDA guidelines for a new drug application (NDA). The FDA process of drug approval can take more than 10 years and cost hundreds of millions of dollars. Obviously, the cosmetic companies are left with compelling incentives to avoid such long delays and exorbitant costs by following the guidelines to keep their products classified as cosmetics. In such cases, even though the companies perform extensive research on such products, their findings are considered proprietary and remain unpublished. This, too, has several implications. The first is that dermatologists and other physicians do not have access to this scientific evidence and are rendered poorly equipped to evaluate the efficacy of the numerous and varied products making it to market. Physicians are taught to practice evidence-based medicine, but without evidence, have little reason to believe that any of these products are efficacious or effective. Consequently, the medical establishment dismisses these products as useless when such formulations may, in fact, offer potential benefits to patients. The second problem is that consumers may often become confused by all the sleek, glitzy marketing. They rarely know how to tell the difference between a reputable company that conducts scientific research and a company of charlatans seeking to capitalize on consumers' dreams of younger and healthier skin. With little guidance given the medical community's lack of information regarding these OTC products, consumers try products and likely feel disappointed with the lack of results. Consumers are also left to operate under the false assumption that you get what you pay for—that is, the more expensive the product, the more likely it is to be effective. This can lead to a general distrust of the entire cosmetic dermatology field. The third problem with cosmetic companies performing internal research and not publishing the results for general review is the circumvention of the peer review process. Peer review has long been considered essential to validate the research findings of scientists. It is difficult to believe or have confidence in the results of a study that has not been subjected to the peer review process.

Also beyond the peer review process, there are individuals outside of companies that attempt to perform research on cosmetic products and procedures without the concern for product classification; however, it is often difficult for these individuals to raise the research funding necessary to perform such studies. There are research grants available from several companies that may help these researchers in their efforts, though. On the other hand, one must consider the dilemma confronting the cosmetic companies: if they support a research study and the product does not work, they lose money and risk their credibility or reputation. If the product does work, the company faces regulation of its product as a drug and the related time lag to market, or they will be unable to use the research findings in their marketing of the product as a cosmetic. Some of the more savvy companies fund research of their products, and inform dermatologists of the results with the hope that the dermatologists will, in turn, become convinced of the product's efficacy and recommend it to patients or other physicians. In this way, the entire marketing problem is avoided because the dermatologist, rather than the company, is promoting the product.

A legal category called cosmeceuticals that includes products shown to have a biologic function but not subjected to the expensive drug approval process would be ideal. However, many companies and individuals oppose such an enactment because it would likely lead to the regulation of most cosmetic products. For example, in Europe, under the European Economic Cosmetic Directive of 1993, the requirements for cosmetic product labeling became formidable and complex.[2] In contrast, companies in the US do not have to demonstrate either efficacy or safety prior to marketing their products. Of course, all reputable companies ensure the safety of their products before distributing them; however, astonishingly, they are technically not required to do so.

What should cosmetic dermatologists do to protect patients and themselves in an atmosphere in which companies are not required to research, or to release their research, on the efficacy and safety of cosmetic products? Fortunately, many individuals are beginning to independently investigate these products and their claims and to publish the findings in peer-reviewed journals. Poster presentations at meetings are also a helpful source of information. Companies seem more likely to present their findings in a poster format; however, it is important to remember that these posters are often not peer reviewed. Some companies will provide unpublished research data on request to interested physicians. The Cosmetic Toiletry and Fragrance Association (CTFA) publishes a helpful guide called the Cosmetic Ingredient Review. It is designed to review and document the safety of cosmetic ingredients. An expert scientific panel examines worldwide published and unpublished safety data in an independent and unbiased manner. Finally, all cosmetic dermatologists who hope to preserve and enhance the integrity of the field should insist that manufacturers of cosmetic products and procedures supply well-controlled published studies to support their claims. If these dermatologists and, later, consumers refuse to buy products lacking an evidence-based medicine approach, the studies will eventually be performed and certainly lead to exciting new developments in the field of cosmeceuticals.

SELF-REGULATION: THE NATIONAL ADVERTISING DIVISION

The National Advertising Division (NAD) of the Council of Better Business Bureaus (http://www.nadreview.org/) is a self-monitoring society to which companies can report other companies for making false claims about products. The NAD renders a decision, with the intention of objectively, quickly, and privately reaching a settlement. The goal is to promote truth in advertising and, in the process, keep government from getting involved in the process and avoid costly litigation. The US Federal Trade Commission (FTC) also can play a role and sanction companies that lack the data to support its claims. Of dermatologic interest, the NAD recently recommended that Skin Doctors Cosmeceuticals alter its claims regarding its "Eyetuck AntiBag Technology," particularly its favorable comparisons to plastic surgery. The NAD deemed that it was inappropriate for manufacturers of a product that works only on the skin surface compare, without substantiating evidence, their cream/serum to plastic surgery procedures that penetrate into the skin.[3]

ORGANIC SKIN CARE

History

The term "organic" can be traced back to 1940. J.I. Rodale, who founded the Rodale book and magazine publishing empire with the modest publication *Organic Farming and Gardening*, coined the expression.[4] From then through 1992, when the US Department of Agriculture (USDA) approved the "organic" label and its accompanying standards, organic has mostly applied to agricultural foods and practices. Today, there are government-regulated standards only for organic food and topical products, but clothing and even pet food are now available in organic varieties. Currently, organic milk is far and away the most popular organic product.[5]

Organic plants are never grown with commercial pesticides or hormones, owing to concerns about human health and environmental impact. Although research has yet to prove that organics are healthier than nonorganic products, evidence has been uncovered to indicate why exposures to certain substances in nonorganic products could be harmful. For example, investigators found in a recent study that exposure to a compound derived from pesticides may be associated with male infertility since it lowered circulating testosterone levels in adult men.[6] Other studies have shown that pesticides in the soil, water, and air are harmful to wildlife. Environmentally conscious consumers take this kind of information into account in their product selections, and often opt for certified organic products when available.

Organic Skin and Body Products

Between 1998 and 2004, the use of natural and organic skin and body products rose by 51% according to "Packaged Facts" provided on www.MarketResearch.com. As recently as 2005, there were no rules regarding the use of terms such as organic or natural. Consequently, the use of these labels has typically caused significant confusion. For example, prior to regulation, manufacturers could call their product organic even if it was composed of 90% water (a so-called organic ingredient), with no other organic active ingredients. To rectify this misleading situation (at the request of numerous manufacturers of natural and organic topical products), the USDA enacted new organic standards for skin and body care products in August 2005. Consumers can now purchase skin, body, and hair products with the USDA Organic Seal. A product that contains at least 95% organic ingredients can be legally labeled as organic. A product that contains at least 75% and up to 94% organic ingredients can be labeled as "made with organic ingredients."

The Rules of Organic Production

In organic farming, of food crops or those intended for topical products, farmers eschew synthetic pesticides, hormones, genetic modification of crops, and chemical products. Organic farming also follows traditional agricultural practices intended to enrich the soil, use resources in an environmentally sound manner, and treat livestock humanely. Specifically, a grower of organic ingredients must meet these basic criteria in order for the products to be certified as organic:

1. Abstain from the application of prohibited materials (including synthetic fertilizers, pesticides, and sewage sludge) for 3 years prior to certification and then continually throughout their organic license.
2. Prohibit the use of genetically modified organisms and irradiation.
3. Employ positive soil building, conservation, manure management, and crop rotation practices.
4. Avoid contamination during the processing of organic products.
5. Keep records of all operations (*courtesy of the Organic Consumers' Association*).

Organic Topical Products

While there are no long-term studies documenting the effects of using topical organic products or ingredients, consumers of organic products are usually as interested in what products *do not* contain, as in what they *do* contain. The organic label assures that the key cleansing and conditioning ingredients are derived from organically grown plant products, rather than conventionally grown plants, synthetic chemicals, or petroleum by-products. In addition, topical organic products exclude or minimize any ingredients that could be considered potentially harmful to people, animals, waterways, or the environment.

The Precautionary Principle

Sometimes certain ingredients are excluded from products based on research. In other cases, exclusions are based on the "precautionary principle," which stipulates that until the cumulative impacts and exposures to a broad range of ingredients can be fully assessed, it is best to err on the side of *caution* and limit use. For example, though many chemical ingredients used in cosmetics are widely considered safe for use, some safety factors have not been fully studied. It is virtually impossible to evaluate the *cumulative effects* of repeated exposures from multiple sources. This is important because consumers, especially women, use several skin, hair, and beauty products per day. The ingredients in these products can potentially interact, or lead to a higher combined rate of exposure to certain ingredients than is usually assessed by studying the safety of a single ingredient in the laboratory. Further, to accurately establish the baseline of the chemical exposures people can safely tolerate, it is necessary to account for *all* chemical exposures from food, urban smog, industrial waste, and other sources.

Obviously, the costs of testing for such exposures are too high for individuals and are not part of routine tests at this time. Consequently, it is impractical for each of us to determine our own particular health care risks. In response to such an uncertainty, many consumers who choose organic foods and topical products prefer to limit chemical exposures as a precaution whenever feasible. People with allergies and illnesses may also choose to be more cautious.

Ingredient Cautions

While not all widely used synthetic ingredients are considered problematic, certain ones represent a source for special concern. For example, the parabens (alkyl esters of p-hydroxybenzoic acid) are used as preservatives in many cosmetics as well as skin, hair, and body care products, and can sometimes provoke allergic reactions[7,8] (see Chapters 18 and 37). Parabens can be absorbed via the skin and migrate into the bloodstream and bodily tissue. One controversial study even found high concentrations of parabens in breast cancer tissue.[9] Products containing parabens should be avoided by most people who know they are allergic to parabens. (This can be determined by patch testing.) There are no cogent data to indicate that parabens pose a risk to those not allergic to this group of compounds. Nevertheless, many people opt to abstain from using products containing this type of preservative ingredient.

Toluene, which is found in several nail polish brands, has been associated with deleterious effects on males in utero. Therefore, major companies such as L'Oréal and Revlon as well as manufacturers of natural and organic products have taken steps to eliminate toluene from their nail polishes. Toluene can also induce a skin rash, typically on the eyelids, in people who use toluene-containing nail polishes. There are several other ingredients that warrant caution, but it is important to know that even organic products can cause problems. For example, coconut oil, a popular organic ingredient, can cause acne. Allergies to many essential oils and botanicals can also develop. In addition, because companies were not able to label their products as organic until recently, there have not been sufficient clinical research trials on the organic products on the market. In fact, it is plausible, if not likely, that most of the American manufacturers of organic brands are just using the label for marketing purposes without proof that their products are efficacious. In particular, the organic sunscreens available in the US are remarkably suboptimal.

Natural Ingredients

It is important to note that a product that is touted as natural is not necessarily organic. The product may contain aloe, vitamin E, or other natural ingredients, but it may also contain chemicals intended to act as preservatives or to improve its texture. Only products that are truly organic are legally permitted to use the organic seal.

Of course, problems or allergic responses can be associated with ingredients that are natural, and/or organic. For instance, many natural and organic brands contain certain fragrances and essential oils that can cause dermatitis. Oil of bergamot and balsam of Peru are both highly allergenic, so even an organic product containing them could irritate sensitive individuals. Organic products that include strong essential oils such as peppermint or rosemary can also irritate or inflame sensitive skin. Chamomile, generally considered a gentle and soothing herb, can induce allergies in some people (who may also tend to be allergic to wheat). Furthermore, conventional products as well as some natural ones contain a "perfume mix" to mask their odor. Components of the perfume mix are rarely listed on the product label since each company uses its own proprietary blend. Even a product listed as 95% organic could contain a perfume mix that might provoke allergic reactions in some people.

Skin Type and Product Choice

Although patients may express preferences among organic, natural, and conventional product options, such considerations should be superseded, from a practitioner's perspective, by identifying a patient's skin type and making appropriate product recommendations. For example, an organic body lotion containing whole soy oil could be suitable for a patient with nonpigmented skin. But, for a patient with pigmented skin, that same product could exacerbate the propensity to melasma and pigmentation. For such patients, opting for a soy product with the estrogenic components removed, thus not considered organic because it has been altered, is preferable to a naturally occurring soy product. Fractionated soy, also known as "active soy," has had the estrogenic components removed. Active soy is contained in several Neutrogena products and in Aveeno's Positively Radiant line. As another example, a patient with dry, wrinkled skin would benefit from using green tea formulations, of which several product options are organic. However, the Topix product Replenix™ has a higher level of green tea polyphenols than any of the organic products currently on the market. In addition, a patient who strictly uses organic products, but who has oily, wrinkle-prone skin, would benefit from using retinoids, even though they are not organic. There are no organic products that have the actions of retinoids.

Is Organic Better?

There is no question that many natural products have proven benefits when topically applied to the skin. Green tea is a good example of a natural ingredient with demonstrated benefits. However, does it matter whether or not the green tea is organic? Likely, it is the form and concentration of the ingredient that is more important or influential than whether it is organic. In the case of green tea, we know the EGCG form is the strongest. When green tea is placed in skin care products in a high enough concentration to be effective, it turns the product brown. It is likely that organic products in the near future will improve and have increased amounts of active ingredients because consumers have shown that they want this. If a product contains the right ingredients for the patient's skin type, and an organic product is available with active levels of that ingredient, then organic is a better option overall. Using organic products can help the environment as well because they can prevent the build-up of parabens and other substances in the environment. The farming methods used to produce them are better for the environment and the packaging is often biodegradable. Once the organic product manufacturers perform trials showing efficacy of their products, they will likely be embraced by skin care professionals and consumers alike.

What About Synthetic Products?

In many cases, it is only the chemical ingredients, such as retinoids, that confer desired benefits and no analogous organic products are available. It is important for practitioners to guide patients in product selection and explain to them the benefits of nonorganic products such as retinoids. A person using retinoids can supplement with natural and organic products, thereby enhancing exposure to beneficial ingredients while limiting the use of synthetic ingredients to only the ones needed. Jurlique is a great example of a company that, while not currently certified as organic, strives to manufacture a pure product line, especially oriented toward and beneficial to people with sensitive skin. Jurlique comes from Australia, a country that has long embraced the idea of organic or natural products. Aesop, another skin care line from Australia, has a large following of organic product customers. Liz Earle is a natural line from the UK. Clarins and Aveeno have been producing natural products for years. In addition, Origins now has a large organic skin care line, and Stella McCartney markets a few such products.

SUMMARY

It is fair to say that products considered cosmeceuticals fall through the regulatory loopholes in laws governing the testing and labeling of drugs and cosmetics. In turn, such rules affect the kind of information readily accessible to the medical establishment that can be used to guide patients. Whether one is considering the merits of a well-tested drug versus an unregulated cosmeceutical, or an unregulated organic product versus an unregulated synthetic one, dermatologists can best advise their patients with more, not less or hidden, evidence.

Of course, with the proper time and attention, most patients/consumers can find the right blend of products suited to their particular skin type. As a practitioner, it is best to keep such concerns at the forefront of your recommendations, while trying to honor a patient's stated preferences. Now that companies are allowed to label their products as organic, these products may become more sophisticated. In fact, these manufacturers may research their products to establish efficacy and safety. It remains important, though, to indicate the advantages and disadvantages of any products that you might recommend. If a certain ingredient is good for a patient, and it is in an organic product, it is suitable for recommendation. If a patient needs a particular ingredient that cannot be found in organic products, broadening the patient's scope to include the conventional product that will best meet the needs of their skin is warranted. Generally, if an ingredient is right for a patient's skin type and it is found in a sufficient form and concentration in the product, then selecting the natural or organic product is perfectly acceptable. However, there are not many well researched naturals on the market and there are even fewer, if any, well researched organic products at this time. Much more nonproprietary research is needed, particularly in the form of randomized controlled trials, to provide sufficient evidence of the efficacy of organic products. Of course, if such products impart a quantifiable biologic action, the potential marketing outlook might significantly alter the manufacturer's plans. The legal and business morass, which affects patients/consumers, physicians, and manufacturers, requires a concerted effort by legislators and the business community to resolve. Despite the recent improvement in the law governing the labeling of organics, a similar solution for the very broad category of cosemeceuticals does not appear to be in the offing.

REFERENCES

1. Kligman A. Cosmeceuticals: do we need a new category? In: Elsner P, Maibach H, eds. *Cosmeceuticals*. New York, NY: Marcel Dekker Inc; 2000:1.
2. Rogiers V. Efficacy claims of cosmetics in Europe must be scientifically substantiated from 1997 on. *Skin Res Technol.* 1995;1:44.
3. National Advertising Division. Skin doctors cosmeceuticals partcipates in NAD forum. http://www.nadreview.org/NewsRoom.asp?PageContext=18776461033183889&SessionID=1242402. Accessed February 27, 2008.
4. *Organic Gardening,* March 1998;22–25.
5. Severson K. An organic cash cow. *New York Times*. November 9, 2005. http://www.nytimes.com/2005/11/09/dining/09milk.html?_r=1&oref=slogin. Accessed February 27, 2008.
6. Meeker JD, Ryan L, Barr DB, et al. Exposure to nonpersistent insecticides and male reproductive hormones. *Epidemiology*. 2006;17:61.
7. Gilman AG, Goodman LS, Gilman A, eds. *Goodman and Gilman's The Pharmacological Basis of Therapeutics*. 6th ed. New York, NY: Macmillan Publishing Co. Inc; 1980:969.
8. Sax NI. The Butyl, Ethyl, Methy, and Propyl Esters have been found to promote allergic sensitization in humans. In: *Dangerous Properties of Industrial Materials*. 4th ed. New York, NY: Van Nostrand Reinhold; 1975:929.
9. Vince G. Cosmetic chemicals found in breast tumours. *New Scientist.com news service*, 12:24, January 12, 2004. Accessed February 27, 2008.

CHAPTER 29

Sunscreens

Leslie Baumann, MD
Nidhi Avashia, MD
Mari Paz Castanedo-Tardan, MD

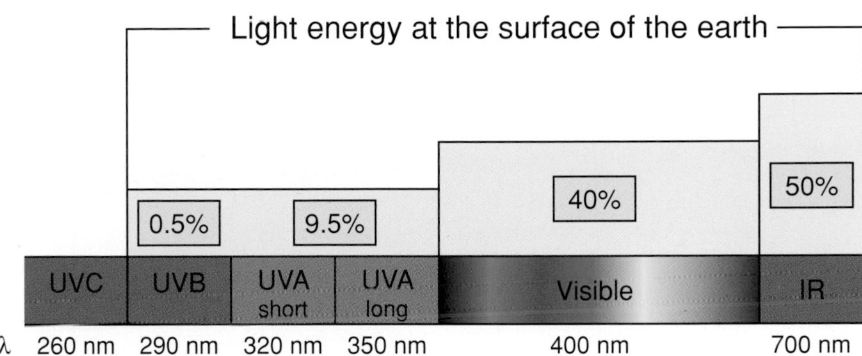

▲ **FIGURE 29-1** Solar wavelengths. On a normal day, UVA is the predominant UV type at the surface of the earth.

For several years, dermatologists have exhorted their patients to avoid or, at the very least, severely limit exposure to the sun since ultraviolet (UV) radiation is the primary cause of skin cancer, exogenous skin aging, wrinkles, and blotchy pigmentation.[1] In spite of these attempts to educate the public, the incidence of skin cancer is increasing at a disturbing rate. In 2005, there were an estimated 60,000 melanoma cases diagnosed in the US. Alarmingly, there are approximately 8000 deaths in the US related to this most potent and fatal of the skin cancers per year.[2] Cosmetic patients offer a captive and interested audience that can be educated about the hazards of the sun and the need for corresponding protective behavior. Of all the skin care advice that is doled out to patients, it is likely that this is the most important, because proper protection from the sun will make a great difference in the patient's future appearance. Patients should be advised that if they do not avoid the sun and practice protective measures, they are wasting their money on cosmetic products and procedures.

Obviously, the daily use of sunscreen is an important adjunct to skin protective behavior. However, because no sunscreen can effectively block all parts of the UV spectrum, sun avoidance, protective clothing and hats, and window shields can all be utilized to lessen acute and cumulative sun exposure. Patients should be instructed about the proper use of sunscreen and asked about sunscreen use at every visit. This constant nagging will help them realize how important it is to protect their skin from the sun. Even if patients claim to use sunscreen and know about the hazards of the sun, studies have shown that they still do not get enough sun protection. In fact, it is known that mothers provide more sun protection to their children than to themselves,[3] and that sun protection attitudes tend to subside from childhood to adolescence.[4] Even well-intentioned sunscreen users can forget the rules. For example, one study found that 98% of 352 family groups applied their sunscreen after arrival at the beach, instead of 30 minutes before as is suggested for optimal sun protection.[5] This chapter discusses the practical aspects of sunscreen formulations and selection, which should enhance the practitioner's ability to help patients find the best sunscreen protection for their skin type and lifestyle as well as answer patients' numerous product questions.

ULTRAVIOLET A AND B

On a typical summer day, UVA comprises about 96.5% of the UV radiation reaching earth, leaving UVB only with the remaining 3.5%.[6] When compared with all kinds of light reaching the earth's surface, UVA makes up 9.5% (Fig. 29-1). While UVA is the predominant UV light reaching the surface of the earth, UVB exposure is more likely to cause squamous cell carcinoma in an experimental setting.[7] This supports the usage of sunscreens intended to block UVB. The first sunscreens that were developed were designed to prevent erythema (skin reddening) and sunburning by blocking UVB, and did little to block UVA. UVA leads to immunosuppression and is thought to play a role in the development of melanoma.[8] Therefore, both UVA and UVB sunscreens should be used. UV light exerts its carcinogenic effect on the skin by inducing mutations in DNA. DNA is considered a chromophore for UV light. Although maximum UV absorption by DNA occurs at 260 nm, UVB is considered a major source of DNA damage.[9] UV irradiation results in DNA damage by formation of two dimers between adjacent pyrimidines, cyclobutane pyrimidine dimers (CPDs), and pyrimidine 6 to 4 photoproducts. Nucleotide excision repair (NER) enzymes are responsible for removal of these carcinogenic products. If not repaired, mutations in the DNA sequence also known as UV "signature mutations" may occur.

UVB is blocked by glass and the amount of UVB that reaches the earth's surface varies by the time of day, with maximal rays reaching the earth from 10 AM to 4 PM. UVA radiation, on the other hand, can pass through glass (Fig. 29-2). Its ability to reach the earth's surface remains more constant regardless of the time of day or the amount of cloud cover (Fig. 29-3). UVA penetrates deeper into the skin, contributing to cutaneous wrinkling and aging. UVA radiation is also known to cause damage to the dermal layer of the skin (Fig. 29-4). In a study performed by Lavker et al., repeated exposures to suberythemic doses of UVA resulted in greater epidermal thickness, in addition to deposition of lysosomes on elastin fibers, as well as decreased Langerhans cells and dermal inflammatory infiltrates.[10] Unfortunately, the sun protection factor (SPF) primarily assesses the protective effects against UVB light, leaving UVA out of the picture. In other words, if SPF 45 is on a

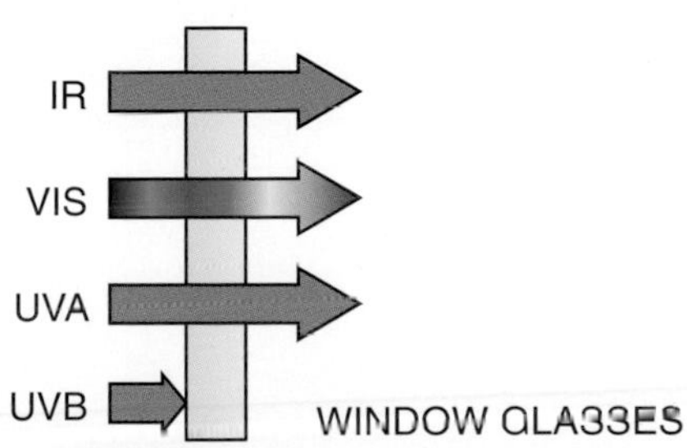

▲ **FIGURE 29-2** UVB is blocked by glass while infrared (IR), visible (VIS), and UVA light can penetrate glass. New plastic coatings are available to coat glass to prevent UVA penetration.

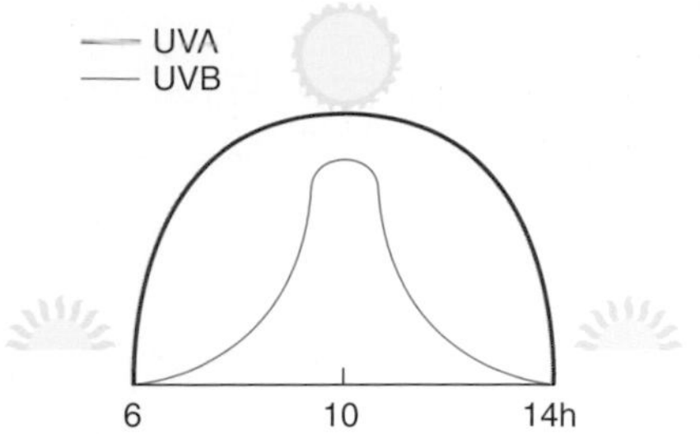

▲ **FIGURE 29-3** UVA rays reach the earth's surface throughout the day, as opposed to UVB, which reaches the earth maximally between 10 AM and 4 PM.

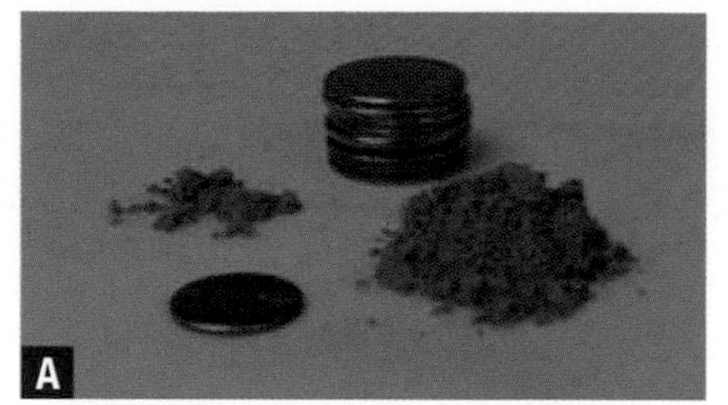

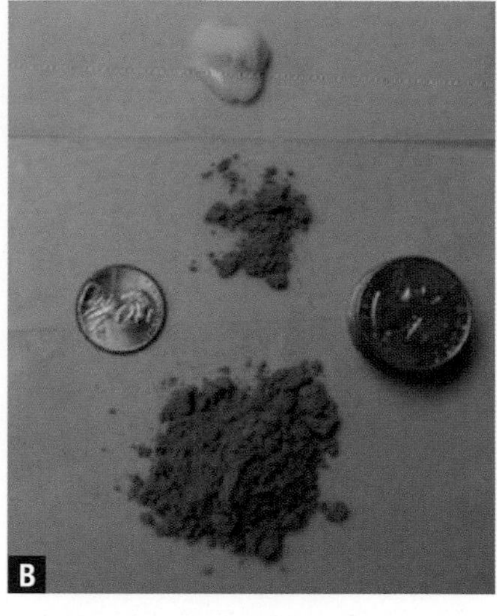

▲ **FIGURE 29-5 A.** The powder on the left is the amount of powder the average woman uses, while the powder pile on the right is the amount of powder necessary to use to meet the SPF on the sunscreen label. The white lotion is the amount of facial lotion required to use on the face to meet the SPF on the label. **B.** The same image viewed from above. In the upper portion of this photo is the amount of facial lotion required to use on the face to meet the SPF on the product label, while the large pile of powder is the amount needed to cover the face with powder to achieve the SPF on the label.

label, this applies to UVB protection only and gives no information about the protection against UVA radiation.

SUN PROTECTION FACTOR

The SPF represents the ability of a sunscreen to delay sun-induced skin erythema, which is a visible sign of damage mainly caused by UVB radiation. SPF is defined technically as the level of sun exposure needed to produce a minimal erythema dose divided by the amount of energy required to produce the same erythema on unprotected skin. In theory, a subject that applies an SPF 10 sunscreen on uncovered skin could stay in the sun 10 times longer without incurring a visible skin erythemal reaction. The SPF is determined through testing on the untanned skin of human volunteers (generally the back or the upper part of the buttocks).

The internationally agreed upon standard quantity of sunscreen per unit of skin surface (i.e., the sunscreen thickness) required to measure the SPF in humans is 2 mg/cm^2 of skin.[11] For an adult to apply this amount of sunscreen to the entire body, 30 mL of sunscreen would be required to obtain that thickness.[12] In most cases people do not apply enough sunscreen.[13] Facial powders, for example, are impossible to apply in an amount sufficient to equal the 2 mg/cm^2 of skin that is used in testing to determine the SPF. The average face is about 600 cm^2; therefore, a person would need to apply about 1.2 g of facial powder to get the SPF stated on the product's label. Most women apply only about 0.085 g of powder at a time. In other words, one would have to apply 14 times the amount of powder normally used to be sufficiently protected against the sun (Fig. 29-5). Facial SPF lotion applications tend to amount to about 0.8 g per average application, as measured in the primary author's practice. Therefore, individuals would need to use about 1.5 times the amount of facial lotion they are accustomed to using in order to achieve the SPF on the label. In fact, a recent study demonstrated that most users probably achieve a mean SPF of between 20% and 50% of that expected from the product label because they do not apply the sunscreen as thickly as is performed in laboratory conditions.[14] The key is applying sufficient amounts of sunscreen evenly across a given area to achieve the intended solar protection.

The notion of inadequate sunscreen application was also suggested by a study of European students that found that the students used approximately one-fifth of the recommended sunscreen quantity.[12] A useful rule-of-thumb is that the protection most people ultimately obtain from a sunscreen is equal to about one-third of the SPF. So applying an SPF-15 sunscreen at a typical application thickness to the face provides about five-fold protection, not 15-fold.[15] While still counseling patients on the proper amount of sunscreen to apply, it is advisable to recommend the highest SPF sunscreen that the patient can tolerate to compensate for this discrepancy.

In the past, the SPF system was based mainly on UVB (280–315 nm) exposure, which is responsible for the immediate reddening seen on the skin. It is important to remember that UVA-associated reddening is seen much later and, therefore, UVA exposure and dose would not be accounted for in the current methods of measuring SPF. UVA light is also responsible for darkening pigment seen after sun exposure. Because of the damaging effects of UVA, there is new

Solar wavelengths

Solar spectrum	UVC	UVB	UVA	VISIBLE	IR
Wavelengths (nm)	200	290	320	400	800
Stratospheric ozone layer					
Solar spectrum reaching the surface of the earth					
Skin outer layer (stratum corneum)					
Epidermis					
Dermis					
Hypodermis					

▲ **FIGURE 29-4** UVA, visible light, and infrared radiation can penetrate into the dermis, while UVB cannot.

research regarding the incorporation of UVA (320–400 nm) into the sun protection index. Globally, there are several UVA rating systems and the FDA is currently trying to decide which rating system to make the standard in the US. Because there is no consensus standard for UVA testing, products in the US do not provide any UVA coverage information on the product label. This is obviously a significant problem.

THE FDA AND SUNCREEN

As this textbook went to press, the FDA was considering the problem of UVA and sunscreen labeling. In August 2007, the FDA proposed the creation of a new rating system for UVA sunscreen products.[16] This system would be based on a scale of one to four stars, with one star representing low UVA protection, two stars, medium protection, three stars, high protection, and four stars, the highest UVA protection available in an OTC sunscreen product. Under this proposal, a sunscreen product that fails to provide at least a low level (one star) of protection would bear a "no UVA protection" marking on the front label near the SPF value. In addition, a warning would be required on labels stating: "UV exposure from the sun increases the risk of skin cancer, premature skin aging, and other skin damage. It is important to decrease UV exposure by limiting time in the sun, wearing protective clothing, and using a sunscreen." It is hoped that this warning will increase awareness that sun avoidance and limiting sun exposure are also necessary. This proposal has not yet been accepted and the star rating system was not yet in place when this chapter was completed. Search www.fda.gov to find out the current sunscreen rulings.

TESTING TO DETERMINE UVA PROTECTION

As suggested above, ascertaining the optimal UVA rating method is difficult and even contentious. Each manufacturer believes that the method they use is the best. L'Oréal developed the persistent pigment darkening (PPD) method,[17] while Johnson & Johnson developed the protection factor UVA (PFA) method.[18] The PPD and PFA are very similar approaches in that they both measure end-result tanning.[19] The FDA has not yet determined which UVA measurement method is best because all methods lack an endpoint measure that is a true surrogate marker for long wavelength (i.e., >340 nm) UVA induced skin damage (i.e., skin cancer or photoaging).[19] The FDA seems to be most seriously considering two methods of UVA testing: the critical wavelength method and the PFA (PA) method. The critical wavelength was developed in 1994 and is an in vitro testing method.[20] It involves placing a certain amount of sunscreen on a slide and exposing the slide to progressively higher wavelengths of light starting at 290 nm, the beginning of the UVB range. When 10% of the incident light passes through the slide, or the protection provided by the sunscreen has dropped to 90%, the corresponding wavelength of light is recorded. For sunscreens with SPF 15 or above, this is a good measure of UVA protection. If one is testing a low-SPF product, below SPF 15, this is thought to be a suboptimal method.

The PFA (PA) method is similar to the UVB SPF rating insofar as it is an in vivo test that measures what is in essence the tanning effect of short wavelength UVA rays (320–350 nm).[21] This is widely used in Europe. However, the PFA (PA) system measures an observed effect (tanning), not the biologic endpoint. It is possible that the FDA will recommend a combination of the critical wavelength and PFA (PA) methods (Tables 29-1 and 29-2 for a brief summary of the three types of tests to ascertain sunscreen efficacy and for related non-US standards).

Another approach to measuring UVA involves the quantitative measurement of free radicals in human skin induced by UV radiation.[22] Reactive free radicals have been correlated with the occurrence of skin damage such as cancer and skin aging. The method of measuring free radicals is known as electron spin resonance (ESR) spectroscopy. This technique incorporates the radical trapping properties of nitroxides. Nitroxides are antioxidant

TABLE 29-1
Three Types of Tests to Determine Sunscreen Efficacy

	Sun Protection Factor (SPF)	UVA Protection Factor (UVAPF)	Broad-Spectrum Protection and Photostability
Goal	To protect skin against UVB (and some UVA) wavelengths	To protect skin from developing persistent pigment darkening (PPD) induced by UVA exposure	To provide broad-spectrum protection against UVB and UVA; to prevent rapid degradation from UV exposure
Method(s)	Testing on humans to compare time of exposure necessary to induce mild skin reddening, or minimum erythema dose (MED), in absence of the product with time needed to induce the same MED in the presence of the product	Testing on humans to compare the time of exposure necessary to induce mild skin darkening in the absence of the product with the time required to induce the same level of darkening in the presence of the product	Laboratory testing to measure the absorbance of light at each wavelength, arriving at a relative ratio of absorbance in the UVB and UVA ranges as well as photostability. The most common measure of broad-spectrum efficacy is critical wavelength (CW).[a] Photostability is measured as the ratio of the absorbance of the formula before irradiation to the absorbance of the formula after irradiation with a particular UV amount.
Result	This ratio = SPF	This ratio = UVAPF	Broad spectrum, if CW ≥370 nm[b]; the photostability value = Beta-value

[a]The FDA may use the same test with a slightly different measurement, considering the ratio of longer wavelength UVA1 (340–400 nm) compared to the total UV (UVA+UVB absorbance).

[b]This is the standard in the European Union (EU) and will be soon adopted in the Association of Southeast Asian Nations (ASEAN).

TABLE 29-2
EU and ASEAN Standards for Sunscreens

SPF	PPD	CW	LABEL
≥6	≥ one-third of the SPF value (e.g., the PPD ≥5 for an SPF 15 product; PPD ≥10 for SPF 30)	≥370 nm	Products that meet all 3 criteria = labeled as broad spectrum; products that do not = labeled as NOT providing UVA protection

and anticancer substances. In a recent study, the nitroxides TEMPO, PCM, and PCA were used because of their known capacity to trap reactive free radicals in skin exposed to UV irradiation. The effects of UV radiation on the nitroxides can be measured because they reduce to hydroxylamines. The nitroxide PCA is found universally in skin and is solely reduced by UV-generated free radicals and reactive oxygen species (ROS) making it possible to estimate the penetration of UVA and UVB irradiation. UV irradiation decreases the PCA intensity, and this reduction has been shown to be engendered mainly by UVA radiation. Therefore, using ESR, the in vivo detection of UV-generated free radicals/ROS via the reduction of the nitroxide PCA in human skin should be possible.[23]

An additional method used to assess UVA radiation damage is comparing the accumulation levels of p53, which is known to be a very important tumor suppressor gene. Mutations in p53 have been noted in more than 90% of squamous cell carcinoma, 50% of basal cell carcinoma, and 60% of actinic keratoses.[24] Expression of p53 is used to quantify skin damage associated with UV-related skin damage and can be used to evaluate the effectiveness of sunscreens.

In a recent study, two sunscreens with identical SPF but varying UVA protection factors were evaluated using the PPD method.[25] The PPD is a measure of the amount of darkening pigment that is present a day or so after sun exposure.[24] The SPF of the sunscreens was 7, while the UVA protection factor (UVA-PF) determined in vivo using the PPD method was 7 for one product and 3 for the other. The amount of p53 was also measured in skin exposed to UV radiation. The results showed that only partial protection was afforded by the two sunscreens with identical SPF, but there was a lower level of p53 in the areas of skin treated with the sunscreen of higher UVA protection factor. The results portrayed a marked increase in the amount of p53 in the skin with increasing exposure to higher levels of UVA radiation. These results confirmed that SPF based on erythemal reaction caused by UVB does not accurately predict the level of protection conferred against UVA damage from sun exposure.[25]

Other Sunscreen Terminology

A sunscreen is considered **water resistant** if the SPF level is determined effective after 40 minutes of water immersion. The testing procedure for these sunscreens is as follows: the subjects must swim in an indoor pool for 20 minutes followed by air drying (not towel drying) the skin. The subjects are then asked to swim for another 20 minutes followed by an air drying period. The water-resistant sunscreen SPF is then measured after the total 40 minutes of water contact.[26] The FDA requires that the SPF listed on the label reflect the SPF that is achieved after this water-resistant testing rather than the SPF value present before testing.

Sunscreens that are labeled **very water resistant** have been shown to exhibit an effective SPF after undergoing the following testing: the subjects swim in an indoor pool for 20 minutes then air dry for 20 minutes. The procedure is repeated for a total of 80 minutes of water immersion. If a sunscreen retains its protective integrity after four 20-minute water immersions, it is considered **very water resistant.** It is important to note that the word "waterproof" is no longer allowed in labeling because it is misleading. No sunscreen is completely waterproof.

The lipophilic base of the vehicle used in these "water-resistant" formulations allows the products to adhere well to the skin, though their typically greasy feel is not often welcome by users. Depending on the ingredients used, the higher SPF formulations tend to be oilier or more opaque.

SUNSCREEN CLASSIFICATION

The two generally recognized major types of sunscreen products are chemical and physical.

Physical Sunscreens

Barrier sunscreens, known more commonly as physical sunscreens, scatter or reflect UV radiation and are rarely associated with allergic reactions. These sunscreens block the widest range of light including UV, visible, and infrared spectra, and are recommended for use especially when intense sun exposure, such as at the beach or at high altitudes, is expected. Patients with sensitive skin are more likely to tolerate this type of sunscreen, as opposed to the chemical variety. Titanium dioxide (TiO_2), magnesium oxide, iron oxide, and zinc oxide (ZnO) are the primary ingredients in physical sunscreens. The older formulations require a thick layer of application, melt in the sun, stain clothing, and can be comedogenic. Some of these agents are so opaque that they are visible and, consequently, often cosmetically unacceptable to most people. Some manufacturers have marketed opaque products in bright colors specifically designed for use by children.

Cosmetically acceptable translucent or colloidal suspensions that consist of micronized preparations of ZnO and TiO_2 have been recently developed. These formulations are popular because they remain on the skin's surface and are not systemically absorbed. This minimizes irritation and sensitization, and maximizes their safety profile.[27] In fact, there have been no reports of contact allergy to these components.[28] In the early 1990s, microfine ZnO became available.[29] Microfine ZnO absorbs appreciably more UV light in the long-wave UVA spectrum from 340 to 380 nm. The only other sunscreen ingredient approved for use in the US that protects against this UVA spectrum is the organic chemical avobenzone. Because avobenzone is photolabile in UV light, its protective ability is uncertain.[30] Notably, ZnO and TiO_2 are not photolabile. However, new photostable formulations of avobenzone have been developed. Formulations containing micronized ZnO or TiO_2 are the most often recommended products for sensitive skin types; however, ZnO or TiO_2 products are not interchangeable. Microfine TiO_2 effectively attenuates UVB (290–320 nm) and UVA2 (320–340 nm); however, it is less effective than ZnO in the UVA1 range (>340 nm).[29] Microfine ZnO has a particle size of less than 0.2 μm. At this size, visible light scattering is minimized and the particles appear transparent in thin films.[31] TiO_2 has a higher refractive index in visible light than ZnO (2.6 for TiO_2 and 1.9 for ZnO); therefore, TiO_2 is whiter and more difficult to incorporate into transparent products than is ZnO.

One problem with metal oxides that contain physical sunscreens, though, is that they may produce oxygen free radicals at their surface when irradiated. The photoreactivity of metal oxides has been extensively studied,[32] and it even has been suggested that photoactive metal oxides may initiate deleterious events in the skin. Generally, TiO_2 is much more photoactive than ZnO as shown in a report by Mitchnick et al.[29] TiO_2 has even been shown to damage DNA in in vitro studies.[33] However, to affect skin, the particles would have to traverse the stratum corneum. Since particles of microfine ZnO and TiO_2 are too large to enter the skin, they would not be expected to be biologically active. Most companies minimize the photoreactivity of these agents by coating the surface with dimethicone or silicone.[34]

Chemical Sunscreens

Chemical sunscreens are usually combined with physical sunscreens or with each other to form high-SPF products that can be used during times of significant sun exposure. However, they have several drawbacks. Chemical sunscreens absorb UV radiation. The absorbed radiation must then be dissipated as either heat or light, or else be used in some chemical reaction. This may result in the creation of ROS or photoproducts that can attack other chemicals in a formulation; if absorbed, such by-products can attack the skin itself (see Chapters. 6 and 34 for a discussion of free radicals and antioxidants). However, in most cases, the radiation simply is emitted again at a longer wavelength and does not lead to free radical formation.[29]

Chemical sunscreens are composed of synthetically prepared organic chemicals that can be broadly labeled as UVB- or UVA-absorbing substances. These colorless, often-odorless agents prevent UV radiation from penetrating the epidermis by acting as filters as they absorb and reflect UV radiation. Many chemical sunscreens have been reported to cause allergic or photoallergic reactions in susceptible patients. Another drawback of chemical sunscreens is that some of them are unstable when exposed to UV radiation. For example, a 15-minute exposure of solar-simulated light has been reported to destroy 36% of avobenzone.[30] Moreover, as avobenzone degrades, other organic sunscreen agents in the formula may be destroyed as well.[35] Some chemical sunscreens are systemically absorbed and levels have been demonstrated in the urine of humans using the product.[36] For this reason, chemical sunscreens should not be used in children younger than 2 years of age. Several popular chemical sunscreen additives will be discussed below.

STABILITY OF SUNSCREENS

One of the main requirements in the development of a sunscreen is that the product be photostable, or maintain its intended protection for a limited time before inevitable breakdown caused by UV exposure. Photostability is characterized by the effect of light on the degradation of certain substances. The photostability of a sunscreen depends on varying factors such as which filters were used, as well as the types of UV filters, solvents, and vehicles. A common means of measuring and quantifying photostability is through the comet assay test. This test is a method to measure DNA damage in cells. It is categorized as a gel-electrophoresis-based test.[37] Recent studies have attempted to evaluate the stability of sunscreens. Avobenzone, a common filter in sunscreens and potent absorber of UV radiation, has been shown to be increasingly photolabile. For this reason, new photostable forms of avobenzone (such as Helioplex™) have been developed. Recent findings have suggested adding Tinosorb, a UVA filter, in conjunction with avobenzone to improve the photostability of avobenzone. When Tinosorb is combined with avobenzone, it prevents avobenzone's degradation caused by UV irradiation.[38] In another study, four different UV filters commonly used in SPF-15 sunscreens were compared using HPLC analysis and spectrophotometry. The following were the UV filter combinations tested: octyl methoxycinnamate (OMC), benzophenone-3 (BP-3), and octyl salicylate (OS) (formulation 1); OMC, avobenzone (AVB), and 4-methylbenzilidene camphor (MBC) (formulation 2); OMC, BP-3, and octocrylene (OC) (formulation 3); and OMC, AVB, and OC (formulation 4). The results showed that all four of the UV filter combinations portrayed varying photostability. The best results were shown by formulation 3 (OMC, BP-3, and OC), followed by, in descending order, formulations 4, 1, and 2. In addition, OC improved the photostability of OMC, AVB, and BP-3.[39] For this reason, many sunscreens on the market contain combinations of sunscreen ingredients.

A novel formulation called UV Pearls utilizes microencapsulation technology to entrap organic sunscreen chemicals in a sol-gel silica glass. This makes it possible to incorporate hydrophobic UV filters into the aqueous phase of sunscreen formulations. The "encapsulation of sunscreens" allows physical separation between organic and inorganic ingredients. This results in an increased overall photostability in sunscreen products. In addition, it is believed that encapsulating UV filters will significantly decrease the dermal uptake of these UV filters, and reduce the amount of free radicals generated by keeping the organic filters on the top layers of the skin. This reduces penetration into the deeper layers and decreases the risk of contact dermatitis.[40]

UVB-ABSORBING SUNSCREEN FORMULATIONS

Para-aminobenzoic Acid

Poorly soluble in water, thus only suitable for alcohol-containing vehicles, para-aminobenzoic acid (PABA) was one of the first commonly used sunscreen ingredients. PABA established a reputation for inducing a stinging sensation in the skin and staining both cotton and synthetic fabrics. Later formulations were labeled as "PABA-free" because of the widespread negative publicity associated with such characteristics. To skirt this problem, manufacturers developed PABA derivatives, which are water soluble and unable to penetrate the stratum corneum. Octyl diethyl PABA or padimate O, a potent absorber of UVB, is the main derivative used. Photoallergic reactions have been reported in association with the use of PABA and its derivatives.

Cinnamates

This category of compounds has largely replaced PABA derivatives. Octyl methoxycinnamate (OMC), with a UV absorption maximum of 310 nm, is the most commonly used. Several cosmetic products, including makeup foundations, lipsticks, and leave-in hair conditioners, contain this compound. The Freeze 24/7 Iceshield uses the UV Pearl technology in which OMC is encapsulated in sol-gel silica glass and formulated into a wash-on sunscreen. In other words, it is a cleanser that deposits sunscreen on the skin with cleansing. This is a great option for people who do not like the greasy feel of sunscreen (men in particular are reputed to complain about greasy formulations). Because cinnamates are poorly soluble in water, they do not wash off with cleansing and are often included in water-resistant and very water-resistant sunscreens. Although allergy to these agents is unusual, photoallergic reactions have been reported in association with the use of formulations containing cinnamates. It is believed that coating the particles with the sol-gel silica glass may decrease the incidence of allergy. Patients allergic to this compound may also be allergic to fragrances and flavorings that contain cinnamic aldehyde and cinnamon oil.[41]

Salicylates

With a UV absorption maximum at 310 nm, salicylates are used to augment the UVB protection in sunscreens. Octyl salicylate (2-ethyl hexyl salicylate) and homosalate (homomenthyl salicylate) are the most popular salicylates in sunscreens. These compounds are stable, nonsensitizing, and water insoluble, yielding high substantivity. The chemical properties of salicylates render them highly suitable for combination with other chemical sunscreen agents, such as benzophenones, in cosmetic formulations. In fact, salicylates are used only in combination with other UV filters because they are too weak to be the sole active filtering ingredients. Contact allergy to salicylates is very rare.

Phenylbenzimidazole Sulfonic Acid

In contrast to other UV filters that are soluble in the oil phase, phenylbenzimidazole sulfonic acid (PSA) is water soluble. As a result, this ingredient imparts a less oily feel to sunscreen formulations. Unfortunately, PSA, like salicylates, is a selective UVB filter and allows almost full UVA transmission. This compound may be more suitable in combination with other filters.

UVA-ABSORBING SUNSCREEN FORMULATIONS

Benzophenones

The absorption range for benzophenones is predominantly in the UVA portion of the light spectrum between 320 and 350 nm. Oxybenzone, which is frequently used to augment UVB protection, has an absorption maximum at 326 nm. This compound is also one of the best blockers of UVA2 (shorter UVA wavelengths) available in the US. Oxybenzone is a very common sunscreen component and it is estimated that 20% to 30% of sunscreens contain this chemical.[42] Unfortunately, oxybenzone is currently the most common sunscreen agent to cause photoallergic contact dermatitis.[41] One case report described a 22-year-old female that developed anaphylaxis after widespread application of a sunscreen containing oxybenzone.[42] The allergy to oxybenzone was later confirmed by skin testing. Further, it has been well established that systemic absorption of oxybenzone occurs. A study in the *Lancet* demonstrated in humans that application of substantial amounts of a sunscreen containing oxybenzone resulted in the oxybenzone being absorbed and subsequently excreted in urine.[36] Oxybenzone has low acute toxicity in animal studies yet little is known about its chronic toxicity and disposition after topical application in humans.[43] For this reason, sunscreens containing this agent are not recommended for use in children.

Menthyl Anthranilate

The absorption peak for this compound is at 340 nm. Consequently, it is a weak UVB filter, but offers effective UVA2 protection. Menthyl anthranilate is less widely used than benzophenone because it is less effective.

Parsol 1789

Parsol 1789 (avobenzone or butyl methoxydibenzoylmethane) has an absorption maximum at 355 nm and provides superior UVA protection. This ingredient was approved by the FDA in the late 1990s. Parsol 1789 has also been frequently reported to cause photoallergic dermatitis.[41] Avobenzone is one of the most commonly used UVA-blocking ingredients. The initial formulations had significant issues with stability. However, since 2007 several stabilized forms of avobenzone have become commercially available, including Helioplex by Neutrogena and Active Photobarrier Complex by Aveeno. Sunscreens made before 2007 should be discarded.

Mexoryl®

The FDA finally approved a new UVA filter after years of negotiations. This sunscreen agent is known as Mexoryl and is owned by L'Oréal. It is found in many L'Oréal brands including La Roche-Posay, Vichy, and Lancôme. Mexoryl SX is the formulation that is approved in the US. It does not block UV light quite as effectively as Mexoryl XL, which is not yet available in the US. However, Mexoryl SX is a water-soluble formulation and therefore feels less greasy on the skin and more suitable for everyday use. On the contrary, Mexoryl XL is oil soluble, making it more suitable as a water-resistant sunscreen. Mexoryl SX is an organic filter that is found to be very effective against shorter UVA wavelengths. These short UVA waves ranging from 320 to 340 nm constitute 95% of UV radiation that reaches the earth. Mexoryl can be added in combination with other UV filters. In contrast to avobenzone, Mexoryl is photostable and does not degrade when exposed to UV radiation.[44]

Sunscreen Combinations

Many sunscreen formulations contain combinations of active sunscreen ingredients to enhance protection and alter the aesthetics of the product. The FDA regulates which sunscreens can be combined with others; this is because of the recognition that certain sunscreen ingredients are incompatible and can actually lower the SPF rating of a product when combined.[26] Combinations are employed to achieve a higher SPF using a lower concentration of sunscreen ingredients.

ROLE OF ANTIOXIDANTS IN SUNSCREENS

Just as the body has its own immune defense system, the skin has its own antioxidant defense system. This system protects the skin from UV-induced oxidative damage. Excess UV radiation can prevent free radicals in the skin from being absorbed by this natural defense mechanism, thus leading to cancer, wrinkling, and aging. This excess of UV exposure calls for the induction and use of antioxidant enzymes.[24] Such enzymes act as UV filters and capture the free radicals before they cause damage. Retinyl esters, a storage form of vitamin A, have been found to absorb UV radiation with a maximum at 325 nm.[45] Along with enzymatic antioxidants, nonenzymatic forms exist as well. GSH, alpha-tocopherol, and beta-carotene are among a few of the nonenzymatic antioxidants administered. Some examples of enzymatic forms include catalase, superoxide dismutase, and GSH peroxidase.[24] Antioxidants can be administered in oral or topical forms (see Chapter 34). Oral forms tend to be more beneficial because they do not wear away from skin by daily rubbing and washing. In addition, topical antioxidants may not have the capacity to be properly absorbed into the skin. Consequently, topical antioxidants do not protect well against UV radiation alone and have a low SPF. Thus, antioxidants should be used in conjunction with a sunscreen to increase their efficiency.

One antioxidant of note is *Polypodium leucotomos*, a botanically-derived compound that belongs to the genus of ferns. It has been used in the treatment of various inflammatory disorders as well as vitiligo. In a study by González et al., the in vivo properties of polypodium were identified. In the study, 21 volunteers were divided into two groups. One group was treated with orally ingested psoralens (8-MOP or 5-MOP) and the other group was not treated. These volunteers were then exposed to solar radiation. The following clinical parameters were evaluated: immediate pigment darkening (IPD), minimal erythema dose (MED), minimal melanogenic dose (MMD), and minimal phototoxic dose (MPD) before and after topical or oral administration of polypodium leucotomos.[46] The results showed that polypodium was photoprotective after topical application as well as oral administration.

ADVERSE EFFECTS OF SUNSCREENS

Current data suggest that adverse effects induced by chemical sunscreens have included no systemic problems but have included local cutaneous manifestations such as contact dermatitis, irritant and allergic, as well as phototoxic and photoallergic reactions. In fact, sunscreens are one of the most common causative agents of photoallergic contact dermatitis in the US.[47] These agents can also cause contact dermatitis in the absence of sun exposure. PABA, benzophenones, cinnamates, and methoxydibenzoylmethane are the most common ingredients in chemical sunscreens implicated in provoking allergic contact dermatitis[48–50] (see Chapter 18). Physical sunscreens containing TiO_2 and ZnO have never been reported to cause contact allergy and, therefore, are suitable for patients with a history of sunscreen hypersensitivity.[28]

It is important to remember that additives to sunscreen preparations such as fragrances and preservatives are also likely to cause allergic reactions in susceptible patients (see Chapters 36 and 37). One study of 603 patients found that although 19% of the subjects complained of some sort of reaction to the sunscreen, none of the subjects were allergic to the sunscreen active ingredients, as revealed by patch testing. In fact, only 10% of the reactions were found to have an allergic component. The majority of adverse responses were consistent with an irritant reaction.[51] Sunscreen vehicles, particularly the oily preparations, can also exacerbate acne, as can acute UV exposure. Research suggests that it is not the individual sunscreen oil but the vehicle that can cause the development of comedones.[52,53]

The misconception that sunscreen offers total protection is insidious insofar as it leads some consumers to increase the length or frequency of their sun exposure. No sunscreen completely blocks the sun. In fact, the FDA no longer allows the term "sunblock" to be used on product labeling. Because the protection offered by many sunscreens is limited to UVB (280–315 nm) and short-wavelength UVA2 (320–340 nm), the use of such products may paradoxically increase exposure to long-wavelength UVA1 (340–400 nm).[54] UVA (320 400 nm) comprises the major portion of UV radiation reaching the surface of the earth and has been shown to play a role in skin carcinogenesis, photodermatosis induction, and other sun-induced skin diseases. UVA has been recognized as a component in the genesis of solar elastosis,[55] and studies by Lavker[10] and Lowe[56] provide evidence that repeated exposure to an artificial source of long-wavelength UVA produces morphologic changes in human skin indicative of photodamage.

In a study by Bissonnette et al., the pigmentation darkening method was used to compare UVA protection afforded by six commercially available sunscreens with an SPF of 20 or more.[57] These products claimed on their labels to offer UVA and UVB protection. Researchers found that the sunscreens that allowed the lowest amount of pigment darkening, and therefore the best UVA coverage, contained Parsol 1789. Interestingly, the sunscreens that protected the least against UVA-induced pigmentation were the sunscreens with the second and third highest SPF (45 and 50), showing that selecting a high SPF sunscreen cannot be used as the only guide to compare UVA protection afforded by sunscreens. Fortunately, many new stabilized avobenzone formulations and Mexoryl have recently entered the market, greatly increasing the UVA protection of easily available sunscreens.

VITAMIN D AND SUNSCREEN

Another current controversy that is far from being resolved pertains to vitamin D and sun exposure. Vitamin D is important for the prevention of many types of cancers. Recent studies have shown that vitamin D prevents cancers such as lung and prostate.[58] Unfortunately, the best method for obtaining a healthy and proper dose of vitamin D is through the sun (Fig. 29-6). Supplements, pills, and fortified milk do not contain the proper recommended dose of daily vitamin D. Lying on a sunny beach for 20 minutes can generate 10,000 IU of vitamin D while a glass of milk produces only 100 IU.[59] Thus emerges the controversy, as the best way of obtaining vitamin D is through sun exposure, yet too much sun exposure is known to cause skin cancer. In addition, sunscreens block most UVB light. It is UVB that promotes the synthesis of vitamin D. UVB is the source of sunburns and suntans as well. Research on this topic is ongoing and a final conclusion has not yet been reached. One study showed that there is no correlation between skin cancer prevention and vitamin D. In this study, 165 melanoma patients and 209 controls were questioned using a food-frequency questionnaire. Investigators controlled for age, hair color, and family history, and the results showed no evidence of vitamin D conferring protection against melanoma or reducing its risk.[60] A parallel study implied that sunscreen application does not decrease vitamin D levels.[61] On the other hand, some studies have found that sunscreen application does in fact decrease vitamin D levels. In one particular study, 20 long-term users of sunscreen with PABA were tested and were found to have significantly lower vitamin D serum levels as compared to normal controls.[62] Although this controversy is far from being settled, most researchers recommend a few minutes in the sun without sunscreen but advise against sun exposure for any significant elapsed amount of time.

Intermittent Use of Sunscreen

Many sunscreen users may have the misconception that intermittent use of a

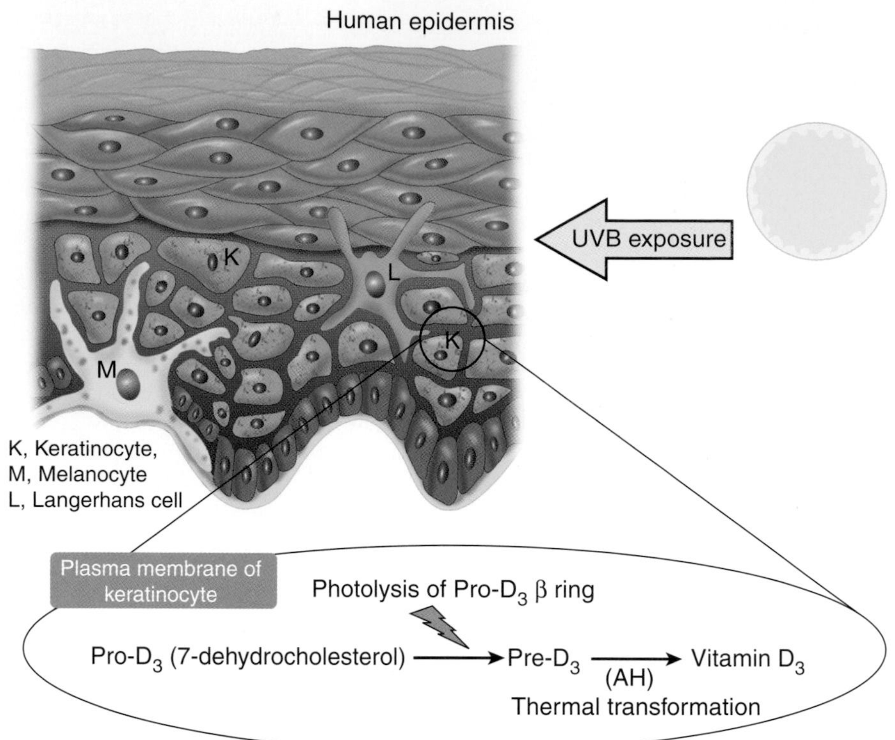

▲ **FIGURE 29-6** Vitamin D conversion in the skin.

high-SPF product is as effective as daily use of a lower-SPF product. For instance, dermatologists are in a position to hear anecdotally that a distinct subset of sunscreen users consider themselves regular users of sunscreen, every time they go to the beach. One study demonstrated that sunscreens must be applied properly, regularly, and in appropriate amounts to be optimally effective in preventing UV-induced skin damage. The findings suggest that missing an application of sunscreen, even a potent one, can have negative consequences for the skin, with regular use of an SPF-15 sunscreen revealed to be more effective than intermittent use of a higher-SPF product in protecting the skin.[63] Therefore, patients should be advised to use sunscreen on a daily basis, even when not planning to go into the sun. This will help protect them from the UVA rays transmitted indoors through glass, and from unanticipated sun exposures.

There are so many different product formulations on the market that an appropriate sunscreen should be available for every patient, though in some cases, identifying one may take some effort. At this point, given the amassed body of research, the benefits of wearing daily sunscreen, at least on exposed areas such as the face, appear to outweigh any risks.

VEHICLE FOR DELIVERY OF ACTIVE INGREDIENTS

Sunscreen product efficacy and aesthetic results are influenced by the manufacturer's choice of vehicle to deliver active ingredients. Emulsions, known as lotions and creams, are the most common sunscreen vehicles. Of course, several kinds of formulations are commercially available and are typically selected according to individual preferences.

Cleansers

One cleanser called IceShield by Freeze 24/7 is available on the market that claims to deposit sunscreen on the skin. This is a great option to use in those who do not like the feel of greasy sunscreens. However, at this time, there is a dearth of data as to how effective these wash-on sunscreens are. While more evidence is needed, it is presently recommended that this product be combined with a more reliable sunscreen when prolonged sun exposure is anticipated.

Lotions and Creams

For people with normal to oily skin, lotions tend to be more preferable because lotions have lower viscosity, spread more easily, and are less greasy. Combination skin is also amenable to lotions, but patients with dry skin typically prefer creams. These products make ideal sunscreens because the most effective active ingredients can be introduced into the lipid phase of an emulsion. Products with a higher SPF contain more sunscreen oil and impart a heavy and greasy feel.[64,65]

Oils

The only advantage to oils is that they spread easily. Unfortunately, they also spread thinly on the skin rendering less sun protection. Consumers tend not to like oils because of the greasy, messy feel on the skin.

Gels

Male patients and those with oily skin tend to prefer gels. For people that are preparing to exercise while wearing sunscreen, water-based gels are appropriate because alcohol-based gels can cause burning and stinging of the eyes.

Sprays

Sprays have become popular in the last few years, especially for use in children. Sprays are a good option for tending to large areas of the body. One must take care to ensure that all exposed body surfaces are covered.

Sticks

Lipid-soluble sunscreen ingredients are contained in sticks. Waxes and petrolatum are added to thicken the formulations. Sticks are effective in protecting narrow and prominent areas such as the lips, ears, nose, and around the eyes. For use during exercise and water activities, sticks are superior to other formulations because they last longer and do not have the tendency to melt, which can irritate the eyes.

PROTECTIVE EFFECTS OF MAKEUP AND OTHER SKIN CARE PRODUCTS

Sunscreen ingredients are now commonly found in many makeup foundations. Most facial foundations provide some sun protection as a result of ingredients such as TiO_2 and the pigments used to color the product. TiO_2 is added specifically to augment the SPF of some of these products, but it does result in a foundation that is more opaque. Consequently, chemical sunscreens are more often added to impart protection. Not every sunscreen ingredient is suitable for inclusion in makeup foundations, however. For example, Parsol effectively blocks UVA, but is inactivated upon exposure to iron oxide and other pigments used in makeup foundations. In addition, as stated above, the SPF on the label of a sunscreen powder and facial foundation is not an accurate reflection of how much sun protection these products offer. This is because the average person applies much less sunscreen product than is used in FDA testing.[13]

Within the last few years, manufacturers have produced hair care products, notably shampoos and conditioners, that contain sunscreen ingredients. Such ingredients are probably rinsed away and rendered ineffective because many sunscreen ingredients are water soluble and many of the hair care products are intended to be rinsed out. Although there are no data establishing their effectiveness, leave-in hair care products are more likely to provide some protection to the hair shaft. The FDA has not recognized any of these products as having protective effects against the sun. Until proper studies have been completed and data made available, including SPF-labeling, one should not rely on these products. The best recommendation is to wear a hat to prevent sun damage to the hair.

Insect Repellent and Sunscreen Combinations

A study by Montemarano et al. found that insect repellent interferes with sunscreen efficacy.[66] However, a subsequent study by Murphy and Montemarano disputed this finding, showing that insect repellent has the same efficacy even when sunscreen is applied with it.[67] At this time, it is advisable to apply these products separately until further information is available.

Sun Protection with Clothing

The UV Protection Factor (UPF) is a useful protection measurement guideline for clothing similar to the SPF that is used for sunscreens.[68] The most common, in vitro, method of ascertaining the UPF of clothing involves the use of a UV radiation source and a photodetector to record the intensity of the UV before and after passing through the fabric. The UPF is simply the ratio of the two measurements. The clothing industry has largely accepted, and embraced in some cases, the concepts of sun protection provided by clothing and the UPF. There is even a British standard for the measurement of UPF.[69] Because clothing is not subject to the wide variation or inconsistency of sunscreen application, a fabric really does provide the level of sun protection that its UPF suggests.[15] Further, it is believed that approximately 90% of summer clothes have a UPF higher than 10 and offer protection equal to that of sunscreens of SPF 30 or higher; the UPF of approximately 80% of such clothing exceeds a reading of 15, and offers nearly complete protection under normal sun exposure patterns.[70,71]

Washing clothes appears to strengthen the UPF. It is well known that cotton clothes shrink from the washing process. Therefore, it is reasonable to infer that the spaces, also known as "pores," between a fabric's threads shrink from washing. In fact, Welsh and Diffey demonstrated such a capacity in their study on the effects of fabric shrinkage (from laundry with water alone and detergent alone) on UPF measurement.[72] The relative size of these "pores" plays a significant role in limiting UV radiation transmission through clothing.[73] Wang et al. compiled fabric porosity data that demonstrated a reduction in the total area of "pores" between threads or yarns in fabrics laundered in various methods.[74] They concluded that the reduction of "pore" size after washing was responsible for the observed increase in UPF measurements and the ensuing decrease in UV transmission through the fabric.

UPF can be further increased by washing fabrics with detergents that contain UV-absorbing agents. Tinosorb, the UV-absorber used in the study by Wang et al., has a stilbene disulfonic acid triazine backbone that, when added to laundry, enables the chemical to vigorously bind to cotton fabric.[74] The result is a reduction in UV transmission through absorption of UV energy onto the ring structures of the compound. The study results showed that the UPF increased significantly after multiple washings with detergent and UV absorber, though there was no noticeable change in the whiteness or texture of the fabric. More UVA was transmitted through the fabrics than UVB, according to the authors.

While clothing obviously plays an integral role in protecting skin exposed to the sun, hats are also useful apparel adjuncts. Wearing a broad-brimmed hat can provide an SPF of about 5.[75] Hats can also add additional protection to the coverage that sunglasses provide by cutting down on the angles of sun exposure (Fig. 29-7).

Window Shields

UVA rays are able to penetrate glass, while UVB rays are not. Because UVB rays are the ones that cause initial reddening, a large amount of UVA exposure can go unnoticed. For patients with photosensitive skin disorders and those who want to go one step further to prevent

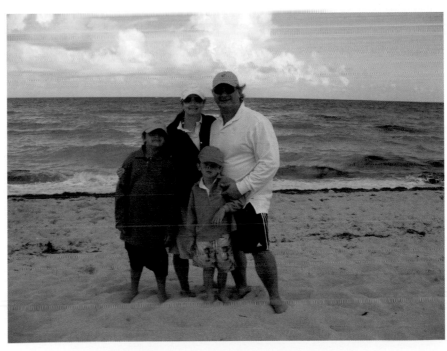

▲ **FIGURE 29-7** In addition to sunscreen, sunglasses, broad-brimmed hats, and sun-protective clothing should be worn when exposed to sunlight for any significant length of time.

UVA exposure, window shields are available that block UVA rays. The Llumar UV Shield is recommended by the Skin Cancer Foundation because it has been shown to block 99.9% of the UVA radiation in the range of 320 to 380 nm. These shields can be placed on car, boat, and house windows to decrease UVA exposure.

Chemoprevention of Photodamage

Chemoprevention is another potential option for protection against sunlight-related skin disorders.[76] Chemoprevention refers to the prevention of disease through dietary manipulation or pharmacologic intervention. Among the agents that have been identified as having potential chemopreventive activities in humans are retinoids[77] and low-fat diets.[78] In addition, a polyphenolic fraction isolated from green tea has been shown to exhibit multiple chemopreventive activities in animal models and in in vitro systems[79–81] (see Chapter 8). Investigations are ongoing regarding the potential chemopreventive properties of several other botanicals and nutritional components.

SUMMARY

There are numerous sunscreen choices on the market. It is important to help patients find the sunscreen that is most suitable for their needs and skin type to increase the likelihood of compliance to a daily sunscreen regimen. It is even more important to emphasize that the daily use of sunscreen is not the first-line defense against the ravages of the sun and that sunscreen use does not indemnify a person from photodamage or give one license to stay out longer because of a coating of sunscreen. The daily use of sunscreens is an important ingredient, though, in the continuing effort to keep the skin looking young and healthy.

REFERENCES

1. Taylor CR, Stern RS, Leyden JJ, et al. Photoaging/photodamage and photoprotection. *J Am Acad Dermatol.* 1990;22:1.
2. Weinstock MA. Cutaneous melanoma: public health approach to early detection. *Dermatol Ther.* 2006;19:26.
3. Autier P, Doré JF, Cattaruzza MS, et al. Sunscreen use, wearing clothes, and number of nevi in 6- to 7-year-old European children. European Organization for Research and Treatment of Cancer Melanoma Cooperative Group. *J Natl Cancer Inst.* 1998;90:1873.
4. Dixon H, Borland R, Hill D. Sun protection and sunburn in primary school children: the influence of age, gender, and coloring. *Prev Med.* 1999;28:119.
5. Robinson JK, Rademaker AW. Sun protection by families at the beach. *Arch Pediatr Adolesc Med.* 1998;152:466.
6. Diffey BL. What is light? *Photodermatol Photoimmunol Photomed.* 2002;18:68.
7. de Gruijl FR. Photocarcinogenesis: UVA vs. UVB radiation. *Skin Pharmacol Appl Skin Physiol.* 2002;15:316.
8. Poon TS, Barnetson RS, Halliday GM. Prevention of immunosuppression by sunscreens in humans is unrelated to protection from erythema and dependent on protection from ultraviolet A in the face of constant ultraviolet B protection. *J Invest Dermatol.* 2003;121:184.
9. Vink AA, Roza L. Biological consequences of cyclobutane pyrimidine dimers. *J Photochem Photobiol B.* 2001;65:101.
10. Lavker RM, Gerberick GF, Veres D, et al. Cumulative effects from repeated exposures to suberythemal doses of UVB and UVA in human skin. *J Am Acad Dermatol.* 1995;32:53.
11. Diffey BL. Sunscreens, suntans and skin cancer. People do not apply enough sunscreen for protection. *BMJ.* 1996;313:942.
12. Autier P, Boniol M, Severi G, et al. Quantity of sunscreen used by European students. *Br J Dermatol.* 2001;144:288.
13. Azurdia RM, Pagliaro JA, Rhodes LE. Sunscreen application technique in photosensitive patients: a quantitative assessment of the effect of education. *Photodermatol Photoimmunol Photomed.* 2000;16:53.
14. Stokes R, Diffey B. How well are sunscreen users protected? *Photodermatol Photoimmunol Photomed.* 1997;13:186.
15. Diffey BL. Sun protection with clothing. *Br J Dermatol.* 2001;144:449.
16. US Food and Drug Administration news. http://www.fda.gov/bbs/topics/NEWS/2007/NEW01687.html. Accessed March 15, 2008.
17. Chardon A, Moyal D, Hourseau C. Persistent pigment darkening response as a method for evaluation of ultraviolet A protection assays. In: Lowe NJ, Shaath MA, Pathak MA, eds. *Sunscreens Development, Evaluation and Regulatory Assays.* 2nd ed. New York, NY: Marcel Dekker; 1997:559-582.
18. Cole C, Van Fossen R. Measurement of sunscreen UVA protection: an unsensitized human model. *J Am Acad Dermatol.* 1992;26:174.
19. Nash JF, Tanner PR, Matts PJ. Ultraviolet A radiation: testing and labeling for sunscreen products. *Dermatol Clin.* 2006;24:63.
20. Cole C. Sunscreen protection in the ultraviolet A region: how to measure the effectiveness. *Photodermatol Photoimmunol Photomed.* 2001;17:2.
21. Moyal D, Chardon A, Kollias N. UVA protection efficacy of sunscreens can be determined by the persistent pigment darkening (PPD) method. (Part 2). *Photodermatol Photoimmunol Photomed.* 2000;16:250.
22. Haywood R, Wardman P, Sanders R, et al. Sunscreens inadequately protect against ultraviolet A induced free radicals in skin: implications for skin aging and melanoma? *J Invest Dermatol.* 2003;121:862.
23. Herrling T, Fuchs J, Rehberg J, et al. UV-induced free radicals in the skin detected by ESR spectroscopy and imaging using nitroxides. *Free Radic Biol Med.* 2003;35:59.
24. Kullavanijaya P, Lim H. Photoprotection. *J Am Acad Dermatol.* 2005;52:937.
25. Seité S, Moyal D, Verdier MP, et al. Accumulated p53 protein and UVA protection level of sunscreens. *Photodermatol Photoimmunol Photomed.* 2000;16:3.
26. Draelos ZD. A dermatologist's perspective on the final sunscreen monograph. *J Am Acad Dermatol.* 2001;44:109.
27. Pinnell SR, Fairhurst D, Gillies R, et al. Microfine zinc oxide is a superior sunscreen ingredient to microfine titanium dioxide. *Dermatol Surg.* 2000;26:309.
28. Rietschel R, Fowler J, eds. *Fisher's Contact Dermatitis.* 5th ed. Philadelphia, PA: Lippincott Williams & Wilkins; 2001:404.
29. Mitchnick MA, Fairhurst D, Pinnell SR. Microfine zinc oxide (Z-cote) as a photostable UVA/UVB sunblock agent. *J Am Acad Dermatol.* 1999;40:85.
30. Deflandre A, Lang G. Photostability assessment of sunscreens. Benzylidene camphor and dibenzoylmethan derivatives. *Intl J Cosmet Sci.* 1988;10:53.
31. Fairhurst D, Mitchnik MA. Particulate sun blocks: general principles. In: Lowe NJ, Shaath NA, Pathak MA, eds. *Sunscreens—Development, Evaluation, and Regulatory Aspects.* New York, NY: Marcel Dekker; 1997:313-352.
32. Wamer WG, Yin JJ, Wei RR. Oxidative damage to nucleic acids photosensitized by titanium dioxide. *Free Radic Biol Med.* 1997;23:851.
33. Hidaka H, Horikoshia S, Serpone N, et al. In vitro photochemical damage to DNA, RNA and their bases by an inorganic sunscreen agent on exposure to UVA and UVB radiation. *Photochem Photobiol.* 1997;111:205.
34. Gillies R, Kollias N. Noninvasive in vivo determination of sunscreen ultraviolet A protection factors using diffuse reflectance spectroscopy. In: Lowe NJ, Shaath NA, Pathak MA, eds. *Sunscreens—Development, Evaluation, and Regulatory Aspects.* New York, NY: Marcel Dekker; 1997:601–610.
35. Sayre RM, Dowdy JC. Avobenzone and the photostability of sunscreen products. *Photodermatol Photoimmunol Photomed.* 1998;14:38.
36. Hayden CG, Roberts MS, Benson HA. Systemic absorption of sunscreen after topical application. *Lancet.* 1997;350:863.
37. Olive P, Banath J. The comet assay: a method to measure DNA damage in individual cells. *Nature Protocols.* 2006;1:23.
38. Chatelain E, Gabard B. Photostabilization of butyl methoxydibenzoylmethane (Avobenzone) and ethylhexyl methoxycinnamate by bis-ethylhexyloxyphenol triazine (Tinosorb S), a new UV broadband filter. *Photochem Photobiol.* 2001;74:401.
39. Gaspar LR, Maia Campos PM. Evaluation of the photostability of different UV filter combinations in a sunscreen. *Int J Pharm.* 2006;307:123.
40. Lapidot N, Gans O, Biagini F, et al. Advanced sunscreens: UV absorbers encapsulated in Sol-Gel glass microcapsules. *J Sol-Gel Sci Tech.* 2003;26:67.
41. Rietschel R, Fowler J, eds. *Fisher's Contact Dermatitis.* 5th ed. Philadelphia,

PA: Lippincott Williams & Wilkins; 2001:403.
42. Emonet S, Pasche-Koo F, Perin-Minisini MJ, et al. Anaphylaxis to oxybenzone, a frequent constituent of sunscreens. *J Allergy Clin Immunol.* 2001;107:556.
43. Cosmetic Ingredient Review. Final report on the safety of benzophenone-1, -3, -4, -5, -9, and -11. *J Am Coll Toxicol.* 1983;2:3577.
44. Moyal D. Prevention of ultraviolet-induced skin pigmentation. *Photodermatol Photoimmunol Photomed.* 2004;20:243.
45. Antille C, Tran C, Sorg O, et al. Vitamin A exerts a photoprotective action in skin by absorbing ultraviolet B radiation. *J Invest Dermatol.* 2003;121:1163.
46. González S, Pathak MA, Cuevas J, et al. Topical or oral administration with an extract of Polypodium leucotomos prevents acute sunburn and psoralen-induced phototoxic reactions as well as depletion of Langerhans cells in human skin. *Photodermatol Photoimmunol Photomedss.* 1997;13:50.
47. Rietschel R, Fowler J, eds. *Fisher's Contact Dermatitis.* 5th ed. Philadelphia, PA: Lippincott Williams &Wilkins; 2001:402.
48. Levy SB. Sunscreens for photoprotection. *Dermatol Ther.* 1997;4:59.
49. Davis S, Capjack L, Kerr N, et al. Clothing as protection from ultraviolet radiation: which fabric is most effective? *Int J Dermatol.* 1997;36:374.
50. González E, González S. Drug photosensitivity, idiopathic photodermatoses, and sunscreens. *J Am Acad Dermatol.* 1996;35:871.
51. Foley P, Nixon R, Marks R, et al. The frequency of reactions to sunscreens: results of a longitudinal population-based study on the regular use of sunscreens in Australia. *Br J Dermatol.* 1993; 128:512.
52. Collins P, Ferguson J. Photoallergic contact dermatitis to oxybenzone. *Br J Dermatol.* 1994;131:124.
53. Funk JO, Dromgoole SH, Maibach HI. Sunscreen intolerance. Contact sensitization, photocontact sensitization, and irritancy of sunscreen agents. *Dermatol Clin.* 1995;13:473.
54. Autier P, Doré JF, Négrier S, et al. Sunscreen use and duration of sun exposure: a double-blind, randomized trial. *J Natl Cancer Inst.* 1999;91:1304.
55. Fourtanier A, Labat-Robert J, Kern P, et al. In vivo evaluation of photoprotection against chronic ultraviolet-A irradiation by a new sunscreen Mexoryl SX. *Photochem Photobiol.* 1992;55:549.
56. Lowe NJ, Meyers DP, Wieder JM, et al. Low doses of repetitive ultraviolet A induced morphologic changes in human skin. *J Invest Dermatol.* 1995;105:739.
57. Bissonnette R, Allas S, Moyal D, et al. Comparison of UVA protection afforded by high sun protection factor sunscreens. *J Am Acad Dermatol.* 2000;43:1036.
58. The Associated Press. Vitamin D research may have doctors prescribing sunshine. *USA Today.* April 20, 2005. http://www.usatoday.com/news/nation/2005-05-21-doctors-sunshine-good_x.htm. Accessed March 2, 2008.
59. Lambert C. Too much sunscreen? *Harvard Magazine.* 2005;108(1):11-12.
60. Weinstock MA, Stampfer MJ, Lew RA, et al. Case-control study of melanoma and dietary vitamin D: implications for advocacy of sun protection and sunscreen use. *J Invest Dermatol.* 1992;98:809.
61. Marks R, Foley PA, Jolley D, et al. The effects of regular sunscreen use on vitamin D levels in an Australian population. Results of a randomized controlled trial. *Arch Dermatol.* 1995;131:415.
62. Matsuoka LY, Wortsman J, Hanifan N, 255et al. Chronic sunscreen use decreases circulating concentrations of 25-hydroxyvitamin D. A preliminary study. *Arch Dermatol.* 1988;124:1802.
63. Phillips TJ, Bhawan J, Yaar M, et al. Effect of daily versus intermittent sunscreen application on solar simulated UV radiation-induced skin response in humans. *J Am Acad Dermatol.* 2000;43: 610.
64. Mills OH, Porte M, Kligman AM. Enhancement of comedogenic substances by ultraviolet radiation. *Br J Dermatol.* 1979;100:699.
65. Mills OH Jr, Kligman AM. Acne aestivalis. *Arch Dermatol.* 1975;111:891.
66. Montemarano AD, Gupta RK, Burge JR, et al. Insect repellents and the efficacy of sunscreen. *Lancet.* 1997;349:1670.
67. Murphy ME, Montemarano AD, Debboun M, et al. The effect of sunscreen on the efficacy of insect repellent: a clinical trial. *J Am Acad Dermatol.* 2000;43:219.
68. Gies HP, Roy CR, Elliott G, et al. Ultraviolet radiation protection factors for clothing. *Health Phys.* 1994;67:131.
69. British Standards Institution. *Method of Test for Penetration of Erythemally Weighted Solar Ultraviolet Radiation Through Clothing Fabrics BS 7914.* London, UK: British Standards Institution; 1998.
70. Gies HP, Roy CR, McLennan A. Textiles and sun protection. In: Volkmer B, Heller H, eds. *Environmental UV-Radiation, Risk of Skin Cancer and Primary Prevention.* Stuttgart, Germany: Gustav Fischer; 1996:213-234.
71. Driscoll C. *Clothing Protection Factors.* Radiological Protection Bulletin. Oxfordshire, England: Chilton National Radiological Protection Board; 2000:222.
72. Welsh C, Diffey B. The protection against solar actinic radiation afforded by common clothing fabrics. *Clin Exp Dermatol.* 1981;6:577.
73. Menzies SW, Lukins PB, Greenoak GE, et al. A comparative study of fabric protection against ultraviolet-induced erythema determined by spectrophotometric and human skin measurements. *Photodermatol Photoimmunol Photomed.* 1991;8:157.
74. Wang SQ, Kopf AW, Marx J, et al. Reduction of ultraviolet transmission through cotton t-shirt fabrics with low ultraviolet protection by various laundering methods and dyeing: clinical implications. *J Am Acad Dermatol.* 2001;44:767
75. Diffey BL, Cheeseman J. Sun protection with hats. *Br J Dermatol.* 1992;127:10.
76. Greenwald P. Chemoprevention of cancer. *Sci Am.* 1996;275:96.
77. DiGiovanna JJ. Retinoid chemoprevention in the high-risk patient. *J Am Acad Dermatol.* 1998;39:S82.
78. Black HS, Herd JA, Goldberg LH, et al. Effect of a low fat diet on the incidence of actinic keratosis. *N Engl J Med.* 1994;330:1272.
79. Katiyar SK, Mukhtar H. Tea in chemoprevention of cancer: epidemiologic and experimental studies. *Int J Oncol.* 1996;8:221.
80. Yang CS, Wang ZY. Tea and cancer. *J Natl Cancer Inst.* 1993;85:1038.
81. Elmets CA, Singh D, Tubesing K, et al. Cutaneous photoprotection from ultraviolet injury by green tea polyphenols. *J Am Acad Dermatol.* 2001;44:425.

CHAPTER 30

Retinoids

Leslie Baumann, MD
Sogol Saghari, MD

Retinoids are a family of compounds derived from vitamin A that includes beta-carotene and other carotenoids, retinol, tretinoin, tazarotene, and adapalene. For many years, retinoids have been used topically and systemically for the treatment of dermatologic diseases, particularly acne. The potential benefits of retinoids for the treatment and prevention of photoaging have also been explored through the last two decades. This research has led to a greater understanding of the etiology of skin aging. Concurrent but unrelated research has also recently demonstrated that doses of ultraviolet (UV) light too low to cause visible skin reddening are still capable of activating the enzymatic machinery that leads to photoaging.[1]

The first anecdotal evidence that retinoids could improve aged skin was seen in female patients being treated for acne. These patients reported that their skin felt smoother and less wrinkled after treatment.[2] This observation was followed by a clinical trial that showed that patients treated with tretinoin demonstrated improvement of sunlight-induced epidermal atrophy, dysplasia, keratosis, and dyspigmentation.[3] A plethora of clinical trials have confirmed such early observations. The data were submitted to the U.S. Food and Drug Administration (FDA), which later approved tretinoin (brand name Renova™) for use against photodamage. Although there are many different topical retinoids on the market today that are also useful against photodamage, Renova and Avage are the only topical agents approved specifically for this purpose. Retinol, the metabolic precursor of tretinoin, is often added to over-the-counter (OTC) cosmetic formulations that are touted as "antiwrinkle" creams. This chapter will focus on the antiaging activity of topical retinoids. It should be noted, though, that oral retinoids are also being used to treat photodamage.

MECHANISM OF ACTION

Chemical Structure

In 1931, the Nobel Prize was awarded to Karrer et al. for determining the structure of retinol.[4] Twelve years later, retinol was successfully synthesized and soon became commercially available. Since that time, the retinoid field has proliferated with compounds, now numbering more than 2500 products.[5] In fact, many generic forms of tretinoin are currently available in the United States and retinoids are even combined with medications such as antibiotics, as in Ziana, and hydroquinone, as in Tri-Luma. Initially, a retinoid was defined as a compound the structure and action of which resembled the parent compound retinol. Through the last several decades, chemists have made extensive modifications to the naturally-occurring molecule that have resulted in the development of three generations of retinoids (Fig. 30-1). The latest retinoids bear little structural resemblance to retinol but still qualify as retinoids because they can exert their biologic action through the same nuclear receptors modulated by the active natural metabolite of vitamin A, retinoic acid.

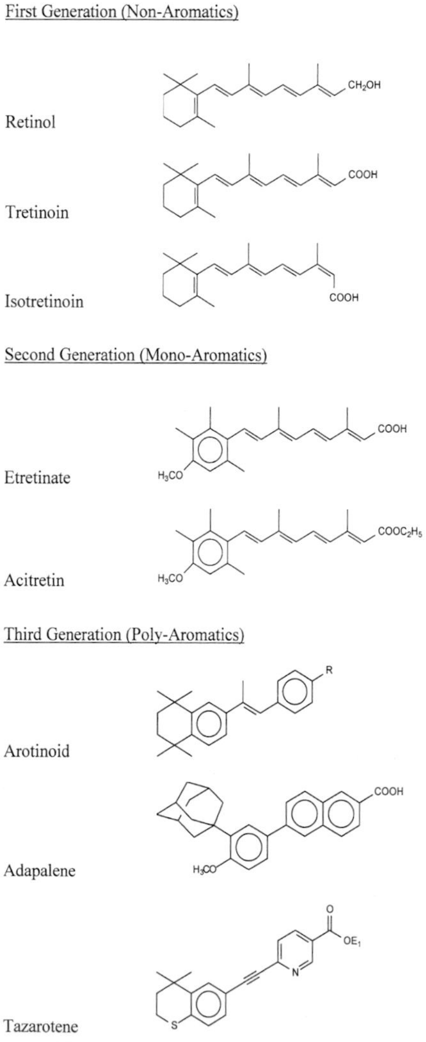

First Generation (Non-Aromatics)

Retinol — CH_2OH

Tretinoin — COOH

Isotretinoin — COOH

Second Generation (Mono-Aromatics)

Etretinate — H_3CO, COOH

Acitretin — H_3CO, $COOC_2H_5$

Third Generation (Poly-Aromatics)

Arotinoid — R

Adapalene — H_3CO, COOH

Tazarotene — S, N, O, OE_t

▲ **FIGURE 30-1** Chemical structures of the three generations of retinoids. Addition of aromatic rings has made third-generation retinoids more stable and more specific for certain receptors.

Retinoic acid is a lipid-soluble molecule known to affect cell growth, differentiation, homeostasis, apoptosis, and embryonic development. In fact, retinoids elicit their effects at the molecular level by regulating gene transcription and affecting activities such as cellular differentiation and proliferation (Fig. 30-2 for the mechanism of action of retinoids in acne). These agents can act directly, by inducing transcription from genes with promoter regions that contain retinoid response elements or indirectly by inhibiting the transcription of certain genes.[6] Three domains within the retinoic acid molecule govern its biologic activity: an acidic function at one extreme and a lipophilic domain at the other, linked by a group that determines their relative spatial orientation.[7] Synthetic retinoids also require an acidic function pointing away from a lipophilic portion for receptor affinity and transcription. The successive generations of retinoids have resulted from modification of the retinoic acid skeleton with structural rigidification, through addition of aromatic rings in place of the vulnerable double bonds found in retinoic acid. This makes the third-generation retinoids more photostable when compared to the first- and second-generation molecules; some compounds within this family have displayed significantly reduced irritation potential.[8]

Retinoid Receptors

Retinoid-binding proteins were first discovered in the 1970s.[9] In 1987, the discovery of retinoic acid receptors led to the realization that tretinoin is a hormone.[10,11] Since that time, much research has been performed to determine the exact roles of these binding proteins and receptors. The biologic effects of retinoic acid are now known to be mediated by several biologic systems: binding proteins such as cellular retinoic acid binding proteins I and II (CRABP I and II); cellular retinol binding protein (CRBP)[2]; and nuclear receptors that are divided into two categories, the retinoic acid receptors (RARs) and the retinoid X receptors (RXRs).[12] All of these nuclear receptors are members of a large superfamily called nuclear hormone superfamily receptors, which includes the

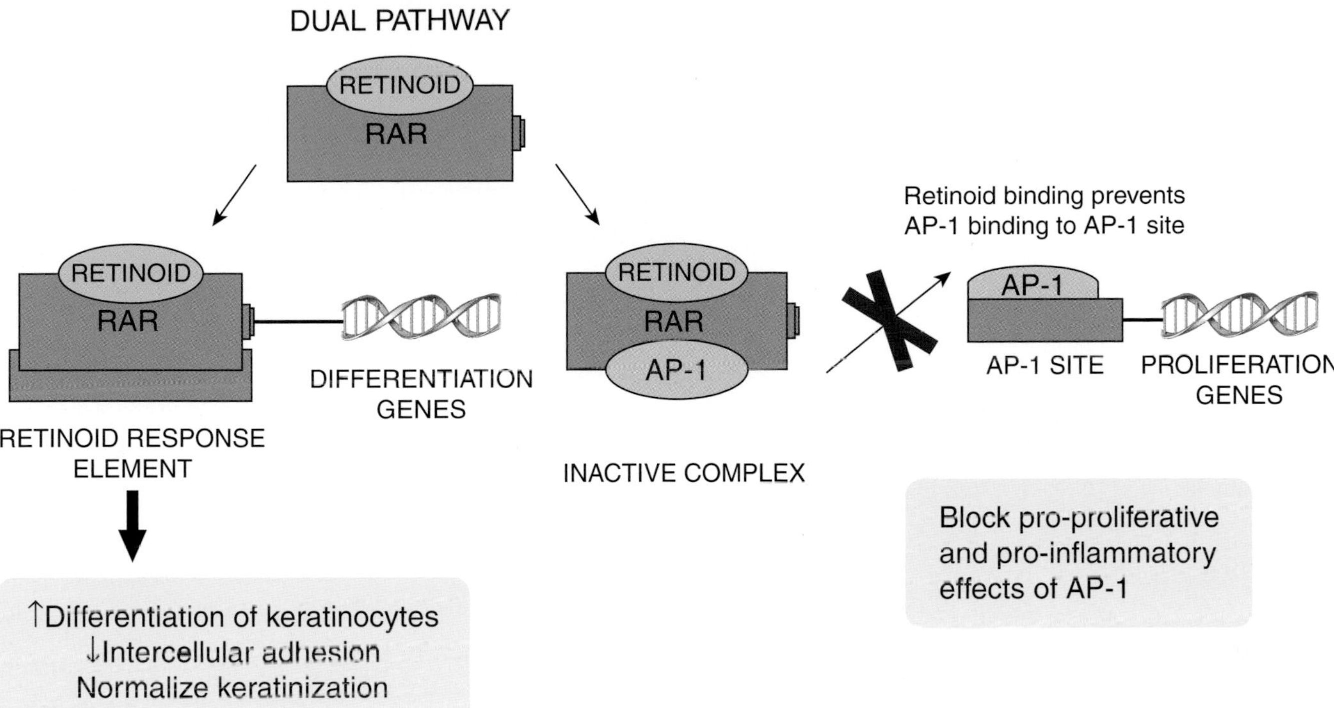

▲ **FIGURE 30-2** Retinoid mechanism of action in acne.

receptors for vitamin D, estradiol, glucocorticoids, and thyroid hormone.[13]

The retinoic acid receptor family is composed of two types of receptors, the RARs and the RXRs. The RARs and the RXRs are divided into α, β, and γ subtypes. The RARα, RARβ, and RARγ genes have been localized to chromosomes 17q21, 3p24, and 12q13, respectively, and the RXRα, RXRβ, and RXRγ genes have been mapped to chromosomes 9q34.3, 6p21.3, and 1q22-23, respectively.[14] These receptors are able to regulate gene expression in two ways: (1) they induce gene expression by binding to specific DNA sequences known as retinoic acid responsive elements (RAREs), or (2) they inhibit gene expression by downregulating the actions of other transcription factors (such as AP-1 and NF-IL6). All the α, β, and γ subtypes exhibit distinct affinities for retinoic acid and show a characteristic tissue distribution. For example, epidermis is a privileged tissue for the expression of RARγ and RXRα, the major isoforms of their respective families in this tissue, whereas RARα is ubiquitous. In the skin, RARβ is primarily found in the dermis, and it is also found in other body tissues.[7] Ninety percent of the RARs in the epidermis and cultured keratinocytes are RARγ, which is the receptor associated with terminal differentiation; therefore, this receptor is the target of the retinoids used in dermatology.[15]

The interactions of the retinoid receptors among themselves and other receptors of the nuclear hormone superfamily are complex. RARs are known to heterodimerize with RXR in order to interact with their RAREs and mediate classic retinoid activity and toxicity. RXRs, however, are more promiscuous, heterodimerizing with several other members of the steroid receptor superfamily including peroxisome proliferator-activated receptors (PPAR), vitamin D receptors, thyroid hormone receptors, and a number of orphan receptors, such as LXR, PXR, and FXR.[16] The interactions of these receptors are being studied intensively; however, more research is necessary to fully delineate the mechanisms of action of retinoid agents.

RETINOIDS AS ANTIAGING AGENTS

Photodamage and Matrix Metalloproteinases

Although tretinoin has been approved for many years for the *treatment* of photoaging, evidence suggests that it also plays a role in the *prevention* of aging. This can be linked to inhibitory effects of retinoids on damaging metalloproteinases. UVB exposure dramatically upregulates the production of several collagen-degrading enzymes known as matrix metalloproteinases (MMPs) (see Chapter 6). Activation of MMP genes results in production of collagenase, gelatinase, and stromelysin, which have been shown to fully degrade skin collagen[17] (Box 30-1). Fisher et al. demonstrated that application of tretinoin inhibits the induction of all three of these harmful MMPs.[1]

In addition to increasing levels of destructive enzymes such as collagenase, UV exposure has also been shown to decrease collagen production. Fisher et al. demonstrated that expression of collagen types I and III is substantially reduced within 24 hours after a single UV exposure.[18] Pretreatment of the skin with all-*trans*-retinoic acid (tretinoin) was shown to inhibit this loss of procollagen synthesis. Therefore, pretreatment of the skin with topical retinoids, when used consistently, is likely to be beneficial in preventing as well as treating photodamage.[19]

Benefits

Retinoids have shown benefits in the treatment of acne (see Chapter 15),

BOX 30-1

Two transciption factors, c-Jun and c-Fos, must combine to produce activator protein-1 (AP-1). AP-1 is able to activate the MMP genes resulting in production of collagenase, gelatinase, and stromelysin. All-*trans*-retinoic acid blocks the UV-induced increase in c-Jun protein. Although high levels of c-Jun mRNA are still present, signifying that the c-Jun gene has been activated, the levels of c-Jun protein are decreased. Topical retinoic acid likely acts to reduce UV induction of c-Jun protein by stimulating its breakdown through the ubiquitin-proteasome pathway19 (Fig. 30-3).

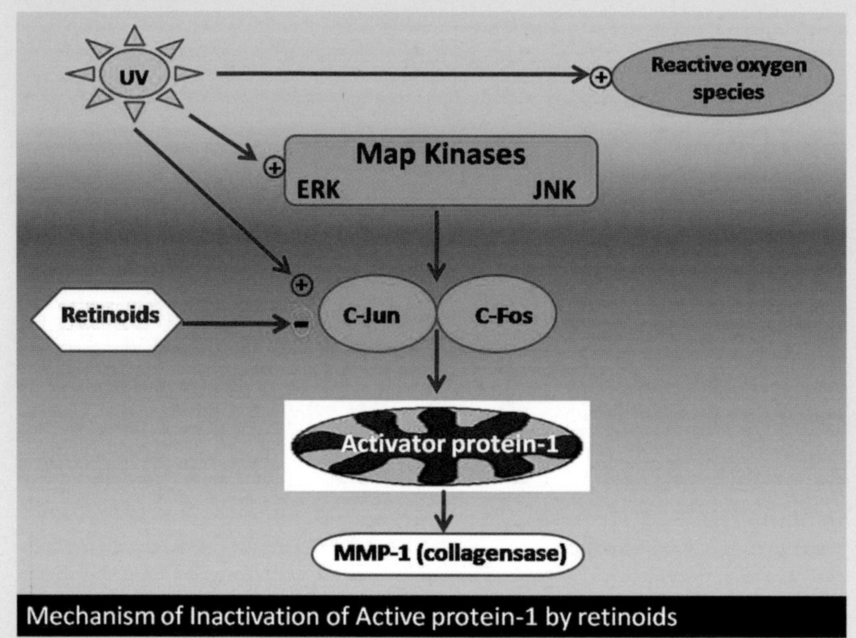

▲ **FIGURE 30-3** Mechanism of inactivation of active protein-1 by retinoids.

psoriasis, ichthyosis, keratoderma, and several other diseases. In fact, there are more than 125 distinct dermatologic disorders for which there is credible evidence of retinoid efficacy.[5] Multiple studies have examined the use of retinoids for the prevention and treatment of photoaging. The first of these clinical trials, using tretinoin, to demonstrate clinical improvement of photoaged skin were published in 1986 and 1988.[3,20] Since then, many other studies and much clinical experience have shown similar results. In one randomized single-center study, 100 subjects were divided into three treatment groups.[21] One group was treated with 0.1% tretinoin, another with 0.025% tretinoin, and the last group with vehicle cream. Treatment with either 0.1% or 0.025% tretinoin resulted in statistically significant improvement of photoaged skin compared with vehicle treatment.

The histologically observed changes with the use of retinoids include abolition of cellular atypia, increased compacting of the stratum corneum, less clumping of melanin in basal cells, and a correction of polarity of keratinocytes, with more orderly differentiation as cells move upward. The ultrastructural changes seen with retinoid use include evidence of hyperproliferation of keratinocytes (e.g., larger nuclei, increased ribosomes, etc.) and a reduction in the size of melanosomes.

As described in Chapter 6, changes in collagen and the ratio of collagen I to collagen III have been found to be important in the photoaging process. Retinoids have been shown to increase collagen synthesis in photoaged individuals.[22] In addition to preventing the breakdown of collagen as described above, topical application of tretinoin 0.1% to photodamaged skin partially restores levels of collagen type I. An increase in anchoring fibrils (collagen VII) is also seen after application of tretinoin 0.1%.[22]

Side Effects

Side effects from retinoid use occur when the product binds undesired receptor subtypes not involved in the expected biologic cascade. The more specific the binding pattern a retinoid exhibits, the fewer side effects it will elicit. The newer generation retinoids destined for dermatologic use have been designed to reduce side effects by making compounds that bind more selectively to the RARγ receptor subtype. However, with these improved molecules, the side effects from topically applied retinoids still persist, likely linked to intrinsic RARγ activation.

The most common side effects of topical retinoids are skin irritation, desquamation, and redness (Fig. 30-4). The increased desquamation and resultant flaking of the skin correspond with increased proliferation of keratinocytes, as indicated by a greater number of mitotic figures and enhanced expression of differentiation markers.[23] These findings seem to be related to the type and dose of the retinoid and usually occur within 2 to 4 days of beginning topical treatment.[24] New studies have suggested that patients may achieve maximum clinical improvement of photoaged skin without developing retinoid dermatitis. In other words, the irritation produced by retinoids is separate from the photoaging benefits of retinoids. This is demonstrated in the study that compared two different strengths of tretinoin (0.1% and 0.025%). Although both strengths were equally efficacious in the treatment of photoaging, the degree of irritation differed markedly between the two treatment groups, with the 0.1% tretinoin-treated group exhibiting approximately a three-fold greater incidence of irritation than the 0.025% tretinoin-treated group.[21] This irritation seems to be receptor mediated as implied by evidence that the topical application of tretinoin to the skin of transgenic mice deficient in RARs does not result in any apparent epidermal hyperplasia or desquamation.[25] This suggests that the development of newer retinoids with specific receptor and pharmacokinetic profiles and relevant dosing may lead to a lower incidence of irritation, flaking, and desquamation.

Erythema is another side effect of topical retinoids, one that elicits noncompliance from patients. This symptom is caused by a different mechanism that appears not to be receptor mediated.[26] Patients with rosacea and naturally pink skin tend to be particularly disturbed by this side effect. Using the techniques described in Table 30-1 may decrease the incidence of all types of skin irritation. A study performed in the late 1990s suggested that after a 48-week regimen of once-daily 0.05% tretinoin emollient cream, the benefits of tretinoin could be sustained by using the treatment only 3 times weekly for an additional 24 weeks.[27] The tretinoin should be used at *least* 3 times a week, however, because the same study showed that once-

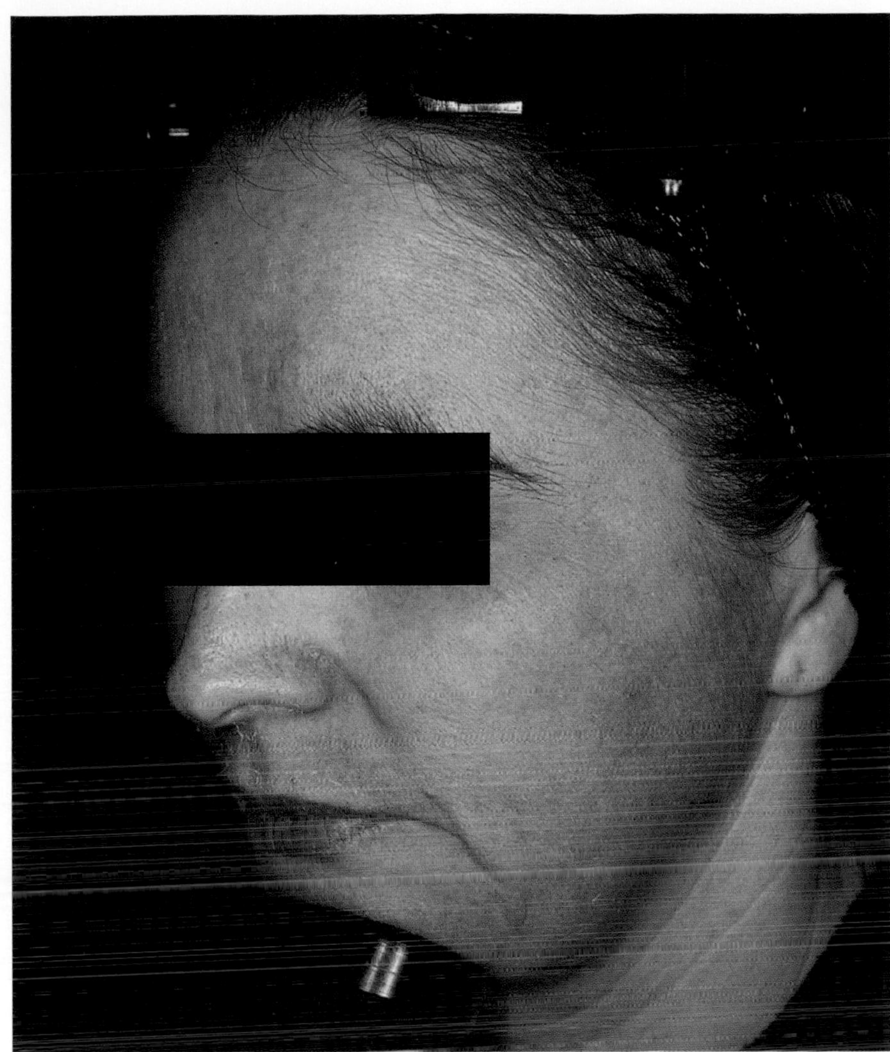

▲ **FIGURE 30-4** Redness, flaking, and tender skin are common symptoms after beginning a retinoid. These symptoms usually improve with time.

weekly treatment with tretinoin was less effective in sustaining the clinical improvement achieved by the initial treatment regimen of tretinoin once daily. The same study also demonstrated reversal of the beneficial effects of tretinoin treatment after discontinuation of therapy for 24 weeks. This indicates that patients must continue tretinoin therapy at least 3 times a week to maintain clinical improvement.

Dry skin is also a common complaint of patients treated with retinoids. The flaking that patients experience when using retinoids often leads them to believe that their skin is dry, although the observed flaking is caused by a different mechanism than those leading to dry skin. The dry skin noted by retinoid users is likely due in part to an increase in transepidermal water loss (TEWL), which accompanies topical retinoid use. The increase in TEWL is an effect typical of topically applied retinoids and is thought to be associated with a perturbation of the stratum corneum water barrier function.[28,29] Although retinoids increase cell proliferation, this leads to a decrease in ceramide biosynthesis (at least in the short term). This decrease in ceramides, a vital component of the water barrier of the stratum corneum, may partly explain the xerosis seen with retinoid use[30] (see Chapter 11).

The side effects commonly seen in patients who have been started on retinoids can usually be lessened by directing the patient to apply small amounts of the retinoids at less frequent intervals. The lowest available dose should be started initially. A topical retinol can be used first. Once the patient is consistently applying the retinol nightly, the strength of the retinol can be increased. Once the maximal retinol strength is reached, the patient can be seamlessly switched to a prescription retinoid. Alternately, a patient can be started on Tri-Luma, which is a combination of hydroquinone, tretinoin, and a mild steroid. The mild steroid prevents irritation while the hydroquinone hastens the resolution of solar lentigos, thereby increasing patient satisfaction and compliance. Whether retinol, Tri Luma, or a less irritating retinoid such as Differin is chosen to start therapy, in individuals with sensitive skin the frequency of use can be slowly ratcheted up as the patient's tolerance increases. Once the patient is using the lowest strength of a particular retinoid every night for 3 months without redness and peeling, the strength of the retinoid can be

TABLE 30-1
Instructions for Patients Using Retinoids (e.g., Atralin Avage, Differin, Tazorac, Retin-A, Renova, Retinol, Tretinoin, Tri-Luma, Ziana) for the First Time

AM: Use cleanser, moisturizer, and sunscreen as directed by your skin care specialist.
PM:
1. Cleanse face.
2. Apply antiaging, acne, or rosacea treatment product.
3. Mix pea size of retinoid product with a pea size of moisturizer. Apply to face. Do this again to neck and chest.

Notes:
1. Use retinoid every third night for the first 2 weeks.
2. If you have no redness, increase to every other night for 2 weeks.
3. If you have no redness, increase to every night.
4. Once you have used it every night for 3 months, ask your physician to give you the next strongest formulation.
5. You may only be able to use the product on your neck twice a week. The neck is more sensitive than the face.
6. Do not apply a moisturizer with glycolic acid or salicylic acid at the same time that you apply the retinoid. If you use these products, apply them and wait 30 minutes before applying the retinoid. Glycolic acid and salicylic cleansers are fine to use.
7. Do not use facial scrubs, microdermabrasion, or at-home chemical peels unless these are prescribed by your skin care specialist.
8. Stop retinoid products 1 week before facial waxing to avoid skin burning from the wax.
9. If you have questions, visit www.SkinTypeSolutions.com.

increased to the next level. In the primary author's experience, patients who are given this regimen along with careful instructions on how to apply the retinoids display increased compliance as well as benefits from the topical retinoids. Table 30-1 lists the instructions that should be given to patients who are beginning retinoids for the first time. It is important not to begin other irritating agents at the same time that a retinoid is started, such as facial scrubs, chemical peels, or microdermabrasion. These can be added later once the retinoid is sufficiently tolerated. However, many dermatologists have observed that patients who have been on hydroxy acids for extended periods before beginning retinoids may exhibit less irritation from the retinoids. The reason for this is currently unclear. However, it is believed that the hydroxy acids enhance the function of the skin barrier, leading to less absorption of the retinoids. Using barrier repair moisturizers in addition to the retinoids can be very helpful to increase tolerability (see Chapters 11 and 32).

Teratogenicity

It is well established that teratogenicity is a significant risk associated with the use of retinoids, especially via oral administration. The advisability of topical retinoid use by women of childbearing age has been the subject of debate because of the potential risk of systemic absorption. As a general rule, great care should be taken when prescribing these drugs to women of childbearing age, and should be restricted to those drugs for which a high safety margin has been clinically demonstrated (e.g., in the courses of treatment for psoriasis or acne). It is recommended to have pregnant and breastfeeding patients cease using topical retinoids, although there are multiple studies that show no effect of some topical retinoids when used during pregnancy. For example, in one controlled study in which 0.025% tretinoin gel was applied daily to the face, neck, and upper part of the chest for 14 days, fluctuations in plasma levels of endogenous retinoids were lower than those of diurnal and nutritional factors.[31] Another study demonstrated no significant increase in the rate of fetal malformation in a large group of patients treated with topical tretinoin during the first trimester of pregnancy, as compared with those who were not exposed to the drug.[32]

Retinoids and Sun Exposure

Many patients and physicians have worried that use of topical tretinoin may lead to increased photosensitivity because the daily use of tretinoin causes the stratum corneum to become thinner and more compact. This concern has been due, at least partially, to the fact that early tretinoin users were warned to apply the product only at night. The precaution stemmed from the product's poor stability when exposed to UV light, though, not to any reported photosensitivity provocation. In fact, it has now been established that there is no decrease of the minimal erythema dose for human skin that has been pretreated with topical tretinoin and irradiated with UV light of a defined energy. This shows that retinoids possess neither phototoxic nor photosensitizing activity.[1]

AVAILABLE TYPES OF TOPICAL RETINOIDS

All retinoids affect RAR receptors, but which RAR receptor subtype they affect may vary (Table 30-2). RARγ and RXRα are located in the epidermis while RARβ is found in the dermis. Although topically applied retinoids seem similar upon cursory inspection, they actually have very important differences that are beyond the scope of this chapter.

First Generation

TRETINOIN Tretinoin, the natural retinoid all-*trans*-retinoic acid, is a first-generation retinoid and was the first available topical retinoid, initially marketed as Retin-A. Once the photoaging benefits of tretinoin were described, a new formulation, Renova, was approved by the FDA and marketed for the treatment of photodamage. Although the other retinoids are also beneficial in treating photodamage, Renova is currently the only retinoid approved specifically for this purpose. Tretinoin is a nonselective retinoid that activates all RAR pathways (α, β, and γ) directly and RXR pathways indirectly through conversion of all-*trans*-retinoic acid to 9-*cis*-retinoic acid (the natural ligand for RXRs).[33] Other brands of tretinoin, such as Avita, are now available, as are generic forms.

Given its availability as a generic drug, tretinoin is currently found in several products. Notably, two combination products have been introduced to the market. Ziana is a medication that contains tretinoin 0.025% and clindamycin 1.2%. It is used at night in patients with acne. This product is ideal for use in adult acne sufferers who can also benefit from an antiaging component in their skin regimen. Tri-Luma combines tretinoin, hydroquinone, and a mild steroid. It has shown utility in pigmentary disorders such as melasma and as a first-line therapy for photoaging (Chapter 33).

RETINOL Retinol, also known as vitamin A, is a first-generation retinoid as well. It must be converted to retinaldehyde and then to all-*trans*-retinoic acid by a dedicated metabolic machinery within the keratinocytes to become active in the epidermis, thus displaying much lower activity than tretinoin.[34] Although it is a precursor to retinoic acid, retinol is classified as a cosmetic rather than a drug; therefore, it is found in many OTC formulations. It is interesting to note that because cosmetic companies cannot claim that their retinol products exert a biologic action, retinol is listed on all cosmetic products as an inactive ingredient. This regulatory quirk, in addition to the fact that early forms of retinol were very unstable and exhibited a brief shelf life, has led many to believe that retinol has minimal, if any, biologic activity. Moreover, homeopathic doses of retinol and its esters are often listed on cosmetic labels, adding to the poor reputation of retinol, while retinol has been shown to have significant biologic action and efficacy at the proper doses.

Although no large multicenter trials have been performed to evaluate the efficacy of retinol, there is much ongoing research evaluating the biologic effects of this product. A recent study

TABLE 30-2
Receptor Selectivity (for Both Receptor Binding, and Gene Transactivation)

	RARs	RXRs
Tretinoin	α, β, γ	$(\alpha, \beta, \gamma)^a$
Isotretinoin	α, β, γ	$(\alpha, \beta, \gamma)^a$
Adapalene	β, γ	—
Tazarotene	β, γ	—

[a]Weak binding because of isomerization to 9-*cis*-retinoic acid

demonstrated that retinol improves the appearance of wrinkles in sun-protected areas.[35] Despite evidence that retinol binds RARs, albeit weakly, and can give rise to tretinoin, its use is not as frequently associated with clinical erythema,[36] and multiple studies have shown it to be less irritating than tretinoin. Although retinol is approximately 20 times less potent than retinoic acid, unoccluded retinol exhibits greater penetration when compared to unoccluded retinoic acid. Retinol at 0.25% may be a useful retinoid-like treatment for application without occlusion because it does not irritate the skin, but does induce cellular and molecular changes similar to those observed with application of 0.025% retinoic acid.[37] A separate study showed that 1.6% retinol induced significant epidermal thickening and other skin changes similar to those produced by retinoic acid but without measurable irritation.[36] However, much higher concentrations of retinol than retinoic acid were needed to achieve similar results. New products with high concentrations of retinol are entering the physician-dispensed market. It will be interesting to see how these perform as compared to the traditional prescribed retinoids.

The application of retinol produces histologic and molecular alterations that are very similar to those seen after application of retinoic acid. However, application of topical retinol results in extremely low systemic levels of retinoic acid. This observation provides evidence that topical retinol has a substantial margin of safety with respect to the potential for systemic absorption.[36]

Although retinol may be an efficacious OTC option for patients, it is important for patients to understand that not all retinol-containing products are equal. Retinol must be manufactured, formulated, and packaged properly to avoid oxidation and loss of potency. Also, the amount of retinol in the product must be high enough to be effective. Unfortunately, manufacturers do not list the concentration of retinol on product packages; therefore, it is difficult for consumers to make an informed purchase. Another obstacle in this area is the inclusion of ineffective esters. Myriad cosmeceutical products contain such compounds, particularly retinyl palmitate, which is topically ineffective.[5] Given the dizzying array of products available, it is important to note that some brands are properly manufactured and packaged, such as RoC Retinol Correxion, Neutrogena Healthy Skin, and Philosophy Help Me. These recommended products are packaged in light-proof aluminum tubes and contain an adequate amount of retinol.

Second Generation

ADAPALENE (DIFFERIN) Adapalene is a third-generation retinoid approved for the treatment of acne. It has selective affinity only for RARγ and RARγ receptors and does not interact with any of the RXR subtypes.[38] The drug was intentionally designed for increased receptor specificity in order to maximize the beneficial effects, and for mitigation of the unwanted effects usually seen with the topical application of retinoids. In fact, adapalene has been demonstrated to be less irritating than tretinoin in several studies.[7] Moreover, it has been shown to possess a comfortable safety margin with regard to teratogenicity, and is the only synthetic retinoid without the X classification (signifying a teratogenic compound). Pharmacologic and preclinical studies of adapalene have revealed the drug to exhibit excellent follicular penetration,[39] comedolytic activity,[40] and anti-inflammatory properties.[41] In addition, adapalene is more chemically stable than tretinoin and does not break down in the presence of light, as does tretinoin.[42] Differin is the only available formulation of adapalene. It is available in a 0.1% and a 0.3% form.

TAZAROTENE (TAZORAC/ZORAC) In 1997, the FDA approved tazarotene for the treatment of both facial acne vulgaris and plaque psoriasis. It is currently available in 0.1% and 0.05% gels and in 0.1% and 0.05% creams. Tazarotene activates the gene expression of RARβ and RARγ, but does not interact with any of the RXR subtypes.[6] Tazarotene, like other retinoids, has been shown to be effective against photoaging. One small double-blind placebo-controlled trial compared the effects of tazarotene 0.1% gel on the forearm to the effects of vehicle alone for a 12-week period.[43] Not surprisingly, tazarotene was associated with improvement in some of the signs of photodamage, such as reduced skin roughness and fine wrinkling, at the end of the study period. Beneficial histologic changes characteristic of retinoid treatment occurred in the epidermis and stratum corneum. There is clinical evidence that tazarotene is well tolerated by acne patients, but there are conflicting data on this subject in the literature. Specifically, a split-face study demonstrated that the tolerability of tazarotene 0.1% gel is clinically comparable to that of tretinoin 0.1% gel microsphere, tretinoin 0.025% gel, and adapalene 0.1% gel,[44] while tazarotene has otherwise been shown to display significantly higher irritation than other retinoids, justifying every-other-day regimens to improve patient compliance. The efficacy of every-other-day tazarotene 0.1% gel was examined in acne patients and was found to offer comparable efficacy to once-daily adapalene 0.1% gel.[45]

AGENTS THAT BIND RXR

RXRs are important in controlling apoptosis. 9-*cis*-retinoic acid (Pan-Retin), which is currently approved by the FDA for the treatment of Kaposi's sarcoma, binds the RXR α, β, and γ receptors. Its use in acne and photoaging has not yet been studied. Targretin gel is another RXR selective retinoid. Targretin selectively binds all three RXRs, α, β, and γ, and is now being reviewed in trials for psoriasis. It can repress AP-1 function, though not as well as retinoids such as retinoic acid or 9-*cis*-retinoic acid (Personal communication. Reid Bissonnette, PhD. Nuclear Receptor Discovery Department of Ligand Pharmaceuticals). The use of RXR ligands in cancer treatments implies that these drugs may have utility in preventing some of the benign neoplasms seen in aging skin; however, this has not yet been studied.

SUMMARY

Retinoids are among one of the most often used classes of agents in the dermatologic armamentarium. Many years of research have led to an ever-widening scope of uses for these products. The promotion of exfoliation, dermal collagen synthesis, and angiogenesis from topical retinoids suggests an important role for these products in the attempt to curtail the cutaneous effects of photoaging.

REFERENCES

1. Fisher GJ, Datta SC, Talwar HS, et al. Molecular basis of sun-induced premature skin ageing and retinoid antagonism. *Nature*. 1996;379:335.
2. Kligman L, Kligman AM. Photoaging—Retinoids, alpha hydroxy acids, and antioxidants. In: Gabard B, Elsner P, Surber C, Treffel P, eds. *Dermatopharmacology of Topical Preparations*, New York, NY: Springer; 2000:383.

3. Kligman AM, Grove GL, Hirose R, et al. Topical tretinoin for photoaged skin. *J Am Acad Dermatol.* 1986;15:836.
4. Karrer P, Morf R, Schopp K. Zur kenntnis des vitamin-a aus fischtranin. *Helv Chim Acta.* 1931;14:1036.
5. Kligman AM. The growing importance of topical retinoids in clinical dermatology: a retrospective and prospective analysis. *J Am Acad Dermatol.* 1998;39:S2.
6. Chandraratna RA. Tazarotene—first of a new generation of receptor-selective retinoids. *Br J Dermatol.* 1996;135:18.
7. Millikan LE. Adapalene: an update on newer comparative studies between the various retinoids. *Int J Dermatol.* 2000; 39:784.
8. Weiss JS. Current options for topical treatment of acne vulgaris. *Pediatr Dermatol.* 1997;14:480.
9. Chytil F, Ong D. Cellular retinoid-binding proteins. In: Sporn MB, Roberts A, Goodman D, eds. *The Retinoids.* Vol. 2. Orlando, FL: Academic Press; 1984: 89–123.
10. Giguere V, Ong ES, Segui P, et al. Identification of a receptor for the morphogen retinoic acid. *Nature.* 1987;330: 624.
11. Petkovich M, Brand NJ, Krust A, et al. A human retinoic acid receptor which belongs to the family of nuclear receptors. *Nature.* 1987;330:444.
12. Pfahl M. The molecular mechanism of retinoid action. Retinoids today and tomorrow. *Retinoids Dermatol.* 1996;44:2.
13. Petkovich M. Regulation of gene expression by vitamin A: the role of nuclear retinoic acid receptors. *Annu Rev Nutr.* 1992;12:443.
14. Chambon P. A decade of molecular biology of retinoic acid receptors. *FASEB J.* 1996;10:940.
15. Nagpal S, Chandraratna RA. Recent developments in receptor-selective retinoids. *Curr Pharm Des.* 2000;6:919.
16. Lippman S, Lotan R. Advances in the development of retinoids as chemopreventive agents. *J Nutr.* 2000;130:S479.
17. Fisher GJ, Wang ZQ, Datta SC, et al. Pathophysiology of premature skin aging induced by ultraviolet light. *N Engl J Med.* 1997;337:1419.
18. Fisher GJ, Datta S, Wang Z, et al. c-Jun-dependent inhibition of cutaneous procollagen transcription following ultraviolet irradiation is reversed by all-trans retinoic acid. *J Clin Invest.* 2000; 106:663.
19. Fisher GJ, Talwar HS, Lin J, et al. Molecular mechanisms of photoaging in human skin in vivo and their prevention by all-trans retinoic acid. *Photochem Photobiol.* 1999;69:154.
20. Weiss JS, Ellis CN, Headington JT, et al. Topical tretinoin improves photoaged skin: a double-blind vehicle-controlled study. *JAMA.* 1988;259:527.
21. Griffiths CE, Kang S, Ellis CN, et al. Two concentrations of topical tretinoin (retinoic acid) cause similar improvement of photoaging but different degrees of irritation. A double-blind, vehicle-controlled comparison of 0.1% and 0.025% tretinoin creams. *Arch Dermatol.* 1995;131:1037.
22. Woodley DT, Zelickson AS, Briggaman RA, et al. Treatment of photoaged skin with topical tretinoin increases epidermal-dermal anchoring fibrils. A preliminary report. *JAMA.* 1990;263:3057.
23. Rosenthal DS, Griffiths CE, Yuspa SH, et al. Acute or chronic topical retinoic acid treatment of human skin in vivo alters the expression of epidermal transglutaminase, loricrin, involucrin, filaggrin, and keratins 6 and 13 but not keratins 1, 10, and 14. *J Invest Dermatol.* 1992;98:343.
24. Griffiths CE, Finkel LJ, Tranfaglia MG, et al. An in vivo experimental model for effects of topical retinoic acid in human skin. *Br J Dermatol.* 1993;129:389.
25. Feng X, Peng ZH, Di W, et al. Suprabasal expression of a dominant-negative RXR alpha mutant in transgenic mouse epidermis impairs regulation of gene transcription and basal keratinocyte proliferation by RAR-selective retinoids. *Genes Dev.* 1997;11:59.
26. Kang S, Voorhees JJ. Photoaging therapy with topical tretinoin: an evidence-based analysis. *J Am Acad Dermatol.* 1998;39:S55.
27. Olsen EA, Katz HI, Levine N, et al. Sustained improvement in photodamaged skin with reduced tretinoin emollient cream treatment regimen: effect of once-weekly and three-times-weekly applications. *J Am Acad Dermatol.* 1997;37:227.
28. Tagami H, Tadaki T, Obata M, et al. Functional assessment of the stratum corneum under the influence of oral aromatic retinoid (etretinate) in guinea-pigs and humans. Comparison with topical retinoic acid treatment. *Br J Dermatol.* 1992;127:470.
29. Effendy I, Kwangsukstith C, Lee LY, et al. Functional changes in human stratum corneum induced by topical glycolic acid: comparison with all-trans retinoic acid. *Acta Derm Venereol.* 1995; 75:455.
30. Griffiths CE, Voorhees JJ. Human in vivo pharmacology of topical retinoids. *Arch Dermatol Res.* 1994;287:53.
31. Buchan P, Eckhoff C, Caron D, et al. Repeated topical administration of all-trans-retinoic acid and plasma levels of retinoic acids in humans. *J Am Acad Dermatol.* 1994;30:428.
32. Jick SS, Terris BZ, Jick H. First trimester topical tretinoin and congenital disorders. *Lancet.* 1993;341:1181.
33. Levin AA, Sturzenbecker LJ, Kazmer S, et al. 9-cis retinoic acid stereoisomer binds and activates the nuclear receptor RXR alpha. *Nature.* 1992;355:359.
34. Kurlandsky SB, Xiao JH, Duell EA, et al. Biological activity of all-trans retinol requires metabolic conversion to all-trans retinoic acid and is mediated through activation of nuclear retinoid receptors in human keratinocytes. *J Biol Chem.* 1994;269:32821.
35. Kafi R, Kwak HS, Schumacher WE, et al. Improvement of naturally aged skin with vitamin A (retinol). *Arch Dermatol.* 2007;143:606.
36. Kang S, Duell EA, Fisher GJ, et al. Application of retinol to human skin in vivo induces epidermal hyperplasia and cellular retinoid binding proteins characteristic of retinoic acid but without measurable retinoic acid levels or irritation. *J Invest Dermatol.* 1995; 105:549.
37. Duell EA, Kang S, Voorhees JJ. Unoccluded retinol penetrates human skin in vivo more effectively than unoccluded retinyl palmitate or retinoic acid. *J Invest Dermatol.* 1997;109:301.
38. Shalita A, Weiss JS, Chalker DK, et al. A comparison of the efficacy and safety of adapalene gel 0.1% and tretinoin gel 0.025% in the treatment of acne vulgaris: a multicenter trial. *J Am Acad Dermatol.* 1996;34:482.
39. Chandraratna RA. Tazarotene: the first receptor-selective topical retinoid for the treatment of psoriasis. *J Am Acad Dermatol.* 1997;37:S12.
40. Burke BM, Cunliffe WJ. The assessment of acne vulgaris—the Leeds technique. *Br J Dermatol.* 1984;111:83.
41. Verschoore M, Bouclier M, Czernielewski J, et al. Topical retinoids. Their uses in dermatology. *Dermatol Clin.* 1993;11:107.
42. Verschoore M, Poncet M, Czernielewski J, et al. Adapalene 0.1% gel has low skin-irritation potential. *J Am Acad Dermatol.* 1997;36:S104.
43. Sefton J, Kligman AM, Kopper SC, et al. Photodamage pilot study: a double-blind, vehicle-controlled study to assess the efficacy and safety of tazarotene 0.1% gel. *J Am Acad Dermatol.* 2000;43:656.
44. Leyden J. Split-face evaluation of the facial tolerability of tazarotene gel compared with tretinoin gels and adapalene gel. Poster presented at the 58th Annual Meeting of the American Academy of Dermatology. San Francisco, CA: March 10-15, 2000.
45. Kakita L. Tazarotene versus tretinoin or adapalene in the treatment of acne vulgaris. *J Am Acad Dermatol.* 2000;43:S51.

CHAPTER 31

Cleansing Agents

Kumar Subramanyan, PhD
K.P. Ananth

Traditionally, the primary purpose of cleansing has been to achieve cleanliness and freshness by removing oily soils, bacteria, and dirt from the face and body. The need to cleanse in order to maintain personal hygiene has been recognized for over a 1000 years. While the use of soap-like materials for cleansing originated as early as 2500 BCE,[1] soap itself is believed to have been invented sometime around 600 to 300 BCE.[2] Interestingly, the steps involved in the soap production process, known as saponification, were a carefully guarded secret until they were published in 1775, which eventually paved the way for the origins of the soap industry.[3] The first industrial manufacturing of soap in an individually wrapped and branded bar form occurred in 1884 in England.[2] Nevertheless, the oldest brand, Yardley, a small-scale perfumery and soap business, was founded in 1770, before the large-scale production of soap was given the boost by the publication of the saponification process. Several current soap producers, including Colgate Palmolive, Dial Corporation, Andrew Jergens, Procter & Gamble, and Unilever, began the manufacturing of soap in the 1800s.[3] The desire for cleanliness and freshness coupled with the sensory pleasures and health benefits drove the growth of the soap industry in the 20th century.[4] Thus, deodorant soaps grew from a need for health and hygiene benefits while the beauty segment, on the other hand, grew from a desire for beautiful skin and the pleasures of cleansing from using bars of different colors, fragrances, and shapes. This chapter will discuss the recent evolution in cleansing agents, focusing on key ingredients, and product types and their interaction with the skin.

THE CLEANSER MARKET

As the cleansing market evolved and use of soaps increased, awareness of soap-induced skin irritation, itching, dry skin, and other potential effects also expanded. This led to an increased desire on the part of the consumer to have mild cleansing bars. The introduction of synthetic detergents into the cleansing arena in 1948 made it possible to develop cleansing bars that were demonstrably milder and hence better for skin than soaps.[4] These bars provided superior skin care benefits as well as unique sensory cues. This was the first step toward providing a skin care benefit from cleansing systems.

The mild-cleanser segment of the market has grown over the years with burgeoning interest in achieving skin functional benefits, especially moisturization, from wash-off systems. The availability of novel chemicals, such as milder surfactants and polymers, coupled with an understanding of cleanser-induced changes in skin have led to novel approaches to deliver skin care benefits from cleansers.[5] The introduction of new product forms, such as liquid cleansers and cleansing cloths, has facilitated the delivery of skin care benefits from cleansers.

Facial and hand cleansing require distinct, specialized approaches. Hand cleansing is an important part of personal hygiene and can help prevent transmission of infectious germs. Health care professionals and food handlers are required to wash their hands frequently for hygienic reasons and they may often wash as many as 20 to 30 times a day. Products used for such applications have regulatory standards in terms of their bactericidal/germicidal activity and often contain specific active ingredients in a cleanser base or an alcohol base for such functions. Frequent washing of the hands can itself lead to dry, damaged, and irritated skin.[6] Use of gentle cleansers and moisturizers is necessary to maintain a healthy skin barrier in such cases.

Facial cleansing is more often associated with achieving freshness as well as enhancing appearance and beauty. Removing "oily" residues (including makeup) without causing any damage to the skin is essential for facial cleansing. Currently available facial cleansing products include foaming (surfactant-containing) and nonfoaming (low- to no-surfactant) systems and towelettes.[3] Nonfoaming cleansers tend to be mild, but somewhat less efficient in cleansing. Cleansing towelettes provide consumers with convenience and ease of use and have been quite popular in the developed markets.

The evolution of skin cleansing technology from the basic soap to synthetic detergent (syndet) bars with moisturizing creams, shower gels that provide positive skin care benefits, and other formats is depicted in Fig. 31-1.

ANATOMY OF A CLEANSER

Figure 31-2 shows the typical anatomy of a skin cleanser. Key ingredients in a cleanser and their roles are discussed below.

Commonly Used Surfactants in Cleansing

Surfactants are the key active ingredients in cleanser formulations and control

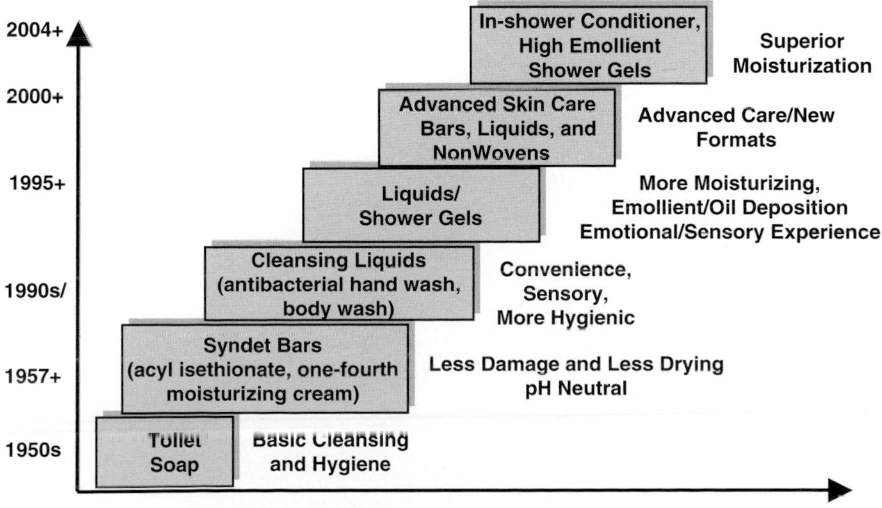

▲ **FIGURE 31-1** Evolution of cleansing products in the market.

Sensory, deposition	Other additives
Occlusion, emolliency	Oils/Lipids
Hydration	Humectants
Sensory	Perfume
Stability	Structurants
Cleansing, foam, lather	Surfactants

▲ **FIGURE 31-2** Typical constituents of a personal cleanser.

the degree of mildness or irritancy associated with the product. Anionic (negatively charged) surfactants, because of their ideal foam and lather characteristics, are typically used as the primary surfactants in cleansers. Because bars have to maintain a "solid" form and the structure has to withstand processing conditions, the number of primary surfactants that can be used in bars is rather limited. In contrast, surfactants for liquid cleansers can exhibit a much wider range of chemistries and can also incorporate higher levels of emollients. The structures of surfactants commonly used in bars and liquids are provided in Table 31-1. A brief review of surfactants used in bar and liquid cleansers follows.

Typical Surfactants Used in Cleansing Bars

The primary surfactant used in most cleansing bars throughout the world is soap (alkyl carboxylate). Soaps, also called natural surfactants, are typically produced by a saponification process that involves a reaction of a triglyceride oil/fat with an alkali. Vegetable oils, such as palm oil, palm oil derivatives (palm stearine, palm olein), rice bran oil, ground nut oil, and castor oil combined with coconut oil or palm kernel oil are typically used in soap production.[3] Nonvegetable ingredients used in soap making usually originate from animal fat such as tallow. Although effective as cleansers, soaps are known to be harsh to the skin. Erythema, xerosis, and pruritus, especially in cold weather, represent the most common cutaneous problems attributed to the use of soap.[3]

Several factors influence the irritancy potential of personal wash products.[7–9] The surfactant type is the main influence. Because they are the most active in solution, surfactants with C_{10} to C_{14} chain lengths are the most aggressive. Soap-based cleansers typically contain surfactants with this chain length distribution. Poor rinsability, which can lead to surfactant residue on the skin, along with a high pH augments the potential irritancy of the product.[3] If the pH of the skin remains increased for more than 4 hours as a result of inadequate rinsing and/or excessive washing, the resulting alkalinity can irritate the skin.[10] Typical soaps are characterized by a pH in the range of 9.5 to 11.0, and are hence alkaline in nature. Attempts to diminish the irritancy of soaps through the addition of secondary components have led to the development of newer classes of soaps such as superfatted soaps, transparent soaps, and combination bars (combars).[3]

SUPERFATTED SOAPS These products are created as a result of incomplete saponification (neutralization) by leaving unreacted fatty acids or oils in the product or by adding fatty alcohols, fatty acids, or esters during the manufacturing process. Superfatting typically enhances various qualities of a soap product, including mildness and moisturization, as well as the lather, mush value, and wear rate characteristics.[3,7,11]

TRANSPARENT SOAPS These products are manufactured with a high level of humectants such as glycerol that tend to solubilize the soaps to yield a transparent, clear appearance. However, these products contain high levels of active soap and an alkaline pH, which tend to promote irritancy. Nevertheless, transparent soaps are typically rendered mild by the presence of glycerin, a humectant, and a low level of total fatty matter.[3]

COMBINATION BARS These products usually contain natural soaps in combination with milder synthetic surfactants. The synthetic surfactants tend to blunt the irritancy of the product, although the pH remains high, at approximately 9.0 to 9.5.[3] Combars are typically less irritating than normal soap bars.

TABLE 31-1
Structure of Commonly Used Surfactants in Cleansing

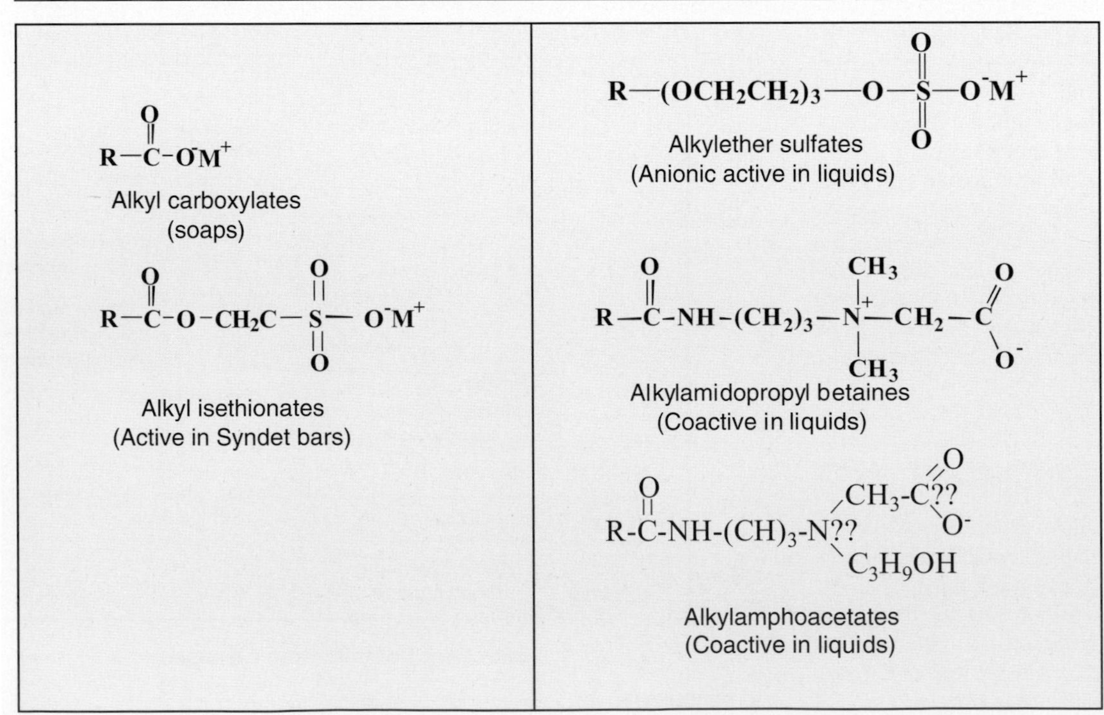

SYNTHETIC DETERGENT BARS Bars composed of synthetic surfactants are often referred to as "syndet bars." Unlike soaps, these surfactants are created via esterification, ethoxylaton, and sulfonation of oils, fats, or petroleum products. Alkyl glyceryl ether sulfonate, alpha olefin sulfonates, betaines, sulfosuccinates, sodium cocoyl monoglyceride sulfate, and sodium cocoyl isethionate are among the commonly included synthetic surfactants in syndet bars.[3] Cleansing bars with soap (alkyl carboxylate) are formulated in the alkaline pH range with pH values as high as 10 to 10.5. In contrast, syndet bars (alkyl isethionate-based bars) are formulated in the neutral pH range. High-melting-point fatty acids, waxes, and esters are among the other ingredients included in syndet bars.[3] Notably, sodium cocoyl isethionate, the most frequently used synthetic surfactant, exhibits unique molecular characteristics that have defined a new dimension in the mildness of cleansing bars as described later in this chapter.

Typical Surfactants Used in Cleansing Liquids

Liquid cleansers often use a combination of anionic and amphoteric (neutral charge) surfactants. Increasingly, nonionic surfactants and amino acid-based surfactants are being included in cleanser systems because of their capacity to enhance mildness. Typical anionic surfactants used in liquid cleansers include soaps (salts of fatty acids) and synthetic surfactants such as alkyl ether sulfate, alkyl acyl isethionates, alkyl phosphates, alkyl sulfosuccinates, and alkyl sulfonates. Amino acid-based anionic surfactants such as acyl glycinates are being used more frequently as primary surfactants in liquid cleansing systems. Commonly used zwitterionic surfactants include cocoamido propyl betaine and cocoamphoacetate. Alkyl polyglucoside is one of the nonionic surfactants found in some cleansers. Amino acid-based surfactants such as alkyl glutamates, sarcosinates, and glycinates are being used with increasing frequency in cleansers. Most liquid cleansers are formulated in the neutral to acidic pH range except those that contain soap (alkyl carboxylate) as the main active ingredient; such products tend to remain in the alkaline range.

Other Elements of a Skin Cleanser

In addition to surfactants, cleansers contain structurants, sensory modifiers, and perfumes. Perfume is probably the single most expensive ingredient in a cleanser and its importance from a consumer perspective cannot be overlooked. In cleansing bars, structurants are required to maintain the "solid format" and to facilitate the rather complex manufacturing process. Commonly used structurants include long-chain fatty acids, waxes, and alkyl esters. In liquids, the role of the structurant is to provide the right rheology/consistency for the product for optimal dispensing and in-use experience. In addition, structurants also ensure physical stability of dispersed/suspended phases and are often included to provide moisturization benefits. Emollients are added to cleansers to minimize the drying effects of the surfactants. Typical emollients/occlusives used in moisturizing shower gels are triglyceride oils, lipids, petrolatum, waxes, and mineral oil. Water-soluble humectants such as glycerol are also used in cleansing systems to impart a moisturizing effect.

Cleansers formulated for specific benefits may contain other functional ingredients. For example, antimicrobial cleansers often contain bactericidal actives such as triclosan or triclocarban. Such ingredients are limited to those approved by the U.S. Food and Drug Administration (FDA) for specific use in cleansing products. The FDA regulates synthetic cleansers and those intended to confer antibacterial or other drug-like effects; the Consumer Product Safety Commission regulates pure soap products. Cleansers designed for frequent hand disinfection among health care workers or food handlers have even more stringent requirements and often contain potent cationic antimicrobials such as chlorohexidine or benzalkonium chloride. Other functional ingredients are also found in facial cleansers designed for "acne" treatment and include actives such as salicylic acid or benzoyl peroxide. These products often have a relatively low pH. With advances in skin care benefit delivery from cleansers, other actives such as antiaging ingredients and skin nutrients are beginning to appear in cleansing formulations.

EFFECTS OF CLEANSERS ON SKIN

The stratum corneum (SC) is the uppermost layer of skin and acts as its protective barrier.[12–14] The SC consists of approximately 70% proteins, 15% lipids, and 15% water and is about 20 μm in thickness (~10+ layers). This membrane prevents extraneous materials from penetrating into the body as well as controls and prevents the loss of materials from within the skin. The SC is characterized by a brick-and-mortar-like structure with protein bricks embedded in a lipid matrix (see Chapter 1). Protein bricks, called corneocytes, are essentially flattened cells (~2 μm in thickness) with a proteinaceous envelope within which keratin bundles are present along with low-molecular-weight water-soluble amino acids. Part of the water in the SC is present within the corneocytes and it is associated with the keratin bundle as well as with the low-molecular-weight amino acids, often referred to as natural moisturizing factor (NMF). The rest of the water resides with the head groups of the lipid layer. Water in the SC is important for maintaining its flexibility, elasticity, and various biologic processes. Corneocytes in one layer are also bound to those in adjacent layers through protein links called desmosomes. Enzymes present in the upper layers of the SC break down the desmosomal proteins allowing the cells to be exfoliated in an orderly manner.[12] During cleansing, the SC is exposed to a relatively high concentration of surfactants (5%–20%). At these concentrations, surfactants have the ability to damage SC proteins and lipids, and increase the leaching/removal of water-soluble amino acids (NMF). The extent of damage depends upon the nature of the surfactant and the cleansing conditions (e.g., water temperature and hardness).

Immediate (Short-Term) Effects of Cleansing

SC hydration increases markedly during cleansing (since the SC absorbs water) and the excess water evaporates off within 10 to 30 minutes after washing. Hypothetical curves of changes to SC hydration immediately after a single wash are depicted in Fig. 31-3. As water evaporates at a rapid rate from the upper layers, a differential stress is created in the SC and this is thought to be the origin of the after-wash-tightness perception. As the evaporation rate reduces to its normal level, the stress is relieved and the tightness disappears. These effects become even more acute under low-humidity and low-temperature conditions. Low humidity will certainly reduce the equilibrium hydration levels in the SC.

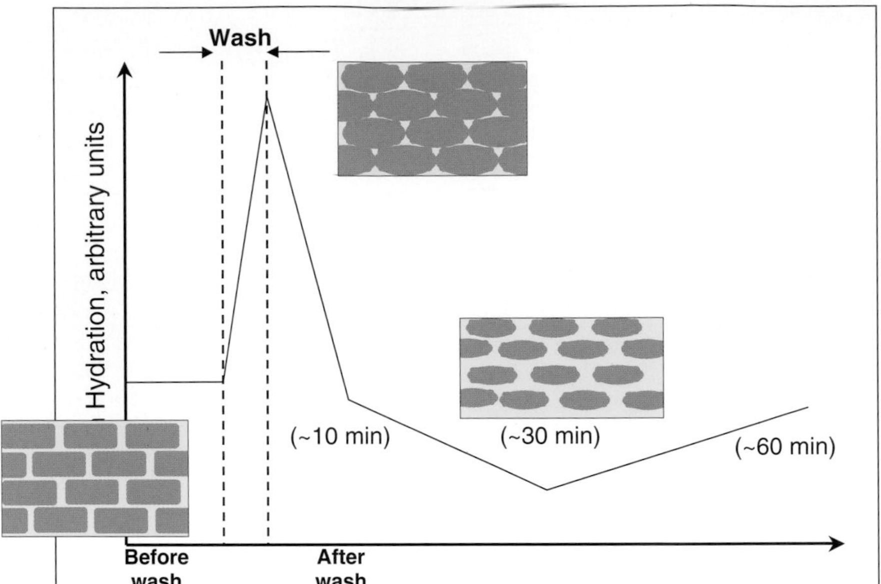

▲ **FIGURE 31-3** Schematic of the relative change in skin water content during a typical cleansing routine. Note the swelling and deswelling of the corneocytes in response to changes in water content. (*Reproduced from Ananthapadmanabhan KP, Subramanyan K, Nole G. Moisturizing cleansers. In: Loden M, Maibach H, eds. Dry Skin and Moisturizers, Chemistry & Function. 2nd ed. Boca Raton, FL: CRC Press; 2006:405-428.*)

Three factors govern how SC hydration changes during and immediately after washing[5]: (1) the amount of water that the SC absorbs during cleansing; (2) the rate of water evaporation immediately after drying; and (3) the equilibrium SC water content as determined by the humidity and temperature conditions immediately after washing. All of these changes are influenced by the nature of the cleanser surfactant through its impact on the SC proteins and lipids as briefly described below.

Effects on Proteins

Most of the water absorbed by the SC during cleansing is present within the corneocytes and results in significant protein swelling. Surfactants increase the swelling further and the extent of surfactant-induced swelling is dependent upon the nature of the surfactant. Increased SC swelling has been shown to increase irritancy and is useful as a predictor of surfactant irritation potential.[15,16] Figure 31-4 provides a comparison of SC swelling in the presence of surfactant active ingredients in a soap and a syndet bar. Results demonstrate that the extent of swelling in the presence of sodium laurate (soap) is significantly higher than in the presence of sodium cocoyl isethionate (syndet). Other factors such as solution pH and temperature can further affect the swelling. For example, high pH solutions (pH 9+) even without the presence of surfactants have been shown to increase SC swelling,[12] further suggesting the benefits of pH-neutral cleansing.

Harsh surfactants have been shown to also remove more NMF from skin.[17] This may be because of the damage to the corneocyte envelope caused by the harsh surfactant that exposes intracellular NMF to leaching. Surfactant binding to proteins may also reduce the water-holding capacity of the proteins. In either case, there is a correlation between harshness of the surfactant and the increasing loss of water-soluble proteins. As can be seen in the results of a porcine skin assay (Fig. 31-5), the higher loss of water-soluble proteins after a single wash with soap versus syndet is consistent with the higher damage/drying potential of the soap.[18]

Effects on Lipids

Among the three classes of lipids in the SC, specifically cholesterol, fatty acids, and ceramides, the latter because of its two-tailed and unusually long alkyl chain is not likely to get solubilized by the surfactants. Cholesterol and lower chain length versions of the fatty acids (e.g., C_{18}, C_{20} fatty acids as opposed to C_{24} and C_{28} fatty acids) may get solubilized in the micelle. Note, however, that even without any solubilization of SC lipids by surfactant micelles, simply by surfactant monomer intercalation into the bilayer, stress and damage can be imparted to the lipid bilayer. Insertion of anionic surfactants into the lipid bilayer can induce a charge in the bilayer and alter membrane packing and permeability. Results with model liposomes indicate that surfactant insertion into the bilayer is usually the first step toward destabilizing the bilayer, eventually leading to the break-up of the bilayer and yielding mixed micelle formation/solubilization of the liposome.[19,20] Even partial/preferential removal of lipids such as cholesterol from the SC can render the bilayer lipid unstable. Results regarding the removal of cholesterol by soap and the syndet bar are provided in Fig. 31-5 and show that soap removes more cholesterol than the syndet. While the exact reasons for this difference are

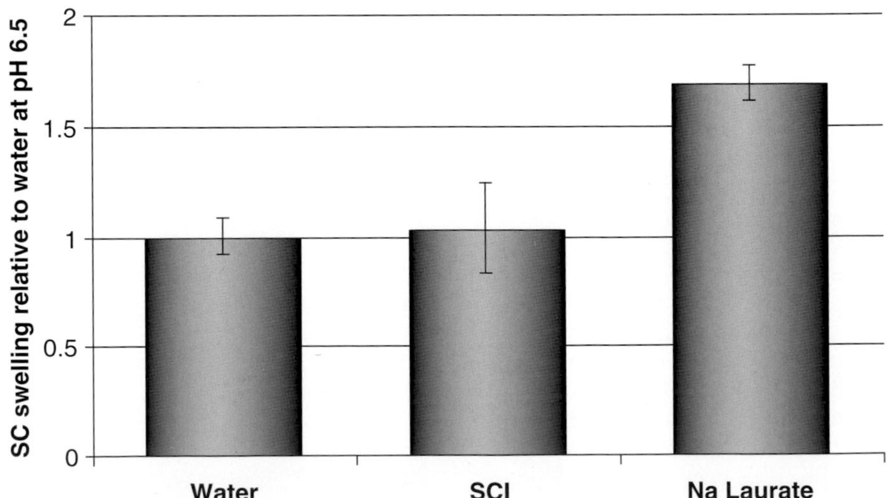

▲ **FIGURE 31-4** Swelling of porcine skin SC in sodium cocoyl isethionate *(SCI, syndet)* and Na laurate *(soap)* solutions (1 wt%). Soap-treated SC shows significantly higher swelling than that treated with syndet. (*Reproduced from Ananthapadmanabhan KP, Subramanyan K, Nole G. Moisturizing cleansers. In: Loden M, Maibach H, eds. Dry Skin and Moisturizers, Chemistry & Function. 2nd ed. Boca Raton, FL: CRC Press; 2006:405-428.*)

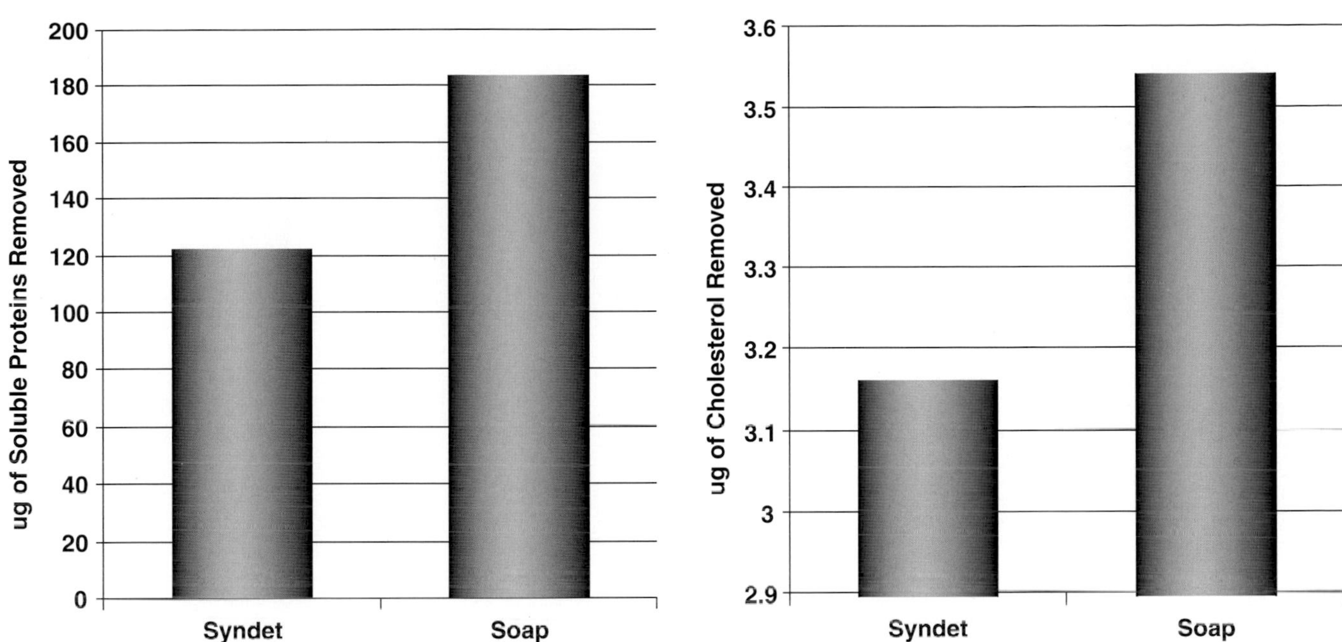

▲ **FIGURE 31-5** The amount of water-soluble free amino acids (*left*) and cholesterol (*right*) removed from porcine skin after a single wash with a syndet bar versus a soap bar. Results show significantly higher removal from the soap-washed site. (*Reproduced from Ananthapadmanabhan KP, Subramanyan K, Nole G. Moisturizing cleansers. In: Loden M, Maibach H, eds. Dry Skin and Moisturizers, Chemistry & Function. 2nd ed. Boca Raton, FL: CRC Press; 2006:405-428.*)

not clear at present, it is likely that the high pH of soap allows ionization of the bilayer fatty acids, facilitating cholesterol extraction from the SC. It is also possible that the increased swelling of soap-damaged SC allows deeper layers of the epidermis to be exposed to the cleansing surfactant.

Cumulative (Longer-Term) Effects of Repeated Exposure to Surfactants

Continued daily use of cleansers that cause short-term damage can lead to skin dryness, scaling, flaking, erythema, and pruritus.[21] While detailed molecular mechanisms involved in these effects have not been fully elucidated, based on current understanding, several possible mechanisms can be hypothesized as detailed below.

Dryness, Scaling, and Flaking

Skin dryness, or xerosis, is more than just a lack of water in the SC (see Chapter 11). It is actually a disruption in the biologic processes underlying healthy normal skin, which affects clinical as well as patient/consumer perception of skin condition. Consumer perception of dryness has both a visible and a tactile component. Visual effects of dryness are manifested by whitening of the skin and the development of visible scaling. Dry skin is also physically tighter, more brittle, and less soft than moisturized skin. Brittle SC can easily crack, leading to chapping and significant barrier damage.

Factors that cause excessive swelling followed by reduced water retention capacity in the SC will allow the corneocytes to swell and shrink repeatedly, and this cycle can create stresses leading to debonding of the corneocytes from the surrounding lipid matrix. With time, the effect may propagate down to deeper cutaneous layers leading to cracking in the SC, a poor barrier, and excessive water loss.

Reduction in the water-holding capacity of the SC can also render the corneocyte proteins brittle and vulnerable to cracking. Keratins in the SC are characterized by a glass transition temperature just below the body temperature,[22] and this is sensitive to humidity levels. The glass transition temperature is the point below which a material becomes brittle. As the humidity/water content of the SC decreases, glass transition temperature increases to values above the body temperature thus leaving the corneocytes brittle at body temperature.

The presence of water in the SC is essential for enzymes to cleave the desmosomes. In dry skin inadequate desmosomal degradation can occur, leading to the accumulation of dry cells. The result is severe xerosis with excessive flakiness in the SC.

Similar to water plasticizing the proteins, fluid lipids in the bilayer lipids are implicated in the elasticity of the SC. Removal of fluid lipids can render the SC brittle. Specifically, solvent treatment of the SC to eliminate fluid lipids has been shown to make the SC brittle.[23] In addition, it has been demonstrated that soap-treated SC acts similarly to solvent-treated SC insofar as both exhibit a brittle fracture under tension. In contrast, syndet bar-treated SC behaves more like water-treated SC, exhibiting a more elastic and pliable structure.

Visible skin dryness has been found to correlate positively with surface hydration, but not necessarily with an increase in transepidermal water loss (TEWL).[24] This suggests that significant barrier breakdown is not a requirement for skin dryness. A continued increase in dryness may, however, lead to scaling, cracking and chapping, barrier breakdown and, eventually, to irritation.

Erythema and Pruritus

Erythema and pruritus are essentially inflammatory responses of the skin when irritants, such as surfactants, penetrate into deeper layers of the SC. In the cleansing context, this is usually because of a breakdown of the barrier for reasons indicated above, leading to penetration of irritant materials. Note, however, that it may not be necessary for the surfactant to penetrate into dermal layers to elicit a response. Communication via production of cytokines in the SC can also elicit a response from the dermis.[21]

Factors that enhance the penetration of surfactants can be expected to increase surfactant-induced irritation. Thus, a swollen SC will allow increased penetration of the surfactant into deeper layers. The ability of a surfactant to swell the SC is an indication of its ability to enhance its own penetration into deeper layers and disrupt the cells in the living layer. This may be the scientific basis for the established correlation between the ability of surfactants to swell the SC and its irritation potential. If the swelling occurs by other mechanisms such as an increase in the protein negative charge because of high solution pH,[25] penetration of surfactants can also be expected to be enhanced under these conditions. Thus, the direct effect of pH 10 by itself on the SC could contribute to increased surfactant irritation. Changes in lipid layers at pH 10 may also impact irritation in that their increased rigidity may render them more vulnerable to cracking and debonding from the corneocytes thereby permitting penetration of irritants.

TECHNOLOGY OF MILD, MOISTURIZING CLEANSING

The first step toward mild cleansing is to minimize the deleterious potential of surfactants to proteins and lipids. The next step is to compensate for the damage and deliver positive benefits by incorporating cutaneously ameliorative agents into the cleanser.

Minimizing Surfactant Protein Damage

As discussed earlier, surfactants that interact potently with SC proteins leading to their swelling and denaturation have an increased potential to cause erythema, and itching.[19,21] The tendency of surfactants to interact with model proteins in vitro has also been associated with their harshness toward human skin. Thus, the greater the tendency of a surfactant to swell the SC,[15,24] model proteins such as collagen[26] and keratin,[27] denature a globular protein such as BSA,[28] or dissolve a water-insoluble hydrophobic protein such as zein,[29, 30] the greater is its tendency to irritate human skin. Results of zein solubilization by several surfactants are provided in Fig. 31-6. As can be seen, the proclivity of surfactants to interact with proteins follows the order: anionic > amphoteric > nonionic. This is consistent with the published results revealing the protein-damaging predispositions of various classes of surfactants. Figure 31-6 also shows the syndet bar active ingredient sodium cocoyl isethionate to have significantly less interaction with proteins than soap. This can be attributed to its larger head group area and lower micellar charge density as compared to sodium soaps. Similarly, the commonly used surfactant system for liquid cleansers, a combination of sodium lauryl ether sulfate (SLES) and cocoamido propyl betaine (CAPB), is significantly milder than soap. Table 31-2 displays a list of commonly used cleanser surfactants classified as relatively harsh or mild.

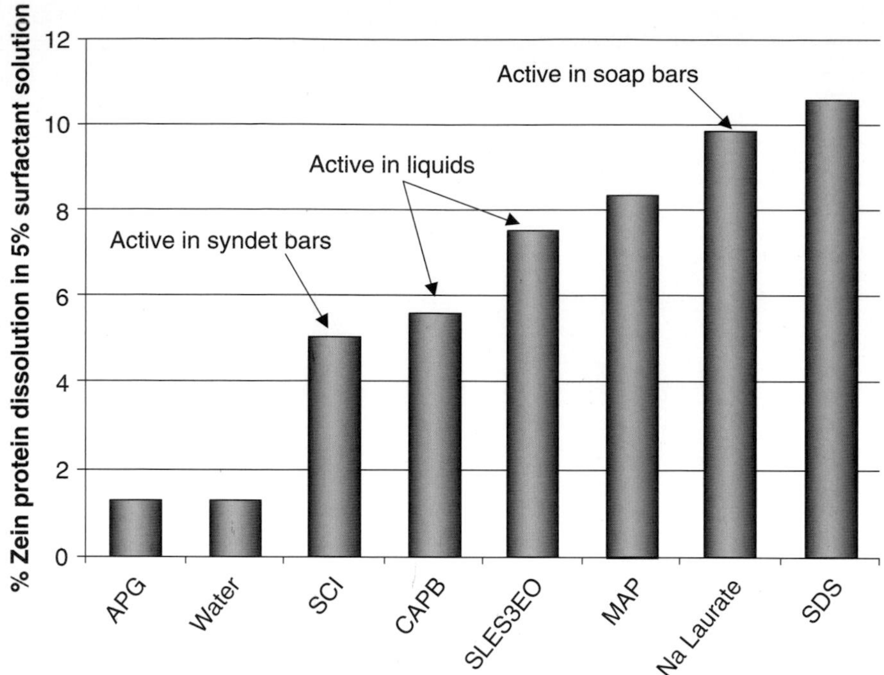

▲ **FIGURE 31-6** Protein damage potential of a number of surfactants determined using the zein dissolution test. The higher the zein dissolution, the higher is the damage potential of the surfactant. (*Reproduced from Ananthapadmanabhan KP, Subramanyan K, Nole G. Moisturizing cleansers. In: Loden M, Maibach H, eds. Dry Skin and Moisturizers, Chemistry & Function. 2nd ed. Boca Raton, FL: CRC Press; 2006:405-428.*)

While these empirical correlations are useful as guidelines for formulation work, quantitative associations between surfactant properties and their protein denaturation propensities are most useful as a predictive ruler. Based on the hypothesis that protein denaturation is essentially due to massive cooperative binding of surfactants on the protein backbone and the resultant increase in the charge of the protein, surfactant micellar charge was correlated with the zein dissolution tendencies of various surfactants. Protein denaturation has been shown to scale linearly with the charge density of surfactant micelles.[31] This insight has allowed formulators to develop novel strategies to predict and increase the mildness of cleanser bases. In general, micelle charge density can be lowered by using surfactants of larger head groups, zwitterionic or nonionic head groups, and a synergistic combination of surfactants that allow strong attractive interactions among head groups leading to a reduction in the overall charge density of the micelle.

TABLE 31-2
Commonly Used Cleanser Surfactants Classified Based on their Interactions with Proteins

Harsh Surfactants	Mild Surfactants
SLS (sodium lauryl sulfate)	SLES (sodium lauryl ether sulfate)
Na soap (Na laurate/ cocoate)	SCI (sodium cocoyl/ lauroyl isethionate)
Alkyl phosphates	CAPB (cocamido propyl betaine)
	Alkyl sulfosuccinates
	Alkyl sarcosinates

Minimizing Surfactant Lipid Damage

Long-term surfactant damage to SC lipids extends from the short-term effects resulting in cumulative loss of barrier function and lipid fluidity leading to profound dryness. The results of an assessment of lipid damage potential of surfactants as measured by the solubility of stearic acid and cholesterol in 5% surfactant solutions are shown in Fig. 31-7. It appears that all the surfactants have some proclivity to solubilize critical SC lipids such as cholesterol and fatty acids. Interestingly, APG shows high potential for solubilizing cholesterol in contrast to its relatively low protein swelling tendency. This result shows that mildness toward proteins does not necessarily imply mildness toward lipids, and achieving mildness toward both proteins and lipids simultaneously may require delicate balancing of surfactant properties.

A relatively less understood mechanism, namely, the presaturation of surfactant micelles with lipid mimics so that the micelle will have a reduced likelihood of delipidating the SC during washing, is a novel approach to minimize surfactant–lipid interactions. The hypothesis is that the added fatty acids actually minimize the damage to both proteins and lipids by incorporating into the surfactant micelles thus rendering the micelles milder toward both proteins and lipids.[32] Presaturation of the micelles with fatty acids will reduce the tendency of the micelles to solubilize SC lipids or intercalate into the SC bilayer. Also, the presence of fatty acids can lower the charge density of the surfactant micelles, thus enhancing their mildness toward proteins.

Compensating for Damage: Enhancing Moisturization

The main approach to minimizing visible signs of skin dryness and augmenting skin hydration has been to deposit lipids, emollient oils, and occlusives (such as those used in a lotion) under cleansing conditions. The challenges of incorporating high levels of emollients into a stable cleansing formulation and depositing the emollients on skin during the wash process have been largely surmounted by the use of specially structured surfactant formulations with cationic polymers to aid deposition and retention of oils/occlusives on the skin. Typical emollients and occlusives used in cleansing liquid formulations are vegetable oils (e.g., sunflower seed and soybean) and petroleum jelly. It is a more significant challenge to deliver water-soluble moisturizers such as glycerin and other humectants to skin during the washing process and, therefore, hydrophobic emollients are more commonly used in cleansers.

It has been demonstrated that body washes containing a high level of emollient ingredients do deposit a significant amount of lipid and emollient material to the skin. A commercial product containing sunflower seed oil was shown to deposit 10 to 15 μg/cm^2 of the emollient onto skin during a normal wash.[5] Figure 31-8 depicts the clinical advantage of such deposition on skin during cleansing. Note that the efficiency of deposition (amount of material transferred to skin versus amount contained in the product) from current technologies is still quite low, which presents an opportunity for enhancing the performance of these moisturizing body washes. Another area of opportunity is to deliver effective water-soluble moisturizers such as glycerin or lactates from a cleanser. These humectant materials are

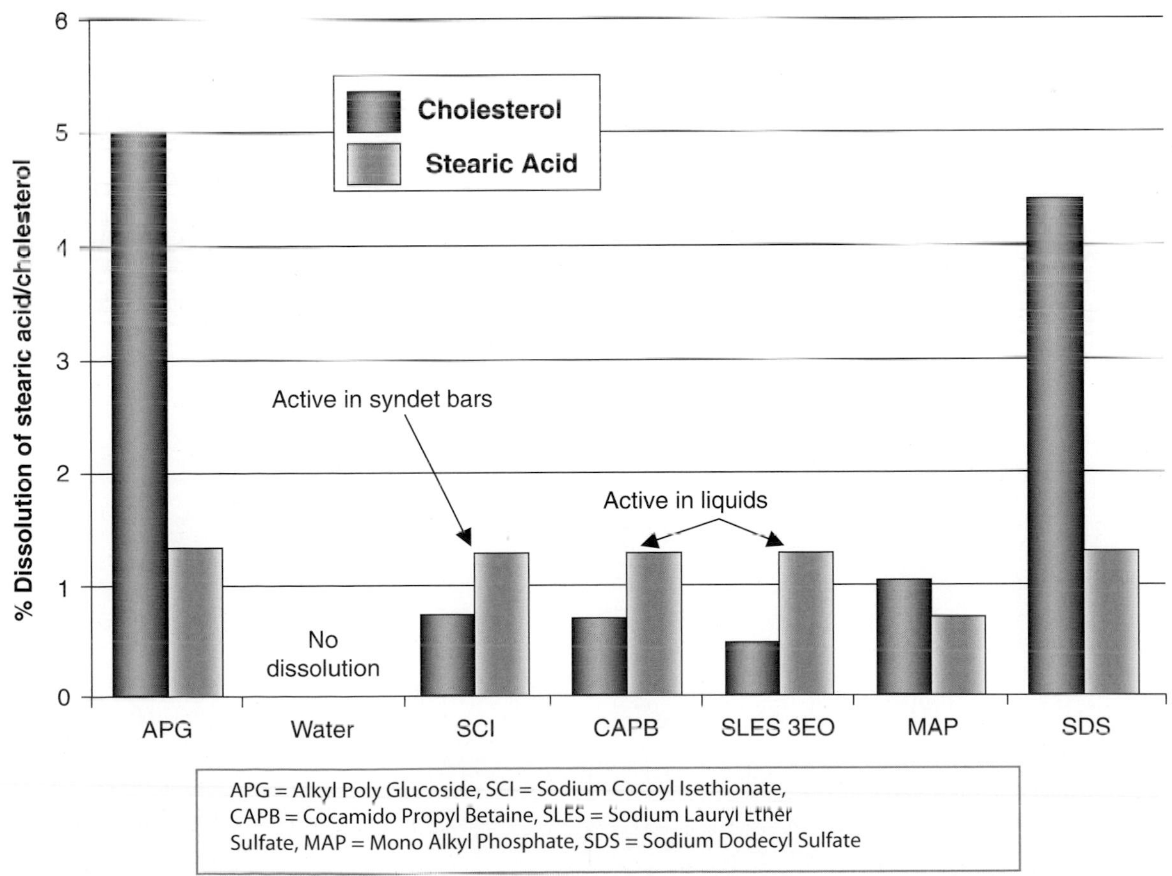

▲ **FIGURE 31-7** Lipid damage potential of a number of surfactants determined by the ability of surfactant micelles to solubilize cholesterol and stearic acid. (*Reproduced from Ananthapadmanabhan KP, Subramanyan K, Nole G. Moisturizing cleansers. In: Loden M, Maibach H, eds. Dry Skin and Moisturizers, Chemistry & Function. 2nd ed. Boca Raton, Fl: CRC Press; 2006:405-428.*)

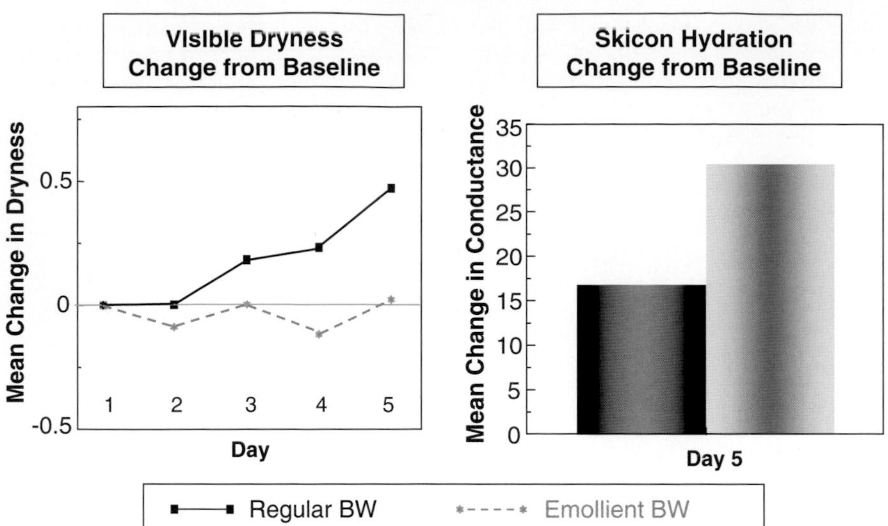

▲ **FIGURE 31-8** Clinical study (*5-day repeat wash*) of regular and emollient body washes shows that emollient body wash induced no visible dryness and significantly improved the hydration state. (*Reproduced from Ananthapadmanabhan KP, Subramanyan K, Nole G. Moisturizing cleansers. In: Loden M, Maibach H, eds. Dry Skin and Moisturizers, Chemistry & Function. 2nd ed. Boca Raton, FL: CRC Press; 2006:405-428.*)

known to increase the water-holding capacity of the skin when imparted from leave-on products.

ROLE OF MILD CLEANSING IN MANAGEMENT OF DERMATOLOGIC DISORDERS

Several common skin disorders such as xerosis, dermatitis, psoriasis, atopic dermatitis, acne, rosacea, and photodamage are linked to varying levels of barrier dysfunctions.[12] Skin cleansing is an essential part of skin care. Its primary role, as mentioned previously, is to remove dirt, oil, other environmental pollutants, and bacteria from the skin. However, it is paradoxical that the act of cleansing typically leads to a weakening of the barrier as described above. Therefore, it appears that for most skin disorders, cleansing with commonly used soap-based products may prove challenging and lead to an exacerbation of patients' skin disorders.

The importance of mild cleansing in the management of compromised skin conditions such as acne, rosacea, atopic dermatitis, and photodamage has been discussed in detail in references 33 and 34. A couple of examples from these references are illustrated here.

Acne Patients: Mild Syndet Bar Versus Soap

In this randomized, double-blind study, 50 patients who were using topical benzamycin or benzamycin plus Differin to treat their moderate acne were recruited to participate in the study. The patients, each under the care of a board-certified dermatologist, were instructed to use either a soap bar or mild syndet bar to cleanse their face for a 4-week period. Patient skin was rated clinically for erythema, peeling, dryness, burning, stinging, itching, and tightness, each using a 4-point scale from 0 = none to 3 = severe. An overall assessment of acne condition was made using a 6-point scale from 1 = very severe to 6 = almost clear.

Figures 31-9 and 31-10 show the changes in skin condition between baseline and week 4, based on the dermatologist's assessment of the patients. It is evident that for the patients using soap, the clinical measures of irritation such as peeling, dryness, and irritation worsened during the 4-week period, while no significant changes in irritation measures were seen for those patients using the syndet bar. The patient self-assessment revealed several advantages for the mild cleansing bar.

Retin-A Photodamage Treatment

Retin-A (tretinoin) is a commonly used topical treatment for acne and other skin disorders, and more recently as a treatment for the lines, wrinkles, and uneven pigmentation characteristic of photodamaged skin. Because Retin-A increases skin susceptibility to irritation, patients using topical Retin-A should use a cleanser that does not exacerbate the state of their weakened barrier.

A 4-week, normal-use study was conducted involving a mild syndet cleansing bar on subjects under maintenance therapy with Retin-A for treatment of photodamaged facial skin. Of the 36 female subjects, aged from 24 to 60 years,

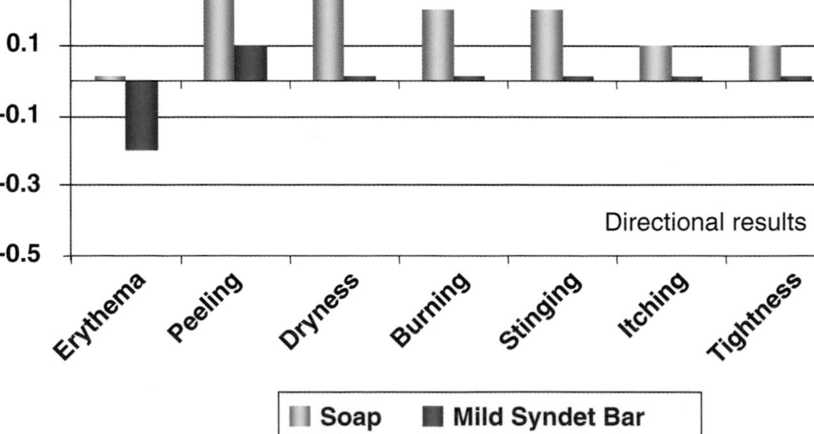

▲ **FIGURE 31-9** Changes in dermatologist assessment of skin condition after 4 weeks of using a mild syndet cleansing bar by patients with moderate acne using a topical Rx acne medication. (*Reproduced from Solodkin G, Chaudhari U, Johnson AW, et al. Benefits of mild cleansing: synthetic surfactant based (syndet) bars for patients with atopic dermatitis. Cutis. 2006;77:317.*)

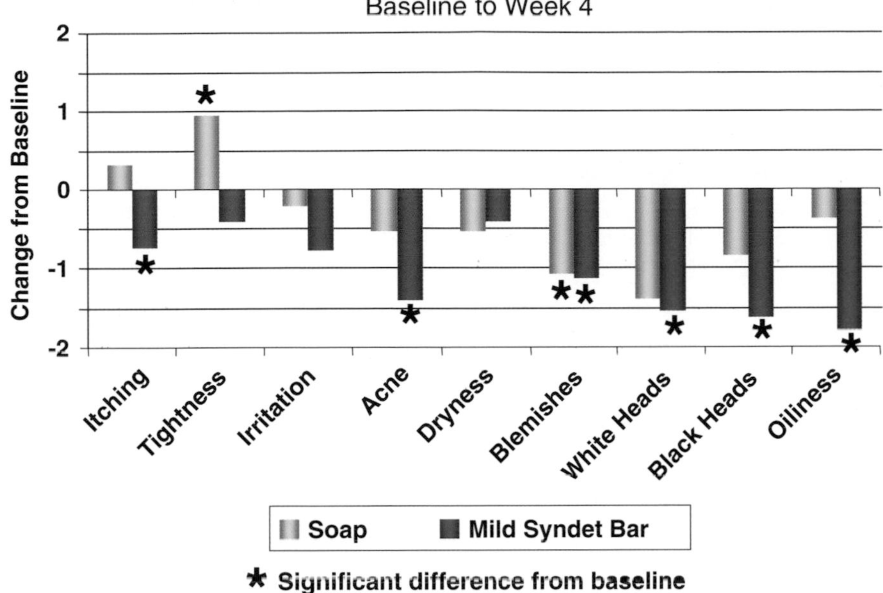

▲ **FIGURE 31-10** Changes in patient self-assessed skin condition after 4 weeks of using a mild syndet cleansing bar by patients with moderate acne using a topical Rx acne medication. (*Reproduced from Solodkin G, Chaudhari U, Johnson AW, et al. Benefits of mild cleansing: synthetic surfactant based (syndet) bars for patients with atopic dermatitis. Cutis. 2006;77:317.*)

who had enrolled, 33 successfully completed the study. On day 1, the subjects were examined by the dermatologist to determine their eligibility for enrollment. The study parameters were evaluated using a 4-point ordinal scoring scale (0 = none to 3 = severe).

In addition to being evaluated by the dermatologist, the subjects were asked to complete a self-assessment questionnaire on the condition of their facial skin at the start of the test. Following enrollment, the subjects were instructed to use the syndet bar (in lieu of their normal facial cleanser) to cleanse their face for the next 4 weeks. A diary was given to the subjects to document daily use routines and any comments concerning skin reactions. The subjects returned to the test facility after 4 weeks. At that time, a final skin examination was performed by the dermatologist. Also, subjects were asked to complete the skin self-assessment questionnaire (as at the beginning of the test) to monitor their perceived change in skin condition over the 4 weeks of product use.

Figures 31-10 and 31-11 show the mean change (from baseline to week 4) in dermatologist-assessed and patient self-assessed skin condition for patients on maintenance Retin-A therapy for treatment of facial photodamage. Significant improvements in dryness, skin health, skin appearance, softness, and smoothness were observed after using the mild cleansing bar for 4 weeks.

Results of the clinical studies reported here clearly show that cleansing with a mild synthetic cleansing bar is beneficial for patients with chronic, as well as "induced," sensitive skin and validate the need for mild cleansing to be a part of routine fundamental skin care.

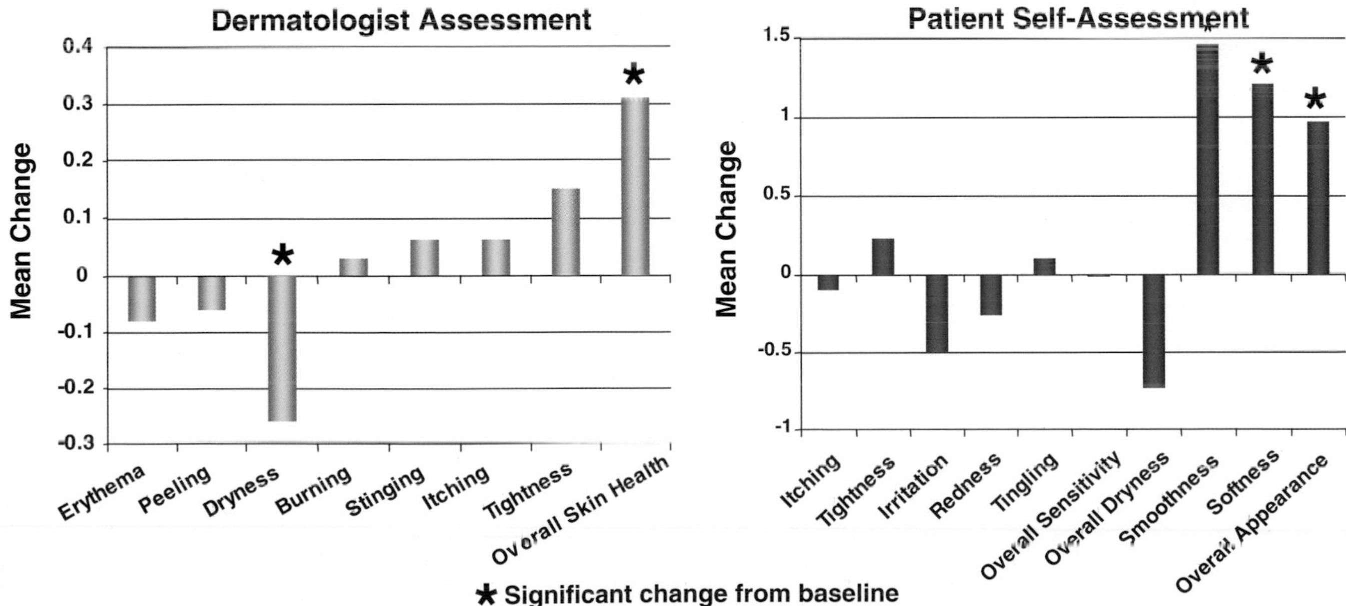

▲ **FIGURE 31-11** Changes in dermatologist-assessed and patient self-assessed skin condition after 4 weeks of using a mild syndet cleansing bar by patients under maintenance Retin-A therapy for photodamage treatment. (*Reproduced from Solodkin G, Chaudhari U, Johnson AW, et al. Benefits of mild cleansing: synthetic surfactant based (syndet) bars for patients with atopic dermatitis. Cutis. 2006;77:317.*)

REFERENCES

1. Spitz L. Soap history, marketing and advertising. In: Spitz L, ed. *Soap Technology for the 1900s*. Champaign, IL: American Oil Chemists' Society; 1990: 1-47.
2. Stanislaus IVS, Meerbott PB. Historical review. In: *American Soap Makers Guide*. New York, NY: Henry Carey Baird; 1928:1-11.
3. Abbas S, Goldberg JW, Massaro M. Personal cleanser technology and clinical performance. *Dermatol Ther*. 2004;17: 35.
4. Frosch PJ, Kligman AM. The soap chamber test: a new method for assessing irritancy of soaps. *J Am Acad Dermatol*. 1979;1:35.
5. Ananthapadmanabhan KP, Subramanyan K, Nole G. Moisturizing cleansers. In: Loden M, Maibach H, eds. *Dry Skin and Moisturizers, Chemistry & Function*. 2nd ed. Boca Raton, FL: CRC Press; 2006: 405-428.
6. Grunewald AM, Gloor M, Gehring W, et al. Damage to skin by repetitive washing. *Contact Dermatitis*. 1995;32:225.
7. Tyebkhan G. Skin cleansing in neonates and infants–basics of cleansers. *Indian J Pediatr*. 2002;69:767.
8. Gabard B, Chatelain E, Bieli E, et al. Surfactant irritation: in vitro corneosurfametry and in vivo bioengineering. *Skin Res Technol*. 2001;7:49.
9. Barel AO, Lambrecht R, Clarys P, et al. A comparative study of the effects on the skin of a classical bar soap and a syndet cleansing bar in normal use conditions and in the soap chamber test. *Skin Res Technol*. 2001;7:98.
10. Morganti P. Natural soap and syndet bars. *Cosmetics and Toiletries*. 1995;110:89.
11. Woollatt E. *The Manufacture of Soaps, Other Detergents and Glycerin*. West Sussex, UK: Ellis Horwood Limited; 1985.
12. Harding CR. The stratum cornuem: structure and function in health and disease. *Dermatol Ther*. 2004;17:6.
13. Elias PM. Epidermal lipids, barrier function, and desquamation. *J Invest Dermatol*. 1983;80:44s.
14. Misra M, Ananthapadmanabhan KP, Hoyberg K, et al. Correlation between surfactant-induced ultrastructural changes in epidermis and transepidermal water loss. *J Soc Cosmet Chem*. 1997; 48:219.
15. Rhein L. In-vitro interactions: biochemical and biophysical effects of surfactants on skin. In: Rieger MM, Rhein LD, eds. *Surfactants in Cosmetics. Surfactant Science Series*. New York, NY: Marcel Dekker; 1997:397-425.
16. Wihelm K, Wolff H, Maibach H. Effects of surfactants on skin hydration. In: Elsner P, Berardesca E, Maibach H, eds. *Bioengineering of the Skin: Water and the Stratum Corneum*. Boca Raton, FL: CRC Press; 1994:257-274.
17. Prottey C, Ferguson T. Factors which determine the skin irritation potential of soaps and detergents. *J Soc Cosmet Chem*. 1975;26:29.
18. Ananthapadmanabhan KP, Moore DJ, Subramanyan K, et al. Cleansing without compromise: the impact of cleansers on the skin barrier and the technology of mild cleansing. *Dermatol Ther*. 2004;17:16.
19. de la Maza A, Coderch L, Lopez O, et al. Permeability changes caused by surfactants in liposomes that model the stratum corneum lipid composition. *J Am Oil Chem Soc*. 1997;74:1.
20. Deo N, Somasundaran P. Mechanism of mixed liposome solubilization in the presence of sodium dodecyl sulfate. *Colloids and surfaces. B Biointerfaces*. 2001; 186:33.
21. Imokawa G. Surfactant mildness. In: Rieger MM, Rhein LD, eds. *Surfactants in Cosmetics*. New York, NY: Marcel Dekker; 1997:427-471.
22. Lévêque JL. Water-keratin interactions. In: Elsner P, Berardesca E , Maibach H, eds. *Bioengineering of the Skin: Water and the Stratum Corneum*. Boca Raton, FL: CRC Press; 1994:13-22.
23. Ananthapadmanabhan K, Subramanyan K, Rattinger G. Moisturising cleansers. In: Leyden LJ, Rawlings AV, eds. *Skin Moisturisation. Cosmetic Science Technology Series*. Vol. 25. New York, NY: Marcel Dekker; 2002:405-432.
24. Rhein L, Robbins C, Kernee K, et al. Surfactant structure effects on swelling of isolated human stratum corneum. *J Soc Cosmet Chem*. 1986;37:125.
25. Ananthapadmanabhan K, Lips A, Vincent C, et al. pH-induced alterations in stratum corneum properties. *Int J Cosmet Sci*. 2003;25:103.
26. Blakehaskins J, Scala D, Rhein L, et al. Determination of surfactant irritancy from the swelling behavior of a collagen membrane. *J Soc Cosmet Chem*. 1985;36: 379.
27. Robbins C, Fernee K. Some observations on the swelling of human epidermal membrane. *J Soc Cosmet Chem*. 1983;34: 21.
28. Cooper E, Berner B. Interaction of surfactants with epidermal tissues: physicochemical aspects. In: Rieger MM, ed. *Surfactants in Cosmetics; Surfactant Science Series*. Vol 16. New York, NY: Marcel Dekker; 1985:195.
29. Gotte E. Skin compatibility of tensids measured by their capacity for dissolving zein. In: *Proceedings of the 4th International Congress on Surface Active Substances;*. 1964:83-90; Brussels.
30. Schwuger M, Bartnik F. Interaction of anionic surfactants with proteins, enzymes, and membranes. In: Gloxhuber C, ed. *Anionic Surfactants, Surfactant Science Series*. Vol. 10. New York, NY: Marcel Dekker; 1980:1-49.
31. Lips A, Ananthapadmanabhan K, Vethamuthu M, et al. On skin protein-surfactant interactions. *Preprint of the Society of Cosmetic Chemists Annual Scientific Seminar.* Washington, DC: 2003: 25.
32. Yang L, Vincent C, Yuan H, et al. Enhancing mildness of Syndet cleansing bars. *Poster presentation at the AAD annual meeting,* New Orleans, LA: February 2005.
33. Subramanyan K. Role of mild cleansing in the management of patient skin. *Dermatol Ther*. 2004;17:26.
34. Solodkin G, Chaudhari U, Johnson AW, et al. Benefits of mild cleansing: synthetic surfactant based (syndet) bars for patients with atopic dermatitis. *Cutis*. 2006;77:317.

CHAPTER 32

Moisturizing Agents

Leslie Baumann, MD

Moisturization research was spearheaded in the 1950s when Blank demonstrated that low moisture content of the skin is a prime factor in dry skin conditions.[1] In the last 50 years, many scientists have devoted their lives to researching moisturization and have begun to unravel the mysteries of skin hydration (see Chapter 11). It is now known that the symptoms of dry skin can be treated by increasing the hydration state of the stratum corneum (SC) with occlusive or humectant ingredients and by smoothing the rough surface with an emollient. Moisturizers represent a multibillion dollar market in the US. Commonly used moisturizers are oil-in-water emulsions, such as creams and lotions, and water-in-oil emulsions such as hand creams. There are two main types of ingredients: occlusives and humectants. A good moisturizer usually contains both components. This chapter will identify and discuss the mechanisms of action of the main components found in popular moisturizers.

MECHANISM OF ACTION OF MOISTURIZERS

There are many moisturizers on the market but they all have the same goal: to increase water content in the SC. This can be accomplished by preventing water evaporation from the skin by using occlusive ingredients or by increasing the integrity of the skin barrier (see Chapter 11). The mainstay of increasing the integrity of the skin's barrier involves providing fatty acids (such as linoleic acid, Fig. 32-1), ceramides, cholesterol, and controlling the calcium gradient. Increasing the skin's ability to hold onto water is another strategy for moisturizing skin. Increasing levels of natural moisturizing factor (NMF), glycerin (glycerol), and other humectants such as hyaluronic acid will help skin hold onto water. Lastly, increasing the ability of the epidermis to absorb important components for the circulation, such as glycerol and water through aquaporin channels, will also aid in increasing skin hydration.

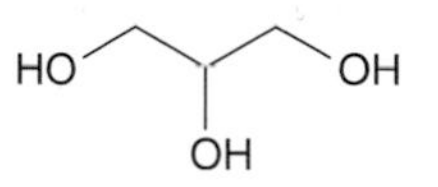

▲ **FIGURE 32-1** Linoleic acid.

OCCLUSIVES

Occlusives coat the SC to retard transepidermal water loss (TEWL). They are usually oily substances that have the ability to dissolve fats and are therefore widely used as a component in skin care cosmetics. An occlusive is one of the best choices to treat dry skin because it provides an emollient effect as well as decreases TEWL. Two of the best occlusive ingredients currently available are petrolatum and mineral oil. Petrolatum, for example, exhibits a water vapor loss resistance 170 times that of olive oil.[2] However, petrolatum has a greasy feeling that may render agents containing it cosmetically unacceptable. Other commonly used occlusive ingredients include paraffin, squalene, dimethicone, soybean oil, grapeseed oil, propylene glycol, lanolin, and beeswax.[3] In addition, "natural" oils such as sunflower oil have been increasing in popularity. Occlusive agents are only effective while present on the skin; once removed, TEWL returns to the previous level. Interestingly, it is not desirable to lower TEWL by more than 40% because maceration with increased levels of bacteria can result.[4] In moisturizers, occlusives are usually combined with humectant ingredients.

Petrolatum

Petrolatum is considered by many, including Kligman,[5] to be one of the best moisturizers. It has been used as a skin care product since 1872. Petrolatum is a purified mixture of hydrocarbons that is derived from petroleum (crude oil). The hydrocarbon molecules present in petrolatum prevent oxidation, giving petrolatum a long shelf life. Because petrolatum is one of the most occlusive moisturizing ingredients known, it is often the gold standard to which other occlusive ingredients are compared.[6] Petrolatum is also well known for being noncomedogenic.[7] Although extremely rare, allergic contact dermatitis to petrolatum has been reported in the literature.[8,9] The possibility of an individual being allergic to petrolatum is so infrequent that some authors believe it to be a nonsensitizing agent.[10] However, when used alone, many find the greasy, oily texture cosmetically inelegant. Therefore, petrolatum is often combined with other ingredients to minimize the greasy feeling.

Lanolin

Lanolin is a complex natural product that cannot be synthesized. The method of refinement used determines the composition and quality of the resulting product, so not all lanolin products display the same properties.[11] Lanolin is derived from the sebaceous secretions of sheep; however, its composition is very different than human sebum.[12] Lanolin shares two important characteristics with SC lipids: (1) lanolin contains cholesterol, an essential component of SC lipids, and (2) lanolin and SC lipids can coexist as solids and liquids at physiologic temperatures. Unfortunately, there is a subset of individuals who develop contact sensitization to lanolin; therefore, it has developed a reputation as a sensitizer that, according to some, may be undeserved.[13] Many moisturizing products are now labeled as "lanolin free." The concern over allergic reactions to lanolin has led to the development of ultra-pure medical grade lanolin products such as Medilan™. Medilan and Medilan Ultra have been shown to be effective in the treatment of xerotic skin and superficial wound healing.[14–16]

Oils

With the surge in popularity of natural and organic ingredients, essential oils are now commonly used in moisturizing products or as moisturizing agents themselves. In addition, moisturizing "cleansing oils" are also commercially available. Oil is a substance that is liquid at room temperature and insoluble in water. It is both hydrophobic and lipophilic. In fact, oils contain copious lipids, which the skin requires for the proper formation and function of cell membranes to prevent TEWL. Vegetable oils are pressed out of seeds and essential oils are steamed from several plant parts, including stems, leaves, and roots. Not all oils are of botanical origin. Mineral oil, or liquid petrolatum, is derived from the distillation of petroleum in the production of gasoline.

Mineral Oil

With a history of cosmetic uses spanning two millennia and inclusion in modern cosmetic agents for more than 100 years, mineral oil is one of the most frequently used oils in skin care products.[17] Nearly 20 years ago, investigators found that an emulsion containing mineral oil was more effective than several linoleic acid emulsions in diminishing skin vapor loss induced in volunteers by the topical application of the surfactant sodium lauryl sulfate.[18] In 2004, a randomized, double-blind, and controlled trial showed that mineral oil and extra virgin coconut oil were equally efficacious and safe as moisturizers in treating mild-to-moderate xerosis in 34 patients, with surface lipid level and skin hydration significantly enhanced in both groups.[19] Because of its source, though, several criticisms, and some myths, have emerged regarding mineral oil. In fact, more than 10 years ago, an epidemiologic review of the relationship between mineral oil exposure and cancer revealed several associations.[20] Importantly, however, any such evidence linking mineral oil exposure (via dermal contact or inhalation) and specific forms of cancer has been derived from cases of protracted exposure to industrial grade mineral oil. Cosmetic grade mineral oil has never been associated with cancer etiology. Furthermore, a recent study suggested that even though industrial grade mineral oil may be comedogenic, cosmetic grade mineral oil patently is not, and, consequently, should not be excluded from appropriate cosmetic formulations because of lingering myths or extrapolations from industrial grade mineral oil regarding comedogenicity.[17]

Natural Oils

Natural oils contain fatty acids that are important in maintaining the skin barrier. Linoleic acid, an omega-6 fatty acid present in sunflower, safflower, and other oils, is an example of an essential fatty acid that must be obtained from the diet or through topical application. In addition to providing structural lipids needed for barrier integrity, linoleic acid is used by the body to produce γ-linolenic acid (GLA). GLA is a polyunsaturated essential *cis* fatty acid important in the production of prostaglandins; therefore, it plays a role in the inflammatory process. Many oils and foods contain linoleic acid (Table 32-1). Several of these oils are found in skin care products that supply fatty acids while functioning as occlusive agents.

TABLE 32-1
Oils and Foods That Contain Linoleic Acid

Oils	Foods
Coconut	Egg yolks
Grape seed	Grass-fed cow milk
Hemp	Lard
Macadamia	Okra
Olive	Soybean
Palm	Spirulina
Peanut	
Pistachio	
Poppy seed	
Rice bran	
Safflower	
Sesame	
Sunflower	
Walnut	
Wheat germ	

SUNFLOWER SEED OIL (*HELIANTHUS ANNUUS*) The primary constituents of sunflower oil, oleic and linoleic acids, are fatty acids that, as suggested above, confer particular benefits to the skin. In a study by Darmstadt et al. intended to identify safe and inexpensive vegetable oils that are effective in enhancing epidermal barrier function and available in developing countries, researchers testing various oils on mouse epidermal barrier function found that mustard, olive, and soybean oils significantly delayed recovery compared to controls or skin treated with Aquaphor, which is used to ameliorate skin barrier function. However, one application of sunflower seed oil significantly accelerated skin barrier function recovery within an hour and sustained this result 5 hours after application.[21] More recently, some of the same investigators compared the effects of the topically applied emollients sunflower seed oil and Aquaphor in the prevention of nosocomial infections in very low birthweight premature infants in Bangladesh. Infants born before week 33 of gestation after hospital admission were randomly assigned to daily massage with either agent (159 subjects in each group) and results were compared with 181 untreated controls by intention-to-treat analysis. Infants treated with sunflower seed oil were 41% less likely to develop nosocomial infections as compared to controls. (Aquaphor performed slightly better than no treatment, but did not significantly reduce infection risk.) This study also fulfilled one of the aims of the earlier study by Darmstadt et al., finding sunflower seed oil an effective, affordable, and available emollient option for patients in developing countries.[22]

EVENING PRIMROSE OIL (*OENOTHERA BIENNIS*) Evening primrose oil (EPO) is rich in omega-6 fatty acids, containing both linoleic and γ-linolenic acids. Indeed, EPO is thought to be the best known source of GLA. Linoleic acid, which helps to maintain SC cohesion and contributes to TEWL reduction, is also used by the body to synthesize GLA.[23] EPO is usually taken as an oral supplement but is also included in topical skin care products. Some studies of EPO have revealed significant effects in the treatment of atopic dermatitis; however, studies have been largely inconsistent regarding such an application.[24] Nevertheless, the presence of linoleic and γ-linolenic acids may justify the use of EPO in patients with dry skin or poor nutrition.

OLIVE OIL (*OLEA EUROPAEA*) Used by the ancient Greeks, Egyptians, and Romans for bathing as well as medicinal purposes, olive oil contains various potent compounds, many with antioxidant properties, such as polyphenols, squalene, fatty acids (particularly oleic acid), triglycerides, tocopherols, carotenoids, sterols, and chlorophylls.[25] In particular, the phenols in virgin olive oil are known to scavenge reactive oxygen [25] and nitrogen species active in human disease; however, it is unknown whether the influence of these compounds extends beyond the extracellular environment.[26] Adverse side effects associated with olive oil are very rare, as this natural oil is generally regarded as safe and very weakly irritant.[27]

JOJOBA (*BUXUS CHINENSIS* OR *SIMMONDSIA CHINENSIS*) Jojoba (pronounced ho-hoba) oil is derived from the cold-pressed peanut- or small olive-sized seeds of the jojoba plant and contains several fatty acids including oleic, linoleic, linolenic, and arachidonic acids.[25] Triglycerides are also among the key components of jojoba oil. Significantly, jojoba oil is similar in consistency with human sebum, which is, in turn, readily compatible with the constituent fatty acids and triglycerides contained in this natural polyunsaturated liquid wax. Consequently considered to be a natural moisturizer, jojoba oil, which is typically used as a humectant, has been found to exhibit significant beneficial properties as an analgesic, antibacterial, anti-inflammatory, antioxidant, antiparasitic, and antipyretic agent.[25]

Essential oils have significantly increased in popularity in recent years. However, it is crucial to realize that these ingredients are common allergens.[28]

Massage therapists and others who are routinely exposed to essential oils should try and limit their exposure in order to lower their risk for developing an allergy to the topically applied oil that can translate to an allergy to the related oil in food products.[29]

HUMECTANTS

Humectants are water-soluble materials with high water absorption capabilities. They have the capacity to attract water from the atmosphere (if atmospheric humidity is greater than 80%) and from the underlying epidermis. Although humectants may draw water from the environment to help hydrate the skin, in low-humidity conditions they may take water from the deeper epidermis and dermis resulting in increased skin dryness.[30] For this reason, they work better when combined with occlusives. Humectants are also popular additives to cosmetic moisturizers because they prevent product evaporation and thickening, thereby extending the shelf life of various moisturizers. Some humectants have bacteriostatic activity as well.[31] Humectants draw water into the skin, causing a slight swelling of the SC that gives the perception of smoother skin with fewer wrinkles. As a result, many moisturizers are touted as "antiwrinkle creams" even though they impart no long-term antiwrinkling effect. Examples of commonly used humectants include glycerin, sorbitol, sodium hyaluronate, urea, propylene glycol, alpha hydroxy acids, and sugars.

Glycerin

Glycerin (glycerol) is a strong humectant and has a hygroscopic ability that closely resembles that of NMF[32] (see Chapter 11). This also allows the SC to retain a high water content even in a dry environment. Recent studies by Choi et al. have shown that glycerol plays an important role in skin hydration because glycerol levels correlate with SC hydration levels.[33]

Appa et al. compared two high-glycerin moisturizers to 16 other popular moisturizers in 394 patients with severely dry skin.[34] The high-glycerin products were superior to all other products tested over this five-year period because they rapidly restored dry skin to normal hydration. They also helped prevent the return to dryness for a longer period than the other formulations, even those containing petrolatum. Ultrastructural analysis of skin treated with "high glycerin" formulations shows that glycerin causes an expansion of the SC because of increased thickness of the corneocytes and expanded spaces between layers of corneocytes.[35] These findings suggest that glycerin appears to create a reservoir of moisture-holding ability that renders the skin more resistant to drying as seen in Appa's study. Glycerin also functions by stabilizing and fluidizing cell membranes and by hydrating enzymes needed for desmosome degradation.[34]

Glycerol can be obtained from topical preparations but can also be transported from the circulation into the epidermis through aquaporin channels (see Chapter 11). Recent studies have shown that normal SC hydration requires endogenous glycerol.[36] Two unrelated inbred mouse models demonstrated the potential importance of endogenous glycerol for normal SC hydration. Knockout mice, which lack the aquaporin-3 (AQP-3) water channel, are unable to transport glycerol from the circulation into the epidermis and they exhibit abnormal SC hydration and reduced SC glycerol levels.[37] This defect in mice is corrected when glycerol is applied topically.[38] Glycerin has been available for many years but this new research suggests that it is here to stay.

Urea

Urea is a component of the NMF. It has been used in hand creams since the 1940s.[39] In addition to being a humectant, urea displays a mild antipruritic effect.[40] Although there is some disagreement in the literature, several studies have shown that the combination of urea with hydrocortisone,[41] retinoic acid,[42] and other agents increases penetration of these agents. In a double-blind experiment, 3% and 10% urea cream were shown to be more effective in dry skin than the vehicle-control. Interestingly, TEWL was unchanged after treatment with the 3% urea cream, while the 10% urea cream caused a decrease in TEWL although the creams were reported clinically to be equally effective.[43]

Hydroxy Acids

Alpha hydroxy acids (AHAs) are a family of naturally-occurring organic acids that function as humectants; they also exhibit exfoliating properties. Glycolic and lactic acids, derived, respectively from sugar cane and sour milk, are the most commonly used AHAs in moisturizing products and were the first ones to reach the market. Other AHAs include malic acid, derived from apples, citric acid, derived from acid fruits, and tartaric acid, derived from grapes.[44] Topical preparations that contain AHAs have long been known to exert significant influence on epidermal keratinization.[45] Salicylic acid, a chemical exfoliant and the lone beta hydroxy acid (BHA), is derived from willow bark, wintergreen leaves, and sweet birch, but is also available in synthetic form.[46]

The cosmetic effects of hydroxy acids include normalization of SC exfoliation resulting in increased plasticization and decreased formation of dry scales on the surface of the skin. AHAs and BHA function by degrading the desmosomes and allowing desquamation to proceed. They also influence corneocyte cohesiveness at the basement levels of the SC,[47] where they affect its pH and improve desquamation.[48] The application of AHAs and BHA in high concentrations leads to detachment of keratinocytes and epidermolysis; application at lower concentrations degrades intercorneocyte cohesion directly above the granular layer, which furthers desquamation and thinning of the SC. A thinner SC is more flexible and compact, giving the skin a more youthful appearance. This increased flexibility obtained from the use of AHAs has been shown to persist even in low-humidity situations.[49] A thinner, more compact SC is also desirable because it better reflects light, making the skin appear more luminous.[48]

A thinner SC, however, does have some purported disadvantages. For instance, exfoliants have been demonstrated to lower the minimal erythema dose (MED) of the skin.[50] Although one study showed that glycolic acid imparted a photoprotective effect,[51] all subsequent studies have revealed increased photosensitivity following the application of AHAs.[52,53] The FDA has reviewed the research on AHAs and now requires that these products include a label warning that they be used in conjunction with sun protection.

Lactic Acid

Lactic acid is unique because it is an AHA as well as a component of the NMF. This means that it confers the same benefit as other AHAs by promoting desquamation, but offers other beneficial effects as well. The benefits of lactic acid on photoaged skin are well understood, as demonstrated by a double-blind vehicle-controlled study that found that an 8% L-lactic acid formula was superior to vehicle for the treatment of photoaged skin. Statistically significant improvements were seen in skin roughness and signs of photodamage (mottled hyperpigmentation and sallowness).[54] However, the benefits of lactic acid in dry skin are just being elucidated. This AHA was first used in 1943 for the treatment of ichthyosis.[55] Lactic acid (especially the L-isomer) has been found in vitro and in vivo to increase the production of ceramides by keratinocytes.[39,56] In addition, application of the L-isomer of lactic acid to keratinocytes not only increased the ceramide content but appeared to increase the ratio of ceramide 1 linoleate to ceramide 1 oleate. This is likely an important finding because a reduced ratio of ceramide 1 linoleate to ceramide 1 oleate is seen in diseases such as atopic dermatitis and acne.[57,58] The increased levels of ceramides, particularly ceramide 1 linoleate, may partly explain why patients treated with the L-isomer of lactic acid exhibited an improved water barrier with less TEWL after a surfactant patch test than did patients treated with vehicle alone. The effect of lactic acid on epidermal turnover is dependent on both pH and concentration. It has been shown that at a fixed lactic acid concentration the pH is the influential factor in epidermal turnover, while at fixed pH the desquamation of the skin is dependent on lactic acid concentration.[59]

Propylene Glycol

Propylene glycol (PG) is an odorless liquid that functions as both a humectant and an occlusive. It displays antimicrobial and keratolytic activity. PG has been shown to enhance the penetration of drugs such as minoxidil and steroids. Although PG is known to be a weak sensitizer itself, it may contribute to contact dermatitis by enhancing penetration by other allergens.[60]

EMOLLIENTS

These are substances added to cosmetics to soften and smooth the skin. They function by filling the spaces between desquamating corneocytes to yield a smooth surface.[61] These products provide increased cohesion causing a flattening of the curled edges of the individual corneocytes.[32] This leads to a smoother surface with less friction and greater light refraction. Many emollients function as humectants and occlusive moisturizers as well. Lanolin, mineral oil, and petrolatum are examples of occlusive ingredients that also confer an emollient effect. As suggested above, lanolin has a reputation as a common sensitizer, prompting several manufacturers to label their products as "lanolin free." This reputation may be unwarranted, though, as it is actually a very weak allergen according to Kligman.[13]

SKIN BARRIER COMPONENTS

For many years, studies have considered the application of the primary skin barrier lipid components, ceramides, cholesterol, and fatty acids, to ameliorate skin barrier function and subsequently skin hydration. In 1993, Man et al. showed that ceramide and fatty acid together, when applied without cholesterol, delayed barrier recovery. In addition, two other mixtures of cholesterol plus fatty acid, or cholesterol plus ceramide delayed barrier repair. These incomplete mixtures produced abnormal lamellar bodies, leading to abnormal SC intercellular membrane bilayers. In contrast, complete mixtures of ceramide, fatty acid, and cholesterol (all three main lipid components) allowed normal barrier recovery.[62] Studies in young mice (<10 weeks) and humans (20–30 years of age) have shown that application of a mixture of cholesterol, ceramides, and essential/nonessential free fatty acids (FFAs) in an equimolar ratio allows normal barrier recovery, whereas any 3:1:1:1 ratio of these four ingredients accelerates barrier recovery.[63] Currently, the goal of the best barrier repair moisturizers is to supply these vital components in a 3:1:1:1 ratio. Several brands such as AtoPalm, Tri Ceram, LBR Lipocream, and Dove are designed with this intention.

COLLAGEN AND POLYPEPTIDE INGREDIENTS

Many expensive moisturizers contain collagen and some manufacturers claim that the collagen in such formulations can replace the collagen lost during the aging process. This claim is unfounded, however, because most of the collagen "extracts" have a molecular weight of 15,000 to 50,000 daltons. Only substances with a molecular weight of 5000 daltons or less can penetrate the SC.[4] The popularity of these products may stem from the fact that the collagen and other hydrolyzed proteins and polypeptides that they contain leave a film on the skin that fills in surface irregularities. This is very similar to the way that hair conditioners work. Once the product dries, the protein films shrink slightly causing a subtle stretching out of fine skin wrinkles. Of course, this effect is *temporary* but can be enhanced with the addition of humectants to further *temporarily* plump out the tiny wrinkles. These products are usually labeled as firming creams as well as moisturizers, although they have little to no effect on TEWL.

HYALURONIC ACID

Hyaluronic acid (HA) is a hygroscopic sugar that can bind over 1000 times its weight in water. It is the most abundant glycosaminoglycan found in the human dermis. The recent popularity of HA fillers for injection into the dermis to correct wrinkles has led to a plethora of HA-containing moisturizers on the market. HA functions as a humectant on the skin's surface. Contrary to many marketing claims, it cannot penetrate the epidermis and enter the dermis when applied topically.[64]

NATURAL INGREDIENTS

Oatmeal

Wild oats (*Avena sativa*) have been used for over 2000 years in traditional folk medicine, particularly as a poultice or soak. Whole oat flour is thought to be protective in nature and to exhibit antioxidant activity, inhibit prostaglandin synthesis, and display a cleansing capacity. Another oat compound, oat beta-glucan, is believed to be immunomodulatory. Oat proteins exert various beneficial effects, including emulsifying activity, fat-binding activity, water-hydration capacity, low foaming potential, and antioxidant activity (courtesy of superoxide dismutase). It is thought that oat lipids influence viscosity and pasting properties and decrease TEWL. For decades, colloidal oat grain suspensions have been used as adjuncts in the treatment of atopic dermatitis.[65] Better benefits are generally seen with the use of oat fractions than whole oatmeal,[25] and colloidal oatmeal has replaced rolled oats and oatmeals in skin care products. Significantly, oatmeal has been shown to have moisturizing and anti-inflammatory properties. In a study on 12 healthy individuals, researchers assessing the anti-inflammatory activity of two topically applied oatmeal extracts (*Avena sativa* and *Avena rhealba*), using the sodium lauryl sulfate irritation model, found that both extracts displayed preventive effects on skin irritation.[66] Interestingly, oatmeal is one of the few botanically derived or natural products labeled by the FDA as an effective skin protectant.

Shea Butter

Used widely in cosmetic products as a moisturizer, particularly as an emollient, shea butter (*Butyrospermum parkii*) is a natural fat derived from the shea or karite tree, which grows naturally across 19 African countries. Recent work has revealed that shea butter manifests anti-inflammatory activity.[67] Composed mainly of oleic and stearic acids, shea butter is also notable for containing a higher percentage of unsaponifiables than other vegetable oils.[68] Shea butter is included and touted in various skin and hair care products, especially high-end skin products, for conferring rich emollient benefits, and is thought to maintain moisture and to provide benefits as an adjuvant moisturizer in the treatment of skin conditions such as atopic dermatitis, dry skin, acne, scars, and striae alba.

OTHER INGREDIENTS

Many moisturizers contain antioxidants such as vitamins C and E, coffeeberry, green tea, and coenyme Q10. These are popular ingredients because antioxidants are thought to reduce the levels of free radicals attacking the skin and related organs, a process that is thought to contribute to skin aging (see Chapter 33). Niacinamide and soy are also popular additives in cosmetic moisturizers (see Chapter 34). Another important ingredient is glycyl-L-histidyl-L-lysine-Cu^{2+} (GHK-Cu), a tripeptide-copper complex found in many moisturizers. Glycyl L histidyl lysine is a naturally-occurring tripeptide with a high affinity to copper, which was initially isolated from human plasma.[69] Copper peptide has been widely used for several years to enhance wound healing. GHK-Cu complex has also been demonstrated to enhance collagen synthesis,[70,71] and to increase levels of sulfated proteoglycans in fibroblast cultures as well as experimental animal wound models.[71,72] In addition, it plays a role in tissue remodeling by increasing the levels of matrix metalloproteinase-2 (MMP-2) and tissue inhibitors of MMPs (TIMP-1 and TIMP-2).[73] The mechanism of action and research behind this complex have led to its popularity in cosmetic products. Although some clinical trials have reported improvement of fine lines and wrinkles with topical use of products containing copper peptide,[74–76] more research is warranted to determine the efficacy of copper peptide as an antiaging agent.

New products that claim to affect calcium and potassium levels have entered the market. Such formulations may play a role in maintaining skin barrier function as fluctuations in Ca^{2+} and potassium levels have been shown to influence skin barrier function.[77] Although these findings are encouraging, they are so recent that no studies evaluating the efficacy of these products had been published as this textbook was being completed. New ingredients continuously enter the market as companies are constantly looking for the "next new thing"; however, clinical trial data are often nonexistent or remain unpublished as proprietary data by the manufacturers.

SIDE EFFECTS

Moisturizers are generally very safe, with few reports of side effects. Allergic contact dermatitis can result from the use of preservatives, perfumes, solubilizers, sunscreens, and other skin care product constituents. Ingredients that may lead to contact dermatitis include fragrances, preservatives, propylene glycol,[78] vitamin E,[79] and Kathon CG (see Chapters 18, 36, and 37 for more information).

SUMMARY

While the ultimate purpose of all moisturizers is to enhance the hydration state of the SC, moisturizing ingredients operate in distinctly specific ways. Occlusives coat the SC and reduce TEWL; humectants attract water from the atmosphere and from the underlying epidermis, hydrating the skin, and emollients soften and smooth the skin. In order to recommend the products most suited to patients' skin, the practitioner should understand the discrete categories of moisturizing ingredients and how the gamut of individual and combination products work.

REFERENCES

1. Blank IH. Factors which influence the water content of the stratum corneum. *J Invest Dermatol.* 1952;18:433.
2. Spruitt D. The interference of some substances with the water vapor loss of human skin. *Dermatologica.* 1971;142:89.
3. Draelos Z. Moisturizers. In: Draelos Z, ed. *Atlas of Cosmetic Dermatology*. New York, NY: Churchill Livingstone; 2000:83.
4. Wehr RF, Krochmal L. Considerations in selecting a moisturizer. *Cutis.* 1987;39:512.
5. Kligman A. Regression method for assessing the efficacy of moisturizers. *Cosm Toiletr.* 1978;93:27.
6. Morrison D. Petrolatum. In: Loden M, Maibach H, eds. *Dry Skin and Moisturizers*. Boca Raton, FL: CRC Press; 2000:251.
7. American Academy of Dermatology Invitational Symposium on Comedoge nicity. *J Am Acad Dermatol.* 1989;20:272.
8. Tam CC, Elston DM. Allergic contact dermatitis caused by white petrolatum on damaged skin. *Dermatitis.* 2006;17:201.
9. Ulrich G, Schmutz JL, Trechot P, et al. Sensitization to petrolatum: an unusual cause of false-positive drug patch-tests. *Allergy*. 2004;59:1006.
10. Schnuch A, Lessmann H, Geier J, et al. White petrolatum (Ph. Eur.) is virtually non-sensitizing. Analysis of IVDK data on 80 000 patients tested between 1992 and 2004 and short discussion of identification and designation of allergens. *Contact Dermatitis.* 2006;54:338.
11. Harris I, Hoppe U. Lanolins. In: Loden M, Maibach H, eds. *Dry Skin and Moisturizers*. Boca Raton, FL: CRC Press; 2000:259.
12. Proserpio G. Lanolides: emollients or moisturizers? *Cosmet Toiletr.* 1978; 93:45.
13. Kligman AM. The myth of lanolin allergy. *Contact Dermatitis.* 1998;39:103.
14. European Society of Contact Dermatitis Congress. 7th edition. Copenhagen, Denmark; 2004:9-12.
15. Clinical study to compare the efficacy of Medilan™ and Petrolatum USP for the treatment of cracked, xerotic skin. Croda Health Care, UK. 2004;V144.
16. Clinical study to compare the effect of Medilan Ultra™ and petrolatum on the rate of healing experimentally-induced blister wounds. Croda Health Care, UK. 2004;142.
17. Dinardo JC. Is mineral oil comedogenic? *J Cosmet Dermatol.* 2005;4:2.
18. Blanken R, van Vilsteren MJ, Tupker RA, et al. Effect of mineral oil and linoleic-aic-containing emulsions on the skin vapour loss of sodium-lauryl-sulphate-induced irritant skin reactions. *Contact Dermatitis.* 1989;20:93.
19. Agero AL, Verallo-Rowell VM. A randomized double-blind controlled trial comparing extra virgin coconut oil with mineral oil as a moisturizer for mild to moderate xerosis. *Dermatitis.* 2004;15:109.
20. Tolbert PE. Oils and cancer. *Cancer Causes Control.* 1997;8:386.
21. Darmstadt GL, Mao-Qiang M, Chi E, et al. Impact of topical oils on the skin barrier: possible implications for neonatal health in developing countries. *Acta Paediatr.* 2002;91:546.
22. Darmstadt GL, Saha SK, Ahmed AS, et al. Effect of topical treatment with skin barrier-enhancing emollients on nosocomial infections in preterm infants in Bangladesh: a randomized controlled trial. *Lancet.* 2005;365:1039.
23. Berbis P, Hesse S, Privat Y. Essential fatty acids and the skin. *Allerg Immunol.* 1990;22:225.
24. Williams HC. Evening primrose oil for atopic dermatitis. *BMJ.* 2003;327:1358.
25. Aburjai T, Natsheh FM. Plants used in cosmetics. *Phytother Res.* 2003;17:987.
26. de la Puerta R, Martínez Domínguez ME, Ruíz-Gutíerrez V, et al. Effects of virgin olive oil phenolics on scavenging of reactive nitrogen species and upon nitrergic neurotransmission. *Life Sci.* 2001;69:1213.

27. Kränke B, Komericki P, Aberer W. Olive oil—contact sensitizer or irritant? *Contact Dermatitis*. 1997;36:5.
28. Boonchai W, Iamtharachai P, Sunthonpalin P. Occupational allergic contact dermatitis from essential oils in aromatherapists. *Contact Dermatitis*. 2007;56:181.
29. Bleasel N, Tate B, Rademaker M. Allergic contact dermatitis following exposure to essential oils. *Australas J Dermatol*. 2002;43:211.
30. Idson B: Dry skin: moisturizing and emolliency. *Cosmet Toiletr.* 1992;107:69.
31. Mitsui T. Humectants. In: Mitsui T, ed. *New Cosmetic Science*. New York, NY: Elsevier; 1997:134.
32. Chernosky ME. Clinical aspects of dry skin. *J Soc Cosmet Chem*. 1976;27:65.
33. Choi EH, Man MQ, Wang F, et al. Is endogenous glycerol a determinant of stratum corneum hydration in humans? *J Invest Dermatol*. 2005;125:288.
34. Orth D, Appa Y. Glycerine. a natural ingredient for moisturizing skin. In: Loden M, Maibach H, eds. *Dry Skin and Moisturizers*. Boca Raton, FL: CRC Press; 2000:217.
35. Orth D, Appa Y, Contard E, et al. Effect of High Glycerin Therapeutic Moisturizers On the Ultrastructure of the Stratum Corneum. Poster presentation at the 53rd Annual Meeting of the American Academy of Dermatology. New Orleans, LA. February; 1995:3-8.
36. Fluhr JW, Mao-Qiang M, Brown BE. et al. Glycerol regulates stratum corneum hydration in sebaceous gland deficient (asebia) mice. *J Invest Dermatol*. 2003; 120:728.
37. Hara M, Ma T, Verkman AS. Selectively reduced glycerol in skin of aquaporin-3-deficient mice may account for impaired skin hydration, elasticity, and barrier recovery. *J Biol Chem*. 2002;277:46616.
38. Hara M, Verkman AS. Glycerol replacement corrects defective skin hydration, elasticity, and barrier function in aquaporin-3-deficient mice. *Proc Natl Acad Sci U S A*. 2003; 100:7360.
39. Harding C, Bartolone J, Rawlings A. Effects of natural moisturizing factor and lactic acid isomers on skin function. In: Loden M, Maibach H, eds. *Dry Skin and Moisturizers*. Boca Raton, FL: CRC Press; 2000:236.
40. Kligman AM. Dermatologic uses of urea. *Acta Derm Venereol*. 1957;37:155.
41. Wohlrab W. The influence of urea on the penetration kinetics of topically applied corticosteroids. *Acta Derm Venereol*. 1984;64:233.
42. Wohlrab W. Effect of urea on the penetration kinetics of vitamin A acid into human skin. *Z Hautkr*. 1990;65:803.
43. Serup J. A double-blind comparison of two creams containing urea as the active ingredient. Assessment of efficacy and side-effects by non-invasive techniques and a clinical scoring scheme. *Acta Derm Venereol Suppl*. 1992;177:34.
44. Lawrence N, Brody HJ, Alt TH. Chemical peeling. In: Coleman W, Hanke W, eds. *Cosmetic Surgery of the Skin*. 2nd ed. St. Louis, MO: CV Mosby; 1997:85-111.
45. Van Scott EJ, Yu RJ. Control of keratinization with alpha hydroxy acids and related compounds. I. Topical treatment of ichthyotic disorders. *Arch Dermatol*. 1974;110:586.
46. Draelos Z. Rediscovering the cutaneous benefits of salicylic acid. *Cosm Derm Supp*. Sept 1997:4.
47. Van Scott EJ, Yu R. Hyperkeratinization, corneocyte cohesion, and alpha hydroxy acids. *J Am Acad Dermatol*. 1984;11:867.
48. Berardesca E, Distante F, Vignoli GP, et al. Alpha hydroxyacids modulate stratum corneum barrier function. *Br J Dermatol*. 1997;137:934.
49. Takahashi M, Machida Y. The influence of hydroxyacids on the rheological properties of the stratum corneum. *J Soc Cosmet Chem*. 1985;36:177.
50. Draelos ZD. Therapeutic moisturizers. *Dermatol Clin*. 2000;18:597.
51. Perricone NV, Dinardo JC. Photoprotective and antiinflammatory effects of topical glycolic acid. *Dermatol Surg*. 1996;22:435.
52. Kaidbey K, Sutherland B, Bennett P, et al. Topical glycolic acid enhances photodamage by ultraviolet light. *Photodermatol Photoimmunol Photomed*. 2003;19:21.
53. Tsen-Fang T, Bowman HP, Shiou-Hwa S, et al. Effects of glycolic acid on light-induced pigmentation in Asian and Caucasian subjects. *J Am Acad Dermatol*. 2000;43:238.
54. Stiller MJ, Bartolone J, Stern R, et al. Topical 8% glycolic acid and 8% L-lactic acid creams for the treatment of photodamaged skin. A double-blind vehicle-controlled clinical trial. *Arch Dermatol*. 1996;132:631.
55. Stern E. Topical application of lactic acid in the treatment and prevention of certain disorders of the skin. *Urol Cutaneous Rev*. 1943;50:106.
56. Rawlings AV, Davies V, Carlomusto M, et al. Effect of lactic acid isomers on keratinocyte ceramide synthesis, stratum corneum lipid levels and stratum corneum barrier function. *Arch Dermatol Res*. 1996;288:383.
57. Yamamoto A, Serizawa S, Ito M, et al. Stratum corneum lipid abnormalities in atopic dermatitis. *Arch Dermatol Res*. 1991;283:219.
58. Wertz P, Miethke M, Long S, et al. The composition of ceramides from human stratum corneum and from comedones. *J Invest Derm*. 1985;84:410.
59. Thueson DO, Chan EK, Oechsli LM, et al. The roles of pH and concentration in lactic acid-induced stimulation of epidermal turnover. *Dermatol Surg*. 1998;24: 641.
60. Hannuksela M. Glycols. In: Loden M, Maibach H, eds. *Dry Skin and Moisturizers*. Boca Raton, FL: CRC Press; 2000:413-415.
61. Draelos Z. Moisturizers. In: Draelos Z, ed. *Atlas of Cosmetic Dermatology*. New York, NY: Churchill Livingstone; 2000: 85.
62. Man MQ, Feingold KR, Elias PM. Exogenous lipids influence permeability barrier recovery in acetone-treated murine skin. *Arch Dermatol*. 1993;129: 728.
63. Zettersten EM, Ghadially R, Feingold KR, et al. Optimal ratios of topical stratum corneum lipids improve barrier recovery in chronologically aged skin. *J Am Acad Dermatol*. 1997;37:403.
64. Rieger M. Hyaluronic acid in cosmetics. *Cosm Toil*. 1998;113:35.
65. Pigatto P, Bigardi A, Caputo R, et al. An evaluation of the allergic contact dermatitis potential of colloidal grain suspensions. *Am J Contact Dermat*. 1997; 8: 207.
66. Vié K, Cours-Darne S, Vienne MP, et al. Modulating effects of oatmeal extracts in the sodium lauryl sulfate skin irritancy model. *Skin Pharmacol Appl Skin Physiol*. 2002;15:120.
67. Thioune O, Ahodikpe D, Dieng M, et al. Inflammatory ointment from shea butter and hydro-alcoholic extract of Khaya senegalensis barks (Cailcederat). *Dakar Med*. 2002;45:113.
68. Lodén M, Andersson AC. Effect of topically applied lipids on surfactant-irritated skin. *Br J Dermatol*. 1996;134:215.
69. Pickart L, Thaler M. Tripeptide in human serum which prolongs survival of normal liver cells and stimulates growth in neoplastic liver. *Nat New Biol*. 1973;243:85.
70. Maquart FX, Pickart L, Laurent M, et al. Stimulation of collagen synthesis in fibroblast cultures by the tripeptide-copper complex glycyl-L-histidyl-L-lysine-Cu^{2+}. *FEBS Lett*. 1988;238:343.
71. Maquart FX, Bellon G, Chaqour B, et al. In vivo stimulation of connective tissue accumulation by the tripeptide-copper complex glycyl-L-histidyl-L-lysine-Cu^{2+} in rat experimental wounds. *J Clin Invest*. 1993;92:2368.
72. Wegrowski Y, Maquart FX, Borel JP. Stimulation of sulfated glycosaminoglycan synthesis by the tripeptide-copper complex glycyl-L-histidyl-L-lysine-Cu^{2+}. *Life Sci*. 1992;51:1049.
73. Simeon A, Emonard H, Hornebeck W, et al. The tripeptide-copper complex glycyl-L-histidyl-L-lysine-Cu2+ stimulates matrix metalloproteinase-2 expression by fibroblast cultures. *Life Sci*. 2000;67:2257.
74. Leyden J, Stephens T, Finkey MB, et al. Skin care benefits of copper peptide-containing facial creams. [Abstract P68], 60th Annual Meeting of the *American Academy of Dermatology Meeting*. New Orleans, LA. February 2002:22-27.
75. Leyden J, Stephens T, Finkey MB, et al. Skin care benefits of copper peptide-containing eye creams. [Abstract P69], 60th Annual Meeting of the *American Academy of Dermatology Meeting*. New Orleans, LA. February 2002:22-27.
76. Appa Y, Barkovic S, Finkey MB, et al. A clinical evaluation of a copper peptide-containing liquid foundation and cream concealer designed for improving skin condition. [abstract taken from P66] 60th Annual Meeting of the *American Academy of Dermatology Meeting*. New Orleans, LA. February 2002:22-27.
77. Denda M, Tsutsumi M, Inoue K, et al. Potassium channel openers accelerate epidermal barrier recovery. *Br J Dermatol*. 2007;157:888.
78. Gonzalo MA, de Argila D, Garcia JM, et al. Allergic contact dermatitis to propylene glycol. *Allergy*. 1999;54:82.
79. Baumann LS, Spencer J. The effects of topical vitamin E on the cosmetic appearance of scars. *Dermatol Surg*. 1999;25:311.

CHAPTER 33

Depigmenting Agents

Leslie Baumann, MD
Inja Bogdan Allemann, MD

Hyperpigmented lesions, whether they are solar lentigos, freckles, or melasma, are the source of frequent complaints by cosmetic patients. In addition, some cosmetic patients develop postinflammatory hyperpigmentation after chemical peels, laser treatments, or even after a bout of acne. Melanin synthesis within melanosomes and their distribution to keratinocytes within the epidermal melanin unit determines skin pigmentation. Hyperpigmentation occurs when this system goes awry (see Chapter 13). But dark spots and patches are unacceptable to cosmetic patients. For this reason, there are hundreds of products on the market that are touted as "lightening creams." Although there are many product choices available, the number of effective agents to treat hyperpigmentation disorders is relatively small. Unfortunately, most of these agents require months of use for improvement to be seen. Combination with retinoids (Chapter 30), sunscreens (Chapter 29), chemical peels (Chapter 20), and lights or lasers (Chapter 24) may enhance the effectiveness of these products. Currently available topical agents used to treat hyperpigmentation include tyrosinase inhibitors, melanosome-transfer inhibitors, melanocyte-cytotoxic agents, retinoids, peeling agents, and sunscreens. This chapter will discuss the ingredients commonly used for the treatment of pigmentary disorders.

TYROSINASE INHIBITORS

Tyrosinase, the enzyme that controls the synthesis of melanin, is a unique product of melanocytes (Fig. 13-1). It is considered to be the rate-limiting enzyme for the biosynthesis of melanin in epidermal melanocytes. Therefore, tyrosinase activity is thought to be a major regulatory step in melanogenesis. Several products on the market contain ingredients that inhibit tyrosinase and thus decrease melanin formation.

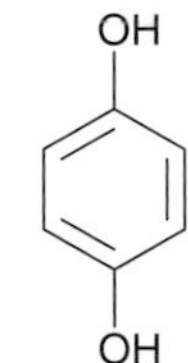

▲ **FIGURE 33-1** The chemical structure of hydroquinone.

Hydroquinone

Hydroquinone (HQ) (Fig. 33-1) is used in over-the counter (OTC) products (2% concentration or less), prescription drugs (4%), and custom pharmacy formulations (2% to ≥10%) as an ingredient to inhibit melanin production and produce skin lightening. The cosmetic products are often labeled as "skin brighteners." HQ also occurs naturally as an ingredient in various plant-derived food and beverage products, such as vegetables, fruits, grains, coffee, tea, beer, and wine.[1] For many years, HQ has been the main treatment modality for postinflammatory hyperpigmentation and melasma. HQ exerts its depigmenting effect by inhibiting tyrosinase and by virtue of its cytotoxicity to melanocytes.[2] It is known to cause reversible inhibition of cellular metabolism by affecting both DNA and RNA synthesis. Also, HQ is an efficient blocker of tyrosinase and has been shown to decrease its activity by 90%.[3] Although useful as a sole agent, HQ is often combined with other agents such as tretinoin, glycolic acid, kojic acid, and azelaic acid.[4]

HQ is currently available as OTC in 2% concentrations and by prescription in 4% concentrations. Although the 4% concentration is more effective than the more conventional 2% concentration, it is more irritating and may be more likely to lead to side effects such as skin redness. Prolonged application of HQ, often 6 weeks or more, is necessary before any improvement becomes noticeable.

Numerous concerns about the safety of HQ have emerged in recent years and, in fact, its use was banned in Europe in 2000 for general cosmetic purposes. In Asia, its use is highly regulated. At the time that this chapter was written, debate was ongoing in the United States as to whether the FDA will ban HQ in OTC formulations. Several companies have removed HQ from their products in anticipation of such a policy change. In addition, many companies with pharmaceutical products containing HQ that have not undergone the FDA approval process fear that the product will soon be banned by the FDA.

Currently, only Tri-Luma™ (Galderma) has been approved by the FDA for use in melasma. The reason for this recent scrutiny is the fact that HQ is a metabolite of benzene and has potential mutagenic properties. Some studies have shown that large doses of HQ delivered systemically—not by topical application—resulted in some evidence of cancer in rats. However, HQ is detoxified in the liver in humans, but metabolized very differently in rats.[5,6] In humans, HQ is probably metabolized to detoxified derivatives, such as glucuronide and sulfate conjugates of HQ.[7] In the 40 years HQ has been on the market, no human cases of cancer have been attributed to its use. The most serious human health effect seen in workers exposed to HQ is pigmentation of the eye and, in a small number of cases, permanent corneal damage.[1] The main concerns of the FDA are the side effects associated with topical use of HQ, which can lead to a condition called exogenous ochronosis.[8] Ochronosis presents as asymptomatic blue-black macules in the area of HQ application, which is basically a more permanent form of hyperpigmentation. It usually occurs after prolonged use of HQ in concentrations of 4% and greater, which are only available by prescription. However, ochronosis has also been reported to have resulted from the use of 2% HQ preparations.[9] Topical HQ products are thought to provoke this disorder by inhibiting the enzyme homogentisic acid oxidase in the skin. This results in the local accumulation of homogentisic acid that then polymerizes to form ochronotic pigment.[10] Exogenous ochronosis seems to occur more commonly among patients with darker skin types. Despite the widespread presence of HQ, only 30 cases of ochronosis have been attributed to its use in North America.[6] Other side effects like skin rashes and nail discoloration may also occur, but can be resolved by simply discontinuing HQ use. The incidence of side effects may also be decreased through the use of lower strengths of HQ, using a test site first to determine the presence of allergy, and taking "hydroquinone holidays" every 3 months. The debate in the FDA about the safety of HQ has increased the need for new depigmenting ingredients.

Many companies are performing research on newer, less controversial skin lighteners.

If a ban on HQ is implemented, there is one product that would remain unaffected: Tri-Luma™. When the FDA solicited safety data on HQ several years ago, only the manufacturers of Tri-Luma™ complied and it has now been approved for the short-term and intermittent long-term treatment of moderate to severe melasma. Tri-Luma™ contains 4% HQ, 0.05% tretinoin, and 0.01% fluocinolone acetonide.

Aloesin

Aloesin (Fig. 33-2) is a *C*-glycosylated chromone naturally derived from aloe vera. It competitively inhibits tyrosinase, by suppressing both the hydroxylation of tyrosine to DOPA and oxidation of DOPA to DOPAchinone, and it inhibits melanin production in cultured normal melanocytes.[11] Aloesin and a few chemically related chromones have been demonstrated to exhibit an even stronger inhibitory effect on tyrosinase than arbutin and kojic acid.[12] Another study on the inhibitory effect of aloesin and/or arbutin (administered 4 times a day for 15 days) on pigmentation in human skin after UV radiation showed suppressed pigmentation by 34% for aloesin, by 43.5% for arbutin, and by 63.3% for the cotreatment with aloesin and arbutin compared with the control group.[13]

Arbutin

Arbutin ($C_{12}H_{16}O_7$) is a naturally-occurring β-D-glucopyranoside that consists of a molecule of HQ bound to glucose (Fig. 33-3). Traditionally used in Japan, arbutin is present in the leaves of pear trees and certain herbs, such as wheat and bearberry. Its depigmenting mechanism involves a reversible inhibition of melanosomal tyrosinase activity rather than suppression of the expression and synthesis of tyrosinase.[14] However, the utility of arbutin as a depigmenting agent is unclear. Nakajima et al. recently reported that although tyrosinase activity was reduced in normal human melanocytes treated with arbutin, an increase of pigmentation occurred.[15] These results have not yet been duplicated and there are currently no published clinical studies evaluating the effects of arbutin on pigmentation disorders. Arbutin serves as an ingredient in various cosmetic products. Deoxyarbutin, a synthetic derivative of arbutin, has shown promising in vitro and in vivo results with a greater inhibition of tyrosinase than the plant-derived compound.[16]

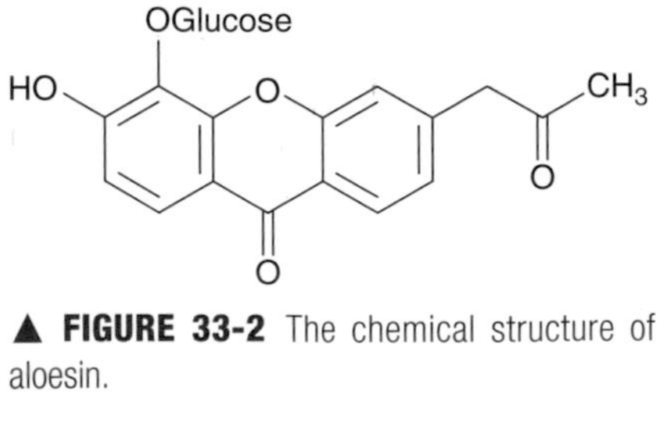

▲ **FIGURE 33-2** The chemical structure of aloesin.

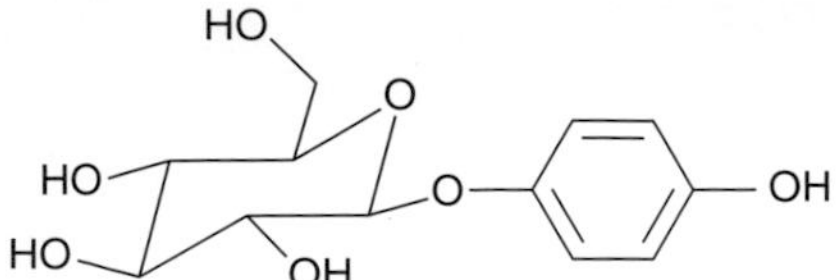

▲ **FIGURE 33-3** The chemical structure of arbutin.

Flavonoids

More than 4000 flavonoids have been identified in leaves, barks, and flowers. All have phenolic and pyrane rings, and are therefore considered benzopyrane derivatives.[17] Many flavonoids display depigmenting effects (Table 33-1). They are classified into six major groups: flavanols, flavones, flavonols, flavanones, isoflavones, and anthocyanidins. These classes differ in the conjugation of rings and the position of hydroxyl, methoxy, and glycosidic groups.[18] Flavonoids exhibit antioxidant properties but they can also directly inhibit tyrosinase and act on the distal part of the melanogenesis oxidative pathway. Resveratrol (Fig. 33-4) falls into the hydroxystilbene derivative group of flavonoids as do oxyresveratrol and gnetol, which are more efficient tyrosinase inhibitors than resveratrol.[19] Resveratrol induces depigmentation also by reducing microphthalmia-associated transcription factor (MITF) and tyrosinase promoter activity—a pathway that will be described in more detail below.[20]

In a recent study aimed at developing a skin whitening agent, investigators assessed the inhibitory effects on tyrosinase of 285 different herbal extracts, and found that *Ramulus mori* extracts performed optimally. This extract contains 2-oxyresveratrol and showed strong inhibition of tyrosinase activity, as well as melanin synthesis in B-16 melanoma cells, and caused no toxicity or irritation in various animal tests.[21]

Ellagic acid is isolated from strawberries, green tea, eucalyptus, and geraniums. It is a tyrosinase inhibitor and has been shown to prevent UV-induced pigmentation. Ellagic acid seems to be more effective than kojic acid or arbutin and it is safer than HQ as it affects melanogenesis without cytotoxic reaction.[22]

TABLE 33-1
Flavonoids and Flavonoid-like Compounds[a] [177]

FAMILY	INHIBITION OF MELANIN FORMATION
Hydroxystilbene derivatives	
Resveratrol	+
Oxyresveratrol	++
Piceatannol (PICE)	+++
Gnetol	++
(4-Methoxy-benzyliden)-(3-methoxy-phenyl)-amine.	+++
4,4-Dihydroxybiphenyl	+++
Rosmarinic acid, rooperol	?
Hydroxyflavanols conjugated to gallic acid	
EGCG [(–)-epigalloc–atechin- 3-*O*-gallate]	+
GCG [(–)-gallocatechin-3-*O*-gallate]	?
Proanthocyanidins	
Grape seed extract	+
Pycnogenol	+
Elaters	
Ellagic acid	+++
Flavonols	
Genistein	–
6,7,4-Trihydroxyisoflavone	+++
Apigenin	+
Quercetin (in onions)	+
Flavanones (Chalcones)	
Isoliquiritigeninchalcone	+++
Butein	+++
Aloesin	+++

[a]Flavonoids and flavonoid-like substances show varying degrees of tyrosinase inhibition. Some of these ingredients also inhibit melanin production through pathways other than tyrosinase inhibition. +, mild inhibition; ++, moderate inhibition; +++, strong inhibition; ?, not enough studies performed to rank.

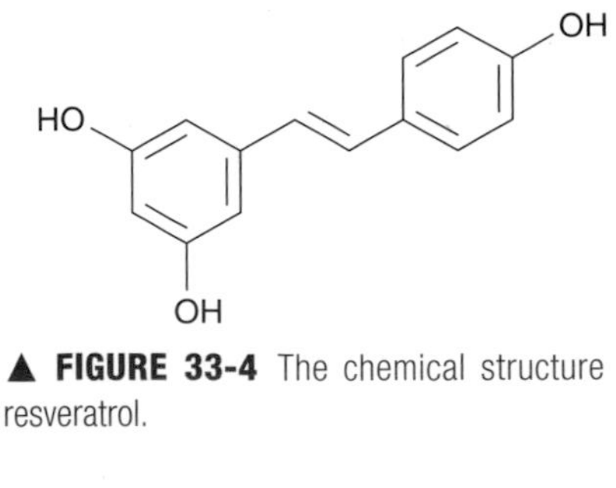

▲ **FIGURE 33-4** The chemical structure of resveratrol.

GENTISIC ACID Gentisic acid (Fig. 33-5) is derived from genetian roots. It has been tested in vitro and in cell cultures proving its inhibitory effect on tyrosinase. However, methyl gentisate seems to be more effective than the free acid. In vitro studies have shown HQ to be less effective and more cytotoxic to melanocytes than methyl gentisate.[23]

Hydroxycoumarins

Coumarins are lactones of phenylpropanoid acid with an *H*-benzopyranone nucleus. They directly interact with tyrosinase. A Japanese group studied the antimelanogenic activity of six hydrocoumarins and alpha-tocopherol in normal human melanocytes. In particular, 7-allyl-6-hydroxy-4,4,5,8-tetramethylhydrocoumarin (hydrocoumarin 4) strongly inhibited melanogenesis and intracellular glutathione (GSH) synthesis in normal human melanocytes. The investigators suggested that hydrocoumarin 4 may be effective in preventing hyperpigmentation and proposed a combined treatment of hydrocoumarins and alpha-tocopherols to enhance the hypopigmenting effect by a free radical-scavenging mechanism.[24]

Kojic Acid

Kojic acid (5-hydroxy-2-hydroxymethyl-γ-pyrone or $C_6H_6O_4$) (Fig. 33-6) is a fungal metabolite commonly produced by various species of *Aspergillus, Acetobacter,* and *Penicillium*.[25] It is widely used as a food additive for preventing enzymatic browning and to promote reddening of unripe strawberries.[26] Kojic acid suppresses tyrosinase activity, mainly by chelating copper. This leads to a whitening effect on the skin.[27] Consequently, manufacturers, particularly in Japan, have used it extensively in cosmetic agents.[28] When used in cosmetic products, kojic acid enhances the product's shelf life through its preservative and antibiotic actions.[29] This stability is one of the advantages of kojic acid when compared to HQ and other depigmenting agents.[30] In two separate studies, kojic acid combined with glycolic acid was shown to be more effective when compared with 10% glycolic acid and 4% HQ for the treatment of hyperpigmentation.[31,32] A study by Lim compared the effect of a gel containing 10% glycolic acid and 2% HQ with and without 2% kojic acid.[33] The result was that the addition of kojic acid to the gel further improved melasma.

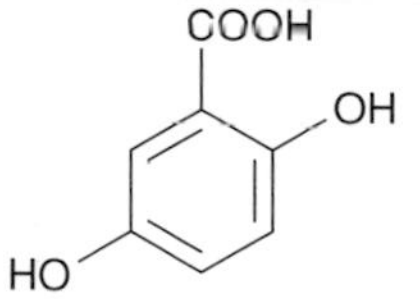

Products that contain kojic acid are usually used twice daily for 1 to 2 months or until the patient achieves the desired effect. Unfortunately, kojic acid has been associated with contact allergy and is considered to have a high sensitizing potential.[34] Because preparations using 2.5% concentrations of kojic acid have resulted in facial dermatitis,[35] a concentration of 1% is usually used. However, there have been reports of sensitization to 1% creams as well.[34] Since it has been extensively used in foods, there have been many reports on its oral safety. Toxicity resulting from an oral dose has been reported in a recent Japanese study recording the occurrence of hepatocellular tumors in p53-deficient mice.[36] Furthermore, convulsions may occur if kojic acid is injected.[30] Lee et al. recently reported on derivatives of kojic acid displaying increased efficiency through increased penetration into the skin.[37]

HO, O, OH, O

▲ **FIGURE 33-5** The chemical structure of gentistic acid.

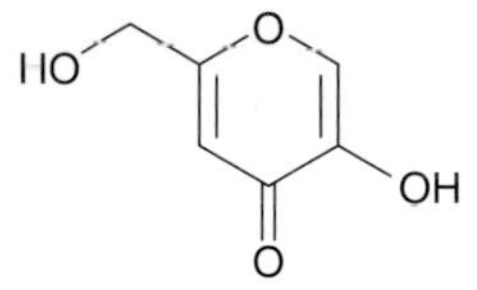

COOH, OH, HO

▲ **FIGURE 33-6** The chemical structure of kojic acid.

Licorice Extract

Glabridin (*Glycyrrhiza glabra*) (Fig. 33-7) is the main ingredient of licorice extract that affects skin. *Gl. glabra* extract has been used to treat dermatitis, eczema, pruritus, cysts, and skin irritation.[38] In addition, *Gl. glabra* has demonstrated antimutagenic, anticarcinogenic, and tumor suppressive capacity against skin cancer in animal models, and the National Cancer Institute has formally recognized the chemopreventive value of its primary constituent glycyrrhizin.[39–41] Glabridin is used in skin lightening products because it inhibits tyrosinase activity in cell cultures without affecting DNA synthesis. Combined analysis of SDS—polyacrylamide gel electrophoresis and DOPA staining on the large granule fraction of these cells has shown that glabridin specifically lowered the activities of T1 and T3 tyrosinase isozymes.

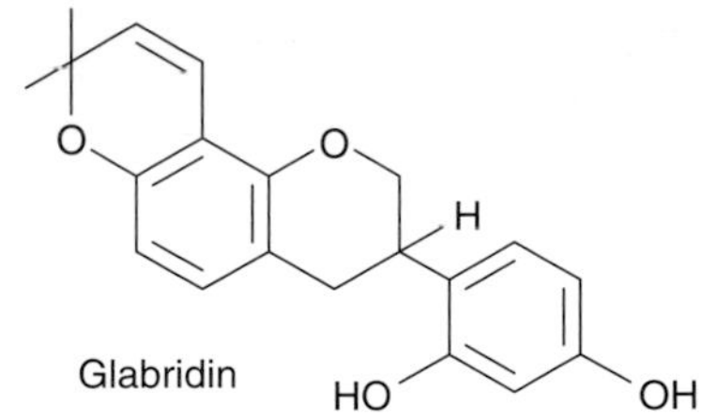

Glabridin

▲ **FIGURE 33-7** The chemical structure of glabridin.

Topical applications of 0.5% glabridin have also been demonstrated to inhibit UVB-induced pigmentation and erythema in the skin of guinea pigs. Furthermore, it has been shown that the inhibition of superoxide anion production and cyclooxygenase activity demonstrated the anti-inflammatory effects of glabridin in vitro.[42] Notably, *Gl. glabra* has shown efficacy in the treatment of melasma.[43] One study suggested that glabridin exhibits a superior depigmenting effect compared to HQ.[44] In Europe, licorice extract is widely used as an anti-inflammatory agent.[45] However, there are no controlled clinical trials in the literature examining the efficacy of this agent to treat inflammation. Forms of licorice extract have been incorporated into skin care products to prevent inflammation. One such ingredient is licochalcone A—an oxygenated retrochalcone that is found in Eucerin Redness Relief™ products. Licochalone has exhibited antiparasitic, antibacterial, and antitumorigenic activity as well as shown efficacy in treating rosacea.[17,46–50]

Paper Mulberry or Mulberry Extract

Paper mulberry is also known as *Broussonetia papyrifera*—an East Asian ornamental deciduous tree. In a study in which 101 plant extracts were evaluated for inhibitory activity against tyrosinase, L-3,4-dihydroxyphenylalanine (L-DOPA) oxidation, and melanin biosynthesis in B16 mouse melanoma cells, investigators noted that the leaves and bark of *B. papyrifera* inhibited both tyrosinase activity and L-DOPA in a concentration-dependent fashion.[51] Although it displays activity as a tyrosinase inhibitor, there are currently no peer-reviewed clinical studies evaluating its use in pigmentary disorders.

Emblicanin

Emblica in an extract from the edible *Phyllantus emblica* fruit and is thus 100% natural. The key components are the tannins emblicanin A and emblicanin B. Emblica combines all the important properties required for a skin lightening ingredient: It acts at several different sites in the melanogenesis pathway, not only as an inhibitor of tyrosinase and/or tyrosinase-related proteins (TRP-1 and 2) and peroxidase/H_2O_2,[52] but also as a broad-spectrum cascading antioxidant (Fig. 33-8). Emblica is thought to have efficacy comparable to HQ and kojic acid, but without provoking similarly harmful side effects. It is photochemically and hydrolytically stable, which facilitates its inclusion in skin care formulations.

MELANOSME-TRANSFER INHIBITORS

Niacinamide

Niacinamide, also known as nicotinamide, is the biologically active amide of vitamin B_3 (Fig. 33-9). Niacinamide has been shown to exhibit anti-inflammatory, antioxidant, and immunomodulatory properties. In addition, it has been demonstrated to inhibit the transfer of melanosomes to epidermal keratinocytes. Clinical trials have shown its ability to inhibit melanosome transfer by up to 68% in an in vitro model and improve unwanted facial pigmentation.[53] Significant effects on hyperpigmentation have been demonstrated by a 5% niacinamide formulation used twice daily for 8 weeks and by 3.5% niacinamide in combination with retinyl palmitate.[54] The effects on pigmentation have been shown to be reversible.[55] Like licorice extract, niacinamide is also an effective anti-inflammatory ingredient (Chapter 35). Niacinamide is found in Olay Total Effects, Olay Regenerist, and Olay Definity skin care lines. NIA24™ products have an ingredient similar to niacinamide.

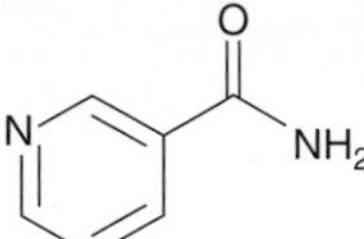

▲ **FIGURE 33-9** The chemical structure of niacinamide.

Soy

The soybean plant belongs to the pea family, *Leguminosae*. Soy is found in tofu products as well as in soybeans and soymilk. Chinese folklore suggests that Chinese women who work in the tofu industry have beautiful skin.[56] As the health benefits of soy have become known, it has been added to many skin care products.

The PAR-2, a G-protein-coupled receptor, has been found to regulate the ingestion of melanosomes by keratinocytes in culture[57] (see Chapter 13). Paine et al. demonstrated that soymilk and the soymilk-derived proteins, namely, soybean trypsin inhibitor (STI) and the Bowman-Birk inhibitor (BBI), are able to inhibit PAR-2 activation and thus induce skin depigmentation.[58] As the inhibition of melanosome transfer is reversible, side effects are negligible with a superb safety profile. The depigmenting activity of these agents and their capacity to prevent UV-induced pigmentation has been demonstrated both in vitro and in vivo. In these studies, dark-skinned Yucatan microswine were treated with soybean extract. Diminished skin color was observed visually and confirmed by F&M staining of histologic sections that demonstrated reduced melanin deposition in the skin biopsies of treated skin. Interestingly, the effect was seen only with fresh soymilk and not seen when pasteurized soymilk preparations were used. This suggests that a heat-labile component of the soymilk, STI, is the active depigmenting agent. Treatments with soymilk were

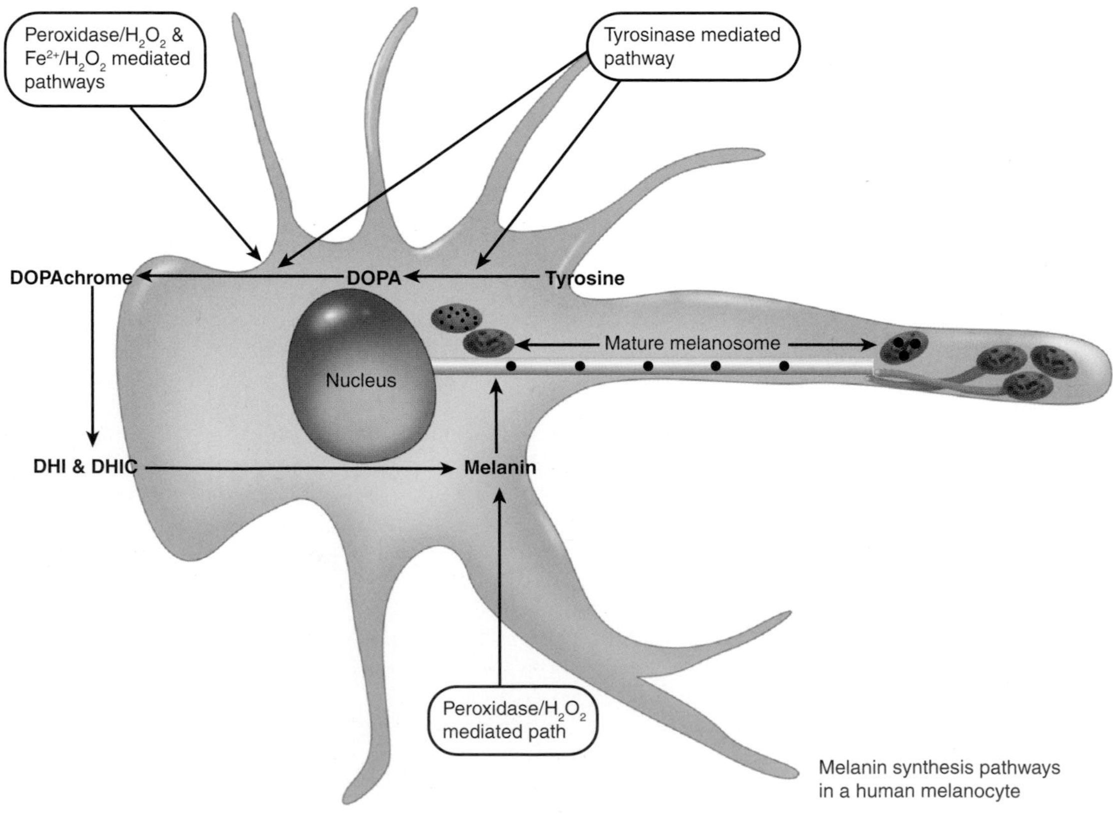

▲ **FIGURE 33-8** Melanin synthesis pathways in a human melanocyte.

also shown to prevent UVB-induced darkening of the swine skin. In addition, human trials have demonstrated lightening of pigmented spots after application of soybean extract.[59]

A recent study examined the efficacy of a novel soy moisturizer containing nondenaturated STI and BBI on pigmentation, the improvement of skin tone, and additional photoaging characteristics. Sixty-five women, aged 30 to 61 with Fitzpatrick phototypes I to III, with moderately severe mottled hyperpigmentation, lentigines, blotchiness, tactile roughness, and dullness were enrolled in the parallel, randomized, double-blind, and vehicle-controlled study. The moisturizer and the vehicle, respectively, were administered twice daily for a period of 12 weeks. By clinical observation, self-assessment, colorimetry, and digital photography, the researchers could show a significant improvement of mottled pigmentation, blotchiness, dullness, fine lines, overall texture, overall skin tone, and overall appearance, versus the vehicle.[60] In addition to these depigmentation properties, soy contains isoflavones, which have antioxidant properties and have been found to confer cancer-preventing benefits (see Chapter 34).

MELANOCYTE-CYTOTOXIC AGENTS

Azelaic Acid

Azelaic acid (Azelex™, Finacea®) (Fig. 33-10) is a naturally-occurring saturated dicarboxylic acid that has been shown to be a useful adjunct in the treatment of postinflammatory pigment alteration (PIPA). While several review articles focus on the use of topical azelaic acid in the management of hyperpigmentary skin disorders and the associated proposed mechanism(s) of action of azelaic acid,[61,62] how azelaic acid exerts its clinical effect is not fully understood. The effect of azelaic acid appears to be attributed to its ability to inhibit the energy production and/or DNA synthesis of hyperactive melanocytes, and partially to its antityrosinase activity.[63] In addition, as it has been reported that hyperpigmentation and lentigo maligna may be related pathogenetically to reactive oxygen species, the clinical effectiveness of azelaic acid is thought to be due in part to its inhibitory action on neutrophil-generated reactive oxygen species, leading to a reduction both in oxidative tissue injury at sites of inflammation and in melanin formation.[64] Research has demonstrated that in vitro azelaic acid is a scavenger of hydroxyl radicals and inhibits oxyradical toxicity in cell cultures.[65,66] Further in vitro studies have demonstrated that azelaic acid is a competitive inhibitor of tyrosinase,[67] the key enzyme for melanogenesis, and a reversible inhibitor of cytochrome-P_{450} reductase activity and 5α-reductase in microsomal preparations supplemented with reduced nicotinamide adenine dinucleotide phosphate (NADPH).[68] The capacity of azelaic acid to reversibly inhibit the activity of mitochondrial respiratory chain enzymes, such as reduced NADH-dehydrogenase, succinic acid dehydrogenase, and reduced ubiquinone cytochrome-*c* oxidoreductase,[69] and to inhibit the synthesis of DNA,[70] responsible for an antiproliferative effect, also appears to be important in hyperpigmentary disorders.

Azelaic acid has been reported to be even more effective than topical HQ for patients with melasma, without the latter's side effects.[63,71,72] In a multicenter, randomized trial lasting 24 weeks, azelaic acid 20% cream produced significantly greater decreases in pigmentary intensity than did its vehicle both subjectively and in the chromameter analysis.[73] Another study demonstrated that the combination of azelaic acid 20% cream and glycolic acid 15% or 20% lotion is as effective as 4% HQ cream in the treatment of hyperpigmentation in darker-skinned patients, with only a slightly higher rate of mild local irritation.[74] In yet another study, in which hyperpigmented lesions visible only with a UVB camera were evaluated, results showed that azelaic acid is superior to glycolic acid in attenuating the subclinical hyperpigmentation when used over a 3-week period.[59] In the United States, topical azelaic acid is available by prescription in concentrations of a 15% gel and a 20% cream for the treatment of rosacea and acne, respectively. The use for hyperpigmentation is off-label. Topically applied azelaic acid is well tolerated, with adverse effects generally limited to mild local cutaneous irritation. Azelaic acid is an excellent alternative for patients who cannot tolerate HQ.

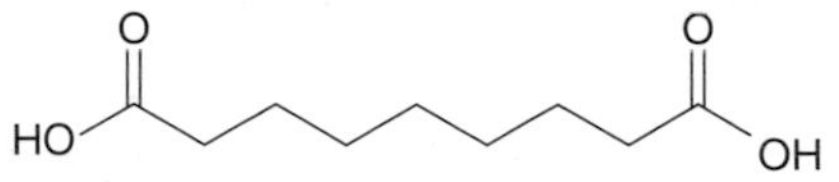

▲ **FIGURE 33-10** The chemical structure of azelaic acid.

Mequinol

Chemically known as 4-hydroxyanisole, mequinol is a derivative of HQ (Fig. 33-11). Its exact mechanism of action is unknown; however, mequinol is a substrate to tyrosinase and acts as a competitive inhibitor of melanogenesis.[75] Notably, 2% mequinol with 0.01% tretinoin has been proven to be effective in the treatment of solar lentigines.[76,77] In a randomized, parallel-grouped, double-masked study with 216 subjects, the effects of 2% mequinol/0.01% tretinoin were compared with those of 3% HQ in the treatment of solar lentigines. With a twice-daily treatment for more than 16 weeks and a follow-up after 24 weeks, a significantly higher proportion of subjects achieved clinical success with 2% mequinol/0.01% tretinoin compared with 3% HQ.[78]

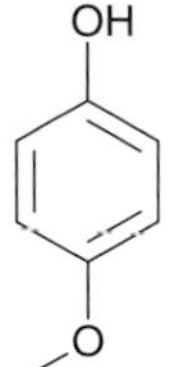

▲ **FIGURE 33-11** The chemical structure of mequinol.

Monobenzone

The monobenzyl ether in HQ is the substance used to cause permanent depigmentation of normal skin. It is often used in vitiligo patients to permanently depigment the skin surrounding depigmented areas when repigmentation is not feasible and the depigmented areas are disfiguring. Monobenzone (Fig. 33-12) is metabolized inside cells into quinine, which acts by permanently damaging the melanocytes.[79] It is usually prepared at a concentration of 20%. Brand names include Monobenzon, Dermochinona, Leucodinine, Carmifal, Depigman, Superlite, and Pigmex. It is applied 2 or 3 times daily on pigmented skin, with depigmentation beginning around 6 to 12 months of treatment. Transfer of the agent can occur to anyone who touches the medication; therefore, contact with others should be avoided for up to 3 hours after application.[80] Potential side effects include contact dermatitis, conjunctival melanosis, skin lightening in untreated areas,[81] the possibility of an unwanted repigmentation starting from

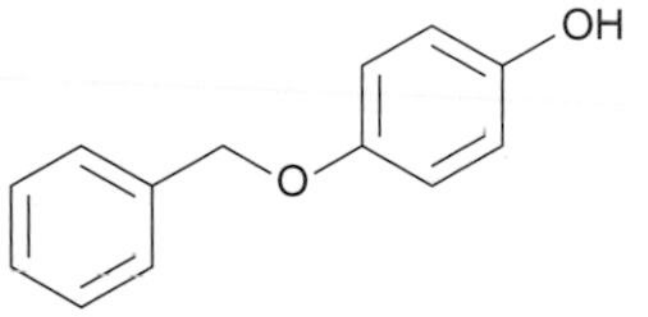

▲ **FIGURE 33-12** The chemical structure of monobenzone—a derivative of hydroquinone.

follicular melanocytes, and the need for lifelong total photoprotection. Because this agent is cytotoxic to melanocytes, it must be stressed that after depigmentation therapy with this agent, future attempts at repigmentation treatment will be completely ineffective.

N-Acetyl-4-*S*-cysteaminylphenol

N-Acetyl-4-*S*-cysteaminylphenol is a melanocytotoxic agent consisting of phenolic and catecholic compounds with potent depigmenting properties. A study in which 12 patients with melasma were treated with a daily application of 4% *N*-acetyl-4-*S*-cysteaminylphenol showed significant reduction in pigmentation, with results being visible as early as 2 to 4 weeks after therapy.[82]

ANTIOXIDANTS

Antioxidants are popular additives in skin care preparations for several reasons. In addition to exhibiting antiaging, anticarcinogenic, and anti-inflammatory activities, they may also decrease pigmentation that occurs after exposure to UV light.[83] This may be useful in the treatment of melasma. Research on vitiligo has shown that antioxidants may affect melanin production. A comparison of normal melanocytes with melanocytes from vitiligo patients has demonstrated lower catalase activity and higher vitamin E and ubiquinone levels in the vitiligo patients suggesting that an imbalance in the antioxidant status and increase in the intracellular peroxide levels could play a role in vitiligo.[84] In addition, antioxidants, including GSH, a naturally-occurring antioxidant involved in regulating melanin synthesis,[85] have been shown to inhibit or delay hyperpigmentation.[86] In support of these findings, a study by Yokozawa and Kim[86] demonstrated that an antioxidant, piceatannol (PICE), could inhibit mushroom tyrosinase. PICE (Fig. 33-13) is a phenolic compound derived from resveratrol, which is found in grapes and red wine. It has antioxidative, antitumorigenic, and apoptosis-inducing effects. In this study, investigators found that PICE inhibited melanogenesis and displayed potent antioxidant properties. The authors concluded that the antioxidant activity played a major role in the inhibition of melanin production. However, some studies have shown that some antioxidants increase skin pigmentation, so the individual properties of each antioxidant should be considered before using them to decrease skin pigmentation.[87]

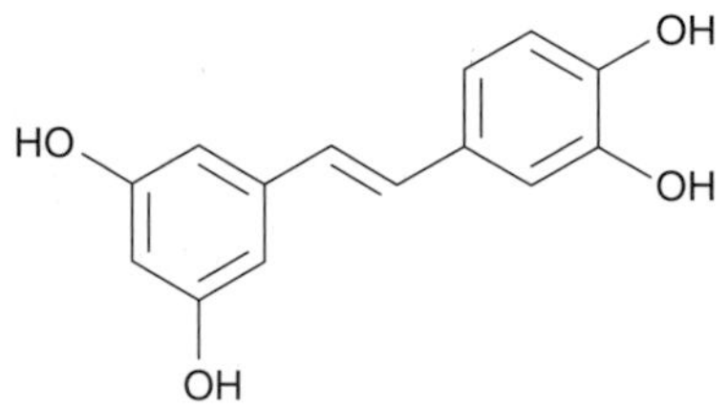

Inflammation has long been known to lead to skin pigmentation, especially in darker skin types. Prostaglandins, which are produced during inflammation, may play a role in skin pigmentation. Indeed, this may be one of the mechanisms by which inflammation can exacerbate melasma. Maeda et al. proposed that *trans*-4-aminomethylcyclohexanecarboxylic acid (*trans*-AMCHA or tranexamic acid), a plasmin inhibitor, decreases tyrosinase activity in the melanocytes via reduction in prostaglandin synthesis, thereby preventing UV-induced pigmentation in guinea pigs. Localized intradermal microinjections of tranexamic acid have been used in an Asian study with some success.[88] However, more studies are needed to determine the efficacy and safety of this treatment.

Latanoprost and Bimatoprost, analogues of prostaglandin $F_{2\alpha}$ ($PGF_{2\alpha}$), are used as intraocular pressure-lowering drugs. Their use has been associated with pigment changes of the iris and the eyelid. Recently, these prostaglandin analogues have become popular for stimulating eyelash growth. However, these should be used with caution by those with darker skin types and those with a history of melasma and other pigmentation disorders. PGF_2 was shown to increase tyrosinase activity, suggesting that prostaglandins may stimulate melanin formation.[89] Antioxidants can prevent the formation of prostaglandins,[90] thereby preventing inflammation and tyrosinase activation.

Inflammation may also play a role in skin pigmentation through the effects of histamine. Histamine is released from mast cells during inflammation and has been found to increase the level of tyrosinase-mediated cAMP via actions on protein kinase A (PKA). The release of histamine stimulates melanogenesis and results in the production of eumelanin rather than pheomelanin.[91] Thus, a possible approach to prevent postinflammatory hyperpigmentation and other pigmentation disorders might be to block histamine action. Yoshida et al. found that blocking H2 receptors with famotidine suppressed the increase in melanogenesis, but antagonists of H1 and H3 do not have any effect.[92] The effect of histamine-related agents is difficult to predict and their use to treat hypo- and hyperpigmentation is still unreliable. However, antioxidants, especially flavonoids, have been shown to inhibit histamine release.[93] Antioxidants likely prevent inflammation and subsequent pigmentation by several other mechanisms including effects on transcription factor nuclear factor-κB (NF-κB), inducible nitric oxide synthase expression, and inhibition of cyclooxygenase.[94]

In spite of the many cited reasons to use antioxidants and free radical scavengers as hypopigmenting agents, the indiscriminate use of these compounds should be weighed with caution. Each antioxidant and its effects should be considered separately and it should not be assumed that all antioxidants will inhibit melanogenesis. In fact, an opposite effect seems to be possible in some cases and unexpected hyperpigmentation can occur. For example, quercetin, an extract of onion, is a tyrosinase inhibitor in vitro[95]; however, this flavonol has been described as a strong inductor of melanogenesis in normal and malignant human melanocytes,[96] and in reconstituted three-dimensional human epidermis models.[97] Glycyrrhizin, another popular antioxidant that is frequently used to inhibit tyrosinase, has been shown to stimulate melanogenesis in B16 melanoma cells.[98] Clinical trials of each individual antioxidant agent, and combinations of agents, are warranted before one can feel confident of their ability to inhibit melanogenesis.

▲ **FIGURE 33-13** The chemical structure of piceatannol (PICE)—a derivative of resveratrol.

Vitamin C

Vitamin C or ascorbic acid (Fig. 33-14) can be found in citrus fruits and green leafy vegetables. It inhibits melanin formation and reduces oxidized melanin because it is able to reduce

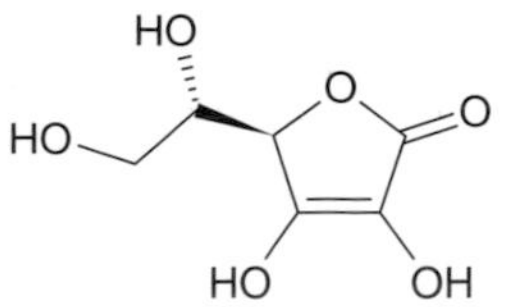

▲ **FIGURE 33-14** The chemical structure of vitamin C (L-ascorbic acid).

o-DOPAquinone back to DOPA, thus avoiding melanin formation.[99] Multiple topical preparations contain vitamin C; however, many of these products have problems with stability and their utility is questionable. Companies like Skinceuticals and La Roche-Posay have developed stabilized vitamin C preparations, which are packaged in a manner intended to minimize inactivation of this easily degraded ingredient. Specifically, the packaging of these products limits UV and air exposure from rapidly oxidizing vitamin C. Magnesium-L-ascorbyl-2-phosphate (VC-PMG) is a stable derivative of ascorbic acid. One study examining the effects of topically applied VC-PMG on patients with melasma or senile lentigos demonstrated a significant lightening effect in 19 of 34 patients.[100] However, percutaneous absorption of magnesium ascorbyl phosphate is marginal because it is a charged molecule, making it difficult to traverse the stratum corneum. In addition to its utility as a depigmenting agent, vitamin C has antioxidant properties and has been shown to stimulate collagen synthesis (see Chapter 34). In a randomized, double-blind, placebo-controlled study, investigators used iontophoresis to enhance the penetration of vitamin C into the skin and significantly decrease pigmentation compared to placebo.[101]

Vitamin E

Oral intake of vitamin E (α-tocopherol or α-T) (Fig. 33-15) has been reported in the Japanese literature to be effective for the treatment of facial hyperpigmentation, especially in combination with vitamin C.[102,103] Studies examining the effects of α-tocopheryl ferulate (a compound composed of α-T and ferulic acid) on melanogenesis in cultured human melanoma cells demonstrated inhibition of tyrosine hydroxylase activity in an indirect manner. The researchers found that this tocopherol derivative was a stronger inhibitor of melanin formation than arbutin and kojic acid.[104] They postulated that α-tocopheryl ferulate could be used to ameliorate and prevent facial hyperpigmentation induced by UV radiation by inhibiting tyrosinase as well through antioxidant mechanisms.[105]

The depigmenting effect of α-T was also examined in normal human melanocytes and investigators showed that 30 μg/mL of α-T dissolved in 150 μg/mL of lecithin inhibited melanization significantly without inhibiting cell growth, and that this phenotypic change was associated with the dose-dependent inhibition of tyrosinase.[106]

Tocopherol employs four homologues (α, β, γ, and δ) with differing numbers and positions of the methyl groups in the chromatin ring. γ-Tocopherol (γ-T) has been found to suppress the expression of tyrosinase melanoma cells.[107] Tocopheryl-dimethyl-glycinate (TDMG) is a novel tocopherol derivative with the dimethylglycine ester linked to the sixth position of the chromanoxyl ring of tocopherol.[108] A Japanese group reported on a novel hydrophilic γ-T derivative known as γ-tocopheryl-*N,N*-di-methylglycinate hydrochloride (γ-TDMG); this derivative converts to the antioxidant γ-T in skin and displays greater bioavailability than γ-T itself. The group examined whether γ-TDMG could reduce UV-induced skin pigmentation in brown guinea pigs. By topically applying 0.1% or 0.5% γ-TDMG to the skin of brown guinea pigs before and after exposure to UVB as well as UVA (3 times/wk for 1 week) and then 10 times/wk for 4 weeks, the investigators could show significant skin lightening with 0.5% γ-TDMG and a dose-dependent inhibition of the melanin synthesis. These data suggest that the topical application of γ-TDMG may be efficacious in preventing photo-induced skin pigmentation in humans.[109]

Green Tea

Green tea is one of the most popular beverages consumed throughout the world. Of all the compounds known to exhibit antioxidant activity, green tea polyphenols (GTPs) are associated with the largest amount of scientific evidence to support their use in dermatology. Consequently, green tea is also a popular ingredient included in various beauty and personal care products, such as moisturizers, cleansers, shower gels, toothpastes, depilatories, shampoos, perfumes, and even soft drinks. Most "green tea-containing" products have minimal amounts of green tea. Products with large amounts of green tea (50%–90% polyphenols) have a tinted brown color. Look for products that have large amounts of green tea, such as Replenix brand by Topix.

A special preparation process of the tea leaves, which involves short steaming and prevents any fermentation, ensures the preservation of the antioxidant polyphenols. Four major polyphenolic catechins can be isolated from the fresh leaves of the green tea plant *Camellia sinensis:* ECG [(–)-epicatechin-3-*O*-gallate], GCG [(–)-gallocatechin-3-*O*-gallate], EGCG [(–)-epigallocatechin-3-*O*-gallate], and EGC [(–)-epigallocatechin][110] (Fig. 33-16). EGCG is the most studied and abundant component and comprises 30% to 40% of the dry weight of green tea leaves.[111,112]

GTPs have been reported to impart numerous health benefits when administered either topically or orally, by dint of their antioxidant, anti-inflammatory, and anticarcinogenic properties.[113–115]

With regard to the skin, there have been several in vitro and in vivo studies. GTPs have been demonstrated to modulate biochemical pathways important in cell proliferation, inflammatory responses, and responses of tumor promoters.[116] These have also been found to be especially potent at suppressing the carcinogenic activity of UV radiation and exerting broad protection against other UV-mediated responses such as sunburn, immunosuppression, and photoaging by inhibiting UV induced elements of the mitogen-activated protein kinase (MAPK) pathways, Ras and activator protein AP-1 and LDH activation, as well as by the upregulation of UVA-suppressed GSH-Px and the inhibition of UVB-induced infiltration of inflammatory cells.[117] GTPs are thus thought to have the potential to protect the skin

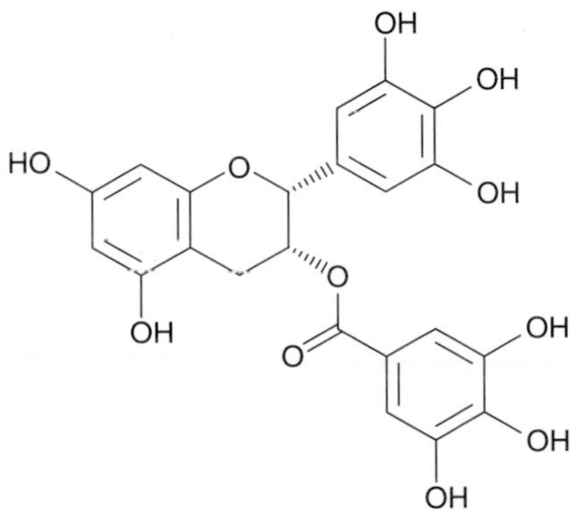

▲ **FIGURE 33-16** The chemical structure of EGCG.

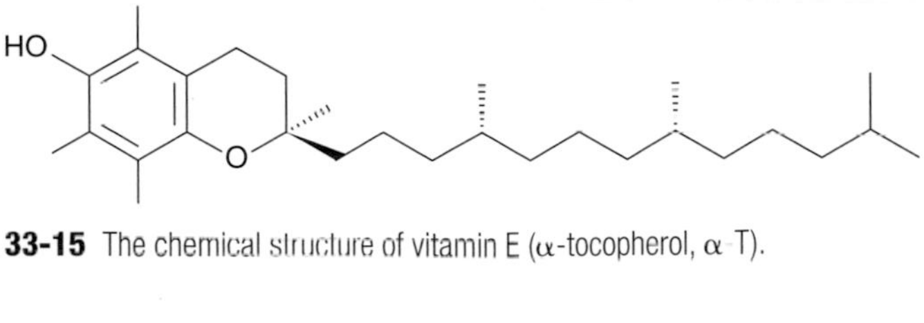

▲ **FIGURE 33-15** The chemical structure of vitamin E (α-tocopherol, α-T).

when used in combination with traditional sunscreens.[118,119]

In a recent study, EGCG was shown to exhibit antiproliferative and proapoptotic effects on human melanoma cells.[120] No et al. examined the tyrosinase inhibitory activity of mushroom tyrosinase in 10 varieties of Korean traditional teas. Of the four major polyphenolic catechins, ECG, GCG, and EGCG proved to be the strongest inhibitors of all. Of these three, GCG showed the strongest inhibitory effect on tyrosinase, competitively inhibiting the enzyme at its active site.[121] Furthermore, EGCG was demonstrated to inhibit melanin synthesis in a concentration-dependent manner, not by cell cytotoxicity but by reducing MITF and tyrosinase protein levels in Mel-Ab cells (a mouse-derived spontaneously immortalized melanocyte cell line that produces large amounts of melanin). EGCG displayed a stronger hypopigmenting effect than kojic acid. Additionally, EGCG inhibited mushroom tyrosinase activity and, to a lesser degree, human tyrosinase.[122]

Studies of GTPs in human skin have been limited in comparison to animal studies. There are two major challenges for the topical use in humans: (1) establishing a standard formulation and delivery systems that ensure the stability of these easily oxidized antioxidants and (2) increasing epidermal penetration of these hydrophilic agents into human skin.

Pycnogenol

Pycnogenol is a standardized pine bark extract that exhibits potent antioxidant, anti-inflammatory, and anticarcinogenic activity.[123–125] The efficacy of pycnogenol in protecting against UV-induced pigmentation was evaluated in a 30-day clinical trial of 30 women with melasma. Patients were given one 25-mg tablet of pycnogenol at each meal, 3 times daily. Investigators found that the average surface area of melasma significantly decreased, revealing pycnogenol to be an effective and safe treatment for this condition.[124] One study has demonstrated that pycnogenol is active when applied topically. In this study, hairless mice exposed to solar-simulated ultraviolet radiation were topically treated, postirradiation, with lotions containing pycnogenol. Dose-dependent reductions in the inflammatory sunburn reaction and immunosuppression were observed as a result of pycnogenol treatment. Tumor formation was delayed and tumor prevalence was also significantly reduced in mice treated with 0.2% pycnogenol. Researchers concluded that topical pycnogenol displays potential as a photoprotective complement to sunscreens, clearly evincing biologic activity when applied after UV exposure.[96] More data are needed to determine the validity of these claims.

Silymarin

Silymarin is a naturally-occurring polyphenolic flavonoid or flavonolignans compound derived from the seeds of the milk thistle plant *Silybum marianum*.[126] Milk thistle has been used for medicinal purposes for more than 2000 years. Today, it is used clinically in Europe and Asia as an antihepatotoxic agent and is available as a supplement in Europe and the United States. The main component of silymarin is silybin (silibinin), which is considered to be its most biologically active constituent in terms of its antioxidant, anti-inflammatory, and anticarcinogenic properties.[91]

Topical application of silybin prior to, or immediately after, UV irradiation has been found to impart strong protection against UV-induced damage in the epidermis by a reduction in thymine dimer-positive cells and an upregulation of p53-p21/Cip1, which researchers believe may lead to the inhibition of cell proliferation and apoptosis. This study suggests that mechanisms other than sunscreen effect are integral to silybin efficacy against UV-caused skin damage.[127] Investigators have also noted that silybin enhances UVB-induced apoptosis and speculated that it acts as a UVB damage sensor to confer its biologic action.[128]

The antioxidant activity of silymarin is well established. Chemoprotective activity against skin cancer has also been reported and continues to be the subject of much investigation.[129,130] In a study to identify the mechanism of photocarcinogenesis prevention in mouse skin by the topical treatment of silymarin, prevention of UVB-induced immunosuppression and oxidative stress were found to be potentially related to the prevention of photocarcinogenesis in mice.[131] The authors concluded from this trial and related data from other recent studies that there are compelling arguments for the inclusion of silymarin in sunscreens or in other products in a skin care regimen. Furthermore, silymarin has been shown to inhibit UV-induced NF-κB activation in keratinocytes. Researchers have hypothesized that the inhibition of NF-κB activation and the consequent inhibition of UV-induced inflammation by silymarin is a result primarily of the inhibition of UV-induced inflammation by free radical scavenging and a modulation of intracellular GSH content.[132]

Most of the milk thistle or silymarin available in the United States comes in the form of oral supplements. The extant evidence on this botanical suggests potent antioxidant strength and great potential as an antiphotodamage, anticarcinogenic component in an improved medical, dermatologic armamentarium. Moreover, silymarin may favorably supplement sunscreen protection and provide additional antiphotocarcinogenic protection.[133]

Alpha Lipoic Acid

Also named thioctic acid, alpha lipoic acid and its reduced form dihydrolipoic acid (DHLA) have both been considered strong antioxidants. Alpha lipoic acid (Fig. 33-17) has been called the universal antioxidant because it is both water and fat soluble and can thus act in the lipid cell membrane and the aqueous compartment of the cell.[134] In addition, alpha lipoic acid has been shown to inhibit the activation of NF-κB transcription factor, modulating the cellular response to UV radiation and preventing UV-induced oxidative injury. It further inhibits tyrosinase by chelating copper and suppressing DOPAquinone-derivative formation.[132] Dihydrolipoic acid shows slightly stronger antioxidant activity by reacting with superoxide and hydroxyl radicals.[135] In addition, alpha lipoic acid elevates intracellular GSH levels by increasing its *de novo* synthesis,[136] which again reduces UV radiation sensitivity.[137]

Both lipoic and dihydrolipoic acids have been proven to block the expression of MITF (a regulator of melanocyte development and survival),[138] consequently inhibiting tyrosinase expression and activity as well as inducing skin lightening.[20] Sodium zinc dihydrolipoylhistidinate (DHLHZn), a compound of Zn^{2+}/dihydrolipoic acid derivate complex, seems to covalently react with DOPAquinone, resulting in a competitive inhibitory effect of DHLHZn on DOPAchrome formation and thus

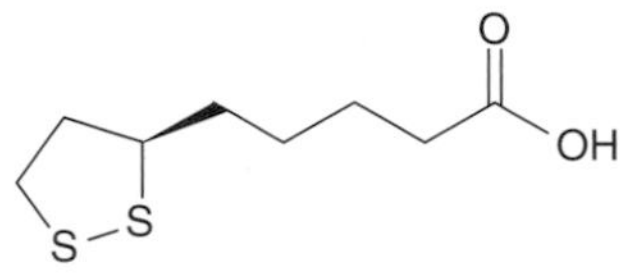

O
OH
S–S

▲ **FIGURE 33-17** The chemical structure of alpha lipoic acid.

potentially serving as an effective skin-lightening agent.[139] Lipoic acid is included in multiple topical cosmetic formulations. However, there has been a report on contact dermatitis to alpha lipoic acid.[140] Further in vivo studies are necessary to verify the above-stated findings. In addition, a recent report has called into question whether the topical antioxidant designation is accurate for alpha lipoic acid.[141]

OTHER AGENTS

Alpha Hydroxy Acids and Beta Hydroxy Acid

Alpha hydroxy and beta hydroxy acid peels have become increasingly prevalent in dermatologic practices. All AHAs have a terminal carboxyl group with one or two hydroxyl groups on the second or alpha carbon and a variable length carbon chain.[142] The two shortest carbon chain acids, glycolic (2-hydroxyethanoic) and lactic (2-hydroxypropanoic), are the most commonly used in dermatology[143] (Figs. 33-18 and 33-19). The former is a very versatile peeling agent causing minimal complications and is used in various strengths ranging from 20% to 70%. People with virtually any skin type can be candidates for AHA and BHA peels, including Asian Americans, African Americans, Hispanics, and others with deeply pigmented skin[144] (see Chapter 20).

Researchers have not yet completely elucidated the exact mechanism of action of AHAs on the skin, but it appears that they exert different effects on the epidermis and the dermis. In the epidermis, the principal effect is diminished corneocyte cohesion.[145] This causes more rapid desquamation of the pigmented keratinocytes with the intention that the newly formed keratinocytes will contain less pigment. It also helps to increase the keratinocyte turnover rate thereby shortening the cell cycle. Recently, it was shown that in melanoma cells alpha hydroxy acids also directly inhibit tyrosinase activity.[146] In 1997, Burns et al. demonstrated that serial glycolic acid peels provide an additional benefit, with minimal adverse effects, for the treatment of postinflammatory hyperpigmentation in individuals with dark complexions.[147] Patients who receive a chemical peel in addition to a topical treatment demonstrate a greater and more rapid improvement of pigmented lesions compared to topical treatment alone with a slight lightening of their normal facial skin tone.[148] In a recent study, lactic acid in a concentration of 92% was used to treat melasma. Patients treated every 3 weeks for a maximum of 6 times showed significant improvement in their melasma area and severity index (MASI) scores.[149] Lactic acid was further shown to be as effective in decreasing pigmentation as Jessner's solution.[150] When treating PIPA with peels, it is initially important to use lower concentrations of AHA and slowly increase the strength to avoid irritating the skin, causing even more hyperpigmentation.[151] The use of topical HQ preparations pre- and postpeel decreases the chances of aggravating PIPA.

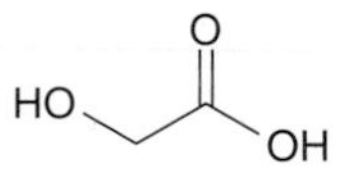

O
HO OH

Glycolic acid
(2-Hydroxyethanoic acid)

▲ **FIGURE 33-18** The chemical structure of gylcolic acid.

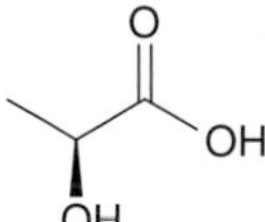

▲ **FIGURE 33-19** The chemical structure of lactic acid.

Octadecenedioic Acid

Octadecenedioic acid is a skin-whitening agent with a similar structure to azelaic acid. It has been demonstrated to be an efficient skin whitener in clinical studies; however, its mechanisms of action were unclear at that time.[152] Recently, Wiechers et al. were able to show that the known whitening activity of octadecenedioic acid is mediated by the stimulation of the peroxisome proliferator-activating receptor (PPAR). The binding to PPAR leads to reduced melanin production through the reduction of the synthesis of tyrosinase mRNA.[153]

PPARs are members of the nuclear receptor superfamily, regulating important cellular functions, including cell proliferation and differentiation, as well as inflammatory responses.[154] It was reported that three subtypes of PPAR (designated α, β, and γ) are expressed in human melanocytes.[155] The above-mentioned study showed that octadecenedioic acid is a PPAR-γ agonist, with a 10-fold higher affinity for this receptor than the other two PPAR receptors.[153] This suggests a novel mechanism of skin pigmentation and consequently a novel approach for the therapy of skin pigmentation disorders.

Pyruvic Acid

Pyruvic acid is an alpha-keto-acid with keratolytic, antimicrobial, and sebostatic properties in addition to the ability to stimulate new collagen production and elastic fiber formation. It is successfully used in the treatment of acne.[156] A treatment with 50% pyruvic acid, employed for four peeling sessions performed every 2 weeks has been shown to effectively reduce the degree of pigmentation in melasma patients and significantly increase skin elasticity as well as decrease skin wrinkling. No side effects, such as persistent erythema or postinflammatory hyperpigmentation, were observed.[157] Comparable results in terms of safety and efficacy were also shown in 20 patients treated for moderately photodamaged facial skin.[158]

Resorcinol

Resorcinol (*m*-dihydrobenzene) is isomeric with catechol and HQ.[159] This bactericidal agent is soluble in water, ether, and alcohol. The primary indications for its use include postinflammatory hyperpigmentation as well as melasma and acne; secondary indications are sun-damaged skin and freckles. Resorcinol should not be used in pregnancy or in darker skin types (IV–VI). Some authors have mentioned the possibility of an allergic reaction to resorcinol and suggest testing the agent by applying it to the retroauricular area a few days before using it as a peel. However, until recently, predictive methods, both animal and human, have not been successful in identifying resorcinol as a skin sensitizer. A recent study was able to establish that resorcinol has a skin sensitization potential, using a local lymph node assay.[160] Shimizu et al. proved that 4-substituted resorcinols, naturally obtained or synthesized, have potent tyrosinase inhibitory ability.[161] In addition, Tasaka et al. showed a depigmenting effect for a resorcinol derivative with an isopentyl group in position 6 of resorcinol (NKO-09), with a more potent depigmenting effect than HQ by inhibiting tyrosine hydroxylation and DOPA oxidation.[162]

Retinoids

Several different substances comprise the family of retinoids, which are lipophilic vitamin A derivatives that easily penetrate the epidermis. The effect of retinoids on pigmentation seems to involve various mechanisms not yet completely identified. Retinoids apparently exert their depigmenting effects directly by influencing melanocytes as well as indirectly by modulating melanogenesis. Topical retinoids seem to directly affect melanogenesis via tyrosinase, TRP-1, and TRP-2 expression.[163–165] Furthermore, it is suggested that by inhibiting the detoxification of toxic species, retinoic acid enhances the melanocytotoxic effect of depigmenting agents. By accelerating the cell turnover of epidermal keratinocytes, topical retinoids promote a decrease in melanosome transfer to the keratinocytes and induce dispersion of keratinocyte pigment granules leading to a uniform distribution of melanin content in the epidermis. More rapid epidermal turnover also reduces the cohesiveness of corneocytes and thus induces desquamation that consequently leads to an accelerated loss of melanin in the stratum corneum.[166] Indirectly, the changes engendered in the stratum corneum may facilitate the penetration of other/additional depigmenting agents into the epidermis and increase their bioavailability, thereby leading to increased depigmentation.

Tretinoin (Retin-A™, Renova™, Avita™) in concentrations of 0.05% to 0.1% is another agent used to treat PIPA. It is frequently employed as an adjuvant in the treatment of pigmentation disorders even though the mechanism of action is not completely understood. Part of the effect is based on the stimulation of the cell turnover of epidermal keratinocytes, which promotes a decrease in melanosome transfer and accelerates the loss of melanin via epidermopoiesis. Although studies have shown retinoic acid to inhibit the induction of tyrosinase, and subsequently melanogenesis, in mouse melanoma cell cultures,[167] animal studies have demonstrated that topical application of retinoic acid can increase melanogenesis.[168,169] Nevertheless, clinical trials have shown tretinoin to be efficacious for the treatment of melasma.[170,171]

The topical retinoid tazarotene (Avage™, Tazorac™) has also been shown to improve irregular hyperpigmentation associated with photoaging.[172]

Adapalene (Differin Gel™ 0.1% and 0.3%) is a potent synthetic retinoid. In a randomized trial, adapalene 0.1% showed the same effect on reduction in MASI as 0.05% tretinoin, yet the patients treated with adapalene had significantly fewer side effects.[173] Oral 0.05% isotretinoin has exhibited clinically important but not statistically significant results in a randomized trial treating Thai patients with melasma.[174]

The side effects of retinoids, such as dryness, irritation, and scaling, are signs of a damaged skin barrier.[175] This condition allows for other agents to more readily penetrate into the skin and enhance their efficacy, as is the case with HQ, which often is used in combination with retinoids. It is advisable to add a corticosteroid to retinoid therapy to mitigate irritation. First proposed by Kligman in 1975, the combination consisting of 0.1% tretinoin, 5% HQ, and 0.1% dexamethasone was named the Kligman formula and has been the most widely used combination formula to treat melasma.[176] There are numerous additional combination treatments in use. (see Chapter 30 for more information on retinoids.)

Sunscreen

Sun protection also plays a role in the treatment of pigmentary disorders. UV radiation stimulates the synthesis of melanin and promotes the transfer of pigments from melanocytes to keratinocytes thereby increasing pigmentation. The use of a broad-spectrum sunscreen has been shown to improve melasma,[174] and should be a part of any skin-lightening regimen. (see Chapter 29 for a discussion of the different types of sunscreens.)

SUMMARY

The process of skin pigmentation is very complex, and more research is necessary to elucidate this integral aspect of skin and cosmetic dermatology. Tyrosinase inhibition has so far been the most common approach to treat disorders of pigmentation, but only a small selection of tyrosinase inhibitors have practical applications owing to formulation issues, stability, irritation, and ability to penetrate into the skin. Pigmentation disorders are a frustrating problem for many cosmetic patients. Manufacturers have responded by making several depigmenting agents available in both prescription and OTC preparations. These agents seem to work best when used in combination.

REFERENCES

1. DeCaprio AP. The toxicology of hydroquinone—relevance to occupational and environmental exposure. *Crit Rev Toxicol.* 1999;29:283.
2. Penney KB, Smith CJ, Allen JC. Depigmenting action of hydroquinone depends on disruption of fundamental cell processes. *J Invest Dermatol.* 1984;82:308.
3. Nordlund JJ. Postinflammatory hyperpigmentation. *Dermatol Clin.* 1988;6:185.
4. Guevara IL, Pandya AG. Melasma treated with hydroquinone, tretinoin and a fluorinated steroid. *Int J Dermatol.* 2001;40:212.
5. Bates B. Derms react to possible FDA ban of hydroquinone: cite poor scientific reasoning, ethnic bias. *Skin and Allergy News.* 2007;38:1.
6. Nordlund JJ, Grimes PE, Ortonne JP. The safety of hydroquinone. *J Eur Acad Dermatol Venerol.* 2006;20:781.
7. Picardo M, Carrera M. New and experimental treatments of cloasma and other hypermelanoses. *Dermatol Clin.* 2007; 25:353.
8. Lawrence N, Bligard CA, Reed R, et al. Exogenous ochronosis in the United States. *J Am Acad Dermatol.* 1988;18: 1207.
9. Barrientos N, Oritz-Frutos J, Gómez E, et al. Allergic contact dermatitis from a bleaching cream. *Am J Contact Dermat.* 2001;12:33.
10. Kramer KE, Lopez A, Stefanato CM, et al. Exogenous ochronosis. *J Am Acad Dermatol.* 2000;42:869.
11. Jones K, Hughes J, Hong M, et al. Modulation of melanogenesis by aloesin: a competitive inhibitor of tyrosinase. *Pigment Cell Res.* 2002;15: 335.
12. Piao LZ, Park HR, Park YK, et al. Mushroom tyrosinase inhibition activity of some chromones. *Chem Pharm Bull (Tokyo).* 2002;50:309.
13. Choi S, Lee SK, Kim JE, et al. Aloesin inhibits hyperpigmentation induced by UV radiation. *Clin Exp Dermatol.* 2002; 27:513.
14. Maeda K, Fukuda M. Arbutin: mechanism of its depigmenting action in human melanocyte culture. *J Pharmacol Exp Ther.* 1996;276:765.
15. Nakajima M, Shinoda I, Fukuwatari Y, et al. Arbutin increases the pigmentation of cultured human melanocytes through mechanisms other than the induction of tyrosinase activity. *Pigment Cell Res.* 1998;11:12.
16. Boissy RE, Visscher M, DeLong MA. DeoxyArbutin: a novel reversible tyrosinase inhibitor with effective in vivo skin lightening potency. *Exp Dermatol.* 2005;14:601.
17. Solano F, Briganti S, Picardo M, et al. Hypopigmenting agents: an updated review on biological, chemical and clinical aspects. *Pigment Cell Res.* 2006; 19:550.
18. Kim YJ, Uyama H. Tyrosinase inhibitors from natural and synthetic sources: structure, inhibition mechanism and perspective for the future. *Cell Mol Life Sci.* 2005;62:1707.
19. Ohguchi K, Tanaka T, Kido T, et al. Effects of hydroxystilbene derivatives on tyrosinase activity. *Biochem Biophys Res Commun.* 2003;307:861.
20. Lin CB, Babiarz L, Liebel F, et al. Modulation of microphthalmia-associated transcription factor gene expression alters skin pigmentation. *J Invest Dermatol.* 2002;119:1218.
21. Lee KT, Lee KS, Jeong JH, et al. Inhibitory effects of Ramulus mori extracts on melanogenesis. *J Cosmet Sci.* 2003;54:133.

22. Shimogaki H, Tanaka Y, Tamai H, et al. In vitro and in vivo evaluation of ellagic acid on melanogenesis inhibition. *Int J Cosmet Sci*. 2000;22:291.
23. Curto EV, Kwong C, Hermersdörfer H, et al. Inhibitors of mammalian melanocytes tyrosinase: in vitro comparisons of alkyl esters of gentisic acid and other putative inhibitors. *Biochem Pharmacol*. 1999;15:663.
24. Yamamura T, Onishi J, Nishiyama T. Antimelanogenic activity of hydrocoumarins in cultured normal human melanocytes by stimulating intracellular glutathione synthesis. *Arch Dermatol Res*. 2002;294:349.
25. Bhat R, Hadi SM. Photoinactivation of bacteriophage lambda by kojic acid and Fe(III): role of oxygen radical intermediates in the reaction. *Biochem Mol Biol Int*. 1994;32:731.
26. Curtis PJ. Chemical induction of local reddening in strawberry fruits. *J Sci Food Agr*. 1977;28:243.
27. Hira Y, Hatae S, Inoue T, et al. Inhibitory effects of kojic acid on melanin formation. In vitro and in vivo studies in black goldfish. *J Jpn Cosmet Sci Soc*. 1982,6:193.
28. Cabanes J, Chazarra S, Garcia-Carmona F. Kojic acid, a cosmetic skin whitening agent, is a slow-binding inhibitor of catecholase activity of tyrosinase. *J Pharm Pharmacol*. 1994;46:982.
29. Uher M, Brtko J, Rajnlakova O, et al. Kojic acid and its derivatives in cosmetics and health protection. *Parfuem Kosmet*. 1993;74:554.
30. Burdock GA, Soni MG, Carabin IG. Evaluation of health aspects of kojic acid in food. *Regul Toxicol Pharmacol*. 2001;33:80.
31. Ellis DA, Tan AK, Ellis CS. Superficial micropeels: glycolic acid and alphahydroxy acid with kojic acid. *Facial Plast Surg*. 1995;11:15.
32. Garcia A, Fulton JE Jr. The combination of glycolic acid and hydroquinone or kojic acid for the treatment of melasma and related conditions. *Dermatol Surg*. 1996;22:443.
33. Lim JT. Treatment of melasma using kojic acid in a gel containing hydroquinone and glycolic acid. *Dermatol Surg*. 1999;25:282.
34. Nakagawa M, Kawai K, Kawai K. Contact allergy to kojic acid in skin care products. *Contact Dermatitis*. 1995;32:9.
35. Nakayama G, Watanabe N, Nishioka K, et al. Treatment of chloasma with kojic acid cream. *Jpn J Clin Dermatol*. 1982;36:715.
36. Takizawa T, Mitsumori K, Tamura T, et al. Hepatocellular tumor induction in heterozygous p53-deficient CBA mice by a 26-week dietary administration of kojic acid. *Toxicol Sci*. 2003;73:287.
37. Lee YS, Park JH, Kim MH, et al. Synthesis of tyrosinase inhibitory kojic acid derivative. *Arch Pharm Chem Life Sci*. 2006;339:11.
38. Saeedi M, Morteza-Semnani K, Ghoreishi MR. The treatment of atopic dermatitis with licorice gel. *J Dermatolog Treat*. 2003;14:153.
39. Wang ZY, Nixon DW. Licorice and cancer. *Nutr Cancer*. 2001;39:1.
40. Agarwal R, Wang ZY, Mukhtar H. Inhibition of mouse skin tumor-initiating activity of DMBA by chronic oral feeding of glycyrrhizin in drinking water. *Nutr Cancer*. 1991;15:187.
41. Craig WJ. Health-promoting properties of common herbs. *Am J Clin Nutr*. 1999;70:491S .
42. Yokota T, Nishio H, Kubota Y, et al. The inhibitory effect of glabridin from licorice extracts on melanogenesis and inflammation. *Pigment Cell Res*. 1998; 11:355.
43. Amer M, Metwalli M. Topical liquiritin improves melasma. *Int J Dermatol*. 2000; 39:299.
44. Holloway VL. Ethnic cosmetic products. *Dermatol Clin*. 2003;21:743.
45. Rico MJ. Rising drug costs: the impact on dermatology. *Skin Ther Lett*. 2000;5:1.
46. Friis-Moller A, Chen M, Fuursted K, et al. In vitro antimycobacterial and antilegionella activity of licochalcone A from Chinese licorice roots. *Planta Med*. 2002;68:416.
47. Barfod L, Kemp K, Hansen M, et al. Chalcones from Chinese liquorice inhibit proliferation of T cells and production of cytokines. *Int Immunopharmacol*. 2002;2:545.
48. Rafi MM, Rosen RT, Vassil A, et al. Modulation of bcl-2 and cytotoxicity by licochalcone-A, a novel estrogenic flavonoid. *Anticancer Res*. 2000;20:2653.
49. Tsukiyama R, Katsura H, Tokuriki N, et al. Antibacterial activity of licochalcone A against spore-forming bacteria. *Antimicrob Agents Chemother*. 2002; 46:1226.
50. Shibata S, Inoue H, Iwata S, et al. Inhibitory effects of licochalcone A isolated from Glycyrrhiza inflata root on inflammatory ear edema and tumour promotion in mice. *Planta Med*. 1991;57:221.
51. Hwang JH, Lee BM. Inhibitory effects of plant extracts on tyrosinase, L-DOPA oxidation, and melanin synthesis. *J Toxicol Environ Health A*. 2007;70:393.
52. Chaudhuri RK. Emblica cascading antioxidant: a novel natural skin care ingredient. *Skin Pharmacol Appl Skin Physiol*. 2002;15:374.
53. Hakozaki T, Minwalla L, Zhuang J, et al. The effect of niacinamide on reducing cutaneous pigmentation and suppression of melanosome transfer. *Br J Dermatol*. 2002;147:20.
54. Otte N, Borelli C, Korting HC. Nicotinamide—biologic actions of an emerging cosmetic ingredient. *Int J Cosmet Sci*. 2005;27:255.
55. Greatens A, Hakozaki T, Koshoffer A, et al. Effective inhibition of melanosome transfer to keratinocytes by lectins and niacinamide is reversible. *Exp Dermatol*. 2005;14:498.
56. Liu J-C, Seiberg M. Applications of total soy in skin care. In: Baran R, Maibached H, eds. *Textbook of Cosmetic Dermatology*. 3rd ed., New York, NY: Taylor & Francis Informa Healthcare; 2004:115.
57. Seiberg M, Paine C, Sharlow E, et al. Inhibition of melanosome transfer results in skin lightening. *J Invest Dermatol*. 2000;115:162.
58. Paine C, Sharlow E, Liebel F, et al. An alternative approach to depigmentation by soybean extracts via inhibition of the PAR-2 pathway. *J Invest Dermatol*. 2001;116:587.
59. Hermanns JF, Petit L, Martalo O, et al. Unraveling the patterns of subclinical pheomelanin-enriched facial hyperpigmentation: effect of depigmenting agents. *Dermatology*. 2000;201:118.
60. Wallo W, Nebus J, Leyden JJ. Efficacy of a soy moisturizer in photoaging: a double-blind, vehicle-controlled, 12-week study. *J Drugs Dermatol*. 2007;6:917.
61. Nazzaro-Porro M. The use of azelaic acid in hyperpigmentation. *Rev Contemp Pharmacother*. 1993;4:415.
62. Nguyen QH, Bui TP. Azelaic acid: pharmacokinetic and pharmacodynamic properties and its therapeutic role in hyperpigmentary disorders and acne. *Int J Dermatol*. 1995;34:75.
63. Fitton A, Goa KL. Azelaic acid. A review of its pharmacological properties and therapeutic efficacy in acne and hyperpigmentary skin disorders. *Drugs*. 1991;41:780.
64. Akamatsu H, Komura J, Asada Y, et al. Inhibitory effect of azelaic acid on neutrophil functions: a possible cause for its efficacy in treating pathogenetically unrelated diseases. *Arch Dermatol Res*. 1991;283:162.
65. Passi S, Picardo M, Zompetta C, et al. Oxyradicals- scavenging activity of azelaic acid in biological systems. *Free Radic Res Commun*. 1991;15(1):17.
66. Passi S, Picardo M, De Luca C, et al. Scavenging activity of azelaic acid on hydroxyl radicals in vitro. *Free Radic Res Commun*. 1991;11(6):329.
67. Nazzaro-Porro M, Passi S. Identification of tyrosinase inhibitors in cultures of Pityrosporum. *J Invest Dermatol*. 1978; 71:205.
68. Nazzaro-Porro M, Passi S, Picardo M, et al. Possible mechanism of action of azelaic acid on acne. *J Invest Dermatol*. 1985; 84:451.
69. Passi S, Picardo M, Nazzaro-Porro M, et al. Antimitochondrial effect of saturated medium chain length (C8-C13) dicarboxylic acids. *Biochem Pharmacol*. 1984; 33:103.
70. Leibl H, Stingl G, Pehamberger H, et al. Inhibition of DNA synthesis of melanoma cells by azelaic acid. *J Invest Dermatol*. 1985;85:417.
71. Verallo-Rowell VM, Verallo V, Graupe K, et al. Double-blind comparison of azelaic acid and hydroquinone in the treatment of melasma. *Acta Derm Venereol Suppl (Stockh)*. 1989;143:58.
72. Baliña LM, Graupe K. The treatment of melasma. 20% azelaic acid versus 4% hydroquinone cream. *Int J Dermatol*. 1991;30:893.
73. Lowe NJ, Rizk D, Grimes P, et al. Azelaic acid 20% cream in the treatment of facial hyperpigmentation in darker-skinned patients. *Clin Ther*. 1998; 20:945.
74. Kakita LS, Lowe NJ. Azelaic acid and glycolic acid combination therapy for facial hyperpigmentation in darker-skinned patients: a clinical comparison with hydroquinone. *Clin Ther*. 1998; 20:960.
75. Riley PA. Mechanism of pigment cell toxicity produced by hydroxyanisole. *J Pathol*. 1970;101:163.
76. Fleischer AB Jr, Schwartzel EH, Colby SI, et al. The combination of 2% 4-hydroxyanisole (mequinol) and 0.01%

tretinoin is effective in improving the appearance of solar lentigines and related hyperpigmented lesions in two double-blind multicenter clinical studies. *J Am Acad Dermatol*. 2000;42:459.

77. Draelos ZD. The combination of 2% 4-hydroxyanisole (mequinol) and 0.01% tretinoin effectively improves the appearance of solar lentigines in ethnic groups. *J Cosmet Dermatol*. 2006;5:239.
78. Jarratt M. Mequinol 2%/tretinoin 0.01% solution: an effective and safe alternative to hydroquinone 3% in the treatment of solar lentigines. *Cutis*. 2004;74:319.
79. Huang CL, Nordlund JJ, Boissy R. Vitiligo: a manifestation of apoptosis [Review]? *Am J Clin Dermatol*. 2002;3(5): 301-308.
80. Halder RM, Richards GM. Management of dyschromias in ethnic skin. *Dermatol Ther*. 2004;17:151.
81. Canizares O, Jaramillo FU, Kerdel Vegas F. Leukomelanoderma subsequent to the application of monobenzylether of hydroquinone. *Arch Dermatol*. 1958; 77:220.
82. Jimbow K. N-acetyl-4-S-cysteaminylphenol as a new type of depigmenting agent for the melanoderma of patients with melasma. *Arch Dermatol*. 1991;127:1528.
83. Yamakoshii J, Otsuka F, Sano A, et al. Lightening effect on ultraviolet-induced pigmentation of guinea pig skin by oral administration of a proanthocyanidin-rich extract from grape seeds. *Pigment Cell Res*. 2003;16:629.
84. Maresca V, Roccella M, Roccella F, et al. Increased sensitivity to peroxidative agents as a possible pathogenic factor of melanocyte damage in vitiligo. *J Invest Dermatol*. 1997;109:310.
86. Yokozawa T, Kim YJ. Piceatannol inhibits melanogenesis by its antioxidative actions. *Biol Pharm Bull*. 2007; 30:2007.
85. Benathan M, Alvero-Jackson H, Mooy AM, et al. Relationship between melanogenesis, glutathione levels and melphalan toxicity in human melanoma cells. *Melanoma Res*. 1992;2:305.
87. Postaire E, Jungmann H, Bejot M, et al. Evidence for antioxidant nutrients-induced pigmentation in skin: results of a clinical trial. *Biochem Mol Biol Int*. 1997;42:1023.
88. Lee JH, Park JG, Lim SH, et al. Localized intradermal microinjection of tranexamic acid for treatment of melasma in Asian patients: a preliminary clinical trial. *Dermatol Surg*. 2006;32:626.
89. Dutkiewicz R, Albert DM, Levin LA. Effects of latanoprost on tyrosinase activity and mitotic index of cultured melanoma lines. *Exp Eye Res*. 2000;70:563.
90. Staniforth V, Chiu LT, Yang NS. Caffeic acid suppresses UVB radiation-induced expression of interleukin-10 and activation of mitogen-activated protein kinases in mouse. *Carcinogenesis*. 2006;27:1803.
91. Lassalle MW, Igarashi S, Sasaki M, et al. Effects of melanogenesis-inducing nitric oxide and histamine on the production of eumelanin and pheomelanin in cultured human melanocytes. *Pigment Cell Res*. 2003;16:81.
92. Yoshida M, Takahashi Y, Inoue S. Histamine induces melanogenesis and morphologic changes by protein kinase A activation via H2 receptors in human normal melanocytes. *J Invest Dermatol*. 2000;114:334.
93. Kawai M, Hirano T, Higa S, et al. Flavonoids and related compounds as anti-allergic substances. *Allergol Int*. 2007;56:113.
94. Biesalski HK. Polyphenols and inflammation: basic interactions. *Curr Opin Clin Nutr Metab Care*. 2007;10:724.
95. Kubo I, Kinst-Hori I. Flavonols from saffron flower: tyrosinase inhibitory activity and inhibition mechanism. *J Agric Food Chem*. 1999;47:4121.
96. Nagata H, Takekoshi S, Takeyama R, et al. Quercetin enhances melanogenesis by increasing the activity and synthesis of tyrosinase in human melanoma cells and in normal human melanocytes. *Pigment Cell Res*. 2004;17:66.
97. Takeyama R, Takekoshi S, Nagata H, et al. Quercetin-induced melanogenesis in a reconstituted three-dimensional human epidermal model. *J Mol Histol*. 2004;35:157.
98. Yung GD, Yang JY, Song ES, et al. Stimulation of melanogenesis by glycyrrhizin in B16 melanoma cells. *Exp Mol Med*. 2001;33:131.
99. Ros JR, Rodriguez-Lopez JN, Garcia-Canovas F. Effect of L-ascorbic acid on the monophenolase activity of tyrosinase. *Biochem J*. 1993;295:309.
100. Kameyama K, Sakai C, Kondoh S, et al. Inhibitory effect of magnesium L-ascorbyl-2-phosphate (VC-PMG) on melanogenesis in vitro and in vivo. *J Am Acad Dermatol*. 1996;34:29.
101. Huh C-H, Seo K-I, Park J-Y, et al. A randomized, double-blind, placebo-controlled trial of vitamin C iontophoresis in melasma. *Dermatology*. 2003;206:316.
102. Hayakawa R. Clinical research group on a combination preparation of vitamins E and C. Effects of combination preparation of vitamin E and C in comparison with single preparation to the patients of facial hyperpigmentation: a double-blind controlled clinical trial. *Nishinihon J Dermatol*. 1980;42:1024.
103. Takigawa M. YEC-1 clinical research group. Clinical evaluation of YEC-1 (UNKER EC) to female patients with facial hyperpigmentation. *Kiso Rinsho*. 1991;25:312.
104. Funasaka Y, Chakraborty AK, Komoto M, et al. The depigmenting effect of alpha-tocopheryl ferulate on human melanoma cells. *Br J Dermatol*. 1999;141:20.
105. Ichihashi M, Funasaka Y, Ohashi A, et al. The inhibitory effect of DL-alpha-tocopheryl ferulate in lecithin on melanogenesis. *Anticancer Res*. 1999;19:3769.
106. Funasaka Y, Komoto M, Ichihashi M. Depigmenting effect of alpha-tocopheryl ferulate on normal human melanocytes. *Pigment Cell Res*. 2000;8(suppl 13):170.
107. Kamei Y, Ohtsuka Y. *Fragrance J*. 2003;56-63.
108. Takata J, Hidaka R, Yamasaki A, et al. Novel d-gamma-tocopherol derivative as a prodrug for d-gamma-tocopherol and a two-step prodrug for S-gamma-CEHC. *J Lipid Res*. 2002;43:2196.
109. Kuwabara Y, Watanabe T, Yasuoka S, et al. Topical application of gamma-tocopherol derivative prevents UV-induced skin pigmentation. *Biol Pharm Bull*. 2006; 29:1175.
110. Yang C, Wang Z. Tea and cancer. *J Natl Cancer Inst*. 1993;85:1038.
111. Wright TI, Spencer JM, Flowers FP. Chemoprevention of nonmelanoma skin cancer. *J Am Acad Dermatol*. 2006; 54:933.
112. Katiyar SK, Elmets CA. Green tea polyphenolic antioxidants and skin photoprotection [review]. *Int J Oncol*. 2001;18:1307.
113. Khan N, Mukhtar H. Tea polyphenols for health promotion. *Life Sci*. 2007; 81:519.
114. Tipoe GL, Leung TM, Hung MW, et al. Green tea polyphenols as an anti-oxidant and anti-inflammatory agent for cardiovascular protection. *Cardiovasc Hematol Disord Drug Targets*. 2007;7:135.
115. Cabrera C, Artacho R, Giménez R. Beneficial effects of green tea—a review. *J Am Coll Nutr*. 2006;25:79.
116. Katiyar SK, Ahmad N, Mukhtar H. Green tea and skin. *Arch Dermatol*. 136: 989, 2000.
117. Hsu S. Green tea and the skin. *J Am Acad Dermatol*. 2005;52:1049.
118. Yusuf N, Irby C, Katiyar SK, et al. Photoprotective effects of green tea polyphenols. *Photodermatol Photoimmunol Photomed*. 2007;23:48.
119. Wang Z, Agarwal R, Bickers D, et al. Protection against ultraviolet B radiation-induced photocarcinogenesis in hairless mice by green tea polyphenols. *Carcinogenesis*. 1991;12:1527.
120. Nihal M, Ahmad N, Mukhtar H, et al. Anti-proliferative and proapoptotic effects of (–)-epigallocatechin-3-gallate on human melanoma: possible implications for the chemoprevention of melanoma. *Int J Cancer*. 2005;114:513.
121. No JK, Soung DY, Kim YJ, et al. Inhibition of tyrosinase by green tea components. *Life Sci*. 1999;65:241.
122. Kim DS, Park SH, Kwon SB, et al. (–)-Epigallocatechin-3-gallate and hinokitiol reduce melanin synthesis via decreased MITF production. *Arch Pharm Res*. 2004;27:334.
123. Sime S, Reeve VE. Protection from inflammation, immunosuppression and carcinogenesis induced by UV radiation in mice by topical Pycnogenol. *Photochem Photobiol*. 2004;79:193.
124. Ni Z, Mu Y, Gulati O, et al. Treatment of melasma with Pycnogenol. *Phytother Res*. 2002;16:567.
125. Bito T, Roy S, Sen CK, et al. Pine bark extract pycnogenol downregulates IFN-gamma-induced adhesion of T cells to human keratinocytes by inhibiting inducible ICAM-1 expression. *Free Radic Biol Med*. 2000;28:219.
126. Svobodová A, Psotová J, Walterová D. Natural phenolics in the prevention of UV-induced skin damage. A review. *Biomed Papers*. 2003;147:137.
127. Dhanalakshmi S, Mallikarjuna GU, Singh RP, et al. Silibinin prevents ultraviolet radiation-caused skin damages in SKH-1 hairless mice via a decrease in thymine dimer positive cells and an up-regulation of p53-p21/Cip1 in epidermis. *Carcinogenesis*. 2004;25:1459.
128. Dhanalakshmi S, Mallikarjuna GU, Singh RP, et al. Dual efficacy of silibinin

in protecting or enhancing ultraviolet B radiation-caused apoptosis in HaCaT human immortalized keratinocytes. *Carcinogenesis*. 2004;25:99.
129. Singh RP, Agarwal R. Flavonoid antioxidant silymarin and skin cancer. *Antioxid Redox Signal*. 2002;4:655.
130. Gupta S, Mukhtar H. Chemoprevention of skin cancer through natural agents. *Skin Pharmacol Appl Skin Physiol*. 2001; 14:373.
131. Katiyar SK. Treatment of silymarin, a plant flavonoid, prevents ultraviolet light-induced immune suppression and oxidative stress in mouse skin. *Int J Oncol*. 2002;21:1213.
132. Saliou C, Kitazawa M, McLaughlin L, et al. Antioxidants modulate acute solar ultraviolet radiation-induced NF-kappa-B activation in a human keratinocyte cell line. *Free Radic Biol Med*. 1999;26:174.
133. Katiyar SK. Silymarin and skin cancer prevention: anti-inflammatory, antioxidant and immunomodulatory effects. *Int J Oncol*. 2005;26:169.
134. Kagan VE, Shvedova A, Serbinova E, et al. Dihydrolipoic acid—a universal antioxidant both in the membrane and in the aqueous phase: reduction of peroxyl, ascorbyl and chromanoxyl radicals. *Biochem Pharmacol*. 1992;44:1637.
135. Packer L, Witt EH, Tritschler HJ. alpha-Lipoic acid as a biological antioxidant. *Free Radic Biol Med*. 1995;19:227.
136. Han D, Handelman G, Marcocci L, et al. Lipoic acid increases de novo synthesis of cellular glutathione by improving cystine utilization. *Biofactors*. 1997;6:321.
137. Tyrrell RM, Pidoux M. Correlation between endogenous glutathione content and sensitivity of cultured human skin cells to radiation at defined wavelengths in the solar ultraviolet range. *Photochem Photobiol*. 1988;47:405.
138. Fisher DE. Microphthalmia: a signal responsive transcriptional regulator in development. *Pigment Cell Res*. 2000;13 (suppl 8):145.
139. Tsuji Naito K, Hatani T, Okada T, et al. Modulating effects of a novel skin-lightening agent, alpha-lipoic acid derivative, on melanin production by the formation of DOPA conjugate products. *Bioorg Med Chem*. 2007;15:1967.
140. Bergqvist-Karlsson A, Thelin I, Bergendorff O. Contact dermatitis to alpha-lipoic acid in an anti-wrinkle cream. *Contact Dermatitis*. 2006;55:56.
141. Lin JY, Lin FH, Burch JA, et al. Alpha-lipoic acid is ineffective as a topical antioxidant for photoprotection of skin. *J Invest Dermatol*. 2004;123:996.
142. Clark CP III. Alpha hydroxy acids in skin care. *Clin Plast Surg*. 1996;23:49.
143. Brody HJ. Chemical Peeling and Resurfacing. St. Louis, MO: Mosby-Year Book; 1997:90-100.
144. Murad H, Shamban AT, Premo PS. The use of glycolic acid as a peeling agent. *Dermatol Clin*. 1995;13:285.
145. Slavin JW. Considerations in alpha hydroxy acid peels. *Clin Plast Surg*. 1998;25:45.
146. Usuki A, Ohashi A, Sato H, et al. The inhibitory effect of glycolic acid and lactic acid on melanin synthesis in melanoma cells. *Exp Dermatol*. 2003;2(suppl 12):43.
147. Burns RL, Prevost-Blank PL, Lawry MA, et al. Glycolic acid peels for postinflammatory hyperpigmentation in black patients. A comparative study. *Dermatol Surg*. 1997;23:171.
148. Lim JT, Tham SN. Glycolic acid peels in the treatment of melasma among Asian women. *Dermatol Surg*. 1997;23:177.
149. Sharquie KE, Al-Tikreety MM, Al-Mashhadani SA. Lactic acid as a new therapeutic peeling agent in melasma. *Dermatol Surg*. 2005;31:149.
150. Sharquie KE, Al-Tikreety MM, Al-Mashhadani SA. Lactic acid chemical peels as a therapeutic modality in melasma in comparison to Jessner's solution chemical peels. *Dermatol Surg*. 2006;32:1429.
151. Rubin MG. The clinical use of alpha hydroxy acids. *Australas J Dermatol*. 1994;35:29.
152. Wiechers JW, Groenhof FJ, Wortel VAL, et al. Octadecenedioic acid for a more even skin tone. *Cosmetics & Toiletries*. 2002;117:55.
153. Wiechers JW, Rawlings AV, Garcia C, et al. A new mechanism of action for skin whitening agents: binding to peroxisome proliferator activated receptor. *Int J Cosmet Sci*. 2005;27:123.
154. Berger J, Moller DE. The mechanisms of action of PPARs. *Ann Rev Med*. 2002; 53:409.
155. Michalik L, Wahli W. Peroxisome proliferator-activated receptors (PPARs) in skin health, repair and disease. *Biochim Biophys Acta*. 2007;1771:991.
156. Cotellessa C, Manunta T, Ghersetich I, et al. The use of pyruvic acid in the treatment of acne. *J Eur Acad Dermatol Venereol*. 2004;18:275.
157. Berardesca E, Cameli N, Primavera G, et al. Clinical and instrumental evaluation of skin improvement after treatment with a new 50% pyruvic acid peel. *Dermatol Surg*. 2006;32:526.
158. Ghersetich I, Brazzini B, Peris K, et al. Pyruvic acid peels for the treatment of photoaging. *Dermatol Surg*. 2004;30:32.
159. Karam PG. 50% resorcinol peel. *Int J Dermatol*. 1993;32:569.
160. Basketter DA, Sanders D, Jowsey IR. The skin sensitization potential of resorcinol: experience with the local lymph node assay. *Contact Dermatitis*. 2007;56:196.
161. Shimizu K, Kondo R, Sakai K. Inhibition of tyrosinase by flavonoids, stilbenes and related 4-substituted resorcinols: structure-activity investigations. *Planta Med*. 2000;66:11.
162. Tasaka K, Kamei C, Nakano S, et al. Effects of certain resorcinol derivatives on the tyrosinase activity and the growth of melanoma cells. *Methods Find Exp Clin Pharmacol*. 1998;20:99.
163. Ortonne JP. Retinoid therapy of pigmentary disorders. *Dermatol Ther*. 2006;19:280.
164. Nair X, Parah P, Suhr L, et al. Combination of 4-hydroxyanisole and all trans retinoic acid produces synergistic skin depigmentation in swine. *J Invest Dermatol*. 1993;101:145.
165. Orlow SJ, Chakraborty AK, Boissy RE, et al. Inhibition of induced melanogenesis in Cloudman melanoma cells by four phenotypic modifiers. *Exp Cell Res*. 1990;191:209.
166. Kasraee B, Handjani F, Aslani FS. Enhancement of the depigmenting effect of hydroquinone and 4-hydroxyanisole by all-trans-retinoic acid (tretinoin): the impairment of glutathione-dependent cytoprotection? *Dermatology*. 2003;206:289.
167. Orlow SJ, Chakraborty AK, Pawelek JM. Retinoic acid is a potent inhibitor of inducible pigmentation in murine and hamster melanoma cell lines. *J Invest Dermatol*. 1990;94:461.
168. Welsh BM, Mason RS, Halliday GM. Topical all-*trans* retinoic acid augments ultraviolet radiation-induced increases in activated melanocyte numbers in mice. *J Invest Dermatol*. 1999;112:271.
169. Ho KK, Halliday GM, Barnetson RS. Topical retinoic acid augments ultraviolet light-induced melanogenesis. *Melanoma Res*. 1992;2:41.
170. Kimbrough Green CK, Griffiths CE, Finkel LJ, et al. Topical retinoic acid (tretinoin) for melasma in black patients. A vehicle-controlled clinical trial. *Arch Dermatol*. 1994;130:727.
171. Griffiths CE, Finkel LJ, Ditre CM, et al. Topical tretinoin (retinoic acid) improves melasma. A vehicle-controlled, clinical trial. *Br J Dermatol*. 1993;129:415.
172. Phillips TJ, Gottlieb AB, Leyden JJ, et al. Efficacy of 0.1% tazarotene cream for the treatment of photodamage: a 12-month multicenter, randomized trial. *Arch Dermatol*. 2002;138:1486.
173. Dogra S, Kanwar AJ, Parsad D. Adapalene in the treatment of melasma: a preliminary report. *J Dermatol*. 2002;29:539.
174. Leenutaphong V, Nettakul A, Rattanasuwon P. Topical isotretinoin for melasma in Thai patients: a vehicle-controlled clinical trial. *J Med Assoc Thai*. 1999;82:868.
175. Weinstein GD, Nigra TP, Pochi PE, et al. Topical tretinoin for treatment of photodamaged skin. *Arch Dermatol*. 1991; 127:659.
176. Kligman AM, Willis I. A new formula for depigmenting human skin. *Arch Dermatol*. 1975;111:40.
177. Solano F, Briganti S, Picardo M, et al. Hypopigmenting agents: an updated review on biological, chemical and clinical aspects. *Pigment Cell Res*. 2006;19:550.

CHAPTER 34

Antioxidants

Leslie Baumann, MD
Inja Bogdan Allemann, MD

THE FREE RADICAL THEORY OF AGING

The free radical theory of aging, proposed by Harman in 1956,[1] is one of the most widely accepted theories to explain the cause of aging.[2] Free radicals, also known as reactive oxygen species (ROS), are compounds formed when oxygen molecules combine with other molecules yielding an odd number of electrons. An oxygen molecule with paired electrons is stable; however, oxygen with an unpaired electron is "reactive" because it seeks and seizes electrons from vital components leaving them damaged.[3] DNA, cytoskeletal elements, cellular proteins, and cellular membranes may all be adversely affected by activated oxygen species.[4] ROS have not only been implicated in the overall aging process,[5] but are believed to be involved cutaneously in causing photoaging, carcinogenesis, and inflammation. It is known that ultraviolet (UV)-induced damage to the skin is in part mediated by reactive oxygen intermediates.[6] If antioxidants can absorb some of the resulting free radicals, they may be able to mitigate UV-induced damage to the skin. Free radicals may also lead to inflammation, which is believed to play a role in skin aging.[6] Lipid peroxidation, another sequela of free radical production, causes harm to cell membranes and can lead to skin aging, atherosclerosis, and other signs of aging. Free radicals are also thought to contribute to the development of skin cancer. There are multiple studies in the literature describing the role of free radicals and skin cancer. The exact mechanisms for all of the detrimental effects of free radicals have not been completely elucidated, however.

Free radicals also play an important role in intrinsic and extrinsic skin aging. They are formed naturally through normal human metabolism, but can be produced as a result of exogenous factors, such as UV exposure, air pollution, smoking, radiation, alcohol use, exercise, inflammation, and exposure to certain drugs or heavy metals such as iron. In fact, UV radiation, stress, cigarette smoke, pollution, drugs, and diet can be sources of ROS such as superoxide, hydroxyl anion, hydrogen peroxide (H_2O_2), and singlet oxygen. Recent data suggest that free radicals can induce a number of transcription factors, such as activator protein-1 (AP-1) and nuclear factor-κB (NF-κB).[7] Further, ROS increase the expression of matrix metalloproteinases (MMPs), specifically collagenase, which has the ability to degrade skin collagen.[8,9] Collagenase formation occurs as a result of the activation of transcription factors c-Jun and c-Fos, which combine to produce the AP-1 that, in turn, prompts the activity of the MMPs.[10] Additionally, the mitogen-activated protein kinase (MAPK) pathway is also a target of oxidative stress[11] (see Chapter 6).

ANTIOXIDANT THEORY

The body has developed defense mechanisms, known as antioxidants, which protect against the ravages of free radicals by reducing and neutralizing them. Antioxidative enzymes that naturally-occur in the skin include superoxide dismutase, catalase, and glutathione peroxidase (GPX); the nonenzymatic endogenous antioxidative molecules are alpha-tocopherol (vitamin E), ascorbic acid (vitamin C), glutathione, and ubiquinone.[12] As part of the natural aging process, our defense mechanisms diminsh, while the production of ROS increases. This leads to an imbalance and an elevated number of unchecked free radicals that damage DNA, cytoskeletal elements, cellular proteins, and cellular membranes. Moreover, many of the body's antioxidant defense mechanisms are inhibited by UV and visible light.[13,14] Additionally, UV light exposure is known to cause an increase in free radical formation.[15] Researchers are currently studying the potential of using exogenous antioxidants to affect this process and mitigate the damage caused by free radicals. Many believe that topical application and oral consumption of combinations of antioxidants may result in a sustained antioxidant capacity of the skin because of synergistic actions of the combined antioxidants. Antioxidants may be particularly useful in UVA-induced skin alterations that are believed to be determined, in large part, by oxidative processes. In fact, topical application of antioxidants has been shown to raise the minimal UVA dose necessary to induce immediate pigment darkening and diminish the severity of UVA-induced photodermatoses.[15] Although antioxidants appear in vegetables and other foods in addition to the human body, many believe that higher levels can be achieved by supplementation. Consequently, the use of products touting antioxidants as protective ingredients in oral supplements and topically applied agents has become extremely popular.

Topical antioxidants are currently marketed for the prevention of aging and UV-mediated skin damage as well as the treatment of wrinkles and erythema caused by inflammation, such as that induced by laser resurfacing. The free radical theory of aging explains why antioxidants are thought to prevent wrinkles, but this theory does not justify the use of antioxidants to treat wrinkles that are already present. Many companies claim that their antioxidant-containing products "treat" wrinkles; however, this is often an exaggeration. *At this time, vitamin C is the ONLY antioxidant that can treat wrinkles, but this capacity is because of its effects in promoting collagen formation, which is unrelated to its antioxidant effects.* When products such as the combination formulation studied by Cho et al. are associated with amelioration of wrinkles, such a result can be ascribed either to a swelling or hydrating effect of the product, or the vitamin C or retinol contained in the product.[16] It is important to stress to patients that antioxidants *prevent* wrinkles but do not *treat* wrinkles (with the exception of vitamin C).

In addition to their namesake antioxidant effects, all antioxidants exhibit anti-inflammatory properties, which are described in detail in Chapter 35. Some of the antioxidants depicted below also possess depigmenting activities, which are described in more detail in Chapter 33.

Although the theory of antioxidants is a sound one, there are several important factors to consider when evaluating the efficacy of antioxidants. In order to be considered biologically active, orally administered products must be absorbed and shown to raise antioxidant levels in the skin. Topically administered products must be absorbed into the skin and delivered to the target tissue in the active form and remain there long enough to exert the desired effects. Some antioxidants are very unstable; therefore, some ingredients such as vitamin C become oxidized and rendered inactive before reaching the target. Stabilizing ingredients in formulation and packaging them in order to minimize air and light exposure are challenging tasks. Absorption is also important and depends on several factors such as the molecular form of the compound, its pH, whether it is water soluble or fat soluble, and the vehicle that contains the product. This chapter will include a discussion of the most popular types of antioxidants found in cosmetic products or taken orally by cosmetic patients.

ANTIOXIDANT SYNERGY

Although there are hundreds of naturally-occurring antioxidants, most of those currently used in the cosmetic industry are believed to work synergistically to regenerate and "enhance the power" of each other. The antioxidants that have been identified as working cooperatively have been referred to as network antioxidants.[17] For example, after an antioxidant "disarms" a free radical by eliminating the odd number of electrons (by either adding or removing an electron), it is unable to function further as an antioxidant unless it is recycled. The five antioxidants that have been labeled as network antioxidants are vitamins C and E, glutathione, lipoic acid, and Coenzyme Q10 (CoQ10). Vitamin C or CoQ10 can recycle vitamin E, donating electrons to vitamin E to return the nutrient to its antioxidant state. Vitamin C and glutathione can be recycled by lipoic acid or vitamin C. These network antioxidants are being included in an increasing number of cosmetic preparations. It is likely that many antioxidants work synergistically, and that the term "network antioxidant" applies to many more antioxidants than the five identified as the "network."

FAT-SOLUBLE ANTIOXIDANTS

These are found in the lipophilic portion of the cell membrane and include vitamin E, carotenoids, and CoQ10. Further, idebenone, the synthetic analog of CoQ10, and food-derived lycopene are also fat-soluble antioxidants.

Vitamin E

Found in vegetables, oils, seeds, nuts, corn, soy, whole wheat flour, margarine, and in some meat and dairy products, vitamin E, or tocopherol, is actually a universal term for a group of compounds comprising of tocol and tocotrienol derivatives, specifically four pairs of racemic stereoisomers (Fig. 34-1). Of the four tocopherols (alpha-, beta-, gamma-, and delta-), alpha-tocopherol (also known as AT) has the highest activity. Since the discovery that vitamin E is the primary lipid-soluble antioxidant in skin that protects cells from oxidative stress,[18] practitioners have used it to treat a wide variety of skin lesions. The general public has frequently looked to it for treatment of minor burns, surgical scars, and other wounds, even though its use for dermatoses has not been approved by the FDA. In addition, vitamin E is touted as beneficial in protecting against cardiovascular disease because lipid peroxidation is a major contributor to atherosclerosis and cardiovascular disease. Administration of vitamin E is thought to decrease the extent of lipid peroxidation and protect against cardiovascular disease.[19] In the same way that vitamin E protects the cells from lipid peroxidation in the arteries, it protects the cell membranes in the skin from peroxidation.

Authors have shown a correlation between dietary deficiency of vitamin E and an increase in oxidative stress and cell injury.[18] In 1993, Tanaka et al. reported that ROS induce changes in the biosynthesis of collagen and glycosaminoglycans (GAGs) in cultured human dermal fibroblasts.[20] This alteration was prevented with the addition of alpha-tocopherol to the fibroblasts. In addition, vitamin E has been shown to lower prostaglandin E_2 production,[21] and augment interleukin-2 (IL-2) production, leading to anti-inflammatory and immunostimulatory activity. It is believed that this stabilization effect may play a role in collagen biosynthesis.[22] Thus far, in vivo attempts to measure and link changes in collagen production with altered concentrations of vitamin E have proved inconclusive.

A lower incidence of infectious disease and cancer has been observed in studies on elderly subjects that exhibit high plasma tocopherol levels.[23–25] For this reason, vitamin E is considered by many to be a necessary and powerful antioxidant. In addition, vitamin E seems to offer photoprotection when taken orally and applied topically. Numerous reports indicate that the topical application of alpha-tocopherol to animal skin is effective in lowering the production of sunburn cells,[26,27] reducing the damage caused by chronic UVB exposure,[28,29] and inhibiting photocarcinogenesis.[30] Specifically, researchers have found that oral and topical vitamin E supplementation in certain animals diminishes the effects of photoaging, inhibits the development of skin cancer, and counteracts immunosuppression induced by UV radiation.[30–33] In 1992, Trevithick et al. noted that topical d-α-tocopherol acetate diminished erythema because of sunburn, edema, and skin sensitivity in mice when application occurred following exposure to UVB radiation.[34] In a study in which tocopherol 5% was applied to mice prior to UVB exposure, Bissett et al. observed a 75% decrease in skin wrinkling, a rise in tumor latency, and a reduction of cutaneous tumors; however, vitamin E failed to affect UVA-induced skin sagging.[35] In a different study in which subjects applied tocopherol (5%–8%) cream facially for 4 weeks, Mayer observed diminished skin roughness, shorter length of facial lines, and reduced wrinkle depth as compared to placebo.[36]

Oral and topical administration of vitamin E have been demonstrated to inhibit UV-induced erythema and edema in animals.[37] In humans, it has been shown that UV-induced expression of human macrophage metalloelastase, a member of the MMP family involved in degradation of elastin, could be inhibited by pretreatment with vitamin E (5%). In this study, vitamine E was applied to the skin under light-tight occlusion 24 hours before UV treatment.[38]

A double-blind, placebo-controlled study examined the protective effects of orally administered vitamin E [400 international units (IU) per day] against UV-induced epidermal damage in humans. The subjects were followed for a 6-month period. Minimal erythema dose (MED) and histologic response were determined at baseline, 1 month, and 6 months. In this study, there was no significant difference between the placebo group and those treated with vitamin E and the investigators concluded that daily ingestion of 400 IU of oral alpha-tocopherol daily did not provide any

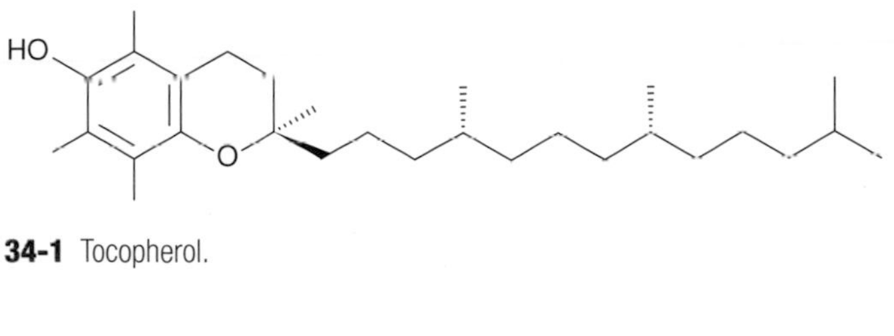

HO

▲ **FIGURE 34-1** Tocopherol.

meaningful photoprotection.[39] Other authors have suggested that if vitamin E provides any photoprotection at all, it may require interaction with other antioxidants, such as vitamin C, to do so.[40] This notion was supported by the study of Lin et al. who showed in Yorkshire pigs that the combined application of 1% α-tocopherol with 15% L-ascorbic acid provided superior protection against erythema and sunburn cell formation compared to either 1% alpha-tocopherol or 15% L-ascorbic acid alone.[41]

WOUND HEALING Oxygen radicals form in response to injury and further inhibit recovery by attacking DNA, cellular membranes, proteins, and lipids. It is believed that antioxidants act to ameliorate wounds by reducing the damage induced by free oxygen radicals, which are released by neutrophils in the inflammatory phase of the healing process.[42] In the late 1960s, Kamimura et al. performed quantitative research demonstrating that topically applied vitamin E penetrates into the deep dermis and subcutaneous tissue.[43] Numerous scientists, as well as many laypersons, have interpreted this to mean that topically applied vitamin E may improve wound healing. Contradictory results have emerged from animal studies undertaken to evaluate the effects of vitamin E on wound healing, however. This may be explained by the fact that unlike other vitamins, tocopherols exhibit species-specific mechanisms of action.[44]

In a prospective, double-blind, randomized study on humans, Jenkins et al. tried to diminish scarring in burn patients following reconstructive surgery by applying topical vitamin E. The researchers observed no difference between the control and treatment groups, however, and nearly 20% of the patients reported local reactions to the vitamin E cream.[45] In another study,[46] the primary author and a collaborator assessed the cosmetic benefit resulting from the use of topically applied vitamin E to surgical scars. In a double-blind fashion, patients applied 320 IU of d-α tocopheryl/gram of Aquaphor to one side of the scar and Aquaphor alone to the other side of the scar. The patients were followed for 6 months. At the conclusion of the study, the vitamin E preparation failed to improve the cosmetic appearance of surgical scars, and even made the scars worse in a few subjects.

FORMS OF VITAMIN E Vitamin E is a family of compounds called tocopherols, including, as mentioned above, alpha-, beta-, gamma-, and delta-tocopherol. Alpha-tocopherol is the most active form and the form on which the recommended daily allowance (RDA) is based. The names of all types of vitamin E begin with either "d" or "dl," designations that refer to differences in chemical structure. The "d" form is the natural form and "dl" is the synthetic form. The natural form is more active and better absorbed. Synthetic vitamin E supplements contain only alpha-tocopherol, while food sources contain several different tocopherols, including alpha-, delta-, and gamma-tocopherol.

Vitamin E forms are listed as either "tocopherol" or the esterified "tocopheryl" followed by the name of the substance to which it is attached, as in "tocopheryl acetate." The two forms are very similar but tocopherol displays better absorption, while tocopheryl forms exhibit slightly better shelf life. In health food stores, the most common oral forms of vitamin E are d-α tocopherol, d-α tocopheryl acetate, and alpha-tocopheryl succinate. The vitamin E forms typically used in cosmetics are alpha-tocopheryl acetate and alpha-tocopheryl linoleate. These compounds are less likely to elicit contact dermatitis than d-α tocopheryl and are more stable at room temperature. However, the tocopherol esters are also more poorly absorbed by the skin than the tocopherol forms,[47] and may not exert the same photoprotective effects. One study demonstrated that alpha-tocopheryl acetate or alpha-tocopheryl succinate not only failed to prevent photocarcinogenesis, but also may have enhanced it.[48] Because the alpha-tocopherol esters are included in many skin lotions, cosmetics, and sunscreens, further studies are needed to determine if the tocopherol esters indeed promote or contribute to photocarcinogenesis.

SIDE EFFECTS The primary author's study[46] as well as the one by Jenkins[45] suggest that the incidence of contact dermatitis because of topical vitamin E application may be relatively high for certain forms of tocopherol.[45] Tocopherol acetate seems to be the worst culprit,[49] but allergy to dl-α-tocopheryl nicotinate has also been reported.[50] In 1992, Swiss researchers evaluated 1000 cases of an atypical papular and follicular contact dermatitis provoked by vitamin E linoleate that was an additive to cosmetics. The conclusion was that oxidized vitamin E derivatives can operate synergistically in vivo as haptens or as irritants.[51] The topical application of vitamin E has also been linked with contact urticaria, eczematous dermatitis, and erythema multiforme-like reactions.[52]

The recommended dose of oral vitamin E is 22 IU per day; however, many physicians recommend 400 IU twice per day. In 1988, a thorough literature review by Bendich and Machlin found extended use of oral vitamin E up to 3000 mg/d to be safe.[53] A subsequent study by Kappus and Diplock established as absolutely safe vitamin E doses up to 400 mg/d, doses between 400 mg and 2000 mg as unlikely to cause adverse reactions, and doses greater than 3000 mg/d over an extended period as a potential source of side effects.[54] Because vitamin E can contribute to a blood-thinning effect, patients on anticoagulant therapy are advised to avoid high doses of vitamin E (>4000 IU).[55] Although there is likely no clinically significant reduction in platelet aggregation in those with normal platelets, patients are frequently advised to suspend vitamin E supplementation prior to surgery. This is essential for patients with abnormal platelets, vitamin K deficiency, or those taking antiplatelet agents.[56]

SUMMARY Vitamin E has been used to treat or protect against various dermatologic conditions including skin cancer, dystrophic epidermolysis bullosa, discoid lupus erythematosus, yellow nail syndrome, granuloma annulare, atopic dermatitis, pemphigus, and lichen sclerosus et atrophicus, among others.[37] Results have varied just as widely as the range of diseases treated. In fact, some authors have reported that the use of oral vitamin E will reduce the side effects of retinoids[57]; however, other studies have not shown this benefit.[58]

The most promising reason for research into the dermatologic use of vitamin E appears to be its antioxidant activity. The potency of vitamin E as an antioxidant can be increased through combination with other antioxidants. Vitamin E also appears to offer a ripe area for research into its potential for therapeutic benefit in the prevention and treatment of skin cancer and photoaging. In addition, vitamin E displays emollient properties, and is stable, easy to formulate, and relatively inexpensive, rendering it a popular additive to antiaging preparations.

Coenzyme Q10 (Ubiquinone)

Coenzyme Q10 (CoQ10) is a naturally-occurring nutrient available through food consumption. Fish and shellfish are good dietary sources of CoQ10. The current recommended oral dose is 90 to 150 mg daily; however, many physicians are recommending 200 to 400 mg/d. CoQ10 is a fat-soluble compound found in all cells as part of the electron transfer chain responsible for energy production. It is estimated that CoQ10 provides 95% of the body's energy (ATP) requirements.[59] CoQ10 has also been found to have antioxidant properties. The "Q" alludes to its membership in the quinone family; the "10" identifies the number of isoprenoid units on its side chain (Fig. 34-2). The biosynthesis of CoQ10 is a complex process that depends on a copious supply of essential amino acids, such as tyrosine, and several vitamins and trace elements. There are several studies on the use of CoQ10 in the cardiology literature.[60]

Researchers have identified an age-related decline of CoQ10 levels in animals and humans.[61] For this reason, many believe that the antioxidant activities of CoQ10 may make it useful as a treatment for aged skin. A study by Hoppe et al. demonstrated that CoQ10 penetrated into the viable layers of the skin and significantly suppressed the expression of collagenase in human dermal fibroblasts following UVA irradiation.[62] It was further shown that prolonged supplementation of CoQ10 in humans reduces wrinkle formation in the corner of the eye. In another study, the same group orally supplemented CoQ10 (0, 1, 100 mg/kg po) daily for 2 weeks and noted that levels of CoQ10 significantly increased in the epidermis, but not in the dermis. They hypothesized that this might be a prerequisite to the reduction of wrinkles and other benefits related to the potent antioxidant and energizing effects of CoQ10 in skin.[63]

Patients taking 3-hydroxy-3-methylglutaryl-coenzyme A (HMG-CoA) reductase inhibitors (statins) to lower their low-density lipoprotein cholesterol have been shown to have decreased mitochondrial CoQ10 levels. This is because statin drugs inhibit the conversion of HMG-CoA to mevalonate, a precursor for cholesterol and CoQ10. In cell culture, decreased mitochondrial CoQ10 levels have been associated with a higher degree of cell death, increased DNA oxidative damage, and a reduction in ATP synthesis. Oral supplementation of CoQ10 has been shown to reduce cell death and DNA oxidative stress, and increase ATP synthesis.[64] For this reason, many physicians recommend that patients taking statins should supplement CoQ10 orally. The most commonly prescribed dose is 200 to 400 mg/d, in the morning. Coenzyme Q10 exhibits caffeine-like effects and can lead to insomnia if taken at night.

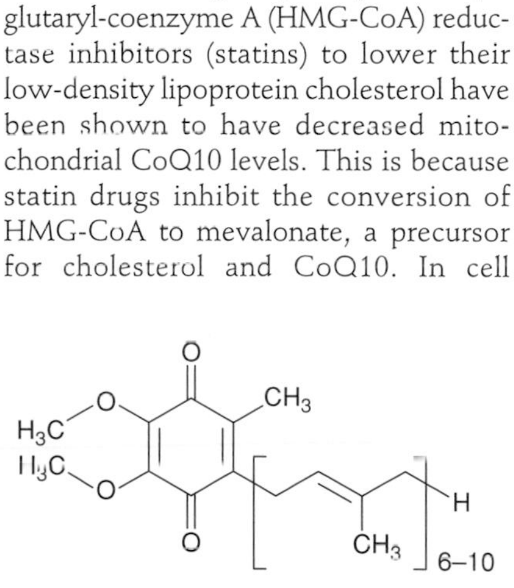

$$\text{Coenzyme Q10: } H_3C\text{–O, } H_3C\text{–O, } CH_3\text{ substituted quinone with } [CH_2CH{=}C(CH_3)CH_2]_{6-10}H$$

▲ **FIGURE 34-2** Coenzyme Q10 (ubiquinone).

COENZYME Q10 LEVELS AND SKIN CANCER Abnormally low plasma levels of CoQ10 have been found in patients with cancer of the breast, lung, or pancreas.[65] A recent study investigated the usefulness of CoQ10 plasma levels in predicting the risk of metastasis and the duration of the metastasis-free interval in melanoma patients. Rusciani et al. showed that CoQ10 levels were significantly lower in melanoma patients than in control subjects and in patients who developed metastases than in the metastasis-free subgroup. They suggested that baseline plasma CoQ10 levels could serve as a prognostic factor to estimate the risk for melanoma progression.[66]

In the adjuvant therapy of melanoma with interferon (IFN), it seems that large amounts of ATP are required for an immune response initiated by IFN to be effective. It has thus been hypothesized that the failure of some patients to respond to IFN therapy may be caused by an inability to meet the excess demand for ATP induced by this medication. However, it is known that CoQ10 plays a key role in the mitochondrial respiratory cycle and production of ATP.[67,68] Therefore, Rusciani et al. conducted a clinical trial in stage I and II melanoma patients examining a postsurgical adjuvant therapy with recombinant IFN alpha-2b in combination with coenzyme Q10 versus IFN alpha-2b alone for the control group. In a 3-year trial, they uninterruptedly treated the patients with low-dose recombinant IFN alpha-2b administered twice daily and coenzyme Q10 (400 mg/d). The control group was treated with only low-dose recombinant IFN alpha-2b in the same dosage and administration. Treatment efficacy was evaluated as incidence of recurrences at 5 years. The group demonstrated that the risk of developing metastases was about 10 times lower in the IFN + CoQ10 patients compared with the IFN-alone group.[69] However, a 10-year follow-up will be needed to provide more significant results.

At the time of publication of this text there were several over-the-counter (OTC) cosmetic products, including Nivea and Eucerin, on the market containing CoQ10. Although they are very popular, more research is needed to examine the long-term preventive effects of these products in order to see if they are truly able to prevent the cutaneous signs of aging. CoQ10 is stable in topical products. Penetration depends on the characteristics of the topical formulation because of the high-molecular-weight of this compound. Formulation with this ingredient leads to a yellow tint in the product.

SIDE EFFECTS Oral CoQ10 supplementation has been associated with a caffeine-like side effect and may cause nervousness or a jittery feeling. So as not to induce insomnia, it is recommended that CoQ10 not be taken at night. Diarrhea, appetite loss, and mild nausea are among the other side effects reported.[70] No side effects have been reported with topical application. CoQ10 has not been reported to cause contact dermatitis.

Idebenone

Idebenone is the synthetic analog of CoQ10, penetrating the skin more efficiently because of its lower molecular weight. Idebenone has been shown to possess superior antioxidant capacity compared to CoQ10, tocopherol, kinetin, ascorbic acid, and lipoic acid in various in vitro and in vivo trials.[71]

TOPICAL APPLICATION McDaniel et al. examined the in vivo efficacy of idebenone in a topical skincare formulation for the treatment of photodamaged skin. In a randomized, blind labeled, nonvehicle control study, 41 female subjects used either 0.5% or 1.0% idebenone formulations twice daily for 6 weeks.[72] After 6 weeks both user groups showed improvement of all examined parameters. A 26% reduction in skin roughness/dryness was measured in the 1.0% user group as was a 29% reduction in fine lines/wrinkles; this group also experienced a 33% improvement in overall global assessment of photodamaged skin. For users of the 0.5% idebenone formulation, reductions in skin roughness/dryness as well as fine lines/wrinkles were 23% and 27%, respectively, and improvement in overall global assessment of photodamaged skin was 30%. It is important to remember that the effects seen on wrinkles in these trials were likely caused by hydration or skin irritation because antioxidants have exhibited no efficacy in treating wrinkles (with the exception of vitamin C), but can help prevent them. Skin care products containing idebenone are commercially available as Prevage MD by Allergan (1% idebenone), and Prevage and Prevage Eye Antiaging Moisturizing Treatment by Elizabeth Arden and Allergan (0.5% idebenone).

SIDE EFFECTS A recent case report of contact dermatitis owing to a facial treatment with an "antiaging" cream in a beauty salon identified the allergen as idebenone 0.5% by patch testing.[73] As idebenone has become more popular, contact allergy to this compound has become more common.[73]

Lycopene

Lycopene is a natural pigment synthesized by plants and microorganisms. It is an open-chain, unsaturated carotenoid that is found in red fruits and vegetables such as tomatoes, pink grapefruit, watermelon, and apricots. In fact, it is lycopene that is responsible for the red pigment we observe in those fruits and vegetables.[74,75] It has been documented that dietary intake of tomatoes and tomato products containing lycopene is associated with decreased risk of chronic disorders such as cancer and cardiovascular diseases.[76–78]

Lycopene has been found to exhibit potent antioxidant properties. Because of its high number of conjugated double bonds, it demonstrates stronger singlet oxygen-quenching ability compared to alpha-tocopherol or beta-carotene.[76] Clinical trials with tomato products suggest a synergistic action of lycopene with other nutrients in lowering biomarkers of oxidative stress and carcinogenesis.[79]

Further, lycopene has been shown to prevent carcinogenesis in various tumor models.[80–83] Reported mechanisms of action are arrest of tumor cell-cycle progression, insulin-like growth factor-1 (IGF-1) signaling transduction, and induction of apoptosis. A recent study suggested that part of the antitumor activity of lycopene might be caused by the trapping activity of lycopene on platelet-derived growth factor (PDGF), suggesting that this antioxidant acts as an inhibitor on tumor stromal cells.[84]

In skin cancer, mouse models have demonstrated its chemopreventive effects against photo-induced tumors.[85,86] Lycopene appears to have the potential to prevent skin cancer and warrants further investigation for such an indication.

Although the clinical data in humans are very limited, lycopene is included in various skin care products, including facial moisturizers, sunscreens, eye creams, and formulations touted for their "antiaging" skin care. Further data in humans are needed to shed more light on the effects of lycopene on human skin.

Curcumin

Curcumin is a yellow pigment found in the root of the tropical turmeric plant, *Curcuma longa,* which belongs to the Zingiberaceae family. Turmeric consists of a water-soluble component, turmerin, and a lipid-soluble component, curcumin.[87] Curcumin has been used for centuries in traditional medicine for various treatments such as inflammatory conditions and other diseases; in Indian cuisine it is used as a spice. Turmeric tubers contain curcuminoids, of which curcumin I (diferuloyl methane) is most abundant, followed by curcumin II (6%) and III (0.3%)[88] (Fig. 34-3). Curcumin has been shown to exhibit a broad array of biologic activities, such as anti-inflammatory, anticarcinogenic, antioxidant, antimicrobial, and wound healing.[89–91] The molecular basis of these effects are mediated through the regulation of various transcription factors, growth factors, inflammatory cytokines, protein kinases, adhesion molecules, apoptotic genes, angiogenesis regulators, and other enzymes.[92,93]

ANTIOXIDANT AND ANTI-INFLAMMATORY ACTIVITIES OF CURCUMIN Curcumin has been identified as a potent scavenger of a variety of ROS, including superoxide anion radicals, hydroxyl radicals, and nitrogen dioxide radicals.[94] Also, curcumin has been shown to downregulate the production of the proinflammatory cytokines IL-1 and tumor necrosis factor-α (TNF-α), and to inhibit the activation of transcription factors NF-κB and AP-1, both regulating the genes for proinflammatory mediators and protective antioxidant genes.[95]

The antioxidant and anti-inflammatory properties of curcumin have been documented in mouse models, proving that curcumin has a beneficial effect against chemo- and photocarcinogenesis. Further studies are needed in order to determine whether topical applications or oral intake of curcumin can inhibit skin carcinogenesis in humans.[96–98] Oral intake of curcumin in humans was recently evaluated and established as nontoxic at doses up to 8 g/d when taken by mouth for 3 months.[99] These are promising developments; further studies are needed to elucidate the role of this antioxidant compound as a photochemopreventive agent.

WOUND-HEALING EFFECTS OF CURCUMIN Sidhu et al. demonstrated that wound closure in curcumin-treated normal and genetically diabetic animals was significantly faster compared to controls. This enhanced healing effect was attributed to the improvement of neovascularization and reepithelialization, the increase of expression and production of transforming growth factor-1 and fibronectin, and the reduction of cell death by curcumin.[100] Curcumin treatment has also improved collagen deposition and increased fibroblast and vascular density, enhancing both normal and impaired wound healing. The observed proangiogenic effect of curcumin in wound healing is believed to be based on inducing transforming growth factor-beta, which in turn induces angiogenesis and the accumulation of extracellular matrix.[101]

CURCUMIN AND SKIN CANCER Curcumin has been demonstrated to inhibit carcinogenesis in several tumor model systems including skin neoplastic models.[95,96,102–104] Its mechanism of action is not precisely known, but it is thought to inhibit initiation, promotion, and progression of cancer.[105] Curcumin was reported to inhibit UVA-induced metallothionein expression and ornithine decarboxylase (ODC) activity, and to induce p53-mediated apoptosis, as well as cell membrane-mediated apoptosis through Fas receptor induction and caspase-8 activation.[96,106,107]

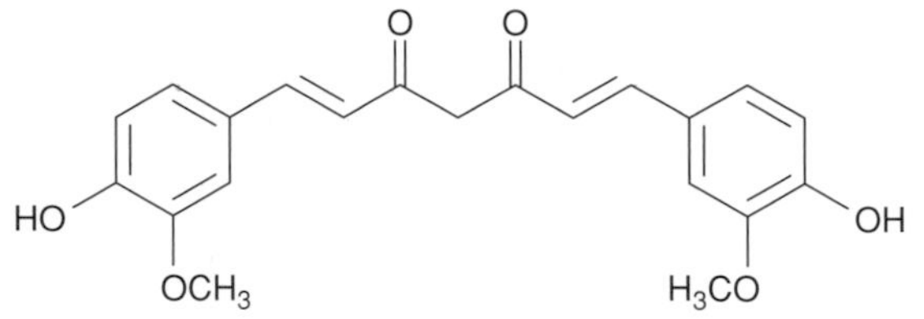

O O
HO OH
OCH_3 H_3CO

▲ **FIGURE 34-3** Curcumin.

Paradoxically, some recent studies have suggested that the anticancer activity of the antioxidant curcumin has actually promoted the generation of ROS.[108] In response, Chen et al. investigated the antioxidant and anticancer activity of curcumin in human myeloid leukemia (HL-60) cells. They determined that the anticancer activity of curcumin was effective in a concentration- and time-dependent manner in reducing the proliferation and viability of leukemia cells, but its effect on ROS was concentration dependent. That is, low concentrations of curcumin decreased ROS generation, but high concentrations had the opposite effect. In additional studies, Chen et al. found that the combination of water-soluble antioxidants amplified the antioxidant and anticancer activity of low curcumin concentrations.[108]

Currently, there are only a few cosmetic products containing curcumin because its distinct and pungent aroma and color make it difficult to formulate into a cosmetically elegant product. More clinical trials are needed to evaluate the effects of curcumin on human skin.

WATER-SOLUBLE ANTIOXIDANTS

These are found in hydrophobic areas of the cell and the serum and include vitamin C and glutathione.

Glutathione

Glutathione is the most abundant antioxidant in the network. It is produced from the amino acids glutamic acid, cysteine, and glycine. Oral glutathione is not well absorbed into the body, so supplementation is difficult—it is not even available in cosmetic products. There are no studies evaluating the efficacy of glutathione as an antioxidant. Significantly, though, lipoic acid can recycle glutathione.

Vitamin C

Vitamin C is historically known for its role in the prevention of scurvy. By the 18th century, sailors knew that eating citrus fruits prevented this condition associated with dental abnormalities, bleeding disorders, characteristic purpuric skin lesions, and mental deterioration. In the 1930s, researchers confirmed that vitamin C is the key ingredient in citrus fruit that prevents scurvy.[109] In contrast to some animals, humans obtain vitamin C solely from food, such as citrus fruits, black currants, red peppers, and leafy green vegetables. Unfortunately oral supplementation of vitamin C does not increase the levels of vitamin C in the skin, as the transport from the gastrointestinal tract is limited. Moreover, sunlight and environmental pollution, such as ozone in city pollution, can deplete epidermal vitamin C.[110,111] Thus, enhancing the levels of vitamin C in the skin is an important goal, as vitamin C is known to be a potent antioxidant.

Today, vitamin C, also known as ascorbic acid, is being studied extensively for its role as an antioxidant. Oral vitamin C has been associated with decreasing the risk of certain cancers, cardiovascular disease, and cataracts, as well as improving wound healing and immune modulation.[112,113] Vitamin C has also been used as a topical antioxidant to prevent sun damage,[26] and for the treatment of melasma,[114] striae alba,[115] and postoperative erythema in laser patients.[116]

CHEMISTRY OF VITAMIN C Vitamin C, or ascorbate, is an alpha-ketolactone that exists as a hydrophilic monovalent hydroxyl anion. Adding one electron to ascorbate creates the ascorbate free radical. This transient form is more stable than other free radicals and can accept other electrons, making it an effective free radical scavenger, and thus a great antioxidant. If the transient form cannot take an electron, it will yield the electron to an enzymatic reaction, thereby becoming an electron donor.

When two electrons are added to ascorbic acid (AA), the reaction forms a new substance called dehydro-L-ascorbic acid (DHAA). Under physiologic conditions, vitamin C predominantly exists in its reduced form, ascorbic acid; it also exists in trace quantities in the oxidized form, DHAA (Fig. 34-4). This substance can be reduced back to ascorbate, but if the lactone ring irreversibly opens, forming diketogulonic acid, the compound is no longer active. Diketogulonic acid is often formed when vitamin C preparations are oxidized. When this occurs, these solutions are rendered ineffective and useless.[112,113] In other words, when vitamin C preparations are exposed to UV rays or to air, the molecule rapidly adds two electrons and converts to DHAA, which contains an aromatic ring. If further oxidized, the ring irreversibly opens and the vitamin C solution becomes permanently inactive.

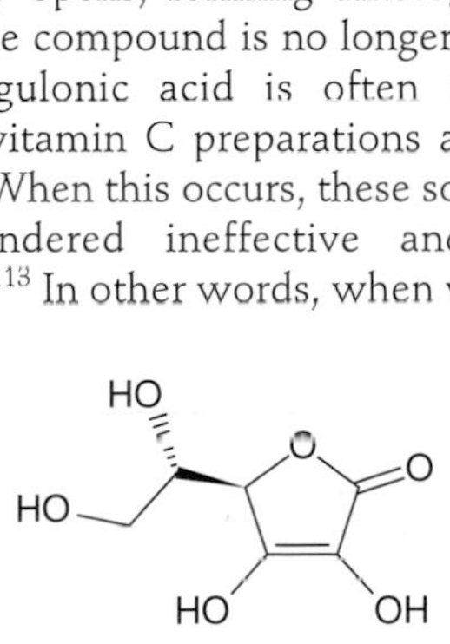

▲ **FIGURE 34-4** Ascorbic acid.

VITAMIN C AS AN ANTIOXIDANT Vitamin C has become a popular addition to "after-sun" products because it has been shown to interfere with the UV-induced generation of ROS by reacting with the superoxide anion[117] or the hydroxyl radical.[118] In fact, vitamin C is known to delay the incidence of UV-induced neoplasms in mice.[119] Topical vitamin C was studied as a photoprotectant first using a porcine skin model.[26] In this study, histologic examination revealed that animals treated with topical ascorbic acid exhibited fewer sunburn cells than those treated with vehicle alone when exposed to both UVA and UVB irradiation. (Sunburn cells are basal keratinocytes undergoing programmed cell death because of irreparable DNA damage and represent a method of quantifying the damaging effects of UV irradiation.) Researchers also observed a significant decrease in erythema in areas treated with vitamin C and decreases in the amount of vitamin C left on the skin after UV irradiation. In a subsequent study, Darr and colleagues discovered that topical vitamin C combined with either a UVA or UVB sunscreen improved sun protection as compared to the sunscreen alone.[120] Vitamins C and E, in combination, also provided notable protection from UVB insult, though the bulk of protection was attributable to vitamin E.

There are multiple studies that demonstrate that mice treated with topical vitamin C have less erythema, fewer sunburn cells, and decreased tumor formation seen in treated skin after UV exposure.[3] Vitamin C, a strong antioxidant itself, also reduces (and therefore recycles) oxidized vitamin E back into its active form so the antioxidant capabilities of vitamin E are amplified or regenerated in this way.[40]

THE EFFECTS OF VITAMIN C ON COLLAGEN AND ELASTIN SYNTHESIS Ascorbate is a cofactor for the enzymatic activity of prolyl hydroxylase, an enzyme that hydroxylates prolyl residues in procollagen, elastin, and other proteins with collagenous domains prior to triple helix formation, and thus is required for collagen synthesis.[121] Consequently, deficiency of ascorbic acid leads to impaired collagen production resulting in scurvy. Elastin also contains hydroxyproline; however, prolyl hydroxylation is not required for the biosynthesis and secretion of elastin,[122] and the role of vitamin C in elastin production is unclear.

The addition of ascorbic acid to fibroblast cultures has been reported to increase collagen production by increasing the transcription rate of procollagen genes and by elevating procollagen mRNA levels.[123] Although the increase of type I collagen production in cells cultured in the presence of ascorbic acid is well known, the effects of ascorbate on other extracellular matrix molecules are still poorly understood.[124]

In fact, studies have suggested that concentrations of ascorbic acid that maximally stimulate collagen biosynthesis act as an antagonist to elastin accumulation.[125] In a series of studies, Bergethon et al.[126] elaborated on these observations by showing that elastin accumulation was sharply diminished in cell cultures treated with vitamin C.[124] In other words, we know that the addition of ascorbic acid to fibroblast cultures increases production of collagen but may decrease production of elastin by an unknown mechanism.

Clinically the relevance of these effects on collagen and elastin are limited. There is one study in the literature that examines the effects of topically applied vitamin C on wrinkles.[127] In this study, Cellex-C was shown to decrease wrinkles when applied topically for a period of 3 months. The patients were evaluated using photography assessments and optical profilometry. Unfortunately, this cannot be considered a blinded study because a large proportion of the patients experienced stinging on the side treated with vitamin C. However, there was a significant difference in the wrinkles on the treated side versus the untreated side. The mechanism of action of this difference is not understood. It might be explained by increased collagen synthesis or by inflammation and irritation induced by the product.

Humbert et al. evaluated the effects of topical vitamin C in healthy photoaged female volunteers in a double-blind, randomized trial. They topically applied cream containing 5% vitamin C over a 6-month period, comparing the action of the vitamin C cream versus excipient on photoaged skin. Clinically, a statistically significant improvement in hydration, wrinkles, glare, and brown spots was noted. A highly significant increase in the density of skin microrelief and a decrease of the deep furrows were also demonstrated. Ultrastructural evidence of the elastic tissue repair was documented. Tissue levels of the inhibitor of MMP-1 were increased, reducing UV-induced collagen breakdown. The mRNA levels of elastin and fibrillin remained unchanged. The topical application of 5% vitamin C cream was well tolerated.[128] However, more clinical trials are necessary to unravel all of the effects of vitamin C on skin and aging.

VITAMIN C AS ANTI-INFLAMMATORY AGENT

Vitamin C has also been shown to possess anti-inflammatory activities. In various cell lines loaded with vitamin C by incubating them with DHA, Carcamo et al. were able to show a significant decrease in TNF-α-induced nuclear translocation of NF-κB, NF-κB-dependent reporter transcription, and IκBα phosphorylation, suggesting that intracellular vitamin C can influence inflammatory, neoplastic, and apoptotic processes via inhibition of NF-κB activation. The decrease of inflammation can lead to a reduction of postinflammatory hyperpigmentation.

TOPICAL VITAMIN C Most of the data available on the effects of vitamin C are derived from studies examining the effects of oral vitamin C or vitamin C applied to tissue cultures. Unfortunately, there are no studies that demonstrate that ingestion of oral vitamin C increases the levels of vitamin C in the skin. Consequently, topical vitamin C preparations have become popular. Ascorbic acid can be formulated into water- or lipid-soluble forms.[129] Topical ascorbyl palmitate, a lipid form, is nonirritating and reportedly photoprotective and anti-inflammatory.[130] Unfortunately, many of the currently available topical preparations are unable to penetrate the stratum corneum and are, consequently, useless. Some manufacturers claim that their products are nonionic and less lipophobic, enhancing the opportunity for percutaneous absorption.[6,131] The aim of these topical products is to deliver higher amounts of vitamin C to a specific local area of the skin. Comparison of the absorption rate of various topical formulations has not yet been performed using human subjects.

Another problem with topically applied ascorbic acid is its lack of stability as described above in the chemistry section. Because few preparations of topical vitamin C are packaged in airtight containers that are protected from UV radiation, most preparations become inactive within hours of opening the bottle.

OTHER COSMETIC APPLICATIONS

Melasma As vitamin C inhibits the enzyme tyrosinase, it can be used as a depigmenting agent[132] (see Chapter 33). In the mid-1990s, Kameyama et al. found that a stable derivative of ascorbic acid produced a significant lightening effect in 19 of 34 patients treated for melasma and senile lentigos.[114] Among patients with normal skin, however, there was no significant lightening.

Postlaser erythema In a study of 10 patients who underwent skin resurfacing with a CO_2 laser, vitamin C topically applied 2 or more weeks after surgery decreased the duration and degree of erythema.[116]

Stretch marks In the late 1990s, Ash et al. compared topical vitamin C in combination with glycolic acid to tretinoin and glycolic acid for the treatment of striae alba.[115] Blinded and unblinded observers determined that both regimens produced an objective improvement in the striae. Although both regimens increased the epidermal thickness, only the tretinoin/glycolic combination augmented the elastin content of the striae.

SIDE EFFECTS The administration of vitamin C, in either oral or topical form, appears to be safe for human use. In the studies reviewed, a small number of patients experienced minimal discomfort (stinging and mild irritation) from the topically applied formulations. The major disadvantages of the various formulations include high cost, questionable efficacy, and the possibility of an adverse effect on elastin production, the clinical significance of which is currently unclear. Ascorbic acid is a great addition to skin care particularly when patients insist on sun exposure, cigarette smoking, or other behavior that contributes to free radical production. The practitioner should advise patients, though, to take the oral form so that they will experience the same antioxidant benefits in the arteries, liver, and other amenable organs. If it really works, why limit its effects to the skin?

SUMMARY Vitamin C preparations are useful in preventing or lessening the harmful effects of UV radiation and ameliorating disorders of hyperpigmentation, striae, and postlaser erythema.

Topical vitamin C products must be formulated properly and stored in airtight, light-resistant containers to be effective. Skinceuticals, Murad, and La Roche-Posay have formulated the most effective vitamin C-containing products.

Green Tea

Green tea has been consumed as a popular beverage in Asian countries, in particular, and throughout the world for many years. It has recently gained greater popularity in western nations, though, because of its purported antioxidant and anticarcinogenic effects. There are numerous in vitro and in vivo studies on the effects of green tea on the skin; in fact, green tea is one of the most studied antioxidants.[133] Besides its antioxidant activity, green tea polyphenols possess anti-inflammatory and anticarcinogenic properties and modulate the biochemical pathways important in cell proliferation, when administered either topically or orally.[134,135]

Polyphenols are a large, diverse family of thousands of chemical substances found in plants. Significantly, many of them are strong antioxidants (Table 34-1). There are four major polyphenolic catechins in green tea: ECG [(-)EpiCatechin-3-O-Gallate], GCG [(-)GalloCatechin-3-O Gallate], EGCG [(-)EpiGalloCatechin -3-O-Gallate], and EGC [(-)EpiGallo Catechin]. EGCG is the most abundant and biologically active component (Fig. 34-5). Special preparation of the tea plant ensures that the antioxidant activities of these polyphenols are preserved. White tea, like green tea, comes from the *Camellia sinensis* plant. However, white tea is more expensive because it is harder to obtain. White tea actually comes from the tips of the green tea leaves or from leaves that are not yet fully open and the buds are still covered by fine white hair. EGCG is the main compound in green and white tea responsible for antioxidant activity.[136,137] When evaluating the utility of a skin care product, it is necessary to know which polyphenols are in the product. EGCG is the most potent form of green tea polyphenols. In addition, it is necessary to know what percent of polyphenols are in the product. The most effective products contain 50% to 90% polyphenols. Such formulations are dark in color and look brown when they contain this high level of polyphenols. The Replenix line by Topix is an example of a product line with a high level of polyphenols.

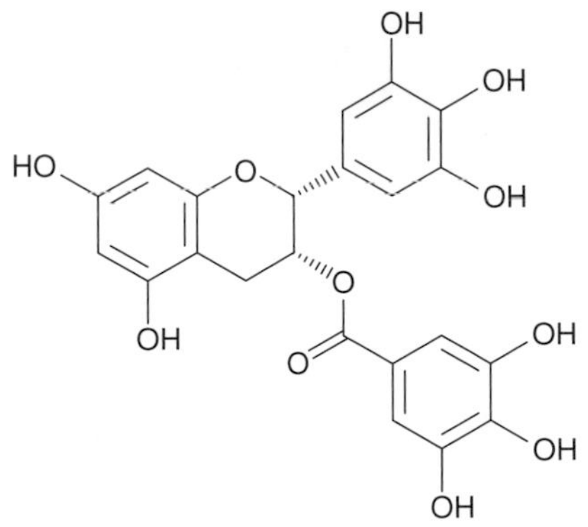

▲ **FIGURE 34-5** Epigallocatechin gallate (EGCG) is the most abundant catechin in tea.

PHOTOPROTECTION BY GREEN TEA In early studies, green tea polyphenols were shown to suppress chemical- and UV-induced carcinogenesis when fed orally or applied topically in hairless or Sencar mice.[138–140] Other studies have confirmed these results and shown EGCG to be a potent suppressor of photocarcinogenesis.[141] The profound photoprotective effects of topically applied green tea polyphenols (GTPs) have also been observed in human skin, demonstrating a dose-dependent reduction of UV-induced erythema, decrease in the number of sunburn cells, protection of epidermal Langerhans cells, and limitation of DNA-damage.[142] Recent studies have demonstrated that GTPs scavenge ROS, stabilizing GPX, catalase, and glutathione, as well as inhibiting nitric oxide synthase, lipoxygenase, COX and xanthine oxidase, and lipid peroxidase. In addition, they act as modulators of different gene groups and signal pathways.

MOLECULAR MECHANISMS OF GREEN TEA Molecular targets of GTPs include among others Ras and AP-1, both of which are involved in the MAPK pathway.[143] The antiapoptotic effects of EGCG on UVB-irradiated keratinocytes seem to be induced by an increase in the expression of the antiapoptotic molecule Bcl-2 and a decrease in the proapoptotic protein Bax.[144] EGCG has further been shown to reduce UV-induced immunosuppression by limiting IL-10 production and increasing IL-12 production, two major cytokines that mediate UV-induced immunosupression.[145] In addition, the EGCG-induced IL-12 increase leads to an augmented synthesis of enzymes that repair UV-induced DNA damage.[146] Also, EGCG seems to reduce UVB-induced immunosuppression by decreasing CD11b, a cell surface marker for activated macrophages and neutrophils in animals treated with UVB.[147] In mice, EGCG has been shown to downregulate UV-induced expression of AP-1 and NF-κB and suppress MMPs, which are known to degrade collagen resulting in photodamage.[148] Prevention of UV-induced oxidative damage and induction of MMPs has been demonstrated in vivo in mouse skin. In the study, GTPs were administered in drinking water to SKH-1 hairless mice, which were thereafter exposed to multiple doses of UVB (90 mJ/cm^2, for 2 months on alternate days). Treatment with GTPs resulted in inhibition of UVB-induced protein oxidation in vivo in mouse skin, which could also be observed in vitro in human skin fibroblast HS68 cells. Further, oral administration of GTPs was shown to inhibit UVB-induced expression of matrix-degrading MMPs in hairless mouse skin, supporting the role of GTPs as antiphotoaging compounds.[148]

GREEN TEA USE IN HUMANS In contrast to the amount of scientific data on GTPs, there are limited studies in human skin examining the topical application of green tea-containing products. This is likely caused by the difficulty of designing a study to measure the preventive effects of green tea on aging skin. Nevertheless, applying topical GTPs in the morning in combination with traditional sunscreens seems to make sense and is thought to have the potential to protect the skin from UV-induced damage. In addition, topical green tea, as is

TABLE 34-1
Polyphenols[a] Classed by Type and Number of Constituents. Examples Appear Below

Phenols	Pyrocatechol	Pyrogallol	Resorcinol	Phloroglucinol	Hydroquinone
Coumaric acid-derived lignins, kaempferol	Catechin, quercetin, caffeic acid- and ferulic acid-derived lignins, hydroxytyrosol esters	Gallocatechins (EGCG), tannins, myricetin, sinapyl alcohol-derived lignins	Resveratrol	Most flavonoids	Arbutin

[a]http://en.wikipedia.org/wiki/Polyphenol; accessed March 10, 2008.

the case with other antioxidants, may improve rosacea, prevent retinoid dermatitis, and play a role in managing pigmentation disorders. There are many products containing green tea that can be obtained OTC. Most of the products, however, have not been tested in controlled clinical trials and the concentration of polyphenols in these products is too low to demonstrate efficacy. It is crucial to know the amount of GTPs in a formulation to judge its efficacy.

Silymarin

Silymarin is a naturally-occurring polyphenolic flavonoid compound derived from the seeds of the milk thistle plant *Silybum marianum*. Milk thistle has been used for medicinal purposes for more than 2000 years. Today, it is used in Europe and Asia as an antihepatotoxic agent and is available as a supplement in Europe and the US. The main component of silymarin is silybin (silibinin), which is considered to be the most biologically active component in terms of its antioxidant, anti-inflammatory, and anticarcinogenic properties[149] (Fig. 34–6).

PHOTOPROTECTION Topical application of silybin prior to, or immediately after, UV irradiation has been found to impart strong protection against UV-induced damage in the epidermis by a reduction in thymine dimer-positive cells and an upregulation of p53-p21/Cip1, which researchers believe may lead to inhibition of cell proliferation and apoptosis. This study suggests that mechanisms other than sunscreen effect are integral to silybin efficacy against UV-caused skin damages.[150] Researchers have also noted that silybin enhances UVB-induced apoptosis and speculated that it acts as a UVB damage sensor to confer its biologic action.[151]

The antioxidant activity of silymarin is well established. Chemoprotective activity against skin cancer has also been reported and continues to be the subject of much investigation.[152–154] In a study to identify the mechanism of photocarcinogenesis prevention in mouse skin by the topical treatment of silymarin, prevention of UVB-induced immunosuppression and oxidative stress were found to be potentially related to the prevention of photocarcinogenesis in mice.[155] Authors concluded from this trial and related data from other recent studies that there are compelling arguments for the inclusion of silymarin in sunscreens or in other products in a skin care regimen.

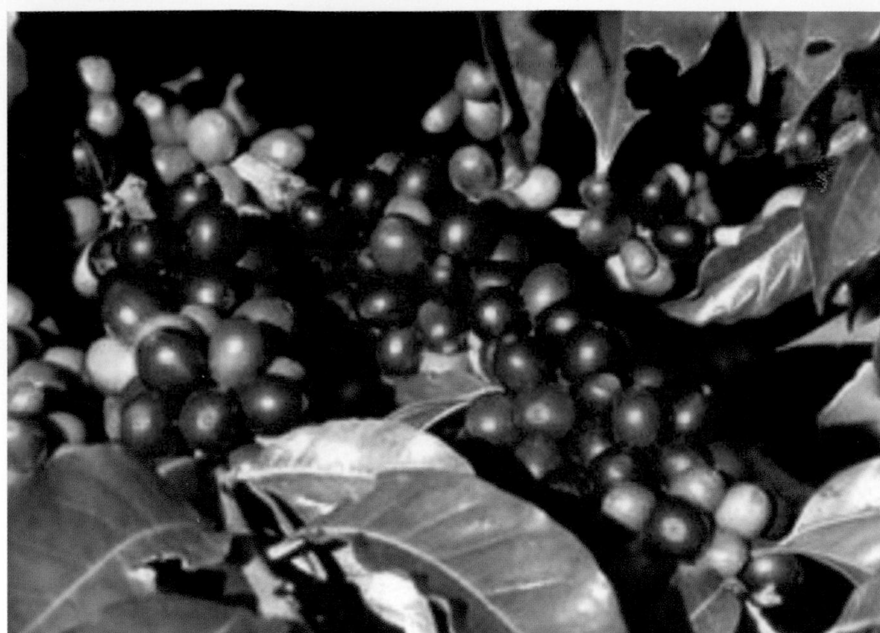

▲ **FIGURE 34-7** The coffee plant *Coffea arabica*.

MODE OF ADMINISTRATION Most of the milk thistle or silymarin available in the US comes in the form of oral supplements. These may inactivate oral contraceptives. Topical formulations are available from SkinCeuticals. Silymarin has been used in topical formulations to treat rosacea.[156]

Coffea Arabica and Coffeeberry Extract

The coffee plant *Coffea arabica* is the source of the globally consumed coffee beverage, originating from Ethiopia and cultivated throughout the world. Extracts of the beans of the coffee plant have been shown to exhibit antioxidant activity after roasting[157] (Fig. 34-7). Besides the coffee beans, the fruit of the coffee plant, especially when harvested in a sub-ripened state, also possesses peak antioxidant activity, by dint of its constituent polyphenols, especially chlorogenic acid, condensed proanthocyanidins, quinic acid, and ferulic acid. Coffeeberry is the proprietary name for the antioxidant that is extracted from the fruit of *Coffea arabica*. In the oxygen radical absorbance capacity assay (ORAC), Coffeeberry has demonstrated higher antioxidant activity than green tea, pomegranate extract, as well as vitamins C and E.[158] Polyphenols, which can be found in coffee beans, green and black tea, various fruits, vegetables and grains, are known to impart multiple health benefits, mainly because of their anti-inflammatory and antioxidant properties.[159,160] In 2007, Stiefel Laboratories launched the product line RevaléSkin, which contains 1% coffeeberry polyphenols. To build on some promising laboratory results, clinical studies assessing the antioxidant effects of topical preparations containing *C. arabica* and coffeeberry extract are needed.

Polypodium Leucotomos

Polypodium leucotomos (PL) is an extract derived from the fern family. It is an oral photoprotectant with strong antioxidant properties. Its major phenolic components have been shown to be 3,4-dihydroxybenzoic acid, 4-hydroxybenzoic acid, vanillic acid, caffeic acid, 4-hydroxycinnamic acid, 4-hydroxycinnamoylquinic acid, ferulic acid, and five chlorogenic acid isomers.[161] In traditional medicine, polypodium leucotomos extract (PLE) has been used for various

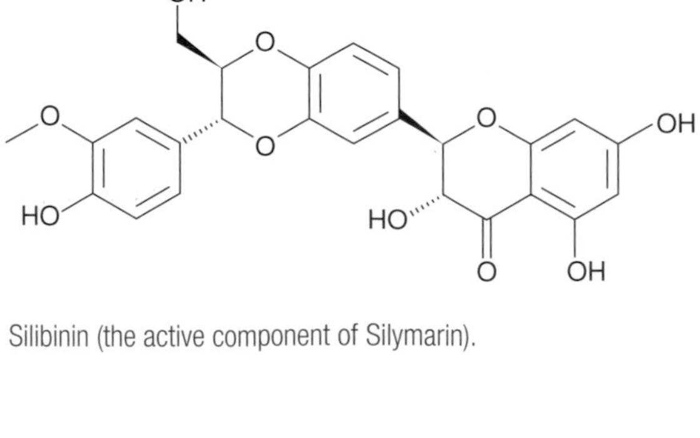

▲ **FIGURE 34-6** Silibinin (the active component of Silymarin).

indications, including psoriasis, atopic dermatitis, vitiligo, rheumatoid arthritis, and tumors and, recently, PLE has been demonstrated to exhibit immunomodulatory activity in vitro and in vivo.[162]

PHOTOPROTECTION The photoprotective effect of PL has been shown for topical or oral administration in various studies.[163] In a study by Gonzáles et al., 21 healthy volunteers, either untreated or treated with oral psoralens (8-MOP or 5-MOP), were enrolled and exposed to solar radiation. Immediate pigment darkening (IPD), MED, minimal melanogenic dose (MMD), and minimal phototoxic dose (MPD) before and after topical or oral administration of PL were evaluated. PL was found to be photoprotective after topical application as well as oral administration showing a prevention of acute sunburn and psoralen-induced phototoxic reactions. Immunohistochemistry revealed photoprotection of Langherhans cells by oral as well as topical PL.[164]

ANTIOXIDATIVE EFFECTS The antioxidant effects of PL have been demonstrated in vitro and in vivo, as well as for the prevention of photoaging.[165,166] Gonzáles et al. showed that PL manifests photoprotective effects in vivo and in vitro by its ability to suppress free radical generation, prevent photodecomposition of both endogenous photoprotective molecules and DNA, and inhibit UV-induced cell death.[167] Oral administration of PLE has proven to have photoprotective effects in various studies. It has been shown to decrease sunburn and UV-induced mast cell infiltration in the skin, and reduce the loss of epidermal Langerhans cells of the skin associated with UV exposure.[168,169] Caccialanza et al. exposed 26 patients with polymorphic light eruption and two with solar urticaria to sunlight while directing them to consume 480 mg/d of PL orally through the study. The response of the skin to sunlight was compared with that occurring previously without administration of PL, and showed statistically significant reduction of skin reaction and subjective symptoms.[170]

MOLECULAR MECHANISM The molecular mechanisms of the photoprotective effects of PL have been investigated in vitro using a solar simulator as UV source in human keratinocytes. The results showed that the photoprotective effects of PL seem to involve inhibition of TNF-α, nitric oxide (NO) production, and inducible nitric oxide synthase (iNOS) upregulation induced by UV light and the modulation of the transcriptional activation of AP-1 and NF-κB, two proinflammatory transcription factors induced by UV-radiation. Finally, it was demonstrated that PL prevents cytotoxic damage and apoptosis induced by UV light in HaCaT cells.[171]

SUMMARY It appears that the dermatologic potential of this tropical plant extract is being harnessed in clinical applications for the treatment of sunburn and the inhibition of the phototoxic reaction, as well as for the prevention of photoaging.[165,172,173] Experimental data support the inclusion of PL extract in sunscreen formulations.[174] This ingredient is currently only available as an oral supplement in the US under the brand name Heliocare and is sold by the company OPKO Health Inc. One to two capsules of Heliocare should be taken 1 hour prior to sun exposure. It should be used in conjunction with a broad-spectrum sunscreen. At this time, there are no topical formulations of this ingredient.

Resveratrol

Resveratrol (*trans*-3,5,4′-trihydroxystilbene) is a polyphenolic phytoalexin compound found in the skin and seeds of grapes, berries, peanuts, red wine, and other foods and has been reported to exhibit a wide range of biologic and pharmacologic properties.[175] It exists in two isoforms: *trans*-resveratrol and *cis*-resveratrol where the *trans*-isomer is the more stable form (Fig. 34-8). Resveratrol is a potent antioxidant with antiproliferative and anti-inflammatory properties.[149,176,177] In vitro and in vivo studies have demonstrated that resveratrol exhibits chemopreventive and antiproliferative activity against various cancers, including skin cancer, by exerting inhibitory effects on diverse cellular events associated with tumor initiation, promotion, and progression and triggering apoptosis in such tumor cells.[178–180]

MOLECULAR MECHANISMS OF PHOTOPROTECTION In recent studies resveratrol has been shown to protect against UVB-mediated cutaneous damages in SKH-1 hairless mice. Topical application of resveratrol to SKH-1 hairless mice prior to UVB irradiation resulted in a significant decrease in UVB-mediated generation of H_2O_2 as well as infiltration of leukocytes and inhibition of skin edema. Also, topical application of resveratrol has been found to significantly inhibit UVB-mediated induction of COX-2 and ODC enzyme activities and protein expression of ODC, which are well-established markers for tumor promotion. Resveratrol further seems to inhibit the UVB-mediated increase of lipid peroxidation, a marker of oxidative stress.[176,181,182] In one study, pretreatment of normal human epidermal keratinocytes (NHEK) with resveratrol inhibited UVB-induced activation of the NF-κB pathway.[177] This protective effect of resveratrol against the damage of multiple UVB-exposure was suggested to be associated with inhibition of the MAPK pathway and mediated via modulation in the expression and function of the cell cycle regulatory protein cki–cyclin–cdk network.[183] Further, in short-term experiments, the topical application of resveratrol to SKH-1 hairless mouse skin prior to UVB irradiation resulted in significant inhibition of cell proliferation and phosphorylation of survivin.[181] Long-term studies have demonstrated that topical application with resveratrol (both pre- and post-treatment) results in inhibition of UVB-induced tumor incidence and delay in the onset of skin tumorigenesis.[102] The posttreatment of resveratrol imparted equal protection to the pretreatment, suggesting that resveratrol-mediated responses may not be sunscreen effects.

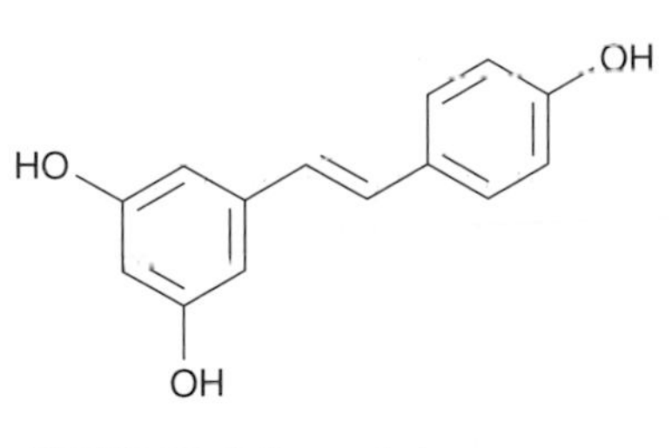

▲ **FIGURE 34-8** Resveratrol.

SUMMARY Data and clinical evidence seem to be promising enough to regard resveratrol as suitable for inclusion in various product types (e.g., emollients, patches, sunscreens, and other skin care products) intended to prevent skin cancer and other conditions thought to be generated by the sun.

Grape Seed Extract

Grapes, also known as *Vitis vinifera,* are globally consumed fruits and the source of wine. The extract prepared from grape seeds is rich in proanthocyanidins, which belong to the polyphenolic flavonoid family. Specifically, grape seed proanthocyanidins are oligomers and polymers of polyhydroxy flavan-3-ol units, such as (+)-catechin and (−)-epicatechin, which are present in large amounts in the polyphenols of red wine and grape seeds. Sixty to seventy percent of the polyphenols are found in the seeds of the grapes.[184,185] Proanthocyanidins are believed to exhibit a wide range of biologic, pharmacologic, chemoprotective, and antioxidant activities.[186]

ANTIOXIDANT ACTIVITY Various studies have reported on the potent antioxidative and free radical scavenging activities of proanthocyanidins.[187–191] Grape seed extract has been shown to be an even stronger scavenger of free radicals than vitamins C and E.[192] Dietary intake of grape seed proanthocyanidins (GSP) has been shown to inhibit UV-induced skin cancer in mice.[193] Mittal et al. demonstrated that oral intake of GSP in SKH-1 hairless mice resulted in prevention of photocarcinogenesis with reduced tumor incidence, multiplicity, and size compared with non-GSP–treated mice following a UVB-induced carcinogenesis protocol. Biochemical analysis revealed that treatment of GSP in in vivo and in vitro systems significantly inhibited UVB- or Fe^{3+}-induced lipid peroxidation, suggesting a possible antioxidant mechanism of photoprotection by GSP.[193] In another study, investigators demonstrated that treatment of NHEK with GPS inhibited UV-induced oxidative stress by inhibiting UVB-induced H_2O_2, lipid peroxidation, protein oxidation, and DNA damage as well as scavenging hydroxyl radicals and superoxide anions in a cell-free system. Moreover, GSP also inhibited UVB-induced depletion of antioxidant defense components, such as GPX, catalase, superoxide dismutase, and glutathione. Treatment of NHEK with GSP further inhibited UVB-induced phosphorylation of ERK1/2, JNK, and p38 proteins of the MAPK family.[194] As UV-induced oxidative stress mediates activation of MAPK and NF-κB signaling pathways, the same group further examined the effect of dietary GSP on these pathways and proved that GSP exhibits the ability to protect the skin from the adverse effects of UVB radiation via modulation of the MAPK and NF-κB signaling pathways. This provides a molecular basis for the photoprotective effects of grape seed extract in an in vivo animal model.[195] Dietary GSP was also shown to modulate UVB-induced immunosuppression by reducing the immunosuppressive cytokine IL-10 while enhancing the production of the immunostimulatory cytokine IL-12, suggesting this to be one of the possible mechanisms by which grape seed extract prevents photocarcinogenesis in mice.[196]

GRAPE SEED EXTRACT APPLICATIONS IN HUMANS Thus far, there are no comparable studies in humans. Grape seed extract is included in topical cosmetic formulations with the intention of imparting an antiaging effect. It is a popular ingredient in "organic" products. However, additional studies are needed to further understand its effects on human skin when used topically.

Pomegranate

Pomegranate (*Punica granatum*) is an edible fruit native to northern India, Iran, Pakistan, and Afghanistan and cultivated in many countries. The fruits are widely consumed in fresh and beverage forms as juice. The pomegranate was one of the first known sources of medicines and has been used extensively in many cultures around the world for various diseases, such as skin inflammation, rheumatism, and sore throats.[197] In Ayurvedic medicine, pomegranates reputedly nourish and restore balance to the skin. The extract of the fruit contains two types of polyphenolic compounds: anthocyanins (such as delphinidin, cyanidin, and pelargonidin), as well as hydrolyzable tannins (such as punicalin, pedunculagin, punicalagin, as well as gallagic and ellagic acid esters of glucose).

ANTIOXIDANT ACTIVITY Extracts can be obtained from various parts of the fruit, such as the juice, seed, and peel and have been reported to have strong antioxidant activity.[198–200] The phenolic components extracted from pomegranate have been shown to possess strong antioxidant properties in several instances.[201] A recent study compared the antioxidant potency of various beverages known to be rich in polyphenols, including pomegranate juice, applying four tests of antioxidant strength. Compared to various fruit juices (apple, açaí, black cherry, blueberry, cranberry, orange), red wines as well as black, green and white tea, pomegranate juice displayed the greatest antioxidant potency and was at least 20% stronger than any of the other beverages tested[202] (Table 34-2). Also, other studies have reported that pomegranate imparts a more potent antioxidant effect than comparable quantities of green tea and red wine.[198,203] With regard to topical application, a methanolic extract of pomegranate peel followed by carbon tetrachloride was demonstrated to restore catalase, peroxidase, and superoxide dismutase enzyme activities in rats.[204]

TABLE 34-2
Antioxidant Potency Composite Index[a], Based on the Ranking of Four Antioxidant Assays[b]

Beverage	Antioxidant Potency Composite Index[a]
Pomegranate juice	95.8
Red wine	68.3
Concord grape juice	61.7
Blueberry juice	50.9
Black cherry juice	46.5
Açaí juice	46.2
Cranberry juice	38.0
Iced green tea	24.2
Orange juice	19.1
Iced white tea	16.8
Apple juice	14.6
Iced black tea	12.2

[a]based on the ranking of all four antioxidant assays (free radical scavenging capacity by 2,2-diphenyl-1-picrylhydrazyl, DPPH; total oxygen radical absorbance capacity, ORAC; ferric reducing antioxidant power, FRAP; Trolox equivalent antioxidant capacity, TEAC) an overall antioxidant potency composite index was calculated by assigning each test equal weight. Antioxidant index score = (sample score/best score) × 100, averaged for all tests for all beverages.
[b]Seeram NP, Aviram M, Zhang Y, Henning SM, Feng L, Dreher M, Heber D. Comparison of Antioxidant Potency of Commonly Consumed Polyphenol-Rich Beverages in the United States. *J Agric Food Chem.* 2008;56(4):1415-1422. Epub 2008 Jan 26.

PHOTOPROTECTION There have been numerous reports on the in vitro and in vivo anticancer properties of pomegranates.[205,206] Pomegranate fruit extract has been demonstrated to exert photochemopreventive properties, ameliorating UVA-mediated damages by modulating cellular pathways.[207] The seed oil of the pomegranate fruit has been shown to possess chemopreventive activity against skin cancer.[208] In a recent study, Afaq et al. showed that topically applied pomegranate fruit extract (PFE) possesses antiskin tumor-promoting effects in a CD-1 mouse model of chemical carcinogenesis.[201] They further studied the effect of PFE on UVB-induced adverse effects in NHEK and showed that PFE protects against the adverse effects of UVB radiation by inhibiting UVB-induced modulations of NF-κB and MAPK pathways.[209] The same group then investigated the effect of polyphenol-rich PFE on UVB-induced oxidative stress and photoaging in human immortalized HaCaT keratinocytes, showing that pretreatment of HaCaT cells with PFE inhibited UVB-mediated reduction in cell viability and intracellular glutathione content as well as an increase in lipid peroxidation. It also inhibited the upregulation of various MMPs, and phosphorylation of MAPKs. These results suggest that PFE protects HaCaT cells against UVB-induced oxidative stress and markers of photoaging and could be a useful supplement in skin care products.[210] This is buttressed by further in vitro studies that suggest that pomegranate peel fractions may promote dermal regeneration while pomegranate seed oil fractions may foster epidermal regeneration, presenting potential additional dermatologic applications.[211] Pomegranate extract is already available OTC in various skin care products.

THE FAT- AND WATER-SOLUBLE ANTIOXIDANT

The sole network antioxidant known to be both water and lipid soluble is lipoic acid.

Alpha Lipoic Acid

Alpha lipoic acid (ALA) is an antioxidant agent used for the treatment and prevention of aging skin.[212] It is different than the other antioxidants because it can be used as a superficial chemical peel to resurface the skin in a manner similar to glycolic acid. ALA is believed to have anti-inflammatory properties that may also make it useful in the treatment of postlaser erythema.[213] This discussion will focus on the science and potential therapeutic applications of ALA in the cosmetic dermatology practice.

CHEMICAL COMPOSITION ALA, formerly called thioctic acid, is an octanoic acid, which means an eight-carbon version of carboxylic acid combined with cysteine (Fig. 34-9). It is an essential cofactor in mitochondrial dehydrogenases.[214] In 1951, it was first discovered that ALA acted as an antioxidant. It is both water- and lipid-soluble and, hence, has been termed the "universal" antioxidant.[215] Other popular antioxidants are either lipophilic, such as vitamin E, or hydrophilic, such as vitamin C.

PENETRATION INTO THE STRATUM CORNEUM Dihydrolipoic acid (DHLA) is formed by reducing ALA. It has a more powerful antioxidative effect than does ALA. DHLA is very unstable, however, and would get oxidized in a matter of minutes after application to the skin. ALA has become popular because it is absorbed in a stable form and after it enters the cells, it is immediately converted to DHLA.[216] Podda et al. studied the capacity of ALA to penetrate the skin in anesthetized hairless mice after application of a 5% solution in propylene glycol for 0.5 to 4 hours. They showed the rate of ALA absorption into the skin to be constant by 30 minutes after application, reaching the maximum concentration by the 2-hour mark.[217]

▲ **FIGURE 34-9** Lipoic acid.

TOPICAL APPLICATION Topical application of 3% ALA in a lecithin base to human skin has been shown to decrease UVB-induced erythema in one-half the time of lesions treated with lecithin base alone.[217] This model indicated that topical application of ALA could prevent free radical damage to skin, and thus prevent photoaging and carcinogenesis.[218] Although ALA is available in topical cosmetic products and in formulations used for office peels, there are no published peer-reviewed clinical trials examining the efficacy of these products.

SYSTEMIC ADMINISTRATION ALA can be used either topically or systemically. When systemically administered, it has been used to influence glucose control and prevent chronic hyperglycemia-associated complications such as diabetes mellitus, Alzheimer's disease, cataracts, HIV activation, and radiation injury.[212,219] ALA has also been used as adjuvant therapy for glaucoma, ischemia-reperfusion injury, amanita mushroom poisoning, cellular oxidative damage,[220] and Chagas disease.[221] There is no currently established RDA but most proponents of ALA supplementation suggest 25 to 500 mg daily.

ANTIOXIDATIVE BENEFITS There are four principal antioxidative properties of ALA: metal chelating capacity, ability to scavenge ROS, ability to regenerate endogenous antioxidants,[222,223] and the ability to repair oxidative damage.[224]

ALA is available in different forms and vehicles and currently marketed in cleansers, moisturizers, and oral supplements. When starting patients on ALA-containing products, they should be warned that they may feel a slight tingling sensation, which decreases after a few seconds and disappears within minutes of application. Topical application of ALA is recommended every other day for the first week, increasing to twice a day for the third week if no side effects occur. ALA can cause a significant amount of inflammation so these patients should be followed closely. Fine skin lines may improve after a few weeks; however, this may be caused by the resultant inflammation. Contact dermatitis to ALA has been reported.[225]

SUMMARY ALA exhibits antioxidant and exfoliating properties that may render it a good choice for resistant skin types with a tendency to wrinkle (see Chapter 9). Please note, though, that the status of ALA as a topical antioxidant has recently been called into question (see Chapter 33).

OTHER ANTIOXIDANTS

Genistein

Genistein (4′,5,7-tri-hydroxyisoflavone), derived from and an active constituent in soybeans, is an isoflavone, thus a member of the polyphenol family. It was first isolated from soybeans in 1931. The recent heightened awareness of this potent compound can mostly be attributed to the fact that in the Asian population various positive beneficial health effects have been at least in part attributed to their increased soy consumption.[226] Most importantly, Asians show significantly lower incidences in breast, colon, and prostate cancers when compared to western populations.[227–230]

Although soybeans contain several ingredients with demonstrated anticancer activities, genistein is its most important component[231] (Fig. 34-10). Genistein is known to possess various biologic activities, such as helping in the treatment and prevention of certain cardiovascular conditions and osteoporosis, as well as enhancing the effects of radiation in the treatment of prostate and breast cancer.[232] Its classification as a phytoestrogen accounts for additional health benefits including the modulation of perimenopausal symptoms without the associated dangers of hormone replacement therapy.[233,234]

▲ **FIGURE 34-10** Genistein.

BIOLOGIC EFFECTS Genistein is a potent antioxidant and its anticarcinogenic effects are well documented on several cancers, including the skin.[235–237] The capacity of genistein to inhibit UV-induced oxidative DNA damage as well as block UV-induced c-Fos and c-Jun proto-oncogene expression has been demonstrated in vitro and in vivo.[238–241] Genistein, either topically applied or orally supplemented, has been shown to inhibit UVB-induced skin carcinogenesis in mice and substantially block the subacute and chronic UVB-induced cutaneous damage and histologic alterations related to photoaging. The possible mechanisms of the anticarcinogenic action include scavenging of ROS, blocking of oxidative and photodynamic damage to DNA, inhibition of tyrosine protein kinase, downregulation of epidermal growth factor (EGF)-receptor phosphorylation and MAPK activation, and suppression of oncoprotein expression in UVB-irradiated cells and mouse skin.[232] In addition, the treatment of human keratinocyte cell line NCTC 2544 with genistein has been documented to limit lipid peroxidation and increases in ROS formation.[242] The potent chemopreventive effect of UVB-induced skin carcinogenesis in human skin was examined by assessing both cutaneous erythema and discomfort, which was significantly inhibited by pre-UVB application of genistein, suggesting that genistein effectively protects human skin against UVB-induced skin photodamage. Genistein has also been demonstrated to protect mouse skin against photodamage induced by psoralen plus UVA (PUVA).

SUMMARY In summary, genistein substantially inhibits skin carcinogenesis and cutaneous aging induced by UV light in mice and photodamage in humans. Supported by extensive data, the soybean isoflavone genistein is thought to offer promising applications in the field of the prevention of UV-induced skin cancer and photoaging. In fact, genistein is already included in various products such as facial moisturizers, sunscreens, and several skin care formulations claiming antiaging effects.

Pycnogenol

Pycnogenol is the patented name for a standardized pine bark extract of the French maritime pine (*Pinus pinaster*). It is rich in condensed flavonoids and monomeric phenolic compounds, including catechin, epicatechin, taxifolin, and procyanidins, also called proanthocyanidins. Proanthocyanidins, as mentioned above (see Grape Seed Extract section), are potent free radical scavengers that can also be found in grape seed, grape skin, bilberry, cranberry, black currant, green tea, black tea, blueberry, blackberry, strawberry, black cherry, red wine, and red cabbage.[243] Pycnogenol is utilized as a nutritional supplement and a phytochemical remedy for various disorders, as it possesses potent antioxidant, anti-inflammatory, and anticarcinogenic properties.[244,245] A large body of literature on the free radical scavenging activity of pycnogenol exists.[246]

In a recent in vitro study, the antioxidative effects of pycnogenol were again confirmed. In addition, the investigators showed statistically significant antimutagenic properties with a correlation between the antioxidant and antimutagenic activities. They thus hypothesized that the antimutagenic effect of pycnogenol is most likely attributable to its antioxidant properties.[247] In humans it has been demonstrated that following oral supplementation with pycnogenol, the antioxidant capacity of plasma was significantly increased, as determined by ORAC.[248] The anticarcinogenic effect of pycnogenol was shown by topical application of 0.05% to 0.2% pycnogenol to the irradiated dorsal skin of Skh:hr hairless mice exposed daily to minimally inflammatory solar-simulated UV radiation. A reduction of the inflammatory sunburn reaction erythema and immunosuppression was observed. Further, tumor formation was delayed and prevalence reduced.[245] The potential of pycnogenol to confer photoprotection for humans has been investigated by Saliou et al. They showed in humans that by oral supplementation of pycnogenol the UV radiation level necessary to reach one MED was significantly elevated. They further suggested that inhibition of NF-κB-dependent gene expression by pycnogenol might possibly contribute to the observed increase in MED.[249] Finally, pycnogenol exerts depigmenting effects, which are described in detail in Chapter 33. Thus, pycnogenol is a safe natural product that is included in various skin care products. Further clinical studies are necessary to elucidate its efficacy when used in humans.

Dehydroepiandrosterone

Dehydroepiandrosterone (DHEA) is believed to be a powerful endogenous antioxidant. However, its antioxidant abilities remain unproven. DHEA purportedly protects against aging and stimulates the immune system. The use of DHEA to combat aging is based on the fact that the secretion and blood levels of DHEA and its sulfate ester (DHEAS) diminish profoundly with age. Although the FDA noted in 1985 that the efficacy and safety of DHEA has never been confirmed, the agent continues to be sold OTC and is discussed in many lay publications.

A study evaluating the safety of oral DHEA and its effects was published in April 2000.[250] In this double-blind, placebo-controlled study, 280 healthy individuals consumed 50 mg DHEA or placebo daily for a year. The subjects given DHEA had slightly elevated levels of testosterone and estradiol. Interestingly, the treated patients exhibited increases in sebum production, skin surface hydration, and epidermal thickness as well as decreased facial pigmentation. No harmful effects of DHEAS were noted. DHEA may protect cells from UV damage as well. A study by Coach et al. assessed whether pretreatment of cells with various doses of DHEA could protect the cells from the damaging effects of UV radiation.[251] Cellular damage, cell counts, and cell morphology were evaluated. They found that the morphologic evaluation of the cells treated with UV radiation showed an increase in degeneration of chromatin and a decrease in cell size as compared to nontreated groups, indicating that DHEA was efficient in protecting the cells from UV damage. Other reported effects of orally administered DHEA in healthy men include reduction of body fat, increase in muscle mass, and reduction of serum low-density lipoprotein cholesterol levels.[252]

Currently, DHEA is available in oral, injectable, and topical forms. It is important to understand that these products are considered nutritional supplements and are not regulated by the FDA. Further studies should be performed to evaluate the safety of DHEA and DHEAS before recommending their use.

SIDE EFFECTS DHEA is a relatively new product in the "antiaging armamentarium"; therefore, little is known about the effects of long-term use. Endogenous DHEA concentrations peak at age 20 to 30 years. Consequently, the use of DHEA in those younger than 35 years may be risky. In fact, there has been a reported case of DHEA being suspected as a contributing factor in a manic episode of a young man.[253] The effects of long-term use of DHEA have not been studied.

Melatonin

Melatonin is a hormone secreted by the pineal gland. Less than 10 years ago, it was discovered to be a direct free radical scavenger. Besides its ability to directly neutralize a number of free radicals and reactive oxygen and nitrogen species, it stimulates several antioxidative enzymes including superoxide dismutase, GPX, and glutathione reductase. This increases its efficiency as an antioxidant.[254] Melatonin has been shown to markedly protect both membrane lipids and nuclear DNA from oxidative damage,[255] and has been shown to reduce skin cancer formation in mice.[256] This may be because of its protective UV absorption effects.[257] Further, various studies in humans have demonstrated that topical melatonin reduces UV-induced erythema (sunburn).[258,259] However, controversial results have been obtained in another study.[260] With regard to photoprotection, melatonin was shown to modulate the expression of apoptosis-related genes in UVB-irradiated HaCaT cells, resulting in increasing cell survival. This suggests that melatonin may be used as a sunscreen substance to reduce cell death of keratinocytes after excessive UVB irradiation.[261]

Melatonin is also used as a medication for sleep disturbance in depression and in people complaining of jet lag. It is currently available in an oral form and has also been added as an ingredient to various topical products, such as facial cleansers and moisturizers, eye creams, and skin lighteners.

Selenium

Selenium (Se) is an essential trace element found in Brazil nuts, walnuts, shellfish, fish, and North American wheat. It is a frequent additive in antidandruff shampoos because it is able to inhibit proliferation of the yeast *Pityrosporum ovale.* The current RDA of selenium is 55 µg/d for both men and women. Selenium behaves both as an antioxidant and anti-inflammatory agent. It is a component of the GPX family of enzymes, which break down peroxides. Therefore, it is able to decrease the amount of free radicals by reducing H_2O_2 and lipid and phospholipid hydroperoxides. Selenium can also reduce hydroperoxide intermediates in the cyclooxygenase and lipoxygenase pathways, thus resulting in a decrease in inflammation.[262] In addition, many studies have suggested that selenium confers an anticancer effect. Low levels of selenium have been associated with an increased incidence of cancer in several studies.[263] Selenium supplementation has been shown to prevent UVB-induced skin tumors in hairless mice.[264,265]

In addition to its antioxidant properties, the protective effects of selenium against skin cancer are enhanced because it prevents the production of inflammatory and immunosuppressive cytokines, which impair immune responses following UV exposure. In fact, selenium has been shown to inhibit the UVB-induction of IL-6, IL-8, IL-10, and TNF-α in a dose-dependent manner.[266] Selenium has also been shown to boost both cellular and humoral immunity.[267] All these actions work synergistically to give selenium its anticancer properties. The anticancer activity was recently demonstrated in a large double-blind, placebo-controlled intervention trial that evaluated whether selenium supplementation could reduce the risk of cancer.[268] In this study, 1312 individuals with a history of nonmelanoma skin cancer were randomized to placebo or 200 µg selenium per day. Although there was no effect on the primary endpoint of nonmelanoma skin cancer, those receiving selenium showed secondary endpoint effects of 50% lower total cancer mortality and 37% lower total cancer incidence with 63% fewer cancers of the prostate, 58% fewer cancers of the colon, and 46% fewer cancers of the lung.

SIDE EFFECTS The Institute of Medicine has set a tolerable upper intake level for selenium at 400 µg/d.[269] Selenium toxicity, or "selenosis," is associated with gastrointestinal upset, hair loss, white blotchy nails, and mild nerve damage.[270] Selenium and other antioxidants should always be taken as part of a balanced diet.[271] Otherwise, selenium can act as a pro-oxidant and cause DNA damage.[272]

SUMMARY Although there is much interest and enthusiasm regarding the use of antioxidants, there is a paucity of clinical trials examining the capacity of antioxidants to prevent or decelerate the aging of skin. One should remember that the theory behind the efficacy of these products is that they function by neutralizing free radicals, thus sparing the organs from the damage caused by these reactive oxygen species. There is no reason to believe that antioxidants treat already formed wrinkles unless it can occur by a different mechanism such as through increased collagen synthesis as seen with vitamin C. Current research suggests that combinations of various antioxidants might have synergistic effects and consequently more efficacy, as each antioxidant is endowed with various properties that distinguish it from other antioxidants.[16,273] Also, some data suggest a cumulative or additive benefit derived from using oral and topical antioxidant products in combination.[274,275] This has resulted in the entry of many antioxidant-containing beverages onto the market. It is unknown if these beverages help prevent aging and inflammation; however, they are harmless and may be beneficial. Further long-term studies in humans are needed to determine the efficacy of both the topical and oral products.

REFERENCES

1. Harman D. Aging: a theory based on free radical and radiation chemistry. *J Gerontol.* 1956;11:298.
2. Pelle E, Maes D, Padulo GA, et al. An in vitro model to test relative antioxidant potential: ultraviolet-induced lipid peroxidation in liposomes. *Arch Biochem Biophys.* 1990;283:234.
3. Werninghaus K. The role of antioxidants in reducing photodamage. In: Gilchrest B, ed. *Photodamage.* London, UK: Blackwell Science; 1995:249.
4. Greenstock CL. Free radicals. In: Alan R, ed. *Aging, and Degenerative Diseases.* New York, NY: Liss Inc; 1986.
5. Rikans LE, Hornbrook KR. Lipid peroxidation, antioxidant protection and aging. *Biochim Biophys Acta.* 1997;1362:116.
6. Black HS. Potential involvement of free radical reactions in ultraviolet light-mediated cutaneous damage. *Photochem Photobiol.* 1987;46:213.
7. Dhar A, Young MR, Colburn NH. The role of AP-1, NF-kappaB and ROS/NOS in skin carcinogenesis: the JB6 model is predictive. *Mol Cell Biochem.* 2002;185:234-235.
8. Kang S, Chung JH, Lee JH, et al. Topical N-acetyl cysteine and genistein prevent ultraviolet-light induced signaling that leads to photoaging in human skin in vivo. *J Invest Dermatol.* 2003;120:835.
9. Fisher GJ, Wang ZQ, Datta SC, et al. Pathophysiology of premature skin aging induced by ultraviolet light. *N Engl J Med.* 1997;337:1419.
10. Baumann L. *Cosmetic Dermatology: Principles & Practice.* New York, NY: McGraw-Hill; 2002:86-87.
11. Kim AL, Labasi JM, Zhu Y, et al. Role of p38 MAPK in UVB-induced inflammatory responses in the skin of SKH-1 hairless mice. *J Invest Dermatol.* 2005; 124:1318.
12. Shindo Y, Witt E, Han D, et al. Enzymic and non-enzymic antioxidants in epidermis and dermis of human skin. *J Invest Dermatol.* 1994;102:122.
13. Fuchs J, Huflejt ME, Rothfuss LM, et al. Acute effects of near ultraviolet and visible light on the cutaneous antioxidant defense system. *Photochem Photobiol.* 1989;50:739.
14. Fuchs J, Huflejt ME, Rothfuss LM, et al. Impairment of enzymic and nonenzymic antioxidants in skin by UVB irradiation. *J Invest Dermatol.* 1989;93:769.

15. Dreher F, Maibach H. Protective effects of topical antioxidants in humans. *Curr Probl Dermatol.* 2001;29:157.
16. Cho HS, Lee MH, Lee JW, et al. Anti-wrinkling effects of the mixture of vitamin C, vitamin E, pycnogenol and evening primrose oil, and molecular mechanisms on hairless mouse skin caused by chronic ultraviolet B irradiation. *Photodermatol Photoimmunol Photomed.* 2007;23:155.
17. Packer L, Colman C. *The Antioxidant Miracle.* New York, NY: John Wiley & Sons; 1999:9.
18. Nachbar F, Korting HC. The role of vitamin E in normal and damaged skin. *J Mol Med.* 1995;73:7.
19. Halliwell B. The antioxidant paradox. *Lancet.* 2000;355:1179.
20. Tanaka H, Okada T, Konishi H, et al. The effect of reactive oxygen species on the biosynthesis of collagen and glycosaminoglycans in cultured human dermal fibroblasts. *Arch Dermatol Res.* 1993;285:352.
21. Diplock AT, Xu G, Yeow C, et al. Relationship of tocopherol structure to biological activity, tissue uptake, and prostaglandin synthesis. In: Diplock AT, Machlin LJ, Packer L, et al., eds. *Vitamin E. Biochemistry and Health Implications.* New York, NY: Academy of Sciences; 1989:72-84.
22. Palmieri B, Gozzi G, Palmieri G. Vitamin E added silicone gel sheets for treatment of hypertrophic scars and keloids. *Int J Dermatol.* 1995;34:506.
23. Knekt P, Aromaa A, Maatela J, et al. Vitamin E and cancer prevention. *Am J Clin Nutr.* 1991;53:283S.
24. Menkes MS, Comstock GW, Vuilleumier JP, et al. Serum beta-carotene, vitamins A and E, selenium, and the risk of lung cancer. *N Engl J Med.* 1986;315:1250.
25. Chevance M, Brubacher G, Herbeth B, et al. Immunological and nutritional status among the elderly. In: Chandra RK, ed. *Nutrition Immunity and Illness in the Elderly.* New York, NY: Pergamon Press; 1985:137-142.
26. Darr D, Combs S, Dunston S, et al. Topical vitamin C protects porcine skin from ultraviolet radiation-induced damage. *Br J Dermatol.* 1992;127:247.
27. Pathak MA, Carbonare MD. Photoaging and the role of mammalian skin superoxide dismutase and antioxidants. *Photochem Photobiol.* 1998;47:7S.
28. Pinnell SR, Murad S. Vitamin C and collagen metabolism. In: Kligman AM, Takase Y, eds. *Cutaneous Aging.* Tokyo, Japan: University of Tokyo Press; 1988:275-292.
29. Bissett DL, Majeti S, Fu JJ, et al. Protective effect of topically applied conjugated hexadienes against ultraviolet radiation-induced chronic skin damage in the hairless mouse. *Photodermatol Photoimmunol Photomed.* 1990;7:63.
30. Gensler HL, Magdaleno M. Topical vitamin E inhibition of immunosuppression and tumorigenesis induced by ultraviolet irradiation. *Nutr Cancer.* 1991;15:97.
31. Jurkiewicz BA, Bissett DL, Buettner GR. Effect of topically applied tocopherol on ultraviolet radiation-mediated free radical damage in skin. *J Invest Dermatol.* 1995;104:484.
32. Slaga TJ, Bracken WM. The effects of antioxidants on skin tumor initiation and aryl hydrocarbon hydroxylase. *Cancer Res.* 1977;37:1631.
33. Meydani SN, Barklund MP, Liu S, et al. Vitamin E supplementation enhances cell-mediated immunity in healthy elderly subjects. *Am J Clin Nutr.* 1990; 52:557.
34. Trevithick JR, Xiong H, Lee S, et al. Topical tocopherol acetate reduces post-UVB, sunburn-associated erythema, edema, and skin sensitivity in hairless mice. *Arch Biochem Biophys.* 1992;296:575.
35. Bissett DL, Chatterjee R, Hannon DP. Photoprotective effect of superoxide-scavenging antioxidants against ultraviolet radiation-induced chronic skin damage in the hairless mouse. *Photodermatol Photoimmunol Photomed.* 1990;7:56.
36. Mayer P. The effects of vitamin E on the skin. *Cosmet Toiletries.* 1993;108:99.
37. Keller KL, Fenske NA. Uses of vitamins A, C, and E and related compounds in dermatology: a review. *J Am Acad Dermatol.* 1998;39:611.
38. Chung JH, Seo JY, Lee MK, et al. Ultraviolet modulation of human macrophage metalloelastase in human skin in vivo. *J Invest Dermatol.* 2002;119:507.
39. Werninghaus K, Meydani M, Bhawan J, et al. Evaluation of the photoprotective effect of oral vitamin E supplementation. *Arch Dermatol.* 1994;130:1257.
40. Chan AC. Partners in defense, vitamin E and vitamin C. *Can J Physiol Pharmacol.* 1993;71:725.
41. Lin JY, Selim MA, Shea CR, et al. UV photoprotection by combination topical antioxidants vitamin C and vitamin E. *J Am Acad Dermatol.* 2003;48:866.
42. Martin A. The use of antioxidants in healing. *Dermatol Surg.* 1996;22:156.
43. Kamimura M, Matsuzawa T. Percutaneous absorption of alpha-tocopheryl acetate. *J Vitaminol (Kyoto).* 1968;14:150.
44. Pehr K, Forsey RR. Why don't we use vitamin E in dermatology? *CMAJ.* 1993;149:1247.
45. Jenkins M, Alexander JW, MacMillan BG, et al. Failure of topical steroids and vitamin E to reduce postoperative scar formation following reconstructive surgery. *J Burn Care Rehabil.* 1986;7:309.
46. Baumann LS, Spencer J. The effects of topical vitamin E on the cosmetic appearance of scars. *Dermatol Surg.* 1999;25:311.
47. Alberts DS, Goldman R, Xu MJ, et al. Disposition and metabolism of topically administered alpha-tocopherol acetate: a common ingredient of commercially available sunscreens and cosmetics. *Nutr Cancer.* 1996;26:193.
48. Gensler HL, Aickin M, Peng YM, et al. Importance of the form of topical vitamin E for prevention of photocarcinogenesis. *Nutr Cancer.* 1996;26:183.
49. Matsumura T, Nakada T, Iijima M. Widespread contact dermatitis from tocopherol acetate. *Contact Dermatitis.* 2004;51:211.
50. Oshima H, Tsuji K, Oh-I T, et al. Allergic contact dermatitis due to DL-alpha-tocopheryl nicotinate. *Contact Dermatitis.* 2003;48:167.
51. Perrenoud D, Homberger HP, Auderset PC, et al. An epidemic outbreak of papular and follicular contact dermatitis to tocopheryl linoleate in cosmetics. Swiss contact dermatitis research group. *Dermatology.* 1994;189:225.
52. Hunter D, Frumkin A. Adverse reactions to vitamin E and aloe vera preparations after dermabrasion and chemical peel. *Cutis.* 1991;47:193.
53. Bendich A, Machlin LJ. Safety of oral intake of vitamin E. *Am J Clin Nutr.* 1988;48:612.
54. Kappus H, Diplock AT. Tolerance and safety of vitamin E: a toxicological position report. *Free Radic Biol Med.* 1992;13:55.
55. Bendich A. Safety issues regarding the use of vitamin supplements. *Ann N Y Acad Sci.* 1992;669:300.
56. Petry JJ. Surgically significant nutritional supplements. *Plast Reconstr Surg.* 1996; 97:233.
57. Dimery IW, Hong WK, Lee JJ, et al. Phase I trial of alpha-tocopherol effects on 13-cis-retinoic acid toxicity. *Ann Oncol.* 1997;8:85.
58. Strauss JS, Gottlieb AB, Jones T, et al. Concomitant administration of vitamin E does not change the side effects of isotretinoin as used in acne vulgaris: a randomized trial. *J Am Acad Dermatol.* 2000;43:777.
59. Ernster L, Dallner G. Biochemical, physiological and medical aspects of ubiquinone function. *Biochim Biophys Acta.* 1995;1271:195.
60. Greenberg S, Frishman WH. Co-enzyme Q10: a new drug for cardiovascular disease. *J Clin Pharmacol.* 1990;30: 596.
61. Beyer R, Ernster L. The antioxidant role of coenzyme Q10. In: Lenaz G, Barnabei O, Rabbi A, eds. *Highlights in Ubiquinone Research.* London, UK: Taylor & Francis; 1990:191-213.
62. Hoppe U, Bergemann J, Diembeck W, et al. Coenzyme Q10, a cutaneous antioxidant and energizer. *Biofactors.* 1999;9:371.
63. Ashida Y, Yamanishi H, Terada T, et al. CoQ10 supplementation elevates the epidermal CoQ10 level in adult hairless mice. *Biofactors.* 2005;25:175.
64. Tavintharan S, Ong CN, Jeyaseelan K, et al. Reduced mitochondrial coenzyme Q10 levels in HepG2 cells treated with high-dose simvastatin: a possible role in statin-induced hepatotoxicity? *Toxicol Appl Pharmacol.* 2007;223:173.
65. Folkers K, Ostemborg A, Nylander M, et al. Activities of vitamin Q10 in animal models and serious deficiency in patients with cancer. *Biochem Biophys Res Commun.* 1997;234:296.
66. Rusciani L, Proietti I, Rusciani A, et al. Low plasma coenzyme Q10 levels as an independent prognostic factor for melanoma progression. *J Am Acad Dermatol.* 2006;54:234.
67. Crane FL. Biochemical functions of coenzyme Q10. *J Am Coll Nutr.* 2001;20:591.
68. Beyer RE, Nordenbrand K, Ernster L. The role of coenzyme Q as a mitochondrial antioxidant: a short review. In: Folkers K, Yamamura Y, eds. *Biomedical and Clinical Aspects of Coenzyme Q.* Amsterdam, The Netherlands: Elsevier Science Publishers B V (Biomedical Division); 1986:17-24.
69. Rusciani L, Proietti I, Paradisi A, et al. Recombinant interferon alpha-2b and

coenzyme Q10 as a postsurgical adjuvant therapy for melanoma: a 3-year trial with recombinant interferon-alpha and 5-year follow-up. *Melanoma Res.* 2007; 17:177.
70. Feigin A, Kieburtz K, Como P, et al. Assessment of coenzyme Q10 tolerability in Huntington's disease. *Mov Disord.* 1996;11:321.
71. McDaniel D, Neudecker B, Dinardo J, et al. Idebenone: a new antioxidant-Part I. Relative assessment of oxidativie stress protection capacity compared to commonly know antioxidants. *J Cosmet Dermatol.* 2005;4:10.
72. McDaniel D, Neudecker B, DiNardo J, et al. Clinical efficacy assessment in photodamaged skin of 0.5% and 1.0% idebenone. *J Cosmet Dermatol.* 2005; 4:167.
73. Sasseville D, Moreau L, Al-Sowaidi M. Allergic contact dermatitis to idebenone used as an antioxidant in an anti-wrinkle cream. *Contact Dermatitis.* 2007;56:117.
74. Britton G. Structure and properties of carotenoids in relation to function. *FASEB J.* 1995;9:1551.
75. Nguyen ML, Schwartz SJ. Lycopene: chemical and biological properties. *Food Technology.* 1999;53:38.
76. Arab L, Steck S. Lycopene and cardiovascular disease. *Am J Clin Nutr.* 2000; 71:1691S.
77. Chan JM, Gann PH, Giovannucci EL. Role of diet in prostate cancer development and progression. *J Clin Oncol.* 2005;23:8152.
78. Willcox JK, Catignani GL, Lazarus S. Tomatoes and cardiovascular health. *Crit Rev Food Sci Nutr.* 2003;43:1.
79. Basu A, Imrhan V. Tomatoes versus lycopene in oxidative stress and carcinogenesis: conclusions from clinical trials. *Eur J Clin Nutr.* 2007;61:295.
80. Giovannucci E, Ascherio A, Rimm EB, et al. Intake of carotenoids and retinol in relation to risk of prostate cancer. *J Natl Cancer Inst.* 1995;87:1767.
81. Kim DJ, Takasuka N, Nishino H, et al. Chemoprevention of lung cancer by lycopene. *Biofactors.* 2000;13:95.
82. Narisawa T, Fukaura Y, Hasebe M, et al. Prevention of N-methylnitrosourea-induced colon carcinogenesis in F344 rats by lycopene and tomato juice rich in lycopene. *Jpn J Cancer Res.* 1998;89:1003.
83. Nagasawa H, Mitamura T, Sakamoto S, et al. Effects of lycopene on spontaneous mammary tumour development in SHN virgin mice. *Anticancer Res.* 1995;15:1173.
84. Wu WB, Chiang HS, Fang JY, et al. Inhibitory effect of lycopene on PDGF-BB-induced signalling and migration in human dermal fibroblasts: a possible target for cancer. *Biochem Soc Trans.* 2007;35:1377.
85. Ahmad N, Gilliam AC, Katiyar SK, et al. A definitive role of ornithine decarboxylase in photocarcinogenesis. *Am J Pathol.* 2001;159:885.
86. Fazekas Z, Gao D, Saladi RN, et al. Protective effects of lycopene against ultraviolet B-induced photodamage. *Nutr Cancer.* 2003;47:181.
87. Cohly HH, Taylor A, Angel MF, et al. Effect of turmeric, turmerin and curcumin on H_2O_2-induced renal epithelial (LLC-PK1) cell injury. *Free Radic Biol Med.* 1998;24:49.
88. Ruby J, Kuttan G, Babu KD, et al. Antitumor and antioxidant activity of natural curcuminoids. *Cancer Lett.* 1995;94:79.
89. Maheshwari RK, Singh AK, Gaddipati J, et al. Multiple biological activities of curcumin: a short review. *Life Sci.* 2006; 78:2081.
90. Ammon HP, Wahl MA. Pharmacology of Curcuma longa. *Planta Med.* 1991;57:1.
91. Sharma OP. Antioxidant activity of curcumin and related compounds. *Biochem Pharmacol.* 1975;25:1811.
92. Aggarwal BB, Kumar A, Bharti AC. Anticancer potential of curcumin: preclinical and clinical studies. *Anticancer Res.* 2003;23:363.
93. Surh YJ, Han SS, Keum YS, et al. Inhibitory effects of curcumin and capsaicin on phorbol ester-induced activation of eukaryotic transcription factors, NF-kappaB and AP-1. *Biofactors.* 2000; 12:107.
94. Conney AH, Lysz T, Ferraro T, et al. Inhibitory effect of curcumin and some related dietary compounds on tumor promotion and arachidonic acid metabolism in mouse skin. *Adv Enzyme Regul.* 1991;31:385.
95. Jagetia GC, Aggarwal BB. "Spicing up" of the immune system by curcumin. *J Clin Immunol.* 2007;27(1):19-35. Epub 2007 Jan 9.
96. Nakamura Y, Ohto Y, Murakami A, et al. Inhibitory effects of curcumin and tetrahydrocurcuminoids on the tumor promoter-induced reactive oxygen species generation in leukocytes in vitro and in vivo. *Jpn J Cancer Res.* 1998;89:361.
97. Huang MT, Smart RC, Wong CQ, et al. Inhibitory effect of curcumin, chlorogenic acid, caffeic acid, and ferulic acid on tumor promotion in mouse skin by 12-O-tetradecanoylphorbol 13-acetate. *Cancer Res.* 1988;48:5941.
98. Cheng AL, Hsu CH, Lin JK, et al. Phase I clinical trial of curcumin, a chemopreventive agent, in patients with high-risk or pre-malignant lesions. *Anticancer Res.* 2001;21:2895.
99. Sidhu GS, Singh AK, Thaloor D, et al. Enhancement of wound healing by curcumin in animals. *Wound Repair Regen.* 1998;6:167.
100. Sidhu GS, Mani H, Gaddipati JP, et al. Curcumin enhances wound healing in streptozotocin induced diabetic rats and genetically diabetic mice. *Wound Rep Regen.* 1999;7:362.
101. Thangapazham RL, Sharma A, Maheshwari RK. Beneficial role of curcumin in skin diseases. *Adv Exp Med Biol.* 2007;595:343.
102. Azuine MA, Bhide SV. Chemopreventive effect of turmeric against stomach and skin tumors induced by chemical carcinogens in Swiss mice. *Nutr Cancer.* 1992; 17:77.
103. Huang MT, Lysz T, Ferraro T, et al. Inhibitory effects of curcumin on in vitro lipoxygenase and cyclooxygenase activities in mouse epidermis. *Cancer Res.* 1991;51:813.
104. Limtrakul P, Lipigorngoson S, Namwong O, et al. Inhibitory effect of dietary curcumin on skin carcinogenesis in mice. *Cancer Lett.* 1997;116:197.
105. Nagabhushan M, Bhide SV. Curcumin as an inhibitor of cancer. *J Am Coll Nutr.* 1992;11:192.
106. Bush JA, Cheung KJ Jr., Li G. Curcumin induces apoptosis in human melanoma cells through a Fas receptor/caspase-8 pathway independent of p53. *Exp Cell Res.* 2001;271:305.
107. Jee SH, Shen SC, Tseng CR, et al. Curcumin induces a p53-dependent apoptosis in human basal cell carcinoma cells. *J Invest Dermatol.* 1998;111:656.
108. Chen J, Wanming D, Zhang D, et al. Water-soluble antioxidants improve the antioxidant and anticancer activity of low concentrations of curcumin in human leukemia cells. *Pharmazie.* 2005; 60:57.
109. Hardman J, Limbird L, eds. *Goodman and Gilman's: The Pharmacological Basis of Therapeutics.* 9th ed. New York, NY: McGraw-Hill; 1996:1568-1672.
110. Shindo Y, Witt E, Han D, et al. Dose-response effects of acute ultraviolet irradiation on antioxidants and molecular markers of oxidation in murine epidermis and dermis. *J Invest Dermatol.* 1994; 102:470.
111. Thiele JJ, Traber MG, Tsange KG, et al. In vivo exposure to ozone depletes vitamins C and E and induces lipid peroxidation in epidermal layers of murine skin. *Free Radic Biol Med.* 1997;23:85.
112. Gey KF. Vitamins E plus C and interacting conutrients required for optimal health. A critical and constructive review of epidemiology and supplementation data regarding cardiovascular disease and cancer. *Biofactors.* 1998; 7:113.
113. McLauren S. Nutrition and wound healing. *Wound Care.* 1992;1:45.
114. Kameyama K, Sakai C, Kondoh S, et al. Inhibitory effect of magnesium L-ascorbyl-2-phosphate (VC-PMG) on melanogenesis in vitro and in vivo. *J Am Acad Dermatol.* 1996;34:29.
115. Ash K, Lord J, Zukowski M, et al. Comparison of topical therapy for striae alba (20% glycolic acid/0.05% tretinoin versus 20% glycolic acid/10% L-ascorbic acid). *Dermatol Surg.* 1998;24:849.
116. Alster TS, West TB. Effect of topical vitamin C on postoperative carbon dioxide laser resurfacing erythema. *Dermatol Surg.* 1998;24:331.
117. Scarpa M, Stevanato R, Viglino P, et al. Superoxide ion as active intermediate in the autoxidation of ascorbate by molecular oxygen. Effect of superoxide dismutase. *J Biol Chem.* 1983;258:6695.
118. Cabelli DE, Bielski BH. Kinetics and mechanism for the oxidation of ascorbic acid/ascorbate by HO_2/O_2 radicals: a pulse radiolysis and stopped flow photolysis study. *J Phys Chem.* 1983;87: 1805.
119. Dunham WB, Zuckerkandl E, Reynolds R, et al. Effects of intake of L-ascorbic acid on the incidence of dermal neoplasms induced in mice by ultraviolet light. *Proc Natl Acad Sci U S A.* 1982;79:7532.
120. Darr D, Dunston S, Faust H, et al. Effectiveness of antioxidants (vitamin C and E) with and without sunscreens as topical photoprotectants. *Acta Derm Venereol.* 1996;766:264.
121. Kivirikko KI, Myllyla R. Post-translational processing of procollagens. *Ann NY Acad Sci.* 1985;460:187.
122. Uitto J, Hoffmann H-P, Prockop DJ. Synthesis of elastin and procollagen by

cells from embryonic aorta. Differences in the role of hydroxyproline and the effects of proline analogs on the secretion of the two proteins. *Arch Biochem Biophys*. 1976;173:187.
123. Geesin JC, Darr D, Kaufman R, et al. Ascorbic acid specifically increases type I and type III procollagen messenger RNA levels in human skin fibroblast. *J Invest Dermatol.* 1988;90:420.
124. Davidson JM, LuValle PA, Zoia O, et al. Ascorbate differentially regulates elastin and collagen biosynthesis in vascular smooth muscle cells and skin fibroblasts by pretranslational mechanisms. *J Biol Chem.* 1997;272:345.
125. Scott-Burden T, Davies PJ, Gevers W. Elastin biosynthesis by smooth muscle cells cultured under scorbutic conditions. *Biochem Biophys Res Commun.* 1979;91:739.
126. Bergethon PR, Mogayzel PJ, Franzblau C. Effect of the reducing environment on the accumulation of elastin and collagen in cultured smooth-muscle cells. *Biochem J.* 1989;258:279.
127. Traikovich SS. Use of topical ascorbic acid and its effects on photodamaged skin topography. *Arch Otolaryngol Head Neck Surg.* 1999;125:1091.
128. Humbert PG, Haftek M, Creidi P, et al. Topical ascorbic acid in photoaged skin. Clinical topographical and ultrastructural evaluation: double-blind study vs. placebo. *Exp Dermatol.* 2003;12:237.
129. Colven RM, Pinnell SR. Topical vitamin C in aging. *Clin Dermatol.* 1996; 14:227.
130. Perricone NV. The photoprotective and anti-inflammatory effects of topical ascorbyl palmitate. *J Geriatric Derm.* 1993;1:5.
131. Darr D, Pinnell S. US Patent. 5,140,043. 1992.
132. Maeda K, Fukuda M. Arbutin: mechanism of its depigmenting action in human melanocyte culture. *J Pharmacol Exp Ther.* 1996;276:765.
133. Hsu S. Green tea and the skin. *J Am Acad Dermatol.* 2005;52:1049.
134. Katiyar SK, Ahmad N, Mukhtar H. Green tea and skin. *Arch Dermatol.* 2000;136:989.
135. Katiyar SK, Elmets CA, Agarwal R, et al. Protection against UVB radiation-induced local and systemic suppression of contact hypersensitivity and edema responses in C3H/HeN mice by green tea polyphenols. *Photochem Photobiol.* 1995;62:855.
136. Shi X, Ye J, Leonard S, et al. Antioxidant properties of (−)-epicatechin-3-gallate and its inhibition of Cr(VI)-induced DNA damage and Cr(IV)- or TPA-stimulated NF-kappaB activation. *Mol Cell Biochem.* 2000;206:125.
137. Wei H, Zhang X, Zhao JF, et al. Scavenging of hydrogen peroxide and inhibition of ultraviolet light-induced oxidative DNA damage by aqueous extracts from green and black teas. *Free Radic Biol Med.* 1999;26:1427.
138. Wang Y, Agarwal R, Bickers D, et al. Protection against ultraviolet B radiation-induced photocarcinogenesis in hairless mice by green tea polyphenols. *Carcinogenesis.* 1991;12:1527.
139. Gensler H, Timmermann B, Valcic S, et al. Prevention of photocarcinognesis by topical administration of pure epigallocatechin gallate isolated from green tea. *Nutr Cancer.* 1996;26:325.
140. Khan WA, Wang ZY, Athar M, et al. Inhibition of the skin tumorigenicity of (±)-7 beta,8 alpha-dihydroxy-9 alpha,10 alpha-epoxy-7,8,9,10-tetrahydrobenzo[a]-pyrene by tannic acid, green tea polyphenols and quercetin in Sencar mice. *Cancer Lett.* 1988;42:7.
141. Mittal A, Piyathilake C, Hara Y, et al. Exceptionally high protection of photocarcinogenesis by topical application of (−)-epigallocatechin-3-gallate in hydrophilic cream in SKH-1 hairless mouse model: relationship to inhibition of UVB-induced global DNA hypomethylation. *Neoplasia.* 2003;5:555.
142. Elmets CA, Singh D, Tubesing K, et al. Cutaneous photoprotection from ultraviolet injury by green tea polyphenols. *J Am Acad Dermatol.* 2001;44:425.
143. Stratton SP, Dorr RT, Alberts DS. The state-of-the-art in chemoprevention of skin cancer. *Eur J Cancer.* 2000;36:1292.
144. Chung J, Han J, Hwang E, et al. Dual mechanisms of green tea extract (EGCG)-induced cell survival in human epidermal keratinocytes. *FASEB J.* 2003;17:1913.
145. Katiyar SK, Challa A, McCormick TS, et al. Prevention of UVB-induced immunosuppression in mice by the green tea polyphenol (−)-epigallocatechin-3-gallate may be associated with alterations in IL-10 and IL-12 production. *Carcinogenesis.* 1999;20:2117.
146. Meeran SM, Mantena SK, Elmets CA, et al. (−)- Epigallocatechin-3-gallate prevents photocarcinogenesis in mice through interleukin-12-dependent DNA repair. *Cancer Res.* 2006;66:5512.
147. Katiyar SK, Bergamo BM, Vyalil PK, et al. Green tea polyphenols: DNA photodamage and photoimmunology. *J Photochem Photobiol B.* 2001;65:109.
148. Vayalil PK, Mittal A, Hara Y, et al. Green tea polyphenols prevent ultraviolet light-induced oxidative damage and matrix metalloproteinases expression in mouse skin. *J Invest Dermatol.* 2004; 122:1480.
149. Svobodová A, Psotová J, Walterová D. Natural phenolics in the prevention of UV-induced skin damage. A review. *Biomed Papers.* 2003;147:137.
150. Dhanalakshmi S, Mallikarjuna GU, Singh RP, et al. Silbinin prevents ultraviolet radiation-caused skin damages in SKH-1 hairless mice via a decrease in thymine dimmer positive cells and an up-regulation of p53-p21/Cip1 in epidermis. *Carcinogenesis.* 2004;25:1459.
151. Dhanalakshmi S, Mallikarjuna GU, Singh RP, et al. Dual efficacy of silibinin in protecting or enhancing ultraviolet B radiation-caused apoptosis in HaCaT human immortalized keratinocytes. *Carcinogenesis.* 2004;25:99.
152. Gupta S, Mukhtar H. Chemoprevention of skin cancer through natural agents. *Skin Pharmacol Appl Skin Physiol.* 2001; 14:373.
153. Afaq F, Adhami VM, Ahmad N, et al. Botanical antioxidants for chemoprevention of photocarcinogenesis. *Front Biosci.* 2002;7:d784.
154. Singh RP, Agarwal R. Flavonoid antioxidant silymarin and skin cancer. *Antioxid Redox Signal.* 2002;4:655.
155. Katiyar SK. Treatment of silymarin, a plant flavonoid, prevents ultraviolet light-induced immune suppression and oxidative stress in mouse skin. *Int J Oncol.* 2002;21:1213.
156. Berardesca E, Cameli N, Cavallotti C, et al. Combined effects of silymarin and methylsulfonylmethane in the management of rosacea: clinical and instrumental evaluation. *J Cosmet Dermatol.* 2008; 7:8.
157. Charurin P, Ames JM, del Castillo MD. Antioxidant activity of coffee model systems. *J Agric Food Chem.* 2002;50: 3751.
158. Farris P. Idebenone, green tea, and Coffeeberry extract: new and innovative antioxidants. *Dermatol Ther.* 2007; 20:322.
159. Chen D, Milacic V, Chen MS, et al. Tea polyphenols, their biological effects and potential molecular targets. *Histol Histopathol.* 2008;23:487.
160. Halder B, Bhattacharya U, Mukhopadhyay S, et al. Molecular mechanism of black tea polyphenols induced apoptosis in human skin cancer cells: involvement of Bax translocation and mitochondria mediated death cascade. *Carcinogenesis.* 2008;29:129.
161. Garcia F, Pivel JP, Guerrero A, et al. Phenolic components and antioxidant activity of Fernblock, an aqueous extract of the aerial parts of the fern Polypodium leucotomos. *Methods Find Exp Clin Pharmacol.* 2006;28:157.
162. Brieva A, Guerrero A, Pivel JP. Immunomodulatory properties of an hydrophilic extract of Polypodium leucotomos. *Inflammopharmacology.* 2002;9: 361.
163. Alcaraz MV, Pathak MA, Rius F, et al. An extract of Polypodium leucotomos appears to minimize certain photoaging changes in a hairless albino mouse animal model. A pilot study. *Photodermatol Photoimmunol Photomed.* 1999;15:120.
164. González S, Pathak MA, Cuevas J, et al. Topical or oral administration with an extract of Polypodium leucotomos prevents acute sunburn and psoralen-induced phototoxic reactions as well as depletion of Langerhans cells in human skin. *Photodermatol Photoimmunol Photomed.* 1997;13:50.
165. González S, Pathak MA. Inhibition of ultraviolet-induced formation of reactive oxygen species, lipid peroxidation, erythema and skin photosensitization by polypodium leucotomos. *Photodermatol Photoimmunol Photomed.* 1996;12:45.
166. Gomes AJ, Lunardi CN, González S, et al. The antioxidant action of Polypodium leucotomos extract and kojic acid: reactions with reactive oxygen species. *Braz J Med Biol Res.* 2001; 34:1487.
167. González S, Alonso-Lebrero JL, Del Rio R, et al. Polypodium leucotomos extract: a nutraceutical with photoprotective properties. *Drugs Today (Barc).* 2007;43:475.
168. Middelkamp-Hup MA, Pathak MA, Parrado C, et al. Orally administered Polypodium leucotomos extract decreases psoralen-UVA-induced phototoxicity, pigmentation, and damage of human skin. *J Am Acad Dermatol.* 2004; 50:41.
169. Middelkamp-Hup MA, Pathak MA, Parrado C, et al. Oral Polypodium leu-

cotomos extract decreases ultraviolet-induced damage of human skin. *J Am Acad Dermatol*. 2004;51:910.
170. Caccialanza M, Percivalle S, Piccinno R, et al. Photoprotective activity of oral polypodium leucotomos extract in 25 patients with idiopathic photodermatoses. *Photodermatol Photoimmunol Photomed*. 2007;23:46.
171. Jańczyk A, Garcia-Lopez MA, Fernandez-Peñas P, et al. A Polypodium leucotomos extract inhibits solar-simulated radiation-induced TNF-alpha and iNOS expression, transcriptional activation and apoptosis. *Exp Dermatol*. 2007;16:823.
172. Alonso-Lebrero JL, Domínguez-Jiménez C, Tejedor R, et al. Photoprotective properties of a hydrophilic extract of the fern Polypodium leucotomos on human skin cells. *J Photochem Photobiol B*. 2003; 70:31.
173. Philips N, Smith J, Keller T, et al. Predominant effects of Polypodium leucotomos on membrane integrity, lipid peroxidation, and expression of elastin and matrix- metalloproteinase-1 in ultraviolet radiation exposed fibroblasts, and keratinocytes. *J Dermatol Sci*. 2003;32:1.
174. Capote R, Alonso-Lebrero JL, García F, et al. Polypodium leucotomos extract inhibits *trans*-urocanic acid photoisomerization and photodecomposition. *J Photochem Photobiol B*. 2006;82:173.
175. Jang M, Cai L, Udeani GO, et al. Cancer chemopreventive activity of resveratrol, a natural product derived from grapes. *Science*. 1997;275:218.
176. Afaq F, Adhami VM, Ahmad N. Prevention of short-term ultraviolet B radiation-mediated damages by resveratrol in SKH-1 hairless mice. *Toxicol Appl Pharmacol*. 2003;186:28.
177. Adhami VM, Afaq F, Ahmad N. Suppression of ultraviolet B exposure-mediated activation of NF-kappaB in normal human keratinocytes by resveratrol. *Neoplasia*. 2003;5:74.
178. Ding XZ, Adrian TE. Resveratrol inhibits proliferation and induces apoptosis in human pancreatic cancer cells. *Pancreas*. 2002;25:e71.
179. Athar M, Back JH, Tang X, et al. Resveratrol: a review of preclinical studies for human cancer prevention. *Toxicol Appl Pharmacol*. 2007;224:274.
180. Delmas D, Rébé C, Lacour S, et al. Resveratrol-induced apoptosis is associated with Fas redistribution in the rafts and the formation of a death-inducing signaling complex in colon cancer cells. *J Biol Chem*. 2003;278:41482.
181. Aziz MH, Afaq F, Ahmad N. Prevention of ultraviolet-B radiation damage by resveratrol in mouse skin is mediated via modulation in survivin. *Photochem Photobiol*. 2005;81:25.
182. Aziz MH, Reagan-Shaw S, Wu J, et al. Chemoprevention of skin cancer by grape constituent resveratrol: relevance to human disease? *FASEB J*. 2005;19: 1193.
183. Reagan-Shaw S, Afaq F, Aziz MH, et al. Modulations of critical cell cycle regulatory events during chemoprevention of ultraviolet B-mediated responses by resveratrol in SKH-1 hairless mouse skin. *Oncogene*. 2004;23:5151.
184. Waterhouse AL, Walzem RL. Nutrition of grape phenolics. In: Rice-Evans CA, Packer L, eds. *Flavonoids in Health and Disease*. New York, NY: Marcel Dekker; 1998:359-385.
185. Carando S, Teissedre P-L. Catechin and procyanidin levels in French wines: contribution to dietary intake. In: Gross GG, Hemingway RW, Yoshida T, eds. *Plant Polyphenols 2: Chemistry, Biology, Pharmacology, Ecology*. New York, NY: Kluwer Academic/Plenum Publishers; 1999:725-737.
186. Bagchi D, Garg A, Krohn RL, et al. Oxygen free radical scavenging abilities of vitamins C and E, and a grape seed proanthocyanidin extract in vitro. *Res Commun Mol Pathol Pharmacol*. 1997; 95:179.
187. Ariga T, Hamano M. Radical scavenging action and its mode in procyanidin B-1 and B-3 from azuki beans to peroxy radicals. *Agric Biol Chem*. 1990;54: 2499.
188. Maffei Facino A, Carini M, Aldini G, et al. Free radicals scavenging action and anti-enzyme activities of procyanidins from Vitis vinifera. A mechanism for their capillary protective action. *Arzneimittelforschung*. 1994;44:592.
189. Ricardo da Silva JM, Darman N, Fernandez Y, et al. Oxygen free radical scavenger capacity in aqueous models of different procyanidins from grape seeds. *J Agric Food Chem*. 1991;39: 1549.
190. Vinson JA, Dabbagh YA, Serry MM, et al. Plant flavonoids, especially tea flavonols, are powerful antioxidants using an in vitro oxidation model for heart disease. *J Agric Food Chem*. 1995; 43:2800.
191. Koga T, Moro K, Nakamori K, et al. Increase of antioxidative potential of rat plasma by oral administration of proanthocyanidin-rich extract from grape seeds. *J Agric Food Chem*. 1999;47:1892.
192. Bagchi D, Bagchi M, Stohs SJ, et al. Free radicals and grape seed proanthocyanidin extract: importance in humn health and disease prevention. *Toxicology*. 2000;148:187.
193. Mittal A, Elmets CA, Katiyar SK. Dietary feeding of proanthocyanidins from grape seeds prevents photocarcinogenesis in SKH-1 hairless mice: relationship to decreased fat and lipid peroxidation. *Carcinogenesis*. 2003;24:1379.
194. Mantena SK, Katiyar SK. Grape seed proanthocyanidins inhibit UV-radiation-induced oxidative stress and activation of MAPK and NF-kappaB signaling in human epidermal keratinocytes. *Free Radic Biol Med*. 2006;40:1603.
195. Sharma SD, Meeran SM, Katiyar SK. Dietary grape seed proanthocyanidins inhibit UVB-induced oxidative stress and activation of mitogen-activated protein kinases and nuclear factor-kappaB signaling in in vivo SKH-1 hairless mice. *Mol Cancer Ther*. 2007;6:995.
196. Sharma SD, Katiyar SK. Dietary grape-seed proanthocyanidin inhibition of ultraviolet B-induced immune suppression is associated with induction of IL-12. *Carcinogenesis*. 2006;27:95.
197. Langley P. Why a pomegranate? *BMJ*. 2000;321:1153.
198. Gil MI, Tomás-Barberán FA, Hess-Pierce B, et al. Antioxidant activity of pomegranate juice and its relationship with phenolic composition and processing. *J Agric Food Chem*. 2000;48:4581.
199. Aviram M, Dornfeld L, Rosenblat M, et al. Pomegranate juice consumption reduces oxidative stress, atherogenic modifications to LDL, and platelet aggregation: studies in humans and in atherosclerotic apolipoprotein E-deficient mice. *Am J Clin Nutr*. 2000;71: 1062.
200. Wang RF, Xie WD, Zhang Z, et al. Bioactive compounds from the seeds of Punica granatum (pomegranate). *J Nat Prod*. 2004;67:2096.
201. Afaq F, Saleem M, Krueger CG, et al. Anthocyanin- and hydrolyzable tannin-rich pomegranate fruit extract modulates MAPK and NF-kappaB pathways and inhibits skin tumorigenesis in CD-1 mice. *Int J Cancer*. 2005; 113:423.
202. Seeram NP, Aviram M, Zhang Y, et al. C1mparison of antioxidant potency of commonly consumed polyphenol-rich beverages in the United States. *J Agric Food Chem*. 2008;56:1415.
203. Schubert SY, Lansky EP, Neeman I. Antioxidant and eicosanoid enzyme inhibition properties of pomegranate seed oil and fermented juice flavonoids. *J Ethnopharmacol*. 1999;66:11.
204. Chidambara Murthy KN, Jayaprakasha GK, Singh RP. Studies on antioxidant activity of pomegranate (Punica granatum) peel extract using in vivo models. *J Agric Food Chem*. 2002;50:4791.
205. Afaq F, Mukhtar H. Botanical antioxidants in the prevention of photocarcinogenesis and photoaging. *Exp Dermatol*. 2006;15:678.
206. Seeram NP, Adams LS, Henning SM, et al. In vitro antiproliferative, apoptotic and antioxidant activities of punicalagin, ellagic acid and a total pomegranate tannin extract are enhanced in combination with other polyphenols as found in pomegranate juice. *J Nutr Biochem*. 2005; 16:360.
207. Syed DN, Malik A, Hadi N, et al. Photochemopreventive effect of pomegranate fruit extract on UVA-mediated activation of cellular pathways in normal human epidermal keratinocytes. *Photochem Photobiol*. 2006;82:398.
208. Hora JJ, Maydew ER, Lansky EP, et al. Chemopreventive effects of pomegranate seed oil on skin tumor development in CD1 mice. *J Med Food*. 2003;6: 157.
209. Afaq F, Malik A, Syed D, et al. Pomegranate fruit extract modulates UV-B-mediated phosphorylation of mitogen-activated protein kinases and activation of nuclear factor kappa B in normal human epidermal keratinocytes paragraph sign. *Photochem Photobiol*. 2005;81:38.
210. Zaid MA, Afaq F, Syed DN, et al. Inhibition of UVB-mediated oxidative stress and markers of photoaging in immortalized HaCaT keratinocytes by pomegranate polyphenol extract POMx. *Photochem Photobiol*. 2007;83:882.
211. Aslam MN, Lansky EP, Varani J. Pomegranate as a cosmeceutical source: pomegranate fractions promote proliferation and procollagen synthesis and inhibit matrix metalloproteinase-1 pro-

duction in human skin cells. *J Ethnopharmacol.* 2006;103:311.

212. Packer L, Witt EH, Tritschler HJ. Alpha-lipoic acid as a biological antioxidant. *Free Radic Biol Med.* 1995;19:227.
213. Egan RW, Gale PH, Beveridge GC, et al. Radical scavenging as the mechanism for stimulation of prostaglandin cyclooxygenase and depression of inflammation by lipoic acid and sodium iodide. *Prostaglandins.* 1978;16:861.
214. Podda M, Tritschler HJ, Ulrich H, et al. Alpha-lipoic acid supplementation prevents symptoms of vitamin E deficiency. *Biochem Biophys Res Commun.* 1994;204:98.
215. Kagan VE, Shvedova A, Serbinova E, et al. Dihydrolipoic acid—a universal antioxidant both in the membrane and in the aqueous phase. Reduction of peroxyl, ascorbyl and chromanoxyl radicals. *Biochem Pharmacol.* 1992;44:1637.
216. Podda M, Han D, Koh B, et al. Conversion of lipoic acid to dihydrolipoic acid in human keratinocytes. *Clin Rec.* 1994;42:41B.
217. Podda M, Rallis M, Traber MG, et al. Kinetic study of cutaneous and subcutaneous distribution following topical application of [7,8-14C]rac-alpha-lipoic acid onto hairless mice. *Biochem Pharmacol.* 1996;52:627.
218. Perricone NV. Pharmacologic cognitive enhancers: dermatologic indications. *Skin & Aging.* 1998;2:68.
219. Hoyer S. Abnormalities of glucose metabolism in Alzheimer's disease. *Ann N Y Acad Sci.* 1991;640:53.
220. Monograph: alpha-Lipoic acid. *Altern Med Rev.* 1998;3:308.
221. Carpintero DJ. Use of thioctic acid forprevention of the adverse effects induced by benznidazole in patients with chronic Chagas' infection. *Medicina (B Aires).* 1983;43:285.
222. Bast A, Haenen GR. Interplay between lipoic acid and glutathione in the protection against microsomal lipid peroxidation. *Biochim Biophys Acta.* 1988;963: 558.
223. Rosenberg HR, Culik R. Effect of alpha-lipoic acid on vitamin C and vitamin E deficiencies. *Arch Biochem Biophys.* 1959; 80:86.
224. Biewenga GP, Haenen GR, Bast A. The pharmacology of the antioxidant lipoic acid. *Gen Pharmacol.* 1997;29:315.
225. Bergqvist-Karlsson A, Thelin I, Bergendorff O. Contact dermatitis to alph-lipoic acid in an anti-wrinkle cream. *Contact Dermatitis.* 2006;55:56.
226. Wet LG, Birac PM, Pratt DE. Separation of the isometric isoflavones from soybeans by high-performance liquid chromatograph. *J Chromatogr.* 1978;150:266.
227. Persky V, Van Horn L. Epidemiology of soy and cancer: perspectives and directions. *J Nutr.* 1995;125:709S.
228. Davis JN, Muqim N, Bhuiyan M, et al. Inhibition of prostate specific antigen expression by genistein in prostate cancer cells. *Int J Oncol.* 2000;16:1091.
229. Lu LJ, Anderson KE, Grady JJ, et al. Decreased ovarian hormones during a soya diet: implications for breast cancer prevention. *Cancer Res.* 2000;60:4112.
230. Lu LJ, Anderson KE, Grady JJ, et al. Effects of soya consumption for one month on steroid hormones in premenopausal women: implications for breast cancer risk reduction. *Cancer Epidemiol Biomarkers Prev.* 1996;5:63.
231. Messina M, Persky V, Setchell K, et al. Soy intake and cancer risk: a review of the in vitro and in vivo data. *Nutr Cancer.* 1994;21:113.
232. Wei H, Saladi R, Lu Y, et al. Isoflavone genistein: photoprotection and clinical implications in dermatology. *J Nutr.* 2003;133:3811S.
233. Albertazzi P, Pansini F, Bottazzi M, et al. Dietary soy supplementation and phytoestrogen levels. *Obstet Gynecol.* 1999;94:229.
234. Albertazzi P, Steel SA, Clifford E, et al. Attitudes towards and use of dietary supplementation in a sample of postmenopausal women. *Climacteric.* 2002; 5:374.
235. Wei H, Bowen R, Cai Q, et al. Antioxidant and antipromotional effects of the soybean isoflavone genistein. *Proc Soc Exp Biol Med.* 1995;208:124.
236. Polkowski K, Mazurek AP. Biological properties of genistein. A review of in vitro and in vivo data. *Acta Pol Pharm.* 2000;57:135.
237. Widyarini S, Husband AJ, Reeve VE. Protective effect of the isoflavonoid equol against hairless mouse skin carcinogenesis induced by UV radiation alone or with a chemical cocarcinogene. *Photochem Photobiol.* 2005;81:32.
238. Wei H, Wei L, Frenkel K, et al. Inhibition of tumor promoter-induced hydrogen peroxide formation in vitro and in vivo by genistein. *Nutr Cancer.* 1993;20:1.
239. Wei H, Barnes S, Wang Y. The inhibition of tumor promoter-induced protooncogene expression mouse skin by soybean isoflavone genistein. *Oncol Rep.* 1995;3:125.
240. Wei H, Cai Q, Rahn RO. Inhibition of UV light- and Fenton reaction-induced oxidative DNA damage by the soybean isoflavone genistein. *Carcinogenesis.* 1996;17:73.
241. Wang Y, Zhang X, Lebwohl M, et al. Inhibition of ultraviolet B (UVB)-induced c-fos and c-jun expression in vivo by a tyrosine kinase inhibitor genistein. *Carcinogenesis.* 1998;19:649.
242. Mazière C, Dantin F, Dubois F, et al. Biphasic effect of UVA radiation on STAT1 activity and tyrosine phosphorylation in cultured human keratinocytes. *Free Radic Biol Med.* 2000;28:1430.
243. Packer L, Rimbach G, Virgili F. Antioxidant activity and biologic properties of a procyanidin-rich extract from pine (Pinus maritima) bark, pycnogenol. *Free Radic Biol Med.* 1999;27:704.
244. Rohdewald P. Pycnogenol®, French maritime pine bark extract. In: Coates PM, Blackman MR, Cragg G, Levine M, Moss J, White J, eds. *Encyclopedia of Dietary Supplements.* New York, NY: Marcel Dekker; 2005:545-553.
245. Sime S, Reeve VE. Protection from inflammation, immunosuppression and carcinogenesis induced by UV radiation in mice by topical Pycnogenol. *Photochem Photobiol.* 2004;79:193.
246. Rohdewald P. A review of the French maritime pine bark extract (Pycnogenol), a herbal medication with a diverse clinical pharmacology. *Int J Clin Pharmacol Ther.* 2002;40:158.
247. Križková L, Chovanová Z, Duračková Z, et al. Antimutagenic in vitro activity of plant polyphenols: Pycnogenol® and Ginkgo biloba extract (EGb 761). *Phytother Res.* 2008;22:384.
248. Devaraj S, Vega-López S, Kaul N, et al. Supplementation with a pine bark extract rich in polyphenols increases plasma antioxidant capacity and alters the plasma lipoprotein profile. *Lipids.* 2002; 37:931.
249. Saliou C, Rimbach G, Moini H, et al. Solar ultraviolet-induced erythema in human skin and nuclear factor-kappa-B-dependent gene expression in keratinocytes are modulated by a French maritime pine bark extract. *Free Radic Biol Med.* 2001;30:154.
250. Baulieu EE, Thomas G, Legrain S, et al. Dehydroepiandrosterone (DHEA), DHEA sulfate, and aging: contribution of the DHEAge Study to a sociobiomedical issue. *Proc Natl Acad Sci U S A.* 2000; 97:4279.
251. Coach C, Benghuzzi H, Tucci M. The effect of ultraviolet radiation and pretreatment of dehydroepiandrosterone on RMK cells in culture. *Biomed Sci Instrum.* 2001;37:31.
252. Nestler JE, Barlascini CO, Clore JN, et al. Dehydroepiandrosterone reduces serum low density lipoprotein levels and body fat but does not alter insulin sensitivity in normal men. *J Clin Endocrinol Metab.* 1988;66:57.
253. Dean CE. Prasterone (DHEA) and mania. *Ann Pharmacother.* 2000;34:1419.
254. Reiter RJ, Tan DX, Osuna C, et al. Actions of melatonin in the reduction of oxidative stress. A review. *J Biomed Sci.* 2000;7:444.
255. Reiter RJ, Tan DX, Cabrera J, et al. The oxidant/antioxidant network: role of melatonin. *Biol Signals Recept.* 1999;8:56.
256. Kumar CA, Das UN. Effect of melatonin on two stage skin carcinogenesis in Swiss mice. *Med Sci Monit.* 2000;6:471.
257. Nickel A, Wohlrab W. Melatonin protects human keratinocytes from UVB irradiation by light absorption. *Arch Dermatol Res.* 2000;292:366.
258. Bangha E, Elsner P, Kistler GS. Suppression of UV-induced erythema by topical treatment with melatonin (N-acetyl-5-methoxytryptamine). A dose response study. *Arch Dermatol Res.* 1996;288:522.
259. Dreher F, Gabard B, Schwindt DA, et al. Topical melatonin in combination with vitamins E and C protects skin from ultraviolet-induced erythema: a human study in vivo. *Br J Dermatol.* 1998;139:332.
260. Howes RA, Halliday GM, Damian DL. Effect of topical melatonin on ultraviolet radiation-induced suppression of Mantoux reactions in humans. *Photodermatol Photoimmunol Photomed.* 2006;22:267.
261. Cho JW, Kim CW, Lee KS. Modification of gene expression by melatonin in UVB-irradiated HaCaT keratinocyte cell lines using a cDNA microarray. *Oncol Rep.* 2007;17:573.
262. Spallholz JE, Boylan LM, Larsen HS. Advances in understanding selenium's role in the immune system. *Ann NY Acad Sci.* 1990;587:123.
263. Yoshizawa K, Willet WC, Morris SJ. Study of prediagnostic selenium level in toenails and the risk of advanced prostate cancer. *J Natl Cancer Inst.* 1998;90:1219.

264. Overvad K, Thorling EB, Bjerring P, et al. Selenium inhibits UV-light-induced skin carcinogenesis in hairless mice. *Cancer Lett.* 1985;27:163.
265. Burke KE, Combs GF Jr, Gross EG, et al. The effects of topical and oral L-selenomethionine on pigmentation and skin cancer induced by ultraviolet irradiation. *Nutr Cancer.* 1992;17:123.
266. Rafferty TS, Beckett GJ, Walker C, et al. Selenium protects primary human keratinocytes from apoptosis induced by exposure to ultraviolet radiation. *Clin Exp Dermatol.* 2003;28: 294.
267. McKenzie RC, Rafferty TS, Beckett GJ. Selenium: an essential element for immune function. *Immunol Today.* 1998; 19:342.
268. Clark LC, Combs GF Jr, Turnbill BW, et al. Effects of selenium supplementation for cancer prevention in patients with carcinoma of the skin. A randomized controlled trial. Nutritional Prevention of Cancer Study Group. *JAMA.* 1996;276:1957.
269. Institute of Medicine, Food and Nutrition Board. *Dietary Reference Intakes: Vitamin C, Vitamin E, Selenium, and Carotenoids.* Washington, DC: National Academy Press; 2000.
270. Koller LD, Exon JH. The two faces of selenium-deficiency and toxicity—are similar in animals and man. *Can J Vet Res.* 1986;50:297.
271. McKenzie RC. Selenium, ultraviolet radiation and the skin. *Clin Exp Dermatol.* 2000;25:631.
272. Stewart MS, Spallholz JE, Neldner KH, et al. Selenium compounds have disparate abilities to impose oxidative stress and induce apoptosis. *Free Radic Biol Med.* 1999;26:42.
273. Pinnell SR, Lin F-H, Lin J-Y, et al. Ferulic acid stabilizes a solution of vitamins A and E and doubles its photoprotection of skin. *J Invest Dermatol.* 2005;125:826.
274. Greul AK, Grundmann JU, Heinrich F, et al. Photoprotection of UV-irradiated human skin: an antioxidative combination of vitamins E and C, carotenoids, selenium and proanthocyanidins. *Skin Pharmacol Appl Skin Physiol.* 2002;15: 307.
275. Passi S, De Pita O, Grandinetti M, et al. The combined use of oral and topical lipophilic antioxidants increases their levels both in sebum and stratum corneum. *Biofactors.* 2003;18:289.

CHAPTER 35

Anti-Inflammatory Agents

Mari Paz Castanedo-Tardan, MD
Leslie Baumann, MD

DEFINING INFLAMMATION

Inflammation, from the Latin word *inflammatio (to set on fire),* is a dynamic vascular and cellular reflexive response of the living tissue to injury; such injury may present in the form of infection, chemical damage (e.g., toxins, irritants), physical damage (e.g., heat, cold, radiation, mechanical trauma), and the binding of antibodies to antigens within the body.[1] Inflammation is therefore a protective mechanism of the organism intended to remove such injurious stimuli as well as to initiate the healing process of the damaged tissue.

Localized vasodilation, increased vascular permeability, extravasation of plasmatic proteins, and migration of leukocytes into the affected tissue produce what Cornelius Celsius defined in the first century as the "cardinal signs" of acute inflammation: *calor* (heat), *dolor* (pain), *rubor* (redness), and *tumor* (swelling).[2] *Functio laesa* (loss of function) was later added to the definition of inflammation by Rudolf Virchow in the 19th century.[3]

A basic sequence of events characterizes virtually all types of inflammatory responses regardless of the provocative stimuli.[4] The initial reaction is vasodilation followed by transient vasoconstriction. The microvascular endothelium then becomes more permeable to plasma proteins, which leak out into the extravascular compartment thus establishing an inflammatory exudate. Inflammatory mediators released in the area induce the expression of selectin-type adhesion molecules on the endothelial cells. Recruited leukocytes then interact with such adhesion molecules, bind to the inflamed endothelium, and extravasate into the tissue where they respond to the insult through phagocytosis and degranulation. Finally, the inflammatory response must be actively terminated when no longer essential to prevent unnecessary damage to tissue.

The process of inflammation, both vascular and cellular, is orchestrated by a large array of inflammatory mediators, which will be reviewed below. These mediators include the following: (1) cellular-derived products, such as vasoactive amines (e.g., histamine), cytokines, eicosanoids (e.g., prostaglandins, thromboxanes, and leukotrienes), enzymes, and oxygen radicals and (2) plasma-derived mediators, which include complement cascade components, kinins, and fibrinopeptides.

CELL-DERIVED INFLAMMATORY MEDIATORS AND THEIR ROLES IN THE INFLAMMATORY PROCESS

Role of Eicosanoids

In reaction to inflammatory stimuli, molecular signaling, or cell destruction, phospholipids contained in the cellular membrane are hydrolyzed by phospholipase A2 (PLA2) thus releasing free arachidonic acid (AA). This fatty acid is the primary precursor of eicosanoids (Fig. 35-1)—important inflammatory mediators that include prostaglandins (PGs), thromboxanes (TXs), and leukotrienes (LTs) among others[5] (Fig. 35-2). Eicosanoids are not stored. Once formed, they act locally at the site of synthesis to regulate autocrine and paracrine functions.[6] Different cell types have particular sets of enzymes for eicosanoid synthesis, which determine their eicosanoid profile. Similarly, different stimuli also influence the eicosanoid profile produced by the cell.[6] There are two different pathways in the synthesis of eicosanoids from AA:

(1) *Cyclooxygenase pathway*: All eicosanoids with ring structures, that is, the PGs, TXs, and prostacyclins, are synthesized via the cyclooxygenase pathway. Two cyclooxygenases have been identified: COX-1 and COX-2. The former is ubiquitous and constitutive, whereas the latter is induced in response to inflammatory stimuli. The products of these and subsequent reactions in this pathway are summarized in Fig. 35-2.

(2) *Lipoxygenase pathway*: Several lipoxygenase enzymes can act on AA to form different peroxidated derivatives (the hydroperoxyeicosatetraenoic [HPETE] acids 5-HPETE, 12-HPETE, and 15-HPETE) depending on which carbon of AA they insert or attach oxygen. HPETEs are then rapidly reduced to hydroxylated derivatives (HETEs), LTs, or lipoxins, depending on the tissue.

Role of Cytokines

Cytokines are intracellular signaling polypeptides produced by activated cells. Most cytokines have multiple sources, targets, and functions[7] (see Chapter 4). The main cytokines that are produced during, and participate in, inflammatory processes[8–10] are given in Table 35-1. These inflammatory-associated cytokines are produced by various cell types, but the most important sources are macrophages and monocytes at inflammatory areas.[7] Chemokines (chemotactic cytokines) are small proteins that direct the movement of circulating leukocytes toward inflamed regions[11]—an essential step for

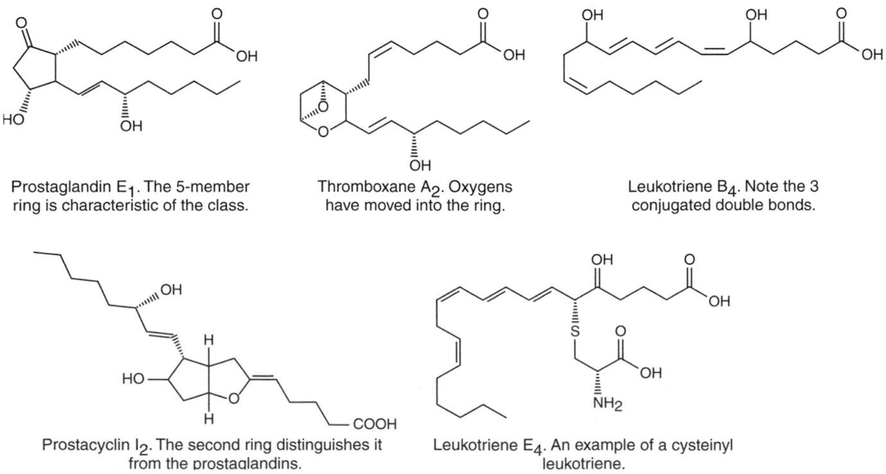

Prostaglandin E_1. The 5-member ring is characteristic of the class.

Thromboxane A_2. Oxygens have moved into the ring.

Leukotriene B_4. Note the 3 conjugated double bonds.

Prostacyclin I_2. The second ring distinguishes it from the prostaglandins.

Leukotriene E_4. An example of a cysteinyl leukotriene.

▲ **FIGURE 35-1** Eicosanoids are signaling molecules made by oxygenation of essential fatty acids. This figure shows the structure of several types of eicosanoids.

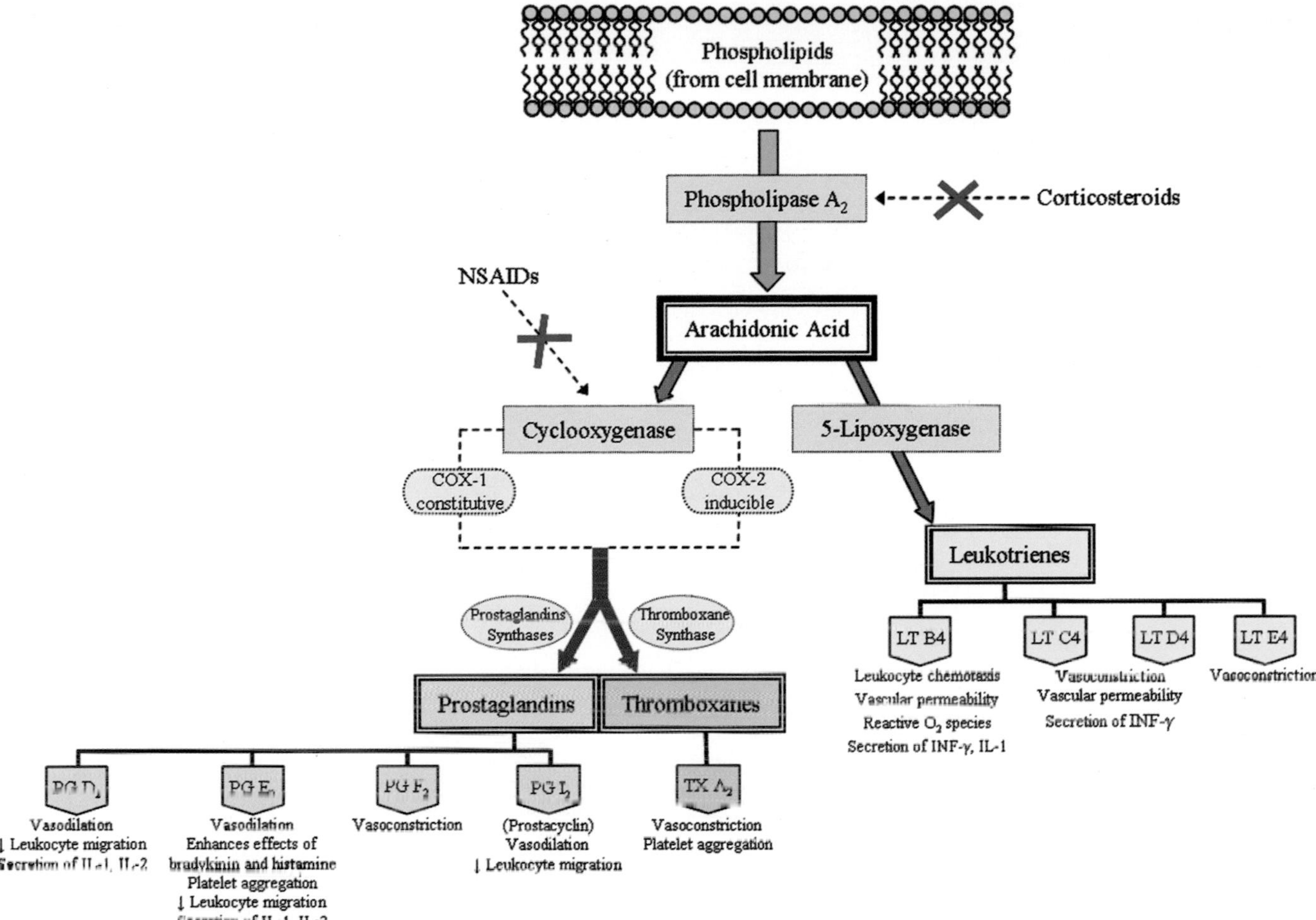

▲ **FIGURE 35-2** The arachidonic acid cascade that leads to inflammation.

the host response to injury. Although a large number of cytokines are found within sites of inflammation, two of these cytokines, namely, interleukin-1 (IL-1) and tumor necrosis factor-α (TNF-α), play a key role in orchestrating the mechanisms responsible for inflammation. These two cytokines induce the production of lipid mediators, proteases, and free radicals, all of which play a direct role in the development of the deleterious effects of inflammation.[8] In fact, certain cytokines, including interferon-γ (INF-γ) and granulocyte colony-stimulating factor (G-CSF), amplify the inflammatory response by increasing the production of IL-1 and TNF-α by macrophages.[8]

Role of Mast Cells

Mast cells, derived from hematopoietic precursors, are found predominantly near blood vessels, nerves, and subepithelial sites, where local immediate hypersensitivity reactions tend to occur.[12,13] These cells can be activated during acute reactions such as allergies through their high-affinity receptors for the Fc portion of immunoglobulin E (IgE) and by several other stimuli including complement components C3a and C5a, which will be briefly explained later in this chapter. Other mast cell stimulators that promote the release of histamine include physical stimuli (e.g., heat, cold, and sunlight), macrophage-derived cytokines, bacterial toxins, venoms, trauma, and the presence of allergens. Mast cells are also present in chronic inflammatory reactions, and may produce cytokines that contribute to fibrosis.[14,15]

When a mast cell armed with IgE antibodies is reexposed to the specific allergen, a series of reactions takes place, leading eventually to the release of various potent mediators responsible for the clinical expression of immediate inflammatory-hypersensitivity reactions. In the first step of this sequence, antigens bind to the IgE antibodies previously attached to the mast cells. The bridging of IgE molecules with the underlying IgE-Fc receptors activates signal transduction pathways that will translate into three outcomes[16]: (1) degranulation, with the secretion of preformed mediators-like vasoactive amines (e.g., histamine), neutral proteases (e.g., chymase, tryptase, hydrolase), and proteoglycans (e.g., heparin, chondroitin sulfate); (2) de novo synthesis of proinflammatory lipid mediators (i.e., LTs C_4, D_4, and B_4, and PG D_2); and finally (3) synthesis and secretion of cytokines (i.e., TNF-α, IL-1, IL-3, IL-4, IL-5, IL-6, and GM-CSF), as well as chemokines, such as macrophage inflammatory protein (MIP)-1β and MIP-1β.[13]

Role of Histamine

Histamine is a naturally-occurring low-molecular-weight amine synthesized by the decarboxylation of the amino acid L-histidine catalyzed by the enzyme histidine decarboxylase. The synthesis of this important vasoactive amine occurs in sites where the former enzyme is expressed, such as basophils and mast cells found throughout the body (including lungs and skin), parietal cells of the gastric-mucosa, and central nervous system neurons.[17,18]

Histamine plays a fundamental role in allergic inflammation,[18] which characterizes certain cutaneous diseases such as allergic contact dermatitis (ACD) and immunologic contact urticaria (ICU). The diverse effects of histamine over human health depend upon four different types of receptors; however, its specific

TABLE 35-1
Inflammatory-Associated Cytokines

Inflammatory Cytokine	Secreted by	Target Cell or Tissue	Activity
IL-1 (α and β)	Monocytes Macrophages B cells Dendritic cells Endothelial cells	TH cells B cells Natural Killer (NK) cells Endothelial cells Hepatocytes Hypothalamus	Targets a wide variety of cells to induce many inflammatory reactions: activation of TH cells; maturation and clonal expansion of B cells; enhancement of the activity of NK cells; production of other cytokines; endothelial gene regulation (increasing the expression of adhesion molecules); chemotaxis of macrophages and neutrophils; leukocyte adherence, synthesis of acute-phase-proteins by the liver; induction of fever
IL-6	Monocytes Macrophages TH2 cells	B cells Plasma cells Hepatocytes	Promotes the terminal differentiation of B cells into plasma cells; stimulates antibodies secretion by plasma cells; induces synthesis of acute-phase proteins.
IL-8	Macrophages Endothelial cells	Neutrophils	Potent chemokine, induces adherence to endothelium and extravasation to tissues.
IL-10	TH2 cells	Macrophages	Also called cytokine synthesis inhibitory factor because it suppresses cytokine production by activated TH1 cells
IL-11	Bone marrow stromal cells Some fibroblasts	T cells B cells Hepatocytes	Stimulation of T cell-dependent B cell immunoglobulin secretion; increased platelet production; induction of IL-6; acute phase protein secretion.
Interferon (INF)-γ	TH1 cells Cytotoxic T cells NK cells	Macrophages Inflammatory cells	Enhances the activity of macrophages, mediates effects important in delayed type hypersensitivity.
TNF-α	Macrophages NK cells	Inflammatory cells	Shares several proinflammatory properties with IL-1. Induces cytokine secretion. Important role in chronic inflammation.
Transforming growth factor-β	Platelets Macrophages Lymphocytes Mast cells	B cells T cells NK cells	Inhibits T cell and NK cell proliferation and activation; attracts monocytes to the site of inflammation; enhances cell adhesion.
Granulocyte colony-stimulating factor (G-CSF)	Macrophages T cells	Neutrophils	Participates in acute inflammation.

role in allergic inflammation mostly occurs through the H_1-receptor.[18,19] Through this receptor, histamine plays a proinflammatory role by inducing the release of cytokines and lysosomal enzymes from macrophages and the expression of cell adhesion molecules.[18,19] Additionally, it influences the activity of basophils, eosinophils, and fibroblasts, causing smooth muscle contraction.[20] Although most of the effects of histamine in inflammatory allergic disease occur through the H_1-receptor, cutaneous itch may occur through both the H_1- and H_3-receptors.[21]

Role of Free Radicals

Oxygen-derived free radicals may be released extracellularly from leukocytes after exposure to pathogens, chemokines, and immune complexes, or following a phagocytic challenge.[22] The physiologic function of these reactive oxygen intermediates is to destroy phagocytized microorganisms. Their production depends on the activation of the nicotinamide adenine dinucleotide phosphate (NADPH) oxidative system, which is a membrane-bound enzyme complex. This system can be found in the plasmatic membrane as well as in the membrane of phagosomes inside the cells. Superoxide anion (O_2^-), hydrogen peroxide (H_2O_2), and hydroxyl radical (OH) are the major species produced within the cell; these metabolites can combine with nitric oxide (NO) to form other reactive nitrogen intermediates[23] (see Chapter 34). Extracellular release of low levels of these potent mediators can increase the expression of chemokines, cytokines, and endothelial leukocyte adhesion molecules, amplifying the cascade that elicits the inflammatory response. At higher levels, the release of these mediators can induce endothelial cell damage, which results in increased vascular permeability, neutrophil degranulation, and inactivation of antiproteases, such as α_1-antitrypsin, leading to increased destruction of the extracellular matrix.[24]

Serum, tissue fluids, and host cells all possess antioxidant mechanisms that protect against these potentially harmful oxygen-derived radicals. These include among others: (1) the copper-containing serum protein ceruloplasmin; (2) the iron-free fraction of serum, transferrin; (3) the enzyme superoxide dismutase, which is found or can be activated in various cell types; (4) the enzyme catalase, which detoxifies H_2O_2; and (5) glutathione peroxidase, another powerful H_2O_2 detoxifier.

The influence of oxygen-derived free radicals in any given inflammatory reaction will always depend on the balance between the production and the inactivation of these metabolites by both cells and tissues.

PLASMA-DERIVED MEDIATORS AND THEIR ROLE IN THE INFLAMMATORY PROCESS

Role of Complement

A complete explanation of the complex complement system is beyond the scope of this chapter. However, when focusing on the inflammatory response, it is necessary to mention the important role of the complement components that are integral to the inflammatory process: C3a and C5a. Both C3a and C5a are plasma-derived mediators that stimulate histamine release by mast cells, thereby inducing vasodilation.[25] Additionally, C5a is able to act as a chemoattractant, directing cells via chemotaxis to the site of inflammation.[25]

Role of Kinins

The kinin-kallikrein system is a network of circulating proteins mainly known for its roles in inflammation, blood pressure control, coagulation, and pain. Furthermore, several recent studies have concluded that this system plays broader roles than those classically described, for example, in rosacea, cancer, cardiovascular, renal, and central nervous system pathologies.[26]

The system consists of proteins, polypeptides, and a group of enzymes that activate and deactivate the compounds. Kinins (bradykinin [BK] and kallidin[KD]) are polypeptides produced from kininogen and broken down by kininases. They are rapidly generated after tissue injury and play a pivotal function in the development and maintenance of the inflammatory process, in which they cause dilation of blood vessels and increased vascular permeability. They act on PLA2 to increase AA release and thus eicosanoid production[27] (Fig. 35-1).

Kinins act by binding to two receptor types, namely B_1, and B_2, which belong to the G-protein coupled receptor family. B_2 receptors are constitutively expressed in various cells under physiologic conditions. On the contrary, B_1 receptors express rapidly under mainly pathologic conditions.[26] Kinins (BK and KD) have a higher affinity to B_2 receptors, the activation of which leads to the release of cytokines and other inflammatory mediators (e.g., PG-E_2).

Since its discovery, BK has been demonstrated to induce the four classical signs of inflammation—heat, redness, swelling, and pain[28]—described at the beginning of this chapter. BK possesses vasoactive properties that enable it to induce vasodilation and increase vascular permeability. Additionally, it causes smooth muscle contraction, induces pain, and has the ability to activate nuclear factor-κB (NF-κB), further contributing to the inflammatory response.

Cutaneous Inflammation

The skin is the primary barrier between our bodies and the environment and therefore the spectrum of insults to which it is exposed are numerous and diverse.[29] The translation of such insults, which include different pathogens and contact-sensitizing antigens, into cutaneous inflammation requires a complex interaction among multiple inflammatory mediators. Notably, NF-κB-mediated inflammation appears to be the final common pathway for the translation of environmental insults into inflammation of the skin. NF-κB, a powerful cellular signaling pathway, can be activated by IL-1, TNF-α,[30] and as mentioned earlier, BK.[26] Interestingly, the epidermis is a "storehouse" of IL-1α and can produce considerable amounts of IL-1β and TNF-α.[31,32] It is known that ultraviolet (UV) radiation from sunlight induces activation of IL-1 and TNF-α,[33] leading to NF-κB-mediated inflammation. NF-κB regulates many genes in skin cells; however, those that are essential to the initiation of cutaneous inflammation include genes for E-selectin, cytokines, defensins (antibacterial peptides), and cell adhesion molecules.[30]

Of special importance for cutaneous immunity is a subgroup of memory T cells with the ability to circulate preferentially to the skin. These memory T cells are identified by a marker known as cutaneous lymphocyte antigen (CLA),[34] and are generated in the lymph nodes that drain the skin. Then, they are specifically recruited back to the skin during inflammation. These unique skin-associated lymphocytes may be positive for either CD4 or CD8, and once activated, may be able to produce either type 1 T-cell cytokines (i.e., INF-γ, IL-2, and lymphotoxin) or type 2 T cell cytokines (i.e., IL-4, IL-5, IL-10 and IL-13).[29] It is the activation of the T cells and the subsequent release of cytokines and other effector molecules that result in clinically apparent T-cell-mediated inflammatory skin diseases.[29]

ANTI-INFLAMMATORY AGENTS FOR THE TREATMENT OF INFLAMMATORY SKIN DISEASES

Topical Corticosteroids

Not so long ago, dermatologic therapy was completely revolutionized with the introduction of corticosteroids in the early 1950s. Spies and Stone, two dermatologists from Alabama, were the first to use topical hydrocortisone to successfully treat a patient with chronic hand dermatitis.[35,36] After this therapeutic success, many dermatologists "seriously wondered if their specialty had come to its end."[37]

Corticosteroids are known to suppress proinflammatory genes that encode cytokines, cell adhesion molecules, and other mediators that interfere with the inflammatory response.[38] They selectively induce annexin I, an anti-inflammatory protein that physically interacts with and inhibits cytosolic phospholipase $A_2\alpha$ (cPL$A_2\alpha$).[39] By inhibiting this phospholipase they block the release of AA and its subsequent conversion to eicosanoids such as PGs, TXs, prostacyclins, and LTs.[40] A second anti-inflammatory protein induced by corticosteroids is MAPK phosphatase-1. Bacteria, viruses, cytokines, and, interestingly, UV radiation are all examples of inflammatory signals that activate the MAPK cascades.[41] Finally, glucocorticoids also induce and antagonize NF-κB, which is known to stimulate the transcription of COX-2, an enzyme essential for PG production.[42]

Since some of the anti-inflammatory mechanisms of glucocorticoids are also involved in physiologic signaling rather than inflammatory signaling, the therapeutic effects of these drugs in inflammation are often accompanied by clinically significant side effects.[40] Therefore, although topical corticosteroids are generally well tolerated for short-term use on inflammatory skin diseases, long-term widespread use can result in serious cutaneous adverse effects that include: skin atrophy, hirsutism, folliculitis, acne, striae, telangiectasia, purpura, and changes in pigmentation.[43,44] Moreover, even more serious systemic side effects such as hypothalamic pituitary axis (HPA) suppression,[45] hyperglycemia,[46] avascular osteonecrosis,[47] glaucoma,[48] and posterior subcapsular cataracts[49] have also been reported in association with the long-term use of topical corticosteroids.

Topical Immune Modulators

Topical calcineurin inhibitors tacrolimus and pimecrolimus have been investigated in the past decade as treatment options for inflammatory skin disorders. These relatively new immunosuppressive drugs act by inhibiting the protein calcineurin, subsequently preventing T cell dephosphorylation of transcription factors. As a result of this inhibition, the signal transduction pathways in such cells are blocked, and inflammatory cytokine production is suppressed.[50]

Between December 2000 and December 2001, topical tacrolimus

ointment and topical pimecrolimus cream received approval by the Food and Drug Administration (FDA) for the treatment of atopic dermatitis.[51] Furthermore, topical tacrolimus has been proven to inhibit other inflammatory skin conditions such as nickel-induced ACD[52,53] as measured by a reduction in erythema, pruritus, vesiculation, induration,[53] and histopathologic pattern.[54] Its inhibitory action has even been found by some researchers to be stronger than the steroid aclometasone dipropionate.[55]

Even though these medicaments are structurally very similar, pimecrolimus has a higher lipophilicity index than tacrolimus (20-fold more lipophilic). Although a higher lipophilicity index has been correlated with a higher affinity for the skin,[43] pimecrolimus is threefold less potent an inhibitor of calcineurin than tacrolimus.[56]

In February 2005, just a few years after these drugs were approved by the FDA, the pediatric advisory committee of the Center for Drug Evaluation and Research of the FDA required that the labeling of tacrolimus and pimecrolimus include the placement of a "black box" warning about the potential cancer risks associated with the systemic administration of these medications.[57] However, although there is a theoretical concern, there has been no evidence to suggest an increased risk of cutaneous or visceral cancer associated with the use of these drugs in their topical form.[58]

Cyclooxygenase Inhibitors

An increasing number of anti-inflammatory agents specifically target bioactive lipids generated from AA, namely, nonsteroidal anti-inflammatory drugs (NSAIDs). Although this group of medicaments is one of the most studied and used throughout medicine, their application for cutaneous disease is somewhat limited.[59] Ibuprofen, however, has been shown to be effective for the treatment of acne, since inflammatory acne lesions are infiltrated with neutrophils and ibuprofen is known to inhibit leukocyte chemotaxis.[60]

More than two decades ago, Wong et al. conducted a double-blind study of 60 male and female patients 15 to 35 years old with acne vulgaris.[61] Patients were randomly assigned to one of four groups: (1) oral ibuprofen (600 mg) plus tetracycline (250 mg) 4 times daily (qid); (2) ibuprofen (600 mg) plus placebo qid; (3) tetracycline (250 mg) plus placebo qid; and (4) two placebos qid. Only the combination therapy had an effect statistically better than the placebo in the improvement of total lesion count. The administration of ibuprofen alone yielded beneficial results comparable to the ones of tetracycline alone but with fewer side effects.

As a follow-up to this study, 1 year later, Funt treated 22 male and female patients aged 14 to 25 years with nodulocystic acne with a combination of minocycline (50 mg) plus oral ibuprofen (400 mg) 3 times daily. After 1 month, all patients apparently responded to the combination therapy with improvement ranging from 75% to 90%. Notably, all 22 patients had a history of unsuccessful oral antibiotic treatment (3-month course of minocycline, 50 mg 3 times daily).[62]

NSAIDs are also applied in dermatology in the treatment of sunburn. Hughes et al. studied the ability to modify skin injury induced by UVB radiation by nonsteroidal drugs (i.e., oral ibuprofen or indomethacin) plus topical betamethasone dipropionate in 24 subjects.[63] Skin responses to UVB (erythema and increased skin blood flow [SBF]) were measured serially and showed a synergistic effect of oral NSAIDs in combination with topical corticosteroids in the reduction of UVB-induced skin injury. In another study, ibuprofen and placebo were compared in a randomized double-blind cross-over study of 19 psoriatic patients receiving UVB phototherapy. Signs and symptoms of UVB-induced inflammation were then assessed. Although a statistical difference was noted for only one variable (i.e., technician's assessment of erythema), results suggest that ibuprofen was more effective than placebo for the symptomatic relief of UVB-induced inflammation after high doses of UVB-phototherapy for psoriasis. The postulated biochemical basis for this result derives from the observation that dermal PGs are elevated after UVB irradiation.[64] Therefore, an NSAID agent that interferes with PG synthesis may reduce UVB-induced inflammation.

Salicylic Acid

Experimental and clinical data indicate that salicylates exhibit a spectrum of activities that include anti-inflammatory and antimicrobial actions.[65] As a member of the aspirin family, salicylic acid achieves its analgesic and anti-inflammatory properties by truncating the AA cascade. Salicylates are active in controlling inflammation by altering gene expressions. They suppress the expression of proinflammatory genes by inhibiting the DNA-binding activities of transcription activators such as NF-κB, activation protein-1 (AP-1) and CCAAT/enhancer-binding protein β (C/EBPβ).[65]

Salicylic acid is known to decrease the frequency and severity of acne eruptions by reducing acne-associated inflammation in addition to imparting an exfoliating action over the pores. It has therefore become a popular ingredient in over-the-counter acne products (see Chapter 20). Salicylic acid is also used to treat rosacea and other superficial inflammatory disorders. In addition, it is found in products intended to treat photoaged skin. Topical salicylic acid in concentrations of up to 30% has been shown to fade age-related pigmented spots, decrease surface roughness, and reduce fine lines.[66] If used in high concentrations or too frequently, salicylic acid may lead to redness, pruritus, scaling, increased skin sensitivity, and even epidermolysis.

Sulfur/Sulfacetamide

The medicinal use of sulfur dates back to the time of Hippocrates, who is believed to have mentioned its use for the treatment of plague.[67] It is currently found in many products including the spa waters and elegant products from the Vichy spa in France. Most of what is known about sulfur was written decades ago, with moderate to little interest evinced in the recent literature. Nevertheless, sulfur continues to be used throughout the world mainly to treat acne, seborrheic dermatitis, rosacea, scabies, and tinea versicolor.[68] Elemental sulfur (a yellow, nonmetallic element) and its various forms (e.g., sulfides, sulfites, and mercaptans) are believed to have antimicrobial, antifungal, and antiparasitic properties. Furthermore, sulfur-containing compounds have proved to be "excellent anti-inflammatory agents."[69] Interestingly, the action of sulfur in the skin depends on its direct interaction with the cutaneous surface; the smaller the particle size, the greater the area available for sulfur—skin interaction and the greater the efficacy.[70] Two sulfur preparations are found as official formulations in the United States Pharmacopoeia: sublimed sulfur and precipitated sulfur. Precipitated sulfur has a smaller particle size and therefore is superior in efficacy to sublimed sulfur; in fact, this is the type of sulfur most widely used.

Sulfur was once the most common active ingredient found in antiacne formulations,[60] but has widely come into disuse mainly because of its malodorousness, resembling rotten eggs. The therapeutic effect of sulfur in acne and seborrheic dermatitis is thought to result from its keratolytic action.[71] The precise mechanism for this effect is unknown but probably depends on its interaction with the cysteine content of keratinocytes, allowing the formation of hydrogen sulfide, which in turn breaks down keratin.[70] In the treatment of acne and seborrheic dermatitis, sulfur is often combined with agents such as salicylic acid, the keratolytic action of which may be synergistic with that of sulfur.[72]

Sulfur is commonly combined with sodium sulfacetamide, a sulfonamide agent with antibacterial activity. It acts as a competitive antagonist to para-aminobenzoic acid (PABA), an essential component for bacterial growth.[73] In fact, sodium sulfacetamide has been demonstrated to be active against *Propionibacterium acnes*.[74] When mixed with sulfur in dermatologic preparations, the combined keratolytic and anti-inflammatory effect of sulfur with the antibacterial effect of sulfacetamide results in an effective topical formulation for the treatment of acne vulgaris, rosacea, and seborrheic dermatitis.[75] This combination is available as a cream, lotion, gel topical suspension, cleanser, and silica-based mask.

Botanicals and Other Natural Ingredients

Natural ingredients have been used in traditional medicine throughout the world for thousands of years; however, it is in the last 15 years that botanically derived products have gained widespread usage and interest among the US population.[76] As a result, botanical products have become highly marketable. This increased popularity has occurred for several reasons: (1) concerns about the adverse effects of chemical drugs; (2) questioning of the approaches and assumptions of allopathic medicine; (3) greater public access to health information; and (4) the growing popularity of organic products. All this translates into a very broad array of botanical products now being used in different medical specialties including dermatology. Fortunately, we are now able to employ scientific methods to prove or question their efficacy and better understand their mechanisms of action. The following discussion focuses on some of the most important botanicals that confer anti-inflammatory properties. Of note, when looking for botanicals as components of personal care products and cosmetics, it is important to consider the names given by the International Nomenclature for Cosmetic Ingredients (INCI), used for ingredient disclosures inside a product's list of ingredients.

Aloe Vera

Aloe vera is one of the most widely used herbal products in the world. It is native to northern Africa and the Arabian Peninsula, but through trade its use extended to most of the ancient civilizations (Egypt, Persia, Greece, Rome, India, and China) where it was used for the treatment of burns and wounds. The Spanish later brought it to America and parts of the Caribbean including Barbados (from which the alternate INCI name *Aloe barbadensis* is derived).[77]

There is a large body of anecdotal evidence attesting to the efficacy of aloe for the treatment of myriad diseases; unfortunately, exaggerated claims are not uncommon and therefore caution is warranted in the interpretation of some of the available information.[70] Explanations of aloe gel efficacy are still varied because it has in fact several active constituents operating through different mechanisms.[79] Its action as a moisturizer, for example, is a popular use that may account for much of its effects.[80] Furthermore, aloe is reputed to exhibit potent anti-inflammatory effects, and the substances that have been proposed as its active anti-inflammatory constituents include salicylates (providing "aspirin like effects"); magnesium lactate, which is believed to inhibit the production of histamine; BK and TX inhibitors, which provide pain reduction; and polysaccharides, particularly acemannan, which has reported immunomodulatory properties.[81,82] Another substance isolated from aloe, *C*-glucosyl chromone, has exhibited topical anti-inflammatory activity equivalent to that of hydrocortisone (200 μg/ mouse ear).[83]

A recent study by Habeeb et al.[84] explored reports of antimicrobial effects associated with aloe.[85] Using a simple in vitro assay, they determined the effect of the inner gel of aloe on bacterial-induced proinflammatory cytokine production (namely, TNF α and IL-1β) from human leukocytes stimulated with *Shigella flexneri*. Results demonstrated the suppression of both bacterial-induced cytokines with the use of aloe inner gel.[84] Further studies are still needed for a deeper and more precise understanding of aloe constituents and their varied biologic activities.

Chamomile

Chamomile is a sweet-scented flower belonging to the Asteraceae (or Compositae) family that has been used as a medicinal herb worldwide for hundreds of years,[86] and is still one of the most widely used medicinal herbs. It has been recognized for its therapeutic properties since the age of Hippocrates (circa 500 BCE). The ancient Greeks and Egyptians used it to treat erythema and dry skin.[87]

There are two primary types of chamomile, Roman chamomile (INCI name: *Chamaemelum nobile*) and German chamomile (INCI name: *Matricaria recutita* or *Chamomilla recutita*). Although both plants have been used for therapeutic applications, the flowers of German chamomile contain a higher concentration of key active ingredients that have shown anti-inflammatory activity in vivo[88]: the terpenoids chamazulene and α bisabolol. Because of this fact, the official medicinal chamomile is German chamomile. In an animal study in which inflammation was induced via the injection of carrageenan and PG E1, German chamomile was found to suppress both the inflammatory effect and leukocyte infiltration.[89] Specifically, chamazulene decreases the inflammatory process by inhibiting LT synthesis.[90] It is believed that chamomile also confers significant beneficial effects to the skin, such as the improvement of texture and elasticity, ameliorating the signs of photodamage.

In addition to reports of anti-inflammatory effects, chamomile is said to possess some antioxidant properties,[90] which are mainly associated with other active ingredients, namely the terpenoid matricine and the flavonoids apigenin and luteolin, all of which have documented antioxidant properties.[91] As a result of its various beneficial properties, chamomile is now included in several cosmetic products intended to improve skin appearance. Of note, chamomile has been reported to cause ACD in susceptible types.[92] Those with known allergies to the compositae plant family (e.g., ragweed) are at the greatest risk.

Cucumber Extract

Cucumber (INCI name: *Cucumis sativus*) has a long history of use in ancient and folk medicine. Reputedly used by Cleopatra to preserve her skin,[93] cucumber extract has found regular usage in modern skin care, with most of its healthy characteristics observed when used topically.

Cucumber extract is known for its emollient and soothing properties, specifically. It contains high amounts of amino acids and organic acids that are beneficial to the skin's acid mantle. In addition, shikimate dehydrogenase, an enzyme extracted from cucumber pulp, has demonstrated anti-inflammatory properties when applied to the skin.[93] More scientific studies are needed, though, to confirm and further expand the limited known cutaneous effects of treatment with cucumber extract.

Feverfew

Feverfew (FF) (INCI name: *Tanacetum parthenium*) is a rapidly growing small bush with citrus-scented leaves and daisy-like flowers (Fig. 35-3). It belongs to the Asteraceae (or Compositae) family, characterized by the star-shaped flower head of its members. Since the first century, FF has been used to reduce fever and pain. The use of this herb as an antipyretic led to the appellation "feverfew"—a corruption of the Latin word *febrifugia* (fever reducer).[94,95] FF acts as a PG antagonist,[96] and one of its extracts, parthenolide, has been reported to inhibit platelet aggregation. Additionally, it has been shown to bind to and inhibit IκB kinase β (IKK-β), the kinase subunit known to play a critical role in cytokine-mediated stimulation of genes involved in inflammation,[97] which may partly explain the anti-inflammatory properties attributed to this herb. Parthenolide is a type of sesquiterpene lactone, an essential oil commonly found in members of the Asteraceae family. Sesquiterpene lactones are known for their anti-inflammatory effects; nevertheless, they also exert the major allergenic effects of this plant family. In fact, FF-derived parthenolide forms part of the Compositae Mix (CM)—a solution of extracts from five plant species that can be applied as a patch test to screen for Asteraceae allergy.[98] The Aveeno Ultra Calming line of skin care products contains FF but with the parthenolide portion removed, thus yielding the anti-inflammatory properties of FF without posing the risk of contact dermatitis. The beneficial effects of this parthenolide-depleted extract of FF were demonstrated in a recent study.[99] In this research, in vitro FF was shown to attenuate the formation of UV-induced hydrogen peroxide and to reduce proinflammatory cytokine release; in vivo, topical FF reduced UV-induced epidermal hyperplasia, DNA damage, and apotosis.[99]

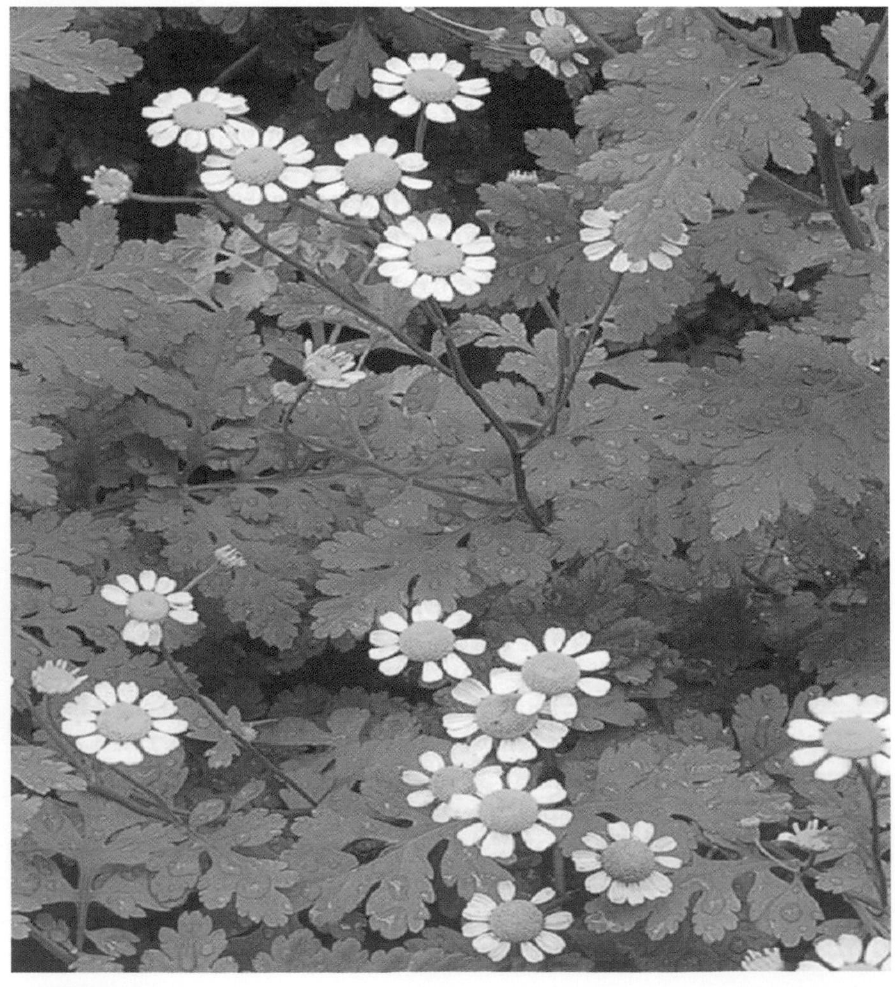

▲ **FIGURE 35-3** Feverfew.

Ginseng

Several types of ginseng are found throughout the world, and all are part of the Araliaceae family in the genus *Panax* (Fig. 35-4). The word *Panax* means "all healing," which describes the traditional belief that ginseng manifests properties that heal all the diseased aspects of the body. There are several different species of ginseng; two of the most commonly used are *P. ginseng* (Chinese ginseng), popular among Asian cultures, and *P. quinquefolius* (American ginseng), commonly used among Native Americans.[100]

Studies indicate that ginseng may exert chemopreventive properties against cancer. Mechanisms behind this assumption include inhibition of DNA damage,[101] induction of apoptosis,[102] and inhibition of cell proliferation.[103] There is also evidence that ginseng has potent effects on the inflammatory cascade and may inhibit the "inflammation-to-cancer sequence." For example, ginsan, a polysaccharide extracted from *P. ginseng*, has been shown to inhibit the release of proinflammatory cytokines in vivo.[104] Furthermore, the ginsenoside Rg3 has been demonstrated to inhibit the NF-κB-mediated induction of the inflammatory process.[105] In addition, BST204, a fermented ginseng extract, can inhibit inducible nitric oxide synthase (NOS) expression and subsequent nitric oxide production in animal models. Finally, ginseng has been proven to inhibit the production of TNF-α and other proinflammatory cytokines by cultured macrophages when exposed to bacterial lipopolysaccharides.[106]

Licorice Extract

Licorice (also known as *Liquiritae officinalis*) is best known in its popular confectionery form of black or red candy. Although it is not often thought of as a plant, it is a botanical source of systemic or topical medications that have been used in herbal medicine for approximately 4000 years.[107] There are different species of licorice; *Glycyrrhiza glabra*

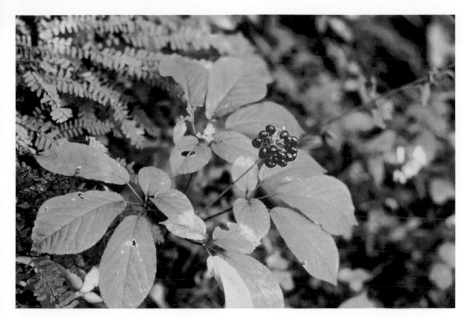

▲ **FIGURE 35-4** Ginseng.

(Fig. 35-5) and *Glycyrrhiza inflata* (Fig. 35-6) are the ones that have displayed the most therapeutic actions, including anti-inflammatory properties. *G. inflata* is actually the Chinese licorice root, while *G. glabra* grows around the Mediterranean Sea, the Middle East, and central and southern Russia.[108]

G. GLABRA Extracts from this more Western species of licorice are an increasingly common ingredient in anti-inflammatory products.[109] Glycyrrhizin is its primary active component, but it also contains polysaccharides and various polyphenols, such as the isoflavone formononetin, which exhibits antioxidant activity.[110] Glycyrrhetic acid (the biologically active metabolite of *G. glabra*) has been reported to have anti-inflammatory activity in subacute and chronic dermatoses, and therefore has been used to treat eczema, pruritus, contact dermatitis, seborrheic dermatitis, and psoriasis.[111] In a double-blind study, Saeedi et al. evaluated the effect of 1% and 2% topical licorice extract preparations on atopic dermatitis in 60 patients. Results indicated that the 2% topical gel was effective in reducing erythema, edema, and pruritus, prompting the researchers to conclude that licorice extract might be effective in treating atopic dermatitis.[111] Studies have shown that glycyrrhetic acid is able to exert a cortisone-like effect, thus inhibiting proinflammatory PGs and LTs.[112] However, licorice (glycyrrhetic acid) has not been demonstrated to be superior to topical corticosteroids in treating acute inflammation, such as atopic dermatitis.[111] The combination of corticosteroids with glycyrrhetic acid has been proven to be effective, however. One study displayed effective potentiation of hydrocortisone activity in skin by the addition of 2% glycyrrhetic acid.[113] In a series of animal studies, Russian scientists found that glyderinine, a derivative of glycyrrhizic acid, exhibited anti-inflammatory, analgesic, as well as antipyretic properties, and concluded that glyderinine is an appropriate ingredient for the treatment of certain skin diseases.[114]

G. INFLATA The primary active ingredient of Chinese licorice root is licochalcone A[115]—a compound that has exhibited anti-inflammatory activity against AA-induced mouse ear edema.[116] It is found in the Eucerin Redness Relief products. In a study assessing the effects of five different chalcones, researchers found that four of the five tested chalcones, including licochalcone A, inhibited the production of proinflammatory cytokines from monocytes and T cells. The investigators concluded that licochalcone A and some of its synthetic analogues may have immunomodulatory effects, potentially rendering them suitable agents for the treatment of infectious and other inflammatory diseases.[117] Chalcones also exhibit activity against oxidative stress. A study assessing their radical scavenging activity revealed that licochalcones B and D potently delay superoxide anion production.[118]

The long history of traditional uses of licorice root and the track record of positive research in the past few decades make licorice one of the most widely researched plants for medicinal purposes. The evidence supporting the medical use of *G. inflata* is slightly less extensive than that of the related species *G. glabra*, but it is similar in terms of the broad range of potential applications.

Mushrooms

Several mushroom species are believed to offer significant potential active ingredients in health-promoting pharmaceutical agents, since these have been used in traditional or folk medicine for thousands of years.[119] In particular, extracts from medicinal mushrooms such as *Ganoderma lucidum* (lingzhi in Chinese, reishi or mannentake in Japanese), *Lentinus edodes* (shiitake in Japanese), *Grifola frondosa* (maitake in Japanese), and *Cordyceps sinensis*, among others, have been used in China, Japan, and Korea to treat

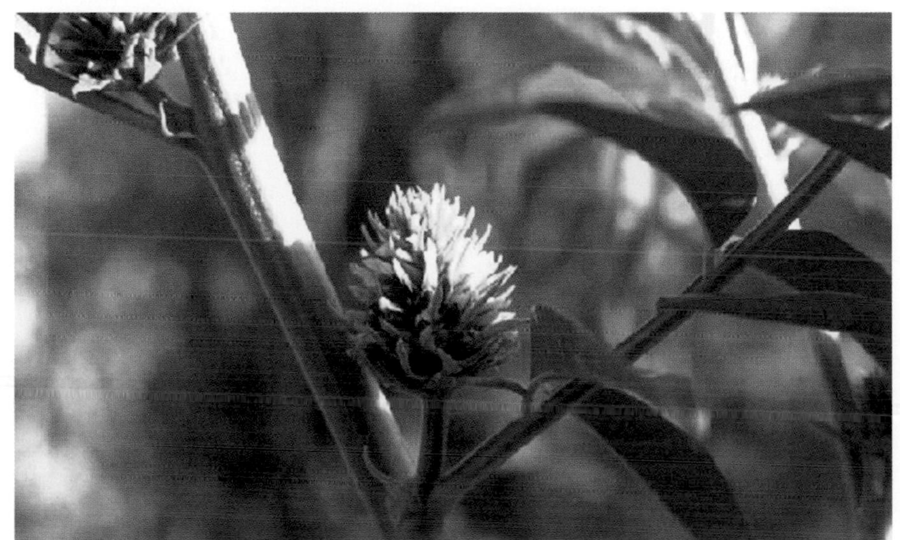

▲ **FIGURE 35-5** Glycyrrhiza glabra is a source of licorice extract. Glabridin is active ingredient.

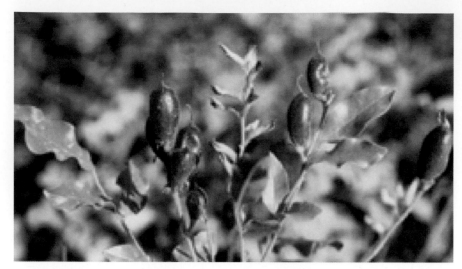

▲ **FIGURE 35-6** Glycyrrhiza inflata from NW China is the source of licochalone.

conditions including allergies, arthritis, bronchitis, gastric ulcer, hepatitis, hyperglycemia, hypertension, inflammation, insomnia, nephritis, neurasthenia, scleroderma, and cancer.[120] Furthermore, these various species have been used in topical dermatologic formulations designed for antiaging purposes.

G. LUCIDUM The dried powder form of Lingzhi has been used since ancient times in China to treat cancer,[120] and currently it continues to be used as a home remedy for the treatment of inflammation and wound healing.[121] Recent research using rats and mice has revealed that the ethanol extract of the mycelium of *G. lucidum* exhibits significant antiperoxidative, anti-inflammatory, antimutagenic,[122] and antioxidant properties.[123] This species of mushroom is one of the most studied botanical treatments in Asia and it has become a popular ingredient in topical skin care products in the West.

C. SINENSIS Mycelium extract of *C. sinensis* has been demonstrated to exhibit immunomodulating activity and the capacity to decrease bacterial growth and dissemination, resulting in improved survival.[124]

G. FRONDOSA Also potentially applicable to dermatology, the extract from *G. frondosa* has been shown to inhibit cutaneous photoaging in UVA-exposed human dermal fibroblasts.[125]

Oatmeal

The skin care application of oats (INCI name: *Avena sativa*) and oat-derived products dates back to 2000 BCE in Egypt and the Arabian Peninsula. In the 19th and early 20th centuries, oatmeal baths were frequently used for the treatment of pruritic inflammatory skin conditions. Somewhat more recently, both Dick and Sompayrac reported in the late 1950s that colloidal oatmeal (CO) baths were demonstrably effective in the management of pediatric atopic dermatitis.[126,127] As a component of the modern dermatologic armamentarium, CO has replaced rolled oats and plain oatmeal. CO is composed of de-hulled oats ground to a fine powder that retains the moisturizing effects of the whole oat grain and disperses more easily in bath water. It can also be added to creams and lotions for use in topical products.

CO consists primarily of polysaccharides (60%–64%), proteins (10%–18%), and lipids (3%–9%). The remaining constituents include enzymes (such as superoxide dismutase), saponins, vitamins, flavonoids, and inhibitors of PG synthesis. Oat lipids contribute to the viscosity of CO and help decrease transepidermal water loss (TEWL), a key factor in skin dryness. In addition, oatmeal proteins exhibit emulsification, hydration, and antioxidant activity. CO proteins and polysaccharides bind to skin and provide a protective barrier to external insults. The proteins further act as a buffer against strong acids and bases.[128]

The combination of components and properties of CO renders it suitable for various uses in the care of inflammatory skin conditions, such as cleaning, moisturizing, protecting (i.e., barrier preservation), and relieving pruritus in inflamed skin. In fact, oatmeal is one of the few natural products recognized by the FDA as an effective skin protectant.[129] As a consequence, CO is one of the few botanicals subject to FDA regulation.[129] The range of dermatologic applications for CO is extensive and includes adjunctive therapy in inflammatory and pruritic skin conditions such as atopic dermatitis; irritant and ACD including contact to poison ivy, oak and sumac; insect bites; diaper dermatitis; cercarial dermatitis; xerosis; ichthyosis; urticaria; and sunburn.[126,128,130,131] CO also prevents and repairs damage caused by environmental insults such as UV radiation, smoke, bacteria, and free radicals.[109]

Published clinical studies of CO have generally yielded positive results that continue to support the therapeutic use of oatmeal. In a clinical model of skin irritation with sodium lauryl sulfate, two different types of CO products significantly reduced the amount of experimentally induced irritation and inflammation.[132] In a different clinical study, two shower gels were evaluated for relief of pruritus in burn patients.[133] Both gels contained liquid paraffin but only one also contained 5% CO. The oatmeal-containing compound was associated with significantly greater reduction in patient-reported pruritus and requests for antihistamines. Furthermore, Boisnic et al. developed a clinical model of cutaneous inflammation involving the effects of an oatmeal extract on tissue fragments exposed to vasoactive intestinal peptide, a proinflammatory neuromediator.[134] The application of vasoactive intestinal peptide increased inflammation, which was significantly ameliorated by treatment with the oatmeal extract.

The therapeutic and cosmetic uses of oatmeal have been enhanced by the isolation and identification of specific oat components. Specifically, avenanthramides, a newly discovered group of polypenolic alkaloids, have been found exclusively in oats. As a group, phenolics display a broad range of biologic activities including prevention of inflammation and oxidation.[135] In fact, phenolics are the strongest antioxidants found in nature,[136] although within this class of compounds, individual substances exert varying levels of antioxidant activity. Oat phenolic compounds including avenanthramides have been identified as potent antioxidants that scavenge reactive oxygen and nitrogen species.[135] Furthermore, they have been reported to inhibit PG biosynthesis nearly as well as the synthetic anti-inflammatory agent indomethacin.[137] Another recent study provided more evidence that avenanthramides evince potent anti-inflammatory activity.[138] In this research, keratinocytes were incubated with an inducer of proinflammatory IL-8 in the presence of vehicle or avenanthramides. The inclusion of avenanthramides reduced the release of the proinflammatory cytokine IL-8 by 10% to 25%. Various other preclinical and preliminary clinical studies have demonstrated a wide range of potential benefits from topical compounds that contain avenanthramides, including: reduction of histamine-induced itch in humans; inhibition of NF-κB, thus inhibiting the activation of inflammatory pathways in the skin; and the amelioration of skin irritation and erythema induced by exposure to UVB irradiation.

Selenium

Selenium is an essential trace element found in the human body, and it is thought to have anticarcinogenic, anti-inflammatory, antioxidant, and therefore antiaging properties. Water, soil, and plant foods are the major sources of selenium in most countries. It is also found in meat, fish, Brazil nuts, shellfish, dairy products, cereals, and cereal products. Selenium is a component of the water used in the La Roche-Posay spa in France that was founded to treat atopic dermatitis patients and psoriasis patients. Many of the La Roche Posay products, including the thermal spring water, contain selenium. The anti-inflammatory role of selenium is very well expressed in one of the reductive metabolic pathways in humans: selenium is the vital antioxidant required to form glutathione peroxidase, one of our most important natural antioxidant defenses. The function of this essential antioxidant enzyme (discussed in section "Role of Free Radicals") is to protect cell membranes from oxidative deterioration, a role that it shares with vitamin E. In fact, studies have concluded that vitamin E and selenium act synergistically to deliver such protection.[139]

Selenium also exerts anti-inflammatory activity in preventing the production of inflammatory cytokines. One study showed that after damage to the skin from UV exposure, inflammatory cytokines inhibited the immune response, thus increasing the number of damaged skin cells.[140] These inflammatory cytokines also lead to the formation of wrinkles and premature aging of the skin. Selenium can decrease production of these cytokines, thereby preventing inflammation. Finally, selenium enhances both humoral and cellular immunity, increasing the host response to infection.[141]

As a result of its antioxidant and anti-inflammatory properties, selenium has been added to topical skin care products as well as natural spring water vaporizers for the skin. The current recommended daily allowance of oral selenium is 55 μg for both men and women. However, cancer researchers are currently considering daily doses as high as 400 μg. It must be noted that selenium toxicity, or selenosis, is possible. High doses of selenium are neurotoxic and can cause hair loss, nail loss, and dermatitis, as well as gastrointestinal upset. Despite advertising claims, most available topical formulations contain very low concentrations of selenium, which are not well absorbed by the skin. Formulated as selenium sulfide, selenium does not penetrate the skin. However, cutaneous selenium absorption can be achieved with L-selenomethionine. Recent animal and human studies have found that when taken orally or applied topically in the form of L-selenomethionine, selenium demonstrated protection against both daily and excessive UV damage. In one study a decade ago, treated patients experienced decreased skin inflammation and pigmentation, plus a delay in the onset and a decrease in the incidence of skin cancer.[142] In a different study performed in the 1990s, researchers at the University of Edinburgh, Scotland, UK, concluded that oral selenium resulted in significant protective effects against UV radiation-induced damage to skin cells. The researchers did not examine topical selenium.[141] Although these early studies of the effects of both oral and topical selenium are promising, more double-blind, placebo-controlled trials are needed to support selenium as an adjunct to the antiaging product market.

Turmeric/Curcumin

Turmeric (INCI name: *Curcuma longa*) is best known as a spice used primarily in Asian cuisine, particularly in curry and prepared mustard. It has a long history in both Chinese and Ayurvedic (Indian) medicine as an anti-inflammatory agent.[143] Curcumin (diferuloylmethane) is the yellow pigment that corresponds to the key biologically active component of turmeric and has been proven to have more acute anti-inflammatory effects when compared to the volatile oil fraction of turmeric.[144] When used orally, this herb inhibits LT formation as well as platelet aggregation and stabilizes neutrophilic lysosomal membranes, thus inhibiting inflammation at the cellular level.[145] A study by Srimal and Dhawan more than 30 years ago showed that the anti-inflammatory activity of curcumin may be superior even to that of ibuprofen.[146] Moreover, it has been demonstrated to exhibit significant wound healing, anticarcinogenic and antioxidant properties. Finally, curcumin produces different effects depending on the dosing level; at low dose it can be a PG inhibitor, while at higher levels it stimulates the adrenal glands to secrete cortisone.[147]

SUMMARY

Inflammation is a multifactorial, convoluted process that plays a vital defensive role in protecting living tissues from an expansive variety of potentially deleterious injuries. However, protracted inflammation itself can pose danger to the very tissues and host organism for which the cascading events of the inflammatory process were launched to protect. Indeed, this is the case in sensitive skin disorders in which inflammation plays a characteristic role, as discussed in Chapter 12. In addition, inflammation is thought to play a role in skin aging. As such, anti-inflammatory agents have a crucial role to play in medicine as a whole, and clearly in the practice of dermatology. Various modalities can help decrease cutaneous inflammation including topical skin care formulations, water used in spas, diet, supplements, as well as prescription and over-the-counter medications.

REFERENCES

1. Gallin JI, Goldstein IM, Snyderman R. Overview. In: Gallin JI, Goldstein IM, Synderman R, eds. *Inflammation: Basic Principles and Clinical Correlates*. 2nd ed. New York, NY: Raven Press, 1991:1–4.
2. Williams RH, Stedman TL. *Stedman's Medical Dictionary*. 25th ed. Philadelphia, PA: Williams & Wilkins; 1990.
3. Cotran RS, Kumar V, Collins T, eds. *Robbins Pathological Basis of Disease*. Philadelphia, PA: WB Saunders Co; 1999:7216–7335.
4. Kimball ES. *Cytokines and Inflammation*. Boca Raton, FL: CRC Press; 1991.
5. Needleman P, Turk J, Jakschik BA, et al. Arachidonic acid metabolism. *Annu Rev Biochem*. 1986;55:69.
6. Smith WL. Prostanoid biosynthesis and mechanisms of action. *Am J Physiol*. 1992;263:F181.
7. Gabay C, Kushner I. Acute-phase proteins and other systemic responses to inflammation. *New Engl J Med*. 1999;340: 448.
8. Cavaillon JM. Contribution of cytokines to inflammatory mechanisms. *Pathol Biol (Paris)*. 1993;41:799.
9. Leirisalo-Repo M. The present knowledge of the inflammatory process and the inflammatory mediators. *Pharmacol Toxicol*. 1994;75(suppl 2):1.
10. Feghali CA, Wright TM. Cytokines in acute and chronic inflammation. *Front Biosci*. 1997;2:d12.

11. Charo IF, Ransohoff RM. The many roles of chemokines and chemokine receptors in inflammation. *N Engl J Med.* 2006;354:610.
12. Kitamura Y. Heterogeneity of mast cells and phenotypic change between subpopulations. *Annu Rev Immunol.* 1989; 7:59.
13. Metcalfe DD, Baram D, Mekori YA. Mast cells. *Physiol Rev.* 1997;77:1033.
14. Galli SJ. Mast cells and basophils. *Curr Opin Hematol.* 2000;7:32.
15. Sayama K, Diehn M, Matsuda K, et al. Transcriptional response of human mast cells stimulated via the Fc(epsilon)RI and identification of mast cells as a source of IL-11. *BMC Immunol.* 2002;3:5.
16. Kawkami T, Galli SJ. Regulation of mast-cell and basophil function and survival by IgE. *Nat Rev Immunol.* 2002;2:773.
17. Mycek MJ, Harvey RA, Champe PC. Autacoids and autacoid antagonists. In: Harvey RA, Champe PC, eds. *Lippincott's Illustrated Reviews: Pharmacology.* 2nd ed. Philadelphia, PA: Lippincott Williams & Wilkins; 2000:419-428.
18. Simons FE. Advances in H1-antihistamines. *N Engl J Med.* 2004;351:2203.
19. Akdis CA, Blaser K. Histamine in the immune regulation of allergic inflammation. *J Allergy Clin Immunol.* 2003;112:15.
20. Simons FE, Simons KJ. The pharmacology and use of H1-receptor-antagonist drugs. *N Engl J Med.* 1994;330:1663.
21. Sugimoto Y, Iba Y, Nakamura Y, et al. Pruritus-associated response mediated by cutaneous histamine H3 receptors. *Clin Exp Allergy.* 2004;34:456.
22. Babior BM. Phagocytes and oxidative stress. *Am J Med.* 2003;109:33.
23. Beckman JS, Koppenol WH. Nitric oxide, superoxide, and peroxynitrite: the good, the bad, and the ugly. *Am J Physiol.* 1996;271:C1424.
24. Guzik TJ, Korbut T, Adamek-Guzik T. Nitric oxide and superoxide in inflammation and immune regulation. *J Physiol Pharmacol.* 2003;54:469.
25. Barrington R, Zhang M, Fischer M, et al. The role of complement in inflammation and adaptive immunity. *Immunol Rev.* 2001;180:5.
26. Costa-Neto CM, Dillenburg-Pilla P, Heinrich TA, et al. Participation of kallikrein-kinin system in different pathologies. *Int Immunopharmacol.* 2008; 8:135.
27. Randal A, Skidgel RA, Erdös EG. Histamine, bradykinin, and their antagonists. In: Brunton L, Lazo J, Parker K, eds. *Goodman & Gilman's The Pharmacological Basis of Therapeutics.* 11th ed. New York, NY: McGraw-Hill; 2006:629–652.
28. Elliott DF, Horton EW, Lewis GP. Actions of pure bradykinin. *J Physiol.* 1960;153:473.
29. Robert C, Kupper TS. Inflammatory skin diseases, T cells, and immune surveillance. *N Engl J Med.* 1999;341: 1817.
30. Barnes PJ, Karin M. Nuclear factor-κB: a pivotal transcription factor in chronic inflammatory diseases. *N Engl J Med.* 1997;336:1066.
31. Kupper TS. Immune and inflammatory processes in cutaneous tissues: mechanisms and speculations. *J Clin Invest.* 1990;86:1783.
32. Lee RT, Briggs WH, Cheng GC, et al. Mechanical deformation promotes secretion of IL-1 alpha and IL-1 receptor antagonist. *J Immunol.* 1997;159:5084.
33. Rosette C, Karin M. Ultraviolet light and osmotic stress: activation of the JNK cascade through multiple growth factor and cytokine receptors. *Science.* 1996;274:1194.
34. Picker LJ, Michie SA, Rott LS, et al. A unique phenotype of skin associated lymphocytes in humans. Preferential expression of HECA-452 epitope by benign and malignant T cells at cutaneous sites. *Am J Pathol.* 1990;136:1053.
35. Steffen C. The introduction of topical corticosteroids. *Skin Med.* 2003;2:304.
36. Spies TD, Stone RE. Effect of local application of synthetic cortisone acetate on lesions of iritis and uveitis, of allergic contact dermatitis, and of psoriasis. *South Med J.* 1950;43:871.
37. Rasmussen N. Steroids in arms science, government, industry, and the hormones of the adrenal cortex in the United States 1930–1950. *Med Hist.* 2002;46:299.
38. Tuckermann JP, Kleiman A, McPherson KG, et al. Molecular mechanisms of glucocorticoids in the control of inflammation and lymphocyte apoptosis. *Crit. Rev Clin Lab Sci.* 2005;42:71.
39. Kim SW, Rhee HJ, Ko J, et al. Inhibition of cytosolic phospholipase A2 by annexin I: specific interaction model and mapping of the interaction site. *J Biol Chem.* 2001;27:15712.
40. Rhen T, Cidlowski JA. Antiinflammatory action of glucocorticoids —new mechanisms for old drugs. *New Engl J Med.* 2005;353:1711.
41. De Bosscher K, Vanden Berghe W, Haegeman G. Interplay between the glucocorticoid receptor and nuclear factor-kappaB or activator protein-1: molecular mechanisms for gene repression. *Endocr Rev.* 2003;24:488.
42. Tanabe T, Tohnai N. Cyclooxygenase isozymes and their gene structures and expression. *Prostaglandins Other Lipid Mediat.* 2002;95:68-69.
43. Cohen DE, Heidary N. Treatment of irritant and allergic contact dermatitis. *Dermatol Ther.* 2004;17:334.
44. Marks R. Adverse side effects from the use of topical corticosteroids. In: Maibach HI, Surger C, eds. *Topical Corticosteroids.* Basel, Switzerland: Karger; 1992:170-183.
45. Walsh P, Aeling JL, Huff L, et al. Hypothalamus-pituitary-adrenal axis suppression by superpotent topical steroids. *J Am Acad Dermatol.* 1993;29: 501.
46. Hengge UR, Ruzicka T, Schwartz RA, et al. Adverse effects of topical glucocorticosteroids. *J Am Acad Dermatol.* 2006;54:1.
47. Gebhard KL, Maibach HI. Relationship between systemic corticosteroids and osteonecrosis. *Am J Clin Dermatol.* 2001; 2:377.
48. Becker B. The effect of topical corticosteroids in secondary glaucomas. *Arch Ophthalmol.* 1964;72:769.
49. Becker B. Cataracts and topical corticosteroids. *Am J Ophthalmol.* 1964;58:872.
50. Bornhovd E, Burgdorf WH, Wollenberg A. Macrolactam immunomodulators for topical treatment of inflammatory skin diseases. *J Am Acad Dermatol.* 2001;45: 736.
51. FDA Public Health Advisory—Elidel (pimecrolimus) Cream and Protopic (tacrolimus) Ointment, March 10, 2005. http://www.fda.gov/cder/drug/advisory/elidel_protopic.htm. Accessed June 5, 2007.
52. Lauerma AI, Stein BD, Homey B, et al. Topical FK506: suppression of allergic and irritant contact dermatitis in the guinea pig. *Arch Dermatol Res.* 1994; 286:337.
53. Saripalli YV, Gadzia J, Belsito D. Tacrolimus ointment 0.1% in the treatment of nickel-induced allergic contact dermatitis. *J Am Acad Dermatol.* 2003;49:477.
54. Lauerma AI, Maibach HI, Granlund H, et al. Inhibition of contact allergy reactions by topical FK506. *Lancet.* 1992; 340:556.
55. Sengoku T, Morita K, Sakuma S, et al. Possible inhibitory mechanism of FK506 (tacrolimus hydrate) ointment for atopic dermatitis based on animal models. *Eur J Pharmacol.* 1999;379:183.
56. Gupta AK, Chow M. Pimecrolimus: a review. *J Eur Acad Dermatol Venereol.* 2003;17:493.
57. Pitts MR. Pediatric Advisory Committee Meeting of the FDA Center for Drug Evaluation and Research. http://www.fda.gov/ohrms/dockets/ac/05/slides/2005–4089s2_01_07_Pitts.ppt. Accessed June 5, 2007.
58. Eichenfield L. Therapeutics in pediatric dermatology. Program and abstracts of the 64th Annual Meeting of the American Academy of Dermatology, Symposium 325: Therapeutics Symposium; March 3–7, 2006; San Francisco, CA.
59. Smith KJ, Selton H. Arachidonic acid-derived bioactive lipids: their role and the role for their inhibitors in dermatology. *J Cutan Med Surg.* 2002;6: 241.
60. Kaminsky A. Less common methods to treat acne. *Dermatology.* 2003;206:68.
61. Wong RC, Kang S, Heezen JL, et al. Oral ibuprofen and tetracycline for the treatment of acne vulgaris. *J Am Acad Dermatol.* 1984;11:1076.
62. Funt LS. Oral ibuprofen and minocycline for the treatment of resistant acne vulgaris. *J Am Acad Dermatol.* 1985;13: 524.
63. Hughes GS, Francom SF, Means LK, et al. Synergistic effects of oral nonsteroidal drugs and topical corticosteroids in the therapy of sunburn in humans. *Dermatology.* 1992;184:54.
64. Black AK, Fincham N, Greaves MW, et al. Time course changes in levels of arachidonic acid and prostaglandin D2, E2, F2 alpha in human skin following ultraviolet-B irradiation. *Br J Clin Pharmacol.* 1980;10:453.
65. Wu KK. Salicylates and their spectrum of activity. *Anti-Inflamm Anti-Allergy Agent Med Chem.* 2007;6:278.
66. Kligman D, Kligman AM. Salicylic acid peels for the treatment of photoaging. *Dermatol Surg.* 1998;24:325.
67. Harvey SC. Antiseptis and disinfectants; fungicides; ectoparasiticides. In: Gilman AG, Goodman LS, Rall TW, Murad F, eds. *Goodman and Gilman's The Pharmacological Basis of Therapeutics.* 7th

ed. New York, NY: MacMillan; 1985: 959-979.

68. Lin AN, Reimer RJ, Carter DM. Sulfur revisited. *J Am Acad Dermatol.* 1988; 18:553.
69. Konaklieva MI, Plotkin BJ. Anti-inflammatory sulfur-containing agents with additional modes of action. *Anti-Inflamm Anti-Allergy Agent Med Chem.* 2007;6:271.
70. Combes FC. Colloidal sulfur: some pharmacodynamic considerations and their therapeutic application in seborrheic dermatoses. *NY State J Med.* 1946; 46:401.
71. McEvoy GK, McQuarrie GM, eds. *Drug information 86, American Hospital Formulary Service.* Bethesda, MD: American Society of Hospital Pharmacists; 1986:1800-1802.
72. Sheard C. *Treatment of Skin Diseases: A Manual.* Chicago, IL: Year Book; 1978: 21-22.
73. Plexion SCT™ (sodium sulfacetamide 10% and sulfur 5%), [package insert]. Scottsdale, AZ, Medicis, The Dermatology Company, 2001.
74. Tarimci N, Sener S, Kilinç T. Topical sodium sulfacetamide/sulfur lotion. *J Clin Pharm Ther.* 1997;22:301.
75. Gupta AK, Nicol K. The use of sulfur in dermatology. *J Drugs Dermatol.* 2004;3: 427.
76. Baumann LS. Less-known botanical cosmeceuticals. *Dermatol Ther.* 2007;20: 330.
77. Baumann LS. Aloe vera. *Skin & Allergy News.* 2003;34:32.
78. Marshall JM. Aloe vera gel: What is the evidence? *Pharm J.* 1990;244:360.
79. Reynolds T, Dweck AC. Aloe vera leaf gel: a review update. *J Ethnopharmacol.* 1999;68:3.
80. Briggs C. Herbal medicine: aloe. *Can Pharm J.* 1995;128:48.
81. Talmadge J, Chavez J, Jacobs L, et al. Fractionation of aloe vera L. inner gel, purification and molecular profiling of activity. *Int Immunopharmacol.* 2004;4: 1757.
82. Lee JK, Lee MK, Yun YP. Acemannan purified from Aloe vera induces phenotypic and functional maturation of immature dendritic cells. *Int Immunopharmacol.* 2001;1:1275.
83. Hutter JA, Salman M, Stavinoha WB, et al. Antiinflammatory C-glucosyl chromone from Aloe barbadensis. *J Nat Prod.* 1996;59:541.
84. Habeeb F, Stables G, Bradbury F, et al. The inner gel component of Aloe vera suppresses bacterial-induced pro-inflammatory cytokines from human immune cells. *Methods.* 2007;42:388.
85. Klein AD, Penneys NS. Aloe vera. *J Am Acad Dermatol.* 1988;18:714.
86. O'Hara M, Kiefer D, Farrell K, et al. A review of 12 commonly used medicinal herbs. *Arch Fam Med.* 1998;7:523.
87. Dockrell TR, Leever JS. An overview of herbal medications with implications for the school nurse. *J Sch Nurs.* 2000; 16:53.
88. Safayhi H, Sabieraj J, Sailer ER, et al. Chamazulene: an antioxidant-type inhibitor of leukotriene B4 formation. *Planta Med.* 1994;60:410.
89. Shipochliev T, Dimitrov A, Aleksandrova E. Anti-inflammatory action of a group of plant extracts. *Vet Med Nauki.* 1981; 18:87.
90. Lee KG, Shibamoto T. Determination of antioxidant potential of volatile extracts isolated from various herbs and spices. *J Agric Food Chem.* 2002;50:4947.
91. Máday E, Szöke E, Muskáth Z, et al. A study of the production of essential oils in chamomile hairy root cultures. *Eur J Drug Metab Pharmacokinet.* 1999;24:303.
92. Paulsen E, Chistensen LP, Andersen KE. Cosmetics and herbal remedies with Compositae plant extracts - are they tolerated by Compositae-allergic patients? *Contact Dermatitis.* 2008;58:15.
93. Borge GI, Vogt G, Nilsson A. Intermediates and products formed during fatty acid alpha-oxidation in cucumber (Cucumis sativus). *Lipids.* 1999;34:661.
94. Isely D. *One Hundred and One Botanists.* Ames, IA: Iowa State University Press; 1994:10–13.
95. Gunther RT, ed. *The Greek Herbal of Dioscorides.* Oxford, UK: Oxford University Press; 1933.
96. Vogler BK, Pittler MH, Ernst E. Feverfew as a preventive treatment for migraine: a systematic review. *Cephalalgia.* 1998; 18:704.
97. Kwok BH, Koh B, Ndubuisi MI, et al. The anti-inflammatory natural product parthenolide from the medicinal herb Feverfew directly binds to and inhibits IκB kinase. *Chem Biol.* 2001;8:759.
98. Hausen BM. A 6-year experience with compositae mix. *Am J Contact Dermat.* 1996;7:94.
99. Martin K, Sur R, Liebel F, et al. Parthenolide-depleted Feverfew (Tanacetum parthenium) protects skin from UV irradiation and external aggression. *Arch Dermatol Res.* 2008;300. 69.
100. Kitts DD, Wijewickreme AN, Hu C. Antioxidant properties of a North American ginseng extract. *Mol Cell Biochem.* 2000;203:1.
101. Park S, Yeo M, Jin JH, et al. Rescue of Helicobacter pylori-induced cytotoxicity by red ginseng. *Dig Dis Sci.* 2005;50:1218.
102. Volate SR, Davenport DM, Muga SJ, et al. Modulation of aberrant crypt foci and apoptosis by dietary herbal supplements (quercetin, curcumin, silymarin, ginseng and rutin). *Carcinogenesis.* 2005; 26:1450.
103. Kang KA, Kim YW, Kim SU, et al. G1 phase arrest of the cell cycle by a ginseng metabolite, compound K, in U937 human monocytic leukamia cells. *Arch Pharm Res.* 2005;28:685.
104. Ahn JY, Choi IS, Shim JY, et al. The immunomodulator ginsan induces resistance to experimental sepsis by inhibiting Toll-like receptor-mediated inflammatory signals. *Eur J Immunol.* 2006;36:37.
105. Keum YS, Han SS, Chun KS, et al. Inhibitory effects of the ginsenoside Rg3 on phorbol ester-induced cyclooxygenase-2 expression, NF-kappaB activation and tumor promotion. *Mutat Res.* 2003;75:523-524.
106. Rhule A, Navarro S, Smith JR, et al. Panax notoginseng attenuates LPS-induced pro-inflammatory mediators in RAW264.7 cells. *J Ethnopharmacol.* 2006; 106:121.
107. Gibson MR. Glycyrrhiza in old and new perspectives. *Lloydia.* 1978;41:348.
108. Agarwal R, Wang ZY, Mukhtar H. Inhibition of mouse skin tumor-initiating activity of DMBA by chronic oral feeding of glycyrrhizin in drinking water. *Nutr Cancer.* 1991;15:187.
109. Aburjai T, Natsheh FM. Plants used in cosmetics. *Phytother Res.* 2003;17:987.
110. Wang ZY, Nixon DW. Licorice and cancer. *Nutr Cancer.* 2001;39:1.
111. Saeedi M, Morteza-Semnani K, Ghoreishi MR. The treatment of atopic dermatitis with licorice gel. *J Dermatolog Treat.* 2003;14:153.
112. Ohuchi K, Kamada Y, Levine L, et al. Glycyrrhizin inhibits prostaglandin E2 production by activated peritoneal macrophages from rats. *Prostaglandins Med.* 1981;7:457.
113. Teelucksingh S, Mackie AD, Burt D, et al. Potentiation of hydrocortisone activity in skin by glycyrrhetinic acid. *Lancet.* 1990;335:1060.
114. Azimov MM, Zakirov UB, Radzhapova ShD. Pharmacological study of the anti-inflammatory agent glyderinine. *Farmakol Toksikol.* 1988;51:90.
115. Friis Møller A, Chen M, Fuursted K, et al. In vitro antimycobacterial and antilegionella activity of licochalcone A from Chinese licorice roots. *Planta Med.* 2002;68:416.
116. Shibata S, Inoue H, Iwata S, et al. Inhibitory effects of licochalcone A isolated from Glycyrrhiza inflata root on inflammatory ear edema and tumour promotion in mice. *Planta Med.* 1991; 57:221.
117. Barfod L, Kemp K, Hansen M, et al. Chalcones from Chinese liquorice inhibit proliferation of T cells and production of cytokines. *Int Immunopharmacol.* 2002;2:545.
118. Haraguchi H, Ishikawa H, Mizutani K, et al. Antioxidative and superoxide scavenging activities of retrochalcones in Glycyrrhiza inflata. *Bioorg Med Chem.* 1998;6:339.
119. Wasser SP. Medicinal mushrooms as a source of antitumor and immunomodulating polysaccharides. *Appl Microbiol Biotechnol.* 2002;60:258.
120. Sliva D. Ganoderma lucidum (Reishi) in cancer treatment. *Integr Cancer Ther.* 2003;2:358.
121. Sliva D, Sedlak M, Slivova V, et al. Biologic activity of spores and dried powder from Ganoderma lucidum for the inhibition of highly invasive human breast and prostate cancer cells. *J Altern Complement Med.* 2003;9:491.
122. Lakshmi B, Ajith TA, Sheena N, et al. Antiperoxidative, anti-inflammatory, and antimutagenic activities of ethanol extract of the mycelium of Ganoderma lucidum occurring in South India. *Teratog Carcinog Mutagen.* 2003;(suppl 1):85.
123. Xie JT, Wang CZ, Wicks S, et al. Ganoderma lucidum extract inhibits proliferation of SW 480 human colorectal cancer cells. *Exp Oncol.* 2006;28:25.
124. Kuo CF, Chen CC, Luo YH, et al. Cordyceps sinensis mycelium protects mice from group A streptococcal infection. *J Med Microbiol.* 2005;54:795.
125. Bae JT, Sim GS, Lee DH, et al. Production of exopolysaccharide from mycelial culture of Grifola frondosa and

its inhibitory effect on matrix metalloproteinase-1 expression in UV-irradiated human dermal fibroblasts. *FEMS Microbiol Lett*. 2005;251:347.
126. Dick LA. Colloidal emollient baths in pediatric dermatoses. *Arch Pediatr*. 1958;75:506.
127. Sompayrac LM, Ross C. Colloidal oatmeal in atopic dermatitis of the young. *J Fla Med Assoc*. 1959;45:1411.
128. Grais ML. Role of colloidal oatmeal in dermatologic treatment of the aged. *AMA Arch Derm Syphilol*. 1953;68:402.
129. US Food and Drug Administration. Title 21: Food and Drugs, Chapter 1: Food and Drug Administration Department of Health and Humans Services, Subchapter D: Drugs for human use, Part 347: Skin protectant drug products for over-the-counter human use. US Dept of Health and Human Services, FDA;21 CFR347. April 1, 2007.
130. Smith GC. The treatment of various dermatoses associated with dry skin. *JSC Med Assoc*. 1958;54:282.
131. Dick LA. Colloidal emollient baths in geriatric dermatoses. *Skin (Los Angeles)*. 1962;1:89.
132. Vié K, Cours-Darne S, Vienne MP, et al. Modulating effects of oatmeal extracts in the sodium lauryl sulfate skin irritancy model. *Skin Pharmacol Appl Skin Physiol*. 2002;15:120.
133. Matheson JD, Clayton J, Muller MJ. The reduction of itch during burn wound healing. *J Burn Care Rehabil*. 2001;22:76.
134. Boisnic S, Branchet-Gumila MC, Coutanceau C. Inhibitory effect of oatmeal extract oligomer on vasoactive intestinal peptide-induced inflammation in surviving human skin. *Int J Tissue React*. 2003;25:41.
135. Chen CY, Milbury PE, Kwak HK, et al. Avenanthramides and phenolic acids from oats are bioavailable and act synergistically with vitamin C to enhance hamster and human LDL resistance to oxidation. *J Nutr*. 2004;134:1459.
136. Tsao R, Akhtar MH. Neutraceuticals and functional foods: I. Current trend in phytochemical antioxidant research. *J Food Agric Environ*. 2005;3:10.
137. Saeed SA, Butt NM, McDonald-Gibson WJ, et al. Inhibitors of prostaglandin biosynthesis in extracts of oat (Avena sativa) seeds. *Biochem Soc Trans*. 1981;9:444.
138. Wallo W, Nebus J, Nystrand G. Agents with adjunctive potential in atopic dermatitis. *J Am Acad Dermatol*. 2007; 56(suppl 2):AB70.tract P712.
139. Vitoux D, Chappuis P, Arnaud J, et al. Selenium, glutathione peroxidase, peroxides and platelet functions. *Ann Biol Clin (Paris)*. 1996;54:181.
140. Leverkus M, Yaar M, Eller MS, et al. Post-transcriptional regulation of UV induced TNF-alpha expression. *J Invest Dermatol*. 1998;110:353.
141. McKenzie RC. Selenium, ultraviolet radiation and the skin. *Clin Exp Dermatol*. 2000;25:631.
142. Stewart MS, Cameron GS, Pence BC. Antioxidant nutrients protect against UVB-induced oxidative damage to DNA of mouse keratinocytes in culture. *J Invest Dermatol*. 1996;106:1086.
143. Rico MJ. Rising drug costs: the impact on dermatology. *Skin Therapy Lett*. 2000;5:1.
144. Arora RB, Kapoor V, Basu N, et al. Anti-inflammatory studies on Curcuma longa (turmeric). *Indian J Med Res*. 1971;59:1289.
145. Srivastava R. Inhibition of neutrophil response by curcumin. *Agents Actions*. 1989;28:298.
146. Srimal RC, Dhawan BN. Pharmacology of diferuloyl methane (curcumin), a non-steroidal anti-inflammatory agent. *J Pharm Pharmacol*. 1973;25:447.
147. Srivastava R, Srimal RC. Modification of certain inflammation-induced biochemical changes by curcumin. *Indian J Med Res*. 1985;81:215.

CHAPTER 36

Fragrance

Edmund Weisberg, MS
Leslie Baumann, MD

Innovative products and procedures inundate medicine and the specialty of dermatology at a dizzying pace. At the same time, the billion-dollar beauty industry continues to expand, with few if any signs of a decline. The global fragrance and flavor market represents a significant and lucrative subdivision of the beauty market and is constantly testing various fragrance ingredients to stay ahead of encroaching regulation and increased rates of sensitization. Indeed, while contact allergy to fragrance is not a presentation seen in the dermatologist's office as frequently as acne, for example, it is a common problem seen often throughout the world. This is not surprising since fragrances are virtually omnipresent in products that come into contact with the skin, for example, soaps, body lotions and moisturizers, shampoos, deodorants, shaving products, cosmetics, perfumes, sunscreens, and dental products, as well as food products, detergents, and even air fresheners. Furthermore, as stated in Chapter 18, fragrances consistently place among the top 10 contact dermatitis allergens and represent the second most common allergen family associated with allergic contact dermatitis, second only to nickel, as well as the most often cited cause of such reactions to cosmetic products. This looms as an especially important realization given the general rise in the incidence of contact allergy to various fragrances and the fact that epidemiologic and human allergen sensitization studies have shown that individuals who are found to be sensitive to one allergen through patch testing are at significantly greater risk of having a second allergen identified.[1–3] Particularly, given the greater expertise expected of cosmetic dermatologists regarding agents intended to beautify the skin, it is incumbent upon such specialists to have a strong working knowledge of the primary fragrances identified as provoking allergic reactions. This chapter will focus briefly on selected problematic fragrances, primarily on the worst offenders found within the Fragrance Mix (FM) I and FM II.

DEMOGRAPHICS AND SIGNIFICANCE

An epidemiologic survey in the United Kingdom published in 2004 reported that 23% of women and 13.8% of men displayed adverse reactions to a personal care product (e.g., deodorants and perfumes, skin care products, hair care products, and nail cosmetics) over the course of 1 year.[4] More recently, in a 1999 to 2006 Brazilian study of 176 patients (154 women and 22 men) seen in a private office who complained of dermatoses resulting from cosmetics, 45% exhibited dermatoses linked to cosmetics and 14% had skin lesions that were found to be caused by inappropriate use of cosmetics.[5] In addition, several studies have demonstrated that approximately 10% of dermatologic patients who are patch tested for 20 to 100 ingredients exhibit allergic sensitivity to at least one ingredient common in cosmetic products.[4] Fragrances and preservatives are the most common allergens and women aged 20 to 60 years represent the demographic group that experiences the majority of these reactions.[6] Individuals who are overexposed to skin care products and patients with an impaired stratum corneum, as manifested by dry skin, reportedly have increased susceptibility to allergic reactions.[7] Contact allergy caused by fragrances is typically seen as axillary dermatitis, dermatitis of the face (including the eyelids) and neck, hand dermatitis, and eruptions in locations where perfume may be dabbed on or sprayed such as the wrists and behind the ears.[8] It is important to note that while the overall risk of allergic reaction to fragrances is low, the absolute numbers of individuals affected by fragrance allergy is significant, and estimated to be 1% of the general population.[8]

FRAGRANCE MIX I

The FM I is composed of eight different substances, including oak moss, isoeugenol, eugenol, cinnamic aldehyde, geraniol, hydroxycitronellal, cinnamic alcohol, and α-amyl cinnamic aldehyde.[9] The FM I (Table 36-1), known simply as the FM for several years, was introduced in 1977 by Larsen and widely adopted.[10] This was a full 20 years after the first report of an allergic reaction to fragrance-based chemicals in 1957.[11]

TABLE 36-1
Fragrance Mix (FM) I

Oak moss
Isoeugenol
Eugenol
Cinnamic aldehyde
Geraniol
Hydroxycitronellal
Cinnamic alcohol
α-Amyl cinnamic aldehyde

In a review of patch test data of 25,545 patients from 1980 to 1996, Buckley et al. found that oak moss was the most common allergen throughout the period. Oak moss contains the potent allergens chloroatranol and atranol.[12,13] Sensitivity to isoeugenol and α-amyl cinnamic aldehyde increased during the 16 year period under review; sensitivity to eugenol and geraniol remained stable; reaction to hydroxycitronellal declined slowly; and precipitous drop offs in sensitivity frequency were associated with cinnamic aldehyde and cinnamic alcohol. Consequently, the authors identified the latter two FM I ingredients as rare fragrance allergens at this juncture.[14] Bruze et al. have subsequently shown, however, that cinnamic aldehyde in the concentration range of 0.01% to 0.32% when applied twice daily on healthy skin induces axillary dermatitis within a few weeks.[15]

Significantly, a recent study of related pairs found in the FM (i.e., cinnamal/cinnamic alcohol and isoeugenol/eugenol) as assessed through records of 23,660 patients patch tested to the FM from 1984 to 1998, indicated that there were substantial isolated reactions to the individual fragrance chemicals, justifying their continued usage as individual constituents in FM I.[16]

In a study intended to evaluate the changing frequencies of sensitization to the FM as well as single compounds *Myroxylon pereirae* (balsam of Peru), and oil of turpentine, investigators analyzed the data amassed by the Information Network of Departments of Dermatology multicenter project that ran from 1996 to 2002. They found significant increases between 1996 and 1998 in the proportions of patients exhibiting sensitivity to both single compounds and the FM. However, a significant decline was observed after 1999 in sensitization to the FM, which the researchers attributed to reduced exposure as a result of the use of

TABLE 36-2
Member Nations of the International Fragrance Association (IFRA)

Australia
Brazil
France
Germany
Indonesia
Italy
Japan
Mexico
Netherlands
Singapore
Spain
Switzerland
Turkey
United Kingdom
United States

less potent allergens in fine fragrances, and the potential lower use of natural ingredient-based cosmetics. Investigators also found the relative share of sensitivity to individual ingredients of the FM to be increased for compounds such as isoeugenol and oak moss that could not be ascribed to their use, which for the top allergen oak moss was reported to be 0.4% as compared to the lower-potency geraniol, thought to be represented in 50% of the product market.[9] In fact, researchers noted that the International Fragrance Association (IFRA) and the Research Institute for Fragrance Materials (RIFM) had recommended the use of lower concentrations of isoeugenol and oak moss (Table 36-2). Such findings helped to illuminate the emerging belief that some ingredients within the FM were much more significant allergens than others and that reevaluation might be warranted, including omission from the FM of some of the less troublesome components. In addition, one of the primary complaints regarding the FM I had been the emergence of false positives and false negatives, and the detection of only approximately 70% of the patients allergic to fragrances.[8]

FRAGRANCE MIX II

In addition to the perceived imbalance in potency of the FM I compounds and the debate over whether certain chemicals continue to merit inclusion, a report in 1993 estimated that the FM I failed to identify at least 15% of perfume allergies.[17] Five years later, Larsen found that as much as 33% of fragrance sensitivity may go undetected if it is tested in isolation, as the only test compound.[18,19]

The incomplete detection of fragrance allergens through the use of the FM I and the identification of additional sensitizing allergens through clinical experience, and subsequent reporting and confirmation of such findings, eventually led to the development of the FM II (Table 36-3). For instance, a multicenter trial in Europe completed in 2002 that evaluated 14 frequently used chemicals laid the groundwork as it identified the six most sensitizing chemicals all of which were ultimately included as the FM II.[20,21] These chemicals—hydroxyisohexyl 3-cyclohexene carboxaldehyde (Lyral®), citral, farnesol, citronellol, α-hexyl-cinnamic aldehyde, and coumarin—were evaluated in 1701 consecutive patients who were patch tested in six European centers. In all six centers, the team of investigators found the numbers of patients who reacted to the three different concentrations of FM II, which would have gone undetected by FM I, to be significant enough to warrant the codification of this new FM. Overall, FM II (14%) elicited a reaction in 2.9% of patients; of these, 33% were negative to FM I. In a more recent study in Germany of 6968 patients, 7.7% reacted to FM I and 4.6% reacted to FM II.

TABLE 36-3
Fragrance Mix (FM) II

Hydroxyisohexyl 3-cyclohexene carboxaldehyde (Lyral®)
Citral
Farnesol
Coumarin
Citronellol
α-Hexyl cinnamal

In 2008, investigators writing on behalf of the European Society of Contact Dermatitis (ESCD) and the European Environmental Contact Dermatitis Research Group (EECDRG), after conducting a literature review, recommended that the FM II at a concentration of 14% w/w (5.6 mg/cm^2) and Lyral, specifically, at 5% w/w (2.0 mg/cm^2) be included in the European baseline patch test series. (The ESCD has delegated the major responsibility for the European patch test series to the EECDRG.) Lyral is the most common sensitizer among the FM II fragrances, followed by farnesol.[19]

Lyral

The synthetic fragrance hydroxyisohexyl 3-cyclohexene carboxaldehyde (HICC, Lyral) is a common allergen that also happens to be used in more than 50% of marketed deodorants.[22] Frosch et al. tested Lyral (5% in petrolatum) along with the FM I and 11 other fragrances on consecutive patients in six European dermatology departments in 1999. Lyral elicited a positive reaction in 2.7% of 1855 patients (range 1.2%–17%) and ranked next to 11.3% with FM allergy, leading the investigators to call for testing of Lyral in patients thought to be suffering from contact dermatitis.[23] Geier et al. reported on a subsequent test of Lyral 5% in petrolatum in 3245 consecutive patch test patients in 20 dermatology departments, with 1.9% reacting to the fragrance. As part of this study, Lyral and FM I were tested in parallel in 3185 patients, with 9.4% reacting to FM and 1.9% to Lyral. A reaction to both occurred in 40 patients, corresponding to 13.3% of those reacting to FM and 67.8% of those reacting to Lyral. As a result of this study, the German Contact Dermatitis Research Group (DKG) opted to include Lyral as part of its standard patch test series.[24] In 2002, Frosch et al. supervised the evaluation of 1855 patients patch tested in six European dermatology centers to determine the frequency of responses to 8% FM and 14 other often used fragrances. The six chemicals displaying the greatest reactivity after FM were, in descending order, Lyral, citral, farnesol, citronellol, hexyl cinnamic aldehyde, and coumarin. As a precursor to the codification of the FM II, they found these six substances worthy of using in patch testing of contact dermatitis patients, with Lyral as the most notable of these chemicals.[21]

In a recent small study, researchers demonstrated that Lyral causes allergic contact dermatitis in a high percentage of sensitized individuals at usage concentrations typically found in deodorants.[22] Previously, Lyral had been found to provoke contact allergic reactions in 2% to 3% of eczema patients undergoing patch testing. In a small study of 18 eczema patients and seven control subjects, Johansen et al. examined a dose-response relationship of Lyral contact allergy. A serial dilution of Lyral in ethanol 6% to 6 ppm was administered to the volar forearm in a 2-week, repeated open application test. Upon no reaction to this dosage, cases were tested for 2 additional weeks at a higher dose. Eleven cases reacted to the low dose, five to the high, and two to neither. There was no reaction to the ethanol vehicle-control. Control subjects failed to react to either Lyral concentration or the ethanol vehicle. With a statistically significant difference between the groups, the investigators concluded that Lyral was causing skin sensitivity. They recommended reductions in usage concentrations to prevent allergic contact dermatitis in response to this fragrance.[25]

In 2006, the North American Contact Dermatitis Group (NACDG) conducted a multicenter study comparing three concentrations of Lyral (5%, 1.5%, and 0.5% in petrolatum) to the NACDG screening tray, which includes FM I, balsam of Peru, cinnamic aldehyde, ylang ylang oil, jasmine absolute, and tea tree oil. Data collected from 1603 patients at six sites identified balsam of Peru (6.6%) and FM I (5.9%) to be the most common patch-test-positive fragrance allergens, followed by cinnamic aldehyde (1.7%), ylang ylang oil (0.6%), jasmine absolute (0.4%), Lyral (0.4% for 5% Lyral, 0.3% for 1.5% Lyral, and 0.2% for 0.5% Lyral), and tea tree oil (0.3%). The investigators concluded that Lyral is an uncommon allergen in North America, and that the 5% concentration should be used in patch tests for patients suspected of having a fragrance allergy.[26]

FM I/II AND THE 26 FRAGRANCES REQUIRED TO BE LABELED IN EUROPE

The creation of the FM II was quickly followed by additional regulation of the fragrance market in Europe. As of March 2005, as mandated by the seventh amendment of the European Union (EU) Cosmetics Directive, all cosmetic products are required to indicate on their labels the presence of 26 individual fragrances if present at >10 ppm in leave-on products and >100 ppm in rinse-off products (Table 36-4). Similar regulations were instituted regarding detergents as of October 2005, with labeling mandated for any of the 26 fragrances present at >100 ppm.[27]

TABLE 36-4
The 26 Individual Fragrances Required by the EU Cosmetics Directive (as of March 11, 2005) to be Labeled on Cosmetic Products if Present at >10 ppm in Leave-On Products and >100 ppm in Rinse-Off Products

A-isomethyl ionone
Amyl cinnamal
Amyl cinnamic alcohol
Anisyl alcohol
Butyl phenyl methyl propional (BPMP, Lilial™)
Benzyl alcohol
Benzyl benzoate
Benzyl cinnamate
Benzyl salicylate
Cinnamal
Cinnamic alcohol
Citral
Citronellol
Coumarin
Eugenol
Farnesol
Geraniol
Hexyl cinnamal
Hydroxycitronellal
Isoeugenol
Limonene
Linalool
Lyral
Methyl heptine carbonate
Oak moss (*Evernia prunastri*)
Tree moss (*Evernia futuracea*)

During the four 6-month periods between January 2003 and January 2005, Schnuch et al. patch tested 21,325 individuals for the 26 fragrances in addition to the standard series of fragrances. Frequencies of sensitization were noted as follows: tree moss (2.4%), Lyral (2.3%), oak moss (2.0%), hydroxycitronellal (1.3%), isoeugenol (1.1%), cinnamic aldehyde (1.0%), farnesol (0.9%), cinnamic alcohol (0.6%), citral (0.6%), citronellol (0.5%), geraniol (0.4%), eugenol (0.4%), coumarin (0.4%), lilial (0.3%), amyl-cinnamic alcohol (0.3%), benzyl cinnamate (0.3%), benzyl alcohol (0.3%), linalool (0.2%), methylheptin carbonate (0.2%), amyl-cinnamic aldehyde (0.1%), hexyl cinnamic aldehyde (0.1%), limonene (0.1%), benzyl salicylate (0.1%), γ-methylionon (0.1%), benzyl benzoate (0.0%), and anisyl alcohol (0.0%). Given such percentages, the investigators concluded that clearly the 26 fragrances range in importance as risks to eliciting contact sensitivity, with some of great concern and others of no significance at all.[28)]

More recently, Buckley evaluated the exposure patterns to fragrances on the UK product market by surveying 300 products including the words "parfum" or "aroma" for any of the 26 listed fragrances. The fragrances that were most frequently identified were linalool (63%), limonene (63%), citronellol (48%), geraniol (42%), butyl phenyl methyl propional (Lilial™) (42%), and hexyl cinnamal (42%). Besides geraniol, all the other FM I ingredients were represented: eugenol (27%), hydroxycitronellal (17%), isoeugenol (9%), cinnamic alcohol (8%), amyl cinnamal (7%), cinnamal (6%), and oak moss absolute (4%). The FM II ingredients, in addition to citronellol and hexyl cinnamal, were also found in the product survey in significant numbers: coumarin (30%), Lyral (29%), citral (25%), and farnesol (8%). Buckley concluded that exposure levels to key allergens in FM I and II continue for the British population. Given the frequent use of the fragrances linalool and limonene, Buckley also suggested that these two chemicals be included in the test series for patients suspected of fragrance allergy.[27]

During the same year, Rastogi et al. conducted a survey of four primary fragrance allergens—isoeugenol, Lyral, atranol, and chloroatranol—included in 22 popular Danish as well as international brands purchased on the Danish retail market. Isoeugenol was identified in 56% of the products, Lyral in 72%, atranol in 59%, and chloroatranol in 36%. While isoeugenol was found to be included in concentrations below the recommended maximum level of 0.02% in each case, Lyral concentration attained a maximum of 0.2%, which is 10-fold higher than the EU Scientific Committee's identification of the safest maximum tolerable concentration. The concentration levels for atranol and chloroatranol were similar to those found in 2003 and the frequency of use of the latter represented a significant reduction.[29]

Noting that the prestige perfumes intended for women have been the products demonstrated to contain the highest concentrations of allergens, Rastogi et al. evaluated 10 fine fragrances, five introduced between 1921 and 1990 and five launched since then by the same companies. They found that the five older perfumes included a mean of 5 allergens in the FM I, whereas the five newer products contained a mean of 2.8 of the FM I allergens. In addition, the mean concentrations of the FM allergens in the old perfumes were 2.6 times higher than the mean for the new products. The investigators concluded that a concerted effort by the fragrance industry to curtail the use of offending ingredients or, perhaps, changes in fashion may have contributed to this decrease in the use of FM I allergens in prestige perfumes.[30]

It is important to note that even in products touted as containing only natural ingredients, fragrance substances represented in the FM I and II, including hydroxycitronellal, coumarin, cinnamic alcohol, and α-amyl cinnamic aldehyde, have been identified. In a study of natural products, Rastogi et al. noted that the presence of hydroxycitronellal and α-hexylcinnamic aldehyde showed that artificial fragrances can be found in products marketed for its natural ingredients.[31]

SUMMARY

Fragrances are ubiquitous chemical constituents in a significant proportion of the products people use on a daily basis. A substantial minority of individuals develop allergic contact dermatitis to at least one of the many hundreds of fragrances used in the wide variety of products that come into contact with the skin. In addition, with the advent of aromatherapy, an increasing number of patients have come to enjoy the olfactory sensation that they experience from using such products. Ironically, the very ingredients that may bring some therapeutic relief by dint of their scents may cause some irritation to the skin. The roster of fragrances in products, as well as the range of products with fragrances added, has expanded as has the list of fragrances included in patch testing for sensitivity since the first allergy to fragrance-based chemicals was identified in 1957. It is important that cosmetic dermatologists and aestheticians be aware of the plethora of chemicals that have been recognized for provoking cutaneous reactions in a distinct but sizable minority of patients.

REFERENCES

1. Heydorn S, Johansen JD, Andersen KE, et al. Fragrance allergy in patients with hand eczema – a clinical study. *Contact Dermatitis*. 2003;48:317.
2. Nielsen NH, Linneberg A, Menné T, et al. Allergic contact sensitization in an adult Danish population: two cross-sectional surveys eight years apart (the Copenhagen Allergy Study). *Acta Derm Venereol*. 2001;81:31.
3. Friedman PS. The immunology of allergic contact dermatitis: the DNCB story. *Adv Dermatol*. 1990;5:175.
4. Orton DI, Wilkinson, JD. Cosmetic allergy, incidence, diagnosis, and management. *Am J Clin. Dermatol*. 2004;5:327.
5. Duarte I, Campos Lage AC. Frequency of dermatoses associated with cosmetics. *Contact Dermatitis*. 2007;56:211.
6. Mehta SS, Reddy BS. Cosmetic dermatitis—current perspectives. *Int J Dermatol*. 2003;42:533.
7. Jovanović M, Poljacki M, Duran V, et al. Contact allergy to Compositae plants in patients with atopic dermatitis. *Med Pregl*. 2004;57:209.
8. de Groot AC, Frosch PJ. Adverse reactions to fragrances: a clinical review. *Contact Dermatitis*. 1997;36:57.
9. Schnuch A, Lessmann H, Geier J, et al. Contact allergy to fragrances: frequencies of sensitization from 1996 to 2002. Results of the IVDK. *Contact Dermatitis*. 2004;50:65.
10. Larsen WG. Perfume dermatitis. A study of 20 patients. *Arch Dermatol*. 1977;113:623.
11. Chatard H. Case of sensitization to perfumes with cutaneous and general reactions. *Bull Soc Fr Dermatol Syphiligr*. 1957;64:323.
12. Johansen JD, Andersen KE, Svedman C, et al. Chloroatranol, an extremely potent allergen hidden in perfumes: a dose-response elicitation study. *Contact Dermatitis*. 2003;49:180.
13. Rastogi SC, Bossi R, Johansen JD, et al. Content of oak moss allergens atranol and chloroatranol in perfumes and similar products. *Contact Dermatitis*. 2004;50:367.
14. Buckley DA, Wakelin SH, Seed PT, et al. The frequency of fragrance allergy in a patch-test population over a 17-year period. *Br J Dermatol*. 2000;142:203.
15. Bruze M, Johansen JD, Andersen KE, et al. Deodorants: an experimental provocation study with cinnamic aldehyde. *J Am Acad Dermatol*. 2003;48:194.
16. Buckley DA, Basketter DA, Smith Pease CK, et al. Simultaneous sensitivity to fragrances. *Br J Dermatol*. 2006;154:885.
17. de Groot AC, van der Kley AM, Bruynzeel DP, et al. Frequency of false-negative reactions to the fragrance mix. *Contact Dermatitis*. 1993;28:139.
18. Larsen W, Nakayama H, Fischer T, et al. A study of new fragrance mixtures. *Am J Contact Dermat*. 1998;9:202.
19. Bruze M, Andersen KE, Goossens A, et al. Recommendation to include fragrance mix 2 and hydroxyisohexyl 3-cyclohexene carboxaldehyde (Lyral) in the European baseline patch test series. *Contact Dermatitis*. 2008;58:129.
20. Frosch PJ, Pirker C, Rastogi SC, et al. Patch testing with a new fragrance mix detects additional patients sensitive to perfumes and missed by the current fragrance mix. *Contact Dermatitis*. 2005;52:207.
21. Frosch PJ, Johansen JD, Menné T, et al. Further important sensitizers in patients sensitive to fragrances. I. Reactivity to 14 frequently used chemicals. *Contact Dermatitis*. 2002;47:78.
22. Jørgensen PH, Jensen CD, Rastogi S, et al. Experimental elicitation with hydroxyisohexyl-3-cyclohexene carboxaldehyde-containing deodorants. *Contact Dermatitis*. 2007;56:146.
23. Frosch PJ, Johansen JD, Menné T, et al. Lyral is an important sensitizer in patients sensitive to fragrances. *Br J Dermatol*. 1999;141:1076.
24. Geier J, Brasch J, Schnuch A, et al. Lyral has been included in the patch test standard series in Germany. *Contact Dermatitis*. 2002;46:295.
25. Johansen JD, Frosch PJ, Svedman C, et al. Hydroxyisohexyl 3-cyclohexene carboxaldehyde—known as Lyral: quantitative aspects and risk assessment of an important fragrance allergen. *Contact Dermatitis*. 2003;48:310.
26. Belsito DV, Fowler JF Jr, Sasseville D, et al. Delayed-type hypersensitivity to fragrance materials in a select North American population. *Dermatitis*. 2006;17:23.
27. Buckley DA. Fragrance ingredient labeling in products on sale in the U.K. *Br J Dermatol*. 2007;157:295.
28. Schnuch A, Uter W, Geier J, et al. Sensitization to 26 fragrances to be labeled according to current European regulation. Results of the IVDK and review of the literature. *Contact Dermatitis*. 2007;57:1.
29. Rastogi SC, Johansen JD, Bossi R. Selected important fragrance sensitizers in perfumes—current exposures. *Contact Dermatitis*. 2007;56:201.
30. Rastogi SC, Menné T, Johansen JD. The composition of fine fragrances is changing. *Contact Dermatitis*. 2003;48:130.
31. Rastogi SC, Johansen JD, Menné T. Natural ingredients based cosmetics. Content of selected fragrance sensitizers. *Contact Dermatitis*. 1996;34:423.

CHAPTER 37

Preservatives

Edmund Weisberg, MS
Leslie Baumann, MD

Preservatives are integral ingredients in various food, pharmaceutical, cosmetic, and skin care formulations. As water is included in the majority of such products, preservatives are added to prevent the growth of microorganisms and the resultant rapid deterioration or decomposition of the product. Indeed, without preservatives, which are biocidal chemicals, these items important to daily life would exhibit little to no shelf life and become quickly invaded and permeated by numerous bacteria, fungi, and molds. As such, preservatives are intended to maintain the integrity of the product and protect the user from infection.[1] While antimicrobial preservatives are essential components in the majority of cosmetics and skin care products, these ingredients have been cited frequently as causes of allergic contact dermatitis.[1-3] Such occurrences are most often associated with topical application on damaged or broken skin. Of greater concern in recent years has been the reports linking the use of some skin care products with cancer incidence. This chapter will focus on the most frequently used class of preservatives, recent data regarding the estrogenic potential of these compounds, and the controversy regarding possible associations between the chronic use of chemical preservatives that make contact with the skin and cancer.

PARABENS

Parabens, alkyl esters of p-hydroxybenzoic acid (PHBA), which are found naturally in some fruits, are common ingredients in food, pharmaceuticals, as well as numerous skin, hair, and body care products, and can sometimes produce allergic reactions.[4] Nevertheless, parabens are the most widely used preservatives in cosmetics,[5] and are used in the vast majority of skin care formulations.[6] In fact, about 25 years ago, it was estimated that at least 90% of personal care products, including deodorants, toothpaste, shampoo, body cream, shower gels, moisturizers, etc., contained one or more parabens as a preservative,[7] because of the strong record of efficacy, safety, and stability exhibited by this group of compounds. The frequency of inclusion of these ingredients has not markedly changed during the last quarter of a century despite the introduction or synthesis of new substances. The use of parabens in pharamaceutical products as preservatives actually dates back to the 1920s.[8] These chemicals have been generally regarded as safe because they are quickly absorbed and hydrolyzed into the less toxic PHBA.[3] It is also worth noting that the metabolism of parabens is influenced by the inclusion in cosmetic preparations of penetration enhancers, which facilitate the rapid absorption of parabens through intact skin.[9,10] There have been several reports of contact sensitivity associated with cutaneous exposure to parabens, but while this mechanism has not yet been fully elucidated, such occurrences, as stated above, are linked to contact with damaged or broken skin.

The family of parabens include methyl paraben (MP), ethyl paraben, butyl paraben, isobutyl paraben, propyl paraben, isopropyl paraben, and benzyl paraben.[11] Methyl, ethyl, propyl, and butyl paraben are the most frequently used parabens in cosmetic formulations[12] (Table 37-1). Notably, these chemicals can be absorbed through the skin and migrate into the bloodstream and bodily tissues.

Methyl Paraben

MP is the most common of the various forms of parabens. It is a stable, nonvolatile substance with a long track record of safe use in foods, drugs, and cosmetics. MP is not considered to be irritating or sensitizing to individuals with normal skin (i.e., people who do not have sensitive skin). A literature review conducted by Soni et al. in 2002 suggested that MP is thought to be absorbed totally and avidly through the skin as well as gastrointestinally metabolized into PHBA, before it is conjugated and eliminated through the urine. Notably, Soni et al. found no evidence of cutaneous or systemic accumulation.[13]

In the wake of the reports postulating a relationship between the chronic use of parabens-containing deodorant and breast cancer incidence (see Parabens and Breast Cancer section), some investigators have undertaken longer-term examination of parabens exposure to the skin. In particular, Ishiwitari et al. considered the effects of daily MP use on human skin. They measured the concentrations of the preservative in the stratum corneum of the human forearm in 12 volunteers after 1 month of twice-daily applications of MP-containing formulations, and also investigated the long-term effects of exposure on keratinocytes in vitro. The investigators found that MP was not completely metabolized, with significant increases in concentrations in the stratum corneum measured after 1 month. MP was also found to have reduced the proliferating capacity of keratinocytes and altered cell morphology. They speculated that the accumulation of MP may be coordinated with the differentiation and aging of keratinocytes, and suggested that further research, especially in vivo study, is warranted to obtain a better understanding of the effects of daily use of MP.[3]

In another recent study, Handa et al. evaluated the effects of ultraviolet-B (UVB) exposure on human keratinocytes treated with MP. Their approach was to culture HaCaT cells in MP-containing medium for 24 hours before exposing the medium to 15 or 30 mJ/cm^2 of UVB, and then culturing for an additional 24 hours. While a 0.003% concentration of MP exhibited no impact on HaCaT cell viability and UVB irradiation alone induced little or no necrosis of keratinocytes, a 0.003% MP concentration was found to significantly enhance UVB-induced apoptosis as well as oxidative stress, nitric oxide synthesis, lipid peroxidation, and transcription factor activation of the keratinocytes. The investigators concluded that the combination of MP and UV may impose deleterious effects on human skin. Consequently, they are investigating

TABLE 37-1
List of the Most Commonly Used Esters of P-Hydroxybenzoic Acid (parabens) As Well As Their Chemical Structures and Molecular Formulas

Paraben	Chemical Structure	Molecular Formula
Methyl paraben	CH_3	$C_8H_8O_3$
Ethyl paraben	CH_2CH_3	$C_9H_{10}O_3$
Propyl paraben	$(CH_2)_2CH_3$	$C_{10}H_{12}O_3$
Butyl paraben	$(CH_2)_3CH_3$	$C_{11}H_{14}O_3$

this potential association in vitro using normal human keratinocytes and are conducting in vivo studies using MP-treated animal skin.[14]

Parabens and Breast Cancer?

A recent study aimed at identifying and characterizing the toxicology of products from the reaction between parabens and singlet oxygen revealed that parabens may engender oxidative stress in the skin following conversion to glutathione conjugates of hydroquinone, through reaction with glutathione and singlet oxygen.[15] While this finding warrants further research, any reaction to it would likely pale in comparison to a controversial study published by Byford et al. in January 2002. In this report, investigators noted high concentrations of parabens in breast cancer tissue, as they identified a weak estrogenic effect exhibited by MP, ethyl paraben, n-propyl paraben, and n-butyl paraben in estrogen-dependent MCF7 human breast cancer cells.[16] Significantly, they concluded that additional research would be needed to ascertain the extent of paraben accumulation in estrogen-sensitive tissues.

Rumors that using antiperspirants could cause breast cancer ensued in mainstream circulation over the Internet and beyond during much of the remainder of the year and may persist in many circles despite the lack of evidence and, in some cases, reports to the contrary. A population-based case–control study published near the end of 2002 evaluated the relationship between underarm antiperspirant/deodorant use and breast cancer risk in women between the ages of 20 and 74 (813 cases and 793 controls). Breast cancer risk was not found to increase based on antiperspirant or deodorant use generally, or use of such products among those who shaved with a blade razor, or use of such products within 1 hour of shaving. Thus, investigators concluded that their results did not support the theory that breast cancer risk is increased by the use of antiperspirant products.[17] A more recent review expressed less certainty as to whether the use of underarm antiperspirant products elevates the risk of human breast cancer.[18] In that study, which was the first study to evaluate the intensity of underarm exposure in a cohort of breast cancer survivors, results from the 437 women assessed revealed that an earlier age of breast cancer diagnosis was associated with frequency and earlier onset of antiperspirant/deodorant usage combined with underarm shaving. Investigators concluded that while underarm shaving with antiperspirant/deodorant usage may contribute to breast cancer, case–control studies are necessary to arrive at appropriate recommendations for alternative axillary hygiene.[19] A review published even more recently states that while no association between parabens in cosmetics and skin care products has been established, this is because the necessary studies have not yet been conducted, not that some effects have not been identified.[20]

Additional Responses to the Controversy

Soni et al. have stated in multiple articles that parabens are virtually nontoxic, and quickly absorbed, metabolized, and excreted in urine.[8,13,21] They have also not found carcinogenic potential to be associated with parabens in reviews of the literature. In reference to the controversy pertaining to the study by Byford et al., they argue that the evidence is ambiguous at best regarding the estrogenic risks of parabens, noting that the available studies do not consider the dose-, route-, and species-dependent metabolism and elimination rates of parabens. They do, however, conclude that a study of reproductive toxicity may be useful.[8]

Darbre responded to the furor over the suggestions of an etiologic connection between underarm cosmetics and breast cancer by noting that the strongest supportive evidence of this contention was the unaccounted for clinical observations revealing a disproportionately high incidence of breast cancer in the upper outer quadrant of the breast, proximate to where these products are applied. He suggested that such data should prompt multidisciplinary research to ascertain the effects of the long-term use of the constituent chemicals of underarm cosmetics.[22] In a commentary on Darbre's article, Harvey acknowledged that while parabens are generally regarded as safe, recent reports have indicated estrogenic effects associated with these preservatives. He echoed Darbre's call for additional research on underarm cosmetics, particularly on components facilitating estrogenic activity, noting the paucity of data on the long-term effects of weakly estrogenic chemicals on human health.[23] In a subsequent article by Harvey and Darbre, the authors suggest that should further data on the influence of topically applied paraben-containing products indicate adverse effects on human health via endocrine disruption, this mode of interruption, given the clarity of exposure, should be more amenable to assessment, measurement, and intervention. Further, they suggest that the potential public health impact and the size of the exposed population should provide incentive for study.[24]

It is important to realize that the presence of parabens in the breast cancer tumors identified in the Byford study is not evidence of a causal link between parabens and breast cancer, cosmetics in general and breast cancer, or even underarm products and breast cancer. If parabens ultimately turn out to be implicated in the etiologic pathway of certain breast cancers or other tumors, it is worth remembering that parabens are used in food products as well,[13] leaving the source of potential causal factors difficult to identify. As yet, no one has any idea (or has evaluated) whether it is the consumption of parabens or their application to the skin that is responsible for their presence in human tissue. In addition, no one knows what the presence of parabens in human tissue means. Nevertheless, such studies raise important questions.

The Estrogenicity of Parabens

Using the uterotrophic assay in immature and adult ovariectomized CD1 mice and in immature Wistar rats, Lemini et al. subcutaneously injected animals for three consecutive days with various doses of parabens or vehicle. They found that uterine weight was increased and all parabens but MP competed with estradiol for estrogen binding sites. The investigators concluded that their in vivo and in vitro data confirm the estrogenicity of parabens.[25] Lemini et al. followed up on these results by presenting a morphometric analysis of the uteri from mice treated with parabens compared with estradiol that confirmed the induction of estrogenic histologic alterations in the uteri of ovariectomized mice.[26]

Acknowledging the various estrogenic effects of parabens seen recently in vivo, Prusakiewicz et al. hypothesized that parabens increase estrogen levels by inhibiting estrogen sulfotransferases (SULTs) in skin. They tested this theory in human skin cytosolic fractions and normal human epidermal keratinocytes (NHEKs). The investigators found that SULT inhibition potency increased with increasing length of the paraben ester chain, with butyl paraben displaying the greatest inhibitory capacity, suppressing cutaneous cytosol sulfation of estradiol, and estrone thus potentially increasing local estrogen levels. They concluded that the estrogenicity of parabens included in topical skin care products and medications may promote or contribute to cutaneous antiaging benefits.[27] The level of estrogenicity bears scrutiny in future studies given the seemingly fine line between the potential salutary, antiaging effects of estrogen, as well as the detrimental, carcinogenic activity.

While acknowledging the weakly estrogenic activity of parabens identified in recent in vitro tests and reported in vivo effects such as increased uterine weight associated with butyl, isobutyl, and benzyl paraben and male reproductive effects linked to butyl and propyl paraben, Golden et al. argued that the parabens with demonstrated activity are several orders of magnitude less active than estrogen and that it is "biologically implausible" that parabens could raise the risk of any estrogen-mediated health effects. Further, they concluded that a worst-case scenario in terms of daily parabens exposure would pose significantly less risk as compared to the risk of exposure to naturally-occurring dietary endocrine-active chemicals (EACs) such as the phytoestrogen daidzein (an isoflavone found in soy).[11]

GENERAL STUDIES

Hussein et al. set out to ascertain the permeation of methyl, ethyl, propyl, and butyl paraben through the epidermal and dermal layers as well as accumulation in the skin layers and/or passage to other bodily tissues. They found that the capacity of the various parabens to penetrate the skin was based on their relative lipophilicity—with the more lipophilic, the less they were likely to penetrate or cross skin layers.[12] Butyl paraben is the most lipophilic of the four, followed by propyl, ethyl, and MP. The most lipophilic paraben, butyl paraben, displayed comparatively weak passage through the skin, and has been shown elsewhere to have the potential for accumulating in the skin, particularly after multiple or frequent applications.[28]

Nicotinamide, the biologically active amide of vitamin B_3, is a hydrophilic molecule used as an active ingredient in cosmetic formulations for its moisturizing and depigmenting activity (see Chapter 33). In a recent study, it has also been shown to have the capacity to influence the transdermal permeation of methyl, ethyl, propyl, and butyl paraben. Specifically, nictotinamide was found to promote the dissolution of parabens in solutions and gels and lower parabens partitioning in the oily phase thus ensuring an effective water-phase concentration in emulsion. Investigators concluded that nicotinamide interacts with parabens by ultimately decreasing transdermal penetration, thereby diminishing the risk or potential for toxicity.[29]

Interestingly, Lee et al. have noted the dearth of studies evaluating the effects of a combination of preservatives in cosmetic formulations even though such products more often include a mixture of preservatives rather than a single preservative. In response, they set out to evaluate the side effects of cosmetic preservatives alone or in combination as product ingredients and to assess objective and subjective sensory skin irritation (representing symptoms such as burning, stinging, and itching absent visual inflammation). The researchers found no significant differences among MP, ethyl paraben, propyl paraben, butyl paraben, phenoxyethanol, and chlorphenesin in objective skin irritation potential at the minimal inhibitory concentration. However, chlorphenesin was found to exhibit greater potential in subjective irritation. They also found that formulation type influenced sensory irritation and that the combination of phenoxyethanol and chlorphenesin significantly increased irritation.[30]

It is worth noting that in a review of the major classes of preservatives as well as newer agents such as Euxyl K 400 and isopropynyl butylcarbamate, Sasseville concludes that while an ideal preservative, effective without potential for provoking irritancy or sensitivity, has not yet been identified, the parabens, which have been used for three-quarters of a century, continue to be the most frequently used preservatives while inducing sensitivity less often than newer biocides.[1]

SUMMARY

In recent years, some concerns have been raised regarding possible links between some cosmetic products and breast cancer incidence. In particular, an estrogenic potential has been reported in association with parabens contained in underarm deodorant, given their frequency of use and proximate location to the human breast and the identification of parabens in breast cancer tissue. It is not uncommon for patients to bring questions to a physician based on mainstream news reports on medical issues. The initial report in 2002 and its reverberating effects in the literature reached public awareness and have prompted some lingering concerns regarding the risks of common skin care product ingredients. Even if patients are not broaching such issues, it is important to be prepared to inform them that nearly all skin care and cosmetic products contain preservatives. While these ingredients are generally regarded as safe, certain risks are associated with their use. In particular, some individuals may be found to be allergic to certain compounds. Damaged or wounded skin may be especially susceptible to some chemical preservatives. In addition, the effects from the chronic use of some products may not be fully understood. This notion could be a pivotal point in the context of recommending daily use of certain products such as sunscreens. It is within this context that the dermatologist should be familiar with preservatives in general and the benefits and risks of the most common preservatives in particular.

Products containing parabens should be avoided by most people who know they are allergic to parabens, which can be determined by patch testing. There are no convincing data that parabens cause harm to those not allergic to these compounds. Because of some sensationalistic reporting in recent years, though, many are choosing to avoid products containing this class of preservative ingredients. Again, for those not allergic to parabens, there are no scientifically established reasons to avoid the plethora of cosmetic and skin care products that contain these preservatives. Much more research is necessary to determine if what appears to be a relatively weak level of estrogenicity in parabens can promote carcinogenesis.

Patients can be directed to health food stores, chains such as Whole Foods, or Internet resources for products that are touted for excluding parabens or other preservatives if they express such interest. It is important to advise them that the efficacy and safety of such products may be questionable and surely not established through randomized, double-blind clinical trials.

REFERENCES

1. Sasseville D. Hypersensitivity to preservatives. *Dermatol Ther.* 2004;17:251.
2. Wilkinson JD, Shaw S, Andersen KE, et al. Monitoring levels of preservative sensitivity in Europe: a 10-year overview

(1991–2000). *Contact Dermatitis*. 2002,46: 207.

3. Ishiwatari S, Suzuki T, Hitomi T, et al. Effects of methyl paraben on skin keratinocytes. *J Appl Toxicol*. 2007;27:1.
4. Gilman AG, Goodman LS, Gilman A, eds. *Goodman and Gilman's The Pharmacological Basis of Therapeutics*. 6th ed. New York, NY: Macmillan 1980:969.
5. Cashman AL, Warshaw EM. Parabens: a review of epidemiology, structure, allergenicity, and hormonal properties. *Dermatitis*. 2005;16:57.
6. Rastogi SC, Schouten A, De Kruijf N, et al. Contents of methyl-, ethyl-, propyl-, butyl- and benzylparaben in cosmetic products. *Contact Dermatitis*. 1995;32:28.
7. Elder RL. Final report on the safety assessment of methyl paraben, ethyl paraben, propyl paraben and butyl paraben. *J Am Coll Toxicol*. 1984;3:147.
8. Soni MG, Carabin IG, Burdock GA. Safety assessment of esters of p-hydroxybenzoic acid (parabens). *Food Chem Toxicol*. 2005;43:985.
9. Dal Pozzo A, Pastori N. Percutaneous absorption of parabens from cosmetic formulations. *Int J Cosm Sci*. 1996; 18:57.
10. Kitagawa S, Li H, Sato S. Skin permeation of parabens in excised guinea pig dorsal skin, its modification by penetration enhancers and their relationship with n-octanol/water partition coefficients. *Chem Pharm Bull (Tokyo)*. 1997;45:1354.
11. Golden R, Gandy J, Vollmer G. A review of the endocrine activity of parabens and implications for potential risks to human health. *Crit Rev Toxicol*. 2005;35:435.
12. El Hussein S, Muret P, Berard M, et al. Assessment of principal parabens used in cosmetics after their passage through human epidermis–dermis layers (ex-vivo) study). *Exp Dermatol*. 2007;16:830.
13. Soni MG, Taylor SL, Greenberg NA, et al. Evaluation of the health aspects of methyl paraben: a review of the published literature. *Food Chem Toxicol*. 2002;40:1335.
14. Handa O, Kokura S, Adachi S, et al. Methylparaben potentiates UV-induced damage of skin keratinocytes. *Toxicology*. 2006;227:62.
15. Nishizawa C, Takeshita K, Ueda J, et al. Reaction of para-hydroxybenzoic acid esters with singlet oxygen in the presence of glutathione produces glutathione conjugates of hydroquinone, potent inducers of oxidative stress. *Free Radic Res*. 2006;40:233.
16. Byford JR, Shaw LE, Drew MG, et al. Oestrogenic activity of parabens in MCF7 human breast cancer cells. *J Steroid Biochem Mol Biol*. 2002;80:49.
17. Mirick DK, Davis S, Thomas DB. Antiperspirant use and the risk of breast cancer. *J Natl Cancer Inst*. 2002;94:1578.
18. Gikas PD, Mansfield L, Mokbel K. Do underarm cosmetics cause breast cancer? *Int J Fertil Womens Med*. 2004;49:212.
19. McGrath KG. An earlier age of breast cancer diagnosis related to more frequent use of antiperspirants/deodorants and underarm shaving. *Eur J Cancer Prev*. 2003;12:479.
20. Darbre PD. Environmental oestrogens, cosmetics and breast cancer. *Best Pract Res Clin Endocrinol Metab*. 2006;20:121.
21. Soni MG, Burdock GA, Taylor SL, et al. Safety assessment of propyl paraben: a review of the published literature. *Food Chem Toxicol*. 2001;39:513.
22. Darbre PD. Underarm cosmetics and breast cancer. *J Appl Toxicol*. 2003;23:89.
23. Harvey PW. Parabens, oestrogenicity, underarm cosmetics and breast cancer: a perspective on a hypothesis. *J Appl Toxicol*. 2003;23:285.
24. Harvey PW, Darbre P. Endocrine disrupters and human health: could oestrogenic chemicals in body care cosmetics adversely affect breast cancer incidence in women? *J Appl Toxicol*. 2004;24:167.
25. Lemini C, Jaimez R, Avila ME, et al. In vivo and in vitro estrogen bioactivities of aklyl parabens. *Toxicol Ind Health*. 2003; 19:69.
26. Lemini C, Hernández A, Jaimez R, et al. Morphometric analysis of mice uteri treated with the preservatives methyl, ethyl, propyl, and butylparaben. *Toxicol Ind Health*. 2004;20:123.
27. Prusakiewicz JJ, Harville HM, Zhang Y, et al. Parabens inhibit human skin estrogen sulfotransferase activity: possible link to paraben estrogenic effects. *Toxicology*. 2007;232:248.
28. Darbre P. Underarm cosmetics and breast cancer. *Eur J Cancer Prev*. 2004;13:153.
29. Nicoli S, Zani F, Bilzi S, et al. Association of nicotinamide with parabens: effect on solubility, partition and transdermal permeation. *Eur J Pharm Biopharm*. 2008 Jan 18 [Epub ahead of print].
30. Lee E, An S, Choi D, et al. Comparison of objective and sensory skin irritations of several cosmetic preservatives. *Contact Dermatitis*. 2007;56:131.

SECTION 6

Other

CHAPTER 38

Bioengineering of the Skin

Leslie Baumann, MD
Mari Paz Castanedo-Tardan, MD

Bioengineering of the skin is a scientific discipline devoted to developing standardized methodologies to measure skin findings in a scientific manner. The International Society for Bioengineering of the Skin has its own journal and there are multiple books published on these methods. It is vital to understand these methodologies in order to effectively evaluate the scientific merit of studies in the dermatology literature. These measurements allow the cosmetic dermatologist to evaluate the efficacy of particular treatments and to objectively measure treatment outcomes. These tests are a necessary addition to cosmetic dermatology clinical trials and they aid cosmetic dermatologists in their pursuit of practicing evidence-based medicine in a cosmetic setting.

SUBJECTIVE MEASUREMENTS

The Lactic Acid Stinging Test

Even when this method lacks objective criteria, this test is widely accepted as a marker of sensitivity and as a standard method for evaluating individuals who report invisible and subjective cutaneous irritation. Stinging is considered to be a variant of pain that develops rapidly and fades quickly any time the appropriate sensory nerves are stimulated[1] (see Chapter 17). In one study, Frosch and Kligman applied 5% lactic acid to the nasolabial fold (a site highly innervated with sensory fibers), when the subject was sweating profusely.[2] Under these conditions, approximately 20% of the research group reported experiencing an unpleasant sensation. In a different study, Seidenari et al. applied 10% lactic acid solution to the nasolabial fold and observed that individuals with "sensitive skin" experienced a much stronger stinging sensation than those in the healthy control group.[3] However, not all studies agree that patients with sensitive skin are more likely to be "stingers." In order to achieve a more reliable response, applying an inert control substance such as saline solution to the contralateral test site is recommended. In addition to lactic acid, other water-soluble substances such as capsaicin can be used.

The Chloroform Methanol and Sorbic Acid Tests

Like the test mentioned above, these may help the practitioner identify patients with sensitive skin. In these procedures, the practitioner applies the substance to the face of the patient to determine if stinging or burning occurs.[4]

Challenge Patch Test

This test uses sodium lauryl sulfate and other detergents that are known to be irritants. The irritants are placed on the skin to determine a patient's sensitivity. In cases of an impaired epidermal water barrier, demonstrated by increased transepidermal water loss (TEWL), the detergents will be more likely to cause irritation. This test is used to examine epidermal barrier function. In one study, the purpose was to discover whether "stingers" (patients with sensitive skin) might represent an easily and rapidly identifiable subpopulation with a more generally increased tendency to manifest skin responses. The response to a 0.3% sodium dodecyl sulfate patch test was assessed in a group of 25 stingers and compared to the response in 25 nonstingers. There was no difference in either the pattern or strength of the irritant response assessed by subjective erythema and dryness scores. The data suggest that there is no correlation between the susceptibility of an individual to a skin stinging response and an irritation reaction.[5]

Evaluation of Itch Response

An itch response can be experimentally induced by topical or intradermal injections of various substances such as vasoactive agents, mast cell degranulators, and proteolytic enzymes. One of the most common procedures to induce itching is the intradermal injection of histamine (100 μg in 1 mL of saline) in the subject's forearm. Information is then obtained by the subject's self-assessment regarding the intensity of the itch using a predetermined grading scale. By using a similar evaluation technique (application of topical 4% histamine in a group of healthy young females), Grove postulated that there is a poor correlation between whealing and itching since the dimensions of a wheal do not correlate with the intensity of pruritus.[6]

Thermal Sensation Test

In dermatology, thermal somatosensory testing is becoming the most utilized quantitative sensory testing (QST) technique.[7] It assesses the function of free nerve endings of both small myelinated and nonmyelinated fibers. By attaching a small device called a *thermode* to the patient's skin, thresholds for warmth, cold, as well as hot and cold pain, are measured quantitatively and then compared with age-matched normal population values. Any deviation from the normal range indicates the existence of peripheral nerve disease.[1] The *thermode* is capable of heating or cooling the skin as needed. In contact with the skin, it produces a stimulus the intensity of which increases or decreases until the subject feels the sensation. The subject is then asked to indicate the intensity of the sensation using a predetermined scale. In the center of the *thermode* a *thermocouple* records the temperature. TSA-II (Medoc Company, Ramat Yishai, Israel) is considered one of the most advanced portable thermal sensory testing devices. It operates between 0°C and 54°C and measures the threshold for four sensory submodalities: Warm sensation, cold sensation, heat-induced pain, and cold-induced pain, of which the last is the most difficult to assess.

Washing Test

In the washing test,[8] subjects are asked to wash their face using a specific foaming agent such as soap or detergent. After washing, subjects are asked to evaluate, according to a point scale, individual sensations of tightness, burning, itching, and stinging. The aim of this test is to identify a subpopulation of people with an increased tendency to produce a skin response.[1]

Exaggerated Immersion Tests

For this test, baseline skin parameters are evaluated. Then, a subject's hands and forearms are soaked in a solution of anionic surfactants such as soap, 0.05% sodium laureth sulfate, or 0.35% paraffin sulfonate at 40°C for 20 minutes. After soaking, hands and forearms are rinsed with tap water and pat dried. Then, the procedure is repeated 2 more times, with a 2-hour period between each soaking for 2 consecutive days. Skin parameters are evaluated 2 hours after the third and sixth soakings and 18 hours after the last soaking. All skin parameters are performed after the subject has rested at least 30 minutes in a 21 ± 1°C environment.[1]

OBJECTIVE MEASUREMENTS

Thermography

This mode of measurement appears to aid in the visualization of the extent of skin damage resulting from bad sunburns or exposure to irritant chemicals.[9] The heat loss detected through thermography can indicate areas of damage on the face. The "hot" areas may correlate with regions demonstrating increased blood flow. Thermography essentially provides a temperature map of skin surface temperature, which in turn is a marker for elevated metabolic rate, signaling skin irritation.

Laser Doppler Velocimetry

This technology uses optical methods to provide a noninvasive and continuous way to record cutaneous blood flow of the superficial skin layers. It is used to evaluate the effects on blood flow of topically applied ingredients. It is also useful in evaluating the degree of skin irritation, given that the degree of the experimentally induced irritant contact dermatitis usually correlates well with the blood flow detected by the laser Doppler velocimetry (LDV).

The Evaporimeter or Tewameter (Transepidermal Water Loss)

This instrument measures water loss from the skin indicating disruption of the stratum corneum (SC) (Fig. 38-1). Of course, TEWL is an important indicator of SC functioning. Diminished function of the SC disrupts the skin barrier resulting in increased TEWL. Maibach et al. showed over a decade ago that TEWL increases at sites of damage, especially in people with a positive dermatologic history as well as hand and facial dermatitis, contact dermatitis, metal dermatitis, and textile itching.[10] Most cutaneous diseases that are characterized by abnormalities in the normal terminal differentiation process of keratinocytes are often associated with high TEWL. Also, high TEWL is correlated with easier, higher permeability by external irritants, hence TEWL implies elevated sensitivity. The evaporimeter test therefore appears to offer high sensitivity but low specificity in diagnosing sensitive skin. (For more information, see Ref. 11.)

The Red-Wine Provocation Test

Patients report a sense of warmth beginning around the head or neck area and moving upward on the face 10 to 15 minutes after ingestion of six ounces of red wine. Within 30 minutes, flushing becomes clinically evident.[9] The disadvantage of this test, though, is that it lacks specificity—it may be positive when other conditions, such as rosacea or alcohol dehydrogenase syndrome, are present.

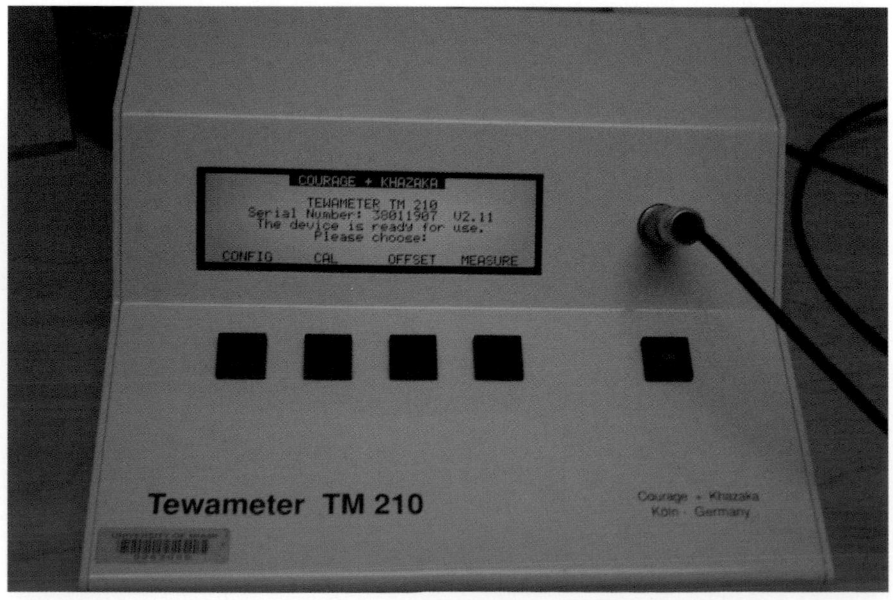

▲ **FIGURE 38-1** The Tewameter is a brand of device similar to an evaporimeter.

Sebutape

This tool allows for the quantitative and objective visualization of sebum excretion. The amount and distribution of sebum vary individually, of course. People with excess sebum (i.e., oily skin) are also more likely to develop acne and, therefore, are probably more sensitive to breakouts when using topical products. This objective assessment of sebum excretion may be superior to the subjective impression of skin type. Manufacturers market product lines and cosmetics for various skin types. The subjective impression of skin type can lead an individual to select an unsuitable product, i.e., one that produces discomfort after application.[9] The Sebumeter is a photometric device whereby a special plastic strip is placed on a patient's skin and then inserted into the instrument. The plastic strip absorbs the lipids on the skin surface and becomes more transparent. The device measures the transparency and therefore sebum based on the light transmission through the strip. The Sebumeter® (SM 815; Courage-Khazaka, Köln, Germany) is commercially available on the market and has been utilized in several studies for the measurement of facial sebum.

SEBUTAPE METHOD This is a more accurate and faster technique using a polymer film to measure lipid absorption. The polymer tape absorbs sebum and becomes transparent to light afterwards. Sebutape can be analyzed in many ways, the easiest of which is the visual scoring of the tapes on a 1 to 5 scale (Fig. 38-2).

The pH Meter

The use of a pH meter with a flat surface glass electrode permits better contact between the probe and the skin surface. Skin itself is slightly acidic, with a pH ranging from 4 to 6, depending on the area of skin and the individual's age. In one study, investigators reported a higher pH in the skin of subjects with eczematous diseases.[3] Bacterial proliferation on the skin is limited by the skin's acidic pH level. Products that raise the cutaneous pH also promote bacterial growth. The physiologic pH value of skin is an average measure of 5.5. Such a pH is essential for maintaining the capacity of the skin for bacteriologic resistance. Buffering substances in the skin, which maintain the cutaneous pH of the skin at its nearly constant level, are able to neutralize small quantities of topically applied acidic or alkaline agents thereby reducing their irritancy.[12] The greater the

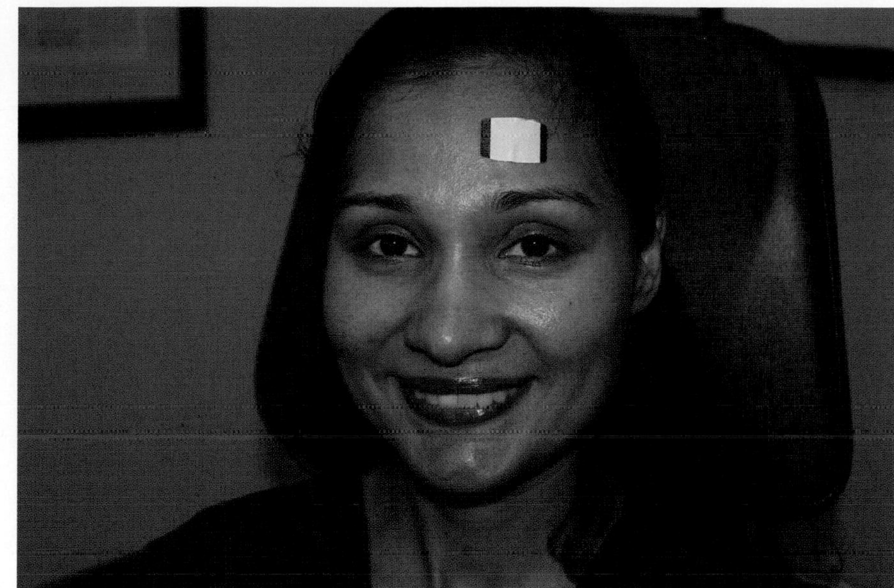

▲ **FIGURE 38-2** Sebutape placed on the forehead to measure sebum secretion.

buffering capacity the smaller the changes in cutaneous pH. The buffering capacity of skin is due especially to the lactic acid/lactate system. Sweat glands produce lactic acid, authorities hypothesize. Since a large amount of eccrine sweat glands are present in the nasolabial fold, one can assume that this quantity accounts for the relatively constant pH values in that area of the skin.

The Chromameter (Colorimetry)

This instrument is useful for assessing skin color, which is expressed in a three-dimensional space. Light from a xenon flash lamp illuminates a 1-cm diameter circular area of the skin and the reflected, tricolor decomposed light is analyzed for its intensity (luminosity, L*) and the color components red–green (a*) and blue–yellow (b*).[13] Erythema is measured on the red–green scale and pigment is measured on the luminosity scale. The chromameter effectively aids the practitioner in looking for increased redness, which is a sign of irritation and sensitivity. The chromameter can also be useful in detecting improvement or worsening of pigmentation disorders such as melasma.

Corneosurfametry

Using reflectance colorimetry, this method studies the interaction between surfactants and the human SC.[14] Cyanoacrylate skin surface stripping (CSSS) is taken from the volar aspect of the subject's forearm and then sprayed with the surfactant to be tested. After 2 hours, the sample is rinsed with tap water and stained with basic fuchsin and toluidine blue dyes for a period of 3 minutes. Once the sample has dried, it is placed on a white reference plate and measured by reflectance colorimetry using, for example, a ChromaMeter CR-200 (Minolta, Osaka, Japan). Then, the index of redness is taken as a parameter of the irritation caused by the surfactant. When water alone is sprayed on the sample, the index has a value of 68 ± 4, and when stronger surfactants are applied, the values decline. Piérard et al. showed that corneosurfametry correlates well with in vivo testing when evaluating surfactant-induced dermatitis in subjects with sensitive skin, and that corneosurfametry shows less interindividual variability than in vivo testing, thus allowing for better discrimination when dealing with mild irritants.[15]

Squamometry

This measurement technique has been postulated to be an effective way to study and quantify nonerythematous irritant dermatitis and a reliable method to investigate the interaction of surfactants with the skin surface.[16] It is a noninvasive, protein-dependent, colorimetric evaluation of the level of alteration in the corneocyte layer collected by adhesive-coated discs, which allow for the quantification of xerotic and inflammatory changes in the SC.[17,18] A short period of applying the discs to the skin (15 s) enables the harvesting of superficial corneocytes (superficial squamometry), while a longer application time (1 hour) collects a thicker layer of corneocytes (deep squamometry).[18,19] The discs are then stained for 30 seconds with a solution of toluidine blue and basic fuchsin in 30% alcohol, followed by rinsing with regular tap water. Measurements of the colors of the sample are made using a reflectance colorimeter. Then, a trained person scores the discs with a microscope at 20x magnification as follows: Intercorneocyte cohesion: 0 = large sheet; 1 = large clusters + a few isolated cells; 2 = small clusters + many isolated cells; 3 = large amount of dye in cells, but uniform; 4 = important staining in all cells, often with grains.[20]

The Corneometer (Corneometry)

This is an effective tool for determining skin surface hydration and it helps to measure the electrical capacitance of the SC. Water exhibits the highest dielectric constant in the skin. A rise in water content causes an increase in capacitance values.[3] Although corneometer measurements are related to water content of the SC, they are not directly related to TEWL. A healthy SC has both a low TEWL (a nonleaky barrier) and a high electrical capacitance (high water content).

The Cutometer

This is a suction device that measures viscoelasticity of the skin (Fig. 38-3). The Cutometer measures the amount of skin elevation caused by the suction force over a defined area of the skin.[21] In order to receive accurate readings with this instrument, the experimental conditions must be well controlled. Various parameters such as load (vacuum), aperture of the suction device, position and pressure of application of the probe, time of application and relaxation, and pretension of the skin must be kept constant. When used properly, the Cutometer provides reproducible and accurate stress-strain and strain-time curves. These data yield quantitative information concerning the purely elastic and viscoelastic properties of the dermis.

The Reviscometer

Using a Reviscometer RVM 600 (Courage & Khazaka Electronic GmbH, Köln, Germany), Ruvolo and his team from the Johnson & Johnson Consumer Companies, Inc. proposed a new methodology for documenting the age-dependent changes of the mechanical properties of the skin.[22] This method is based on determining the directional dependence of the speed of an acoustic shear wave on the skin surface at intervals of 3 degrees. Based on the angular distribution of the resonance running time they defined two

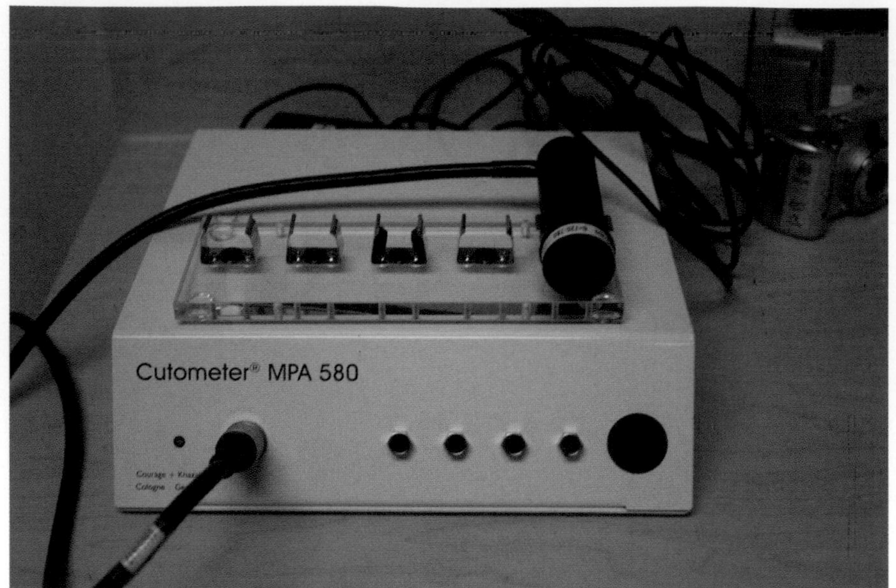

▲ **FIGURE 38-3** The Cutometer. The black suction device is placed on skin to measure elasticity.

parameters: the ansitropy and the angular dispersion width. According to their findings, with increasing age the ansitropy increases, while the angular dispersion width decreases. The ratio of these two values provides a sensitive parameter for the assessment of the behavior of the mechanical properties of the skin, and is also capable of demonstrating the differences in skin viscoelasticity from infants up to adults 75 years of age.

Dermaflex

This instrument also measures the elastic properties of the skin using suction. However, in contrast to the Cutometer, which uses a disproportional superficial strain method, this device uses a proportional full-thickness strain method. The Cutometer is more often used for cosmetic studies and Dermaflex is used more often in dermatologic studies.[21]

Optical Profilometry

This technique requires the use of silicone rubber casts that are made of the skin's surface. These casts are then analyzed using optical profilometry based on digital image processing in the following manner. Tangential lighting is cast across the replicas. The degree of skin surface irregularities is then measured by means of a digital camera to show the fractional area of shadows in the replica. If the surface is smooth, there will be fewer shadows, whereas for a rough and wrinkled surface, the shadowed areas will increase.[23] The values across 10 equally-spaced horizontal segments are plotted to generate profiles reflecting the surface features at these specific locations. Computerized image analysis of skin replicas has been used in several studies.[24–26] A good correlation has been observed between the profilometric results and clinical observations.[27]

Ultraviolet Light

Ultraviolet (UV) light is widely used by dermatologists in diagnosing certain disorders of skin pigmentation. UV lamps usually emit a light spectrum of 300 to 400 nm. The melanin in the epidermis absorbs and accentuates under the light. Wood's light (360 nm) is a useful instrument for assessing patients with melasma. If an epidermal component is present, the hyperpigmented areas are viewed as darker than the surrounding epidermis, while the dermal component will not appear any different than normal epidermis. Conversely, in patients with vitiligo, the hypopigmented spots will light up under the illumination, indicating the lack of melanin.

Photography

Photographic illustrations of skin are becoming more popular in the field of dermatology. In the past, photographs were mainly used in the before and after treatment scenario to monitor the success of therapy. Recently, through different techniques, they have also been used to demonstrate epidermal and dermal changes, including in the superficial vasculature network as well as sun damage and pigment alterations. In addition to helping physicians select the appropriate treatment plan, the patients are afforded the opportunity to visualize the undesired changes of their skin including the adverse effects of sun exposure. By using photography in daily practice, patients feel more involved in their skin care and this may lead to increased compliance with treatment plans and sunscreen application.

UV Light Photography

This method utilizes UV light for evaluating the skin surface. A filter is placed on the camera lens that only allows the transmission of the desired UV light spectrum. Epidermal changes, including the pigment network of the skin surface, are visualized by using this method while the dermal component is eliminated. This allows the physician to evaluate epidermal pigment alterations without the influence of the dermal pigment network.

Polarized Light Photography

The light reflected from the skin consists of two elements: "regular reflectance" (glare) and "back scattered" light.[28] Polarized light photography uses the two mentioned types of reflected light to illustrate epidermal and dermal components of the skin. While the regular reflectance provides assessment of the epidermis, the back-scattered light illustrates the dermal components of the skin.[28] This is handled by the orientation of the filters in the camera. If the lens filter is parallel to the flash filter, only the regular reflectance is allowed to transit through, while the perpendicular orientation permits the transmission of the back-scattered light.[28] This method is useful in assessing the epidermal and dermal components of skin independent of each other.

TruVu Digital Imaging System

Developed by Johnson & Johnson Consumer Companies, Inc., TruVu (Fig. 38-4) is a facial imaging system that accurately provides revealing photos and objective measures of subdermal conditions. It is very useful in a clinical dermatology practice or an aesthetician's office because it has the ability to track improvements in the patient's skin. Over the past decade, the company has conducted more than 100 clinical trials of its skincare products and amassed a database of more than 40,000 consumer images. In the process, the imaging system has been improved, becoming smaller, more flexible, and portable. The current system pinpoints conditions on and below the surface of the skin in a series of five images of each client's face. All five images are captured in approximately 10 seconds. This imaging system

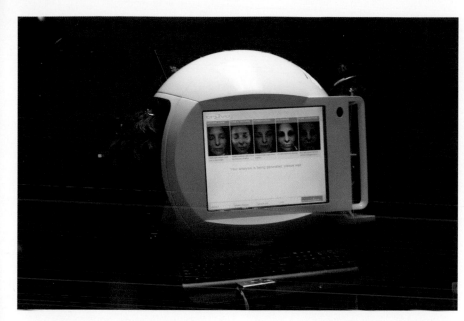

▲ **FIGURE 38-4** TruVu®Digital Imaging Systems.

employs a sophisticated lens and several flashes and filters using two types of polarized lights, as well as fluorescent and ultraviolet lights. The system's four lights include: parallel-polarized light, which highlights fine lines and pores; cross-polarized light, which reveals redness and irritation; blue light, which discloses the presence of bacteria and clogged pores; and an ultraviolet light, which shows sun damage. The images are stored in the system, where they can be easily retrieved when needed.

Canfield Scientific Camera System

These camera systems are specifically designed to meet the needs of the individual physician using the camera. The camera system has an adjustable chin rest and a forehead rest with a fiber optic guide light to ensure proper positioning of the head in before and after pictures. This is necessary to ensure that the before and after pictures are as similar as possible, with the only variable being the finding that is being photographed. Canfield systems come with regular cameras and/or ultraviolet cameras, and may also include digital cameras and software that can measure distances in the before and after pictures. This software is useful, for example, when studying the effects of botulinum toxin on eyebrow shape and height.

Confocal Laser Scanning Microscopy

Confocal Laser Scanning Microscopy (CLSM) is a scanning technique using a diode laser to visualize a three-dimensional image of skin from the SC of the epidermis to the papillary dermis. The commercially available devices are the Vivascope 1000 and the newer version 1500 (Lucid, Rochester, NY). The instrument is a diode laser with a wavelength of 830 nm and a 30× objective lens, providing a high resolution for visualizing skin morphology. Epidermal thickness can be measured and keratinocytes identified via this technique. In addition, melanin has a strong "contrast,"[29] providing information on pigment alteration and melanocyte distribution in the epidermis. CLSM has been used in various applications in dermatology such as for the evaluation of pigmented lesions,[30] melanoma[31,32] and nonmelanoma skin cancers,[33,34] as well as inflammatory skin conditions including psoriasis[35] and contact dermatitis.[36] Of note, CLSM is still considered an experimental device in basic and clinical science and more research is warranted for its application in the diagnosis of skin conditions.

Dermoscopy

Dermoscopy, also known as epiluminescence microscopy, is a noninvasive method useful in evaluation of morphologic features of cutaneous lesions. Although utilized in both pigmented and nonpigmented neoplasms, it is mostly used to differentiate benign pigmented lesions such as seborrheic keratoses and solar lentigines from malignant melanomas. Dermoscopy is based on several criteria including pigment network, structural pattern, lesional border, and symmetry.[28] While benign nevi illustrate symmetry, regular borders, and a pigment network, melanomas are asymmetric and show an irregular pigment network, blue-white hue, and regression. Dermoscopy also helps in the identification of seborrheic keratoses, which are characterized by milia-like cysts and comedo-like openings,[37] also referred to as a "brain-like pattern."

Beau Visage

A skin imaging and consultation system, Beau Visage was developed especially for aesthetic medicine practitioners, beauty clinics, and MediSpas (Fig. 38-5). Beau Visage allows the aesthetician to view up to 2 mm beneath the surface of

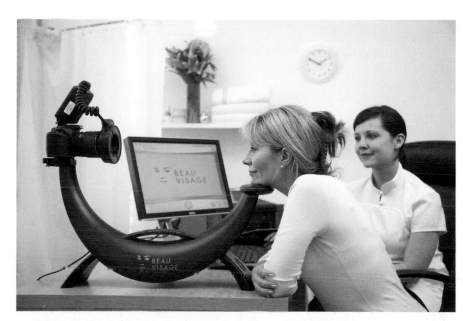

▲ **FIGURE 38-5** The Beau Visage system takes a full-face picture and highlights the hemoglobin and melanin content in the skin. It also compares the facial age versus chronologic age based on other images in its system.

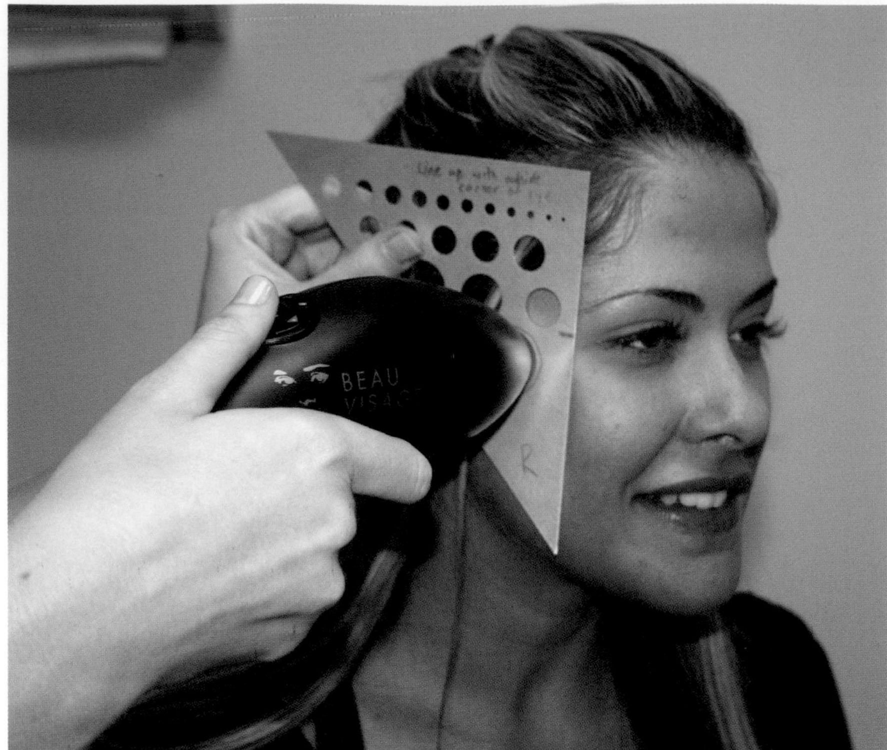

▲ **FIGURE 38-6** The Cosmetrics system uses the same hand device that comes with Beau Visage. This hand-held device is placed against the skin to produce an image used to measure extracellular matrix content, melanin, and hemoglobin. The data are tracked in software that is designed to conduct cosmetic clinical trials. The triangle with the circles is used by the author's practice to ensure that the readings are taken at exactly the same site each time. Marks on this triangle line up with the corner of the eye and other sites on the face.

the skin and to analyze the components responsible for the way their client looks and ages, such as blood, melanin, and sun damage. It also allows for the calculation of skin age based on the health of the client's skin. Beau Visage has been specifically designed to increase revenue from client consultations and to rebook clients for additional treatments. This is a modular system, with add-on elements including wrinkle analysis, spot collagen, and spot dermal melanin. Beau Visage is powered by SIAscopy, a technology that is used globally to help diagnose skin conditions as severe as skin cancer. The Baumann Visage System utilized by Beau Visage contains a module that will help determine the Baumann Skin Type (see Chapter 9).

Cosmetrics

Cosmetrics allows cosmetic formulators to test and accurately quantify the effect of a product by extracting data from live skin (Fig. 38-6). It was developed as a cosmetic trial management solution to the challenge faced by manufacturers in the skin treatment/product markets, whose consumers increasingly demand proof of product claims. Cosmetrics is the only single system currently available that can visualize and accurately measure living hemoglobin, melanin, and collagen up to 2 mm beneath the surface of the skin in vivo. It is powered by SIAscopy™ (the same system that powers Beau Visage), which is a patented skin visualization and measurement technology that provides a view of the structure of the skin.[38]

SUMMARY

This is by no means an exhaustive list of the skin bioengineering techniques that are available. However, these methods are the ones most commonly referred to in the cosmetic dermatology literature. Most of these techniques are simple to use and will help physicians collect data on patients that will help various practitioners evaluate the efficacy of the many new cosmetic procedures and treatments available on the market.

REFERENCES

1. Primavera G, Berardesca E. Sensitive skin: mechanisms and diagnosis. *Int J Cosmet Sci*. 2005;27:1.
2. Frosch PJ, Kligman AM. A method for appraising the stinging capacity of topically applied substances. *J Soc Cosmet Chem*. 197;28:197.
3. Seidenari S, Francomano M, Mantovani L. Baseline biophysical parameters in subjects with sensitive skin. *Contact Dermatitis*. 1998;38:311.
4. Lahti A. *Nonimmunologic Contact Urticaria*. Thesis, Department of Dermatology, University of Oulu and Helsinki, 1980.
5. Basketter DA, Griffiths HA. A study of the relationship between susceptibility to skin stinging and skin irritation. *Contact Dermatitis*. 1993;29:185.
6. Grove GL. Age-associated changes in intertegumental reactivity. In Léveque JL, Agache PG, eds. *Aging Skin: Properties and Functional Changes*. New York, NY: Marcel Dekker; 1993:189-192.
7. Simion FA, Rau AH. Sensitive skin. *Cosmet Toilet*. 1994;109:43.
8. Hannuksela A, Hannuksela M. Irritant effects of a detergent in wash and chamber tests. *Contact Dermatitis*. 1995;32:162.
9. Mills OH, Berger RS. Defining the susceptibility of acne prone and sensitive skin populations to extrinsic factors. *Dermatol Clin*. 1991;9:93.
10. Maibach HI, Lammintausta K, Berardesca E, et al. Tendency to irritation: sensitive skin. *J Am Acad Dermatol*. 1989;21:833.
11. Pinnagoda J, Tupker RA, Agner T, et al. Guidelines for transepidermal water loss (TEWL) measurement. *Contact Dermatitis*. 1990;22:164.
12. Issachar N, Gall Y, Borell MT, et al. pH measurements during lactic acid stinging test in normal and sensitive skin. *Contact Dermatitis*. 1997;36:152.
13. Takiwaki H, Serup J. Measurement of color parameters of psoriatic plaques by narrow-band reflectance spectrophotometry and tristimulus colorimetry. *Skin Pharmacol*. 1994;7:145.
14. Piérard GE, Goffin V, Piérard-Franchimont C. Corneosurfametry: a predictive assessment of the interaction of personal-care cleansing products with human staratum corneum. *Dermatology*. 1994;189:152.
15. Piérard GE, Goffin V, Hermanns-Lê T, et al. Surfactant-induced dermatitis: comparison of corneosurfametry with predictive testing on human and reconstructed skin. *J Am Acad Dermatol*. 1995;33:462.
16. Charbonnier V, Maibach HI. Squamometry. In: Chew AL, Maibach HI, eds. *Irritant Dermatitis*. Berlin, Germany: Springer; 2006:231-235.
17. Piérard GE, Piérard-Franchimont C, Saint-Leger D, et al. *Squamometry: The Assessment of Xerotic by Colorimetry of D-squame Adhesive Discs*. Boca Raton, FL: CRC Press; 1996:.
18. Piérard GE, Piérard-Franchimont C. In: Maibach HI, ed. *Dermatologic Research Techniques: Drug and Cosmetic Evaluations with Skin Strippings*. Boca Raton, FL: CRC Press; 1996:132-149.
19. Piérard GE. EEMCO guidance to the assessment of dry skin (xerosis) and ichthyosis: evaluation by stratum corneum strippings. *Skin Res Technol*. 1996;2:3.
20. Paye M, Morrison BM Jr. Non visible skin irritation. *Proceedings of the fourth World*

Surfactant Congress. Barcelona, Spain. 1996;3:42.
21. Gniadecka M, Serup J. Suction chamber method for measurement of skin mechanical properties: The dermaflex. In: Serup J, Jemec G, eds. *Handbook of Noninvasive Methods and the Skin.* Boca Raton, FL: CRC Press; 1995:329.
22. Paye M, Mac-Mary S, Elkhyat A, et al. Use of the reviscometer for measuring cosmetics-induced skin surface effects. *Skin Res Technol.* 2007;13:343.
23. Grove G, Grove M, Leyden J. Optical profilometry: an objective method for quantification of facial wrinkles. *J Am Acad Dermatol.* 1989;21:631.
24. Grove GL. Dermatological applications of the magiscan image analysing computer. In: Marks R, Payne PA, eds. *Bioengineering and the Skin.* New York, NY: MTP Press; 1976:173-80.
25. Grove GL, Grove MJ. Objective methods for assessing skin surface topography noninvasively. In: Lévêque JL, ed. *Cutaneous Investigations in Health and Disease.* New York, NY: Marcel Dekker; 1988:1-32.
26. Grove GL, Grove MJ. Effects of topical retinoids on photoaged skin as measured by optical profilometry. In: Packer L, ed. *Methods in Enzymology.* New York, NY: Academic Press; 1990:360-71.
27. Olsen EA, Katz HI, Levine N, et al. Tretinoin emollient cream for photodamaged skin: results of 48-week, multicenter, double-blind studies. *J Am Acad Dermatol.* 1997;37:217.
28. Taylor S, Westerhof W, Im S, et al. Noninvasive techniques for the evaluation of skin color. *J Am Acad Dermatol.* 2006;54:S282.
29. Rajadhyaksha M, Grossman M, Esterowitz D, et al. In vivo confocal scanning laser microscopy of human skin: melanin provides strong contrast. *J Invest Dermatol.* 1995104:946.
30. Langley RG, Burton E, Walsh N, et al. In vivo confocal scanning laser microscopy of benign lentigines: comparison to conventional histology and in vivo characteristics of lentigo maligna. *J Am Acad Dermatol.* 2006;55:88.
31. Marghoob AA, Charles CA, Busam KJ, et al. In vivo confocal scanning laser microscopy of a series of congenital melanocytic nevi suggestive of having developed malignant melanoma. *Arch Dermatol.* 2005;141:1401.
32. Busam KJ, Charles C, Lohmann CM, et al. Detection of intraepidermal malignant melanoma in vivo by confocal scanning laser microscopy. *Melanoma Res.* 2002;12:349.
33. Torres A, Niemeyer A, Berkes B, et al. 5% imiquimod cream and reflectance-mode confocal microscopy as adjunct modalities to Mohs micrographic surgery for treatment of basal cell carcinoma. *Dermatol Surg.* 2004;30:1462.
34. Horn M, Gerger A, Koller S, et al. The use of confocal laser-scanning microscopy in microsurgery for invasive squamous cell carcinoma. *Br J Dermatol.* 2007;156:81.
35. Gonzalez S, Rajadhyaksha M, Rubinstein G, et al. Characterization of psoriasis in vivo by reflectance confocal microscopy. *J Med.* 1999;30:337.
36. Gonzalez S, Gonzalez E, White WM, et al. Allergic contact dermatitis: correlation of in vivo confocal imaging to routine histology. *J Am Acad Dermatol.* 1999;40:708.
37. Braun RP, Rabinovitz HS, Krischer J, et al. Dermoscopy of pigmented seborrheic keratosis: a morphological study. *Arch Dermatol.* 2002;138:1556.
38. Astron Clinica Web site. http://www.astronclinica.com/. Accessed March 8, 2008.

CHAPTER 39

Scales Used To Classify Skin

Mari Paz Castanedo-Tardan, MD
Leslie Baumann, MD

TABLE 39-1
Fitzpatrick's Skin Phototyping System

Skin Type	Typical Features	Tanning Ability
I	Pale white skin, blue/hazel eyes, blond/red hair	Always burns, does not tan
II	Fair skin, blue eyes	Burns easily, sometimes tans
III	Darker white/medium skin	Sometimes burns, always tans
IV	Light brown skin	Burns minimally, tans easily
V	Brown skin	Rarely burns, always tans
VI	Dark brown or black skin	Never burns, always tans darkly

Skin type classifications are not only important in patient evaluation and treatment, but also play a key role in the assessment of patients in clinical trials. Some classifications such as Fitzpatrick skin phototyping are mostly used for treatment plans and response. Others, on the other hand, are primarily used in clinical studies to assess the severity of the cosmetic disorder and evaluate and follow-up the treatment response. In order to understand and assess the treatment response, physicians greatly benefit from the use of structural measurement scales. Both types of classifications will be discussed in this chapter.

FITZPATRICK CLASSIFICATION

Fitzpatrick skin classification became the initial skin typing system when it was introduced in 1975 by Dr. Thomas B. Fitzpatrick to measure skin sensitivity to ultraviolet (UV) light (Table 39-1). It was originally designed to classify patients in order to determine the correct dose of UV light for treating psoriasis. Notably, this classification was not intended to define skin color; rather, it is based on patients' skin responses to UV light. Although not an indicator of patients' ethnicity, it provides an idea of subjects' skin color and complexion. For many years, Fitzpatrick's skin classification was the predominant skin typing system used in the literature. Currently, dermatologists use this classification approach for planning treatments with UV light in addition to predicting skin response to different laser treatments.

BAUMANN SKIN TYPE CLASSIFICATION

The Baumann Skin Typing System was introduced in 2005 in the book *The Skin Type Solution* (New York, Bantam 2005). This approach to classifying skin type and tailoring corresponding treatments is discussed at length in Chapter 9 and can be used for patients regardless of their age, gender, or ethnicity. It is based on evaluating the skin according to four major parameters: oily versus dry (O/D), sensitive versus resistant (S/R), pigmented versus nonpigmented (P/N), and wrinkled versus tight (W/T). To obtain one's four-letter skin type code, patients take a self-administered questionnaire known as the Baumann Skin Type Indicator (BSTI), which provides a score correlating with an individual's prevailing cutaneous tendencies along the four descriptive spectra. The various permutations of the four parameters yield 16 different skin types (Table 39-2). The questionnaire to determine Baumann Skin Type can be found at www.skinIQ.com

SKIN SENSITIVITY

Acne Quality of Life Scale

The psychosocial effects of acne are very well known among dermatologists (see Chapters 15 and 40). The Acne-Specific Quality of Life Questionnaire (Acne-QoL) was specifically designed to assess the psychologic impact of acne on patients affected with this condition.[1] The test contains 19 questions in four major categories: self-perception, role-social, role-emotional, and acne symptoms (Table 39-3). The questions are asked about the patient's feelings and concerns within the "last week" prior to answering the questionnaire. The answers are assessed on a seven-point scale ranging from "0" correlating with "extremely" or "extensive" to "6" representing "not at all" or "none." The values are then totaled, with a higher score indicating a better quality of life. This system provides physicians with a universal approach to assessing patients with psychosocial impacts of acne both in clinical practice and trials.

PIGMENTATION

The Melasma Area and Severity Index

The Melasma Area and Severity Index (MASI) was introduced by Kimbrough-Green et al. to quantify the severity and treatment response in patients with melasma (Fig. 39-1). The MASI score evaluates facial skin based on three variables: area (A) of involvement, darkness (D) of melasma, and homogeneity (H) of hyperpigmentation (Table 39-4A).

TABLE 39-2
Baumann Skin Typing System

ORNT—oily, resistant, nonpigmented, and tight	ORNW—oily, resistant, nonpigmented, and wrinkled	ORPT—oily, resistant, pigmented, and tight	ORPW—oily, resistant, pigmented, and wrinkled
OSNT—oily, sensitive, nonpigmented, and tight	OSNW—oily, sensitive, nonpigmented, and wrinkled	OSPT—oily, sensitive, pigmented, and tight	OSPW—oily, sensitive, pigmented, and wrinkled
DRNT—dry, resistant, nonpigmented, and tight	DRNW—dry, resistant, nonpigmented, and wrinkled	DRPT—dry, resistant, pigmented, and tight	DRPW—dry, resistant, pigmented, and wrinkled
DSNT—dry, sensitive, nonpigmented, and tight	DSNW—dry, sensitive, nonpigmented, and wrinkled	DSPT—dry, sensitive, pigmented, and tight	DSPW—dry, sensitive, pigmented, and wrinkled

TABLE 39-3
Acne-Specific Quality of Life Questionnaire System

SELF-PERCEPTION	ROLE-SOCIAL	ROLE-EMOTIONAL	ACNE SYMPTOMS
Feel unattractive	Concern about going out in public	Concern about not looking best	Bumps on face
Feel embarrassed	Concern about meeting new people	Concern about medication not working fast enough	Bumps full of pus on face
Feel self-conscious	Problem in interacting with opposite sex (same sex if homosexual)	Feel upset about facial acne	Scabbing from facial acne
Negative self-confidence	Problem with socializing	Annoyed about spending time to treat and clean face	Oily facial skin
Dissatisfied with self-appearance		Bothered by the need to have medication or cover-up available	Concern about scarring on face

Four facial areas, the forehead, right and left malar regions, and chin are considered in this assessment, with the following subdivisions and designations: right frontal (RF), left frontal (LR), right malar (MR), left malar (ML), and chin (C). These correspond to 15% (right frontal), 15% (left frontal), 30% (right malar), 30% (left malar), and 10% (chin) of facial surface area. Melasma involvement is evaluated in each of the four areas by assigning a numerical value of involvement between 0 and 6. They are defined as 0 = no involvement; 1 = <10%; 2 = 10% to 29%; 3 = 30% to 49%; 4 = 50% to 69%; 5 = 70% to 89%; and 6 = 90% to 100% (Table 39-4B). Darkness and homogeneity of hyperpigmentation are assessed on a scale of 0 (absent) to 4 (maximum). The score is calculated based on the MASI formula. The calculation can be performed using scores for each half face and summed up, or be completed from scores for the full face. The value for each half face is calculated between 0 and 24 and then added to the other half for the total facial score between 0 and 48. The equations for half face and full face are as follows:

$$\text{MASI (half face):} = 0.15(D_{RF} + H_F)A_F + 0.3(D_{RM} + H_{RM})A_{RM} + 0.05(D_{RC} + H_{RC}).$$

$$\text{MASI (full face)} = 0.3(D_F + H_F)A_F + 0.3(D_{MR} + H_{MR})A_{MR} + 0.3(D_{ML} + H_{ML})A_{ML} + 0.1(D_C + H_C).$$

Taylor Hyperpigmentation Scale

The Taylor Hyperpigmentation Scale is a visual scale introduced by Taylor et al. in 2005.[2] This assessment is composed of 15 colored plastic cards that are applicable to Fitzpatrick skin classification types I to VI. Each card has 10 progressively darker bands of skin color gradations, demonstrating the increasing level of hyperpigmentation. The combination of 15 cards each with 10 increasingly darker bands provides the dermatologist with a wide range of skin hues by which to render an evaluation. This system is an inexpensive and effective approach to patient follow-up and assessment of treatment response. However, there is a significant intra and interindividual difference of grading among the investigators[2] (see Figure 14-1 in Chapter 14).

Forehead R.Malar L.Malar Chin
MASI = 0.3A (D+H) + 0.3A (D+H) + 0.3A (D+H) + 0.1A (D+H)

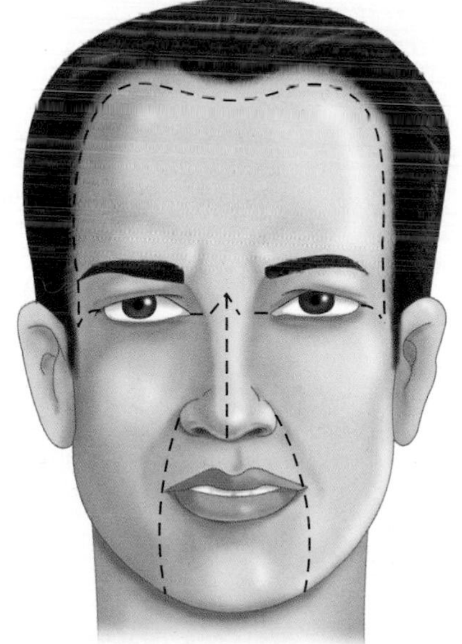

▲ **FIGURE 39-1** Melasma Area and Severity Index (MASI) score—division of facial areas. *(Adopted from Pandya A, Berneburg M, Ortonne JP, et al. Guidelines for clinical trials in melasma. Pigmentation Disorders Academy. Br J Dermatol. 2006;156(suppl1):21; Kimbrough-Green CK, Griffiths CE, Finkel LJ, et al. Topical retinoic acid (tretinoin) for melasma in black patients. A vehicle-controlled clinical trial. Arch Dermatol. 1994; 130:727.)*

TABLE 39-4
Melasma Area and Severity Index (MASI)

A.

	FOREHEAD (F), RT FOREHEAD (RF), LT FOREHEAD (LF)	RIGHT MALAR REGION (MR)	LEFT MALAR REGION (ML)	CHIN (C)
Area value (A)	A_F ($A_{RF} + A_{LF}$)	A_{MR}	A_{ML}	A_C
Darkness (D	D_F ($D_{RF} + D_{LF}$)	D_{MR}	D_{ML}	D_C
Homogeneity (H) of hyperpigmentation	H_F ($H_{RF} + H_{LF}$)	H_{MR}	H_{ML}	H_C

B.

	AREA (A)	DARKNESS (D)	HOMOGENEITY (H)
0	No involvement	Absent	Minimal
1	<10%	Slight	Slight
2	10%–29%	Mild	Mild
3	30%–49%	Moderate	Moderate
4	50%–69%	Severe	Maximum
5	70%–89%		
6	90%–100%		

Area of involvement is scored from 0 to 6. Darkness and homogeneity are scored from 0 to 4.

WRINKLES AND PHOTOAGING SCALES

Glogau Photoaging Classification

The Glogau Classification, known in the lay media as "The Wrinkle Scale," was designed for the assessment of generalized facial photoaging. It is based on four major criteria consisting of no wrinkles (Type I), wrinkles in motion (Type II), wrinkles at rest (Type III), and only wrinkles (Type IV) (Table 39-5).

TABLE 39-5
Glogau Photoaging Classification

TYPE I NO WRINKLES	TYPE II WRINKLES IN MOTION	TYPE III WRINKLES AT REST	TYPE IV ONLY WRINKLES
Usually ages 20s–30s	Usually ages late 30s–40s	Usually age 50 or older	Usually age 60 or above
Early photoaging	Early to moderate photoaging	Advanced photoaging	Severe photoaging
Mild pigmentary changes	Early senile lentigines	Obvious dyschromias, telangiectasias	Yellow-gray skin
No keratoses	Palpable but not visible keratoses	Visible keratoses	Prior skin malignancies
Minimal wrinkles	Parallel smile lines beginning to appear lateral to mouth.	Persistent wrinkling	No normal skin

Adapted from Glogau RG. Chemical peeling and aging skin. *J Geriatric Dermatol.* 1994;2(1):31.

Fitzpatrick's Classification of Facial Wrinkling (Perioral and Periorbital)

Dr. Richard E. Fitzpatrick's classification of facial wrinkling is directed toward skin elasticity and generalized wrinkling and was designed for perioral and periorbital rhytides (Table 39-6). It was originally designed for establishing the effects of laser resurfacing of wrinkled skin.

TABLE 39-6
Fitzpatrick's Classification of Facial Wrinkling

CLASS	SCORE	WRINKLING	DEGREE OF ELASTOSIS
I	1–3	Fine wrinkles	Mild (fine textural changes with subtly accentuated skin lines)
II	4–6	Fine to moderate-depth wrinkles, moderate number of lines	Moderate (distinct papular elastosis, individual papules with yellow translucency, dyschromia)
III	7–9	Fine to deep wrinkles, numerous lines, with or without redundant skin	Severe (multipapular and confluent elastosis, thickened, yellow, and pallid cutis rhomboidalis)

Adapted from Fitzpatrick RE, Goldman MP, Satur NM, et al. Pulsed carbon dioxide laser resurfacing of photo-aged facial skin. *Arch Dermatol.* 1996;132:395.

Hamilton Scale

Hamilton described a classification of contour changes of facial skin. It is based on four variables: clinical morphology (laxity, furrows, or wrinkles); tissue location (muscular, musculocutaneous, or cutaneous); clinical location (cheeks, neck, eyelids, forehead, etc.); and etiology (genetic, repeated facial expression, or photoaging). Each type of change is then presented with a proper procedural treatment, such as rhytidectomy, soft tissue augmentation, resurfacing with lasers or chemical peels, or a combined approach (Tables 39-7A and B).

Lemperle Scale

The Lemperle Scale is another approach to assessing facial wrinkles[3] (Table 39-8). It was originally designed to evaluate treatment response with injectable fillers. This classification addresses specific wrinkles on different anatomical areas. The wrinkles assessed on this scale are horizontal forehead furrows, glabellar frown lines, periorbital lines, periauricular lines, cheek lines, nasolabial folds, radial upper lip lines, radial lower lines, corner of the mouth lines, marionette lines, the labiomental crease, and horizontal neck folds.

Larnier Photographic Scale

The Larnier Photographic Scale was designed to rate photoaging of skin based on photographs.[4] It is a six-point photographic scale, with each point consisting of three separate photos to illustrate each level of severity. Therefore, the scale consists of six grades of photoaging severity, with grade 1 corresponding to mild and grade 6 to very severe. Larnier's scale has been validated for assessing photodamage in Caucasian subjects, but not other ethnic groups.

TABLE 39-7A
Hamilton Classification—Changes in Facial Contours Occurring with Age

FACIAL AGING	CLINICAL MORPHOLOGY	TISSUE LOCATION	CLINICAL LOCATION	ETIOLOGY	OPTIMAL TREATMENT
A	Folds	Muscular	Nasolabial folds, neck, eyelids	Loss of tone, gravity	Rhytidectomy, blepharoplasty
B	Furrows	Musculocutaneous	Forehead, smile lines	Repeated facial expressions	Filler substances, injectables, implants
C	Wrinkles	Cutaneous	Cheeks, crow's feet, perioral	Intrinsic aging, photoaging	Resurfacing, laser, chemical peel
D	Combination				Combined approach

Adapted from Hamilton DG. A classification of the aging face and its relationship to remedies. *J Clin Dermatol.* Summer. 1998:35.

TABLE 39-7B
Appropriate Treatments According to Hamilton Classification

TYPE OF CHANGE	OPTIMAL TREATMENT
A	Rhytidectomy (with or without implants); blepharoplasty
B	Filler substances: injectables/ implants
C	Resurfacing: laser, chemical peel
D	Combined approach

Adapted from Hamilton DG. A classification of the aging face and its relationship to remedies. *J Clin Dermatol.* Summer. 1998:35.

The Wrinkle Severity Rating Scale

The Wrinkle Severity Rating Scale (WSRS) is a five-grade photographic scale assessing the nasolabial folds.[5] Physicians are provided with photographs that help them in ascertaining the severity of nasolabial folds and evaluating the outcomes of cosmetic procedures. The grading is defined as absent, mild, moderate, severe, and extreme, corresponding with grades 1 to 5, respectively.

TABLE 39-8
Lemperle Scale

CLASS	DESCRIPTION
0	No wrinkles
1	Just perceptible wrinkles
2	Shallow wrinkles
3	Moderately deep wrinkles
4	Deep wrinkles, well-defined edges
5	Very deep wrinkles, redundant fold

Adapted from Lemperle G, Holmes RE, Cohen SR, et al. A classification of facial wrinkles. *Plast Reconstr Surg.* 2001;108:1735.

Griffith's Photonumeric Scale

This is a nine-point photonumeric scale for assessing facial photodamage. It is illustrated by five sets of photographs depicting five of the nine scaling grades (0–8), with the odd number grading points not illustrated. Each set consists of two photographs (*en face* and 40-degree oblique). They are graded as 0, 2, 4, 6, and 8, correlating with no damage, mild, moderate, moderate/severe, and severe damage, respectively.[6]

L'Oréal Scale

L'Oréal has published an atlas that has a wide array of photographs that can be used to grade the aging of the skin of men and women.[7] Volume 1 covers what the company refers to as Caucasian type skin. These photos are useful in both the research and clinical settings to evaluate the performance of the actions undertaken; compare the effects of different products and treatments; and measure their effectiveness, using a standardized visual evaluation criterion. A few examples appear in Figs. 39-2 and 39-3.

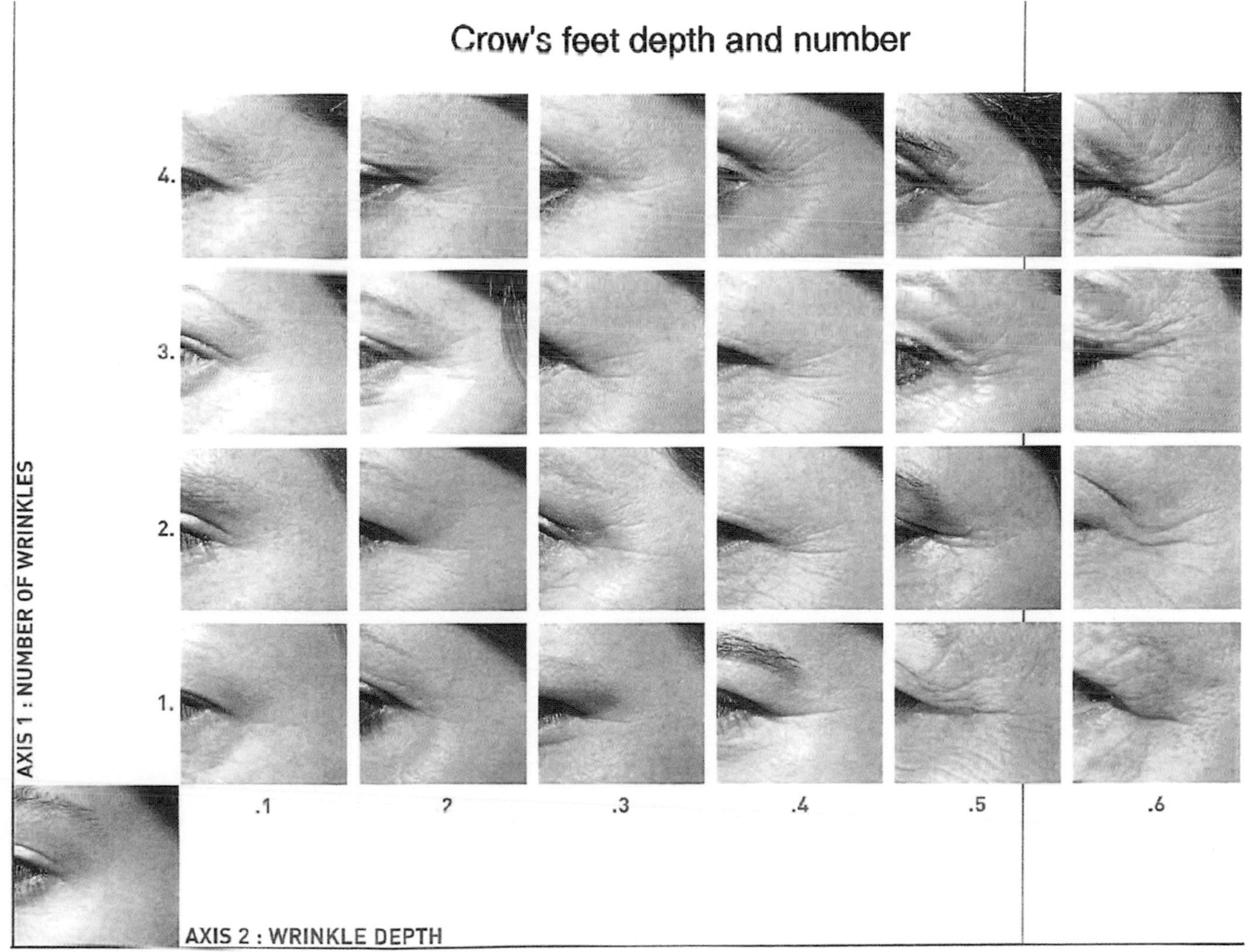

▲ **FIGURE 39-2** L'Oréal Visual Scale for the evaluation of Caucasian type, female crow's feet depth and number.

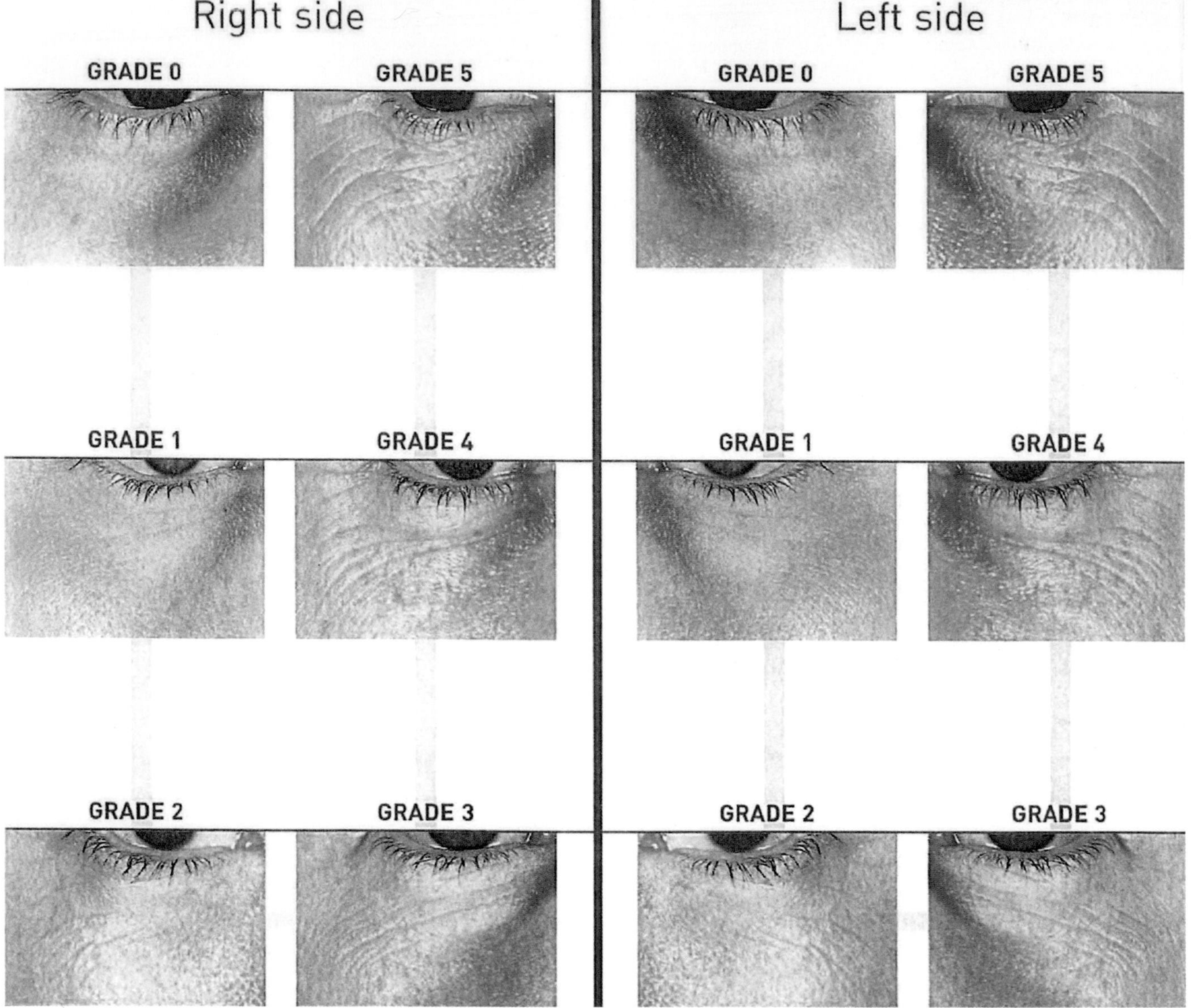

▲ **FIGURE 39-3** L'Oréal Visual Scale for the evaluation of Caucasian type, female underneath eye.

SUMMARY

There are several scales available in the practice of cosmetic dermatology for the purposes of classifying and evaluating the skin prior to and after ameliorative procedures. The ideal scale is uncomplicated, easy to use, and reliable with well-defined categories. An ideal scale should also be reliable for use in daily practice in addition to clinical trials. Finally, the best scales are intelligible to patients, as patients prefer and benefit from understanding and following the scaling system, allowing them to feel more involved in their treatment plan and progress.

REFERENCES

1. Girman CJ, Hartmaier S, Thiboutot D, et al. Evaluating health-related quality of life in patients with facial acne: development of a self-administered questionnaire for clinical trials. *Qual Life Res.* 1996;5:481.
2. Taylor SC, Arsonnaud S, Czernielewski J, et al. The Taylor Hyperpigmentation Scale: a new visual assessment tool for the evaluation of skin color and pigmentation. *Cutis.* 2005;76:270.
3. Lemperle G, Holmes RE, Cohen SR, et al. A classification of facial wrinkles. *Plast Reconstr Surg.* 2001;108:1735.
4. Larnier C, Ortonne JP, Venot A, et al. Evaluation of cutaneous photodamage using a photographic scale. *Br J Dermatol.* 1994;130:167.
5. Day DJ, Littler CM, Swift RW, et al. The wrinkle severity rating scale: a validation study. *Am J Clin Dermatol.* 2004; 5:49.
6. Griffiths CE, Wang TS, Hamilton TA, et al. A photonumeric scale for the assessment of cutaneous photodamage. *Arch Dermatol.* 1992;128:347.
7. Bazin R, Doublet E. *Skin Aging Atlas.* Vol. 1. Paris, France: Caucasian Type. MED'-COM; 2007.

CHAPTER 40

The Psychosocial Aspects of Cosmetic Dermatology

Edmund Weisberg, MS

In an ideal world, people would base their sense of self-esteem only on the content of their character and not their outward appearance; there would be no discernible disparity in hiring rates among those considered attractive and those deemed unattractive; and the cultural emphasis on or obsession with beauty would be relegated to a level of focus much closer to its actual importance. Needless to say, we do not live in an ideal world. Certainly, there is ample evidence to suggest that across a wide swathe of the population, one's own appearance is important on the individual level and has wider social implications. The American Society of Plastic Surgery reports that nearly 11 million cosmetic procedures (comprising cosmetic surgery and minimally-invasive but not reconstructive procedures) were performed by board-certified physicians in the United States in 2006, which represented a 7% increase over the previous year, and a 48% increase from 2000. In turn, the 2005 total represented a 151% increase from 2000 and a 775% increase from 1992 (the first year for which the 76-year-old organization has detailed statistics). In 2006, Botox injections, chemical peels, laser hair removal, microdermabrasion, and hyaluronic acid, in descending order, were the five most popular procedures.[1] In total, soft tissue filler procedures (also including calcium hydroxylapatite, collagen, fat, and polylactic acid) collectively represented the second most popular type of procedure. The top five cosmetic surgical procedures, also in descending order, were breast augmentation, nose reshaping, liposuction, eyelid surgery, and tummy tuck. According to psychiatric studies, the number of "healthy" people seeking aesthetic surgery has increased steadily since 1980, indicating greater public acceptance, wider diversity in those seeking the procedures, and an evolution in the psychiatric definition of "healthy."[2]

As with most of the topics covered in this text, a full book could be devoted to the psychosocial aspects of cosmetic dermatology and, in particular, the billion-dollar beauty industry as well as the historic, philosophic, and theoretical investigation of beauty itself. This chapter will discuss some of the underlying reasons for the ever-increasing incidence of elective aesthetic procedures in the developed world and what motivates people to undergo these procedures. Specifically, this chapter will focus on the influence and significance of beauty in society and its implications for the field of cosmetic dermatology. The significant social and psychic consequences that disorders such as psoriasis, alopecia, hirsutism, melasma, rosacea, vitiligo, and others have on individual's health-related quality of life are generally beyond the scope of this chapter, though such effects related to acne are briefly considered as is the role of stress as an initiating or mediating factor in cutaneous conditions that may, in turn, induce anxiety over the effects on one's skin, fostering the desire for remedial cosmetic treatment.

THE VIEW OF EVOLUTIONARY PSYCHOLOGY: PULCHRITUDE TO THE MULTITUDE

In the United States, more than twice as much money is spent on personal care than on reading material. In 2000, North America represented 80% of the market of the 45 billion-dollar global cosmetics and toiletries industry with Europe accounting for 34.9%, Japan, 18.9%, and other countries comprising the remaining 16.2%.[3] Since then, the industry has at least trebled, with US $150 billion earned in 2004.[4] According to Global Cosmetics and Toiletries 2006, the United States and Japan are the top two individual markets, with China recently moving into third place ahead of France and Germany.[5] In addition to China, Russia, Argentina, and Brazil have shown high rates of recent growth in the cosmetics and toiletries market.[4] Although expendable income seems an integral part of the consumer equation, plenty of money is spent on cosmetics in the developing world as well. For instance, for at least the last decade, there have been more Avon ladies in Brazil than there are members of the military, with Avon ladies now outnumbering military personnel 1 million + to ~400,000 (Personal communication with the Brazilian Embassy. 3006 Massachusetts Avenue: Washington, DC; 2008).[6–8]

The usage of personal care or "cosmetic" products dates back at least 40,000 years, suggesting a lengthy history of human fascination and concern with appearance.[3,9] In fact, through the thousands of years of recorded human history, concepts of beauty have continually evolved and, in the modern age, come under close scientific scrutiny.

Evolutionary psychology purports to explain the human interest in and attraction to beauty. Although there has long been an aversion among academics to seriously investigate the subject of beauty, an explosion of research in the last three decades has challenged the assumption that beauty is merely an arbitrary cultural concoction.[10] Regardless of ethnic origin of the observer or the object of observation, studies across culture have shown a consistent basis for ascribing beauty.[11] In fact, numerous researchers now believe that while culture and individual history may influence assessments of human beauty, the general geometric facial features that form the perception of beauty might be universal.[12] Further, there is widespread support for the theory that such a universal standard for facial beauty follows the divine proportion (1:1.618),[13] which is also known as the golden ratio among several other expressions, and is also applied to overall human dimensions, additional forms in nature, as well as manifestations of human creativity, particularly architecture (Figs 40-1,

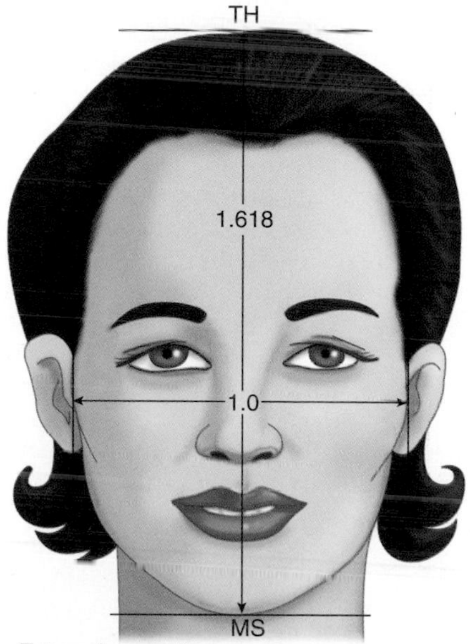

▲ **FIGURE 40-1** Facial beauty and the golden ratio.

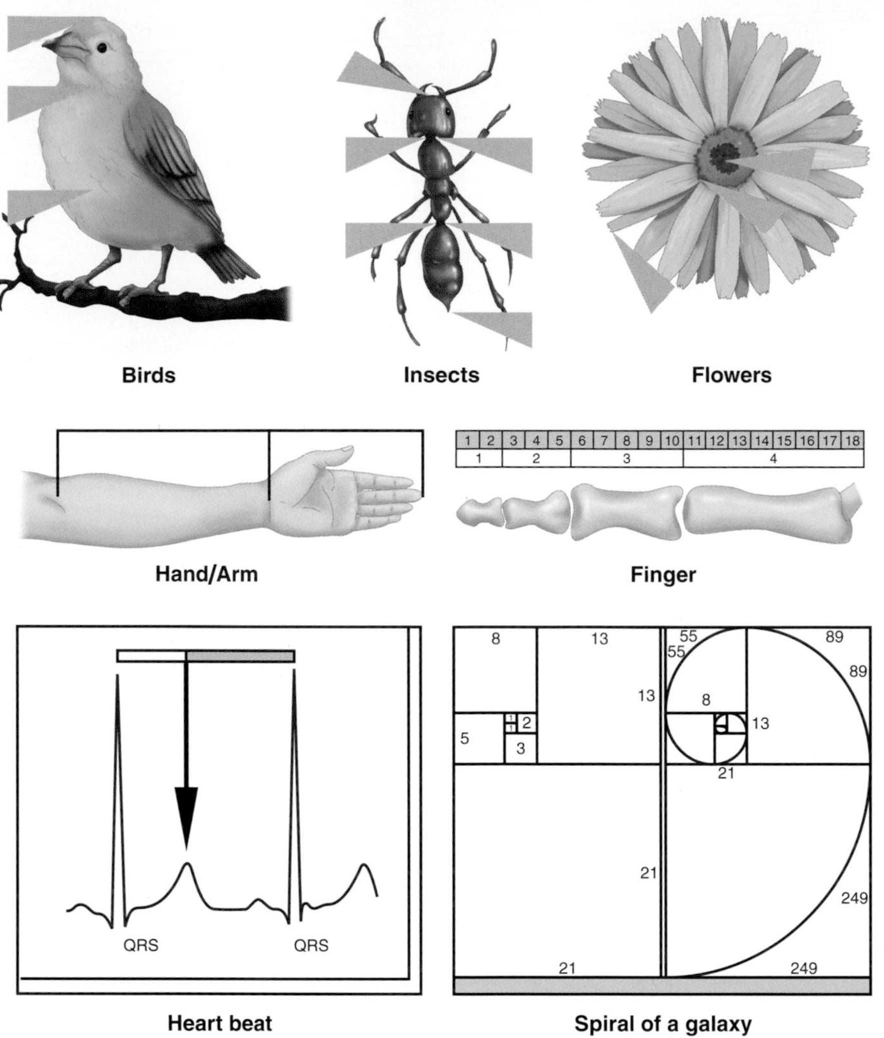

▲ **FIGURE 40-2** Manifestations of the golden ratio in nature.

40-2, and 40-3*A&B*). The argument of evolutionary psychology is that beauty is a biologic adaptation, a species-wide aspect of the human condition that elicits pleasure, compels attention, and propels activity that leads to the continuation of the gene pool. Natural selection, so the theory goes, has molded human brain circuitry to appreciate smooth skin, thick shiny hair, curved waists, and symmetric bodies because the people who, through evolution, responded to these signals had more reproductive success.[14] Etcoff suggests in her book *Survival of the Prettiest* that the human response to beauty is automatic even though thoughts and behavior are within conscious control. Further, Olson and Marshuetz have shown that facial attractiveness is assessed quickly based on few visual cues, which makes beauty difficult to ignore, they conclude, and may explain the significant social status of beauty.[15] The following discussion focuses on the human definitions of and responses to beauty, particularly the concept of facial appearance, attractive-

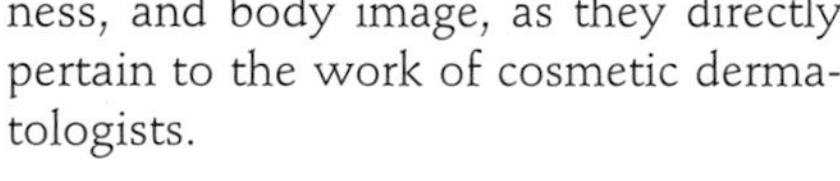

ness, and body image, as they directly pertain to the work of cosmetic dermatologists.

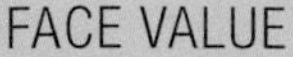

FACE VALUE

Though other areas are treated, the face is the primary locus for minimally-invasive cosmetic procedures performed by dermatologists and plastic surgeons, as well as a frequent cite for cosmetic surgical procedures. Given that the face is the most frequently and prominently displayed bodily area, it is reasonable that greater anxiety and concern would be focused on facial appearance.

The importance of the face and the frequency at which parts of the face represent the primary treatment site are a given in cosmetic practices. But is there one ideal that physicians should envision or use as a model when working to cosmetically improve a patient's face? Research has suggested that there just might be such a paragon of facial beauty. Classical musings on beauty from pre-Socratic philosophers onward to the present day appear to contain a common thread. In fact, these theories have converged on clarity, symmetry, harmony, and vivid color as important characteristics that impart beauty.[16] Ideal proportions of the face are viewed even more specifically by plastic surgeons (Fig. 40-4). Overall, more recent research has also revealed averageness, sexual dimorphism, and youthfulness along with symmetry to be significant determinants of attractiveness.[17] A provocative analysis by Langlois et al. found that subjects both within and across cultures agreed regarding those who are and are not attractive.[18] Rhodes et al., working with Chinese and Japanese study participants, have also demonstrated that

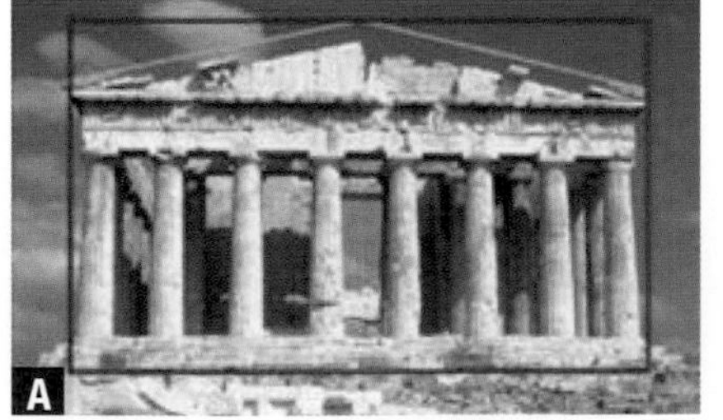

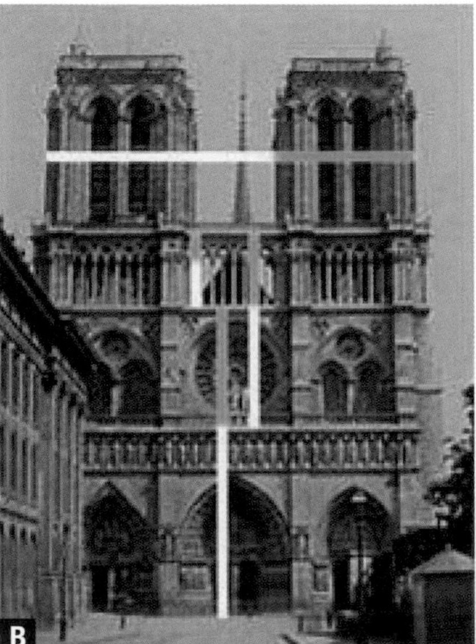

▲ **FIGURE 40-3A and 40-3B** The ancient Greeks attributed the discovery of the golden ratio to Pythagoras (*560–480 BCE*). Here, the golden ratio is expressed in the dimensions in the Parthenon at the Acropolis **A** and Notre Dame de Paris **B**.

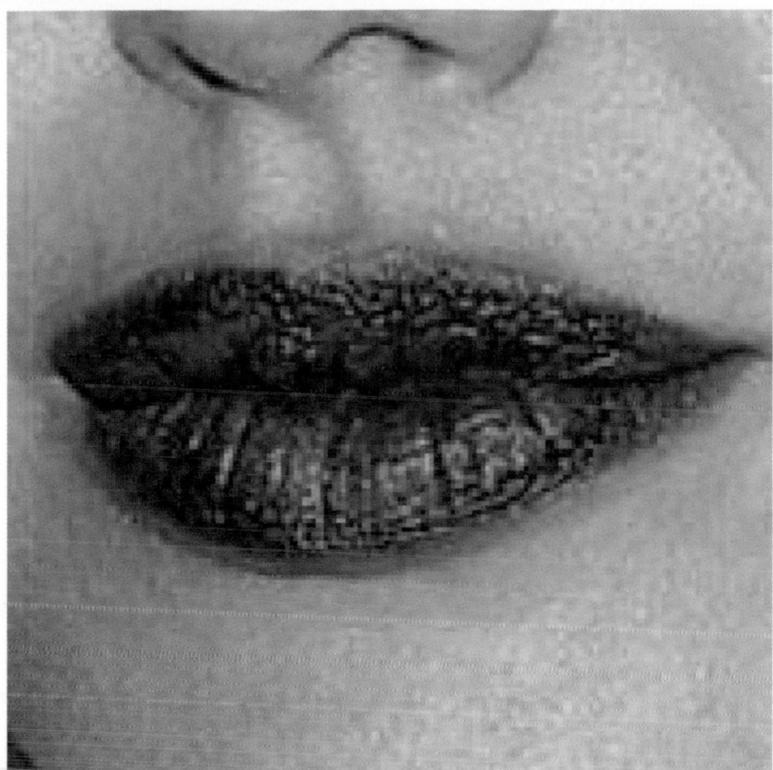

▲ **FIGURE 40-4** What is considered to be the "ideal" mouth is characterized by fullness, a well-defined philtrum, and a lower lip twice as long as the upper lip.

preferences for facial averageness and symmetry are not limited to Western cultures, buttressing the theory that such perceptions are based in biology.[19] Therefore, the "ideal face" *may* be considered ideal in any and every culture. This is important for the cosmetic dermatologist because the techniques used in one country and culture would be applicable in other cultures as well.

Despite the identification of universal notions of attractiveness, variations across cultures and among individuals in the perceptions of beauty, as well as in the particular target areas for enhancement, do persist, however. For example, a recent survey study of 50 Korean women and 50 Japanese women revealed that Korean women sought a larger fold parallel to the lid margin and epicanthal fold elimination, whereas Japanese women were primarily interested in thinner lips and generally more delicate facial characteristics.[20] Furthermore, not all theorists agree that a universal beauty ideal exists. Armstrong contended that no single principle can adequately explain the concept of beauty.[21] Hönekopp bucks the near-consensus even further by suggesting that the data that have led to the support and promulgation of universal standards of attractiveness have been misinterpreted and that, in fact, private taste is as potent as shared taste in terms of facial attractiveness perceptions.[22] On the other hand, Rubenstein argues that because different standards are employed to evaluate dynamic versus static faces and perceived emotion may play a greater role in assessing attractiveness in dynamic faces compared with static faces, a deeper understanding of the factors involved in the human perception of facial attractiveness might be achieved by more fully exploring the differences between dynamic and static faces.[23] Rhodes suggests that no gold standard for facial beauty prevails, possibly because of variable interpretations of "attractiveness" among those surveyed on the topic.[24] She does acknowledge averageness, symmetry, and sexual dimorphism as significant components of biologically based preferences, however. Such qualities can serve as important guidelines for patients as well as practitioners regardless of whether one clings to the dominant view of a universal beauty ideal.

It has been argued that the perception of beauty is a learned behavior dependent on the environment in which one is raised rather than an inherent ability to perceive beauty. Indeed, Perrett et al. have shown that the learning of parental characteristics can influence perceptions of facial attractiveness.[25] In their study, women born to parents older than 30 years of age were more attracted to male faces with visual age signals as compared to women born to parents younger than 30 years of age. Mother's age, but not the father's age, influenced men's attraction to particular female faces only when long-term relationships were considered. Humans with no preconceived notions and little or no environmental influence, in other words, babies, are perhaps the most instructive on this subject. In a study by Langlois, hundreds of slides of people's faces from a diverse population were collected and shown to adults who were asked to rate the attractiveness of the individuals. The same slides were then shown to 6-month-old babies who stared significantly longer at the same faces that the adults found most attractive.[26] These results suggest that babies can distinguish beauty and that human faces may possess universal features of beauty across different racial and individual features.[27] It is important to note that relative beauty does not affect how babies feel or interact toward their caregivers; this study dealt only with reactions to unfamiliar faces. A more recent study demonstrated that 6-month-old infants categorized pictures of female faces into attractive and unattractive groups, which the investigators suggest may reveal the foundation for the "beauty is good" stereotype.[28]

Infants have also been shown to prefer looking at symmetric as opposed to asymmetric patterns. A study of monozygotic twins who are genetically but not developmentally identical revealed that participants consistently selected the more symmetric twin of the pair as more attractive.[29] In addition, female facial attractiveness as determined by male judges has been found to be best exemplified by symmetry and averageness as well as features such as thin eyebrows, large eyes, small nose, salient cheekbones, thick lips, and a small chin.[30] These findings demonstrate that symmetry of the face is significant in the perception of beauty.

Of course, the majority of people do not have symmetric faces. In fact, it appears that natural asymmetry is an evolutionary adaptation. In one study by Zaidel et al., the investigators selected straight head-on pictures of professional models and obtained beauty ratings of these photographs from one group of subjects.[31] A different group of participants were shown left-left and right-right composites along with the original pictures, with significant differences in the ratings between the original and the symmetric composites indicating to the authors that functional asymmetry can occur within faces that are deemed beautiful. Recently, in a different study, Zaidel and other colleagues found an association between symmetry and health, but not a strong relationship between symmetry and attractiveness.[32] The researchers concluded that facial symmetry may be a potent factor in conveying health but is not essential in communicating attractiveness. If desired, asymmetric features can often be easily remedied by the adept cosmetic dermatologist or plastic surgeon, however (Fig. 40-4).

As implied above, facial symmetry is not the only important facial characteristic that factors into the human perception of a beautiful visage. Baby faces in general trigger tender emotions in adults who find the soft skin and hair, large eyes and pupils, fat cheeks, and small noses irresistible.[33] Etcoff asserts that this is another useful adaptation since defenseless infants must arouse nurturing behavior from adults on whom they are dependent for sustenance. These "baby face" facial features are often irresistible in adult faces as are slightly feminized faces. In a cross-cultural study of Japanese and Scottish subjects, participants preferred feminized shapes for both female and male faces, which may indicate a selection pressure limiting sexual dimorphism and promoting neoteny.[34] In a recent study of 400 British men and women asked to judge pictures of male faces (excluding hair, ears, neck, shoulders, etc.) digitally altered to appear more masculine or more feminine, women, on average, associated the more feminine faces with warmer, more faithful, and better parenting personalities, as well as better mate options.[35] This study appears to reinforce previous work by Rhodes et al. as well as the above work by Perrett et al. that found feminized faces to be preferred over average or masculinized faces.[36] The fact that babies and adults appear to find the same facial features attractive is compelling evidence pointing toward the biologic adaptation argument. Anthropologists have contended that facial preferences for attractive traits may indeed be adaptations because such traits may indicate important qualities in the mate, such as health. Does this mean that dermatologists and plastic surgeons should strive toward the universally admired geometric features? If so, what are the implications for those patients whose features cannot quite meet the ideal? If such universal standards exist, do they exert significant pressure on people to correct perceived imperfections? Or is the race against time the primary motivator behind cosmetic procedures?

The popularity of the billion-dollar cosmetics and toiletries industry as well as that of cosmetic procedures suggests that the seemingly relentless barrage of beauty ideals can influence people across various demographic spectra. The pervasiveness of media images of attractiveness has been shown, in fact, to exert a negative impact on women's self-perceptions, particularly the facial satisfaction levels of women who are already sensitive about their appearance.[37] Such media exposure certainly contributes to the continually escalating drive to alter one's appearance. Further, the particular images held up as iconic examples of beauty, along with their ubiquity, may even negatively affect those already considered attractive. In a study of 203 young women, researchers rated participants on facial attractiveness and obtained subjects' self-reports on perfectionism, weight preoccupation, and neuroticism.[38] After controlling for body size and neurotic perfectionism, investigators found attractiveness and weight preoccupation to be positively related, suggesting that facial beauty may pose a risk for the development of eating disorders.[38] Obviously, some attractive people yearn and strive to be perceived as even more attractive. It is important for the cosmetic dermatologist to be cognizant of this phenomenon because it is not unusual for patients to request a cosmetic procedure that is not only inappropriate for them but could actually do them harm. An example of this is a young woman in the primary author's practice who wanted CO_2 laser resurfacing for her 30th birthday. This patient was counseled and treated with a topical retinoid that resolved the imperfection with much less risk.

BODY IMAGE

Eleanor Roosevelt once said, "No one can make you feel inferior without your consent."[39] Some would have us believe that the cosmetics and toiletries industry makes a valiant attempt. In fact, there are those who would characterize the advertising of the billion-dollar beauty industry as an outright assault. Although a near-consensus regarding beauty standards seems to have emerged, the judgment of attraction is heavily influenced by mass media, art, literature, television, movies, and other media.[40] Unless one is able to steadfastly avoid television, the Internet, billboards, bus advertisements, magazines, and the like, it is virtually impossible not to encounter the plethora of beauty images virtually omnipresent in our culture today. Scanning the magazine racks, paying attention to advertisements, and watching television can leave a person feeling bombarded with what society seems to deem the ideal images of a healthy, beautiful person.

Through art history, beginning with the classical images of beauty, particularly female beauty, as depicted in ancient times, through the Medieval and Baroque periods, especially the generously-proportioned figures painted by Peter Paul Rubens, the Renaissance and on into contemporary times, it is clear that beauty ideals wax and wane. This is more patently clear when one considers the apparent changes in modern female iconography as represented by so-called supermodels, pin-up models, or centerfolds. Larger, more curvaceous women, such as Marilyn Monroe and Jayne Mansfield, were considered ideal a half century ago, while considerably thinner models, such as Kate Moss, are more typical now. Changes have also been noted and quantified regarding centerfolds during the last half century.

A recent study by Seifert that considered the height, weight, breast, waist, and hip measurements of 559 *Playboy* centerfold models over the last 50 years revealed a subtle, gradual trend toward slimness, with very thin models rarely seen until this century.[41] Greater specificity was achieved in a fascinating study that included economic conditions as a variable in facial and body feature preferences. Pettijohn and Jungeberg explored the relationships of United States social and economic factors to facial and body characteristics of *Playboy* Playmates of the Year from 1960 to 2000. They found that older, heavier, taller models with a larger waist and waist-to-hip ratio, smaller bust-to-waist ratio, smaller body mass index (BMI), and smaller eyes were chosen during periods when social and economic conditions were measurably difficult, and concluded that environmental security conditions can influence perceptions of attractiveness.[42]

In a broader study considering idealized female body images represented by *Playboy* Playmates of the Year, Miss America Pageant winners, fashion models, and young women in general spanning eight decades, Byrd-Bredbenner et al. reported that the general trend in all groups changed from a less curvaceous figure during the early 20th century to a more curvaceous shape by mid-century, returning to a less curvaceous body by the end of the century. In addition, they found a significant decline in BMI in the idealized groups over time, with an opposite trend in young women, and a markedly wider divergence between the typical body sizes of young women and the idealized images depicted in the media.[43] A smaller previous study by Katzmaryzyk and Davis that considered the changes in body weight and shape of 240 *Playboy* centerfolds from 1978 to 1998, a cohort tacitly understood as "ideal," found that 70% of the models were underweight, which underscores the nature of the social pressures for thinness that women face and helps to explain their body dissatisfaction and increased risks for eating disorders.[44]

Currently, the idealized female profile is tall and thin but sporting an hourglass figure, large eyes, prominent cheek bones, and large forehead. Other features associated with attractiveness for females include a smaller than average chin, smaller than average nose, and higher than average forehead.[45] The typical male image is also tall, muscular with little body fat, and features large eyes, prominent cheekbones, and a large chin.[46] When juxtaposed, the female has lighter hair than the male, who typically has dark hair, to match documented preferences.[40] However, negative self-esteem or body image effects on both women and men are seen more often as increasingly narrow and nearly unattainable gender stereotypes are emphasized with ideal images of physical beauty.[47]

Although women have long been described as victims of this onslaught of idealized images of feminine beauty, there is evidence to suggest that men are even starting to feel the implied pressure of such masculine imagery. Purchases of fitness equipment and even pectoral and other implants may very well be manifestations of Western cultural norms for presentations of the ideal male body that are growing increasingly muscular.[48] It is generally accepted that men spend significantly more money now than 10 to 15 years ago on aesthetic surgery, cosmetics, fitness equipment, and hair products, including dyes, weaves, and transplants. Nevertheless, 90% of the patients who underwent cosmetic surgery or minimally-invasive procedures in 2006, as tracked by the American Society of Plastic Surgeons (which measures procedures performed by physicians of all disciplines), were women.[1] This suggests that women remain more drastically and measurably influenced by beautification pressures. In a study of 246 medical students in Austria, answers to a questionnaire on weight and attitudes toward personal body weight indicated that both men and women, but women in particular, characterize their weight according to current beauty ideals as opposed to the BMI definition.[49] Researchers observed significant body dissatisfaction among women, much more than among men, and concluded that the females in the study group were more profoundly influenced by current ideals of slenderness.

Further evidence of the effects of body image on individual self-esteem is found from a study by Pinhas et al. in which 51 female subjects were shown slides of fashion models and 67 control subjects were shown slides with no human figures. The researchers found that the study group members were more depressed and angry following exposure to the slides of female fashion models, indicating that such images have an immediate negative impact on women's moods.[50] These findings are particularly noteworthy because body dissatisfaction is considered a potent risk for the development of eating disorders and can contribute to depression. A more recent meta-analysis also supports these results regarding female body image. In considering data from 25 studies, Groesz et al. observed that body image of female subjects was significantly worse after subjects saw media images of thin women as compared to average-size models, plus-size models, or inanimate objects.[51]

Although the beauty industry is frequently blamed for stimulating women's desire to appear younger and more attractive, the industry itself might not be culpable. Instead, these longings may be a reflection of preferences hard-wired into human brain circuitry through evolution. The billion-dollar beauty industry exists because women want to attract men, and men are often attracted to younger women. Etcoff argues that this attraction has occurred because of evolutionary pressure. Men remain attracted to nulliparous women who abundantly exhibit signs of fertility because this leads to propagation of the species.[52] The beauty industry, represented by the physical fitness branch, aesthetic surgery, cosmetics, and advances in beauty technology, allows people to indulge in the illusion of an extended youth and continued membership in the visually preferred age group.

Nevertheless, the advertising branch of the business might still be presenting a skewed view of what most people find desirable or acceptable. In a study on acceptable body sizes, 303 children, 427 adolescents, 261 young adults, and 326 middle-aged adults were shown several line drawings of human figures ranging in age grouping and size.[53] Participants were instructed to evaluate sets of drawings that were divided by age group—infant, children, young adult, middle-aged adult, and older adults. Each subject group preferred similar ideal body sizes across all arrays, choosing the midrange of fatness, and eschewing both the obese and very thin body sizes. Although a medically healthy range for a particular height for adults would translate to four or five of the nine body sizes depicted in the study, participants demonstrated acceptance for an average of three or fewer body sizes. This suggests that the ideal imagery exhibited in various media may filter into people's internal ideations and that midrange models might better reflect what people typically find acceptable or desirable. Further, very different images of the ideal body form continue to exist in non-Western cultures such as the Inuit, Maori, Tibetans, and Bushmen of the Kalahari Desert.[54]

The notion of the power of visual media is reinforced by a study on body dissatisfaction and abnormal eating attitudes among congenitally blind women, women who were blinded later in life, and sighted women. Baker et al. found that congenitally blind women had the lowest body dissatisfaction scores and the most positive eating attitudes while sighted women exhibited the highest level of body dissatisfaction and the most negative eating attitudes.[55] The external pressures exerted on the psyche are inestimable and provide an important backdrop for consultation with a physician prior to any decision for cosmetic alteration.

BODY DYSMORPHIC DISORDER

Body dysmorphic disorder (BDD) is a psychiatric condition defined in the Diagnostic and Statistical Manual of Mental Disorders IV (DSM-IV) as a preoccupation with an imagined defect in appearance.[56] The preoccupation causes impairment in social, occupational, or other important areas of functioning. BDD is frequently associated with significant psychologic distress and may lead to suicidal ideation and suicide attempts.[57] In fact, a study in the *British Journal of Dermatology* reported that most dermatology patients who committed suicide had acne or BDD.[58] BDD often leads to unnecessary cosmetic procedures. The most common areas that concern these patients are the skin, hair, and nose.[59] For several obvious reasons, it is important for the cosmetic dermatologist or plastic surgeon to identify these patients during history and prescreening. BDD can lead to significant morbidity as well as a disproportionately high number of risks for unnecessary procedures. In addition, these patients can be difficult to treat because they are often dissatisfied with the outcomes of the treatments they do receive.[60,61]

Phillips et al. screened 268 patients from two different environments: a general dermatology outpatient practice in a community setting and a dermatologic cosmetic surgery outpatient practice at a university teaching hospital.[59] They found that 11.9% of patients screened positive for BDD. Interestingly, the patients treated in the cosmetic surgery practice had a lower rate of BDD (10.0%) than did those in the general dermatology practice (14.4%); however, one-third of eligible subjects in the cosmetic practice refused to complete the questionnaire. This may have affected the study results, which also revealed that BDD is as common in men as it is in women. In an investigation of female college students' body images as well as their experiences and attitudes regarding cosmetic surgery, Sarwer et al. found that two-thirds of the 559 participants surveyed knew someone who had received cosmetic surgery (with approximately one-third reporting that a family member had undergone surgery), 5% had undergone cosmetic surgery themselves, and 2.5% screened positive for BDD.[62] Cosmetic dermatologists and plastic surgeons should be aware of the possibility that this syndrome is affecting some patients and should encourage such patients to receive psychiatric help. BDD can be successfully treated with serotonergic antidepressants and cognitive-behavioral treatments.[63] Of course, confronting these patients is very difficult and the approach used must be individualized for each patient. In the study by Sarwer et al., it is worth noting that participants expressed an overall favorable attitude regarding cosmetic surgery, with an association found between such favorable attitudes and greater psychologic stock placed in physical appearance as well as internalization of beauty imagery absorbed from various mass media.[62]

MOTIVATIONS FOR SEEKING COSEMTIC PROCEDURES

The media often cite the disproportionate number of overweight people in the United States, an epidemic of obesity, which invariably leads to recitations of the importance of exercise and good health, usually associating these qualities with youthfulness and beauty. The implication is that one's social acceptance and even professional success hinge on these qualities.[64] Clearly, body dissatisfaction, exogenous criticism, and the feeling that one fails to measure up to cultural standards of appearance and beauty propel people to change their behavior, lifestyles, and appearance. In a study by Santor and Walker, 75 people were examined for the degree to which their appraisals of self-worth were linked to the appraisals of how interested other people were in them. The investigators found a strong association between the degree to which people measure certain attributes of self-worth and the degree to which individuals believed others were interested in them.[65] In other words, the amount of interest one thought others showed them mediated the study subjects' expression of confidence in their own physical attributes, attractiveness, and sense of social self-worth. With ideal imagery playing a greater role in daily life, the chances that individuals will internalize such iconography and use the implications against themselves and others grows immeasurably. This is why motivations for cosmetic enhancement, while always personal, can include social and even professional elements.[66] Studies have shown, for instance, that attractive children and adults are judged and treated more positively than unattractive children and adults, even by those who know them, and such advantages persist into every age category.[18,67]

As others have noted, the reasons to undergo cosmetic procedures are always personal, based on an individual's psychologic constitution, and inextricably linked to body image, which is based on a convoluted interplay of factors both outward and inward, objective and subjective. The essential value of the procedure, though, is derived from the patient's opinion and reaction to the result and not from the general perception of the visible change as determined by those in a patient's life.[68] Of course, a patient's assessment of the result may be tempered by the reactions of her or his family and friends. Research does show that enhancing a physical characteristic and improving physical attractiveness positively affects personality and, thus, interpersonal interactions, the results of which are internalized, exerting a positive effect on self-esteem.[69]

An interesting recent study of cosmetic surgery in adolescents is illustrative, practically by definition, of the social and internalized pressures regarding appearance that can drive teenagers to seek cosmetic enhancement, as well as the potential psychologic and physical boosts that such procedures can deliver. The responses to 12 survey questions administered to 86 of 165 adolescents who underwent surgery between January 2001 and June 2005 revealed no statistically significant differences between males and females regarding postoperative satisfaction, with an overall satisfaction rate of 93.83%. Further, postoperative satisfaction was found to be strongly related to overall life satisfaction, self-esteem, and body image.[70]

Youth Movement

Beauty is a powerful springboard propelling millions of people toward the motivations that underlie the pursuit of cosmetic enhancement—the conscious desire, perhaps driven by potent, subconscious genetic impulses, to look younger. From movies to music to other forms of entertainment and advertising, society seems to increasingly cater to the young or youthful. The beauty industry, too, is youth-oriented, only it aims to assist the consumer in achieving the universally sought-after youthful appearance. Aesthetics and the search for youth apply most directly to the skin, as the largest and most visible organ of the body (though, of course, body shape or contour is also an important aspect of appearance). As skin ages, the perpetual cycle of cell turnover, which pushes fresh, young-looking skin cells to the stratum corneum during youth, slows considerably. But women of all ages strive throughout their lives to maintain the fair skin of youth. In mimicking nubile adolescent beauty, older women join in the universal obsession with clear skin and the numerous ploys and attempts to recapture and display it.[71] In that regard, it is of course worth noting that an increasing number of men are striving to improve the appearance of their skin.

It is not surprising, then, to consider the results of a study of 132 young adults (with an average age of 19 years) and 142 elderly adults (with an average age of 74 years) who were enlisted to evaluate 35 different aspects of their own bodies.

The elderly subjects expressed attitudes that were less positive as compared to those of their young counterparts regarding body functioning (e.g., physical coordination, agility, sex drive, and health) and facial attractiveness (e.g., lips, appearance of eyes, and cheeks/cheekbones).[72] The investigators noted that these results hew closely to the physical changes that take place in the body and face through aging, which distance people further from cultural beauty standards. Men had more positive body attitudes than women, but this gender difference was not nearly as pronounced among the elderly in this study.

Although the elderly have lower opinions of their own attractiveness than do young people, Kligman and Graham have found that attractiveness stereotypes persist into middle age and later years, showing that the elderly viewed as attractive have advantages over the elderly deemed unattractive.[67] Kligman and Graham suggest that cosmetics can make a crucial difference for the elderly, helping them to receive some of the benefits of the attractive through improvement in care for their appearance. Makeup has long been used as a tool to camouflage blemishes, highlight fertility signals and, later, mask age. With increasing frequency, cosmetic facial procedures have become another such instrument. However, the illusions of youth, and even fertility, play an important role in the formation of unreasonable expectations as many cosmetic patients delude themselves into believing that, after a cosmetic procedure, they will appear as they did 20 years ago. This is one of the most important notions that a physician must be alert to and prepared to dispel. Whether it is counteracting the effects of chronic sun exposure, smoking, other unhealthy behavior, or simple chronologic aging, there is a limit to how far a physician can turn back the clock.

COMMON SKIN DISEASES AND THEIR PSYCHOSOCIAL CONSEQUENCES

The forces that motivate individuals to seek cosmetic enhancement are compelling enough when a person is healthy, but an illness, particularly one that disfigures in even a minor fashion, can wreak havoc with a person's self-esteem and confidence level. Indeed, cosmetic dermatologists and plastic surgeons not too infrequently encounter patients who seek to alter their appearance because of the effects of cutaneous disorders or trauma, as well as the more standard impetus–age. The notions that stress can exacerbate dermatologic conditions and that dermatologic disorders can engender significant distress, particularly when the face is involved, may seem to be obvious accepted dogma to the modern practitioner. After all, given the status that appearance has in our society, it is no wonder that any disease process that disfigures or negatively alters one's appearance could be a source of significant anxiety. The existence of the wide variety of quality of life indices (e.g., Acne Disability Index, Psoriasis Disability Index, Dermatology Life Quality Index, Skindex, Dermatology Quality of Life Scales, Dermatology Specific Quality of Life, and the Children Dermatology Life Quality Index)[73] related to dermatology is testament to the fact that clinicians are well aware of the nexus between the appearance and condition of the skin and an individual's psychologic state. Nevertheless, investigators conducting a Medline review of the dermatologic and psychiatric literature, as well as other pertinent journals, from 1966 to 2000 found that the psychosocial effects (e.g., anxiety and depression) that can result from dermatologic problems have the potential to seriously impact individuals' lives but that these effects are underappreciated.[74] Indeed, it is estimated that in at least 30% of dermatologic conditions, psychologic and psychiatric factors play significant roles, with the psychiatric comorbidity associated with disorders such as acne or psoriasis (e.g., suicidal ideation or attempts) serving as a key gauge to the patient's overall disability.[75]

Stress and the Skin

The most common skin disorder, acne vulgaris, which afflicts approximately 17 million people in the United States alone,[76] is also a common source of emotional stress, self-consciousness, and great personal dissatisfaction. A recent review of case–control, cross-sectional population surveys, and cohort studies of acne patients has buttressed previous observational or anecdotal evidence that acne provokes significant psychosocial morbidity and psychologic distress.[77] A more recent cross-sectional study screening for BDD symptoms using a validated self-report questionnaire and single-observer assessment of acne severity among acne patients offers additional support. This study revealed that a significant proportion of patients (ranging from 14.1% to 21.1% depending on the stringency of the criteria used to evaluate acne) exhibited notable preoccupation and anxiety regarding their facial appearance.[70] Of course, distress in response to a cutaneous condition can be associated with the wide range of dermatologic disorders that can affect the face, including rosacea, melasma, vitiligo, and others.

While stress may result as a reaction to the emergence of a skin disorder, stress can also precipitate or contribute to the etiologic pathway of a cutaneous manifestation. Elias has shown that the cutaneous homeostatic permeability barrier as well as the protective action of the stratum corneum is disrupted by stress.[79] Studies have also demonstrated that glucocorticoids, which are generated in response to stress, inhibit lipid production thereby reducing the synthesis and secretion of lamellar bodies, thus contributing to disruption of the skin barrier.[80,81] Indeed, psychologic stress appears to aggravate, or even initiate, various dermatologic disorders including psoriasis and atopic dermatitis[82] (see Chapter 11).

Although the nature of the association between stress and the exacerbation of certain skin conditions has not been fully elucidated, two traditional explanations have been offered. That is, the activation of two stress axes, the hypothalamic-pituitary-adrenal (HPA) axis, which elevates cortisol levels, and the sympathetic nervous system axis, which increases adrenaline levels, are thought to alter immune balance and facilitate cutaneous inflammation.[83] Recently, a third stress axis has been suggested. Specifically, Pavlovic et al. have demonstrated that peripheral neuropeptidergic nerve fibers transmit stress to the skin, exacerbating cutaneous inflammation. The investigators showed that the number of cutaneous nerve fibers containing the stress neuropeptide substance P was increased significantly by sound stress and atopic dermatitis-like allergic dermatitis in mice. They concluded that AD is aggravated by stress by dint of substance P-dependent cutaneous neurogenic inflammation and ensuing local cytokine movement, warranting consideration as a therapeutic target.[84]

Just as the identification of a third stress axis suggests the potential for novel therapeutic approaches to mitigating the effects of stress on certain skin conditions, additional recent research appears to suggest the potential for eventual clinical impact. Aberg et al. have shown that the severity of group A

Streptococcus pyogenes skin infection in mice was augmented by psychologic stress, which led to elevated synthesis of endogenous glucocorticoids. In particular, they found that increased glucocorticoid production reduced epidermal lipid synthesis and lamellar body secretion, specifically lowering the level of expression of two pivotal antimicrobial peptides and their delivery into the lamellar bodies.[85] In an article in the same issue of *The Journal of Clinical Investigation* in which the findings of Aberg et al. were published, Slominski, a specialist in dermatopathology and neuroendocrinology of the skin, commented on the work of Aberg and colleagues, suggesting the potential for clinical impact in various forms, including systemic and topical selective receptor antagonists for HPA axis peptide and steroid messengers, topical agents that promote cortisol metabolism inactivation, and the development of agents that inhibit steroidogenesis (thereby enhancing cutaneous antimicrobial and barrier protection activity).[86]

As discussed previously, stress can also be an influential factor in pigmentary disorders (see Chapter 13). Melanocyte-stimulating hormone (MSH) levels have been shown to be influenced by a rise in adrenocorticotropic hormone (ACTH) levels, which increase with stress. Through this pathway, MSH may play a role in aggravating melasma and other dyspigmentations in stressed patients.[87]

The Skin and the Mind

The intimate, complex relationship between the status of one's appearance and the emotional reaction to it, or the relationship between the skin and the mind, is clearly important to assess in screening patients before cosmetic procedures. Indeed, Jafferany, the author of a review of the dermatologic and psychiatric literature in Medline from 1951 to 2004, concluded that consideration of related psychosocial factors is an integral part of effectively managing the cutaneous conditions of most patients who present to dermatologists.[88] Further, the identification of psychiatric or psychosocial comorbidity would likely contraindicate cosmetic treatment until the satisfactory resolution of the symptoms, perhaps through cooperative efforts of dermatologists and psychiatrists (of course, psychiatric conditions may also lead to some dermatologic problems, but such scenarios are beyond the scope of this chapter). The potential motivations that lead a patient to seek cosmetic enhancement, as understood through the filter of the psychosocial framework that informs our perceptions and feelings about appearance, are important to consider, even passively, as one screens patients to determine their suitability for cosmetic treatment.

SUMMARY

For better of for worse, appearance matters in our society. It matters to the observer and the observed. That is, people are concerned about their own appearance and that of others, particularly the appearance of a prospective mate. Interest in appearance matters enough to form the foundation of the multibillion-dollar beauty industry and its concomitant but lucrative advertising. Appearance also matters enough to propel millions of people each year to seek cosmetic enhancement at the hands of dermatologists and plastic surgeons as well as other body alterations from nonmedical specialists. But it is important to realize that appearance is hardly all that matters. For those who are not visually impaired, appearance is central in the first impression made to the world. What matters more, though, is the content of character, as well as the life choices and actions one pursues. Appearance is clearly a component in self-esteem, but it is just as clearly a relative component, it matters much more to some than others. Indeed, for many, though, beauty is a controversial, inflammatory subject.

Cosmetic dermatologists and plastic surgeons can play a unique role in patients' lives by performing procedures that impart a more youthful appearance, and by educating these patients on techniques to prevent aging, thereby providing an additional avenue for patients to improve self-esteem. In addition, practitioners have a unique opportunity to be involved in pivotal changes in a patient's psyche. Making patients feel good about themselves is certainly one of the perks of being a cosmetic dermatologist or plastic surgeon.

There is an apparently inexhaustible, cross-cultural search for and obsession with "beauty." The concept of beauty has evolved, perhaps, throughout the centuries as attempts to define, understand, or capture it have persisted. Indeed, the search for beauty appears universal and timeless. As such, when the notion is associated with enhancing or making modifications to one's natural endowment (to become more "beautiful"), and it seems there is a steady supply of people who will seek to do so, such a procedure is best left in the hands of professionals who are expert in the physiology and health of the areas to be altered. Essentially, it is better that cosmetic dermatologists and plastic surgeons meet the steady demand and, in so doing, apply medical knowledge and expertise toward the redevelopment and enhancement of the psyche as well as the skin. Perhaps it is true that "no one can make you feel inferior without your consent"; but it may be equally true that patients are giving consent to their physicians to make them feel superior—superior to their recent selves or simply on a par with their earlier selves. Physicians should handle this power responsibly and wisely. Practitioners must recognize that there are countless influences on the aesthetic judgments of individuals and strive to educate patients to make the proper choices that will enhance their self-esteem and ameliorate their quality of life, without causing harm.

REFERENCES

1. American Society of Plastic Surgery Web site. http//www.plasticsurgery.org. Accessed August 21, 2007.
2. Etcoff N. *Survival of the Prettiest: The Science of Beauty*. New York, NY: Anchor Books; 2000:19-20.
3. Etcoff N. *Survival of the Prettiest: The Science of Beauty*. New York, NY: Anchor Books; 2000:95-96.
4. Cosmetics Design-Europe.com. Developing markets still head growth in global cosmetics and toiletries market. http://www.cosmeticsdesign-europe.com/news/ng.asp?id=61158-kline-global-cosmetics. Accessed August 21, 2007.
5. Global Cosmetics and Toiletries 2006. Kline and Company: China surpasses France in global cosmetics and toiletries sales rankings. http://www.klinegroup.com/news/china_ct_042007.asp. Accessed August 21, 2007.
6. Brooke J. Who braves piranha waters? Your Avon lady! *New York Times*. July 7, 1995 http://query.nytimes.com/gst/fullpage.html?res=990CE2D9113FF934A35754C0A963958260&sec=&spon=. Accessed March 15, 2008.
7. Etcoff N. *Survival of the Prettiest: The Science of Beauty*. New York, NY: Anchor Books; 2000:6.
8. Williams J. *50 Facts That Should Change the World*. Cambridge, UK: Icon Books Ltd; 2005.
9. Blanco-Davila F. Beauty and the body: the origins of cosmetics. *Plast Reconstr Surg*. 2000;105:1196.
10. Etcoff N. *Survival of the Prettiest: The Science of Beauty*. New York, NY: Anchor Books; 2000:22.
11. Drury NE. Beauty is only skin deep. *J R Soc Med*. 2000;93:89.
12. Etcoff N. *Survival of the Prettiest: The Science of Beauty*. New York, NY: Anchor Books; 2000:23.
13. Jefferson Y. Facial beauty—establishing a universal standard. *Int J Orthod*. 2004;15:9.
14. Etcoff N. *Survival of the Prettiest: The Science of Beauty*. New York, NY: Anchor Books; 2000:24.

15. Olson IR, Marshuetz C. Facial attractiveness is appraised in a glance. *Emotion*. 2005;5:498.
16. Etcoff N. *Survival of the Prettiest: The Science of Beauty*. New York, NY: Anchor Books; 2000:15.
17. Bashour M. History and current concepts in the analysis of facial attractiveness. *Plast Reconstr Surg*. 2006;188:741.
18. Langlois JH, Kalakanis L, Rubenstein AJ, et al. Maxims or myths of beauty? A meta-analytic and theoretical review. *Psychol Bull*. 2000;126:390.
19. Rhodes G, Yoshikawa S, Clark A, et al. Attractiveness of facial averageness and symmetry in non-Western cultures: in search of biologically based standards of beauty. *Perception*. 2001;30:611.
20. Dobke M, Chung C, Takabe K. Facial aesthetic preferences among Asian women: are all oriental Asians the same? *Aesthetic Plast Surg*. 2006;30:342.
21. Armstrong J. *The Secret Power of Beauty: Why Happiness is in the Eye of the Beholder*. London, UK: Allen Lane; 2004.
22. Hönekopp J. Once more: is beauty in the eye of the beholder? Relative contributions of private and shared taste to judgments of facial attractiveness. *J Exp Psychol Hum Percept Perform*. 2006;32: 199.
23. Rubenstein AJ. Variation in perceived attractiveness differences between dynamic and static faces. *Psychol Sci*. 2005;16:759.
24. Rhodes G. The evolutionary psychology of facial beauty. *Annu Rev Psychol*. 2006;57:199.
25. Perrett DI, Penton-Voak IS, Little AC, et al. Facial attractiveness judgements reflect learning of parental age characteristics. *Proc Biol Sci*. 2002;269:873.
26. Langlois JH, Ritter JM, Roggman LA, et al. Facial diversity and infant preferences for attractive faces. *Dev Psychol*. 1991;27:79.
27. Etcoff N. *Survival of the Prettiest: The Science of Beauty*. New York, NY: Anchor Books; 2000:32.
28. Ramsey JL, Langlois JH, Hoss RA, et al. Origins of a stereotype: categorization of facial attractiveness by 6-month-old infants. *Dev Sci*. 2004;7:201.
29. Mealey L, Bridgstock R, Townsend GC. Symmetry and perceived facial attractiveness: a monozygotic co-twin comparison. *J Pers Soc Psychol*. 1999;76:151.
30. Baudouin JY, Tiberghien G. Symmetry, averageness, and feature size in the facial attractiveness of women. *Acta Psychol (Amst)*. 2004;177:313.
31. Zaidel DW, Cohen JA. The face, beauty, and symmetry: perceiving asymmetry in beautiful faces. *Int J Neurosci*. 2005;115:1165.
32. Zaidel DW, Aarde SM, Baig K. Appearance of symmetry, beauty, and health in human faces. *Brain Cogn*. 2005;57:261.
33. Etcoff N. *Survival of the Prettiest: The Science of Beauty*. New York, NY: Anchor Books; 2000:34.
34. Perrett DI, Lee KJ, Penton-Voak I, et al. Effects of sexual dimorphism on facial attractiveness. *Nature*. 1998;394:884.
35. Boothroyd LG, Jones BC, Burt DM, et al. Partner characteristics associated with masculinity, health and maturity in male faces. *Pers Individ Dif*. 2007;43:1161.
36. Rhodes G, Hickford C, Jeffery L. Sex-typicality and attractiveness: are supermale and superfemale faces super-attractive? *Br J Psychol*. 2000;91:125.
37. Newton JT, Minhas G. Exposure to 'ideal' facial images reduces facial satisfaction: an experimental study. *Community Dent Oral Epidemiol*. 2005;33:410.
38. Davis C, Claridge G, Fox J. Not just a pretty face: physical attractiveness and perfectionism in the risk for eating disorders. *Int J Eat Disord*. 2000;27:67.
39. Etcoff N. *Survival of the Prettiest: The Science of Beauty*. New York, NY: Anchor Books; 2000:87.
40. Melli C, Giorgini S. Aesthetics in psychosomatic dermatology. I. Cosmetics, self-image, attractiveness. *Clin Dermatol*. 1984;2:180.
41. Seifert T. Anthropomorphic characteristics of centerfold models: trends towards slender figures over time. *Int J Eat Disord*. 2005;37:271.
42. Pettijohn TF II, Jungeberg BJ. Playboy playmate curves: changes in facial and body feature preferences across social and economic conditions. *Pers Soc Psychol Bull*. 2004;30.1186.
43. Byrd-Bredbenner C, Murray J, Schlussel YR. Temporal changes in anthropometric measurements of idealized females and young women in general. *Women Health*. 2005;41:13.
44. Katzmarzyk PT, Davis C. Thinness and body shape of Playboy centerfolds from 1978 to 1998. *Int J Obes Relat Metab Disord*. 2001;25:590.
45. Cellerino A. Psychobiology of facial attractiveness. *J Endocrinol Invest*. 2003; 26.45.
46. Cunningham MR, Barbee AP, Pike CL. What do women want? Facialmetric assessment of multiple motives in the perception of male facial physical attractiveness. *J Pers Soc Psychol*. 1990;59:61.
47. Kilbourne J. Killing us softly: gender roles in advertising. *Adolesc Med*. 1993; 4:635.
48. Leit RA, Pope HG Jr, Gray JJ. Cultural expectations of muscularity in men: the evolution of playgirl centerfolds. *Int J Eat Disord*. 2001;29:90.
49. Kiefer I, Leitner B, Bauer R, et al. Body weight: the male and female perception. *Soz Praventivmed*. 2000;45:274.
50. Pinhas L, Toner BB, Ali A, et al. The effects of the ideal of female beauty on mood and body satisfaction. *Int J Eat Disord*. 1999;25:223.
51. Groesz LM, Levine MP, Murnen SK. The effect of experimental presentation of thin media images on body dissatisfaction: a meta-analytic review. *Int J Eat Disord*. 2002;31:1.
52. Etcoff N. *Survival of the Prettiest: The Science of Beauty*. New York, NY: Anchor Books; 2000:74.
53. Rand CS, Wright BA. Continuity and change in the evaluation of ideal and acceptable body sizes across a wide age span. *Int J Eat Disord*. 2000;28:90.
54. Loefler IJ. Female beauty. *J R Soc Med*. 2000;93:334.
55. Baker D, Sivyer R, Towell T. Body image dissatisfaction and eating attitudes in visually impaired women. *Int J Eat Disord*. 1998;24:319.
56. American Psychiatric Association. *Diagnostic and statistical manual of mental disorders (DSM-IV)*. 4th ed. Washington, DC: American Psychiatric Association; 1994.
57. Phillips KA. Body dysmorphic disorder: the distress of imagined ugliness. *Am J Psychiatry*. 1991;148:1138.
58. Cotterill JA, Cunliffe WJ. Suicide in dermatological patients. *Br J Dermatol*. 1997;137:246.
59. Phillips K, Dufresne R, Wilkel C, et al. Rate of body dysmorphic disorder in dermatology patients. *J Am Acad Dermatol*. 2000;42:436.
60. Cotterill JA. Body dysmorphic disorder. *Dermatol Clin*. 1996;14:457.
61. Koblenzer CS. The dysmorphic syndrome. *Arch Dermatol*. 1985;121:780.
62. Sarwer DB, Cash TF, Magee L, et al. Female college students and cosmetic surgery: an investigation of experiences, attitudes, and body image. *Plast Reconstr Surg*. 2005;115:931.
63. Castle DJ, Morkell D. Imagined ugliness: a symptom which can become a disorder. *Med J Aust*. 2000;173:205.
64. Pitanguy I. Evaluation of body contouring surgery today: a 30-year perspective. *Plast Reconstr Surg*. 2000;105:1499.
65. Santor DA, Walker J. Garnering the interest of others: mediating the effects among physical attractiveness, self-worth and dominance. *Br J Soc Psychol*. 1999;38:461.
66. Pitanguy I. Facial cosmetic surgery: a 30-year perspective. *Plast Reconstr Surg*. 2000;105:1517.
67. Kligman AM, Graham JA. The psychology of appearance in the elderly. *Dermatol Clin*. 1986;4:501.
68. McGrath MH, Mukerji S. Plastic surgery and the teenage patient. *J Pediatr Adolesc Gynecol*. 2000;13:105.
69. Patzer GL. Improving self-esteem by improving physical attractiveness. *J Esthet Dent*. 1997;9:44.
70. Kamburo_lu HO, Ozgür F. Postoperative satisfaction and the patient's body image, life satisfaction, and self esteem: a retrospective study comparing adolescent girls and boys after cosmetic surgery. *Aesthetic Plast Surg*. 2007 May 25;[Epub ahead of print].
71. Etcoff N. *Survival of the Prettiest: The Science of Beauty*. New York, NY: Anchor Books; 2000:104.
72. Franzoi SL, Koehler V. Age and gender differences in body attitudes: a comparison of young and elderly adults. *Int J Aging Hum Dev*. 1998;47:1.
73. Chuh A, Wong W, Zawar V. The skin and the mind. *Aust Fam Physician*. 2006; 35:723.
74. Barankin B, DeKoven J. Psychosocial effect of common skin diseases. *Can Fam Physician*. 2002;48:712.
75. Gupta MA, Gupta AK. Psychiatric and psychological co-morbidity in patients with dermatologic disorders: epidemiology and management. *Am J Clin Dermatol*. 2003;4:833.
76. Berson DS, Chalker DK, Harper JC. Current concepts in the treatment of acne: report from a clinical roundtable. *Cutis*. 2003;72:5.
77. Tan JK. Psychosocial impact of acne vulgaris: evaluating the evidence. *Skin Therapy Lett*. 2004;9:1.
78. Bowe WP, Leyden JJ, Crerand CE, et al. Body dysmorphic disorder symptoms

among patients with acne vulgaris. *J Am Acad Dermatol.* 2007;57:222.
79. Elias PM. Stratum corneum defensive functions: an integrated view. *J Invest Dermatol.* 2005;125:183.
80. Kao JS, Fluhr JW, Man MQ, et al. Short-term glucocorticoid treatment compromises both permeability barrier homeostasis and stratum corneum integrity: inhibition of epidermal lipid synthesis accounts for functional abnormalities. *J Invest Dermatol.* 2003;120:456.
81. Choi EH, Brown BE, Crumrine D, et al. Mechanisms by which psychologic stress alters cutaneous permeability barrier homeostasis and stratum corneum integrity. *J Invest Dermatol.* 2005;124:587.
82. Arck PC, Slominski A, Theoharides TC, et al. Neuroimmunology of stress: skin takes center stage. *J Invest Dermatol.* 2006;126:1697.
83. Hendrix S: Neuroimmune communication in skin: far from peripheral. *J Invest Dermatol.* 2008;128:260.
84. Pavlovic S, Daniltchenko M, Tobin DJ, et al. Further exploring the brain—skin connection: stress worsens dermatitis via substance P-dependent neurogenic inflammation in mice. *J Invest Dermatol.* 2008;128:434.
85. Aberg KM, Radek KA, Choi EH, et al. Psychological stress downregulates epidermal antimicrobial peptide expression and increases severity of cutaneous infections in mice. *J Clin Invest.* 2007;177:3339.
86. Slominski A. A nervous breakdown in the skin: stress and the epidermal barrier. *J Clin Invest.* 2007;177:3166.
87. Inoue K, Hosoi J, Ideta R, et al. Stress augmented ultraviolet-irradiation-induced pigmentation. *J Invest Dermatol.* 2003; 121:165.
88. Jafferany M. Psychodermatology: a guide to understanding common psychocutaneous disorders. *Prim Care Companion J Clin Psychiatry.* 2007;9:203.

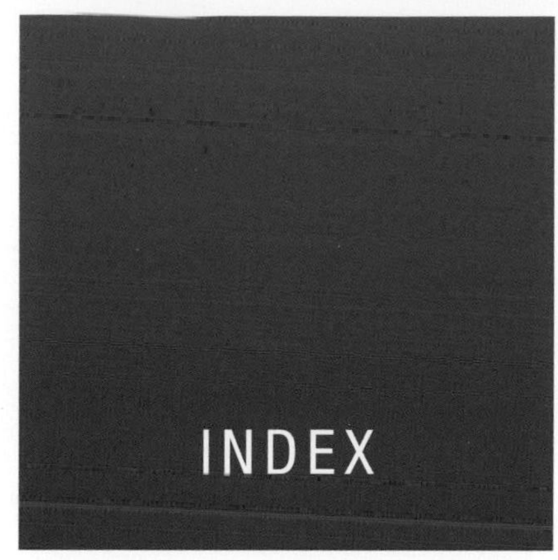

INDEX

T